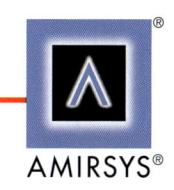

DIAGNOSTIC PATHOLOGY
NORMAL HISTOLOGY

DIAGNOSTIC PATHOLOGY
NORMAL HISTOLOGY

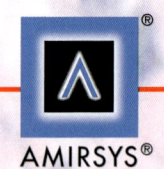

Laura W. Lamps, MD
Professor and Vice-Chair for Academic Affairs
Department of Pathology
University of Arkansas for Medical Sciences
Little Rock, Arkansas

Charles Matthew Quick, MD
Assistant Professor
Director of Gynecologic Pathology
Department of Pathology
University of Arkansas for Medical Sciences
Little Rock, Arkansas

Jesse K. McKenney, MD
Associate Head, Surgical Pathology
Pathology and Laboratory Medicine Institute
Department of Anatomic Pathology
Glickman Urological and Kidney Institute
Cleveland Clinic
Cleveland, Ohio

Matthew R. Lindberg, MD
Assistant Professor
Department of Pathology
University of Arkansas for Medical Sciences
Little Rock, Arkansas

Jonathan B. McHugh, MD
Associate Professor of Pathology
Clinical Associate Professor of Surgery
Section of Oral Surgery
University of Michigan Medical School
Ann Arbor, Michigan

Anthony Chang, MD
Associate Professor of Pathology
The University of Chicago Medicine
Chicago, Illinois

Roni Michelle Cox, MD
Assistant Professor
Department of Pathology
University of Arkansas for Medical Sciences
Little Rock, Arkansas

Dylan V. Miller, MD
Associate Professor
University of Utah School of Medicine
Director of Electron Microscopy and Immunostains
Intermountain Central Laboratory
Salt Lake City, Utah

Alexandros D. Polydorides, MD, PhD
Associate Professor of Pathology
Mount Sinai School of Medicine
New York, New York

David Cassarino, MD, PhD
Consultant Dermatopathologist
Southern California Permanente Medical Group
Los Angeles, California
Clinical Professor of Dermatopathology
University of California, Irvine
Irvine, California

Jeremy C. Wallentine, MD
Staff Hematopathologist and Director of
Molecular Diagnostics
Intermountain Healthcare and Utah Pathology
Services, Inc.
LDS Hospital
Salt Lake City, Utah

Kathryn Foucar, MD
Professor and Vice Chair of Clinical Affairs
Department of Pathology
The University of New Mexico School of Medicine
Albuquerque, New Mexico

Brenda L. Nelson, DDS, MS
Head of Anatomic Pathology
Naval Medical Center San Diego
San Diego, California

Cyril Fisher, MD, DSc, FRCPath
Consultant Histopathologist
The Royal Marsden NHS Foundation Trust
Professor of Tumor Pathology
Institute of Cancer Research
University of London
London, United Kingdom

David G. Hicks, MD
Director of Surgical Pathology
Professor of Pathology and Laboratory Medicine
University of Rochester Medical Center
Rochester, New York

Jerome B. Taxy, MD
Professor
Department of Pathology
The University of Chicago Medicine
Chicago, Illinois

Peter Pytel, MD
Associate Professor of Pathology
Department of Pathology
The University of Chicago Medicine
Chicago, Illinois

AMIRSYS®
Names you know. Content you trust.®

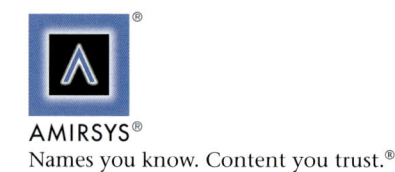

First Edition

© 2013 Amirsys, Inc.

Compilation © 2013 Amirsys Publishing, Inc.

All rights reserved. No portion of this publication may be reproduced, stored in a retrieval system, or transmitted, in any form or media or by any means, electronic, mechanical, optical, photocopying, recording, or otherwise, without prior written permission from the respective copyright holders.

Printed in Canada by Friesens, Altona, Manitoba, Canada

ISBN: 978-1-931884-66-2

Notice and Disclaimer

The information in this product ("Product") is provided as a reference for use by licensed medical professionals and no others. It does not and should not be construed as any form of medical diagnosis or professional medical advice on any matter. Receipt or use of this Product, in whole or in part, does not constitute or create a doctor-patient, therapist-patient, or other healthcare professional relationship between the copyright holders and any recipient. This Product may not reflect the most current medical developments, and the copyright holders (individually and jointly), make no claims, promises, or guarantees about accuracy, completeness, or adequacy of the information contained in or linked to the Product. The Product is not a substitute for or replacement of professional medical judgment. The copyright holders, and their affiliates, authors, contributors, partners, and sponsors, individually and jointly, disclaim all liability or responsibility for any injury and/or damage to persons or property in respect to actions taken or not taken based on any and all Product information.

In the cases where drugs or other chemicals are prescribed, readers are advised to check the product information currently provided by the manufacturer of each drug to be administered to verify the recommended dose, the method and duration of administration, and contraindications. It is the responsibility of the treating physician relying on experience and knowledge of the patient to determine dosages and the best treatment for the patient.

To the maximum extent permitted by applicable law, the copyright holders provide the Product AS IS AND WITH ALL FAULTS, AND HEREBY DISCLAIMS ALL WARRANTIES AND CONDITIONS, WHETHER EXPRESS, IMPLIED OR STATUTORY, INCLUDING BUT NOT LIMITED TO, ANY (IF ANY) IMPLIED WARRANTIES OR CONDITIONS OF MERCHANTABILITY, OF FITNESS FOR A PARTICULAR PURPOSE, OF LACK OF VIRUSES, OR ACCURACY OR COMPLETENESS OF RESPONSES, OR RESULTS, AND OF LACK OF NEGLIGENCE OR LACK OF WORKMANLIKE EFFORT. ALSO, THERE IS NO WARRANTY OR CONDITION OF TITLE, QUIET ENJOYMENT, QUIET POSSESSION, CORRESPONDENCE TO DESCRIPTION OR NON-INFRINGEMENT, WITH REGARD TO THE PRODUCT. THE ENTIRE RISK AS TO THE QUALITY OF OR ARISING OUT OF USE OR PERFORMANCE OF THE PRODUCT REMAINS WITH THE READER.

The respective copyright holders, individually and jointly, disclaim all warranties of any kind if the Product was customized, repackaged or altered in any way by any third party.

Library of Congress Cataloging-in-Publication Data

Diagnostic pathology. Normal histology / [edited by] Laura W. Lamps. -- 1st ed.
   p. ; cm.
Normal histology
ISBN 978-1-931884-66-2
I. Lamps, Laura W. (Laura Webb) II. Title: Normal histology.
[DNLM: 1. Histological Techniques--methods--Atlases. QS 17]

616.8'4--dc23

2012047353

For my dear husband, Paul Ward, who helps me maintain polarity.
I would also like to thank my coauthors for their excellent contributions, and Dave Chance, Kellie Heap, Katherine Riser, and Laura Sesto from the Amirsys team for their dedication to creating wonderful books
LWL

To Dexter, Shelly, Chuck, and Jeanne Quick – Thank you for everything
CMQ

To my family, Amy, Madeleine, Hannah Jane, and Ennis
JKM

To my wife, Rani, for her love and support
MRL

To my parents and brothers, who have taught me many valuable life lessons. To Carly for her unyielding support. To all of the students, residents, fellows, and colleagues I have worked with who have taught me so much about pathology and histology
JBM

To my wife, Brittany, and children, Brandon and Brianna, for your endless love and support
AC

To my family and friends
RMC

For Tonya, with gratitude for her boundless tolerance
DVM

To all my mentors, past and present, for teaching me the art and science of pathology and to all students, residents, and fellows, present and future, to whom I hope to pass that on
ADP

To my wonderful wife and children for their support and inspiration
DC

To my wife, Crystal, for her unwavering support, love, and dedication
JCW

To my family, Elliott, Jim, Charlie, and Morgan Foucar
KF

To my husband, Dave, and my son, Adam. Thank you for all your love and support!
BLN

To my extended family
CF

To my awesome wife, Patti, and my wonderful family for all of your love and support
DGH

To my residents and fellows, teachers, and family
JBT

Thanks to Fritz and Mariele
PP

vi

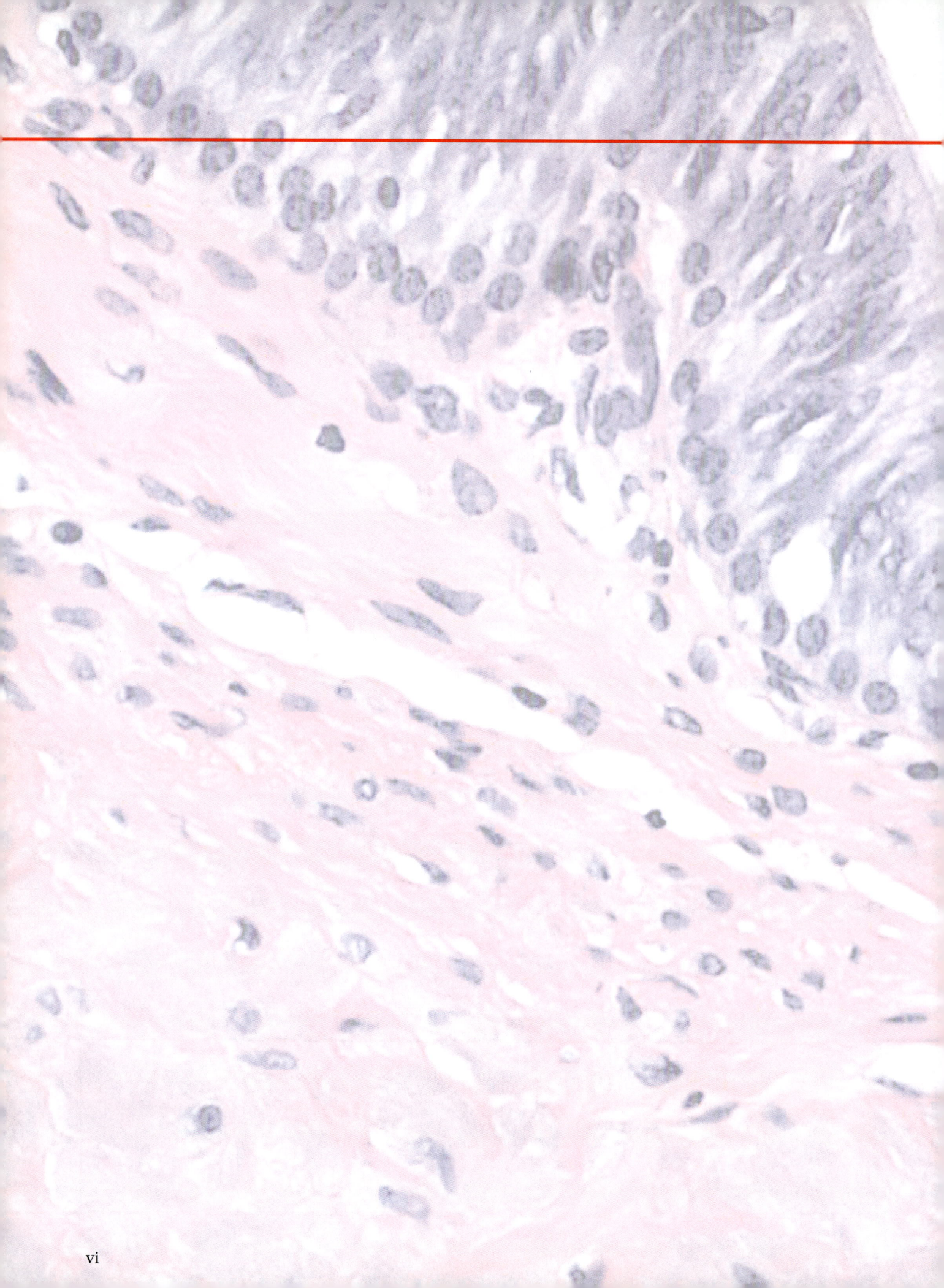

PREFACE

A thorough knowledge of normal histology, in all of its wonderful variation, is essential to the study of disease. *Diagnostic Pathology: Normal Histology* is designed for practicing pathologists, pathologists in training, medical students, and students of histology in any setting as they strive to learn about the spectrum of normal.

This reference provides clear, concise information on the normal histology of every organ system. It also features nearly 1,800 images, including photomicrographs, spectacular gross images, electron micrographs, and medical illustrations. There are introductory chapters on electron microscopy, immunofluoresence, immunohistochemistry and histochemistry, the cell, and the basic organization of tissues. As with all books in the *Diagnostic Pathology* series, the key facts pertaining to each diagnosis are highlighted in a box for ease of use.

On behalf of all of the authors of this book, we hope that *Diagnostic Pathology: Normal Histology* becomes a mainstay of your library and that it is a favorite reference to which you return on a regular basis.

Laura W. Lamps, MD
Professor and Vice-Chair for Academic Affairs
Department of Pathology
University of Arkansas for Medical Sciences
Little Rock, Arkansas

viii

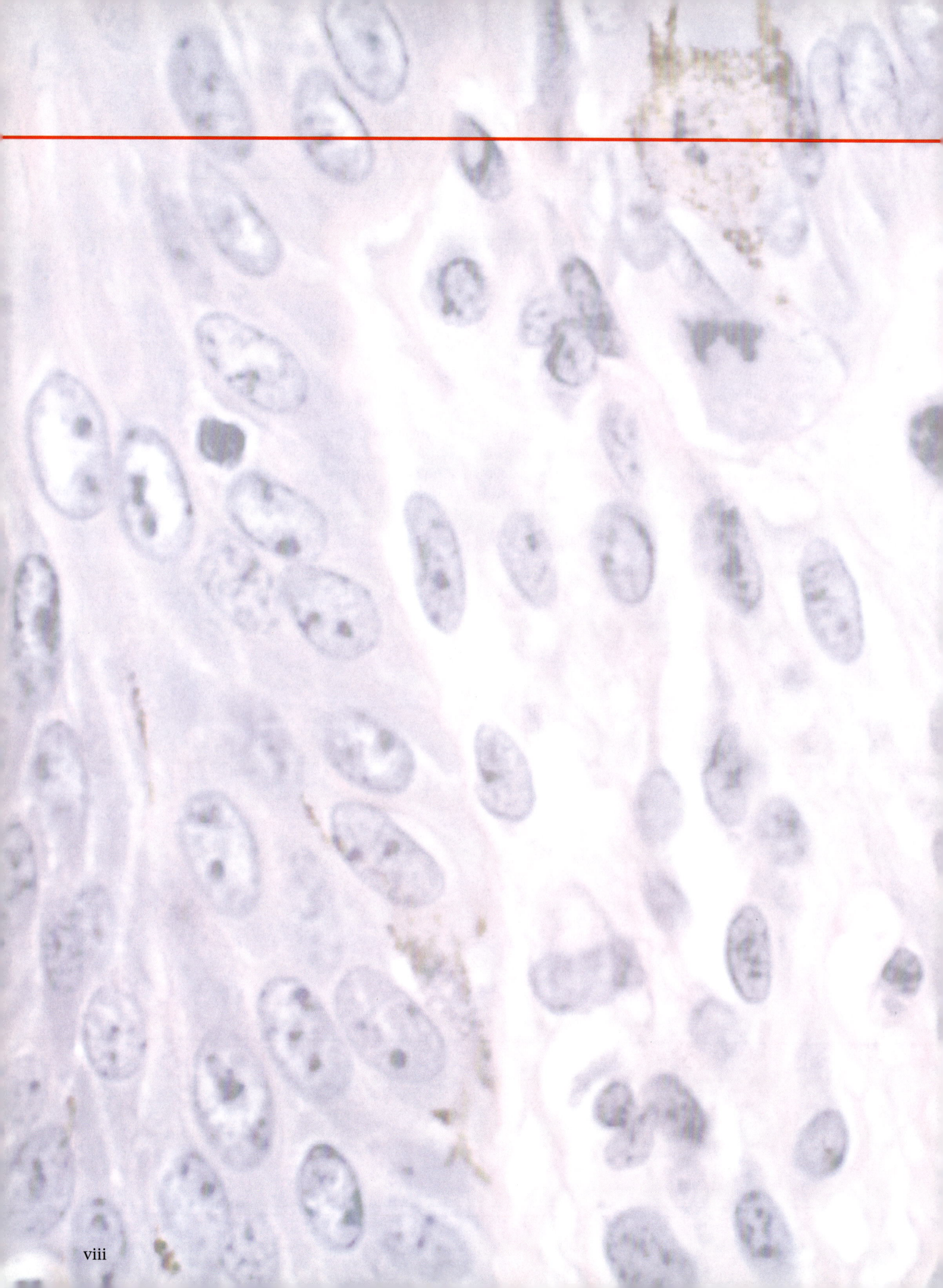

ACKNOWLEDGMENTS

Text Editing
Arthur G. Gelsinger, MA
Lorna Kennington, MS
Rebecca L. Hutchinson, BA
Angela M. Green, BA
Kalina K. Lowery, MS

Image Editing
Jeffrey J. Marmorstone, BS
Lisa A. M. Steadman, BS

Medical Text Editing
Kristin Mitchell Dishongh, MD
Katherine Sherman Blevins, PhD

Illustrations
Laura C. Sesto, MA
Lane R. Bennion, MS
Richard Coombs, MS
Brenda L. McArthur, MA

Art Direction and Design
Laura C. Sesto, MA
Lisa A. M. Steadman, BS

Lead Editor
Dave L. Chance, MA

Production Lead
Katherine L. Riser, MA

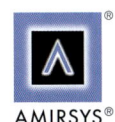

AMIRSYS®
Names you know. Content you trust.®

x

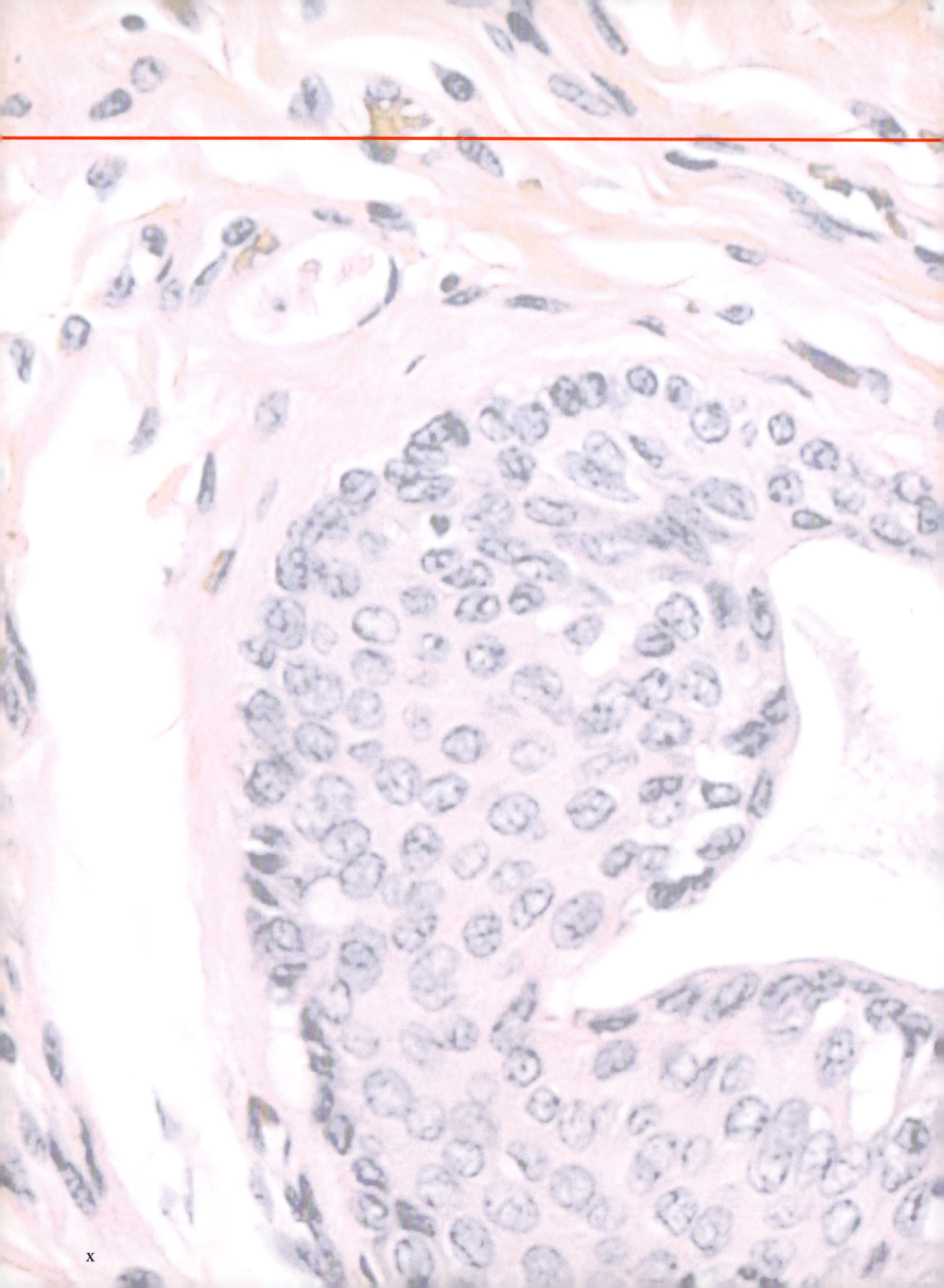

SECTIONS

Introduction to Histology and Basic Histological Techniques

Integument

Musculoskeletal System

Circulatory System

Nervous System

Hematopoietic and Immune Systems

Head and Neck

Respiratory System

Breast

Tubular Gut and Peritoneum

Hepatobiliary Tract and Pancreas

Genitourinary and Male Genital Tract

Female Genital Tract

Endocrine

TABLE OF CONTENTS

SECTION 1
Introduction to Histology and Basic Histological Techniques

Introduction to Special Stains and 1-2
Immunohistochemistry of Normal Tissues
Laura Webb Lamps, MD

Immunofluorescence 1-4
Anthony Chang, MD

Electron Microscopy 1-8
Anthony Chang, MD
Peter Pytel, MD & Jerome Taxy, MD

Introduction to the Cell 1-12
Jerome Taxy, MD & Anthony Chang, MD

Introduction to Histology 1-20
Laura Webb Lamps, MD

SECTION 2
Integument

Epidermis (Including Keratinocytes and 2-2
Melanocytes)
David Cassarino, MD, PhD

Dermis 2-6
David Cassarino, MD, PhD

Adnexal Structures 2-10
David Cassarino, MD, PhD

Nail 2-14
David Cassarino, MD, PhD

SECTION 3
Musculoskeletal System

Bone and Cartilage 3-2
Matthew R. Lindberg, MD

Connective Tissue 3-8
Matthew R. Lindberg, MD

Adipose Tissue 3-10
Cyril Fisher, MD, DSc, FRCPath

Skeletal Muscle 3-14
Cyril Fisher, MD, DSc, FRCPath

SECTION 4
Circulatory System

Heart 4-2
Dylan Miller, MD

Cardiac Valves 4-6
Dylan Miller, MD

Cardiac Conduction System 4-8
Dylan Miller, MD

Arteries 4-12
Dylan Miller, MD

Capillaries, Veins, and Lymphatics 4-16
Dylan Miller, MD

SECTION 5
Nervous System

Peripheral Nervous System 5-2
Alexandros D. Polydorides, MD, PhD

Central Nervous System 5-6
Alexandros D. Polydorides, MD, PhD

Meninges 5-10
Alexandros D. Polydorides, MD, PhD

Choroid Plexus 5-12
Alexandros D. Polydorides, MD, PhD

SECTION 6
Hematopoietic and Immune Systems

Overview of the Immune System 6-2
Jeremy C. Wallentine, MD

Lymph Nodes 6-6
Jeremy C. Wallentine, MD

Spleen 6-10
Jeremy C. Wallentine, MD

Bone Marrow 6-14
Kathryn Foucar, MD

Peripheral Blood 6-22
Kathryn Foucar, MD

Thymus 6-26
Matthew R. Lindberg, MD

SECTION 7
Head and Neck

Eye and Ocular Adnexa 7-2
Charles Matthew Quick, MD

Oral Mucosae 7-12
Brenda L. Nelson, DDS, MS

Gingivae 7-14
Brenda L. Nelson, DDS, MS

Minor Salivary Glands 7-16
Brenda L. Nelson, DDS, MS

Teeth 7-18
Brenda L. Nelson, DDS, MS

Tongue 7-22
Jonathan B. McHugh, MD

Tonsils/Adenoids 7-26
Jonathan B. McHugh, MD

Ear 7-30
Jonathan B. McHugh, MD

Nose and Paranasal Sinuses 7-34
Jonathan B. McHugh, MD

Pharynx 7-38
Jonathan B. McHugh, MD

Larynx 7-40
Jonathan B. McHugh, MD

Major Salivary Glands 7-44
Jonathan B. McHugh, MD

SECTION 8
Respiratory System

Trachea 8-2
Matthew R. Lindberg, MD

Lung 8-4
Matthew R. Lindberg, MD

Mesothelium 8-10
Matthew R. Lindberg, MD

SECTION 9
Breast

Breast 9-2
David G. Hicks, MD

SECTION 10
Tubular Gut and Peritoneum

Esophagus 10-2
Matthew R. Lindberg, MD

Stomach 10-8
Laura Webb Lamps, MD

Small Intestine 10-14
Laura Webb Lamps, MD

Large Intestine 10-18
Matthew R. Lindberg, MD

Appendix 10-24
Matthew R. Lindberg, MD

Anus and Anal Canal 10-28
Laura Webb Lamps, MD

Peritoneal Membranes 10-32
Matthew R. Lindberg, MD

SECTION 11
Hepatobiliary Tract and Pancreas

Liver 11-2
Laura Webb Lamps, MD

Gallbladder 11-10
Laura Webb Lamps, MD

Extrahepatic Biliary Tract 11-14
Laura Webb Lamps, MD

Vaterian System 11-16
Laura Webb Lamps, MD

Pancreas 11-18
Laura Webb Lamps, MD

SECTION 12
Genitourinary and Male Genital Tract

Kidney 12-2
Anthony Chang, MD

Ureter and Renal Pelvis 12-12
Jesse K. McKenney, MD

Bladder 12-16
Roni Michelle Cox, MD

Urethra 12-22
Jesse K. McKenney, MD

Prostate: Regional Anatomy With Histologic Correlates 12-28
Jesse K. McKenney, MD

Prostate: Benign Glandular and Stromal Histology 12-38
Jesse K. McKenney, MD

Penis   12-48
Roni Michelle Cox, MD

Testis and Associated Excretory Ducts   12-52
Roni Michelle Cox, MD

SECTION 13
Female Genital Tract

Vulva   13-2
Jesse K. McKenney, MD

Vagina   13-6
Jesse K. McKenney, MD

Uterus   13-10
Charles Matthew Quick, MD

Fallopian Tube   13-24
Charles Matthew Quick, MD

Ovary   13-30
Charles Matthew Quick, MD

Placenta   13-40
Charles Matthew Quick, MD

SECTION 14
Endocrine

Adrenal Gland   14-2
Roni Michelle Cox, MD

Paraganglia   14-6
Jesse K. McKenney, MD

Thyroid   14-8
Jonathan B. McHugh, MD

Parathyroid   14-12
Jonathan B. McHugh, MD

Pineal Gland   14-16
Alexandros D. Polydorides, MD, PhD

Pituitary   14-18
Alexandros D. Polydorides, MD, PhD

DIAGNOSTIC PATHOLOGY
NORMAL HISTOLOGY

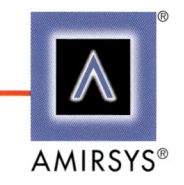

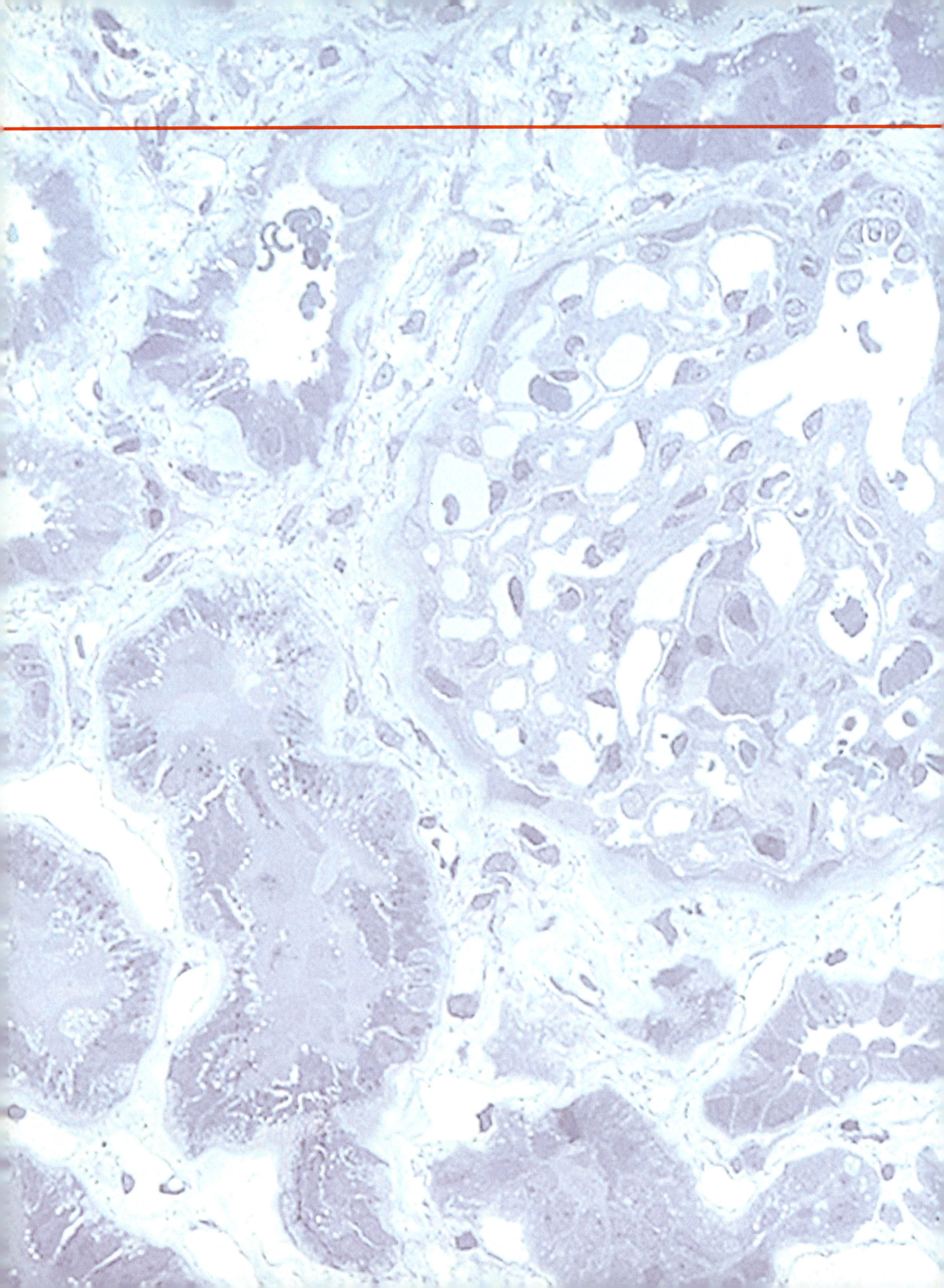

Introduction to Histology and Basic Histological Techniques

Introduction to Special Stains and Immunohistochemistry of Normal Tissues	1-2
Immunofluorescence	1-4
Electron Microscopy	1-8
Introduction to the Cell	1-12
Introduction to Histology	1-20

INTRODUCTION TO SPECIAL STAINS AND IMMUNOHISTOCHEMISTRY OF NORMAL TISSUES

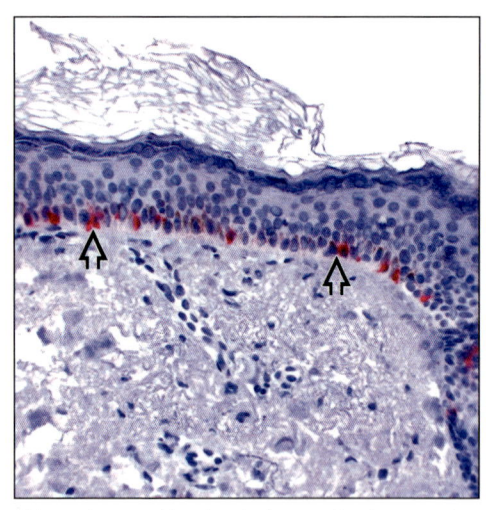

This immunohistochemical antibody against melanocytes highlights normal melanocytes in skin (red chromagen).

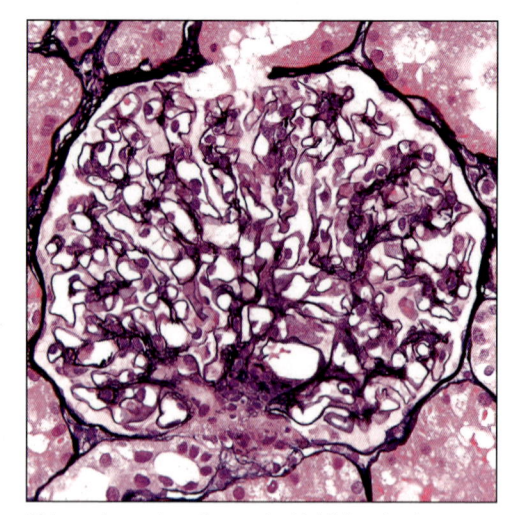

This methenamine silver stain highlights the basement membrane of the glomerulus. The basement membrane stains black with this stain.

TERMINOLOGY

Fixation
- Alteration of proteins in tissue so that tissue is made resistant to further changes

Processing
- Process of preparing tissue so that microscopic sections can be made
  - Dehydration, clearing, infiltrating tissue with wax, embedding, cutting tissue sections for microscopic slides

Histochemical Staining
- Use of chemical reactions to highlight or differentiate various components of tissue on a slide

Immunohistochemical Staining
- Use of labeled antibody of known specificity to detect antigen in tissue
  - Antibody is labeled with chromagen so that positive reaction is identified by visualizing color
- Technical considerations
  - Most antibodies suitable for use in formalin-fixed, paraffin-embedded routinely processed tissue
    - Fixation may impair antigenicity due to protein cross-linking
  - Epitope retrieval may be required to unmask antigens (antigen retrieval) using heat or enzymes

NUCLEAR AND CYTOPLASMIC STAINING

Hematoxylin and Eosin
- Routine H&E stain used most commonly in examination of tissues; stains nuclei blue and cytoplasm pink

Feulgen Stain
- Stains nuclear DNA reddish purple

Methyl Green-Pyronin Y
- Differentiates between DNA and RNA; nuclear DNA stains blue to green, cytoplasmic RNA stains pink to rose
- Used to detect plasma cells and immunoblasts

Romanowsky (e.g., Wright, Giemsa)
- Differentiates between hematopoietic cells based on staining properties

CARBOHYDRATE STAINS

PAS (Periodic Acid-Schiff)
- Polysaccharides, neutral mucins, basement membranes: Stains them bright pink

PAS With Diastase
- Demonstrates glycogen (pink); glycogen washes out of section with use of diastase

Mucicarmine
- Stains acid mucin, typically in epithelia (bright pink)

Alcian Blue (pH 2.5)
- Stains acid mucopolysaccharides bright blue, including sulfated and carboxylated acid mucopolysaccharides and sulfated and carboxylated sialomucins

Alcian Blue (pH 1.0)
- Stains sulfated mucins (pale blue)

Alcian Blue/Hyaluronidase
- Differentiates epithelial and connective tissue mucins
  - Acid mucopolysaccharides and sialomucins stain deep blue; substances containing hyaluronic acid and chondroitin sulfates A and C lose staining with digestion

Alcian Blue/PAS
- Differentiates between neutral and acidic mucins; acid mucosubstances blue; neutral polysaccharides magenta

INTRODUCTION TO SPECIAL STAINS AND IMMUNOHISTOCHEMISTRY OF NORMAL TISSUES

Colloidal Iron
- Stains carboxylated and sulfated mucopolysaccharides and glycoproteins (deep blue)

CONNECTIVE TISSUE STAINS

Masson Trichrome
- Differentiates between collagen (blue) and smooth muscle or parenchyma (red)

Elastic Stain
- Demonstrates elastic fibers; stain black or dark purple depending on method of staining

Pentachrome Stain
- Demonstrates 5 tissue types: Collagen (yellow), muscle (red), elastic fibers (black), mucins (blue), fibrin (intense red)

Reticulin Stain
- Demonstrates reticulin fibers (black)

MUSCLE STAINS

PTAH (Phosphotungstic Acid-Hematoxylin)
- Stains muscle cross striations and fibrin; both stain blue, along with nuclei

FAT STAINS

Oil Red O
- Stains neutral lipids (red) in frozen sections

Sudan Black B
- Stains neutral lipids (black)

NERVE

Silver Nitrate
- Stains nerve fibers and neurofibrils black

Mallory PTAH (Phosphotungstic Acid)
- Stains glial fibers blue, neurons salmon pink, myelin blue

Cajal Stain
- Stains astrocytes black

Weil Stain
- Stains myelin blue/black

Luxol Fast Blue
- Stains myelin blue

PIGMENTS, MINERALS, AND GRANULES

Prussian Blue
- Stains ferric iron blue

Fontana-Masson
- Stains melanin black

Calcium Stain (von Kossa)
- Stains calcium black

Copper (Rhodanine)
- Stains copper rust brown

MISCELLANEOUS STAINS

Toluidine Blue
- Stains mast cells deep violet

Methenamine Silver
- Stains glomerular basement membranes black

GENERAL CATEGORIES OF IMMUNOHISTOCHEMICAL ANTIBODIES AND EXAMPLES

Epithelial Markers
- Examples: Keratins AE1/AE3 (broad spectrum keratin), CK7 (lung, breast), CK20 (GI tract), EMA, calretinin

Muscle Markers
- Examples: Actin, desmin (smooth muscle); myogenin, MYOD1, desmin (skeletal muscle)

Myoepithelial Markers
- Examples: Calponin, p63

Vascular Markers
- Examples: CD34, CD31
  - Lymphatic epithelial markers: Podoplanin, D2-40

Neural Markers
- Examples: S100, CD57, NFP, GFAP

Melanocyte Markers
- Examples: S100, Melan-A, HMB45

Neuroendocrine Markers
- Examples: CD56, chromogranin, synaptophysin

Hematopoietic/Lymphoid Markers
- Examples: LCA (lymphocytes); CD20 (B cells); CD3, CD4, CD8 (T cells); CD163 (histiocytes); CD138 (plasma cells)

Hormones
- Examples: ACTH, parathyroid hormone, insulin, HCG, glucagon, somatostatin, gastrin

Enzymes
- Examples: Chymotrypsin, trypsin

Mucins
- Examples: MUC2, MUC3 (intestinal); MUC6 (gastric)

RELATED REFERENCES

1. Carson FL: Histotechnology: A Self-Instructional Text. 2nd ed. Chicago: ASCP Press, 1997
2. Bancroft JD et al: Theory and Practice of Histological Techniques. New York: Churchill Livingstone, 1992
3. Luna LG: Histopathologic Methods and Color Atlas of Special Stains and Tissue Artifacts. Gaithersburg: American Histolabs Inc. Publications Division, 1992

IMMUNOFLUORESCENCE

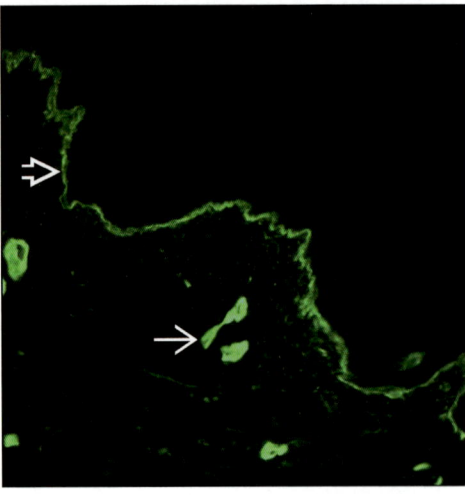

The α-1 chain of collagen IV shows normal, strong, continuous staining of the epidermal basement membrane ⇨ and capillary basement membranes ⇨ in this skin biopsy.

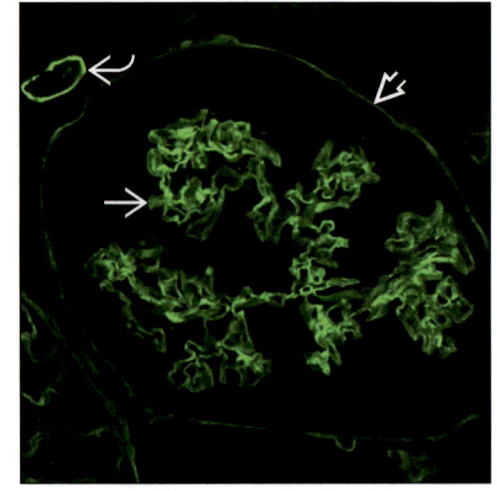

The α-5 chain of collagen IV shows normal, strong, and continuous linear staining of the glomerular ⇨ and distal tubular basement membrane ⇨ and Bowman capsule ⇨.

TERMINOLOGY

Abbreviations
- Immunofluorescence (IF)

Definitions
- IF uses fluorescently labeled antibodies to detect antigens of interest with a fluorescence microscope
  - Direct IF
    - Primary antibody directly conjugated with a fluorescent dye, typically fluorescein isothiocyanate (FITC), for detection using a fluorescence microscope
  - Indirect IF
    - Primary antibody not conjugated with fluorescent dye and requires adding a secondary antibody conjugated with a fluorescent dye for detection using a fluorescence microscope

METHODOLOGY

Transport Media
- Michel or Zeus
  - These media must be kept refrigerated until use
  - Once placed in media, tissue can be kept at room temperature for up to 5 days prior to processing
  - These are transport media and not fixatives

Fresh Tissue
- Embed and freeze tissue in optimal cutting temperature (OCT) medium
- Generally more sensitive than IF or immunohistochemistry that is performed using formalin-fixed tissue sections

Formalin-fixed, Paraffin-embedded Tissue
- An important salvage technique when fresh frozen tissue is not available for IF
  - In general, formalin fixation reduces sensitivity of antigen detection by IF compared with fresh frozen tissue
- Requires digestion of tissue for antigen retrieval
- Digestion enzymes include the following
  - Pronase
  - Proteinase XXIV
  - Trypsin
  - Pepsin
  - Protease
  - Proteinase K

Antibodies
- Primary antibodies often directly conjugated with FITC
- Antibodies used in clinical evaluation of nonneoplastic biopsies (particularly kidney) include
  - IgG
    - IgG$_1$
    - IgG$_2$
    - IgG$_3$
    - IgG$_4$
    - IgG subclass testing **not** needed on a routine basis
  - IgA
  - IgM
  - Complement component C3
  - Complement component C1q
  - Fibrinogen or fibrin
  - Kappa light chain
  - Lambda light chain
  - Albumin
  - Complement component C4d
    - Tested in transplant allografts, typically kidney or heart
    - Strong and diffuse capillary endothelial staining is suggestive of antibody-mediated rejection
    - Normal granular staining of glomerular mesangial cells
  - α-3 and α-5 chains of collagen IV

Slide Storage
- Ambient light causes photobleaching
  - Store slides in dark

IMMUNOFLUORESCENCE

ASSESSMENT OF CLINICAL SPECIMENS

Kidney
- Glomerulus
  - Normal glomeruli show no immunoglobulin or complement component staining
- Mesangium
  - Granular C4d staining **not** considered pathologic
  - C4d IF tested on renal allograft specimens
- Podocyte (visceral epithelial cell)
  - Normal podocytes show no immunoglobulin or complement component staining
  - Protein resorption droplets can be prominent in some proteinuric states
    - Globular appearance and **not** to be mistaken for immune complexes, which are granular
- Glomerular basement membrane
  - Normal linear staining of the α-3 and α-5 chains of collagen IV
    - **Absence** of staining for the α-3 and α-5 chains of collagen IV in the X-linked inheritance pattern of Alport syndrome in **males**
    - **Segmental** staining for the α-3 and α-5 chains of collagen IV in the X-linked inheritance pattern of Alport syndrome in **females**
- Bowman capsule
  - Normal expression of α-5 and α-6 chains of collagen IV
- Tubule
  - C3 synthesized in proximal tubular epithelial cell cytoplasm
  - Kappa and lambda light chains and albumin highlight protein reabsorption droplets in proximal tubular epithelial cell cytoplasm
    - May be pronounced in proteinuric states
    - Monoclonal light chain staining observed in light chain proximal tubulopathy
- Tubular basement membrane
  - Normal linear staining of the α-1 chain of collagen IV
  - Normal linear staining of the α-3 and α-5 chains of collagen IV in distal tubules
- Arterioles
  - Normal granular C3 staining of endothelial cells due to cell synthesis in cytoplasm
- Interstitial inflammatory cells
  - Kappa &/or lambda light chain cytoplasmic staining can demonstrate monoclonal or polyclonal nature

Skin
- Normal skin shows no significant immunoglobulin or complement component staining
  - Abnormal staining in various vesiculobullous skin diseases
- Epidermal basement membrane
  - Normal linear staining for α-1 and α-5 chains of collagen IV
    - **Absence** of staining for the α-5 chain of collagen IV in the X-linked inheritance pattern of Alport syndrome in **males**
    - **Segmental** staining for the α-5 chain of collagen IV in the X-linked inheritance pattern of Alport syndrome in **females**
  - α-3 chain of collagen IV **not** expressed
    - Autosomal inheritance pattern of Alport syndrome (α-3 or α-4 chain of collagen IV mutations) **cannot** be excluded using a skin specimen

Oral Mucosa
- Normal oral mucosa shows no significant immunoglobulin or complement component staining
  - Abnormal staining in various vesiculobullous diseases

Lung
- Normal basement membranes show no significant immunoglobulin or complement component staining
  - Strong linear staining for IgG and kappa and lambda light chains observed in pulmonary involvement by anti-glomerular basement membrane disease (Goodpasture syndrome)

Transplant Allografts
- C4d capillary staining is suggestive of antibody-mediated rejection
  - Typically tested in heart and renal allografts
    - Interstitial C4d staining is a nonspecific finding in heart allografts
    - Tubular basement membrane C4d staining of atrophic tubules is nonspecific and can mimic peritubular capillaries

RELATED REFERENCES

1. Haas M: Alport syndrome and thin glomerular basement membrane nephropathy: a practical approach to diagnosis. Arch Pathol Lab Med. 133(2):224-32, 2009
2. Wagrowska-Danilewicz M et al: Immunofluorescence on paraffin-embedded sections in evaluation of immune complex deposits in renal biopsy specimens. Pol J Pathol. 60(1):3-9, 2009
3. van der Ven K et al: Immunofluorescence on proteinase XXIV-digested paraffin sections. Kidney Int. 72(7):896, 2007
4. Nasr SH et al: Immunofluorescence on pronase-digested paraffin sections: a valuable salvage technique for renal biopsies. Kidney Int. 70(12):2148-51, 2006
5. Zhou W et al: Intrarenal synthesis of complement. Kidney Int. 59(4):1227-35, 2001
6. Fogazzi GB et al: Comparison of immunofluorescent findings in kidney after snap-freezing and formalin fixation. Pathol Res Pract. 185(2):225-30, 1989
7. Miura M et al: Evaluation of the staining findings of immunofluorescence in unfixed or fixed renal biopsy specimens from patients with IgA nephropathy and membranous nephropathy. Acta Pathol Jpn. 35(2):315-21, 1985
8. Qualman SJ et al: Immunofluorescence of deparaffinized, trypsin-treated renal tissues. Preservation of antigens as an adjunct to diagnosis of disease. Lab Invest. 41(6):483-9, 1979

IMMUNOFLUORESCENCE

Normal Glomerulus

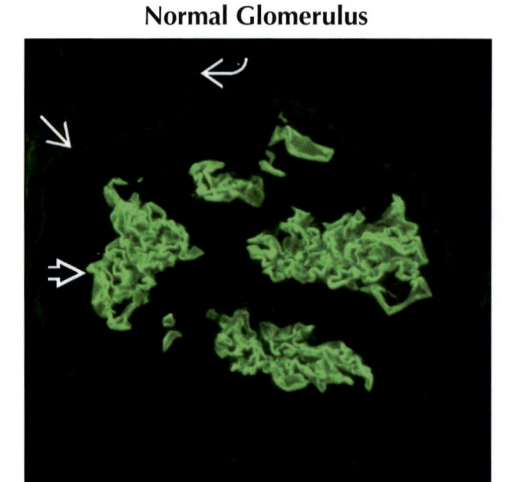

Normal Distal Tubules

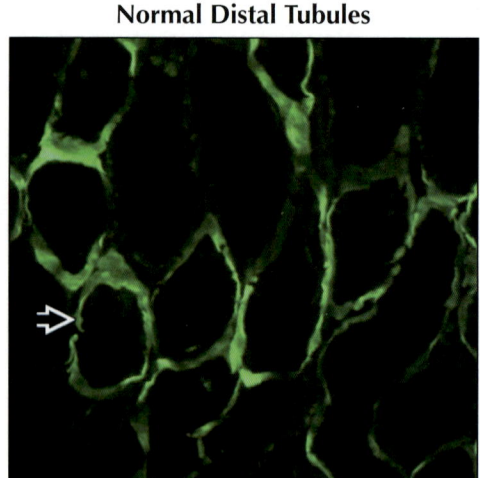

(Left) This glomerulus shows normal linear staining of the glomerular basement membranes ➡ for the α-3 chain of collagen IV. Bowman capsule ➡ consists of only α-5 and α-6 chains of collagen IV and shows no staining. The adjacent proximal tubular basement membranes ➡ show no staining for the α-3 chain of collagen IV. *(Right)* The distal tubules in this medullary ray demonstrate strong linear staining of the tubular basement membranes ➡ for α-3 chain of collagen IV.

Normal C3 Synthesis in Tubular Epithelial Cells

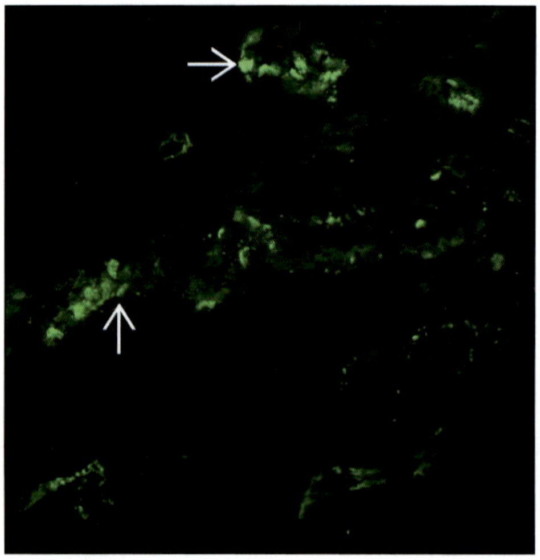

C3 in Endothelial Cells

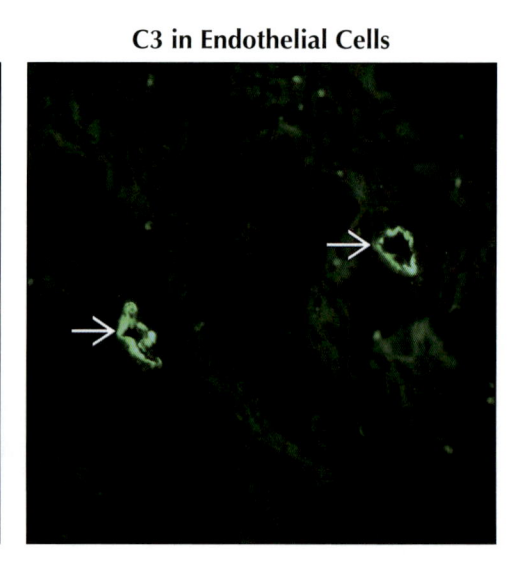

(Left) IF for C3 reveals this protein within the tubular epithelial cell cytoplasm ➡, which is due to normal synthesis. Linear C3 staining of tubular basement membranes (not shown) may be present and is of uncertain significance. *(Right)* C3 is synthesized in endothelial cells ➡ of several arterioles and this is a useful internal positive control. Granular C3 staining of the vessel walls along with C1q and other immunoglobulins can be observed in lupus nephritis and would be consistent with immune complexes.

C4d in Glomerulus

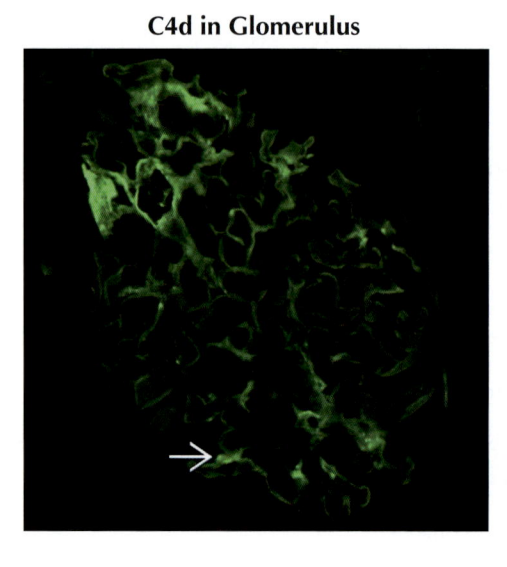

Albumin in Tubular Epithelial Cells

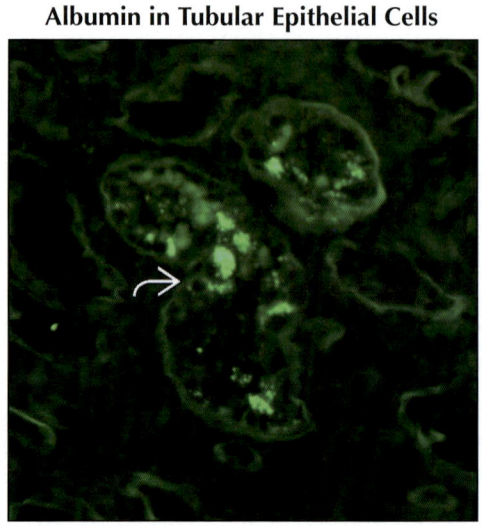

(Left) Granular mesangial ➡ C4d staining is a useful internal control and not considered a pathologic finding. The presence of C4d deposition of peritubular capillaries (not shown) in a kidney transplant biopsy would be suggestive of antibody-mediated rejection. *(Right)* IF reveals normal reabsorption for albumin within the proximal tubular epithelial cell cytoplasm ➡. Tubular resorption droplets may be increased in proteinuric states. Kappa and lambda light chains often stain these droplets.

IMMUNOFLUORESCENCE

Normal Skin

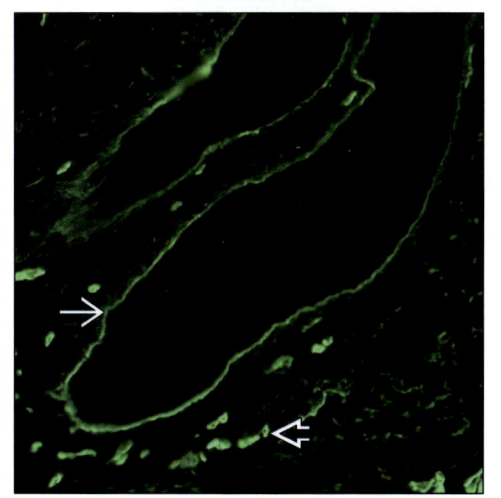

Normal Skin

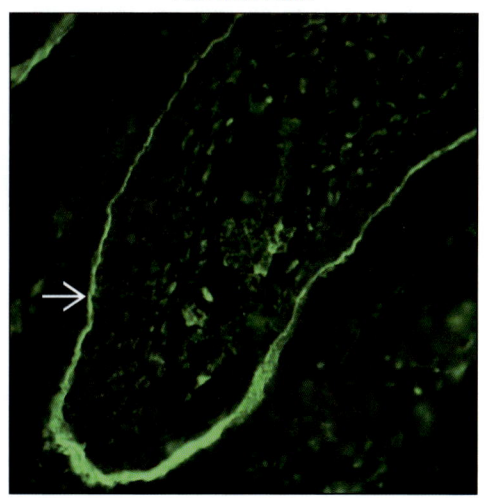

(Left) The epidermal ➡ and capillary ➡ basement membranes from this normal skin biopsy demonstrate strong linear staining for the α-1 chain of collagen IV. **(Right)** The epidermal basement membrane ➡ from this normal skin biopsy reveals strong linear staining for the α-5 chain of collagen IV. Significant background staining of the epidermis (not shown) may be present in some specimens and should not be mistaken for the epidermal basement membrane.

X-linked Alport Syndrome Skin Biopsy in Male Patient

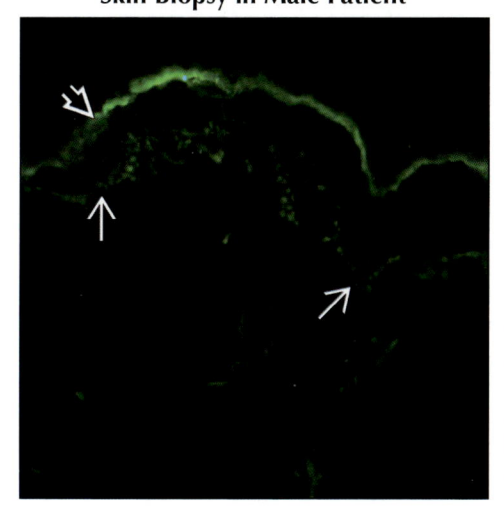

X-linked Alport Syndrome Skin Biopsy in Female Patient

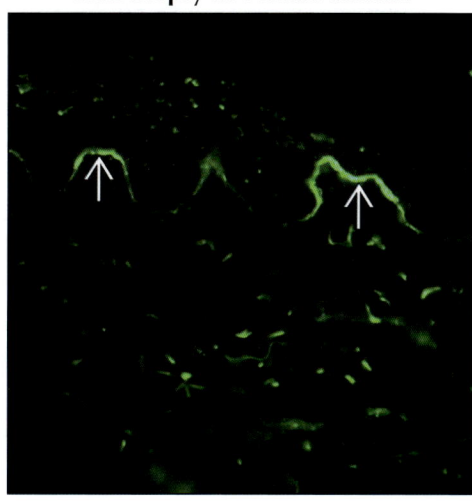

(Left) The α-5 chain of collagen IV shows no staining of the epidermal basement membrane ➡, which is diagnostic of the X-linked inheritance pattern of Alport syndrome (hereditary nephritis). There is a blush of staining in the overlying cornified layer (stratum corneum) ➡ that should not be mistaken as a positive result. **(Right)** Segmental staining ➡ of the epidermal basement membrane for the α-5 chain of collagen IV is diagnostic of Alport syndrome in a female patient.

Pulmonary Basement Membranes

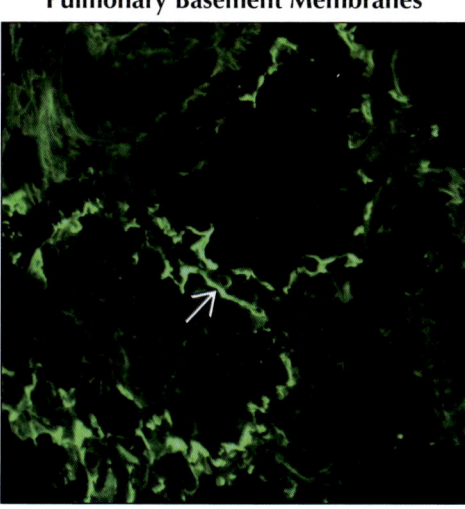

C4d in Heart Allograft

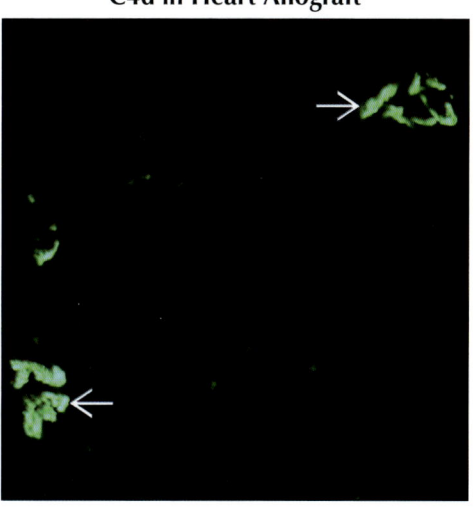

(Left) IgG linear staining of the basement membranes ➡ is observed in a patient with pulmonary hemorrhage (Goodpasture syndrome) and anti-glomerular basement membrane nephritis. The epithelial and capillary basement membranes are normally irregularly fused as shown in these alveoli, but a normal lung would not reveal any IgG deposition. **(Right)** C4d stains several necrotic myocytes ➡ but the capillaries are negative, which argues against antibody-mediated rejection.

ELECTRON MICROSCOPY

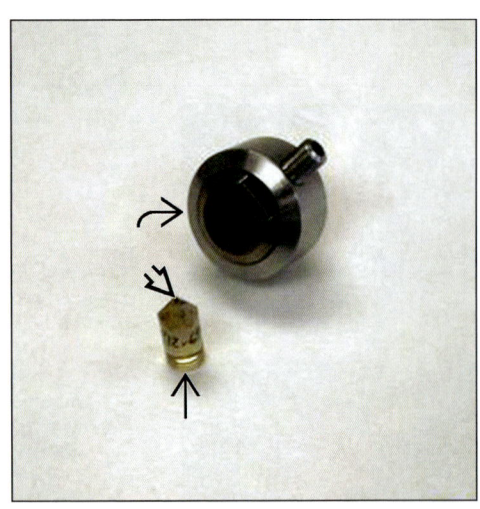

The tissue measures 1 mm in width at the tip of the epoxy resin block with the specimen label. The block is subsequently placed in the microtome holder for sectioning. (Courtesy J. Brainer, MS.)

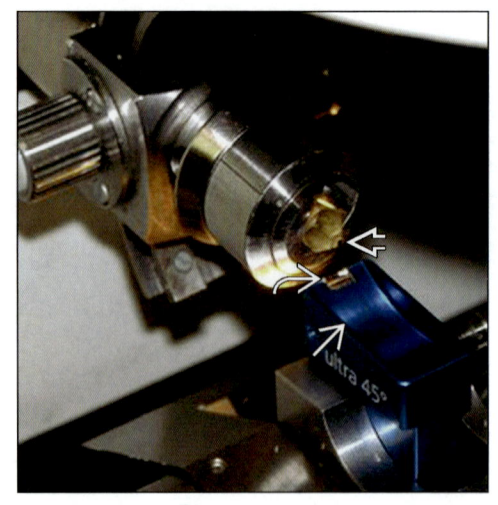

The EPON block is in the microtome. The knife trough collects the tissue sections as they come off the diamond knife. These sections are placed on grids for EM evaluation. (Courtesy J. Brainer, MS.)

TERMINOLOGY

Abbreviations
- Electron microscopy (EM)

Definitions
- Transmission EM
  - Resolution of 0.2 nm compared to 200 nm for light microscope
  - Clinically useful in certain settings
- Scanning EM
  - Electron beam scans surface of (not through) examined specimen
  - Provides 3D image of surfaces and topography

SPECIMEN HANDLING

Tissue Handling
- Place tissue in fixative immediately

Fixatives
- Karnovsky
  - 2% formaldehyde and 2.5% glutaraldehyde
- Glutaraldehyde
- 10% buffered formalin
  - Tissue may not have been initially submitted for EM after gross examination
    - Tissue fixed in formalin may be subsequently placed in glutaraldehyde or Karnovsky media for EM processing
  - Processing formalin-fixed, paraffin-embedded tissue results in poor preservation of fine cellular structures

Post Fixation
- Osmium tetroxide
  - Heavy metal that reacts with phospholipids to increase electron density for imaging

SPECIMEN PROCESSING

Embedding Media
- Methacrylate/acrylate
- Epoxy resin/EPON

Sectioning Blocks and Staining Sections
- 1 μm thick (or semi-thin) sections are generated from plastic-embedded tissue
  - Light microscopic examination with the following special stains
    - Toluidine blue
    - Methylene blue
- Thin sections (~ 100 nm thickness) are placed on special grids for definitive EM evaluation
  - Thicker sections (> 100 nm) may be visualized with more recently developed electron microscopes
  - Grids stained with uranyl acetate and lead citrate

Immunolabeling
- Primary or secondary antibodies labeled with particles (e.g., gold) of uniform size may detect antigens of interest

EM ASSESSMENT OF CLINICAL SAMPLES

Kidney
- Glomerular basement membrane
  - Consists of lamina rara externa (region between podocyte and lamina densa), lamina densa, and lamina rara interna (region between lamina densa and endothelial cell)
  - Range for 9 years or older: 264-460 nm
    - < 264 nm considered thin basement membrane disease by World Health Organization
  - Lamellation or "basket-weave" appearance characteristic of Alport syndrome (hereditary nephritis)
- Podocyte (visceral epithelial cell)
  - Intact foot processes
    - Effacement of foot processes correlates with proteinuria
  - Absence of inclusions or crystals
    - Crystals present in light chain Fanconi syndrome
    - Myelin bodies present in Fabry disease

ELECTRON MICROSCOPY

- Endothelial cell (fenestrated)
  - Swelling of cytoplasm (endotheliosis) in preeclampsia
  - Tubuloreticular inclusions
    - Observed in states of high interferon, including systemic lupus erythematosus and human immunodeficiency virus infection
- Mesangial matrix
  - Increased in diabetic nephropathy
- Proximal tubular epithelial cell
  - Brush border or microvilli at apical surface
    - Loss or blunted in acute tubular injury
  - Basolateral interdigitations
    - Loss in acute tubular injury
- Peritubular capillary
  - Multilayering of basement membrane in renal allografts with chronic antibody-mediated rejection

Muscle

- Syncytial multinucleated myofibers develop through fusion of mononucleated myoblasts
- Cell membrane (sarcolemma) surrounded by continuous basement membrane
- Neuromuscular junction
  - Ultrastructural changes with myasthenia gravis and other myasthenic syndromes
- T-tubules
  - Tubular invaginations of sarcolemma allowing uniform spread of depolarization throughout myofibers
  - Sandwiched between endoplasmic reticulum ("sarcoplasmic reticulum") as "triad"
  - Triad essential for electromechanical coupling
    - Uniform calcium release in response to depolarization triggering contraction
- Sarcomeres
  - Contractile filaments are arranged into myofibrils
    - Serially arranged sarcomeres; each ~1 μm in diameter and 2-3 μm in length
  - Z discs anchor thin actin filaments
  - M line marks the anchorage of thick myosin filaments
  - Disorganized or disrupted arrangement of sarcomere elements, e.g., intensive care unit (ICU) myopathy or nemaline myopathy
- Organelles
  - Peripheral subsarcolemmal nuclei
  - Mitochondria, glycogen, and other organelles between myofibrils
    - Increased numbers of and morphologically abnormal mitochondria with mitochondrial disease
  - Abnormal accumulations of glycogen or lipid with some storage diseases
- Blood vessels between myofibers may show endothelial cell inclusions (tubuloreticular inclusions) with autoimmune conditions like dermatomyositis

Nerve

- Axons arranged into fascicles
- Fascicles surrounded by perineurial cells (long thin processes, continuous basement membrane, and prominent pinocytotic vesicles)
- Myelinated axons
  - 1 Schwann cell myelinates a single internode of a single axon
  - Myelin thickness proportional to axonal diameter
- Unmyelinated axons
  - 1 Schwann cell surrounds segments of several axons
- Axonal density decreased with axonal disease
- Thinned myelin sheath with demyelinating disease or axonal regeneration

Sinonasal Mucosa

- Cilia
  - Normal 9+2 structure of microtubules
    - Absence of dynein arms in Kartagener syndrome or primary ciliary dyskinesis

Heart

- Adriamycin (doxorubicin) toxicity
  - Swelling of myocyte sarcoplasmic reticulum
  - Disruption or loss of myofibrils
  - Possible focal involvement

Small Intestinal Mucosa

- Intact microvilli
  - Microvillus inclusion disease
    - Absence of apical microvilli
    - Accumulation of secretory granules
  - Tufting enteropathy
    - Increased length and number of desmosomes between small intestinal epithelial cells

Neoplasm

- EM may reveal ultrastructural clues to the cell type, such as
  - Premelanosomes and melanosomes in melanocytes
  - Weibel-Palade bodies in endothelial cells
  - Birbeck granules in Langerhans cells
  - Neuroendocrine granules in neuroendocrine tumors
  - Fibrillary background in neuroblastoma
  - Muscle filaments and Z band material in rhabdomyosarcoma
  - Immunohistochemistry has largely supplanted EM for cellular characterization

RELATED REFERENCES

1. Sterling C et al: Pathology of Skeletal Muscle. 2nd edition. Oxford University Press, 2001
2. Haas M: A reevaluation of routine electron microscopy in the examination of native renal biopsies. J Am Soc Nephrol. 8(1):70-6, 1997
3. Erlandson RA: Diagnostic Transmission Electron Microscopy of Tumors. Philadelphia: Lippincott, 1994
4. Hayat MA: Principles and Techniques of Electron Microscopy: Biological Applications. Vol 1. New York: Van Norstrand Rheinhold, 1975

ELECTRON MICROSCOPY

(Left) Semi-thin or thick (1 μm) sections are evaluated to assess if additional thin sections should be obtained for ultrastructural evaluation. Significant histologic information can be obtained by light microscopic examination. **(Right)** This low-magnification photograph (150x) demonstrates the grid upon which the thin tissue section sits. Occasionally, the gridlines ➡ may obstruct a specific structure of interest, but several tissue sections are often available on the grid for ultrastructural evaluation.

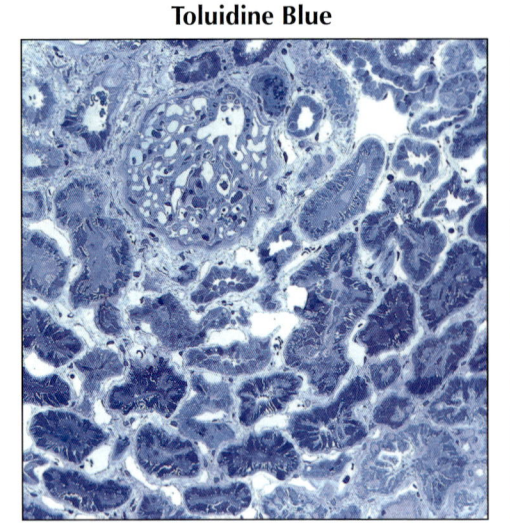

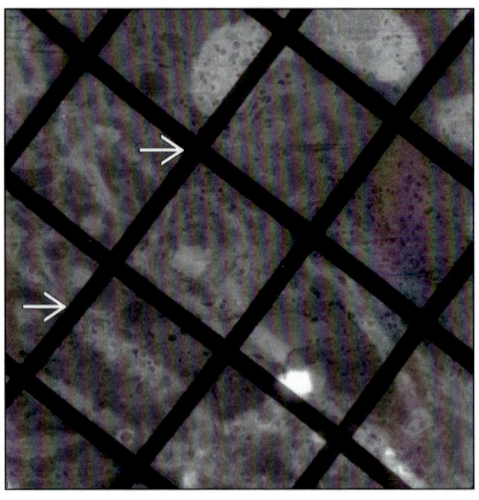

Toluidine Blue

EM Grid

(Left) The glomerular basement membranes ➡ of several capillaries are of normal thickness and are covered by podocytes ➡ with intact foot processes ➡. A mesangial cell nucleus ➡ is present. **(Right)** This normal proximal tubular epithelial cell contains many mitochondria ➡. There is an intact brush border with microvilli ➡ at the apical surface, with basolateral interdigitations ➡. In acute tubular injury, the microvilli are blunted and there is loss of the basolateral interdigitations.

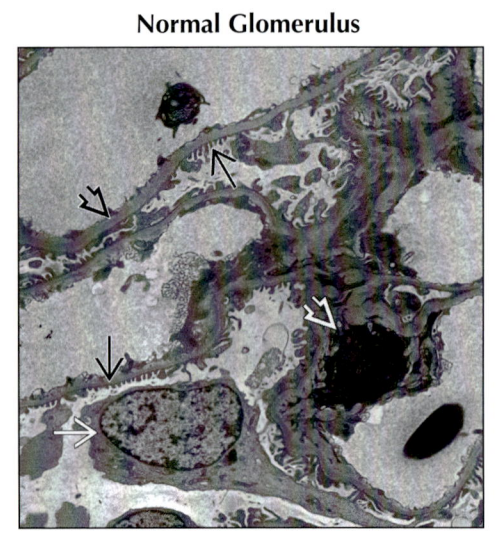

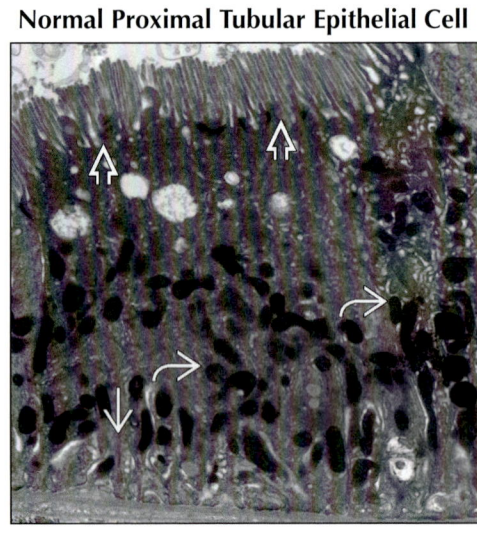

Normal Glomerulus

Normal Proximal Tubular Epithelial Cell

(Left) The cilia ➡ in this sinonasal biopsy, captured in the correct plane, demonstrate the normal 9+2 configuration of microtubules with dynein arms ➡, which excludes the diagnosis of Kartagener syndrome. (Courtesy E. Sengupta, MD.) **(Right)** Numerous villi ➡ are present at the apical surface of this normal small intestinal epithelial cell from a pediatric patient with diarrhea, which excludes the diagnosis of microvillus inclusion disease. (Courtesy E. Sengupta, MD.)

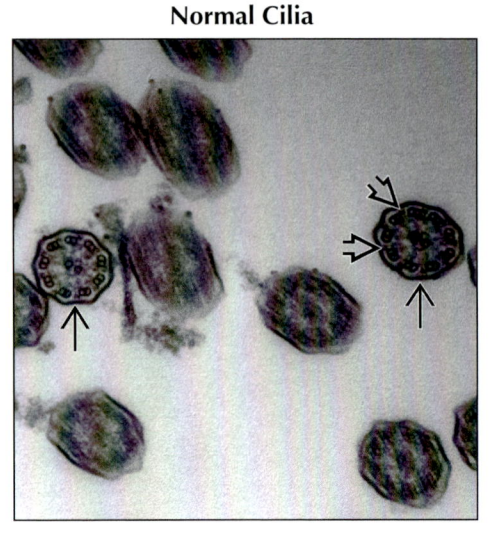

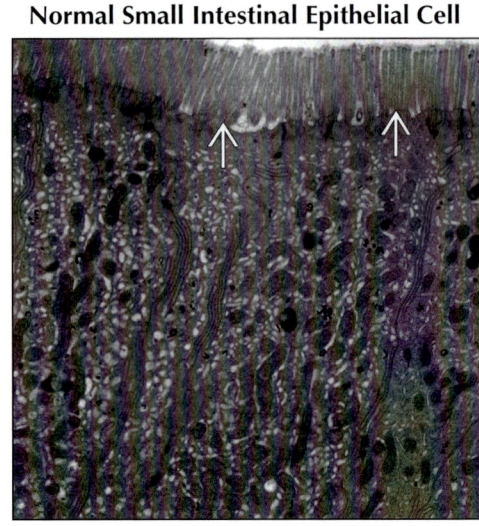

Normal Cilia

Normal Small Intestinal Epithelial Cell

ELECTRON MICROSCOPY

Normal Skeletal Muscle

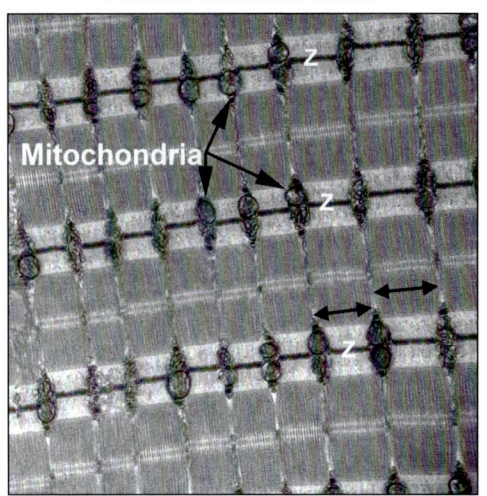

Normal Skeletal Muscle: Sarcomere

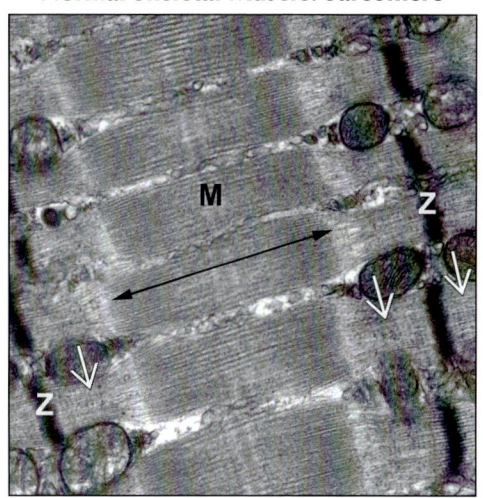

(Left) The characteristic arrangement of contractile filaments and organelles appear as cross-striations on light microscopy. Myofibrils consist of sarcomeres, defined as the area between adjacent Z discs (Z). Double arrows mark the diameter of myofibrils. Mitochondria are found between myofibrils. *(Right)* A sarcomere is bordered by 2 Z discs (Z), which also are the I band midline. The M line (M) anchors myosin filaments at the sarcomere midline. The A band (double arrow) is separated by I bands ➡.

Normal Skeletal Muscle: T-Tubule

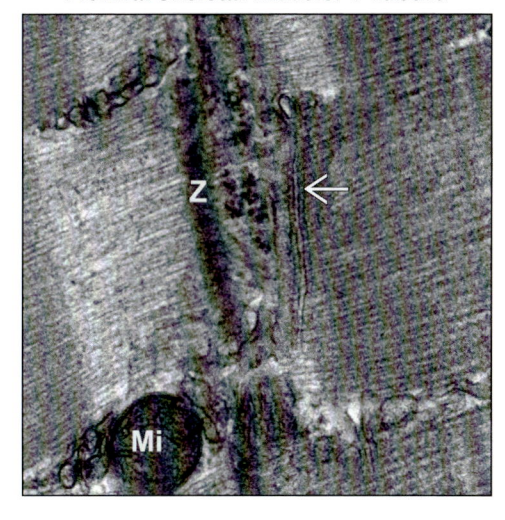

Malignant Neoplasm

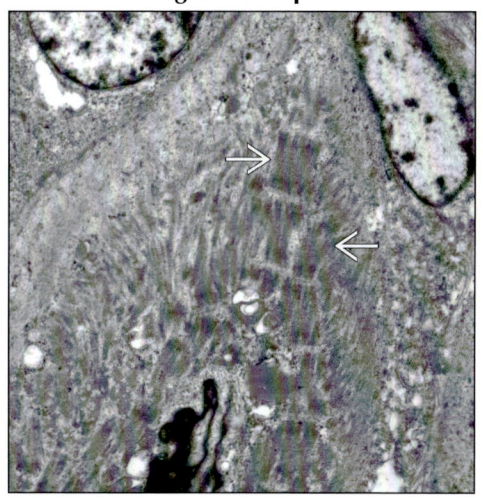

(Left) The T-tubule ➡ is the membranous structure running perpendicular to the orientation of the sarcomere. A Z disc (Z) and a mitochondrion (Mi) are present. *(Right)* Skeletal muscle differentiation is established based on the distinct sarcomeres ➡ that are identified within the cell cytoplasm of this neoplasm. This finding in the setting of a malignant peripheral nerve sheath tumor indicates a triton tumor, which often has an aggressive clinical course.

Normal Nerve

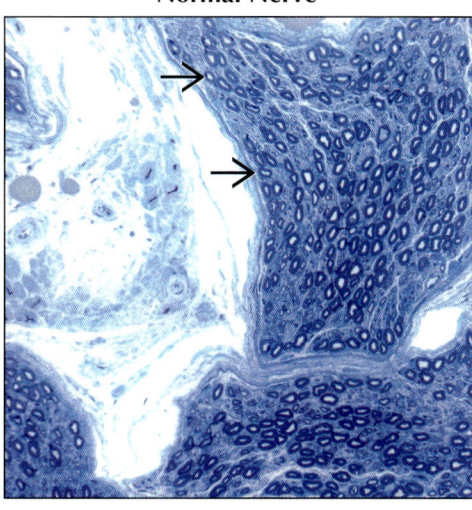

Normal Nerve

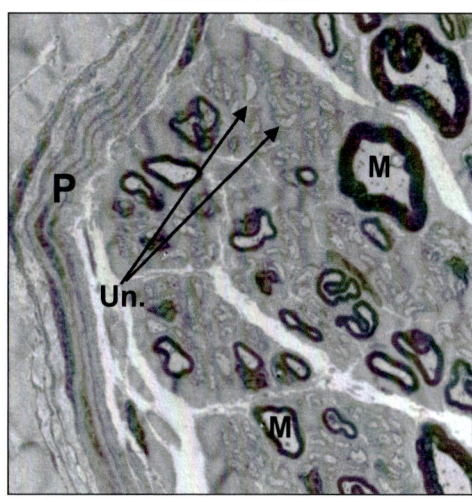

(Left) The embedding process nicely preserves the lipid-rich myelin layer ➡ around axons in this normal nerve, which is better visualized with the toluidine blue stain than on a paraffin section. *(Right)* Cross section of peripheral nerve shows perineurium marking the outer border of a fascicle (P). Myelinated axons of varying diameter are seen (M). The thickness of the myelin sheaths correlates with the diameter of the axons. Thin, unmyelinated axons are found in the background (Un.).

INTRODUCTION TO THE CELL

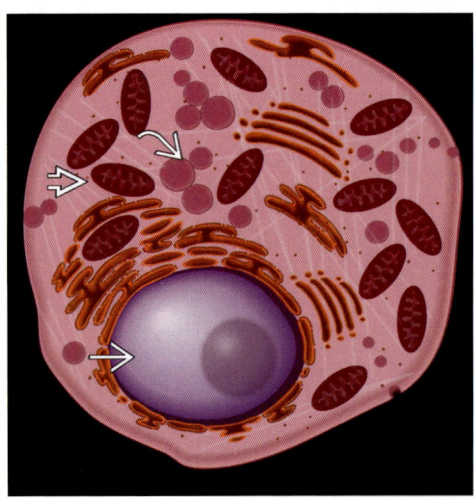

This depiction of organelle distribution within a cell shows a basally placed nucleus ➡, mitochondria ➡, endoplasmic reticulum, and variably sized granules ➡ (mucin or other proteins).

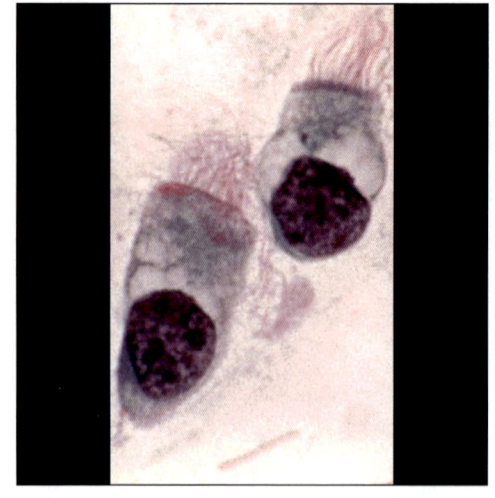

Endocervical cells from a Pap smear show typical cellular organization (basal nucleus, variable chromatin clumping, terminal bar with cilia, granular cytoplasm, and vacuoles, probably Golgi with mucin droplet formation).

TERMINOLOGY

Definitions
- Cell: Basic structural unit of all tissue
- Organelles: Intracellular heterogeneous interactive substructures best resolved by transmission electron microscopy

OVERALL CELL ORGANIZATION

Membrane
- Major unit of organization
- Membranes appear as single linear structure by light microscopy and low-magnification electron microscopy
- Phospholipid bilayer: Hydrophilic surface, hydrophobic center with interspersed variable-sized protein globules

Membrane-Bound Organelles
- Plasma membrane, nucleus, endoplasmic reticulum (rough and smooth), Golgi apparatus, mitochondria, various types of secretory/neuroendocrine granules, mucin droplets, lysosomes
- Plasma membrane surface specialization: Microvilli

Non-Membrane-Bound Organelles
- Nuclear chromatin, nucleolus, intracytoplasmic contractile and anchoring filaments, cytoskeletal tubules, free ribosomes, glycogen, fat globules, desmosomes, attachment plaques, centrioles, and basal bodies

Extracellular Elements
- Basal lamina, collagen, matrix proteoglycans

NUCLEUS

Chromatin
- Electron-dense aggregates representing DNA
  - Heterochromatin: Clumped, electron-dense DNA, biologically inactive
  - Euchromatin: Dispersed DNA, biologically active
- Individual chromosomes not apparent without cell culture

Chromosomes
- 46 total chromosomes per human cell

Nucleolus
- Focus of variable prominence in nucleus
- Filamentous and granular nucleolonema composed of histones, RNA, and regulatory cell cycle proteins

Cytoplasmic Interactions
- Via
  - Nuclear pores
  - Nuclear blebs
  - Cisternal space contiguous with endoplasmic reticulum (ER)
  - Dissolution of nuclear membrane during mitosis

CYTOPLASM

Endoplasmic Reticulum
- Definition
  - Parallel arrangement of membranes adjacent to and contiguous with nucleus
- Rough ER (rER)
  - Ribosomes are free, small granular aggregates of cytoplasmic RNA which, when attached to ER membranes, constitute rER
  - Messenger RNA (mRNA) attaches at junction of 2 ribosomal regions
  - Transfer RNA (tRNA) sequentially attaches 1 end to mRNA with opposite end bearing amino acid
  - Protein synthesis accumulates in cistern of rER for cell membrane maintenance or for secretory export
- Smooth ER (sER)
  - Same membrane complex but no associated ribosomes
  - Often contiguous with rER
  - Involved in detoxification, synthesis of steroids, lipid absorption, and metabolism

INTRODUCTION TO THE CELL

  - Also known as sarcoplasmic reticulum in cardiac and skeletal muscle

Golgi Apparatus
- Receives proteins from rER for post-translational modification and packaging
- Delivers enzymes to lysosomes
- Histologic appearance is clear area adjacent to nucleus (hof in typical plasma cell)

Mitochondria
- Complex of internal membranes (cristae) bound by external membrane
- Energy source for cell through adenosine triphosphate (ATP) production
- High numbers impart granular eosinophilic cytoplasm, e.g., oncocytes

Lysosomes
- Membrane bound, round, protein-containing bodies
- May contain hydrolytic enzymes
- Involved in cell maintenance by degrading membranes and obsolescent organelles
- End stage is "residual body"

Cell Membrane Specializations
- Microvilli
  - Apical foldings protruding into gland lumen
  - Increase surface area of cell for absorption from gland lumen
- Pinocytotic vesicles
  - Tiny plasma membrane invaginations
  - Facilitate exchange or movement of fluid
  - Prominent in endothelial cells and smooth muscle cells

CYTOSKELETON

Thin Filaments (Actin)
- Actin biochemically ubiquitous
- In muscle cells, organized into short wavy bundles held together by "dense bodies"
- Best seen in smooth muscle, myoepithelial cells, myofibroblasts
- Contractile function

Thick Filaments
- Predominantly myosin, most prominent in skeletal and cardiac muscle
- Organized with actin filaments and Z bands giving "striated" appearance by light microscopy
- Contractile function

Microtubules
- Long, hollow cylindrical structure
- Consists of tubulin
- Anchored to centrosome

Intermediate Filaments
- Cytokeratin: Short, wavy bundles often inserting on desmosomes or plasma membrane plaques, best seen in squamous epithelium
- Vimentin: Widespread in mesenchymal cells
- Desmin: Contractile protein in muscle cells
- Glial fibrillary acidic protein: Predominant in glia of CNS
- Neurofilament: Predominant in CNS, peripheral nervous system, and neuroendocrine cells

Centrioles
- Basal bodies: Anchoring structures, usually at apex of epithelial cells
- Cilia: Tubular doublets arranged 9 (peripheral) + 2 (central)

CELL ADHESION

Desmosomes (Macula Adherens)
- Attachment of epithelial cell to another epithelial cell
- Zonula occludens
- Zonula adherens
- Terminal bar is light microscopic structure composed of desmosomes linked by horizontal filaments near apex beneath numerous microvilli

Hemidesmosomes
- Attachment of epithelial cell to connective tissue

EXTRACELLULAR SUBSTANCES

Basal Lamina
- Cell product forming interface between cell and underlying connective tissue
- Epithelial cells (principally glandular), myoepithelial cells, endothelial cells, pericytes, smooth muscle, Schwann cells
- Composed of type IV collagen
- Basement membrane is light microscopic structure composed of basal lamina and underlying polymerized collagen fibers, best seen by PAS staining

Collagen
- Major protein product of some cells
- Organized as fibrils with periodicity of 64 nm

RELATED REFERENCES
1. Ross MR et al: Histology: A Text and Atlas With Correlated Cell and Molecular Biology. 6th ed. Philadelphia: Lippincott Williams & Wilkins, 2011
2. Alberts B et al: Molecular Biology of the Cell. 4th ed. New York City: Garland Sciences, 2002

INTRODUCTION TO THE CELL

Nucleus and Nucleoli

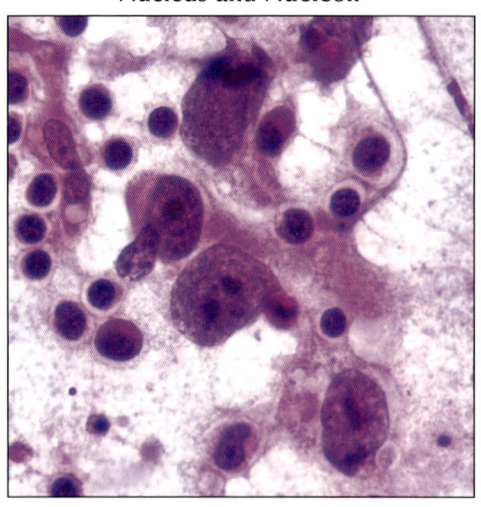

Nucleus, Nucleolus, and Unit Membrane

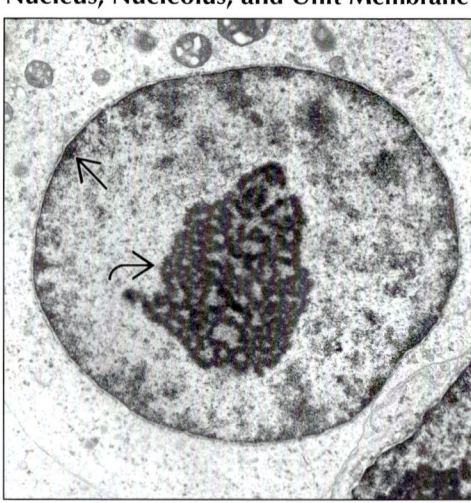

(Left) This touch imprint from a seminoma of the testis with a cluster of tumor cells and background lymphocytes demonstrates well-defined, enlarged nuclei, each with at least 1 prominent nucleolus. (Right) The nuclear membrane appears as a single linear structure on this EM. There is both heterochromatin ⇨ (clumped along the nuclear membrane) and euchromatin (dispersed), the latter reflecting metabolic activity. The central prominent nucleolus ⇨ is composed of filamentous nucleolonema.

Unit Membrane

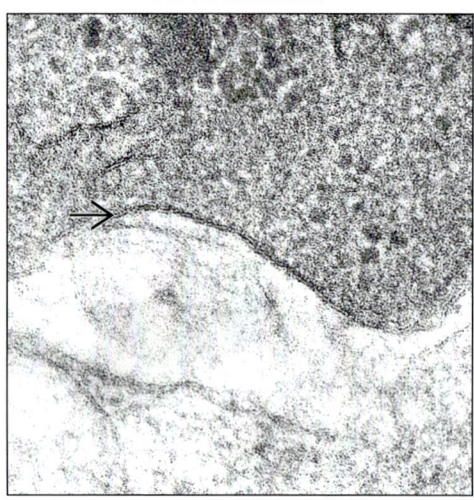

Nuclear-Cytoplasmic Interactions

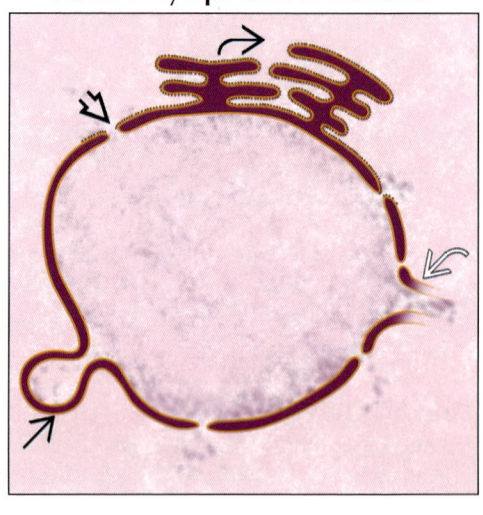

(Left) This high magnification EM of nuclear membrane demonstrates a trilaminar structure ⇨ with 2 fine parallel densities separated by a lucent region. The top half of the image is represented by heterochromatin. (Right) This diagram highlights the nuclear-cytoplasmic communication that occurs through the following structures: (1) nuclear blebs ⇨, (2) nuclear pores ⇨, (3) communication between perinuclear space and rER ⇨, and (4) dissolution of the nuclear membrane during mitosis ⇨.

Nuclear Blebs: EM

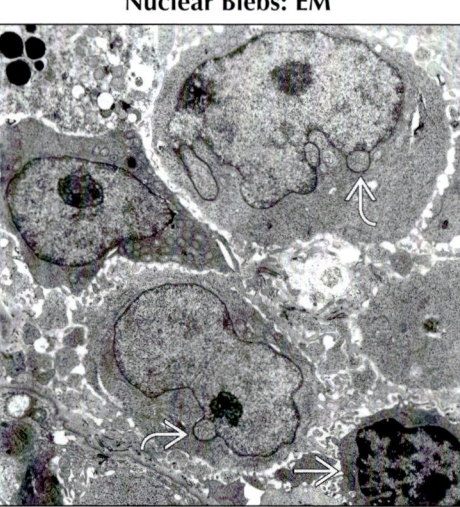

Rough Endoplasmic Reticulum

(Left) EM shows there are several lymphoid cells in various stages of activation. A mature lymphocyte ⇨ is in the lower right. Each of the remaining nuclei has a prominent nucleolus. The nuclear membranes of the 2 center cells are convoluted and show occasional thin circular extensions ⇨ entrapping cytoplasms. (Right) Apposing membranes of the endoplasmic reticulum create a flattened compartment for protein synthesis. The attached external granules are ribosomes.

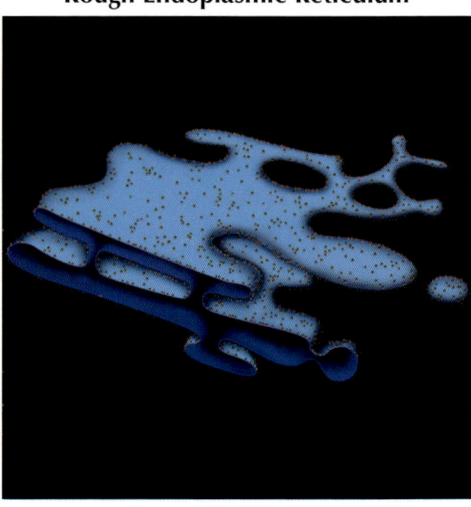

INTRODUCTION TO THE CELL

Plasma Cells

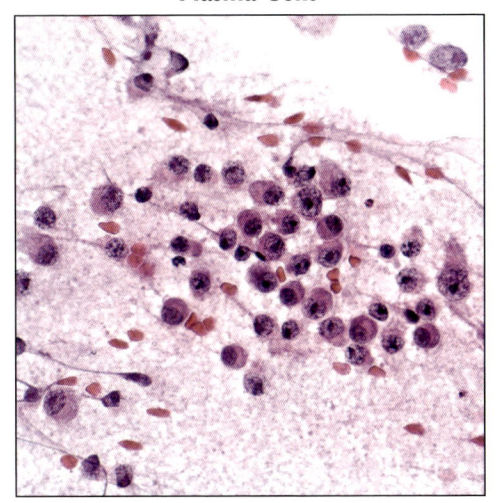

Plasma Cell

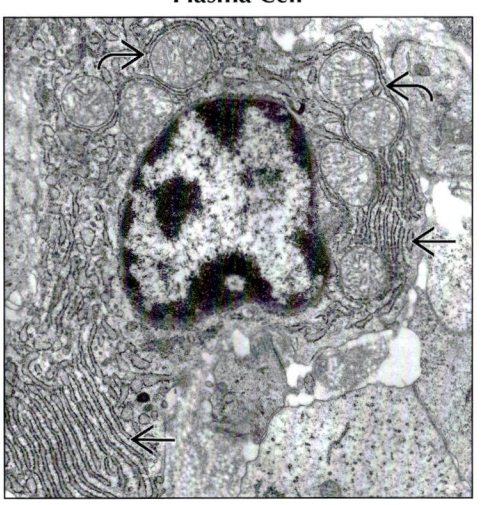

(Left) Touch imprint of a cluster of reactive plasma cells shows the displaced, clock-faced nucleus adjacent to a cleared area of cytoplasm (hof) that corresponds ultrastructurally to the location of the Golgi apparatus, mitochondria, & assorted organelles. Basophilic cytoplasm corresponds to distribution of rER. (Right) In this EM of mature plasma cell, the area next to the nucleus is occupied by mitochondria ➔. Most of the cytoplasm is occupied by flat cisterns of endoplasmic reticulum ➔.

Plasma Cell

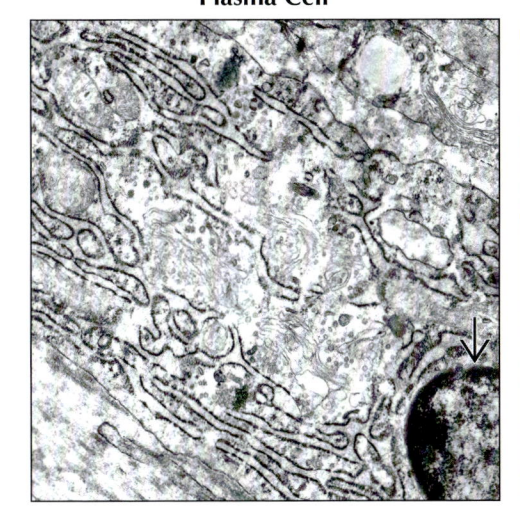

Free Ribosomes and rER

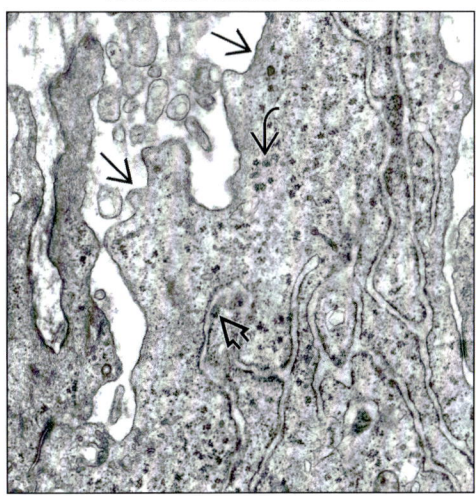

(Left) EM shows that in the perinuclear area of this plasma cell, the nucleus ➔ is apposed to flat cisterns of the Golgi apparatus, all of which are surrounded by flattened rough endoplasmic reticulum (rER). (Right) This portion of a cell periphery on EM shows convoluted plasma membranes ➔ and scattered intracytoplasmic ribosomes ➔, some of which attach to rER ➔.

Smooth ER (sER)

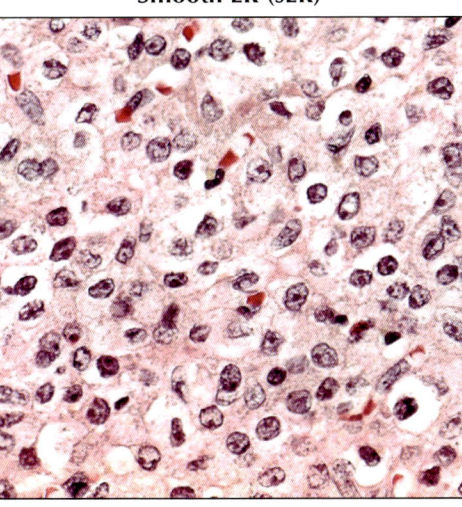

Smooth Endoplasmic Reticulum

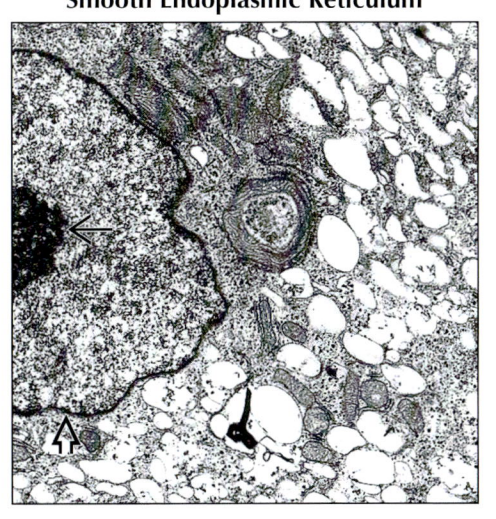

(Left) In this portion of an adrenal cortical adenoma, the tumor cells have abundant foamy cytoplasm reflective of prominent smooth endoplasmic reticulum. (Right) EM shows a portion of an adrenal cortical tumor cell with cytoplasm is filled with rounded, clear spaces of smooth endoplasmic reticulum (sER). Note the large nucleus ➔ with dispersed chromatin and part of a prominent nucleolus ➔. The prominent sER correlates with steroid production.

INTRODUCTION TO THE CELL

Salivary Gland Ducts and Acini

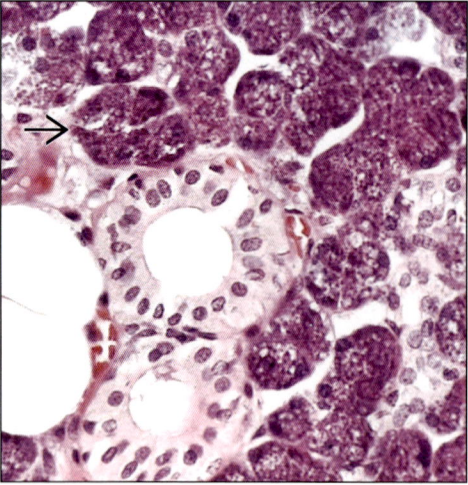

Acinar Cell

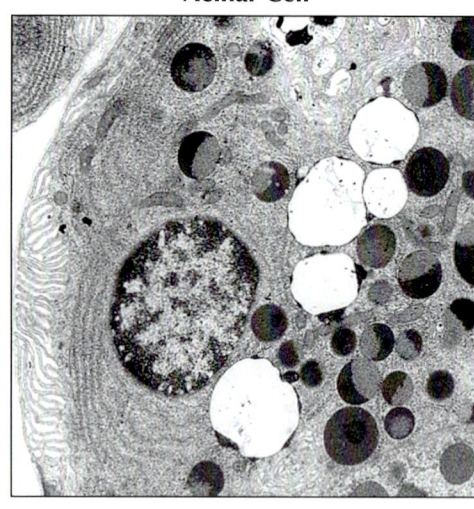

(Left) A salivary gland lobule with 2 ducts is surrounded by acini with cytoplasm ➡ filled with enzymatic granules, which is indicative of an active Golgi system. (Right) Electron microscopy shows an acinar cell with a basal nucleus and apical variably sized granules of heterogeneous electron density. Flat rER surrounds the bottom and sides of the nucleus. Basally, there are numerous folds of plasma membrane abutting the stroma and outlined by a basal lamina.

Mast Cell Granules

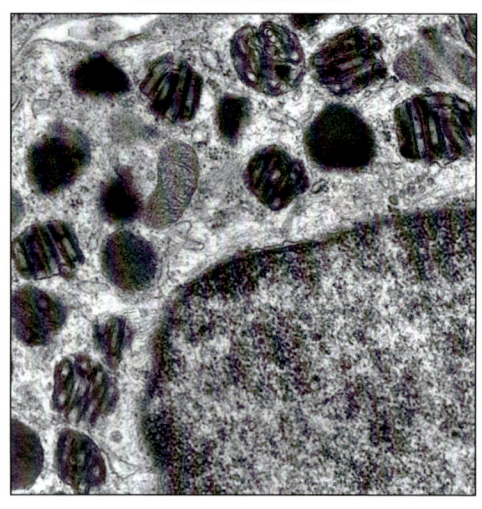

Neuroendocrine Granules and Centriole

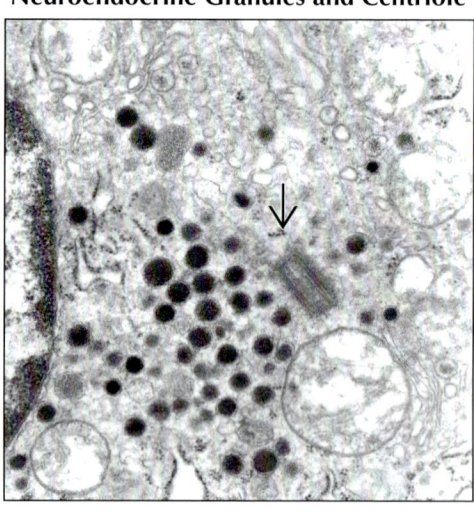

(Left) Secretory granules may contain mucin or digestive enzymes, be lysosomal as in lipofuscin, or be specialized. These granules have a scroll-like structure and are characteristic of mast cells. (Right) This juxtanuclear collection of neuroendocrine granules is from a paraganglioma. These small granules contain mixtures of peptides and amines. There is a centriole ➡ adjacent to the cluster of granules.

Lipofuscin Granules

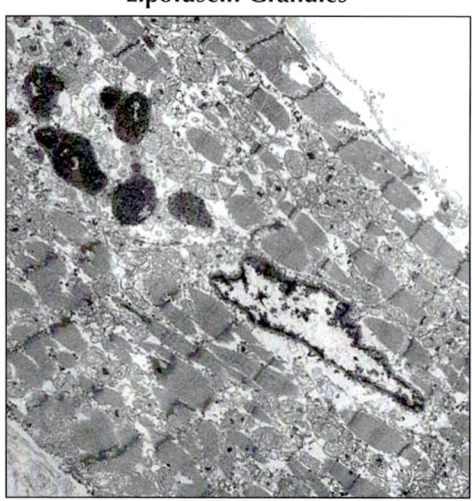

Lysosomes

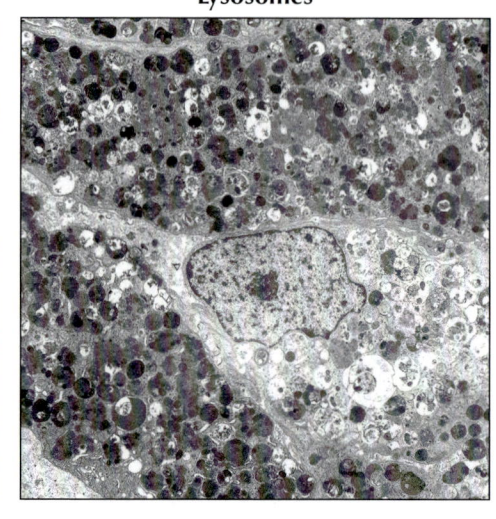

(Left) EM shows this portion of a cardiac muscle cell contains paranuclear clusters of variably sized, dark, membrane-bound granules. Histologically, these granules are brown and similar to those seen in the liver. (Right) EM shows several tumor cells from a granular cell tumor contain intracytoplasmic granules, which are of variable size, density, and internal complexity. These are characteristic of lysosomes.

INTRODUCTION TO THE CELL

Oncocytes

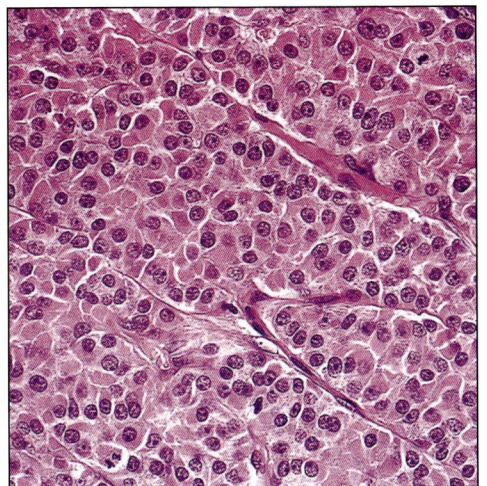

Oncocytoma

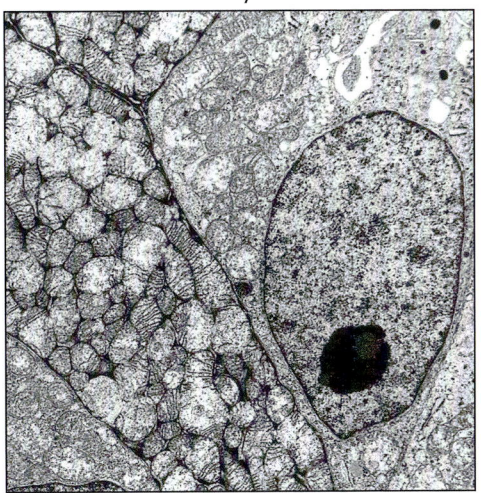

(Left) The cells of an oncocytoma have granular, eosinophilic cytoplasm reflecting numerous intracytoplasmic mitochondria. *(Right)* EM shows the cytoplasm is filled with mitochondria, to the exclusion of most other organelles. The internal substructure of cristae is clearly visible.

Fat, Glycogen, and Lipofuscin

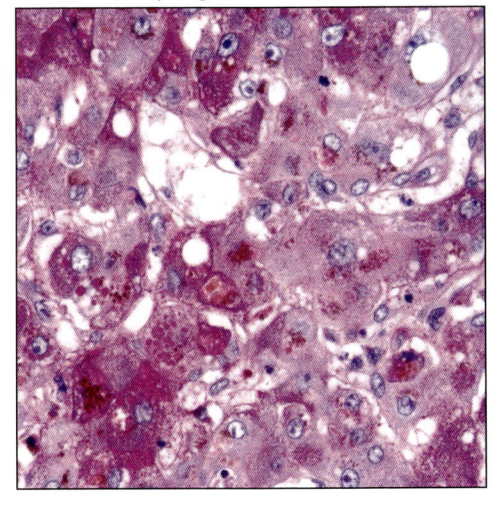

Glycogen and Fat

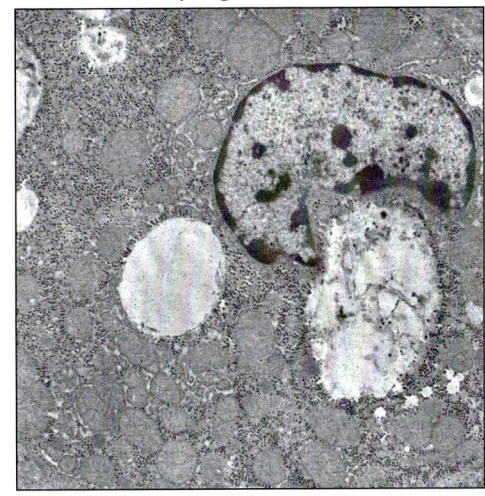

(Left) A section of liver stained with PAS before diastase digestion reveals scattered fat globules and intracytoplasmic brown pigment (lipofuscin) coexisting with numerous dark-staining glycogen granules. *(Right)* EM shows this liver cell contains numerous mitochondria, dispersed granules of glycogen, and scattered globules of fat. Glycogen granules may occasionally be confused with free ribosomes.

Skeletal Muscle

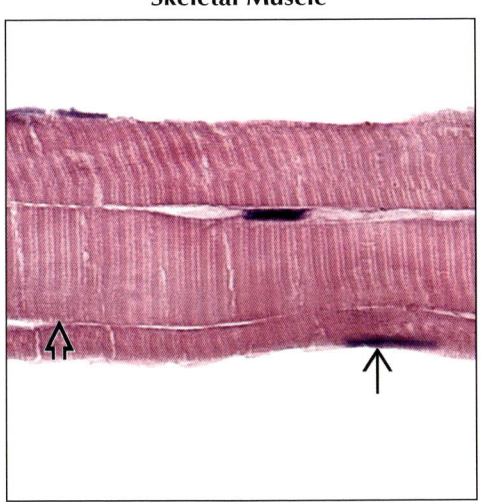

Skeletal Muscle Contractile Filaments

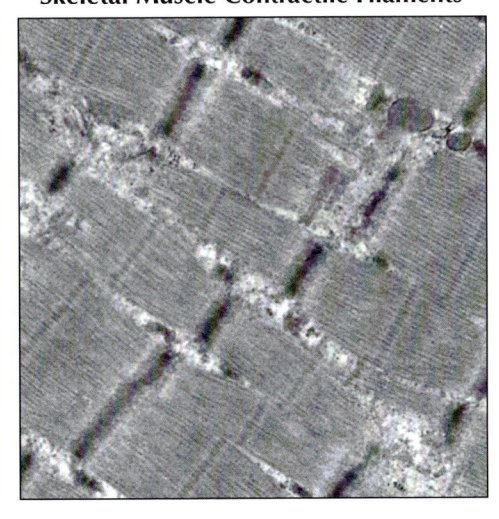

(Left) Normal skeletal muscle demonstrates peripheral elongated nuclei ➡. Typical cross striations ➢ of the cytoplasm are present. *(Right)* EM Shows the skeletal muscle cytoplasm is organized into dark Z bands, which receive thick and thin myofilaments responsible for contractile function. These correlate directly with the light microscopic striations.

INTRODUCTION TO THE CELL

Smooth Muscle Cells

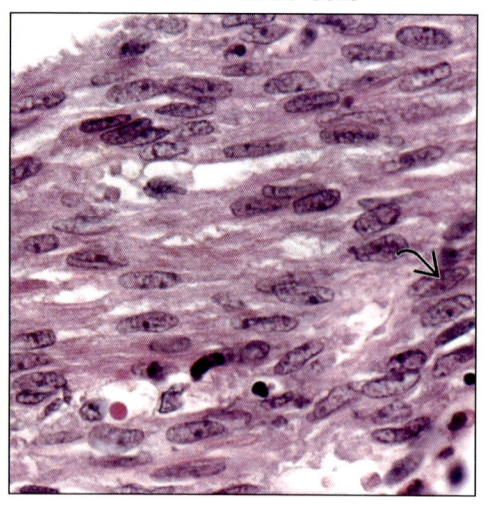

Smooth Muscle Cell

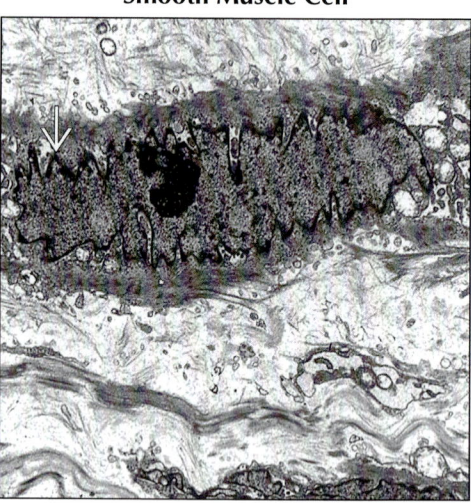

(Left) Smooth muscle cells demonstrate elongated nuclei that are blunted at the ends and have occasional transverse lines perpendicular to the long axis ➔, reflecting deep nuclear folds. The cytoplasm is fibrillar and eosinophilic. The cell borders are distinct. (Right) Em shows smooth muscle cell with a corrugated nuclear contour ➔ corresponds to transverse lines histologically. The cytoplasm is filled with fine actin filaments and dense bodies. The collagen fibers are extracellular.

Smooth Muscle Cell

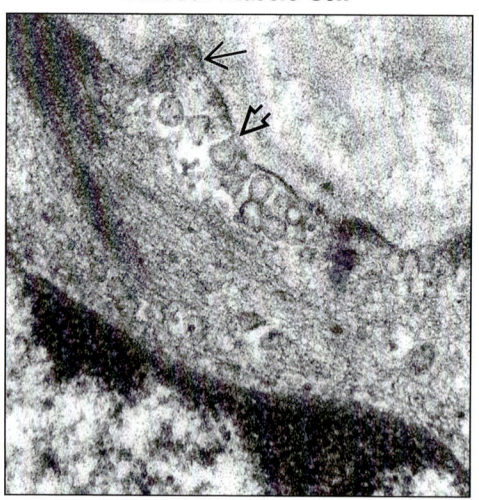

Intercellular Bridges in Squamous Epithelium

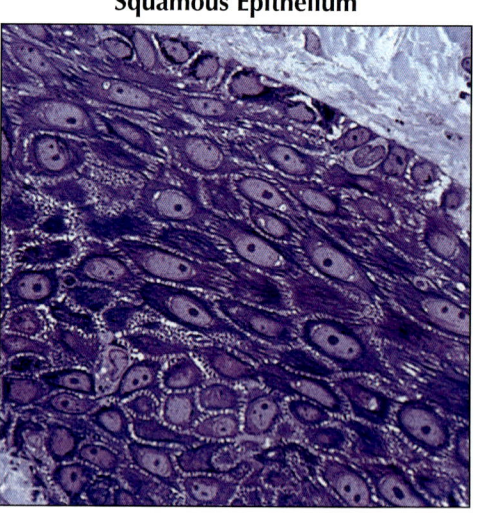

(Left) On EM the edge of a smooth muscle cell shows actin filaments parallel to and inserting on the plasma membrane ➔ from which pinocytotic vesicles invaginate ➔. Thin basal lamina parallels the plasma membrane. (Right) A Toluidine blue-stained tangential section through the mid epidermis demonstrates stratified squamous epithelium with numerous intercellular bridges.

Intercellular Bridges, Tonofilaments, and Squamous Epithelium

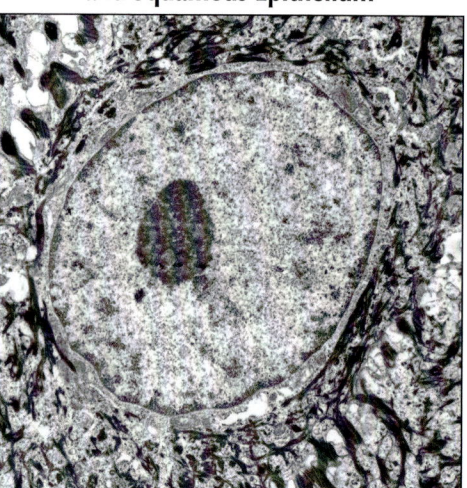

Tonofilaments Inserting on Desmosome

(Left) EM shows the cytoplasm of this squamous epithelial cell is filled with wavy fascicles of tonofilaments inserting on desmosomes. Cytoplasmic extensions of these complexes form the intercellular bridges. (Right) This high-magnification electron micrograph shows an intercellular bridge consisting of a central desmosome ➔ (thickened apposing segments of plasma membrane and a central intervening linear density), onto which wavy tonofilaments insert.

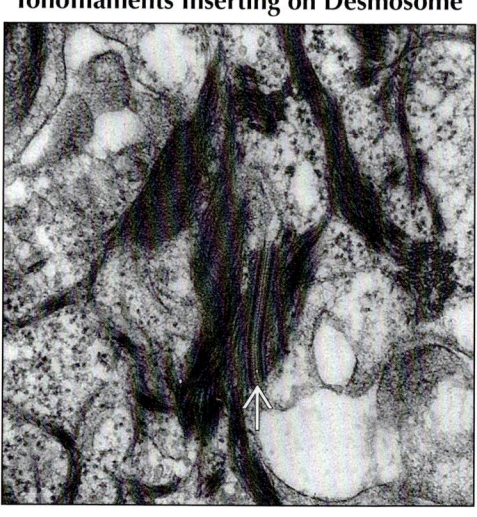

INTRODUCTION TO THE CELL

Small Bowel Epithelium

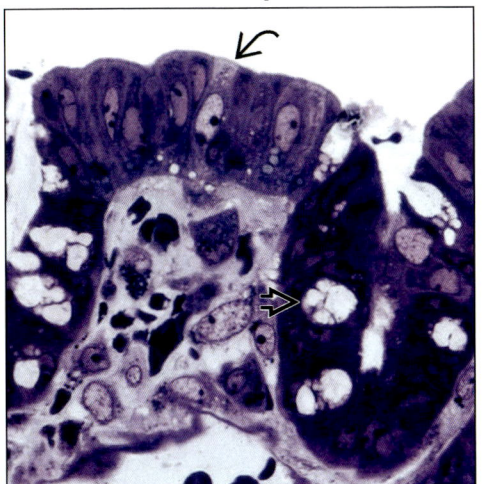

Small Bowel Apex

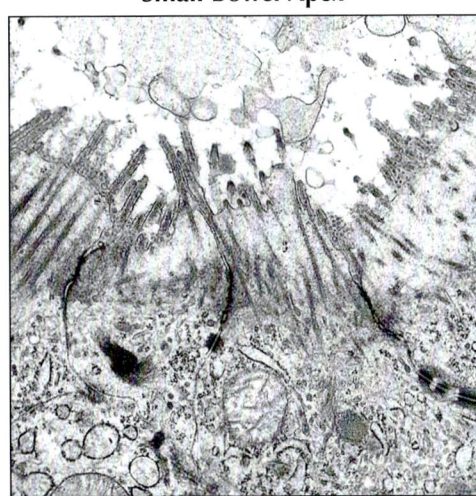

(Left) Toluidine blue stain shows glandular epithelium of the small bowel demonstrates mucinous vacuolization ⇨ and a dense apical terminal bar ➔. *(Right)* The apical region of several adjacent glandular cells of the small bowel is visualized by electron microscopy. The terminal bar by light microscopy is represented by numerous microvilli anchored into the apical cytoplasm by thin filaments. The cells are joined by desmosomal complexes.

Glandular Space

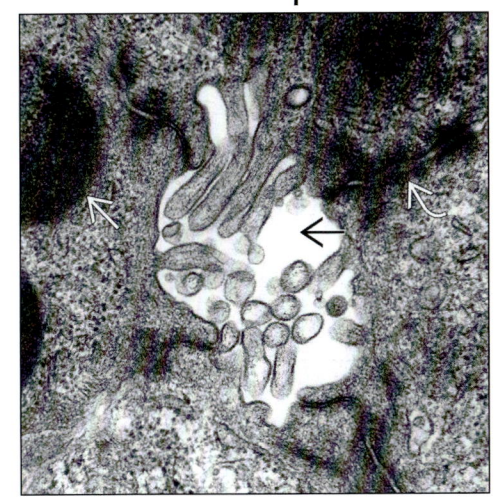

Cilia

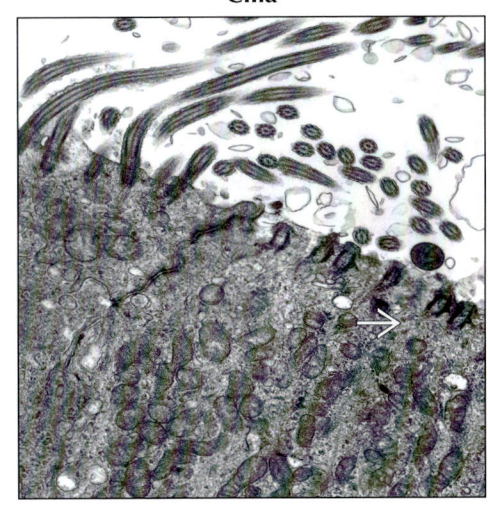

(Left) EM shows a glandular lumen ⇨ is formed by several salivary gland acinar cells and filled with microvilli. A secretory granule is present ➔. The apical portion of the cells is held together by junctional complexes ➔. *(Right)* Electron microscopy shows a portion of 2 ciliated respiratory epithelial cells. The cilia are modified centrioles with the same tubular substructure. They are anchored into the cytoplasm by angled striated blepharoplasts ➔.

Capillary, Basal Lamina, and Collagen

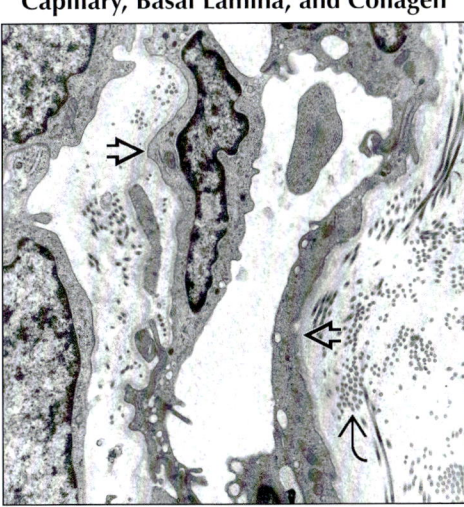

Extracellular Collagen

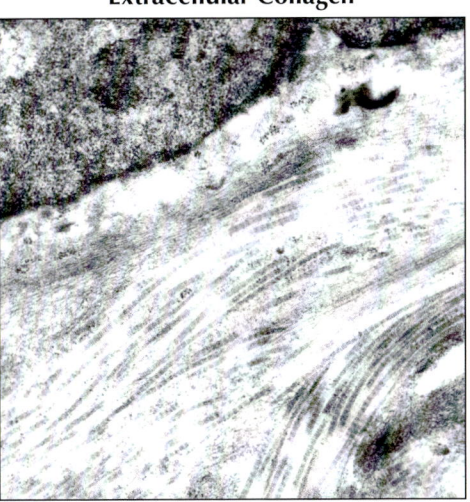

(Left) EM shows a thin-walled capillary is lined by endothelial cells. A thin single layer of basal lamina ⇨ surrounds and runs parallel to the outer plasma membrane. Collagen fibers ➔ in varying stages of cross section are in the stroma. *(Right)* Extracellular collagen fibers exhibit the characteristic periodicity of 64 nm, which is visualized by electron microscopy.

INTRODUCTION TO HISTOLOGY

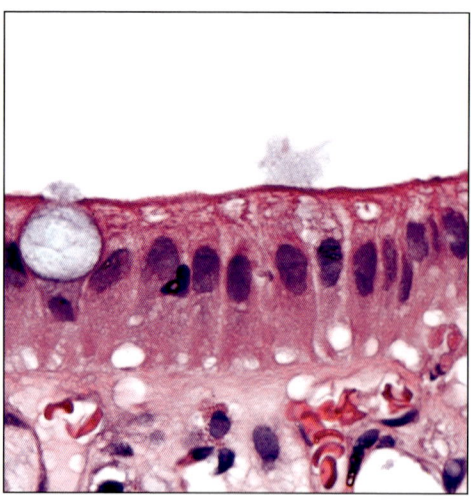

Epithelium consists of sheets of tightly bound contiguous cells that cover the external surfaces of the body and line the internal surfaces. Epithelial cells are bound to the underlying connective tissue by a basement membrane.

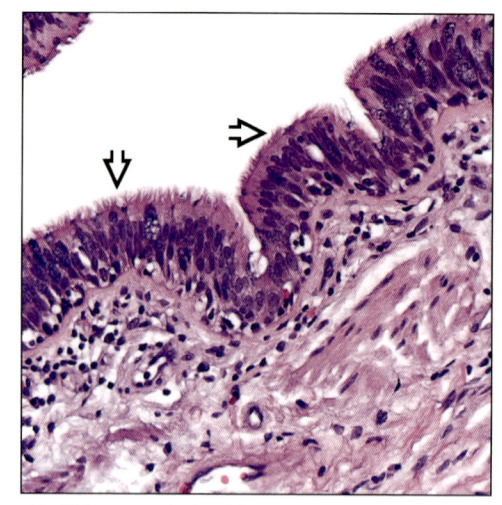

Cilia ▷ are motile, hair-like projections on the surfaces of some epithelial cells that are used to propel substances along the lumen, as seen here in the bronchus.

HISTOLOGY

Definition
- The study of tissues
  - All tissues are composed of cells and extracellular matrix
  - Tissue types are grouped together to form organs
  - Organs are grouped together to form organ systems
- In humans, histology is used synonymously with microscopic anatomy
- 4 basic tissue types are epithelium, connective tissue, muscle, and nerve

TISSUES

Cells
- Basic functional unit of complex organisms
- Cells are grouped together to form tissues

Epithelium
- Sheets of tightly bound contiguous cells
  - Cover external surface of body and line internal surfaces
  - Epithelial cells are bound together by junctional complexes
  - Little intercellular space between cells
- Derived from all 3 embryonic germ layers (ectoderm, mesoderm, and endoderm) although mostly from ectoderm and endoderm
- Separated from underlying connective tissue by extracellular matrix called basal lamina
  - Extracellular matrix is made by epithelial cells
- Epithelium is avascular
  - Derives nourishment and oxygen from underlying connective tissue
- Functions of epithelium
  - Protection
  - Lining of surfaces
  - Transport of molecules across epithelial layers and between body compartments
  - Absorption
  - Detection/sensation
  - Excretion
  - Secretion
- Classification of epithelium is by number of cell layers as well as morphology
  - Number of cell layers between basal lamina and free surface
    - **Simple epithelium**: Composed of single layer of tightly packed cells; functions as lining or limiting membrane as well as for fluid transport, gas exchange, lubrication, absorption
    - **Stratified epithelium**: Composed of > 1 cell layer; used for protection, absorption, secretion
    - **Pseudostratified epithelium**: Appears stratified but is actually a single layer of cells, e.g., trachea, primary bronchi, auditory canal, nasal cavity, epididymis, lacrimal sac
  - Morphology
    - **Squamous** (flat): Polygonal cells
    - **Simple squamous**: Thin, plate-like cells arranged in a single layer, e.g., pulmonary alveolar lining, loop of Henle, mesothelium
    - **Stratified squamous**: Layers of squamous epithelium that provide toughness, e.g., skin, esophagus, larynx, vagina; may be keratinized or nonkeratinized
    - **Cuboidal**: Short and square with centrally placed round nuclei
    - **Simple cuboidal**: Lining of ducts, external surface of ovary, some renal tubules
    - **Stratified cuboidal**: Lines sweat gland ducts
    - **Columnar**: Tall and rectangular with ovoid, usually basally located nuclei
    - **Simple columnar**: e.g., lining of gut, some large ducts; may have cilia or microvilli at luminal border
    - **Stratified columnar**: e.g., conjunctiva, some large ducts, portions of male urethra
    - **Transitional**: Originally believed to be intermediate between stratified squamous and stratified columnar, now known to be a special distensible epithelium that lines bladder and much of urinary tract

INTRODUCTION TO HISTOLOGY

- Polarity and specialized structures
  - Most epithelial cells have apical domain and basolateral domain that differ according to cell function
  - Apical domain faces a lumen
  - Microvilli: Finger-like projections of cytoplasm extending from free surface of cell into lumen; critical for absorption
  - Glycocalyx: Carbohydrate coating overlying luminal surface of microvilli; for protection, cell recognition; combination of glycocalyx and microvilli make up brush border of intestines
  - Stereocilia: Long microvilli found only in epididymis and on sensory hairs cells of cochlea; increase surface area (epididymis) and aid in signal generation (cochlea)
  - Cilia: Motile, hair-like projections on surfaces of some epithelial cells, used to propel substances along lumen and for sensation
  - Basolateral domain: In contact with basal lamina
  - Lateral membrane specializations (terminal bars, junctional complexes) hold cells together
  - Basal membrane specializations (basal lamina, plasma membrane enfoldings, hemidesmosomes) anchor cell to underlying connective tissue

Glands

- Epithelial structures that originate from invaginated epithelial cells
- Secretory units and accompanying ducts make up parenchyma of gland
- Underlying supporting connective tissue is known as stroma
  - In some larger glands, connective tissue subdivides gland into lobules
  - Connective tissue lobules contain vessels, lymphatics, nerves
- Formation
  - Epithelial cells proliferate and invade underlying stroma
    - If contact with surface maintained: Exocrine gland
    - No contact with surface: Endocrine gland
  - Differentiate further into specific type of gland
- Function
  - Secrete mucus, hormones, enzymes, etc.
  - Manufacture products intracellularly
  - Products usually stored in vesicles called secretory granules
- **Exocrine** glands
  - Secrete their products onto external or internal surface from which they originated, via ducts
    - **Mucous** glands: Secrete mucinogens that ultimately become mucus (e.g., goblet cells of GI tract, minor salivary glands, mucous glands of stomach, genital tract, respiratory tract)
    - **Serous** glands: Secrete watery fluid rich in enzymes (e.g., exocrine pancreas)
    - **Mixed serous and mucinous** glands: Produce both mucous and serous secretions (e.g., minor salivary glands)
  - 3 different mechanisms for releasing secretory products
    - Merocrine: Released by exocytosis; cell membranes/cytoplasm not part of secretion (e.g., parotid gland)
    - Apocrine: Small portion of apical cytoplasm released with product (e.g., lactating mammary gland; ironically, apocrine sweat glands are believed to use the merocrine mechanism of secretion release)
    - Holocrine: Mature secretory cell dies and becomes secretory product (e.g., sebaceous gland)
  - Unicellular
    - Simplest type of exocrine gland
    - Isolated cells within an epithelium (e.g., goblet cells of GI tract)
  - Multicellular
    - Organized clusters of secretory cells
    - Majority of glands are multicellular
    - Simple: Consist of 1 unbranched duct
    - Compound: Consist of branching ducts
    - Further classified according to morphology: Tubular, acinar (or alveolar), tubuloacinar (tubuloalveolar)
    - Multicellular glands typically have capsule
  - Myoepithelium
    - Cells with features of both smooth muscle and epithelium
    - Located between basal lamina and basal pole of duct or secretory cell of many multicellular glands
    - Help express secretions
    - Can be identified by myoepithelial markers such as actin, calponin
    - Examples: Sweat, mammary, lacrimal, salivary glands
- **Endocrine** glands
  - Secrete their products into blood or lymphatics
    - Secrete hormones, including peptides, proteins, glycoproteins, steroids
  - Do not have ducts that connect them to originating epithelium
    - Contact with originating epithelium lost during formation
  - Major endocrine glands: Adrenal, pituitary, thyroid, parathyroid, pineal
  - 2 major structural forms
    - Cords: Anastomosing cords around capillaries or sinusoids (e.g., adrenal, parathyroid)
    - Follicles: Glandular cells surround a cavity that receives the hormone (e.g., thyroid)
  - Ovaries, testes, placenta, pancreas also have significant endocrine component
    - Ovary: Granulosa cells, thecal cells, interstitial cells, hilus cells
    - Testes: Sertoli cells, Leydig cells
    - Pancreas: Islets of Langerhans
    - Placenta: Syncytiotrophoblast, decidua
- Some glands are **mixed endocrine and exocrine**
  - e.g., pancreas has both exocrine acini and endocrine Islets of Langerhans

Connective Tissue

- Connective tissue proper
  - 4 types
    - Loose
    - Dense

INTRODUCTION TO HISTOLOGY

- - - Reticular
    - Adipose
  - Loose
    - Right beneath skin, below mesothelium, around blood vessels, around glands, lamina propria
  - Dense
    - Dermis, nerve sheaths, organ capsules, tendons, ligaments, aponeuroses, in blood vessels
  - Reticular
    - Framework of hepatic sinusoids, bone marrow, lymph nodes, spleen, islets of Langerhans
  - Adipose tissue
    - White or brown fat
- Specialized connective tissue
  - Cartilage
    - Hyaline, elastic, or fibrocartilage
  - Bone
- Composed of cells and extracellular matrix
- Functions
  - Structural support
  - Medium for exchange
  - Fat storage
  - Defense/protection
- Cell types: Fibroblasts, adipocytes, pericytes, white blood cells, mast cells, macrophages

Muscle
- Striated
  - Skeletal
  - Cardiac
- Smooth
  - Walls of blood vessels and viscera; dermis of skin

Nerve
- Central nervous system
  - Brain
  - Spinal cord
- Peripheral nervous system
  - Cranial nerves
  - Spinal nerves
  - Ganglia

Extracellular Matrix
- Complex of nonliving macromolecules manufactured by cells and exported into extracellular space
  - Ground substance: Amorphous gel-like material composed of glycoproteins, proteoglycans, glycosaminoglycans
  - Fibers: Collagen, elastin, reticulin
    - Provide strength and elasticity
  - Basement membrane
    - Interface between epithelium and underlying connective tissue
- Integrins and dystroglycans
  - Transmembrane proteins that serve as receptors and facilitate formation of basal lamina

ORGAN SYSTEMS

Blood
- Red blood cells
- White blood cells
- Plasma

Circulatory System
- Cardiovascular system
  - Arteries
  - Capillaries
  - Veins
  - Heart
  - Cardiac valves
- Lymphatic System

Lymphoid (Immune) System
- Lymph nodes
- Bone marrow
- Thymus
- Spleen
- Mucosa-associated lymphoid tissue
- Tonsils

Endocrine System
- Glands
  - Pituitary
  - Thyroid
  - Parathyroid
  - Adrenal
  - Pineal
- Dispersed neuroendocrine cells
- Paraganglia

Integumentary System
- Epidermis
- Dermis
- Skin appendages and fingernails

Breast
- Nipple
- Glandular tissue
- Adipose tissue

Respiratory System
- Nasal cavity
- Sinuses
- Nasopharynx
- Larynx
- Trachea
- Lungs/bronchial tree

Oral Cavity
- Oral mucosa
- Tongue
- Gingiva
- Teeth
- Palate
- Minor salivary glands

Digestive System: Alimentary Canal
- Esophagus
- Stomach
- Small bowel
- Appendix
- Large bowel
- Anus

Digestive System: Viscera/Glands
- Major salivary glands
- Pancreas
- Liver

INTRODUCTION TO HISTOLOGY

- Gallbladder and biliary tree

Genitourinary System
- Kidneys
- Urinary bladder
- Ureters
- Urethra
- Prostate
- Ovaries
- Fallopian tubes
- Uterus/cervix
- Vagina
- Vulva/external genitalia
- Prostate
- Testes
- Penis
- Genital ducts and glands

Special Sensory Organs
- Eye
- Nose
- Ear
- Tongue/taste buds

RELATED REFERENCES

1. Eroschenko V: diFiore's Atlas of Histology with Functional Correlations, 10th Ed. Philadelphia: Lippincott, Williams, and Wilkins, 2004
2. Kanitakis J: Anatomy, histology and immunohistochemistry of normal human skin. Eur J Dermatol. 12(4):390-9; quiz 400-1, 2002
3. Gartner LP et al: Epithelium and Glands. In: Color Textbook of Histology, 2nd ed, W.B. Saunders Co. 85-108, 2001
4. Morrison EE et al: Morphology of olfactory epithelium in humans and other vertebrates. Microsc Res Tech. 23(1):49-61, 1992
5. Levine DS et al: Normal histology of the colon. Am J Surg Pathol. 13(11):966-84, 1989
6. Martinez-Madrigal F et al: Histology of the major salivary glands. Am J Surg Pathol. 13(10):879-99, 1989
7. Githens S: The pancreatic duct cell: proliferative capabilities, specific characteristics, metaplasia, isolation, and culture. J Pediatr Gastroenterol Nutr. 7(4):486-506, 1988
8. Bron AJ et al: The normal conjunctiva and its responses to inflammation. Trans Ophthalmol Soc U K. 104 (Pt 4):424-35, 1985
9. Martinez-Hernandez A et al: The basement membrane in pathology. Lab Invest. 48(6):656-77, 1983
10. Lim DJ: Normal and pathological mucosa of the middle ear and eustachian tube. Clin Otolaryngol Allied Sci. 4(3):213-32, 1979
11. McDowell EM et al: The respiratory epithelium. I. Human bronchus. J Natl Cancer Inst. 61(2):539-49, 1978
12. Skerrow CJ: Intercellular adhesion and its role in epidermal differentiation. Invest Cell Pathol. 1(1):23-37, 1978
13. Pitts JD et al: Permeability of junctions between animal cells. Intercellular transfer of nucleotides but not of macromolecules. Exp Cell Res. 104(1):153-63, 1977
14. Puchtler H et al: Investigation of staining, polarization and fluorescence microscopic properties of myoepithelial cells. Histochemistry. 40(4):281-9, 1974
15. Fisher ER et al: Ultrastructure of human normal and neoplastic prostate. Pathol Annu. 5:1-26, 1970
16. Fawcett DW et al: The ultrastructure of endocrine glands. Recent Prog Horm Res. 25:315-80, 1969
17. Leblond CP et al: Structures corresponding to terminal bars and terminal web in many types of cells. Nature. 186:784-8, 1960

INTRODUCTION TO HISTOLOGY

Simple Squamous

Simple Squamous

(Left) The mesothelium consists of a single layer of squamous epithelial cells ⇨.
(Right) The epithelial cells are anchored to underlying stroma by the basement membrane, as seen in this high-power view of mesothelium. Epithelium is avascular, so it derives nourishment and oxygen from underlying connective tissue.

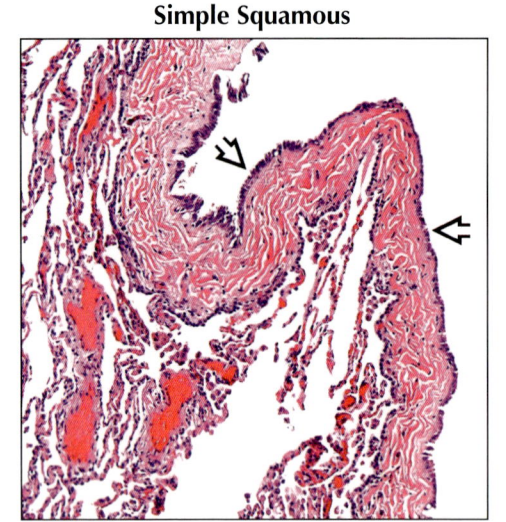

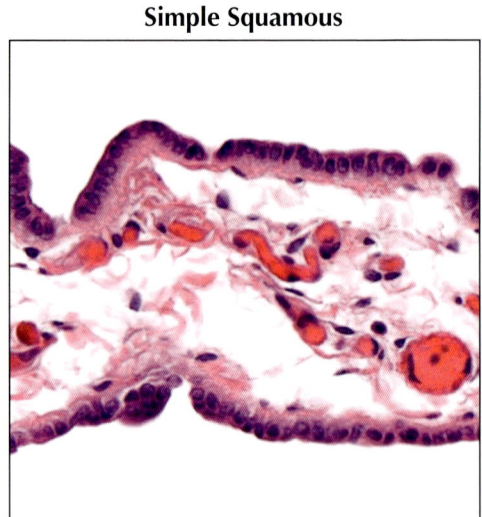

Stratified Squamous, Nonkeratinizing

Stratified Squamous, Nonkeratinizing

(Left) Stratified squamous epithelium consists of multiple layers of polygonal squamous cells, as seen here in the esophagus. This stratified squamous epithelium is nonkeratinizing because the top layers have nuclei.
(Right) This example of nonkeratinizing squamous epithelium is from the conjunctiva; it consists of multiple layers of polyhedral squamous cells. The nuclei extend to the surface. This type of epithelium is usually moist and found on mucous membranes.

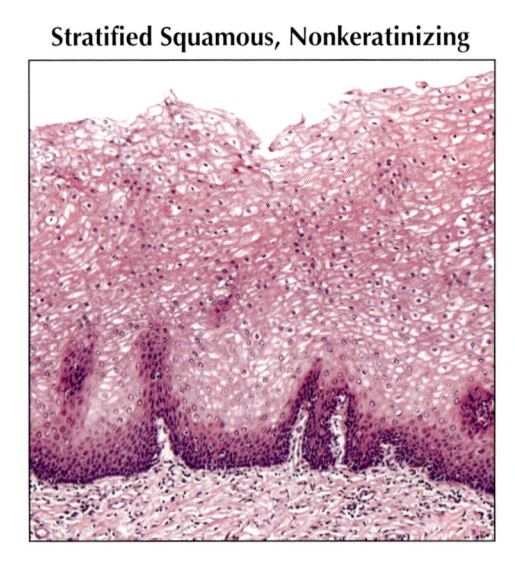

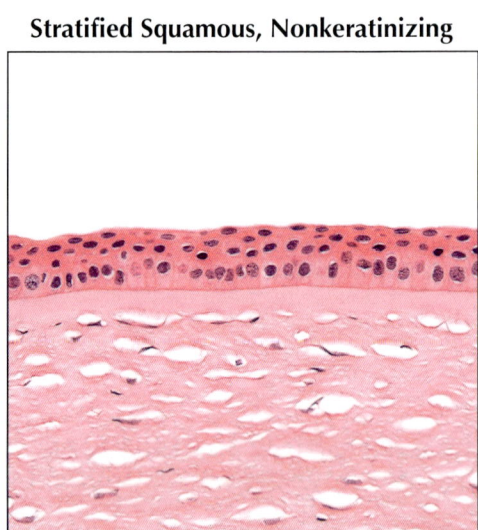

Stratified Squamous

Simple Cuboidal

(Left) In keratinizing stratified squamous epithelium, the superficial layers are composed of dead cells that have been replaced with keratin ⇨, providing toughness, as in the skin.
(Right) Cuboidal epithelial cells are short and square, with centrally placed round nuclei ⇨. This example is a small pancreatic duct. Examples of simple cuboidal epithelium include the linings of ducts, the external surface of the ovary, and some renal tubules.

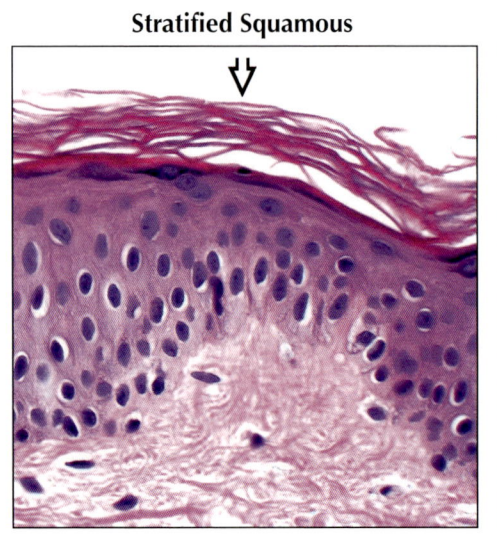

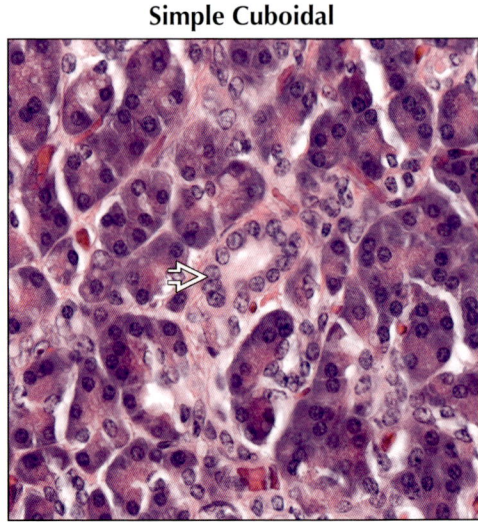

INTRODUCTION TO HISTOLOGY

Stratified Cuboidal

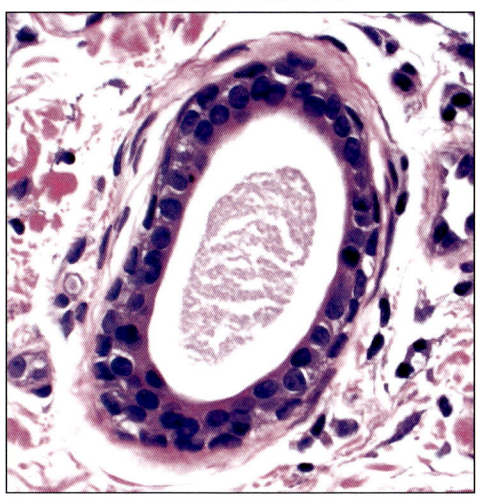

Simple Columnar

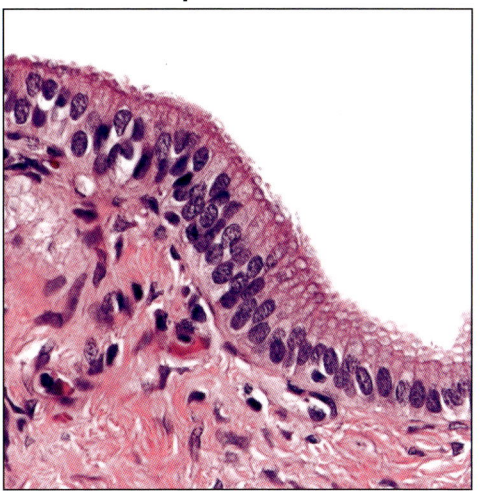

(Left) This sweat gland duct is lined by multiple layers of cuboidal epithelium. Stratified cuboidal epithelium is rare. *(Right)* Simple columnar epithelium consists of tall, rectangular cells with ovoid, basally located nuclei. This example is from the pancreatobiliary tree. Other examples include the lining of the gut, and other large ducts. Cilia or microvilli may be present at the apical border.

Stratified Columnar

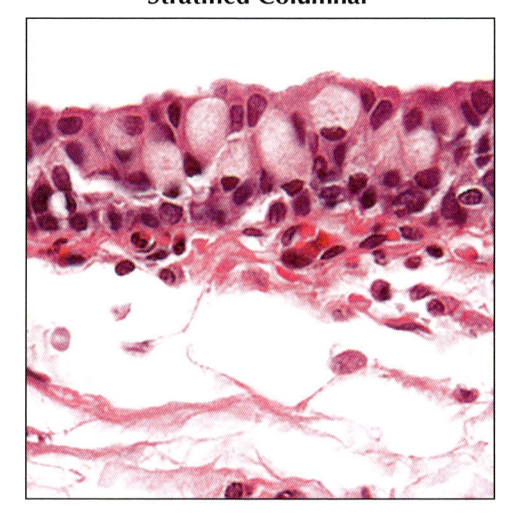

Transitional

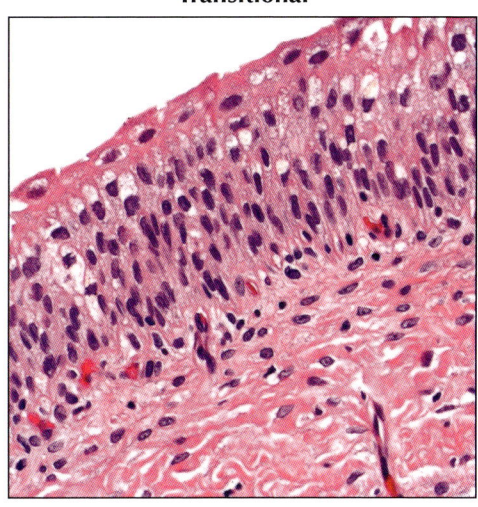

(Left) Stratified columnar epithelium is seen in some portions of the conjunctiva, as well as in some large ducts and portions of the male urethra. *(Right)* Transitional epithelium is a specialized multilayered epithelium with basal low columnar or cuboidal cells, overlying intermediate cells, and large, sometimes dome-shaped surface or umbrella cells. It allows structures of the urinary tract to expand when distended with urine and collapse when empty.

Transitional

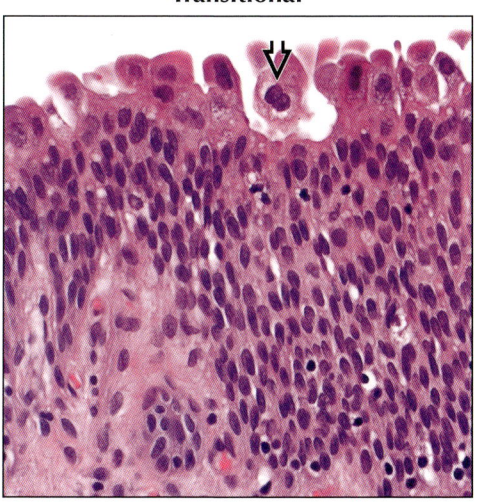

Pseudostratified

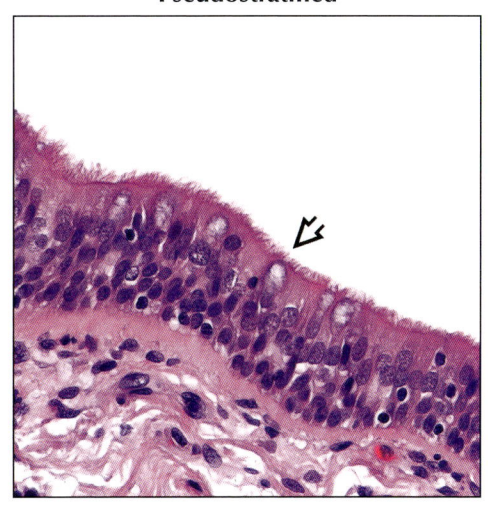

(Left) The umbrella cells may be binucleate ⇨ and may bulge into the luminal space. *(Right)* This example of pseudostratified epithelium is from the trachea. All cells rest on the basement membrane, but not all reach the surface. Since the nuclei are at different heights, it imparts the appearance of stratification. Most pseudostratified epithelia are ciliated, as seen here ⇨. Functions of this type of epithelium include secretion, absorption, lubrication, protection, and transportation.

INTRODUCTION TO HISTOLOGY

Glands

Glands

(Left) The secretory units and their ducts make up the parenchyma of a gland (as shown here by this example of lactating breast). **(Right)** The connective tissue surrounding a gland constitutes the supporting stroma. Here, peribiliary mucous glands are surrounded by lobular connective tissue stroma.

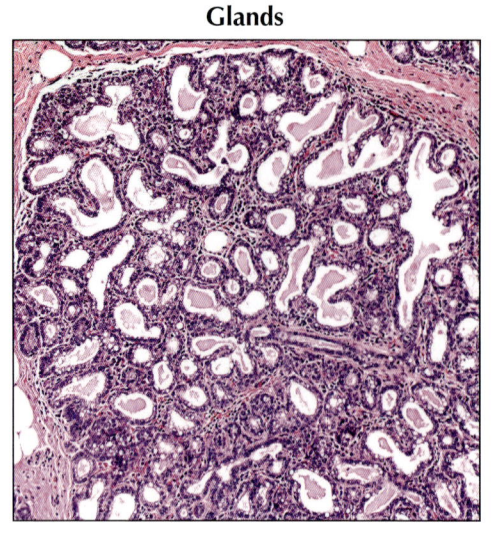

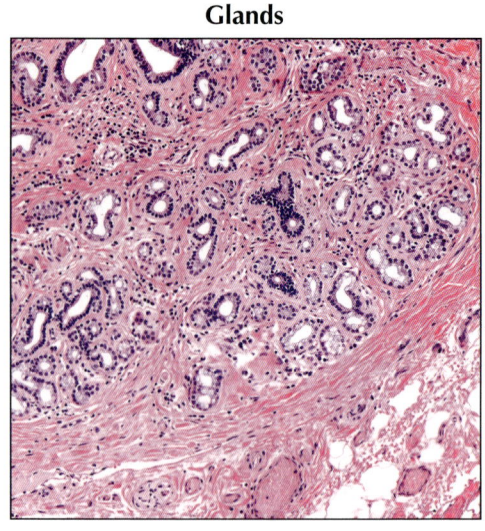

Mucous Glands

Serous Glands

(Left) Mucous glands, as seen here in this example from a minor salivary gland, are exocrine glands that secrete mucinogens, which ultimately become mucus. Note that the secretory unit is surrounded by connective tissue stroma ➡.
(Right) Serous glands, such as the exocrine pancreatic acini shown here, are exocrine glands that secrete a watery, enzyme-rich fluid. The products of glands are often stored in secretory granules.

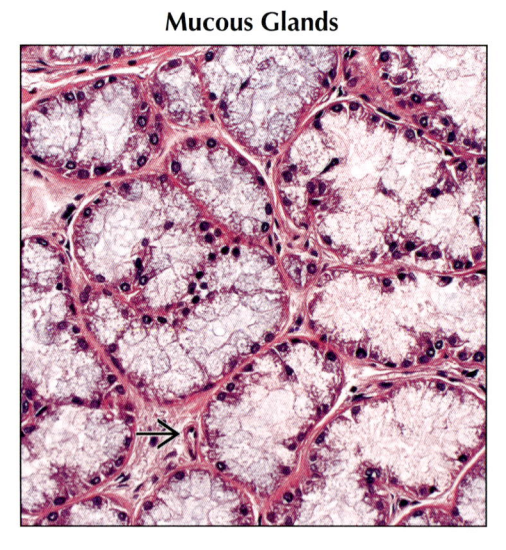

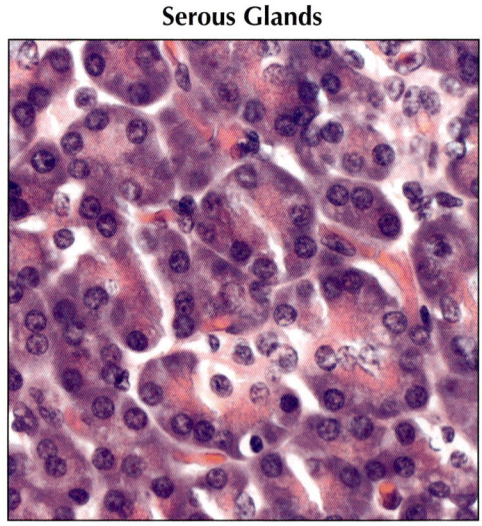

Mixed Mucinous and Serous Gland

Sebaceous Exocrine Gland

(Left) Mixed serous and mucinous glands, illustrated here in a minor salivary gland, are exocrine glands that produce both mucous and serous secretions. The distinct mucous cells ➡ are filled with basophilic mucin, with overlying granular serous demilunes ➡. **(Right)** Sebaceous glands have abundant clear-staining cytoplasm due to abundant lipid. This sebaceous gland is attached to an adjacent hair follicle and empties its contents into the follicle via the sebaceous duct.

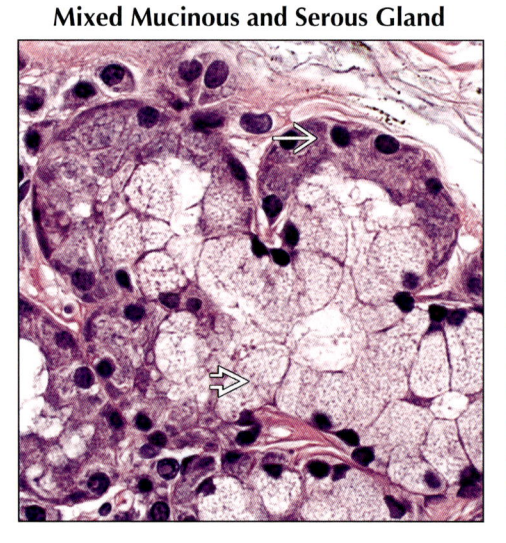

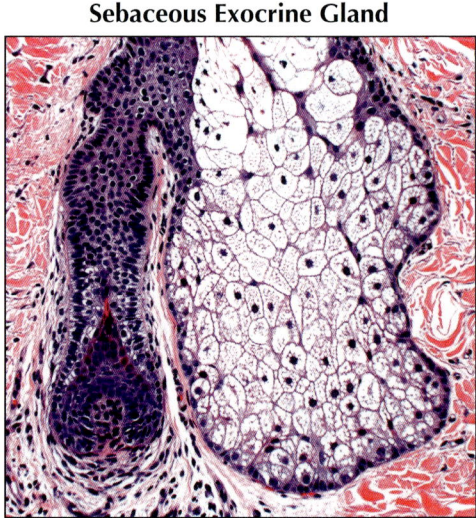

INTRODUCTION TO HISTOLOGY

Myoepithelium

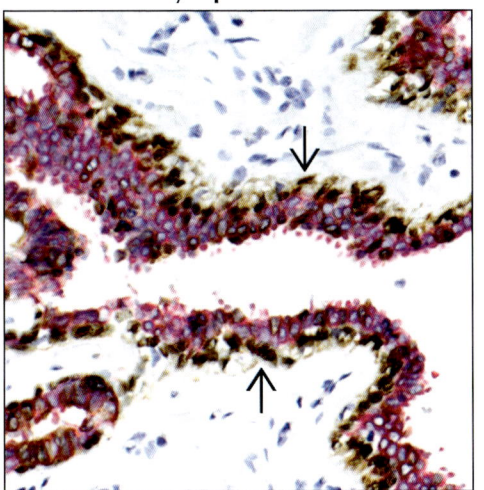

Endocrine Gland

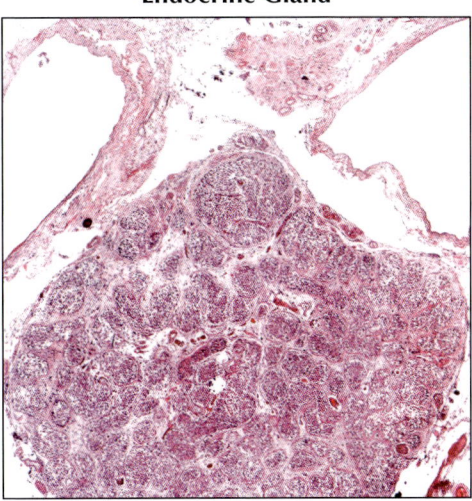

(Left) Myoepithelial cells have features of both smooth muscle and epithelium, and they help express secretions. In this section of breast, the epithelial cells mark with keratin (red chromagen), and the myoepithelial cells mark with calponin ➡ (brown chromagen). (Right) Endocrine glands (such as the pineal gland shown here) have no ducts, as they have lost the connection to the originating epithelium during formation. They secrete their products directly into blood or lymphatics.

Endocrine Gland

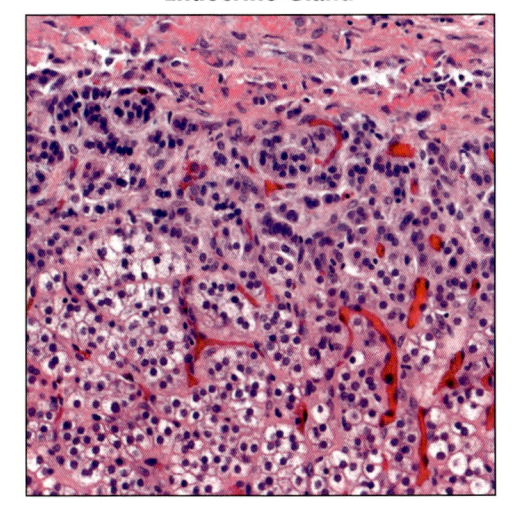

Endocrine Gland

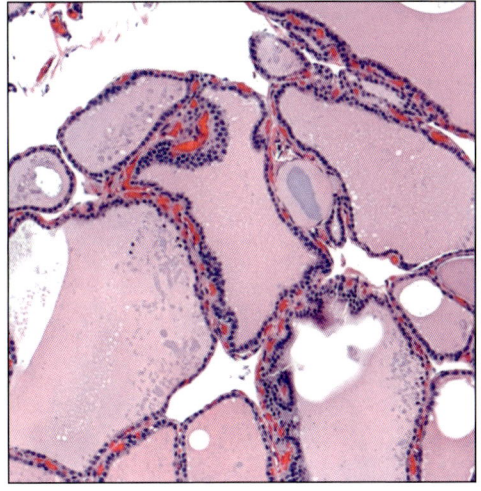

(Left) The adrenal gland is an endocrine gland arranged in cords of endocrine cells surrounding capillaries. (Right) Some endocrine glands are arranged in follicles, or glandular cells that surround a cavity, which receive the hormone. (Courtesy J. Hunt, MD.)

Mixed Glands

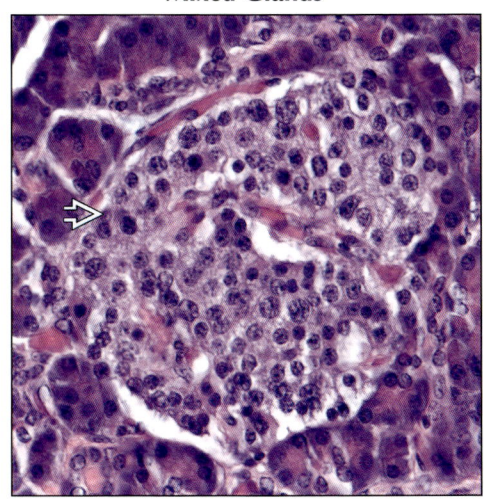

Endocrine Cells

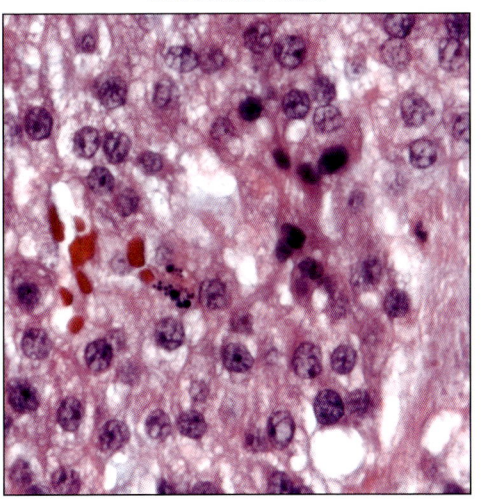

(Left) Some glands, such as the pancreas, are mixed endocrine and exocrine. This photomicrograph of pancreas shows the endocrine islet of Langerhans ➡ surrounded by exocrine acinar parenchyma. (Right) The granulosa cells of the ovary, shown here, are an example of a collection of endocrine secretory cells that exist within an organ that contains multiple tissue types. The testis, pancreas, and placenta are other examples.

INTRODUCTION TO HISTOLOGY

Diffuse Neuroendocrine System

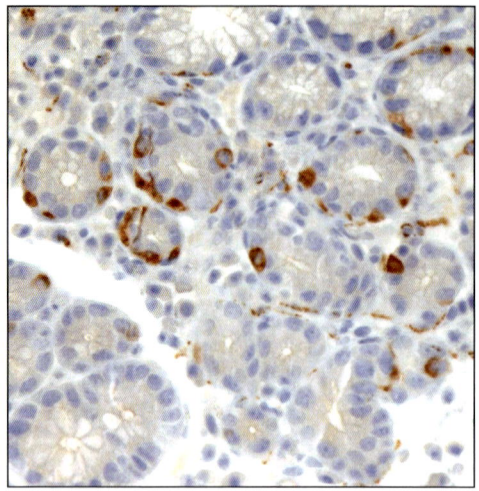

Loose Connective Tissue

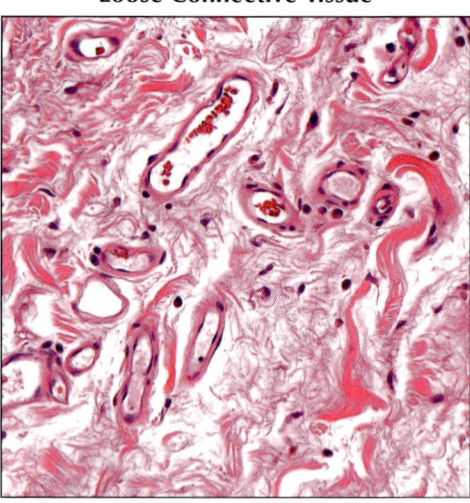

(Left) The diffuse neuroendocrine system is present throughout the digestive tract and respiratory tract. These cells make many different types of hormones. They are also known as APUD cells (amine precursor uptake and decarboxylation). These neuroendocrine cells in the stomach are highlighted by CD56. **(Right)** Loose connective tissue consists of a loose arrangement of fibers with abundant ground substance and extracellular fluid. It also contains scattered collagen, reticulin, and elastic fibers.

Dense Connective Tissue

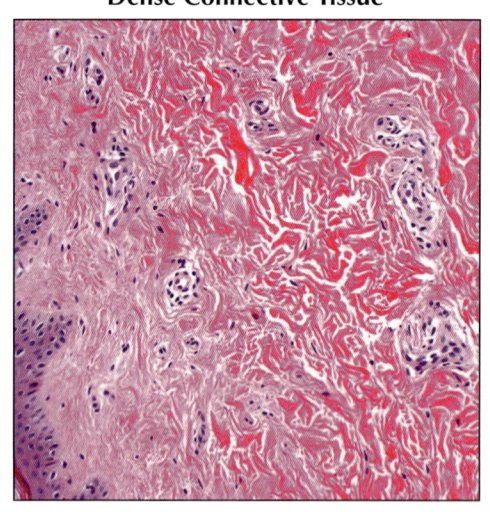

Reticular Connective Tissue

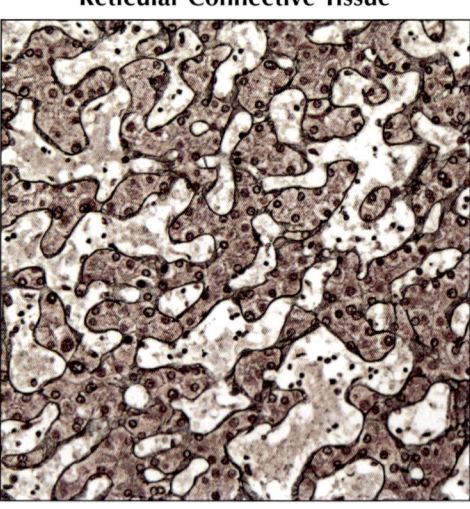

(Left) Dense connective tissue, seen here in the dermis, contains more fibers than loose connective tissue. Note the dense eosinophilic collagen fibers. **(Right)** Reticular connective tissue is composed of type III collagen, which forms a network that makes the framework for many organs and glands. A reticulin stain shows the reticular network in the liver, which supports the sinusoids and hepatic cell plates.

Adipose Tissue

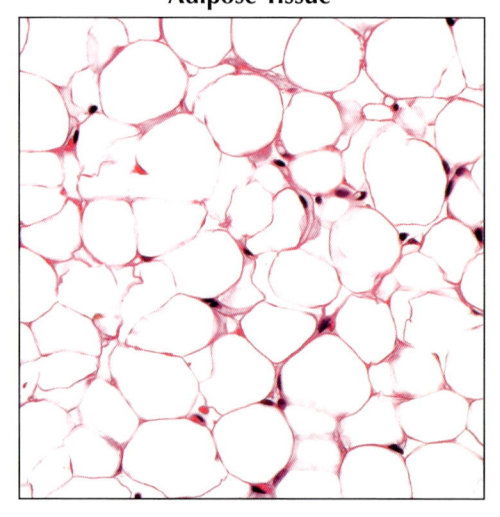

Bone

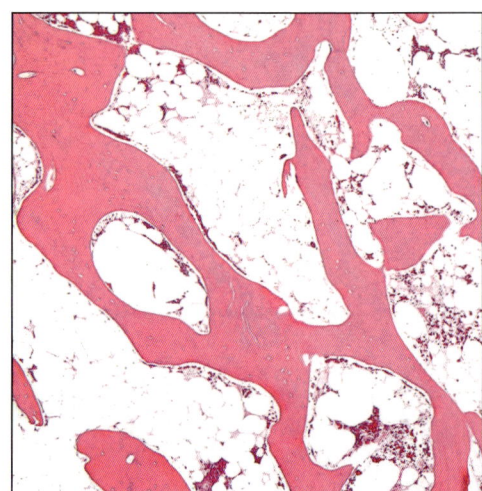

(Left) Adipose tissue is a type of connective tissue that stores fat. It also contains receptors for many substances, including glucocorticoids, growth hormone, and insulin. It is present in the subcutaneous tissue, omentum, and mesentery. **(Right)** Bone is a type of specialized connective tissue that comprises the primary structural framework for the body (skeleton). Its extracellular matrix is calcified and surrounds the cells that secreted it.

INTRODUCTION TO HISTOLOGY

Cartilage

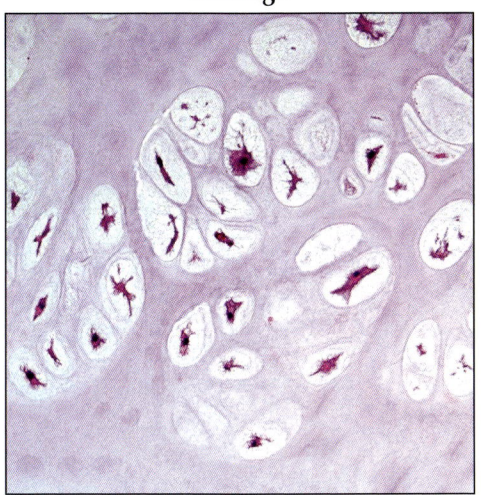

Skeletal Muscle

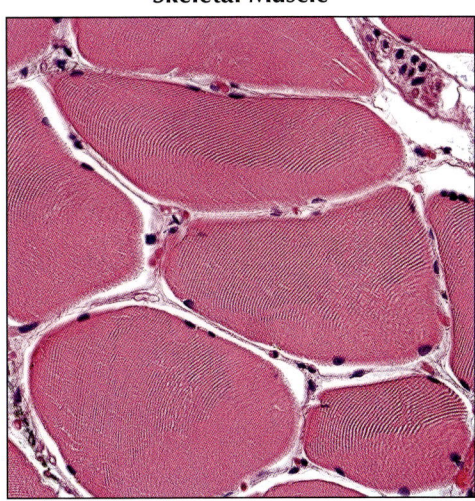

(Left) Cartilage is a specialized connective tissue that is very flexible. It lines the articulating surfaces of the bones, serves as a template for endochondral bone formation, and is part of many organs such as the ear, larynx, and intervertebral discs. *(Right)* Skeletal muscle is a type of striated muscle that comprises the majority of the voluntary muscle mass in the body. The cells are long and cylindrical (shown here in cross section) and have peripheral nuclei.

Cardiac Muscle

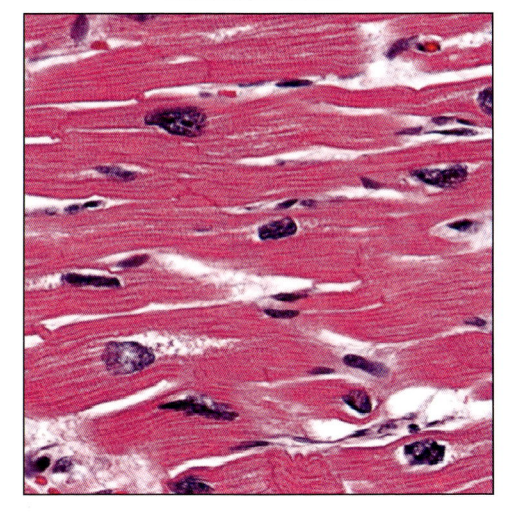

Smooth Muscle

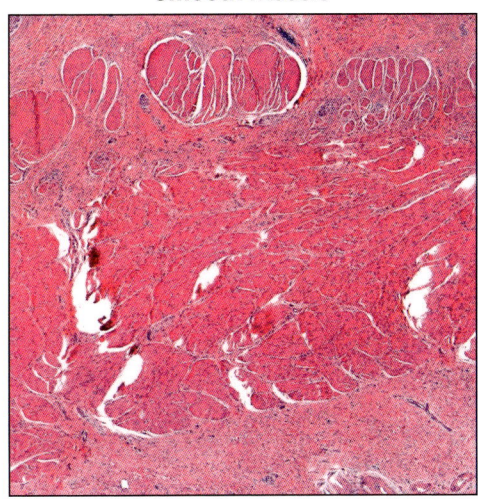

(Left) Cardiac muscle is a nonvoluntary, striated muscle that is present only in the heart and proximal segments of the pulmonary veins where they join the heart. The muscle fibers are striated, and the nuclei are centrally located. *(Right)* Smooth muscle is present in the walls of the viscera, such as in this example of the wall of the stomach.

Peripheral Nerve

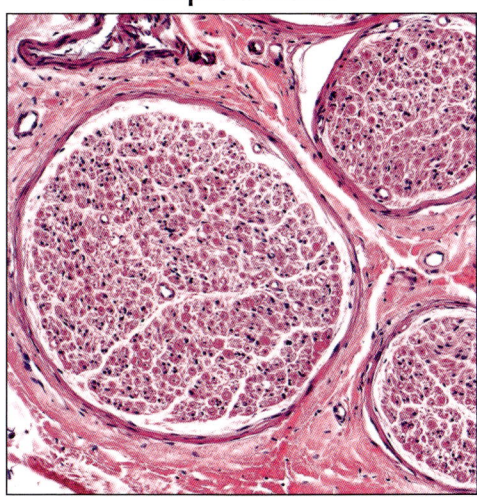

Ganglia

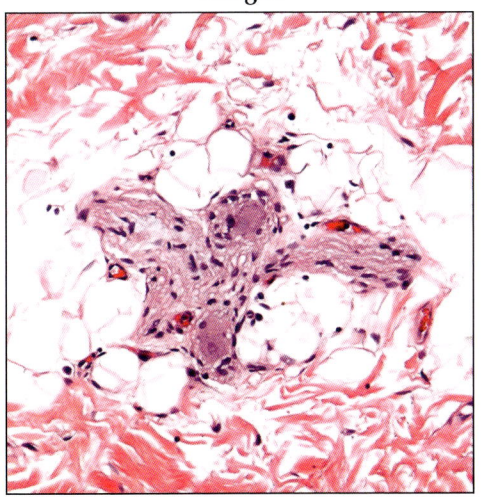

(Left) Peripheral nerves are composed of multiple bundles (or fascicles) of nerve cells, each enclosed by connective tissue known as perineurium. The peripheral nervous system includes cranial and spinal nerves. (Courtesy P. Burger, MD.) *(Right)* Ganglia are located throughout the body. They are aggregates of neurons within the peripheral nervous system that contain the cell bodies of sensory and postganglionic autonomic neurons.

IMMUNOHISTOCHEMICAL AND SPECIAL STAINS

Immunohistochemical Stains

IHC Stain	Clones/Alternate Names	Chapter(s)
ACTH		Pituitary
AE1/AE3		Kidney; Mesothelium
B72.3	TAG72, CC49, TAG-72, BRST-3	Mesothelium
BCL-2	ONCL2, BCL2/100/D5, 124, 124.3	Lymph Nodes
BER-EP4	AUA1, VU-1D9, EPCAM, C10, HEA125	Mesothelium
C-Kit	CD117, C-19, 104D2, 2E4, C-KIT, A4502, H300, CMA-767	Esophagus
Calcitonin	Calbindin 28	Thyroid
Calponin	N3, 26A11, CALP, CNN1, SMCC, Sm Calp	Introduction to Histology
Calretinin	DAK-CALRET, 5A5, CAL 3F5, DC8, AB149	Mesothelium
CD1a	JPM30, CD1A, O10, NA1/34	Epidermis (Including Keratinocytes and Melanocytes)
CD3	F7238, A0452, CD3-P, CD3-M, SP7, PS1	Lymph Nodes; Tonsils/Adenoids
CD4	IF6, 1290, 4B12, 1F6, CD04	Overview of the Immune System
CD5	NCL-CD5, 4C7, 54/B4, 54/F6	Lymph Nodes
CD8	M7103, C8/144, C8/144B	Overview of the Immune System
CD10	NCL-270, CALLA, neprilysin, neutral endopeptidase, NEP	Kidney
CD15	VIM-2, 3C4, LEU-M1, TU9, VIM-D5, MY1, CBD1, MMA, 3CD1, C3D1, Lewis X, SSEA-1	Mesothelium
CD20	BER-H2, KI-1, TNFRSF8	Lymph Nodes; Spleen; Tonsils/Adenoids
CD25	2A3, 4C9	Overview of the Immune System
CD31	JC/70, JC/70A, PECAM-1	Adipose Tissue; Kidney
CD34	MY10, IOM34, QBEND10, 8G12, 1309, HPCA-1, NU-4A1, TUK4, clone 581, BI-3c5	Breast; Kidney
CD42b	glycoprotein Ib, GP lb	Bone Marrow
CD56	MAB735, ERIC-1, 25-KD11, 123C3, 24-MB2, BC56C04, 1B6, 14-MAB735, NCC-LU-243, MOC-1, NCAM	Stomach
CD61	Integrin, beta 3 (platelet glycoprotein IIIa), ITGB3, GP3A, GPIIIa, Y2/5, HPA	Bone Marrow
CD68	PG-M1, KP-1	Central Nervous System; Liver
CD71	Transferrin receptor protein 1 (TfR1)	Bone Marrow
CD95	FAS, APO-1, UB2, B-10, FAS	Overview of the Immune System
CD117	C-19 (C-KIT), 104D2, 2E4, C-KIT, A4502, H300, CMA-767	Bone Marrow; Dermis
CD138	B-B4, AM411-10M, MI15	Bone Marrow
CD163	10D6	Kidney
Chromogranin A	PHE-5, PHE5, E001, DAK-A3	Bladder; Parathyroid
CK5/6	D5/16 B4	Breast; Epidermis (Including Keratinocytes and Melanocytes); Kidney; Mesothelium
CK7	K72.7, KS7.18, OVTL 12/30, LDS-68, CK07	Anus and Anal Canal; Breast; Kidney
CK20	KS20.8	Adnexal Structures; Epidermis (Including Keratinocytes and Melanocytes); Kidney; Pancreas
Cytokeratin, NOS		Discussed generally in: Anus and Anal Canal; Bladder; Breast; Kidney; Mesothelium; Paraganglia; Parathyroid; Prostate: Benign Glandular and Stromal Histology
D2-40	podoplanin, M2A	Capillaries, Veins, and Lymphatics; Kidney; Mesothelium
Desmin	M760, DE-R-11, D33, DE5, DE-U-10, ZC18	Mesothelium
E-cadherin	36B5, ECH-6, ECCD-2, CDH1, 5H9, NCH 38, clone 36, 4A2 C7, E9, 67A4, HECD-1, SC-8426	Breast
EMA	GP1.4, 214D4, MC5, E29, MUC1, EMA/MUC1	Kidney

IMMUNOHISTOCHEMICAL AND SPECIAL STAINS

Immunohistochemical Stains

IHC Stain	Clones/Alternate Names	Chapter(s)
ER	1D5, 6F11, SP1, 15D, H222, TE111, ERP, ER1D5, NCLER611, NCL-ER-LH2, PGP-1A6	Breast
FasL	CD95L, G247-4, CD95-L, FAS-L, TNFSF6	Overview of the Immune System
GFAP	6F2, M761, GA-51, GFP-8A	Central Nervous System
Glycophorin A	CD235a, JC159	Bone Marrow
HBME-1		Mesothelium
HMB-45		Epidermis (Including Keratinocytes and Melanocytes)
Ki-67	MMI, KI88, IVAK-2, MIB1	Lymph Nodes
LYVE-1		Capillaries, Veins, and Lymphatics
Melan-A	M2-7C10, CK-MM, MART-1	Epidermis (Including Keratinocytes and Melanocytes)
MITF	34CA5, D5, C5+D5	Epidermis (Including Keratinocytes and Melanocytes)
MOC-31		Mesothelium
Myeloperoxidase	MPO	Bone Marrow
NeuN	A60	Central Nervous System
Neurofilament protein	NFP, TPNFP-1A3, SMI31, SMI33, NFP, SMI32, TA-51, 2F11	Central Nervous System; Peripheral Nervous System
p16	Cyclin dependent kinase inhibitor p16 antibody, INK4, INK4a, MLM, MTS1, multiple tumor suppressor 1 antibody, p12, p14, p16 γ, p16 INK4, p16 INK4a, INK4 p19, TP16, P16_INK4A, E6H4, sc1661, JC8, ZJ11, G175-405, F-12, DCS-50, 6H12, 16P07, 16P04	Anus and Anal Canal
p63	P63-P53 homologous nuclear protein; delta-NP63, 4A4, P63, H-137, 7JUL	Breast; Epidermis (Including Keratinocytes and Melanocytes); Prostate: Benign Glandular and Stromal Histology; Skeletal Muscle; Thyroid
pax-8		Prostate: Benign Glandular and Stromal Histology
Podoplanin	D2-40, M2A	Breast
PR	PRP, 10A9, PGR-1A6, KD68, PGR-ICA, PRP-P, PRI, 1A6, 1AR, HPRA3, PGR-636, 636, PR88, NCL-PGR	Breast
PSA	PSA-M, ER-PR8, PSA-P, F5	Prostate: Benign Glandular and Stromal Histology
PSAP		Prostate: Benign Glandular and Stromal Histology
PTH		Parathyroid
S100	S-100, A6, 15E2E2, Z311, 4C4.9, S100 protein	Adipose Tissue; Adnexal Structures; Epidermis (Including Keratinocytes and Melanocytes); Kidney; Paraganglia; Peripheral Nervous System
Somatostatin		Pancreas
Synaptophysin	SVP38, SY38, SNP-88, SYP, SYPH, Sypl, Syn p38	Bladder; Central Nervous System; Pancreas; Paraganglia; Pineal Gland
Thrombomodulin	1009, 15C8	Mesothelium
Tryptase		Bone Marrow
Tyrosinase	NCL-TYROS, T311	Epidermis (Including Keratinocytes and Melanocytes)
Vimentin	43BE8, 3B4, V10, V9, VIM-3B4, VIM	Connective Tissue
WT1		Mesothelium

IMMUNOHISTOCHEMICAL AND SPECIAL STAINS

Special Stains

Special Stain	Chapter(s)
Alcian Blue	Breast; Pancreas
Bielschowsky silver stain	Central Nervous System
Elastic van Gieson	Arteries; Capillaries, Veins, and Lymphatics; Cardiac Valves; Connective Tissue; Lung
Jones methenamine silver	Kidney
Luxol fast blue	Central Nervous System; Peripheral Nervous System
Luxol fast blue + H&E	Central Nervous System
Mucicarmine	Minor Salivary Glands
Myeloperoxidase	Bone Marrow
Oil red O	Parathyroid
Papanicolau	Introduction to the Cell
PAS-diastase	Epidermis (Including Keratinocytes and Melanocytes); Liver
PAS-light green	Adnexal Structures; Epidermis (Including Keratinocytes and Melanocytes)
Periodic acid-Schiff	Breast; Esophagus; Eye and Ocular Adnexa; Introduction to the Cell; Kidney; Liver; Pancreas; Spleen
Phosphotungstic acid	Skeletal Muscle
Prussian blue	Bone Marrow; Liver
Reticulin	Introduction to Histology; Liver; Pituitary; Spleen
Toludine blue	Electron Microscopy; Introduction to the Cell; Peripheral Nervous System
Trichrome	Cardiac Conduction System; Heart; Kidney; Liver; Ovary; Peripheral Nervous System; Skeletal Muscle
Wright stain	Bone Marrow; Peripheral Blood

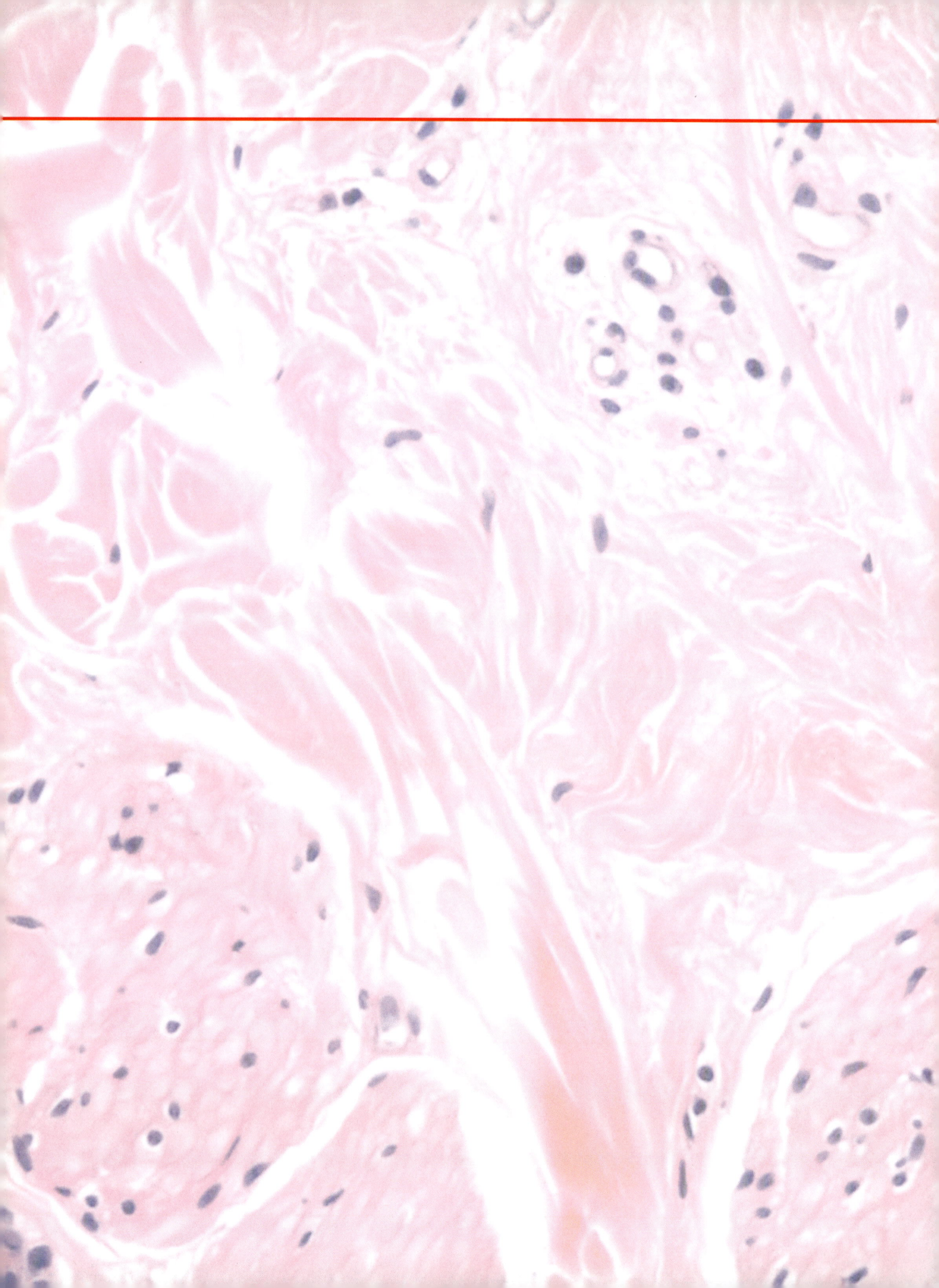

Integument

Epidermis (Including Keratinocytes and Melanocytes)	2-2
Dermis	2-6
Adnexal Structures	2-10
Nail	2-14

EPIDERMIS (INCLUDING KERATINOCYTES AND MELANOCYTES)

Key Facts

Macroscopic Anatomy
- Thin, most superficial layer of skin
- Appears white-gray or brown grossly
  - Color depends on amount of melanin pigment (ethnic variations)
- Function
  - Prevents pathogens from entering body; regulates body temperature and electrolytes
- Thickness varies based on anatomic location and is thinnest on eyelids and thickest on palms/soles

Microscopic Anatomy
- Stratified squamous epithelium
- **Multiple levels**
  - Stratum corneum: Surface layer of epidermis composed of multiple layers of anucleate keratinocytes that often intertwine to give basketweave appearance
  - Stratum granulosum: 1-3 layers of cells under corneum, composed of flattened cells oriented parallel to skin surface with basophilic keratohyalin granules
  - Stratum spinosum: 5-10 layers of keratinocytes connected by desmosomes under stratum granulosum
  - Stratum basalis: Deepest layer of epidermis, composed of proliferating keratinocytes and melanocytes, attached to basement membrane by desmosomes
  - Basement membrane separates epidermis from dermis; composed of collagens and laminins
- **Cell types**
  - Keratinocytes: Main cell of epidermis, comprising the stratified squamous epithelium with round to oval nuclei and cell-to-cell bridges (desmosomes); positive for CK5/6 and p63 by immunohistochemistry
  - Melanocytes: Melanin-producing cells in stratum basalis with hyperchromatic round to oval nuclei and cleared-out cytoplasm; positive for S100, HMB-45, Melan-A, tyrosinase, and microphthalmia transcription factor (MITF)
  - Langerhans cells: Dendritic cells with kidney bean-shaped nuclei, usually in stratum spinosum; contain Birbeck granules, express CD1a, S100, and Langerin
  - Merkel cells: Oval, clear cells in stratum basalis associated with underlying sensory nerve endings; express CK20 (not identifiable by routine histology)
- Rete ridges
  - Epidermal areas that extend downward between dermal papillae
- Acrosyringium
  - Most superficial part of eccrine glands; acrosyringium is the intraepidermal eccrine duct, which spirals through epidermis in a corkscrew pattern
- Follicular Ostia
  - Intraepidermal hair follicle opening with lamellated keratin
- Melanin pigment
  - There is more melanin pigment in darker skinned individuals due to increased accumulation of pigment in basilar keratinocytes
- Acral skin
  - Often shows thick stratum corneum with a prominent granular layer; epidermis is also thicker than at other locations

Pitfalls/Artifacts
- Reactive keratinocytic atypia may be seen in inflammatory conditions; acute inflammation, erosions, &/or ulceration typically present

Age Variation
- There are more melanocytes and more Langerhans cells in children and fewer in elderly
  - Sun-damaged skin in adults can have increased numbers of junctional melanocytes

Hyperplasia
- Often seen in association with chronic inflammatory conditions (i.e., chronic spongiotic dermatitis, psoriasis, lichen simplex chronicus, lichen planus, etc.)

(Left) This graphic of normal thick skin (palm or sole) shows the layers of the epidermis, including the stratum basalis ⤴, stratum spinosum ➡, stratum granulosum ⤵, and a thickened stratum corneum ➡. *(Right)* The keratinocytes in normal epidermis form the normal stratum basalis ⤴, stratum spinosum ➡, stratum granulosum ⤵, and stratum corneum ➡, which has associated orthokeratosis (anuclear keratin layer).

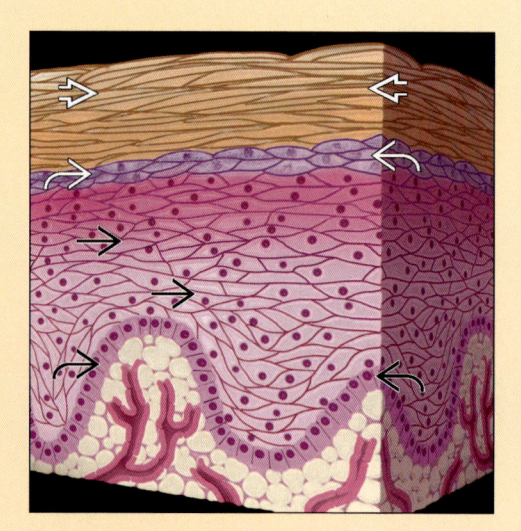

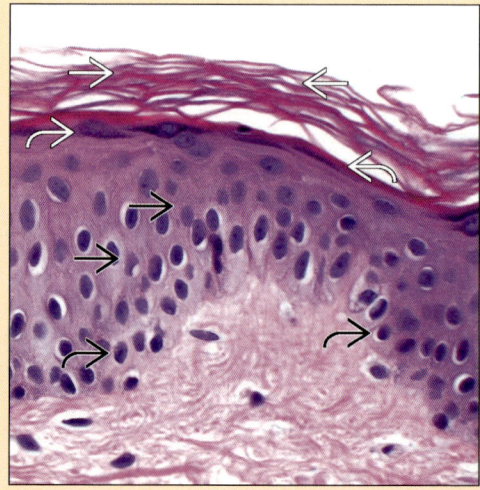

EPIDERMIS (INCLUDING KERATINOCYTES AND MELANOCYTES)

Normal Epidermis and Superficial Dermis

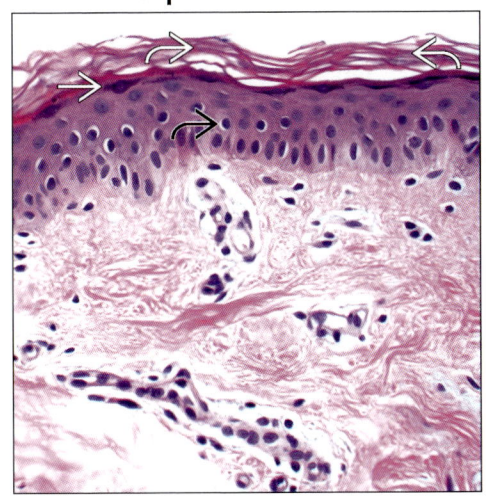

Normal Epidermis

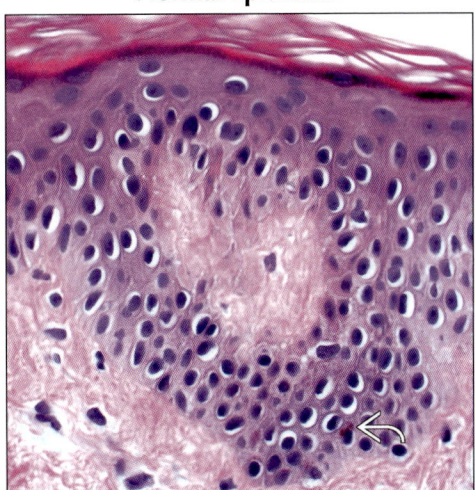

(Left) Normal thin skin on the arm features epidermis composed of 4-5 layers of bland-appearing keratinocytes with round to oval, hyperchromatic nuclei ➔. The granular layer ➔ is well formed, and there is overlying basketweave stratum corneum ➔. The superficial dermis is underneath the epidermis. *(Right)* This photograph shows fused rete ridges, which can be seen occasionally in normal skin. Focal cytoplasmic melanin pigment is also seen ➔ in a keratinocyte.

Acral Skin

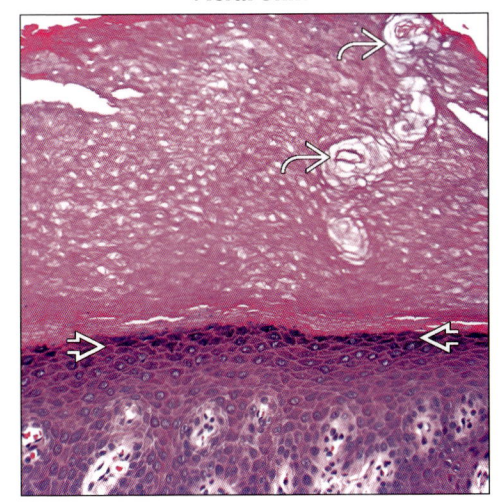

Acral Skin

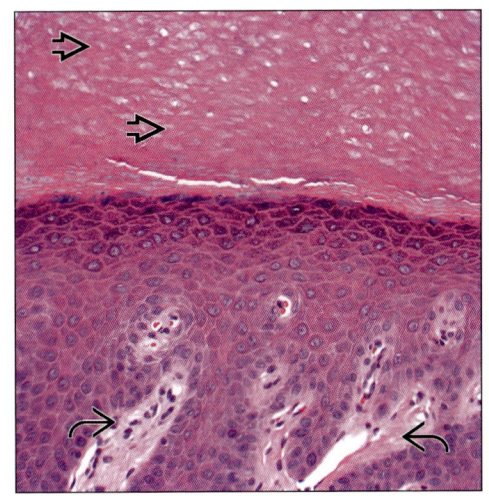

(Left) Acral-type skin contains prominent, dense keratin in the stratum corneum, with an intracorneal acrosyringium ➔. The epidermis also has a prominent granular layer ➔. *(Right)* Higher magnification of acral skin shows a thickened stratum corneum ➔. The epidermis is also thicker than at other sites and the dermis displays mild dermal fibrosis ➔.

Epidermis With Focal Parakeratosis

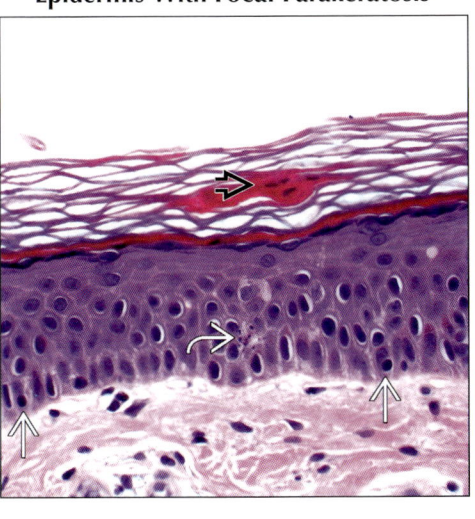

PAS Stain in Normal Epidermis

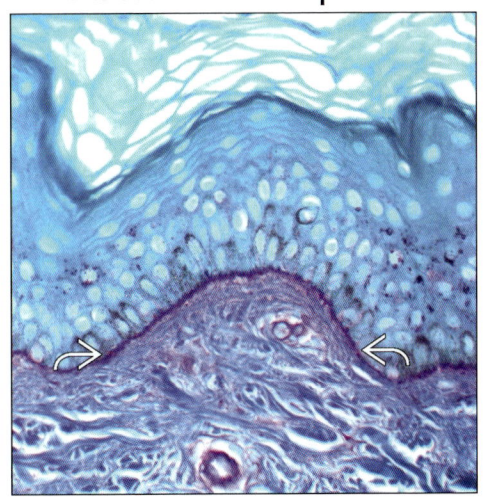

(Left) This high magnification of the epidermis in a case of resolving spongiotic dermatitis (which can be mistaken for normal skin) shows focal parakeratosis ➔, rare lymphocytes ➔ in the basilar layer, and focal apoptotic bodies ➔. These mild reactive changes indicate a previous inflammatory insult. *(Right)* PAS stain will highlight the normal basement membrane ➔. It can be thickened or reduplicated in pathologic processes such as lupus and lichen sclerosus et atrophicus.

EPIDERMIS (INCLUDING KERATINOCYTES AND MELANOCYTES)

Epidermis With Follicular Ostia

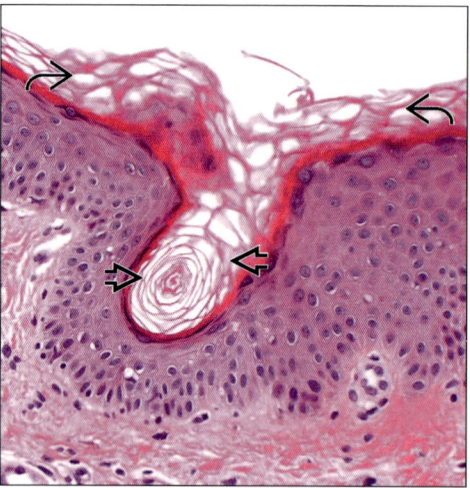

Acrosyringium

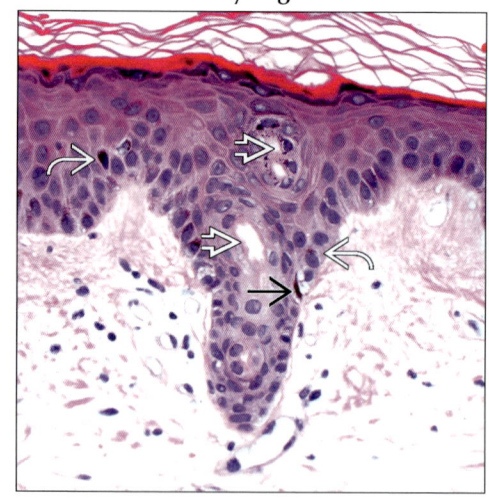

(Left) The follicular ostia (intraepidermal opening of a hair follicle) is composed of an invagination of the epidermis containing laminated keratin ⇨. The adjacent stratum corneum shows basketweave orthokeratosis ➔. *(Right)* Histologic section of an intraepidermal eccrine duct (acrosyringium) shows a small ductal lumen ⇨ within the epidermis. Melanin pigment is seen in the cytoplasms of basilar keratinocytes ➔ and a melanocyte ➔.

Moderately Pigmented Skin

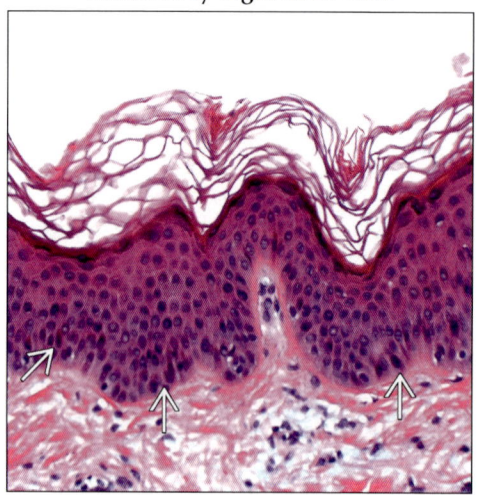

Darkly Pigmented Skin

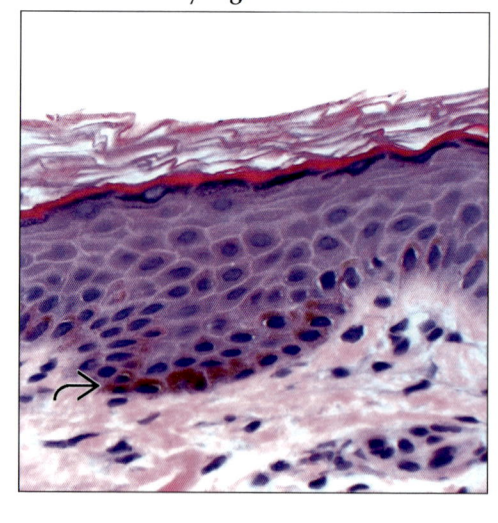

(Left) The normal epidermis in a darker-skinned (i.e., Hispanic or Southeast Asian) patient shows increased melanin pigment in the basilar keratinocytes ➔. *(Right)* Normal epidermis from a dark-skinned (i.e., African origin) patient shows prominent basilar keratinocytic pigmentation ➔. The increased pigment is due to greater accumulation in keratinocytes, not an increased number of melanocytes.

Normal Epidermis With Melanocytes

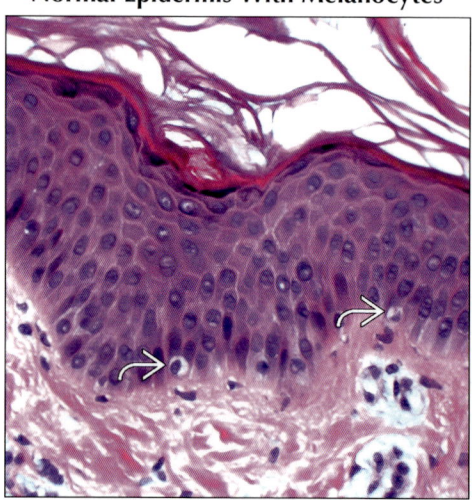

Normal Epidermis With Melanocytes

(Left) High magnification of the epidermis in a Caucasian patient shows a few basilar melanocytes with clear cytoplasm ➔. *(Right)* Higher magnification section of the epidermis in a Caucasian patient shows several basilar melanocytes, which display hyperchromatic nuclei and cleared-out cytoplasm ➔.

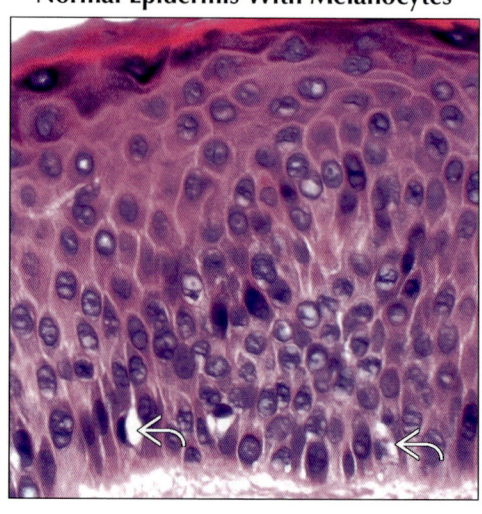

EPIDERMIS (INCLUDING KERATINOCYTES AND MELANOCYTES)

Junctional Melanocytes in Sun-Damaged Skin

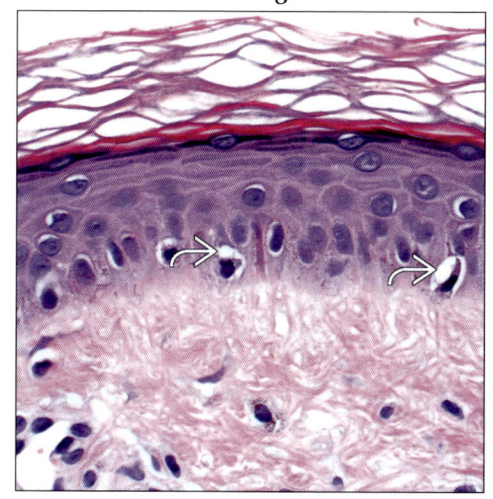

Melan-A Immunohistochemistry in Sun-Damaged Skin

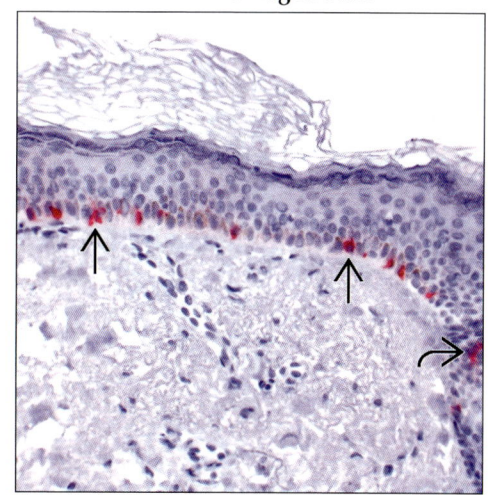

(Left) This epidermis from sun-damaged skin shows several junctional melanocytes with clear spaces ⇨ separating them from the keratinocytes. While the nuclei are hyperchromatic, there is no significant cytologic atypia or pagetoid spread. *(Right)* This Melan-A/Mart-1 immunohistochemical-stained section shows mildly increased numbers of small, normal-appearing junctional melanocytes ⇨ in the basilar epidermis and focally in the superficial portion of a hair follicle ⇨.

Intraepidermal Langerhans Cells

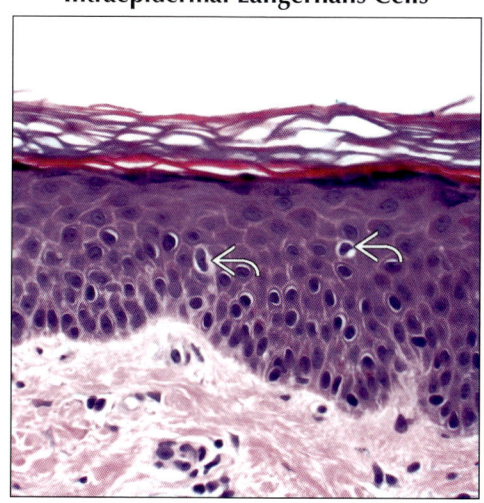

CD1a Immunohistochemical Stain for Langerhans Cells

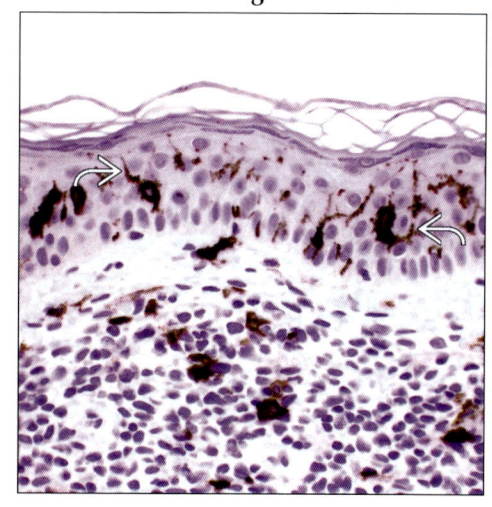

(Left) The normal epidermis contains scattered Langerhans cells ⇨ with somewhat curved to kidney bean-shaped nuclei. There is overlying orthokeratosis present as well. *(Right)* CD1a immunohistochemical stain for Langerhans cells shows very strong cytoplasmic staining of multiple intraepidermal cells with elongated, branching cytoplasmic processes ⇨, typical of Langerhans cells.

Miliaria Crystallina

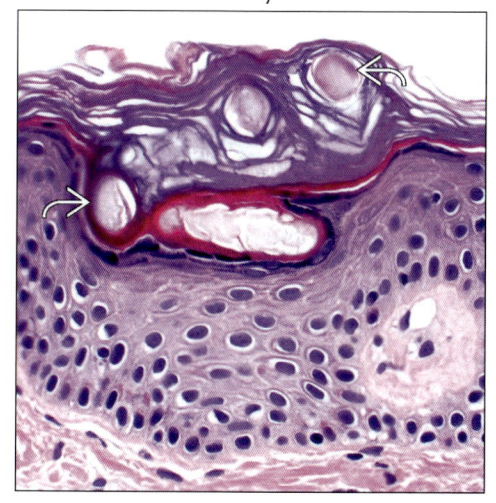

PAS Stain in Miliaria Crystallina

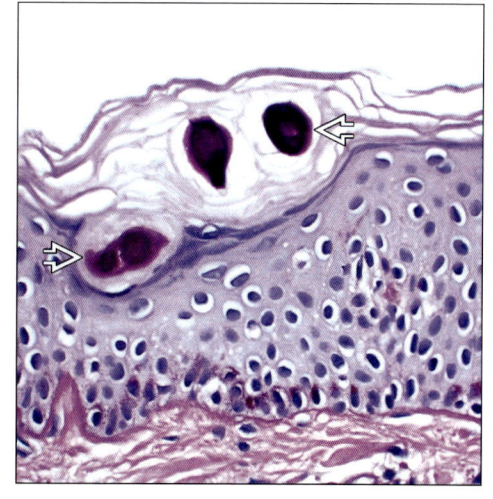

(Left) Histologic section of the epidermis in miliaria crystallina shows amorphous mucinous secretions ⇨, which plug the acrosyringium. These biopsies can appear very similar to normal skin, especially at low-power examination, and the diagnosis can be easily missed if the sections are not examined closely. *(Right)* PAS-stained section shows strong purplish staining of the intracorneal secretions ⇨ in miliaria crystallina.

DERMIS

Key Facts

Macroscopic Anatomy
- Firm, white-yellow appearance

Microscopic Anatomy
- **Papillary dermis**
  - Collagen: Loose, thinner fibers (mostly type I, less type III collagen) than in reticular dermis, with associated mucin
  - Elastic fibers: Typically sparse, thin, and branching
  - Blood vessels: Small, capillary type; numerous vessels present at papillary/reticular dermis interface (superficial plexus) and capillary beds also form beneath epidermis
  - Nerve fiber endings and Meissner corpuscles (encapsulated nerve endings; function as touch receptors) present in acral skin
  - Dermal papillae: Finger-like projections of dermis pushing into overlying epidermal basement membrane, surrounded by epidermal rete ridges
- **Reticular dermis**
  - Collagen: Denser fibers (mostly type I), with less mucin; much more dense and sclerotic-appearing on the back
  - Elastic fibers: More numerous and thicker than papillary dermis
  - Blood vessels: Small and medium-sized vessels (arterioles and venules, lymphatics) form deep plexus
  - Nerves: Typically associated with vessels (neurovascular bundles); pacinian corpuscles (encapsulated nerve endings surrounded by circumferential lamellae; function as pressure receptors in acral skin)
  - Pilar muscles: Small muscle bundles associated with hair follicles; insert below level of sebaceous glands
  - Smooth muscle bundles present in dermis in genitalia and areola
- **Stromal cells**
  - Fibroblasts and myofibroblasts: Normal component of dermis; often sparsely distributed, bland spindle-shaped hyperchromatic nuclei with inconspicuous nucleoli
  - Mast cells (tissue basophils): Scattered mast cells normally present; show central round to oval nuclei, abundant basophilic-staining granular cytoplasm
  - Lymphocytes: At least a few small perivascular lymphocytes physiologically present
  - Plasma cells: Normally a few present in mucosal sites, and often seen in scalp skin
  - Histiocytes (tissue macrophages) and dendritic cells: Normally sparsely distributed; show indented nuclei with vesicular chromatin, abundant lightly staining cytoplasm

Pitfalls/Artifacts
- Fixation: Poor fixation leads to suboptimal staining
- Processing: Artifactual clefts often present in dermis; tissue may be fragmented, portions may be missing
- Cautery: Leads to homogenization of collagen fibers and streaming effects on nuclei

Age Variation
- Embryonal: Cellular dermis, hypoplastic adnexal structures (except for eccrine glands)
- Infants and children: Dermis is less cellular, adnexal structures are typically developed (except for apocrine glands)
- Adults: Dermal atrophy can be seen with aging, due to loss of mucin and stromal cells
  - Solar elastosis often present in older adults (in non-sun-protected sites)
  - Elastic fibers are enlarged, thickened, and appear light bluish on H&E
  - Hemorrhage commonly seen in elderly patients' biopsies, due to fragility of vessels
  - Decreased numbers of fibroblasts, dendritic cells, mast cells

Hyperplasia
- Epidermal hyperplasia very common (i.e., lichen simplex chronicus, prurigo nodularis, psoriasis, etc.), but dermal hyperplasia is rare
  - Typically part of a pathologic process (i.e., scar or morphea, scleroderma) associated with increased collagen production

(Left) The dermis is composed of connective tissue, blood vessels ⇒, and nerves ⇒. Multiple adnexal structures, including eccrine glands ⇒, apocrine glands ⇒, Pacinian corpuscles (blue oval), and hair follicles ⇒ are present. (Right) Normal skin shows epidermis ⇒, papillary dermis ⇒ with thin, lightly-eosinophilic-staining collagen, and reticular dermis ⇒ with thicker, denser collagen bundles.

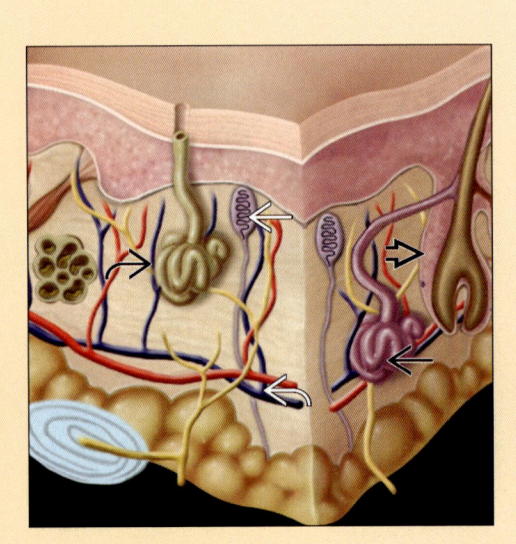

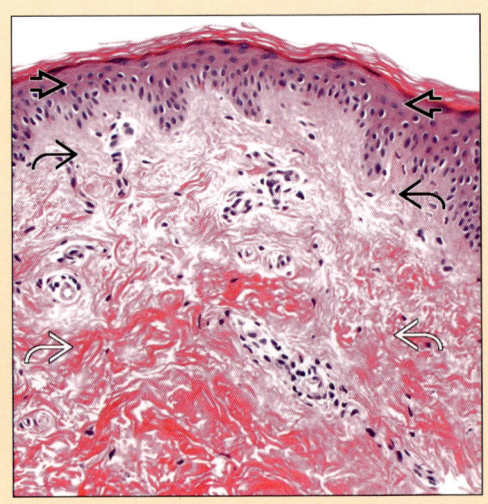

DERMIS

Papillary Dermis

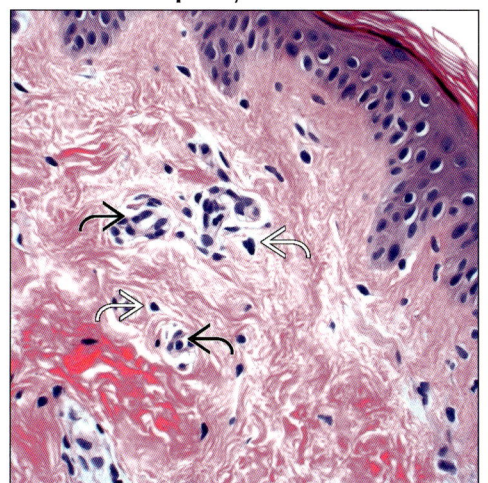

Papillary Dermis

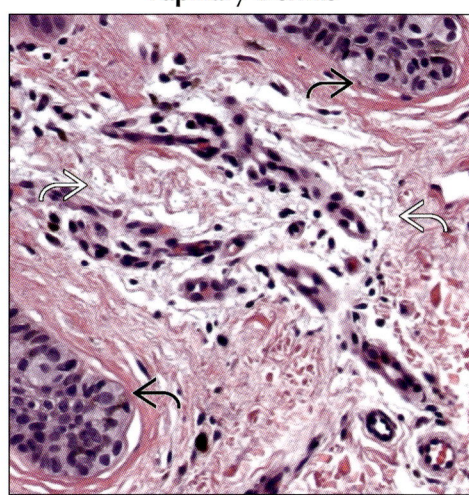

(Left) High magnification photo of the papillary dermis shows loose collagen and multiple small, capillary-type blood vessels ⇨. A few stromal lymphocytes ⇨ are normally present. (Right) The papillary dermis between rete ridges ⇨ normally contains multiple small, capillary-type blood vessels and a loose collagen matrix with mucinous material ⇨.

Severe Solar Elastosis in Superficial Dermis

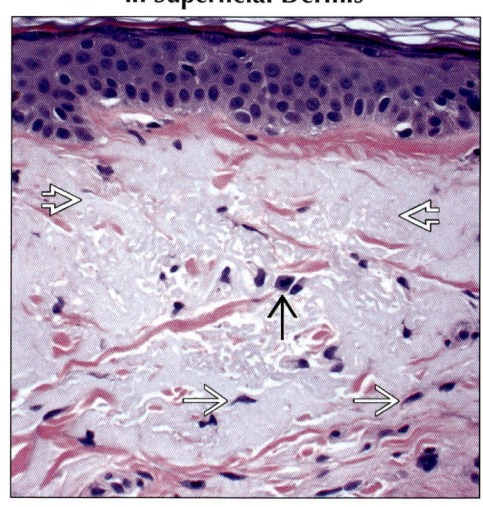

Papillary Dermal Melanin Pigment

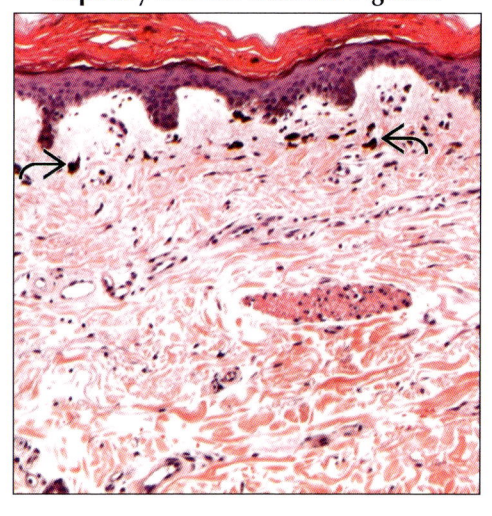

(Left) Solar elastosis is a common finding in sun-damaged skin of the elderly. It consists of degenerating elastic fibers ⇨ in the papillary dermis and superficial reticular dermis that stain blue-gray. Note the few scattered mast cells ⇨ and fibroblasts ⇨. (Right) Pigment is often seen in the dermis in skin that has previously been inflamed. In this case, there is no residual inflammation, but prominent melanin pigment deposits ⇨ are seen in the papillary dermis.

Interface Between Papillary and Reticular Dermis

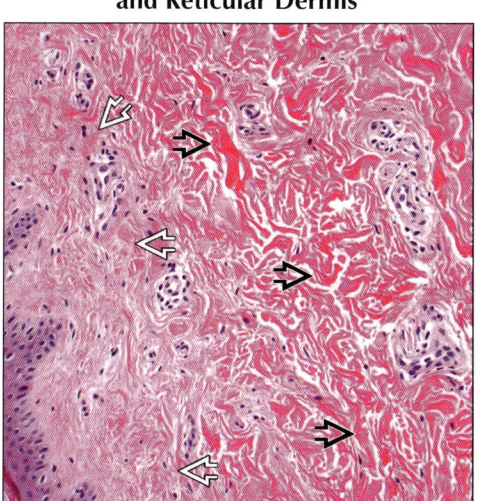

Reticular Dermis

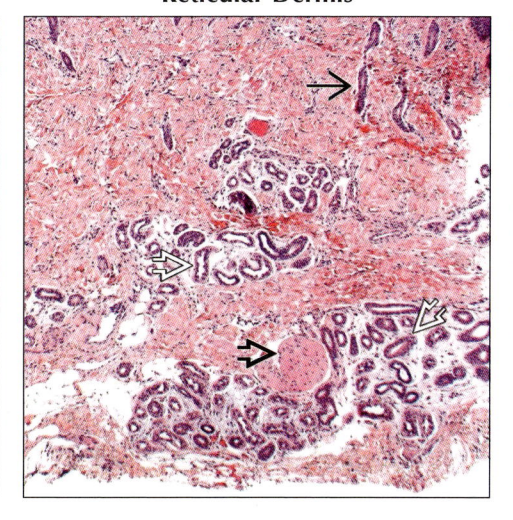

(Left) In this low magnification photo of the papillary dermal/reticular dermal interface, the papillary dermis on the left is composed of thinner, lighter staining collagen bundles ⇨, whereas the reticular dermis on the right is composed of thicker, more eosinophilic-appearing collagen bundles ⇨. (Right) The reticular dermis contains multiple adnexal structures including eccrine ducts ⇨, eccrine and apocrine glands ⇨, and a pilar muscle ⇨ in the deeper dermis.

DERMIS

Reticular Dermis

(Left) The reticular dermis from the back shows a dense arrangement of thickened eosinophilic collagen bundles. Note the eccrine ducts at the top of the field ➡. *(Right)* The deep reticular dermis contains dense, sclerotic-appearing, hyalinized collagen bundles. This finding is usually abnormal except for the skin of the back, which typically has this appearance. Note the cluster of deep pilar muscles ➡.

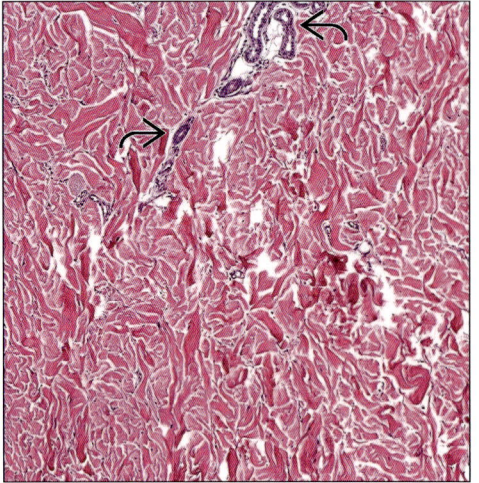

Deep Dermis

Neurovascular Bundle and Apocrine Glands

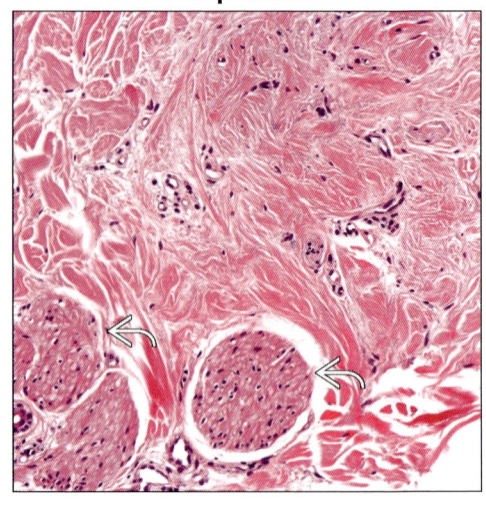

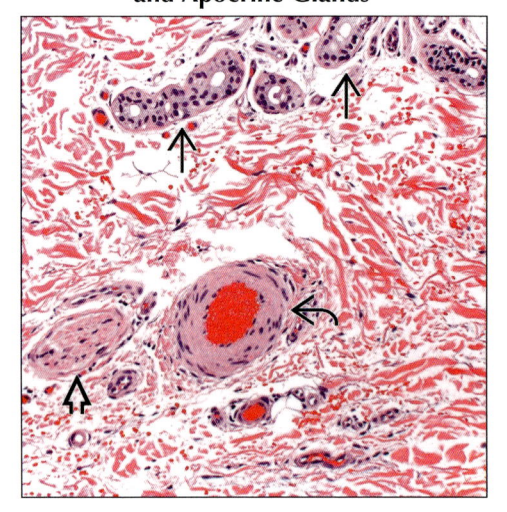

(Left) This photo illustrates a neurovascular bundle and a small muscular vessel ➡ on the right, and a small nerve on the left ➡. A more superficial cluster of apocrine glands is also seen ➡. *(Right)* This photo shows a deep dermal blood vessel with a thin muscular lining, consistent with a venule. Note the small adjacent arteriole ➡ and lymphatics ➡.

Dermal Blood Vessels and Lymphatics

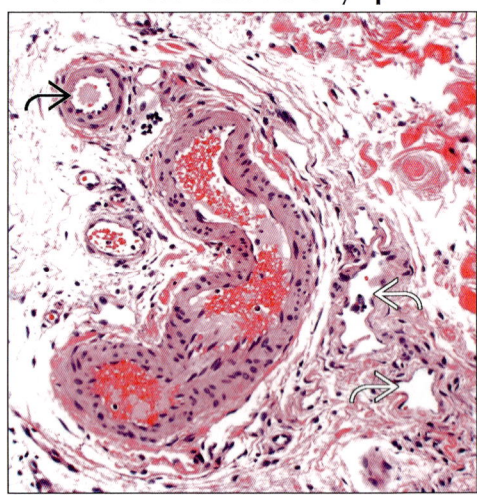

Blood Vessels and Collagen Bundles

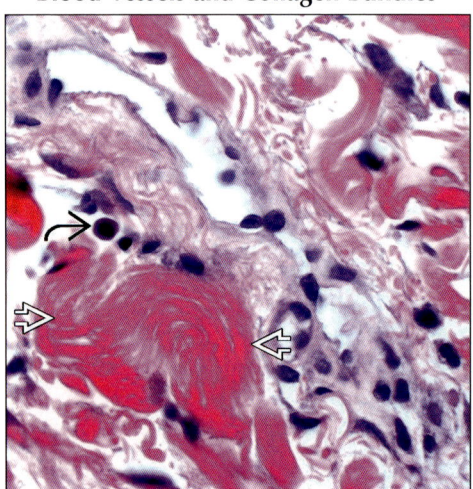

(Left) This high-magnification photo shows small blood vessels and prominent, thickened collagen bundles ➡. A few lymphocytes and a mast cell ➡ are seen in the stroma. *(Right)* This deep neurovascular bundle at the dermal/subcutaneous junction ➡ consists of a small nerve on the left ➡ and the vessels on the right ➡.

Deep Neurovascular Bundle

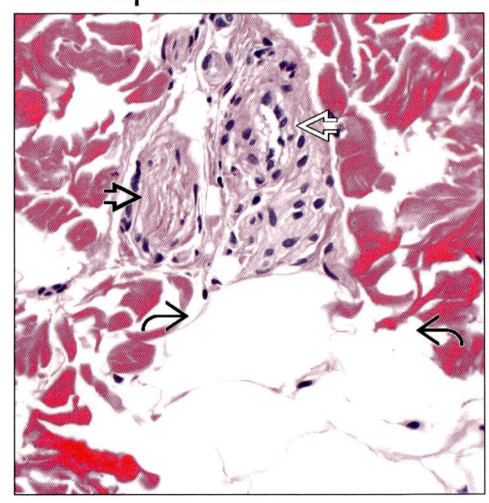

DERMIS

Deep Dermal Nerve

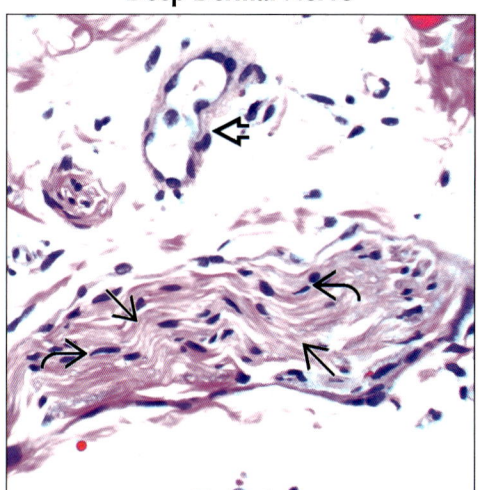

Pacinian Corpuscle

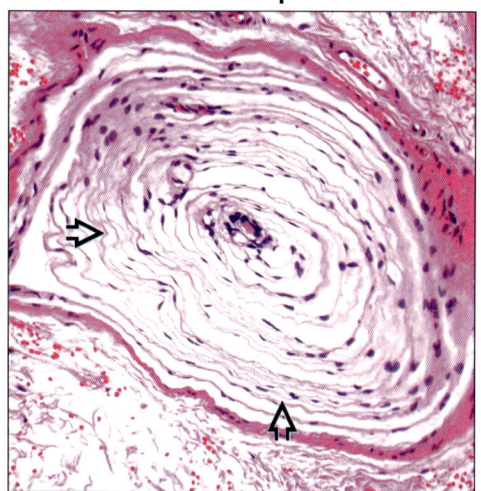

(Left) A medium-sized nerve in the deep dermis is composed of a collection of spindle-shaped cells with angulated nuclei ➔ and wispy, lightly eosinophilic-staining cytoplasm ➔. A few small blood vessels are also present superior to the nerve ➔. *(Right)* This photo of a pacinian corpuscle on acral skin illustrates the distinctive concentric laminated pattern ➔ of nerve sheath fibers.

Sebaceous Gland and Pilar Muscles

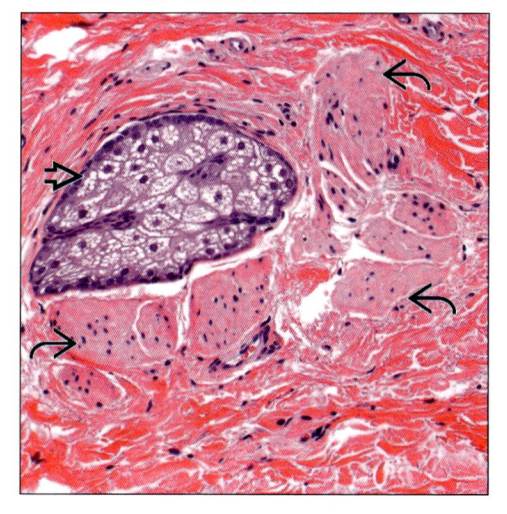

Pilar Muscle

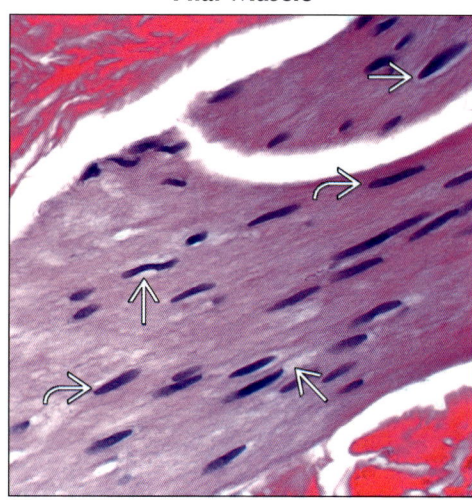

(Left) This section shows a sebaceous gland ➔ and surrounding pilar muscles ➔ in the reticular dermis. *(Right)* This pilar muscle at high magnification features elongated, spindle-shaped nuclei with a "cigar-shaped" (or blunt-ended) ➔ appearance and abundant eosinophilic-staining cytoplasm. Note the perinuclear clearing in some cells ➔.

Mast Cells at Deep Dermis/ Subcutaneous Junction

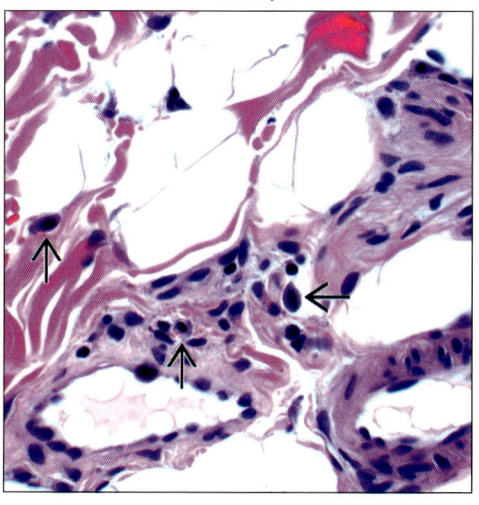

Mast Cells

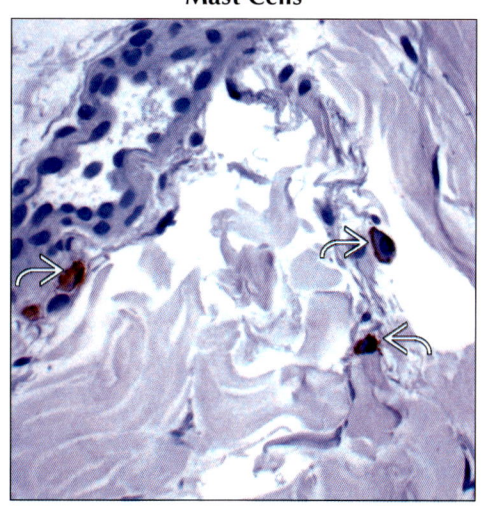

(Left) This photograph of the deep dermis/subcutaneous junction shows multiple mast cells that are normally present ➔ in the perivascular stroma. The mast cells show hyperchromatic-staining oval nuclei and abundant basophilic-staining granular cytoplasm. *(Right)* CD117 immunohistochemistry prominently highlights the cytoplasmic membranes ➔ of mast cells in the deep dermis.

ADNEXAL STRUCTURES

Key Facts

Macroscopic Anatomy
- Only hair follicles typically visible grossly
  - May show dilated lumen filled with keratin and hairs
  - Hairs may be fine/vellus (arms, legs, face, back) or coarse (scalp, genital)
- Sebaceous glands may be seen if hyperplastic
  - Appear yellow

Microscopic Anatomy
- **Hair follicles**
  - Bulb: Base of follicle, composed of small basaloid cells forming the matrix, often with cytoplasmic melanin pigmentation
  - Papillary mesenchymal body: Invagination of cellular stroma into bulb
  - Inner root sheath: Eosinophilic-staining cells around hair matrix in suprabulbar region (includes Huxley layer and Henle layer)
  - Outer root sheath: Clear-staining cells (due to cytoplasmic glycogen) surrounding inner root sheath in suprabulbar region
  - Isthmus: Above suprabulbar region; bulge delineates lower portion of isthmus; upper portion defined by insertion of sebaceous duct; keratinization without a granular layer (pilar/trichilemmal keratinization) seen in upper portion of isthmus
  - Bulge region: Insertion of pilar muscle and proposed origin of follicular stem cells
  - Infundibulum: Uppermost region of follicle (above insertion of sebaceous duct); keratinization with a granular layer (infundibular/epidermoid keratinization)
  - Ostia: Opening of follicle at epidermal surface; often contains keratin, small collections of bacterial organisms, and may show a few *Malassezia* (*Pityrosporum*) organisms
- **Sebaceous glands**
  - More abundant in facial and eyelid areas
  - Lobular collections of large, central clear cells with abundant multivacuolated cytoplasm and small, vesicular nuclei with indentations
  - Peripheral layer of small, cuboidal basaloid cells (may show mitotic activity)
  - Glands empty lipids and entire necrotic cells ("holocrine necrosis") into sebaceous duct, which attaches to follicular lumen
- **Apocrine glands**
  - More abundant in axillary, groin, breast, and eyelid areas
  - Clusters of glands in deep dermis or superficial subcutis
  - Composed of cuboidal to columnar cells with eosinophilic cytoplasm; may show apical snouts and secretions
  - Apocrine duct connects to follicle; ductal cells appear identical to eccrine ductal cells
- **Eccrine glands**
  - Concentrated on acral surfaces, but present in all cutaneous sites
  - Clusters of glands in deep dermis or superficial subcutis
  - Composed mostly of cuboidal cells with pale eosinophilic to clear cytoplasm (clear cells)
  - Eccrine ducts connect directly to epidermis (acrosyringium is intraepidermal duct)

Pitfalls/Artifacts
- Fixation &/or processing artifact can make it difficult to discern small glands and follicles from tumors, especially basal cell carcinoma (BCC)
- Tangentially sectioned hair bulbs can be mistaken for BCC, especially in frozen sections

Age Variation
- Adnexal structures are hypoplastic in infancy
- Hair follicles and sebaceous glands mature during puberty, especially in axillary, facial, and genital areas

Metaplasia
- Squamous metaplasia may be seen in adnexal ducts; typically associated with inflammation or scarring (i.e., previous biopsy or excision site)

(Left) Normal cutaneous adnexal structures include hair follicles ➡ with associated apocrine ➡ and sebaceous glands ➡. The eccrine gland attaches directly to the epidermis ➡. *(Right)* This is a small (vellus) hair follicle and sebaceous gland. The follicle shows a papillary mesenchymal body ➡ invaginating into the bulb. The sebaceous gland is composed of large clear cells.

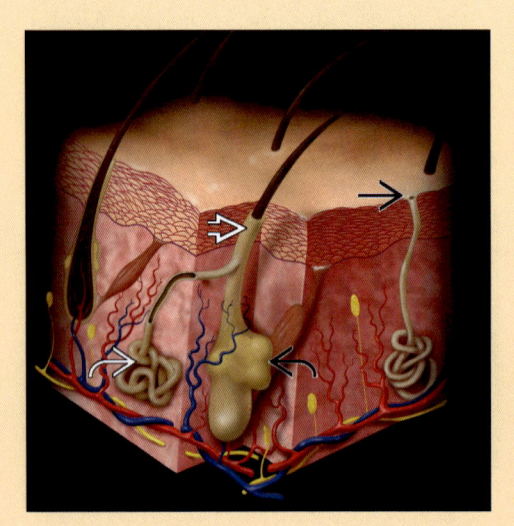

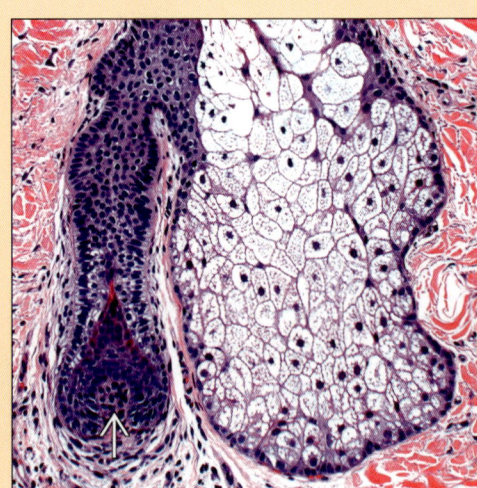

ADNEXAL STRUCTURES

Bulb and Suprabulbar Region of Vellus Follicle

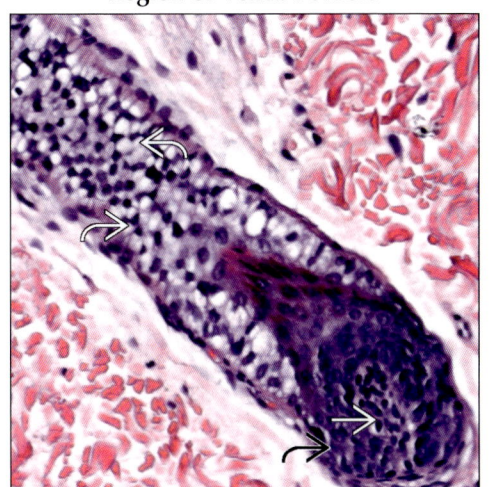

Cross Section of Hair Bulb

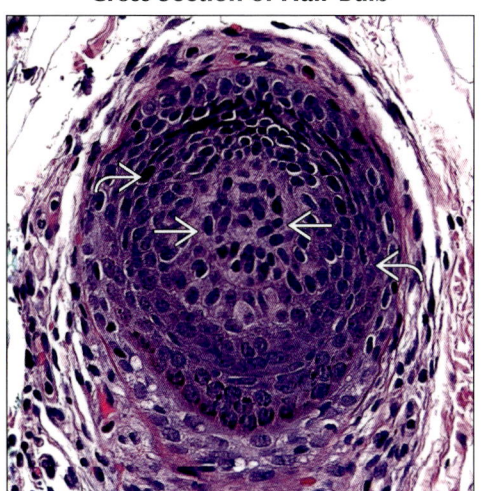

(Left) H&E shows a hair follicle at the bulbar region with the papillary mesenchymal body ➡ surrounded by small basaloid cells ➡ with scant amounts of cytoplasm. Note the more superficial outer root sheath cells with clear cytoplasm ➡. (Right) Cross section of a hair follicle at the bulbar region shows the papillary mesenchymal body ➡ surrounded by small basaloid cells ➡ with scant amounts of cytoplasm.

Cross Section of Suprabulbar Region

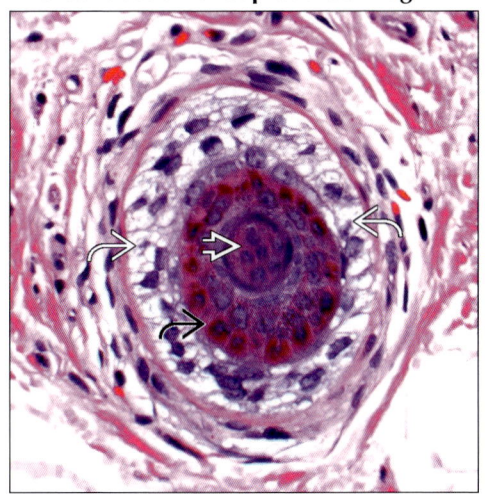

Cross Section of Anagen-Phase Hair Follicle

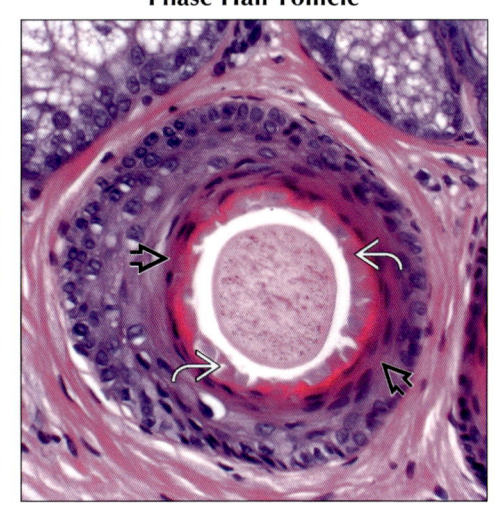

(Left) Cross section of an anagen (growth phase) follicle in the suprabulbar region shows the follicle with clear outer root sheath cells ➡ surrounding eosinophilic-staining inner root sheath cells ➡ and the central hair matrix ➡. (Right) This cross section of an anagen-phase follicle at the level of the isthmus shows a central hair shaft, presence of the inner root sheath ➡, and keratinization without a granular layer ➡.

Cross Section of Telogen-Phase Hair Follicle

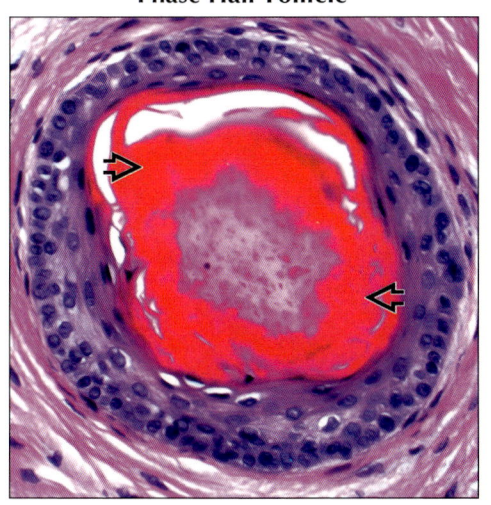

Isthmus of Hair Follicle With Sebaceous Glands

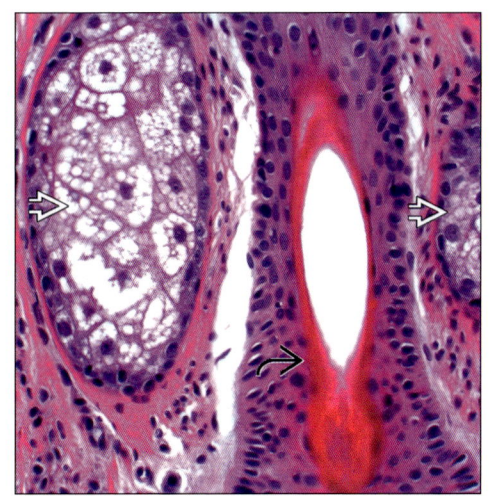

(Left) This cross section of a telogen-phase follicle (resting phase) at the level of the isthmus shows absence of the inner root sheath and brightly eosinophilic-staining keratinous material ➡. Note the absence of a granular layer (which is not present until the level of the infundibulum). (Right) This longitudinal section of a telogen hair follicle at the level of the isthmus shows keratinization without a granular layer ➡. Adjacent sebaceous glands ➡ are present.

ADNEXAL STRUCTURES

Vellus Follicle With Sebaceous Glands

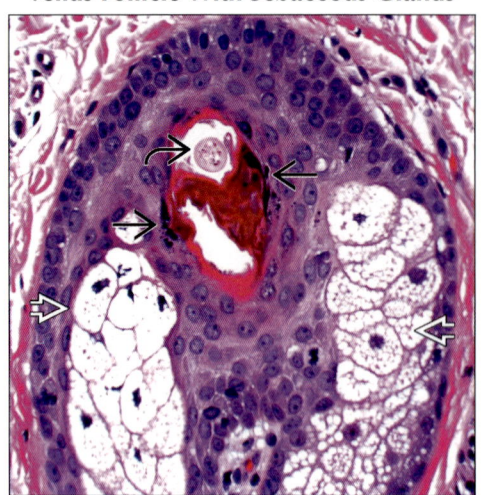

Infundibular Region of Follicles With Demodex

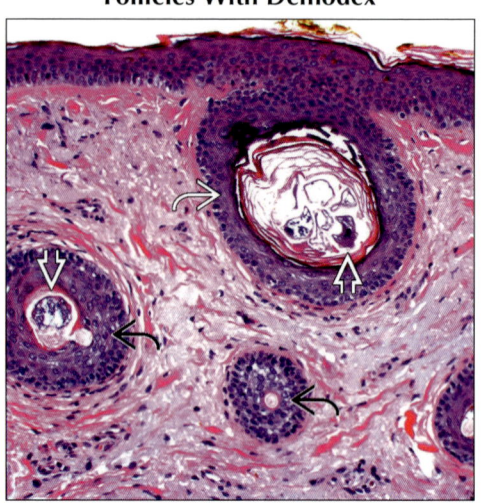

(Left) This cross section of a vellus (fine, light-colored) hair follicle at the lower level of the infundibulum shows the miniaturized hair shaft ➡ and adjacent small sebaceous glands ➡. Note the focal presence of a granular layer ➡. *(Right)* This section of superficial dermis contains multiple follicles (including a terminal hair ➡ and several vellus hairs ➡), with multiple intrafollicular Demodex organisms present ➡ (these are common in adult skin).

Epidermis With Follicular Ostia

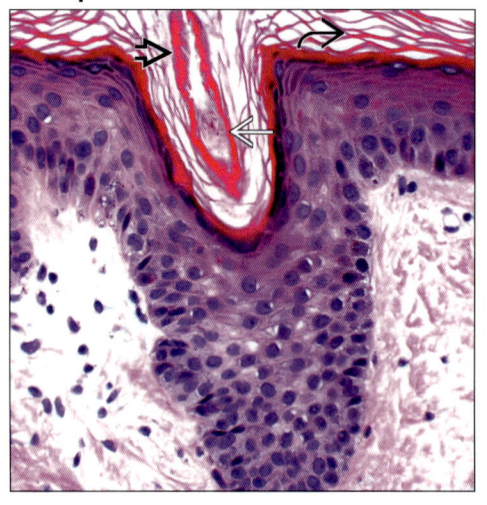

CK20(+) Merkel Cells in Hair Follicle

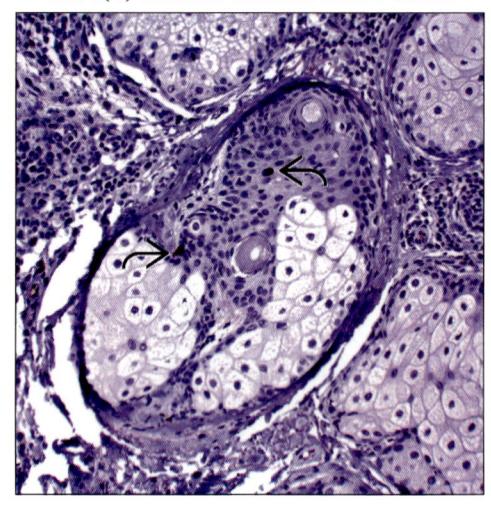

(Left) The follicular ostia (intraepidermal opening of the hair follicle) is composed of an invagination of the epidermis containing laminated keratin ➡ and the hair shaft ➡. The adjacent stratum corneum shows basket-weave orthokeratosis ➡. *(Right)* Immunohistochemical stain for CK20 shows a few normal Merkel cells ➡ in a hair follicle. Merkel cells are not identifiable by routine histology, but are easily identified by CK20 in both the epidermis and hair follicles.

Sebaceous Glands Attached to Hair Follicle

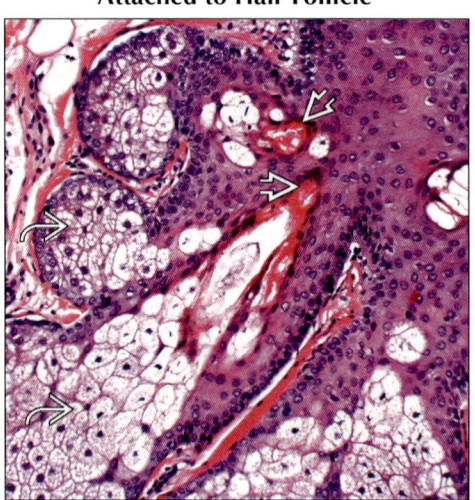

Sebaceous Gland at High Magnification

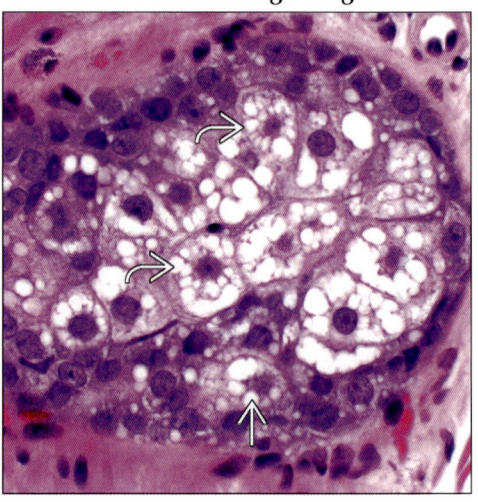

(Left) Vertical section of a hair follicle shows multiple attached mature sebaceous glands ➡, which empty directly into the follicle via sebaceous ducts ➡. *(Right)* High-magnification cross section of a sebaceous gland shows cells with abundant, multivacuolated, clear-staining cytoplasm ➡. The nuclei are round to oval, with vesicular to hyperchromatic-appearing chromatin. Some show indentations ➡ due to the cytoplasmic lipid.

ADNEXAL STRUCTURES

Apocrine Glands

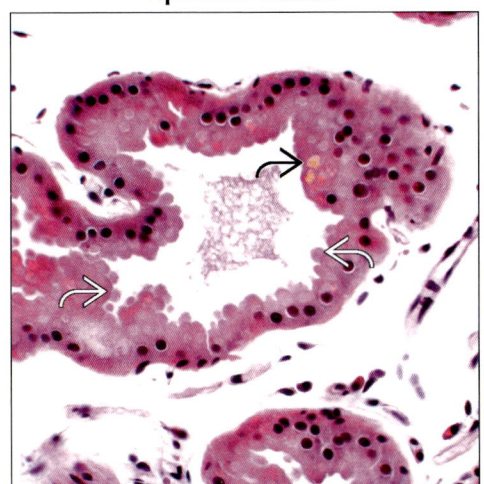

High Magnification of Apocrine Glands

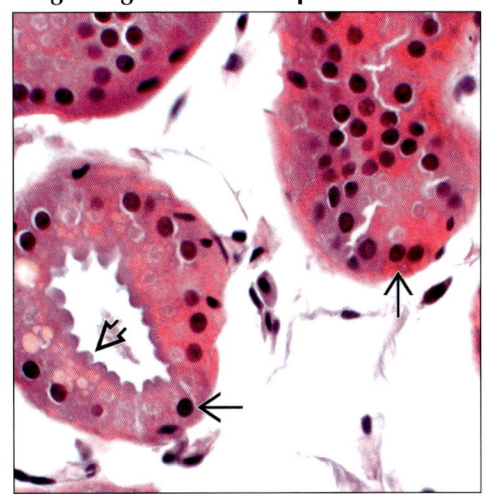

(Left) Apocrine glands are characterized by large epithelial cells with abundant eosinophilic-staining cytoplasm and numerous apical cytoplasmic snouts and secretions ⇨. Focal lipofuscin ⇨ is also present in some of the cells. **(Right)** High-magnification view of apocrine glands shows a population of large columnar cells with hyperchromatic nuclei ⇨, abundant eosinophilic-staining cytoplasm, and apical snouts ⇨.

PAS Stain in Apocrine Glands and Ducts

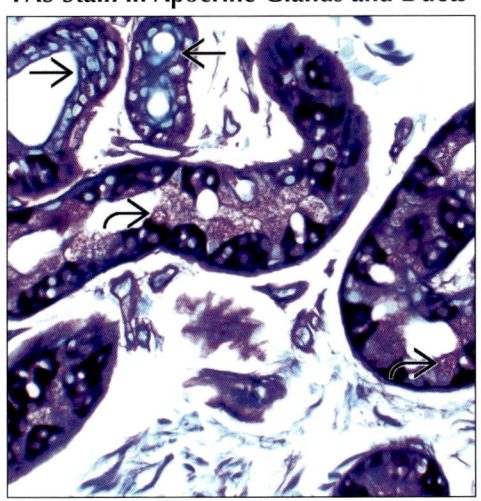

Eccrine Glands and Ducts

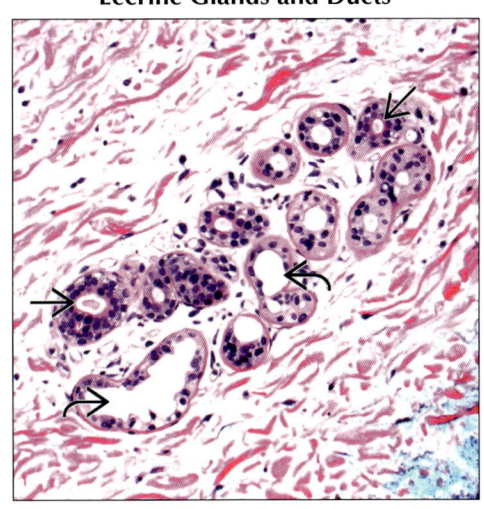

(Left) PAS stain in apocrine glands strongly stains the cytoplasm of most of the cells and highlights small granules in many of the luminal cells ⇨. Note that the apocrine ducts ⇨ do not show strong staining. **(Right)** Eccrine glands and ducts, here in the deep dermis, are characterized by a proliferation of small, bland-appearing epithelial cells with abundant clear cytoplasm surrounding central lumina ⇨. The ducts show smaller lumina with focal intraluminal secretions ⇨.

Eccrine Duct

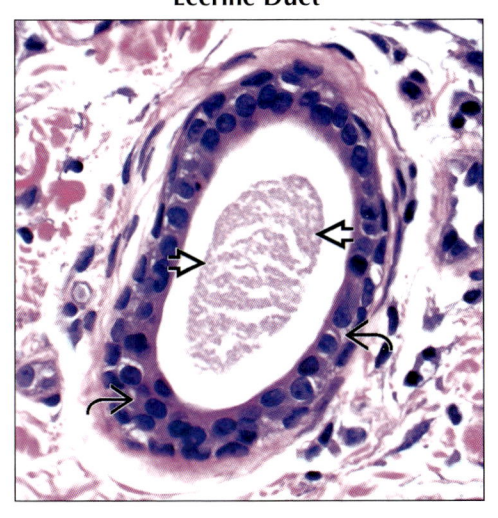

Superficial Dermal Eccrine Duct

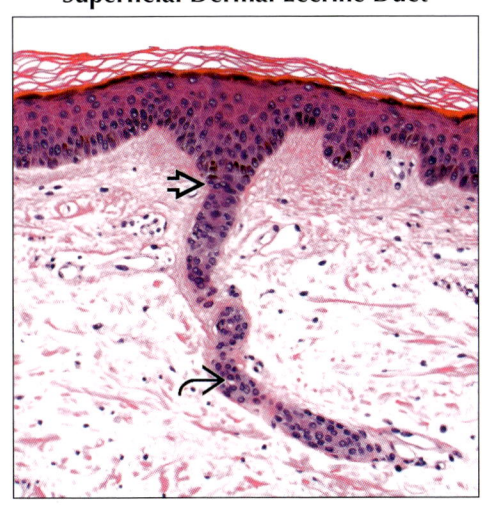

(Left) This cross section of an eccrine duct in the dermis shows a well-formed lumen with proteinaceous debris ⇨ surrounded by a 2-3 cell-thick layer of small, cuboidal-shaped epithelial cells ⇨ with eosinophilic-staining cytoplasm. **(Right)** Histologic section of an intradermal eccrine duct entering into the epidermis ⇨ (which contains the acrosyringium) shows a small ductal lumen ⇨ within the dermal portion.

NAIL

Key Facts

Macroscopic Anatomy
- Keratin plate and associated epithelium covering dorsal parts of terminal phalanges of fingers and toes
  - Consists of convex to flat/rectangular white/pink hard nail plate, which lies on nail bed
  - Translucent, but appears pink from underlying vasculature
  - Color may change when diseased
- The part of the nail that grows is at proximal end of nail, beneath epidermis
- Protects fingertips and toes from injury and enhances sensation of fingertips

Microscopic Anatomy
- **Nail plate**
  - Consists of nail proper or body of nail; composed of dense keratin material
  - Composed of layers of interdigitating polyhedral keratinocytes that lack nuclei or organelles
  - Contains calcium bound by phospholipids as well as small amounts of copper, iron, manganese, and zinc
  - **Free margin** is distal edge or anterior margin of nail plate (cutting edge of nail)
  - **Onychodermal band** is a 0.5-1.5 mm distal transverse band (glassy/gray color) proximal to free margin of nail
  - Onychodermal band forms a seal between nail plate and hyponychium
- **Proximal nail fold**
  - Wedge-shaped skin fold on dorsum of digit that overlies nail plate
  - Made of 2 layers of epidermis: Dorsal and ventral
  - **Dorsal proximal nail fold** continues epidermis on digit; cuticle is part of dorsal proximal nail fold and protects nail base/matrix
  - **Ventral proximal nail fold** overlies newly formed base of nail; eponychium is epithelium of ventral part of proximal nail fold
  - Eponychium and cuticle form a protective seal over proximal nail
  - Perionyx is projecting edge of eponychium covering proximal lunula
- **Matrix**
  - Tissue upon which proximal nail rests
  - Produces cells that form nail plate
  - Consists of acanthotic squamous epithelium without a granular layer, under proximal nail fold
  - Basaloid cells progress to larger squamoid keratinocytes, which form nail plate after flattening, losing nuclei, and condensing cytoplasm
  - Matrix contains small numbers of normal melanocytes, Merkel cells, and Langerhans cells
  - Lunula is the distal portion of matrix: Whitish crescent-shaped base of the visible nail
  - **Nail bed** is epithelium underlying remainder of nail plate: Flat epithelium, ~ 3 cells thick without melanocytes
  - **Hyponychium** Is distal nail bed epithelium under nail plate between free edge and skin of finger tip
  - Hyponychium is a thick keratin layer, acanthotic squamous epithelium, and transverse papillae that forms a seal that protects nail bed

Pitfalls/Artifacts
- Due to dense keratin material, nails are difficult to process, and histologic sections of nail often show processing &/or fixation artifact
- Artifactual staining or entrapped air bubbles may make it difficult to assess for pigment (melanin or hemosiderin) deposition

Age Variation
- Nail increases in thickness with advancing age
- Adults have larger dorsal nail keratinocytes compared to children

Hyperplasia
- Verrucous epithelial hyperplasia may be seen in subungual verrucae
  - Acanthosis, papillomatosis, and tiers of parakeratosis underlying nail plate
- Irregular thickening (dystrophy) of nail may be seen in infections (i.e., bacterial and fungal)

(Left) This histologic section shows the proximal nail fold ➟ and cuticle ➥ overlying the proximal nail plate ➟, and the nail matrix ➟ in an infant. Note the underlying immature bone ➟. *(Right)* Higher magnification of the proximal nail fold shows keratinizing eponychium ➟, as well as the cuticle ➥ overlying the nail plate. The nail matrix shows elongated rete ridges ➟ composed of bland squamous cells.

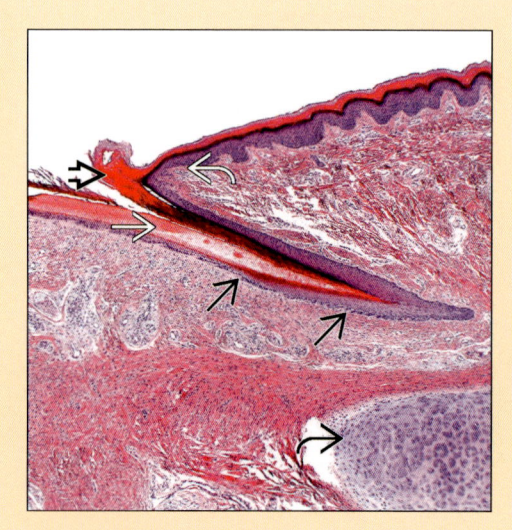

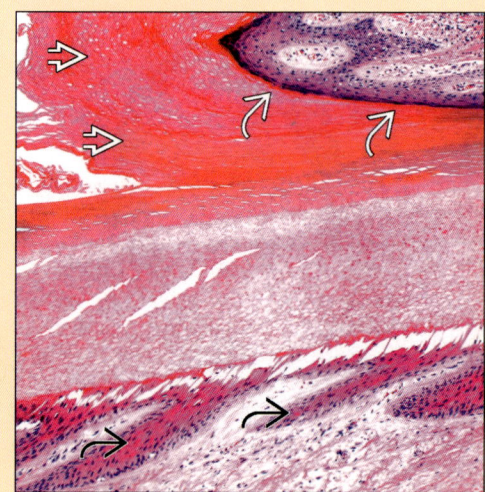

NAIL

Proximal Nail Matrix

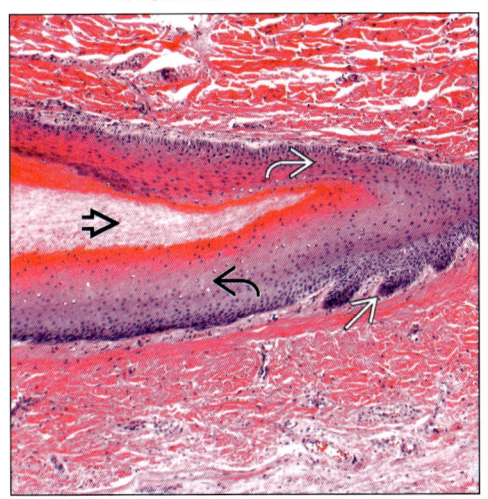

Matrix Angle Epithelium

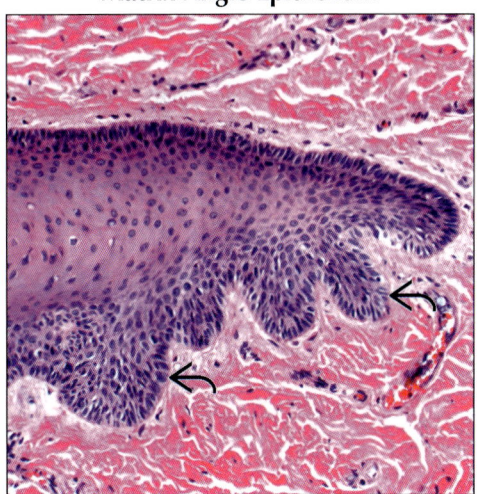

(Left) The proximal nail matrix (both dorsal ⇨ and ventral/intermediate ⇨) shows keratinizing squamous epithelium forming the proximal nail plate ⇨. Note the focal elongated rete ridges of the most proximal area of the ventral matrix ➡. (Right) This photo illustrates the most proximal portion of the matrix (matrix angle/dorsal and intermediate matrix). The matrix in this region is formed by proliferating basaloid cells ⇨ that lead to the production of the nail plate.

Higher Magnification of the Intermediate Matrix

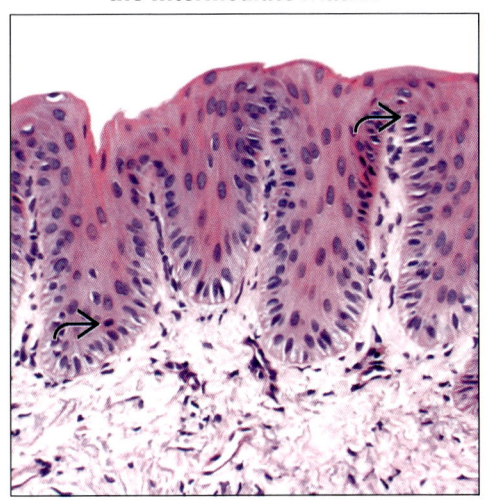

Hyponychium

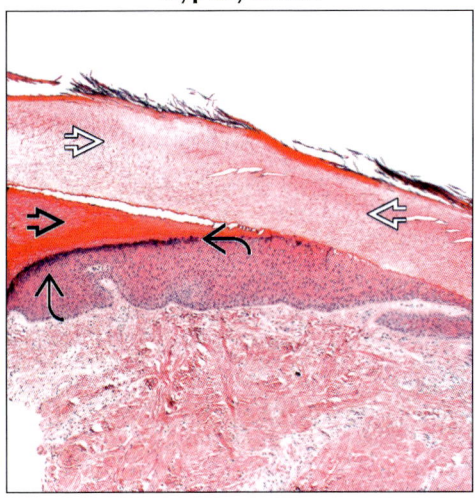

(Left) The intermediate matrix shows an acanthotic epithelium composed of bland-appearing squamous cells with eosinophilic cytoplasm and rare intraepithelial lymphocytes ⇨. No increase in melanocytes or melanin pigment is present. (Right) This is a view of the hyponychium, which is the distal nail bed epithelium under the nail plate ⇨ between the free edge and the skin of the finger tip. Note the very dense keratin layer ⇨ and prominent granular layer ➡.

Higher Magnification of the Hyponychium

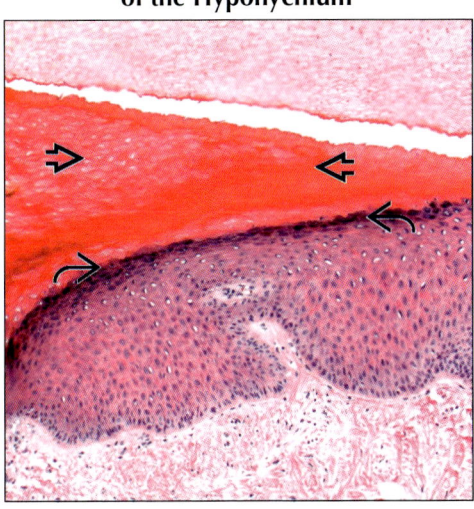

Melanocytes in the Proximal Nail Fold

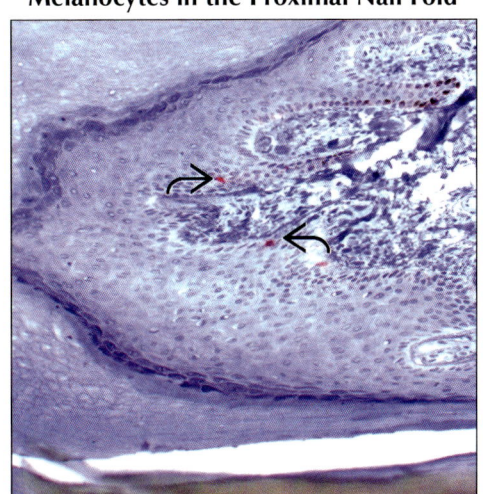

(Left) The hyponychium at higher magnification shows epithelial acanthosis with a thickened layer of mature squamous keratinocytes. There is marked overlying hypergranulosis ⇨ and dense hyperkeratosis ⇨. (Right) Immunohistochemical stain for Mart-1/Melan-A highlights scattered normal melanocytes ⇨ in the proximal nail fold and the eponychium. Normally, only a few scattered single melanocytes should be present in this region.

SELECTED REFERENCES

EPIDERMIS (INCLUDING KERATINOCYTES AND MELANOCYTES)

1. Kanitakis J: Anatomy, histology and immunohistochemistry of normal human skin. Eur J Dermatol. 12(4):390-9; quiz 400-1, 2002
2. Smack DP et al: Keratin and keratinization. J Am Acad Dermatol. 30(1):85-102, 1994
3. Boot PM et al: The distribution of Merkel cells in human fetal and adult skin. Am J Dermatopathol. 14(5):391-6, 1992
4. Foster CA et al: Ontogeny of Langerhans cells in human embryonic and fetal skin: cell densities and phenotypic expression relative to epidermal growth. Am J Anat. 184(2):157-64, 1989
5. Gould VE et al: Neuroendocrine (Merkel) cells of the skin: hyperplasias, dysplasias, and neoplasms. Lab Invest. 52(4):334-53, 1985
6. Tarnowski WM: Ultrastructure of the epidermal melanocyte dense plate. J Invest Dermatol. 55(4):265-8, 1970

DERMIS

1. Chang E et al: Aging and survival of cutaneous microvasculature. J Invest Dermatol. 118(5):752-8, 2002
2. Pasquali-Ronchetti I et al: Elastic fiber during development and aging. Microsc Res Tech. 38(4):428-35, 1997
3. Labat-Robert J et al: Aging of the extracellular matrix and its pathology. Exp Gerontol. 23(1):5-18, 1988
4. Smith LT et al: Structure of the dermal matrix during development and in the adult. J Invest Dermatol. 79(Suppl 1):93s-104s, 1982

ADNEXAL STRUCTURES

1. Niemann C: Differentiation of the sebaceous gland. Dermatoendocrinol. 1(2):64-7, 2009
2. Poblet E et al: The contribution of the arrector pili muscle and sebaceous glands to the follicular unit structure. J Am Acad Dermatol. 51(2):217-22, 2004
3. Sanders DA et al: The isolation and maintenance of the human pilosebaceous unit. Br J Dermatol. 131(2):166-76, 1994
4. Cotton DW: Immunohistochemical staining of normal sweat glands. Br J Dermatol. 114(4):441-9, 1986
5. Fenske NA et al: Structural and functional changes of normal aging skin. J Am Acad Dermatol. 15(4 Pt 1):571-85, 1986
6. Rechardt L et al: Innervation of human axillary sweat glands. Histochemical and electron microscopic study of hyperhidrotic and normal subjects. Scand J Plast Reconstr Surg. 10(2):107-12, 1976
7. Fusaro RM et al: The normal human eccrine and apocrine glands. J Invest Dermatol. 36:79-82, 1961

NAIL

1. Baran R et al: Hair and nail relationship. Skinmed. 4(1):18-23, 2005
2. De Berker D et al: Keratin expression in the normal nail unit: markers of regional differentiation. Br J Dermatol. 142(1):89-96, 2000
3. Fuchs E: Keratins and the skin. Annu Rev Cell Dev Biol. 11:123-53, 1995
4. Johnson M et al: Nail is produced by the normal nail bed: a controversy resolved. Br J Dermatol. 125(1):27-9, 1991
5. Omura EF: Histopathology of the nail. Dermatol Clin. 3(3):531-41, 1985
6. Runne U et al: The human nail: structure, growth and pathological changes. Curr Probl Dermatol. 9:102-49, 1981
7. Lewin K: The normal finger nail. Br J Dermatol. 77(8):421-30, 1965

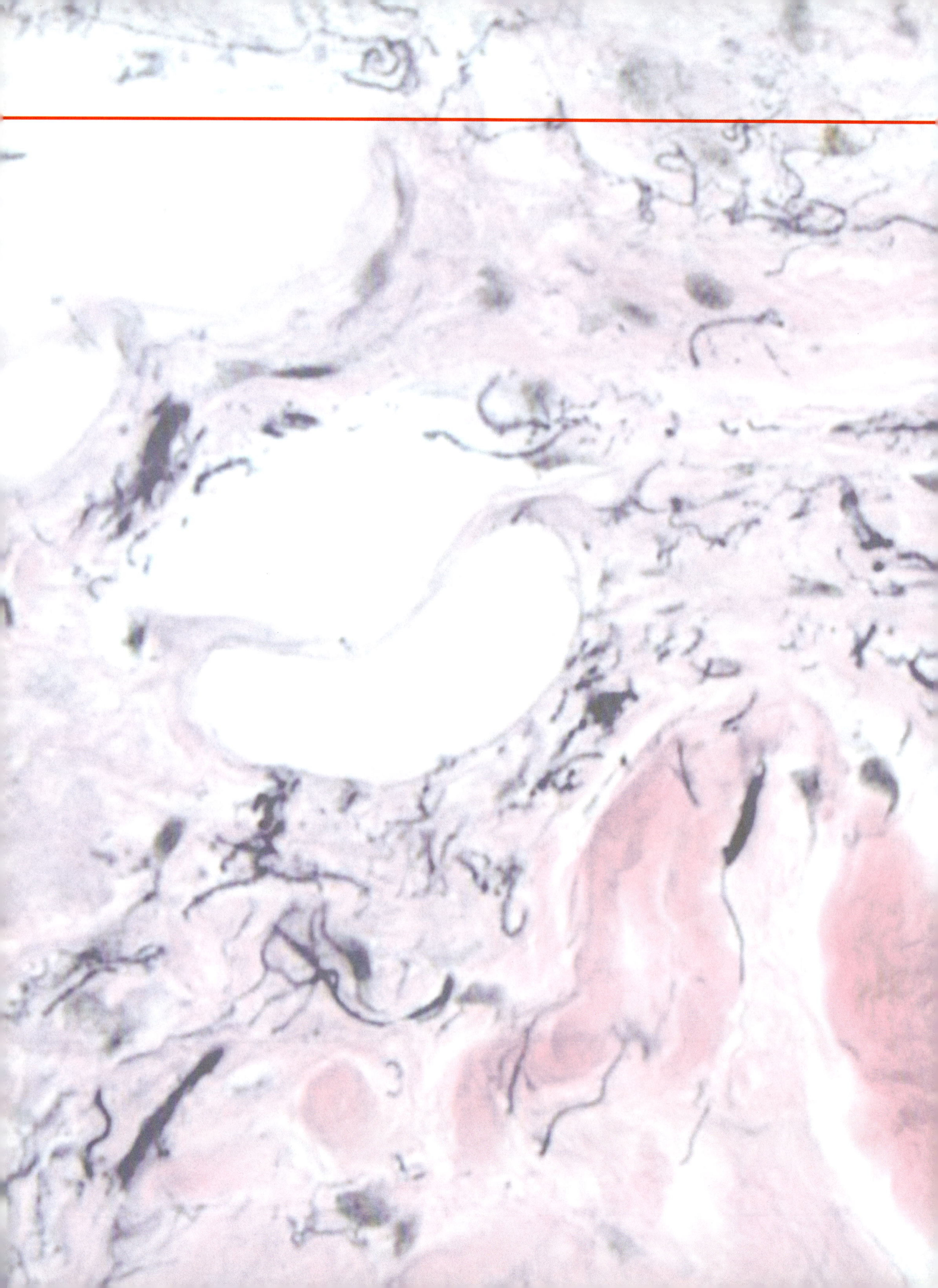

Musculoskeletal System

Bone and Cartilage   3-2

Connective Tissue   3-8

Adipose Tissue   3-10

Skeletal Muscle   3-14

BONE AND CARTILAGE

Key Facts

Macroscopic Anatomy
- Bones classified into 3 general groups: Flat, cuboid, and tubular
- Tubular bones have 3 regions: Epiphysis, metaphysis, and diaphysis
  - Epiphysis: Extends from articular surface to growth plate
  - Metaphysis: Extends from growth plate to diaphysis
  - Diaphysis (shaft): Narrowest portion of the bone
- Individual bones have unique apophyses (bumps, protuberances) for tendinous/ligamentous attachment
- Cartilage
  - Hyaline cartilage is most common and covers articular surfaces of all long bones
  - Glassy and blue to gray-white in color
  - Also found in growth plate (physis) during active growth

Microscopic Anatomy
- Periosteum: Lines outer surface of cortical bone
- Endosteum: Lines inner surfaces of cortical bone and cancellous bone
- 2 basic types of bone, which can be present in any location
  - Woven bone (immature bone): Irregular collagen fibrils, hypercellular, large osteocytes and lacunae in haphazard distribution
  - Lamellar bone (mature bone): Parallel collagen fibrils, hypocellular, small osteocytes and lacunae in organized distribution
- Cortex: Composed of cortical (compact) bone
  - 3 architectural patterns: Circumferential (outermost layer of cortex), concentric (around osteons), and interstitial (everything else)
- Haversian system (osteon): Composed of Haversian canals filled with blood vessels, nerves, and mesenchymal cells and surrounded by concentric lamellar bone
  - Canal of Volkmann: Connects Haversian canals to other Haversian canals, as well as to external cortical surface and medullary cavity
- Medullary cavity: Contains cancellous (trabecular) bone and bone marrow
  - Cancellous or spongy bone: Interconnecting trabeculae of bone within medullary cavity
  - Bone marrow: Contains a mixture of hematopoietic elements and adipose tissue
- Osteoblasts: Elongated mononuclear cells with eccentric nuclei, prominent nucleoli, and perinuclear halos; often form thin line around trabecular bone
- Osteocytes: Small, mature osteoblasts with high nuclear:cytoplasmic ratio found within lacunae
- Osteoclasts: Large, multinucleated cells, often found in Howship lacunae
- Cartilage
  - Hyaline cartilage: Abundant glassy extracellular matrix containing chondrocytes in variable cellularity
  - Tidemark: Sharp demarcation between cartilage and bone that represents site of previous growth plate
  - Other much less common cartilage types are fibrocartilage and elastic cartilage
  - Chondrocytes: Generally small cells with eosinophilic cytoplasm and dark, round nuclei; reside in lacunae

Pitfalls/Artifacts
- Irregular fragments of woven bone with prominent osteoblastic rimming can mimic osteosarcoma
- Markedly increased cellularity at growth plate (physis) can be mistaken for a chondroblastic neoplasm
- Enchondral ossification can be mistaken for a cartilaginous tumor

Age Variation
- Bony trabeculae often become thinner as a result of age- or hormone-related osteopenia (osteoporosis)
- Growth plate (physis) disappears after long bone growth ceases

(Left) This graphic demonstrates the 3 regions of a long bone: The epiphysis, metaphysis, and diaphysis. Also highlighted are the cortex ➡, medullary cavity ➡, and articular surfaces ➡. (Right) This graphic illustrates the cross sectional anatomy of a long bone. Note the peeled-back periosteal layer ➡, as well as the Haversian system (osteon) ➡ containing a central Haversian canal.

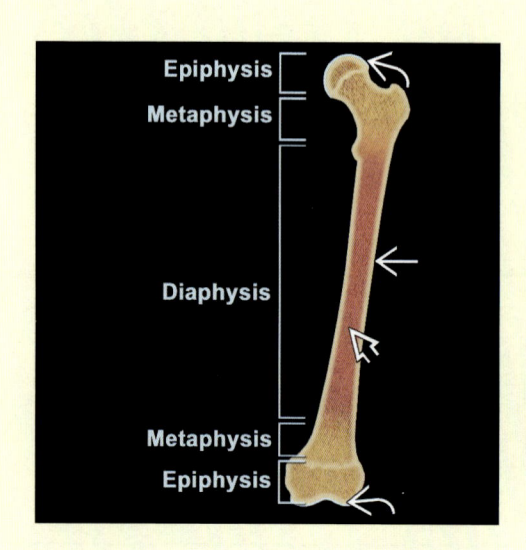

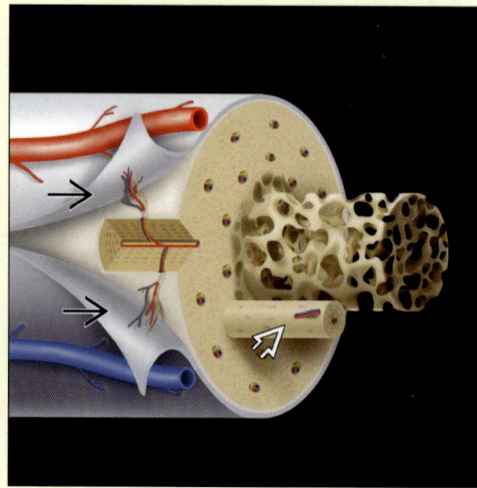

BONE AND CARTILAGE

Periosteum

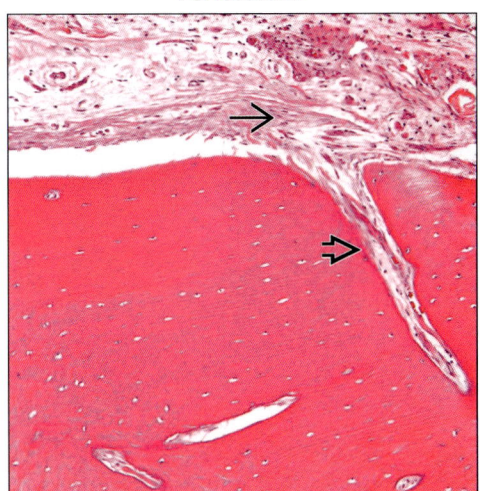

Cortical (Compact) Bone

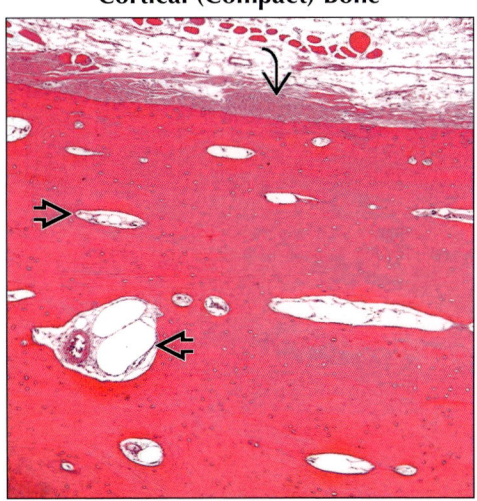

(Left) The periosteum ➔ is a thin layer of connective tissue that is present on the outer surface of cortical bone. Note the presence of a periosteal vessel ➔, which is seen penetrating the outer cortex. These small vessels are thought to provide nutrients to the outer cortical bone. *(Right)* Cortical bone is very dense and lacks bone marrow. Haversian canals ➔ are circular or tubular structures within the bone that contain nutrient vessels. Note the periosteal layer ➔.

Cortical (Compact) Bone

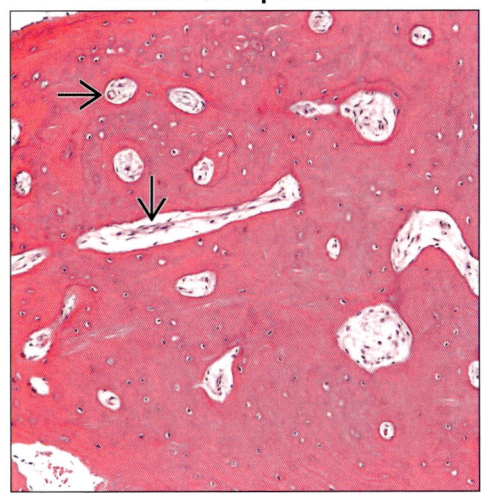

Cancellous (Trabecular) Bone

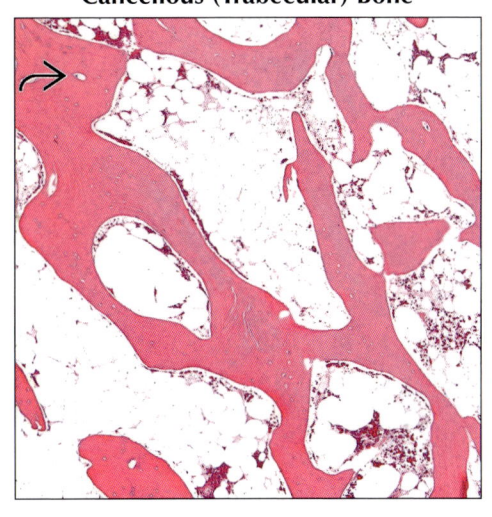

(Left) Haversian canals are easily identified as round or tubular spaces within otherwise solid-appearing cortical bone. Note the small blood vessels ➔ seen within some of the canals. *(Right)* Cancellous (or trabecular) bone is found in the medullary cavity of long bones and appears as interanastomosing trabeculae. Unlike cortical bone, there is marrow and fat present in cancellous bone. Haversian systems are also seen ➔.

Cancellous (Trabecular) Bone

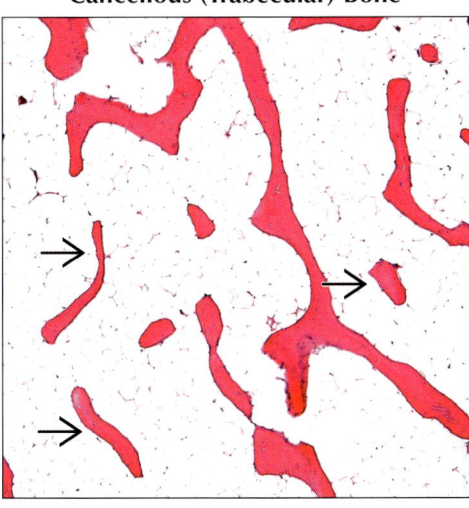

Lamellar Bone

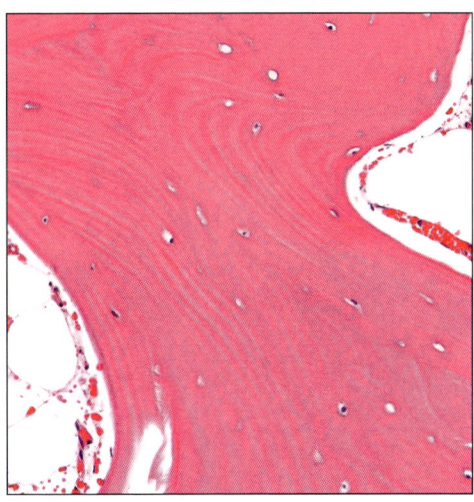

(Left) In elderly patients, particularly those with osteoporosis, it is common to see thinning of the bony trabeculae, also referred to as osteopenia. This thinning also leads to the illusion that some trabeculae are "floating" in adipose tissue ➔. *(Right)* Lamellar (or mature) bone is composed of an orderly, parallel arrangement of type I collagen fibers, giving it a "topographic" or plate-like appearance. It is seen in both cortical and medullary bone.

BONE AND CARTILAGE

Lamellar Bone

(Left) The parallel arrays of collagen fibers in lamellar bone are readily apparent on routine H&E sections. This type of lamellar architecture is also referred to as interstitial lamellar bone. **(Right)** One of the 3 architectural patterns of lamellar bone, concentric, is displayed in this image. Note the concentric arrays of collagen ➔ and localization around a Haversian canal ➔. The remaining bone architecture seen elsewhere in this image is interstitial lamellar bone.

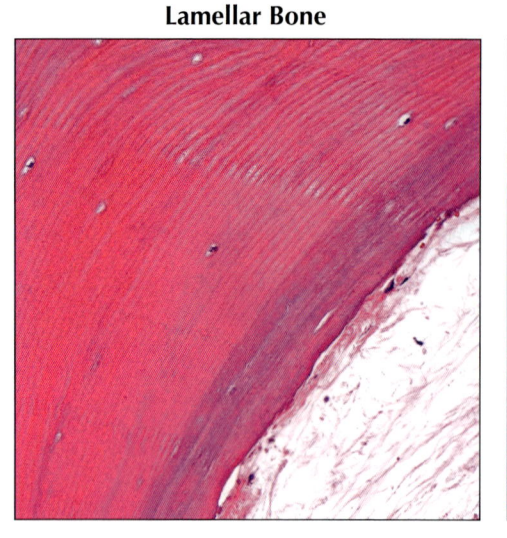

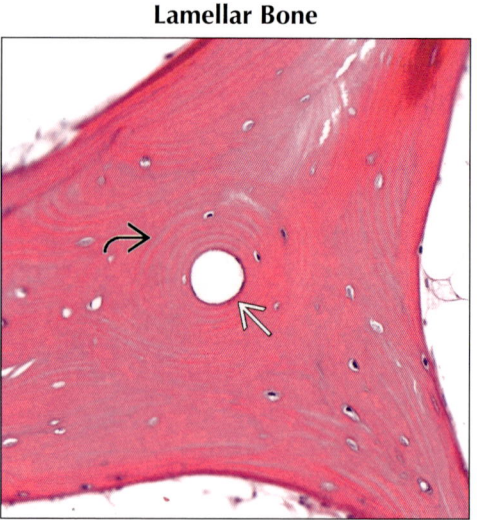

Lamellar Bone / Haversian System

(Left) Under polarized light, the parallel collagen arrays of lamellar bone are brilliantly depicted. Note the concentric lamellae around the small Haversian canal ➔. **(Right)** This image shows 2 tubular Haversian canals ➔ running lengthwise, each containing nutrient vessels. The smaller channel ➔ that runs perpendicularly and connects the 2 Haversian canals is known as a Volkmann canal.

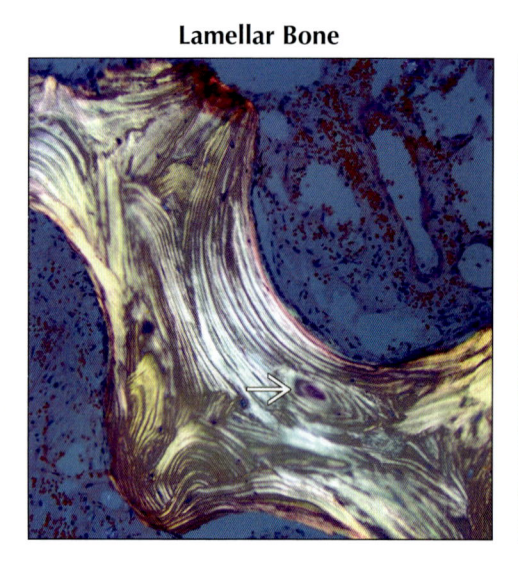

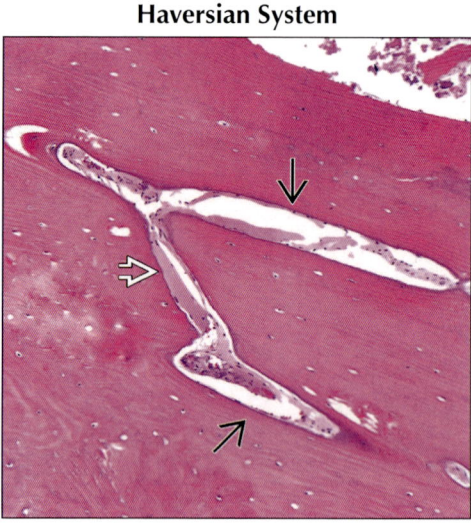

Lamellar Bone

(Left) Often, lamellar bone can take on a purple hue ➔ in routine histologic preparations. This is due to the fact that the bone is mineralized and has not been decalcified completely. This finding usually varies from focal to diffuse. **(Right)** During the process of enchondral ossification (a part of bone growth), bone is laid down on top of a cartilage framework ➔. This can lead to the appearance of cartilage trapped in bone and should not be confused with a cartilaginous tumor.

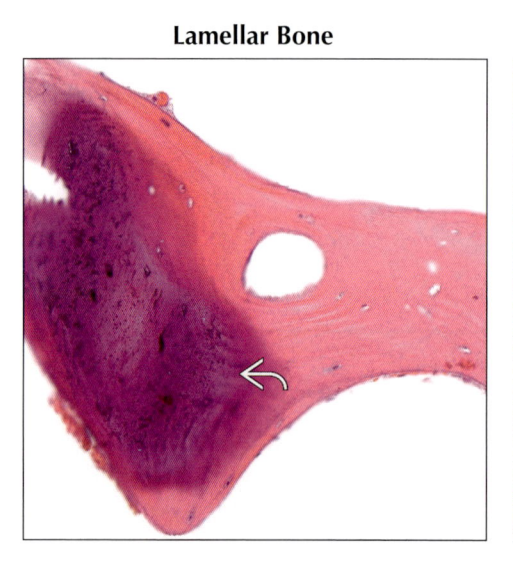

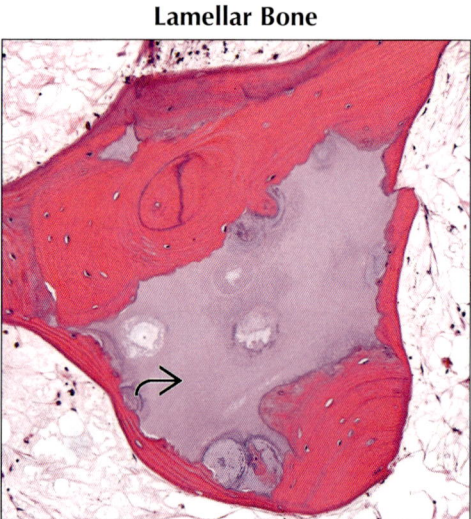

BONE AND CARTILAGE

Woven Bone

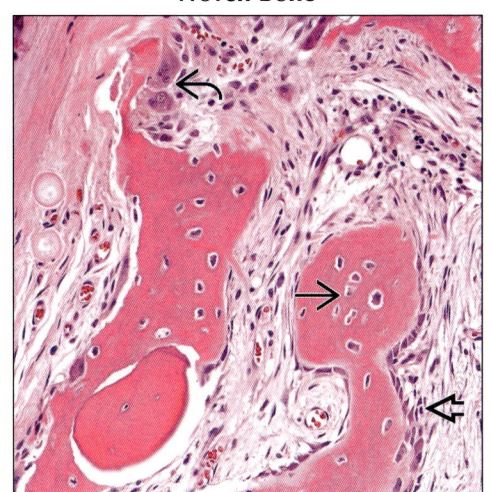

Woven Bone

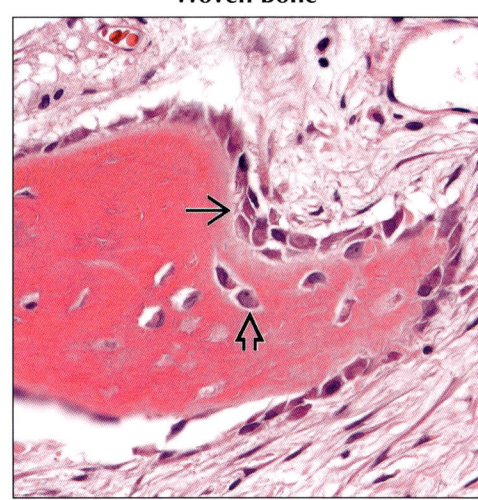

(Left) Compared to lamellar bone, woven (immature) bone is more irregularly shaped, less organized, and contains more osteocytes ⇨ per unit area. Osteoblasts ⇨ and osteoclasts ⇨ are commonly seen near or around the periphery. (Right) Woven bone often shows a prominent lining of activated osteoblasts ⇨, which are responsible for producing the bone. Osteoblasts can become trapped in the bony matrix ⇨ and mature into osteocytes.

Woven Bone

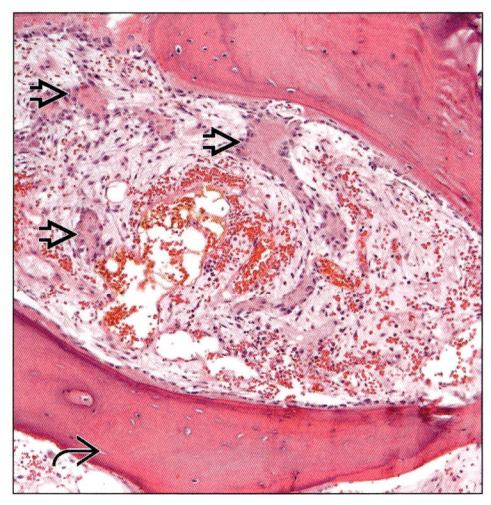

Osteoblasts

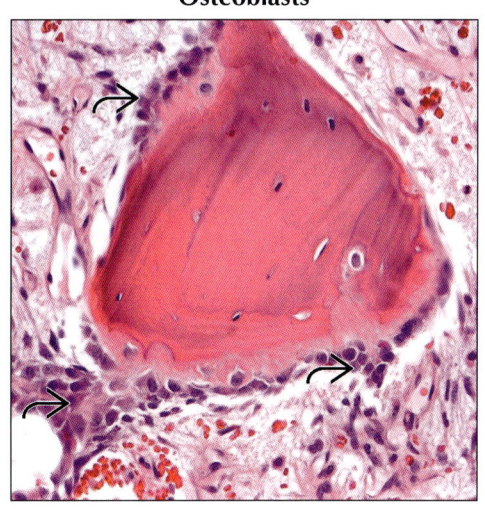

(Left) Following a fracture, it is common to see irregular tongues ⇨ of woven bone being formed between larger, mature bony trabeculae ⇨. This appearance can be alarming and may be confused with an osteosarcoma; however, the osteoblasts in normal woven bone formation are not cytologically abnormal. (Right) Osteoblasts ⇨ are small, elongated cells with pink cytoplasm and single nuclei. They are readily identified around woven bone but can also be seen around lamellar bone.

Osteoblasts

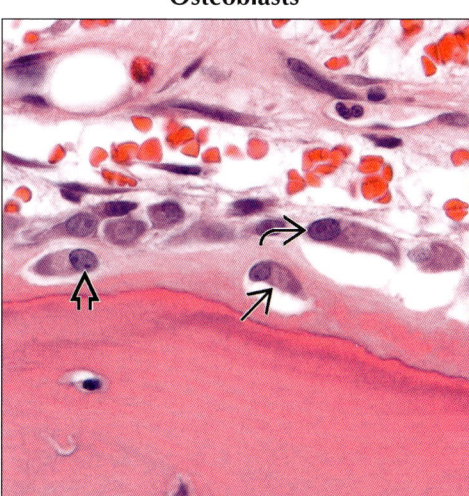

Osteoblasts

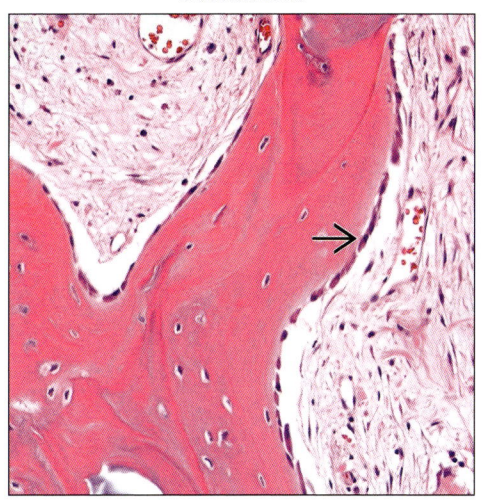

(Left) Osteoblasts characteristically contain a single nucleus that is eccentrically located at 1 pole ⇨ of the cell. Note the paler cytoplasm ⇨ near the nucleus. This region contains the Golgi apparatus. Activated osteoblasts can show 1 or 2 prominent nucleoli ⇨ within the nucleus. (Right) Although more commonly associated with woven bone, osteoblasts ⇨ can be found lining lamellar bone. However, this layer is usually more subtle and the osteoblasts are smaller.

BONE AND CARTILAGE

Osteocytes

(Left) Osteocytes are mature osteoblasts that have become enveloped by the bony matrix. Each one resides in a small cavity called a lacuna. Note that not all lacunae contain an osteocyte in any given section, which is often a function of viewing a 3D object in a 2D plane. *(Right)* Due to the small size of the osteocyte, the nucleus is often the only visible part of the cell. Nuclear detail cannot be appreciated. Note the Haversian canal.

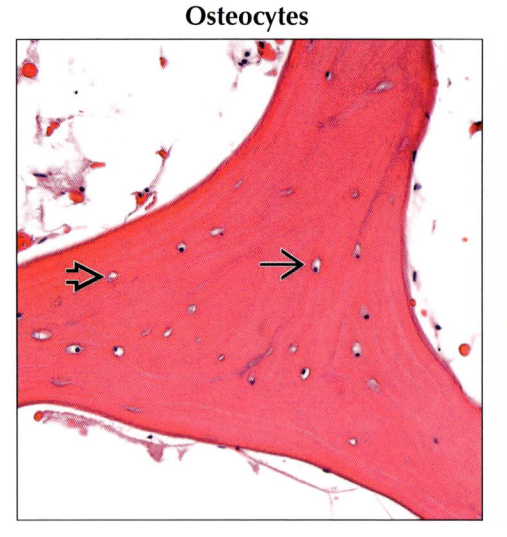

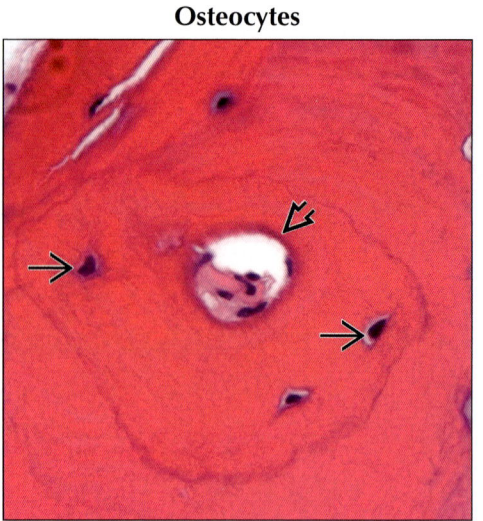

Osteoclasts

(Left) Osteoclasts are large, multinucleated cells with eosinophilic cytoplasm and variably prominent nucleoli. They are often found clustered together and are responsible for bone resorption. Note the woven (immature) bone. *(Right)* Osteoclasts can sometimes be seen "chewing" or "burrowing" through bony trabeculae. This tunneling is what ultimately leads to the formation of Haversian canals.

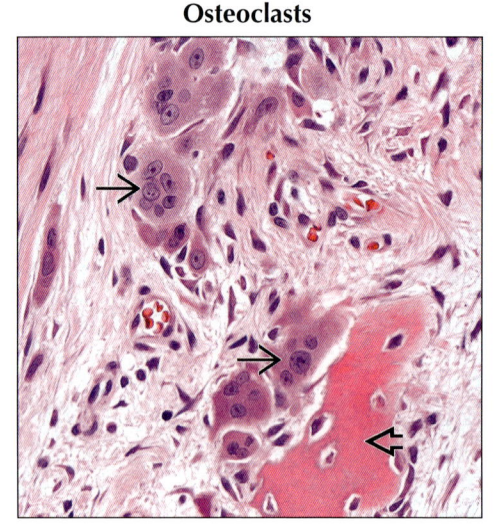

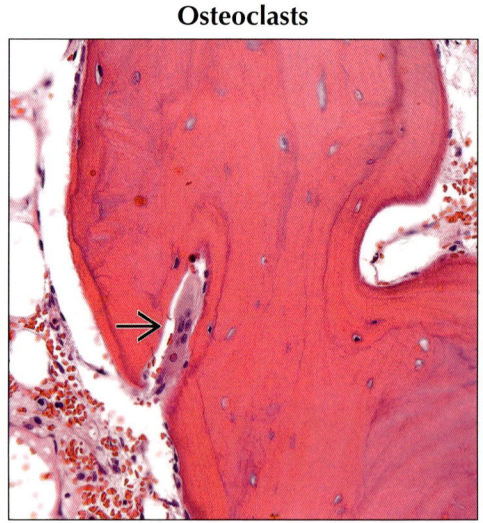

Osteoclasts / Hyaline Cartilage

(Left) During the resorption process, osteoclasts often cluster together in a concave space known as a Howship lacuna. These lacunae form as a result of bony matrix digestion. *(Right)* Hyaline cartilage is the most common type of cartilage in the human body. It is found on the articular (joint) surfaces of all long bones. It has a glassy appearance and ranges from blue to pink in color, depending on stain preparations.

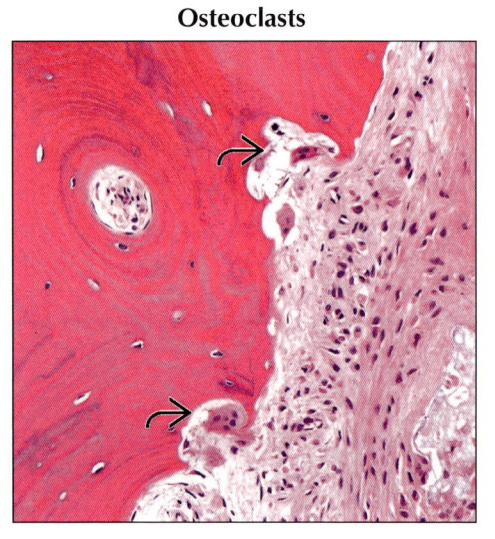

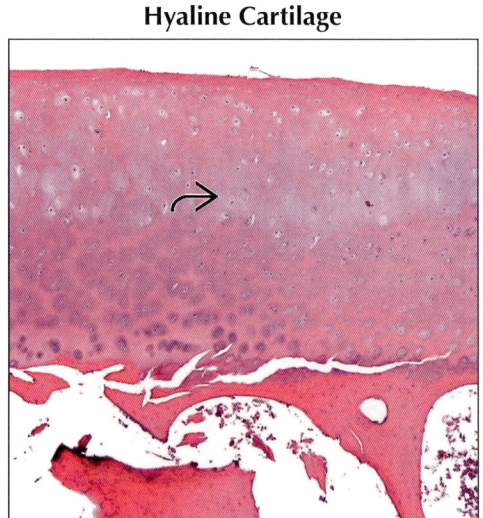

BONE AND CARTILAGE

Hyaline Cartilage

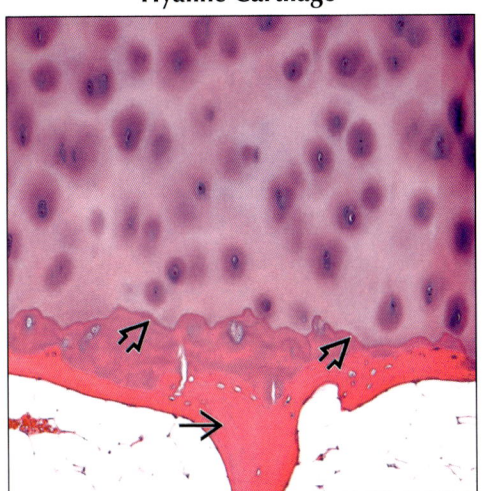

Chondrocytes

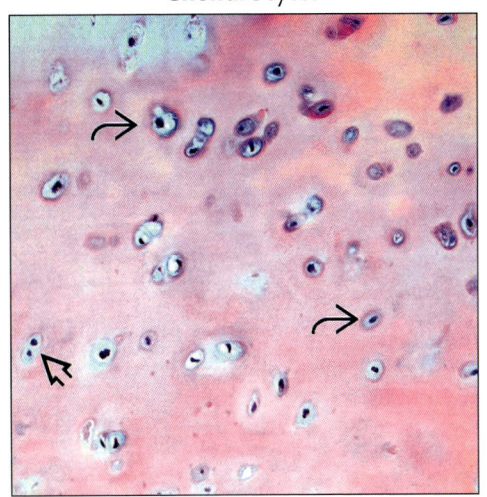

(Left) At the base of the articular cartilage is a conspicuous undulating line known as a tidemark ➢. The tidemark separates unmineralized articular cartilage from the underlying subchondral lamellar bone ➢. It is a remnant of a previously active growth plate (physis). *(Right)* Chondrocytes ➢ are often evenly distributed throughout the extracellular matrix of hyaline cartilage. It is not uncommon to see an occasional lacuna filled with more than 1 chondrocyte ➢.

Chondrocytes

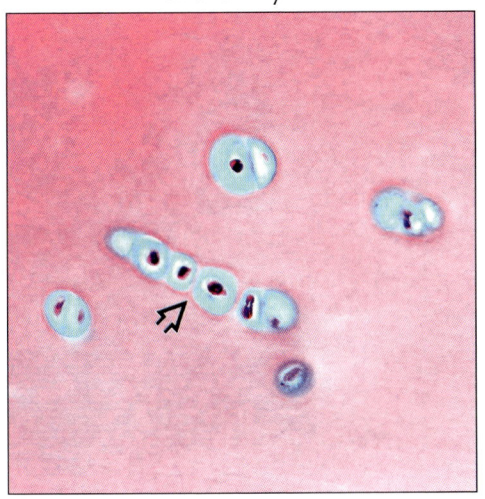

Chondrocytes

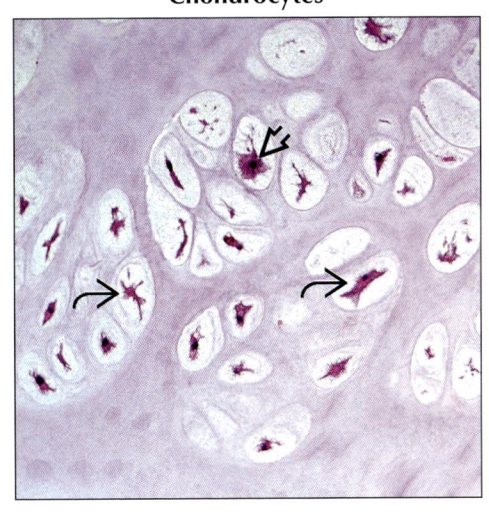

(Left) Chondrocytes are typically small and cytologically bland. In fact, they often appear much smaller than the lacunae in which they reside. They can be seen in clusters, as single cells, or in linear arrays ➢. *(Right)* This image shows clusters of chondrocytes. Sometimes chondrocytes can appear larger and more stellate ➢ than usual (a processing artifact). However, even though the cytoplasm is larger, the nuclei ➢ are still small and bland.

Chondrocytes

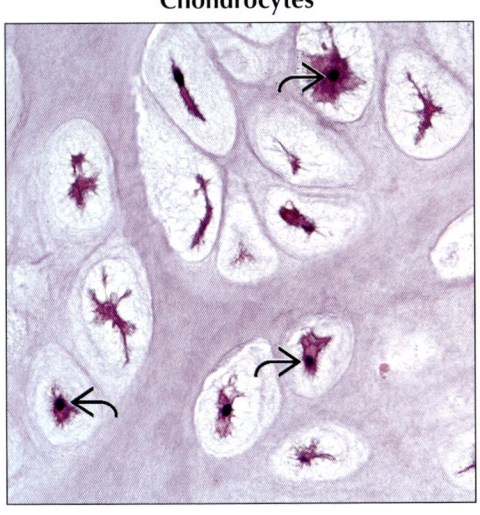

Fracture Callus

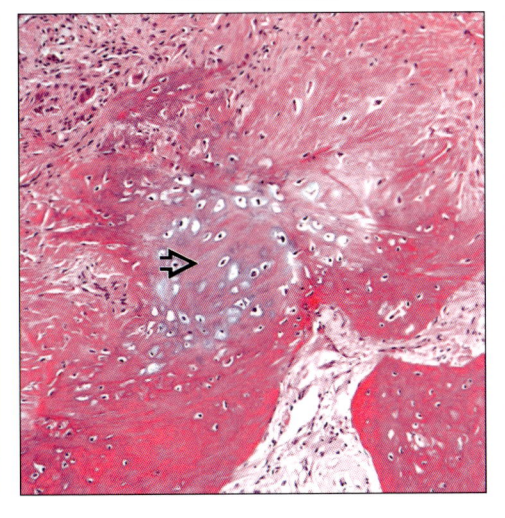

(Left) Higher magnification illustrates the consistently small size of the chondrocyte nuclei ➢, despite the large, pink, and stellate appearance of the cytoplasm. Enlarged chondrocyte nuclei are atypical, and this is a common feature of cartilaginous neoplasms. *(Right)* In addition to woven bone formation, irregular nodules of hypercellular cartilage ➢ are commonly seen within a fracture callus. The cellularity can sometimes lead to a mistaken diagnosis of chondrosarcoma.

CONNECTIVE TISSUE

Key Facts

Microscopic Anatomy
- Variable composition consisting of myofibroblasts, collagen, elastic fibers, chronic inflammatory cells, fat, vessels, and nerves
  - Myofibroblast: Spindled to stellate cell with amphophilic cytoplasm and single elongated nucleus with 1 or 2 conspicuous nucleoli
  - Collagen: Eosinophilic, acellular fibrillar bundles of varying thickness
  - Elastic fibers: Very thin, small fibers that provide tissue flexibility
- Exact composition of connective tissue depends upon site and physiologic state
- Variations in certain conditions
  - Granulation tissue: Reactive myofibroblasts with prominent capillary proliferation, fibrin, and acute and chronic inflammatory cells
  - Desmoplasia: Loose blue-gray myofibroblastic reaction to an invasive neoplasm
  - Myxoid change: Decreased cellularity with light blue tinge to the stroma
- Typical myofibroblastic immunophenotype
  - Commonly expresses smooth muscle actin in a characteristic peripheral cytoplasmic ("tram-track") pattern
  - Diffuse strong vimentin expression (nonspecific)

Pitfalls/Artifacts
- Reactive myofibroblasts often have prominent nucleoli
- Exuberant granulation tissue can mimic a neoplasm
- Myofibroblasts can show a high level of mitotic activity in reactive states

(Left) The composition of connective tissue varies depending upon the site and physiologic state of the tissue. This image shows dense connective tissue with an abundance of pink collagen ⇨ and scattered myofibroblasts, identifiable by their dark nuclei ⇨. (Right) This image shows loose connective tissue with more extracellular matrix between the collagen fibers ⇨. Note the myofibroblastic nuclei ⇨ and blood vessels ⇨.

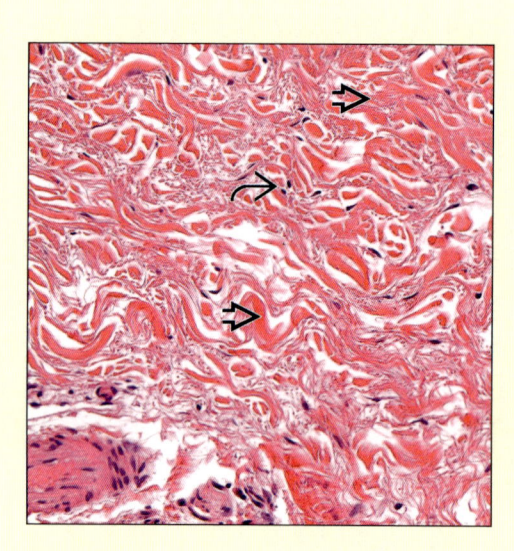

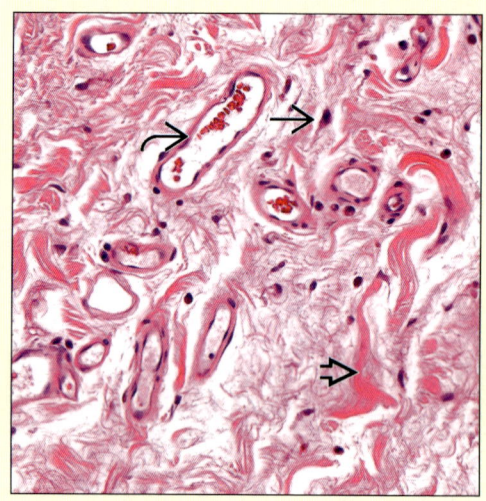

(Left) Myofibroblasts ⇨ often show amphophilic, spindled to stellate cytoplasm with prominent nuclei. In reactive conditions, it is not unusual for these cells to show very eosinophilic cytoplasm and prominent central nucleoli. (Right) Collagen is an eosinophilic acellular protein that constitutes a variable proportion of the connective tissue or stroma. Upon closer inspection, the individual fibers that make up the collagen bundles are often wavy ⇨. Note the myofibroblasts ⇨.

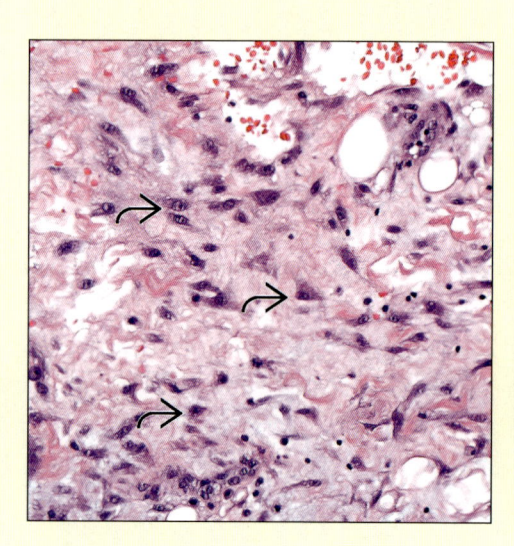

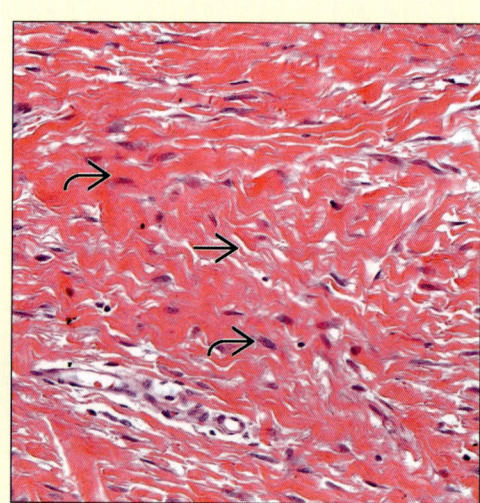

CONNECTIVE TISSUE

Elastic Fibers

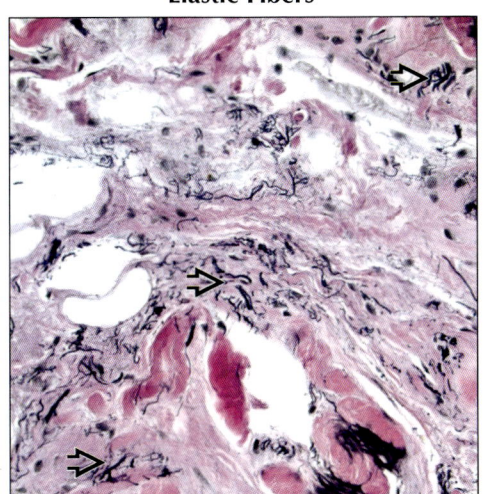

Granulation Tissue

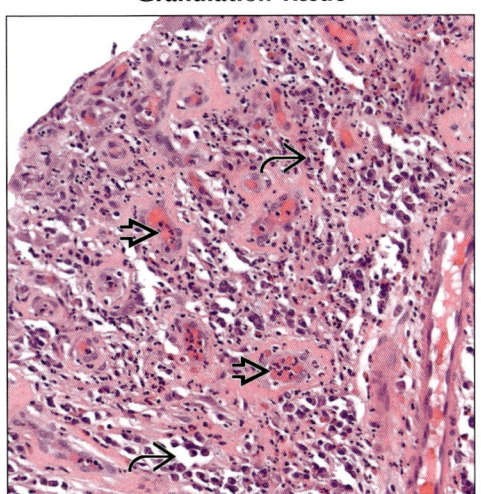

(Left) Wavy elastic fibers are often difficult to see with the naked eye, but they can be highlighted ⇒ by an elastin-specific histochemical stain (elastic fibers appear black). These fibers provide flexibility and support to the connective tissue. **(Right)** Granulation tissue is often seen in areas of ulceration. It is composed of a reactive capillary proliferation ⇒ associated with numerous acute and chronic inflammatory cells ⇒ and scattered reactive myofibroblasts.

Myxoid Stromal Change

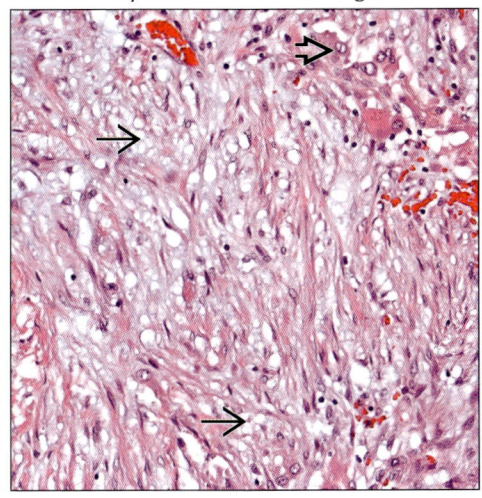

Desmoplasia

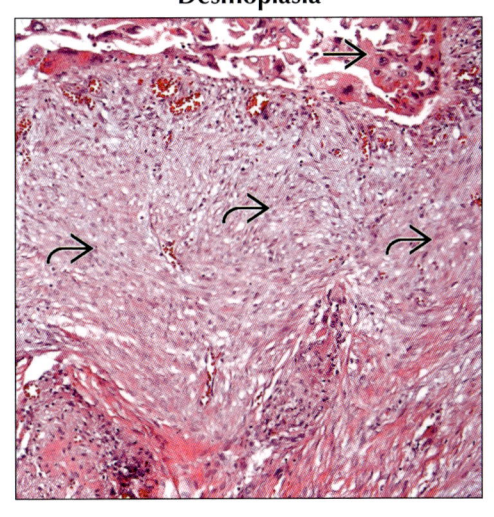

(Left) Myxoid stromal change can be seen in either reactive or neoplastic states and imparts a light blue or gray tinge to the connective tissue, sometimes with a bubbly ⇒ appearance. Note the plump reactive myofibroblasts ⇒. **(Right)** Desmoplasia ⇒ is a reactive stromal (host) myofibroblastic proliferation in response to invasive epithelial malignancy (carcinoma) ⇒. It often has a blue or pink myxoid appearance and contains a cellular population of myofibroblasts.

Reactive Myofibroblasts

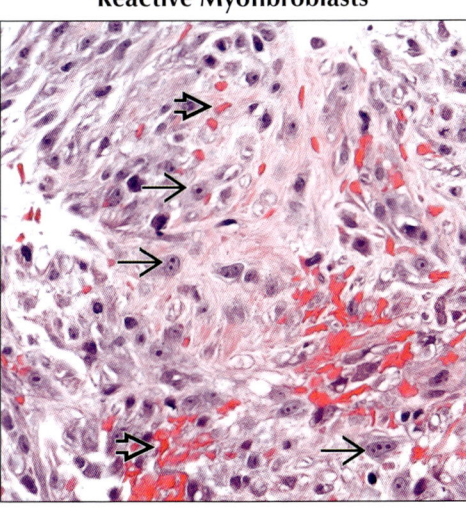

Myofibroblastic Immunophenotype

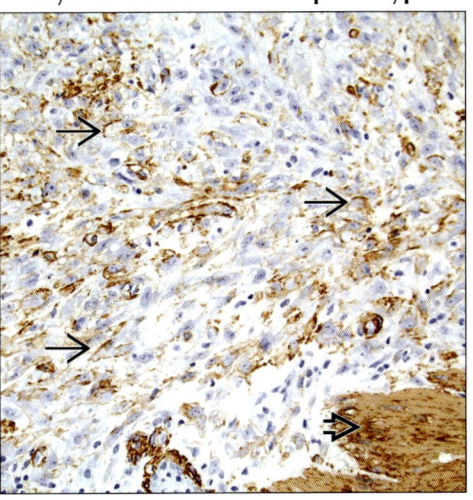

(Left) Myofibroblasts often demonstrate 1 or a few central nucleoli ⇒, which may be prominent in exuberant reactive states. This appearance can look atypical and may result in misidentification as a neoplastic process. Note the extravasated blood cells ⇒, a common finding in reactive states. **(Right)** Myofibroblasts are characteristically positive for smooth muscle actin in a fine peripheral cytoplasmic distribution ⇒. Compare to diffuse staining in true smooth muscle ⇒.

ADIPOSE TISSUE

Key Facts

Macroscopic Anatomy
- White fat
  - Yellow soft tissue
  - Lobulated by fine fibrous septa
  - Widely distributed
  - In subcutis, intraabdominal sites
  - Can replace normal muscle in pathological processes
  - Component of several organs in health or disease
  - Has insulation, energy-storage, and endocrine function; produces leptin, adiponectin, resistin, and cytokines
- Brown fat
  - Pale brown lobulated tissue
  - In neck, mediastinum, paravertebral, paraaortic, and other retroperitoneal locations
  - Cells are thermogenic; uncoupling protein (UCP1) on sympathetic stimulation uncouples fatty oxidation from ATP production, producing heat
  - Subset in brown fat areas derive from MYF5-positive precursors, possibly sharing origin with muscle cells
  - MYF5-negative brown adipocytes occur in white fat

Microscopic Anatomy
- White fat
  - Lobular architecture, with fatty lobules separated by thin collagenous septa with blood vessels
  - Mature adipocyte is polygonal-spherical
  - Intranuclear vacuole can be present
  - Cytoplasm forms very thin peripheral layer
  - Fatty vacuole fills most of cell
  - Mitotic activity absent
  - Nuclei and cytoplasm are S100 protein positive
  - Blood vessels scanty
- Brown fat
  - Lobular architecture
  - Cells smaller than mature white adipocytes
  - Nucleus rounded, often centrally located
  - Variable numbers of lipid vacuoles
  - Cytoplasm between vacuoles is granular due to numerous mitochondria
  - Mitotic activity absent
  - Immunoreactive for CD31
  - More vascular than white fat and has nerves
  - Univacuolated white adipocytes can be admixed

Pitfalls/Artifacts
- Intranuclear vacuole (termed Lochkern) can mimic lipoblasts
- Atrophy
  - Seen with starvation
  - Lobular architecture is maintained and accentuated
  - White adipocytes smaller, contain less fat, can be epithelioid
- Fat necrosis
  - Variably-sized adipocytes
  - Macrophages with finely vacuolated or "foamy" cytoplasm
  - Regenerating fat can mimic lipoblasts
- Fat can accumulate in other cell types
  - Liver, heart

Age Variation
- White fat
  - Cells enlarge in first 6 months of life
  - Number of cells increases in childhood
  - Number and size of cell increases during puberty
- Brown fat
  - Maximal in childhood
  - Gradual shrinkage and loss with age, with replacement by white fat
  - Persists mostly in neck, mediastinum, and around aorta

Metaplasia
- Fat can replace a variety of normal tissues with advancing age and pathologic conditions
  - Thymus, parathyroid, pancreas
  - Bone marrow, lymph nodes
  - Skeletal muscle, heart, cardiac valve

Hyperplasia
- Size of fat cells increases (hypertrophy) in obesity
- Number of fat cells increases (hyperplasia) in obesity
  - Mitotic activity not seen
- Number of fat cells can increase in fatty infiltration of organs

(Left) Normal subcutaneous adipose tissue is lobulated by slender fibrous septa ➔. There is a finely nodular pattern, and the fat ➔ is largely homogeneous in appearance and color. (Right) Lipocytes vary in size and appear empty because lipid is removed during processing. Nuclei ➔ are inconspicuous; peripheral cell membranes are sharply defined. Some cells have a thin layer of cytoplasm.

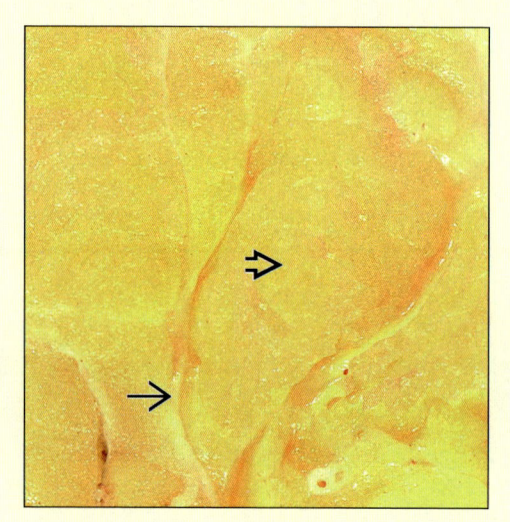

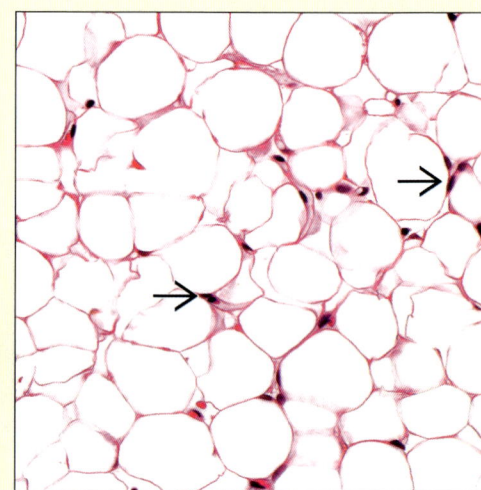

ADIPOSE TISSUE

Fetal Fat

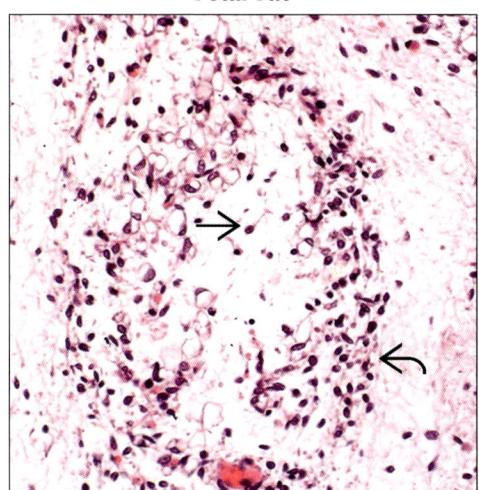

Fetal Fat

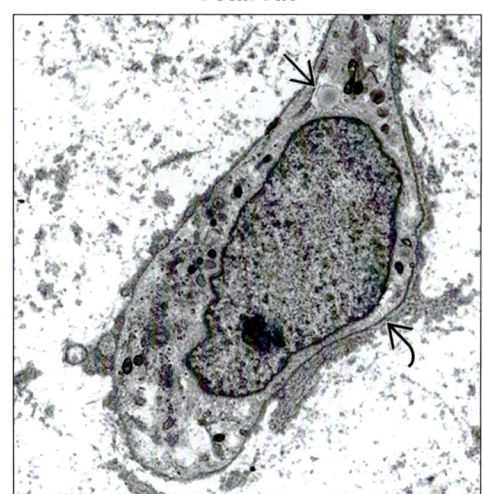

(Left) Primordial fat lobules consist of myxoid stroma and pericyte-derived, S100-positive spindle cells ➡. These adipocyte precursors (preadipocytes) condense around lobules of proliferating capillaries ➡ by the 14th gestational week. (Right) Preadipocytes are spindle cells with incomplete basement membranes ➡. As the cell matures, small paranuclear lipid droplets ➡ appear, enlarge, and coalesce as a vacuole. CHOP gene controls differentiation of fibroblasts into adipocytes.

Fetal Fat

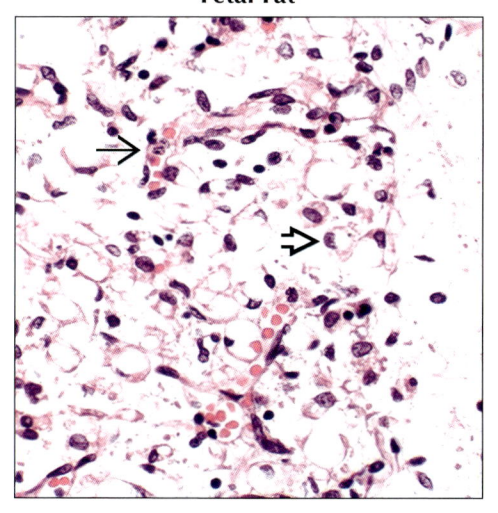

S100 Protein in White Fat

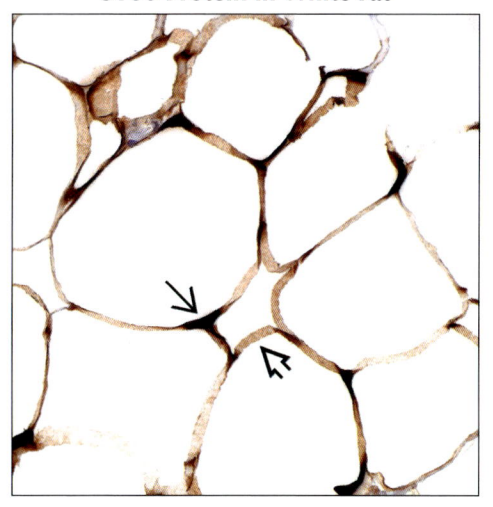

(Left) Multilocular adipocytes predominate at first and then become unilocular. Continued proliferation results in vacuolated fat cells ➡ within a rich capillary network ➡. At 24 weeks, the lobules are enclosed within fibrous septa. (Right) Immunostaining for S100 protein is strong and diffuse in adipocytic nuclei ➡ and also highlights the rim of cytoplasm ➡ in some cells. Demonstration of this antigen can sometimes be useful in the diagnosis of liposarcoma.

Normal White Adipose Tissue

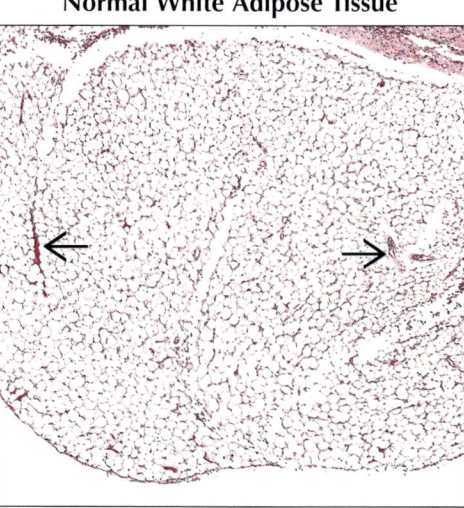

White Fat in Omentum

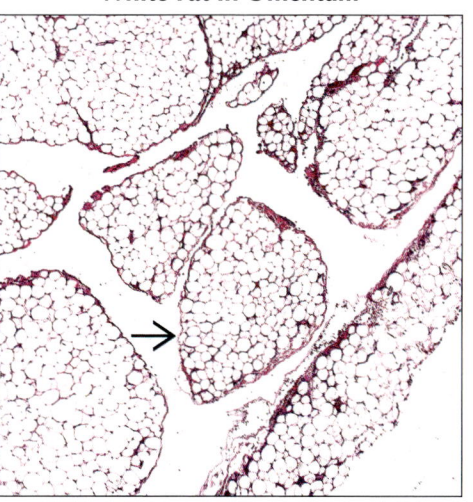

(Left) Normal white fat in the subcutis forms lobules divided by delicate fibrovascular septa. The adipocytes and nuclei are uniform. Nuclear atypia is not seen in normal fat, and if seen on low magnification suggests an atypical lipomatous tumor. Fat is relatively hypovascular but occasional small-caliber blood vessels are seen ➡. (Right) The omentum is one of the storage sites of normal white fat. It forms variably sized lobules within the mesothelial surface layer ➡.

ADIPOSE TISSUE

Lochkern

(Left) Normal adipocytes in white fat can have 1 or more intranuclear rounded, clear vacuoles ⇨, termed Lochkern. These should not be mistaken for lipoblasts, which have cytoplasmic vacuoles that push the nucleus to 1 side and indent it with a scalloped appearance.

(Right) These nuclei have multiple Lochkern ⇨ that vary in size. However, each Lochkern is contained within a rim of nuclear chromatin and the "empty" appearance of cytoplasmic lipid vacuoles is lacking.

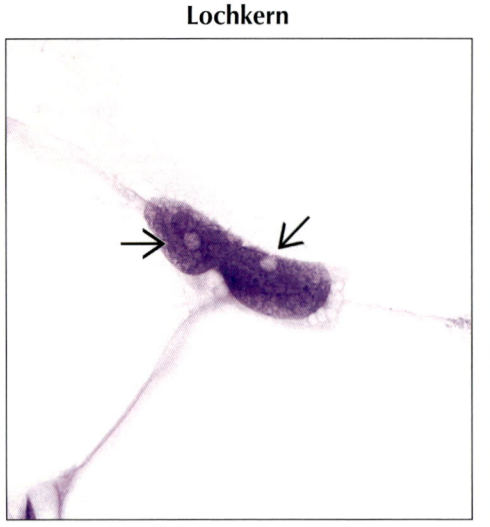

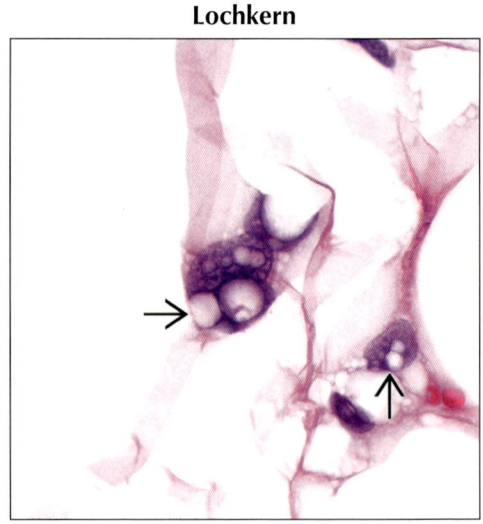

Brown Fat

(Left) In adults, brown fat exists as small islands in supraclavicular, mediastinal, and retroperitoneal sites, especially in the paraaortic, paravertebral, and periadrenal areas. The variably sized lobules ⇨ are separated by loose fibrous tissue. *(Right)* There are variable numbers of brown fat cells and white fat cells showing mild variation in diameter. The 2 types are admixed within the cellular lobules. Thin-walled blood vessels ⇨ are congested but sparse.

Brown Fat

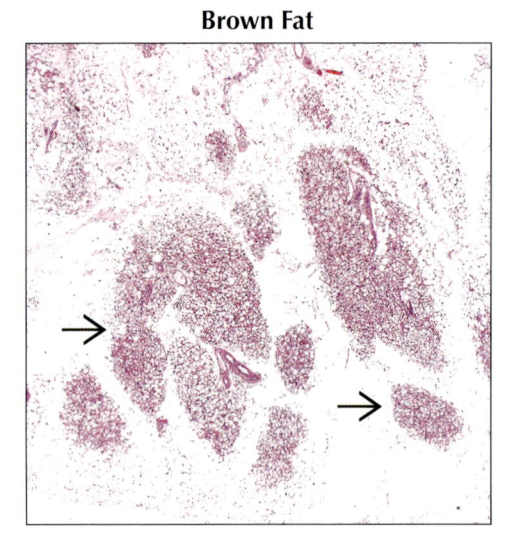

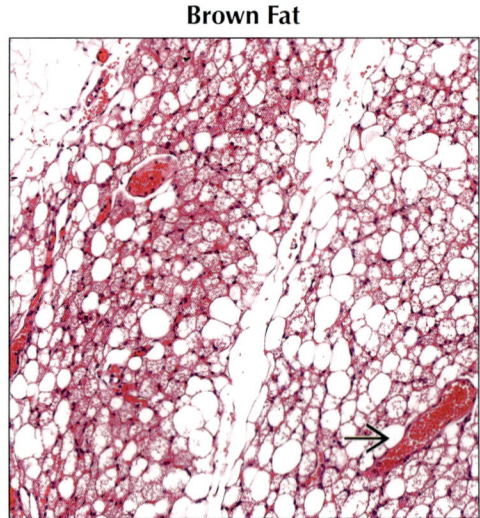

(Left) Brown fat is composed of closely packed rounded cells with numerous small intracytoplasmic vacuoles. The nucleus is rounded and located centrally or eccentrically. Nuclear atypia and mitoses are absent. An occasional white fat cell ⇨ is seen. *(Right)* An electron micrograph of the cytoplasm in a brown fat cell in a hibernoma shows numerous mitochondria displaying prominent transverse cristae ⇨ as well as electron-dense forms ⇨ and lipid droplets ⇨.

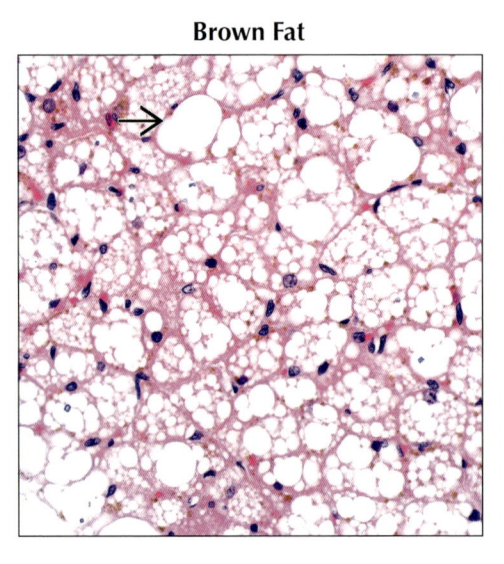

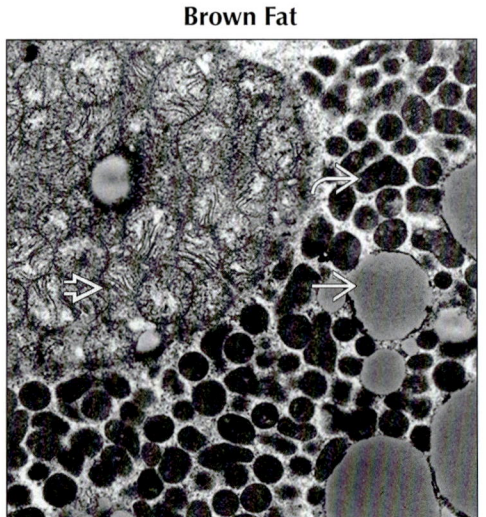

ADIPOSE TISSUE

Fatty Replacement in the Parathyroid Gland

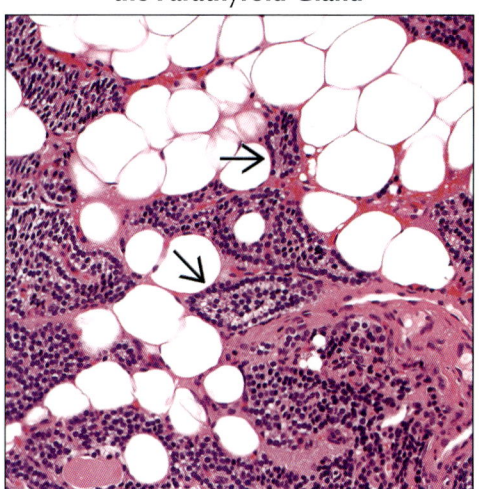

Fatty Replacement in the Thymus

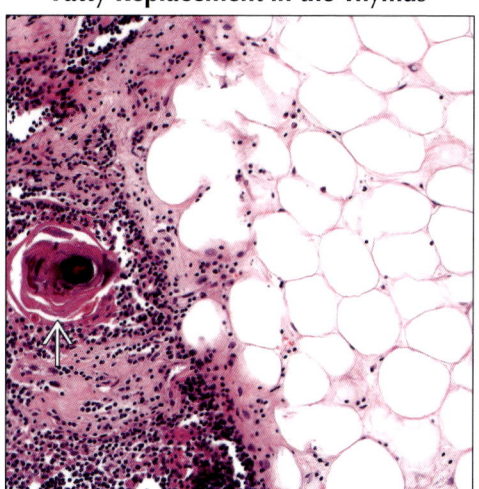

(Left) Islands of parathyroid tissue ⇒ are admixed with fat. With advancing age, parathyroid glandular tissue is gradually replaced by normal adipose tissue. Fatty replacement usually reaches a maximum between 40 and 60 years of age. The amount of fat can be different in each of the 4 parathyroid glands. *(Right)* With increasing age, the thymus undergoes involution, a process in which the gland is replaced by normal white adipose tissue. Residual thymic tissue including a Hassall corpuscle ⇒ is seen.

Atrophy of White Fat

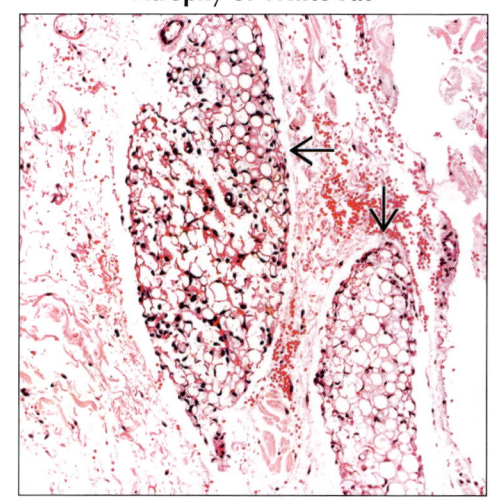

Atrophy of White Fat

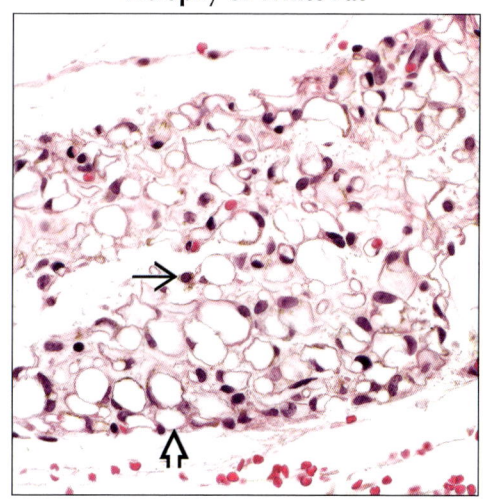

(Left) White adipose tissue can undergo atrophy in starvation and severe systemic illness. The fatty tissue shrinks so that lobules ⇒ become smaller and discrete. The intervening tissue shows myxoid change. *(Right)* Individual adipocytic cells are smaller than normal ⇒ due to reduction of intracytoplasmic lipid, resulting in more prominent appearance of nuclei ⇒. The lobular configuration is maintained and nuclear atypia is absent. Lipofuscin pigment is sometimes seen.

Fat Necrosis

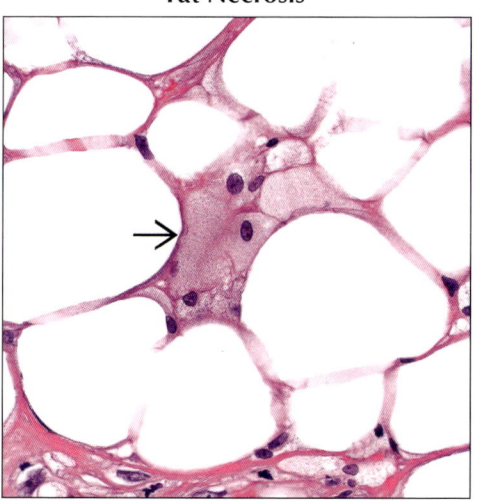

Fat Necrosis

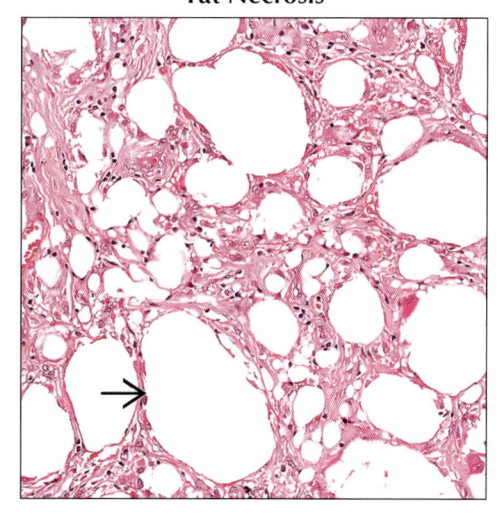

(Left) In fat necrosis, fatty spaces become enlarged when the cell membranes break down and macrophages phagocytose the escaped lipid substance, resulting in "foamy" cells with finely vacuolated cytoplasm ⇒. *(Right)* In later stages, there is inflammation, fibrosis, and focal calcification. No significant nuclear atypia is seen, which helps to exclude sclerosing and inflammatory variants of well-differentiated liposarcoma. Note the large empty spaces ⇒ due to coalescence of cells.

SKELETAL MUSCLE

Key Facts

Microscopic Anatomy
- Muscles are composed of bundles of fibers
  - Each fiber is an elongated tube with polygonal cross section 25-90 μm in diameter
  - Fibers are larger in males and in proximal muscles
  - 406 nuclei per cell; peripheral beneath sarcolemma
  - Fiber types can be distinguished by histochemistry
  - Type 1 is faster (aerobic), type 2 is slower (anaerobic)
- Cytoplasm has cross striations on light microscopy
  - Striations due to alignment of actin (thin) and myosin (thick) filaments and related structures
  - Highlighted by immunostaining for desmin
  - A band: Dark thick and thin filaments; has lighter H zone and central M line linked to myosin
  - I band: Light thin filaments; has Z bands (discs) delineating sarcomere
- Endomysium: Thin fibrous layer around single fibers
- Perimysium: Encloses several fibers to form fascicles
  - Contains nerves and blood vessels
- Epimysium: Encloses entire muscle

- In contraction, calcium binds to troponin, exposing actin site that interacts with myosin head
  - Thick and thin filaments slide past each other with loss of I and H bands; A bands stay constant
- Adenosine triphosphate releases myosin from actin, relaxing muscle

Pitfalls/Artifacts
- Regenerating muscle
  - Small and variably sized fibers
  - Multiple or hyperchromatic nuclei
- Vacuolar change due to poor fixation

Age Variation
- Loss of muscle volume with age (partly neurogenic)

Metaplasia
- Adipose tissue can replace muscle fibers
  - In atrophy or focal myositis
  - Around infiltrating angiomas or other tumors

Hyperplasia
- Muscle fibers can enlarge in width after exercise

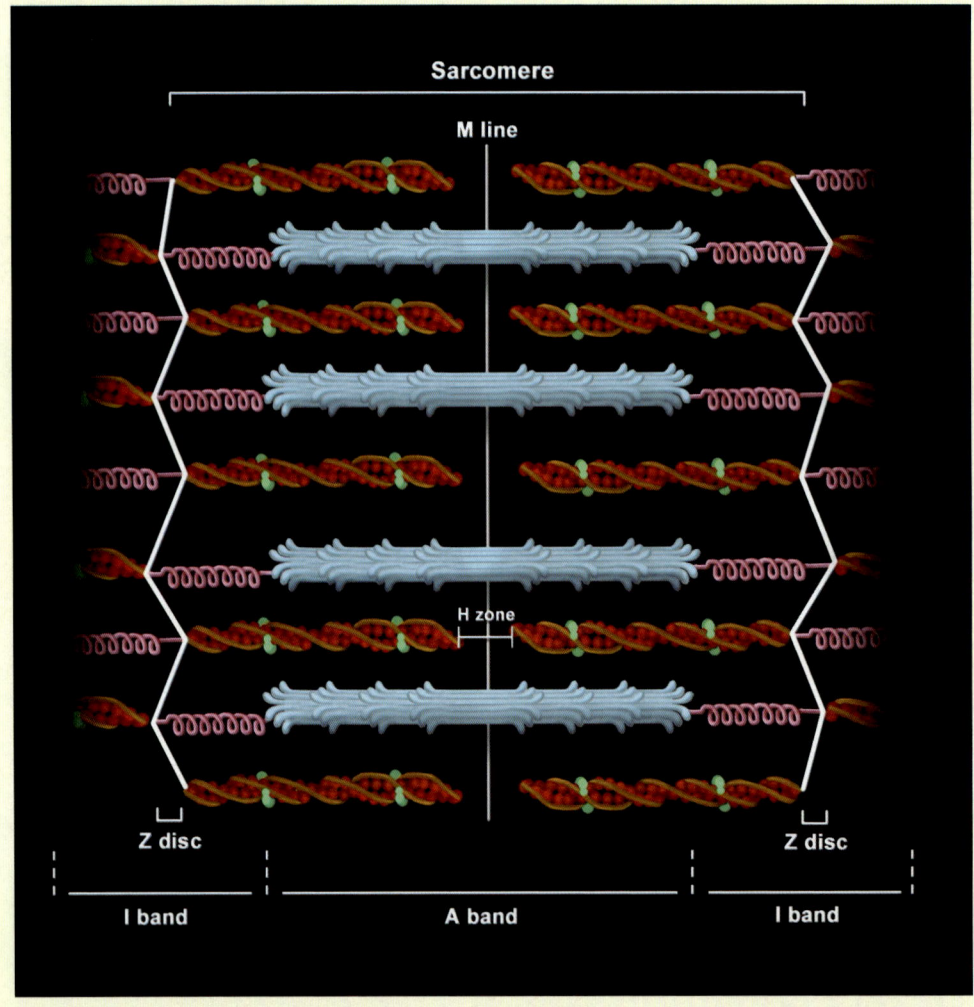

This graphic depicts the A band. The red protein denotes the thin actin contractile proteins. The blue protein demonstrates the arrangement and morphology of the thick myosin contractile proteins. In light microscopy or electron microscopy, I bands are lighter and A bands are darker because more protein is arranged in the A band. The lightest area in the A band is the H zone. The center of each H zone is a dark M line. Z discs bisect the I bands. The basic contractile unit of the skeletal muscle fibers is the sarcomere, and a sarcomere is defined as the length between adjacent Z discs.

SKELETAL MUSCLE

Embryonic Skeletal Muscle

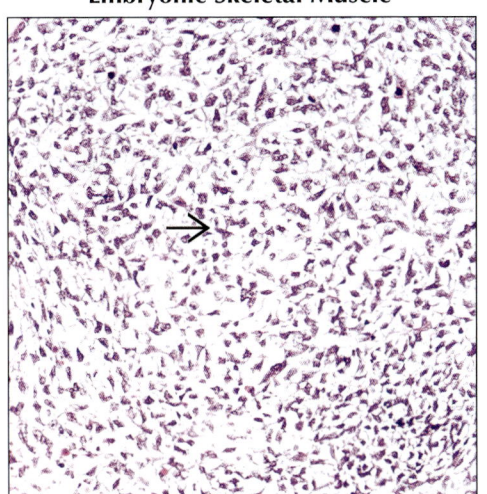

Fetal Skeletal Muscle

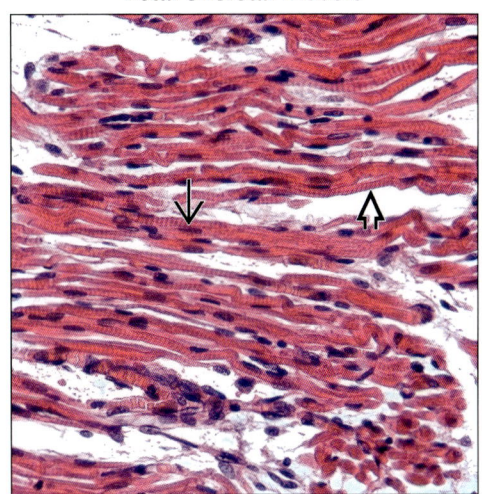

(Left) During embryogenesis, skeletal muscle develops within the paraxial mesoderm of somites as a proliferation of primitive spindle and stellate mesenchymal cells ➔ within myxoid stroma. Myogenesis is controlled in stages by myogenic regulatory factors including MYOD1, myogenin, and PAX7. (Right) Myoblasts proliferate and then form into multinucleated myotubes with central ➔ and later peripheral nuclei. Myofilaments appear in the 9th week, then develop cross-striations ➔.

Transverse Section

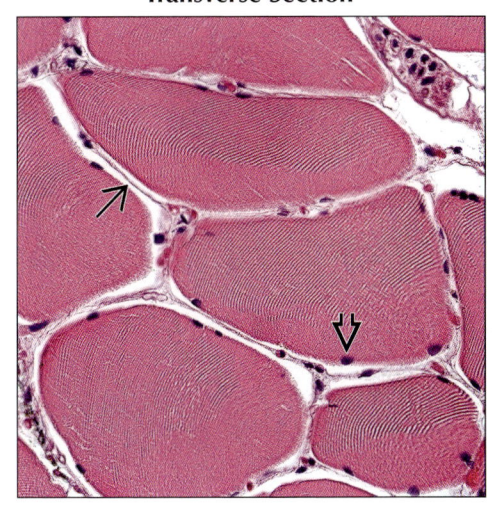

Transverse Section

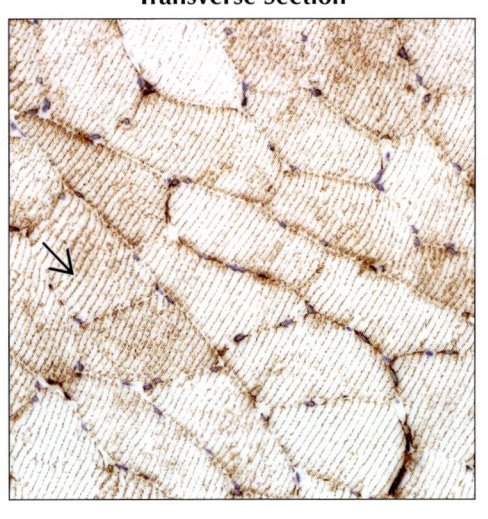

(Left) These skeletal muscle fibers are shown in cross section. Because skeletal muscle cells are cylindrical and very long, there is little variation in cross sectional fiber diameter. This image also demonstrates peripherally located nuclei ➔ of skeletal muscle and eosinophilic contractile filaments that completely fill the cytoplasm. Endomysium ➔ is located around individual skeletal muscle fibers outside the basement membrane. (Right) Immunostaining for desmin shows cross striations ➔ spaced regularly within each fiber.

Cross Striations

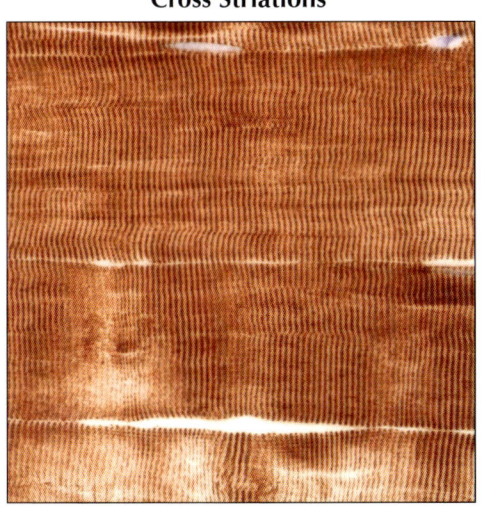

Ultrastructure

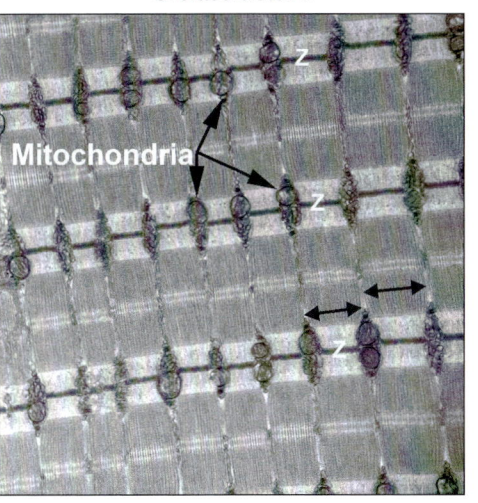

(Left) Desmin immunohistochemistry shows striations in longitudinal section. This feature is diagnostic of skeletal muscle and can also be seen on H&E stain, special stains such as phosphotungstic acid hematoxylin, and p63 immunohistochemistry. (Right) This electron micrograph shows several sarcomeres arranged in consistent bands. The sarcomere is the area between adjacent Z discs (Z). Double-pointed arrows mark the diameter of myofibrils. Mitochondria lie between myofibrils. (Courtesy P. Pytel, MD.)

SKELETAL MUSCLE

Ultrastructure of Sarcomere

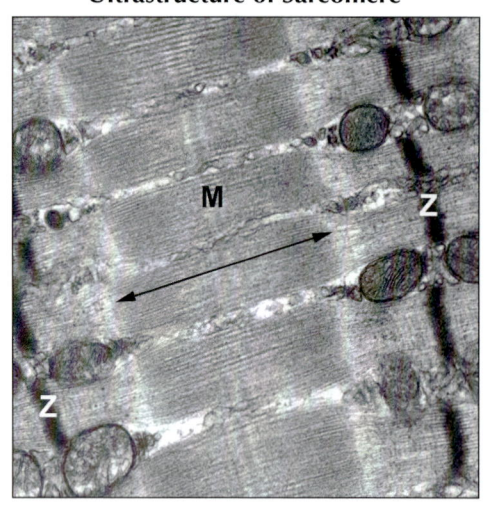

Structure of Sarcomeric A Band

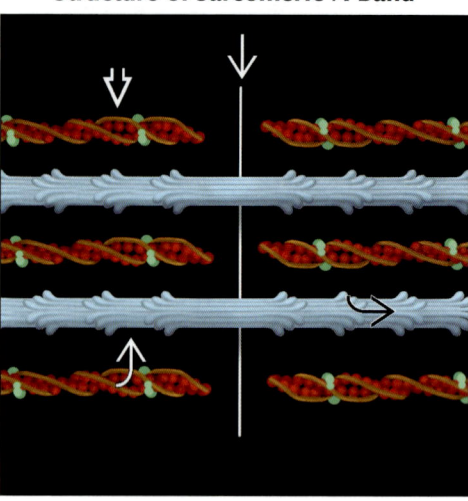

(Left) A sarcomere is bordered by 2 Z discs (Z). The M line (M) is a thin midline band that anchors myosin filaments. The double arrow marks the width of an A band. (Courtesy P. Pytel, MD.) **(Right)** This graphic shows an A band that is dark because both thin (actin) ⇒ and thick (myosin) ⇒ myofilaments with characteristic "heads" ⇒ are present. In cross section, a thick filament lies within a hexagonal array of thin filaments. The M line ⇒ is in the lighter H zone at the center of the A band.

Perimysium and Epimysium

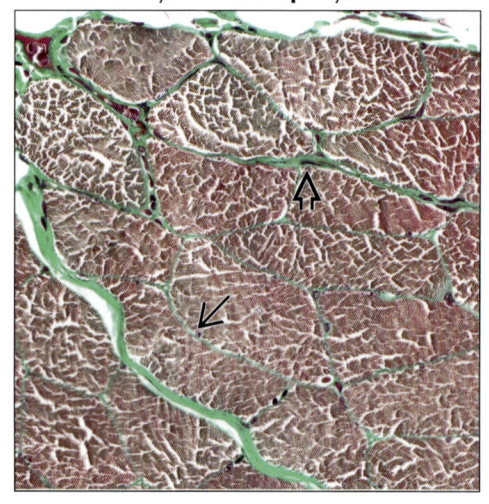

Perimysium

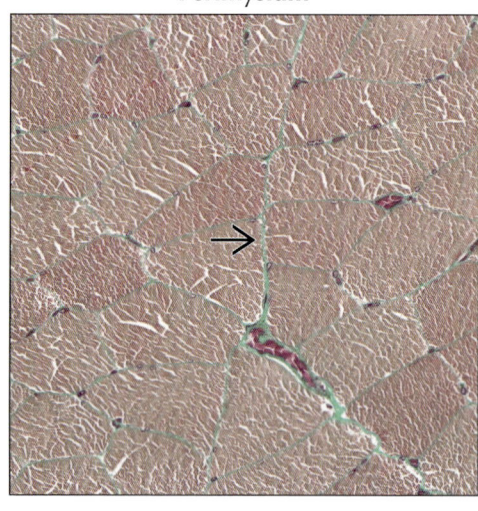

(Left) The endomysium ⇒, a thin layer of collagen-stained green in this trichrome preparation, encloses individual muscle fibers. Several fibers enclosed within a thicker layer of connective tissue, termed perimysium ⇒, form a fascicle. The fibrous layer enclosing the entire muscle is termed epimysium. **(Right)** The perimysium ⇒ encloses several muscle fibers. The connective tissue layers within the muscle contain and channel the contractile force of the muscle fibers (trichrome).

Innervation of Skeletal Muscle

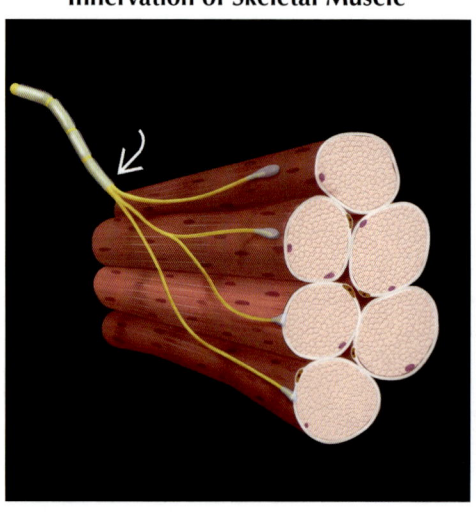

Innervation of Skeletal Muscle

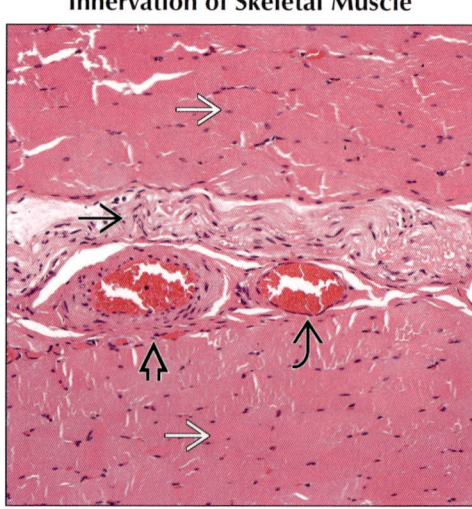

(Left) Nerves branch ⇒ to supply individual muscle fibers. A motor unit, the functional unit of muscle contraction, comprises a motor neuron and all of the skeletal muscle fibers it innervates. The size of the motor unit relates to the muscle's functional requirements. **(Right)** A nerve branch ⇒, along with an artery ⇒ and a vein ⇒, lies between muscle fascicles ⇒ in the connective tissue forming the perimysium. Mechanoreceptors are also located in this plane.

SKELETAL MUSCLE

Atrophic Fibers in Skeletal Muscle

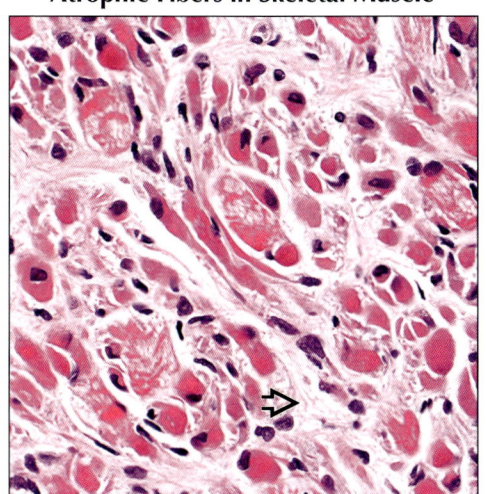

Fiber Atrophy of Skeletal Muscle

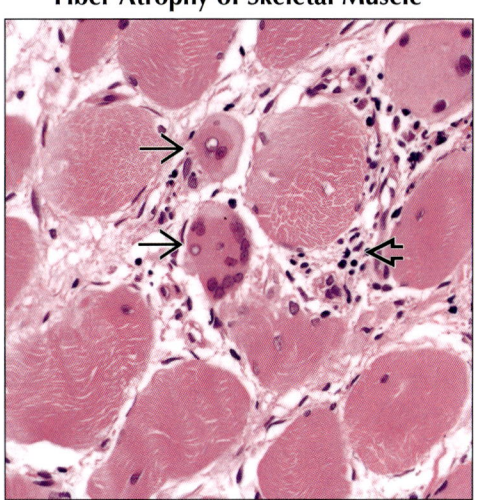

(Left) This skeletal muscle has shrunken muscle fibers with hyperchromatic nuclei (some central) and eosinophilic cytoplasm. There is interstitial fibrosis ⊳ that can result in scarring. *(Right)* This is a biopsy from a case of focal myositis. Damaged muscle fibers ➡ in the center of the image are smaller than their neighbors. Nuclei appear to be increased in number, and some are located within the cytoplasm rather than lying at the periphery of the fiber. There are adjacent inflammatory cells ⊳.

Fatty Replacement of Muscle

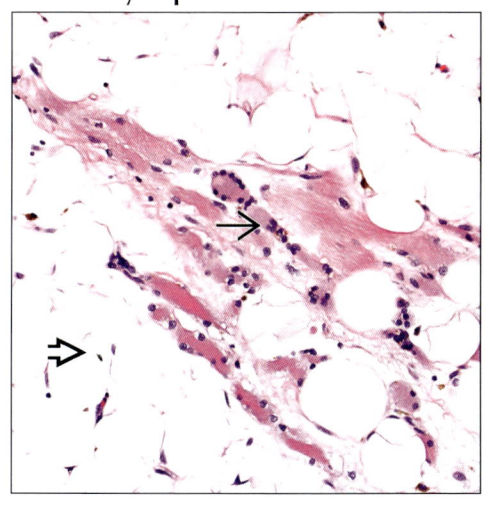

Fatty Replacement of Muscle

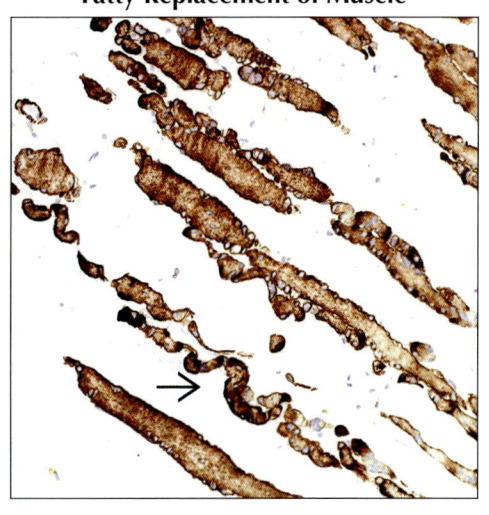

(Left) Atrophic muscle is often replaced by fat. This skeletal muscle, located in the lower limb close to a degenerative hip joint, was atrophied due to inactivity. The skeletal muscle fibers have been extensively replaced by mature fatty tissue ⊳. The residual muscle fibers are smaller than normal and exhibit condensation of nuclei ➡. *(Right)* Immunohistochemistry for desmin shows atrophic muscle fibers of variable diameter but mostly thinner than normal and sometimes wavy ⊳. The usual pattern of cross striations is indistinct.

Regenerating Muscle Fibers

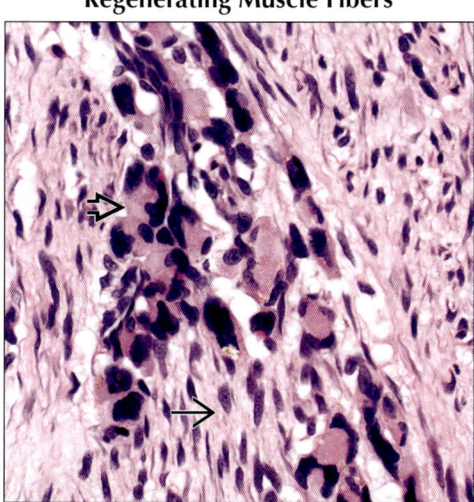

Regenerating Muscle Fibers

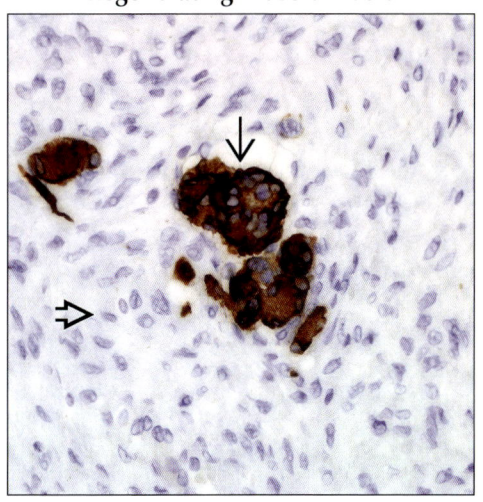

(Left) This is an example of fibromatosis, a myofibroblastic neoplasm, infiltrating skeletal muscle. The muscle fibers are not separated by the infiltrating spindle cells ➡ but show damage and regenerative changes with clumping of nuclei and cytoplasmic eosinophilia ⊳. This should not be mistaken for malignancy. *(Right)* The abnormal muscle fibers ➡ can be highlighted by immunohistochemistry for desmin, which sharply delineates them from the cells of fibromatosis ⊳, which do not stain.

SELECTED REFERENCES

BONE AND CARTILAGE

1. Adler CP: Bones and bone tissues. In Bone Diseases. New York: Springer-Verlag. 1-12, 2000
2. Adler CP: Normal anatomy and histology. In Bone Diseases. New York: Springer-Verlag. 13-30, 2000
3. McCarthy EF: Anatomy and physiology of bone. In McCarthy EF et al: Pathology of Bone and Joint Disorders. Philadelphia: W. B. Saunders. 25-50, 1998
4. Athanasou NA: Cellular biology of bone-resorbing cells. J Bone Joint Surg Am. 78(7):1096-112, 1996
5. Marks SC Jr et al: Bone cell biology: the regulation of development, structure, and function in the skeleton. Am J Anat. 183(1):1-44, 1988
6. Nijweide PJ et al: Cells of bone: proliferation, differentiation, and hormonal regulation. Physiol Rev. 66(4):855-86, 1986

CONNECTIVE TISSUE

1. Eyden B: The myofibroblast, electron microscopy and cancer research. Int J Cancer. 125(7):1743-5; author reply 1746, 2009
2. Ushiki T: Collagen fibers, reticular fibers and elastic fibers: a comprehensive understanding from a morphological viewpoint. Arch Histol Cytol. 65(2):109-26, 2002
3. Leblond CP: Synthesis and secretion of collagen by cells of connective tissue, bone, and dentin. Anat Rec. 224(2):123-38, 1989
4. Seemayer TA et al: The myofibroblast: biologic, pathologic, and theoretical considerations. Pathol Annu. 15(Pt 1):443-70, 1980

ADIPOSE TISSUE

1. Nedergaard J et al: Three years with adult human brown adipose tissue. Ann N Y Acad Sci. 1212:E20-36, 2010
2. Seale P et al: PRDM16 controls a brown fat/skeletal muscle switch. Nature. 454(7207):961-7, 2008
3. Tang W et al: White fat progenitor cells reside in the adipose vasculature. Science. 322(5901):583-6, 2008
4. Nedergaard J et al: Unexpected evidence for active brown adipose tissue in adult humans. Am J Physiol Endocrinol Metab. 293(2):E444-52, 2007
5. Cannon B et al: Brown adipose tissue: function and physiological significance. Physiol Rev. 84(1):277-359, 2004
6. Atanassova P: Immunohistochemical expression of S-100 protein in human embryonal fat cells. Cells Tissues Organs. 169(4):355-60, 2001
7. Obara T et al: Stromal fat content of the parathyroid gland. Endocrinol Jpn. 37(6):901-5, 1990
8. Dufour DR et al: The normal parathyroid revisited: percentage of stromal fat. Hum Pathol. 13(8):717-21, 1982
9. Hull D: The structure and function of brown adipose tissue. Br Med Bull. 22(1):92-6, 1966

SKELETAL MUSCLE

1. Martin SE et al: Cytoplasmic p63 immunohistochemistry is a useful marker for muscle differentiation: an immunohistochemical and immunoelectron microscopic study. Mod Pathol. 24(10):1320-6, 2011
2. Sanger JM et al: The dynamic Z bands of striated muscle cells. Sci Signal. 1(32):pe37, 2008
3. Luther PK et al: Muscle Z-band ultrastructure: titin Z-repeats and Z-band periodicities do not match. J Mol Biol. 319(5):1157-64, 2002
4. Jarosch R: Muscle force arises by actin filament rotation and torque in the Z-filaments. Biochem Biophys Res Commun. 270(3):677-82, 2000
5. Schroeter JP et al: Three-dimensional structure of the Z band in a normal mammalian skeletal muscle. J Cell Biol. 133(3):571-83, 1996

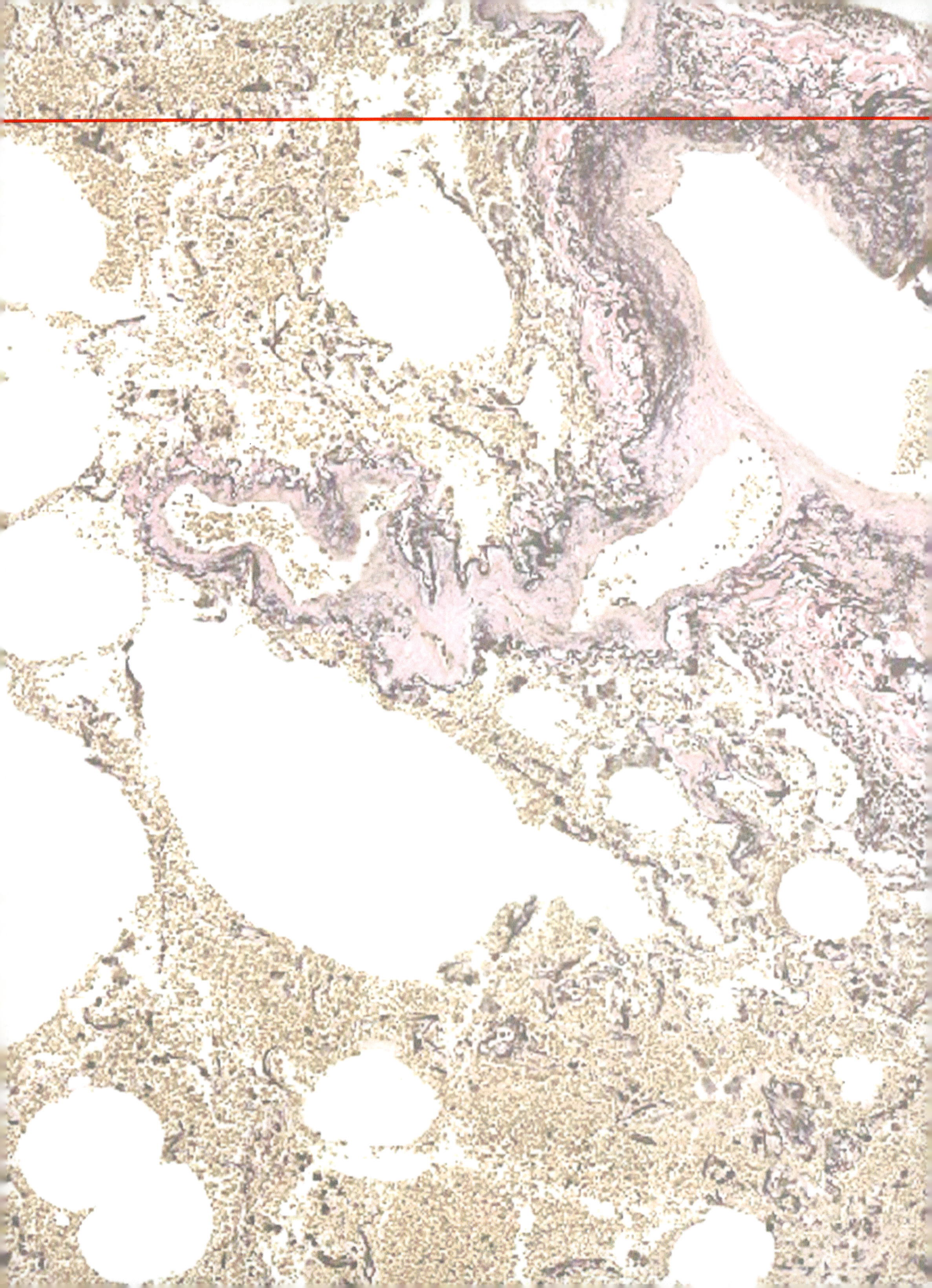

Circulatory System

Heart	4-2
Cardiac Valves	4-6
Cardiac Conduction System	4-8
Arteries	4-12
Capillaries, Veins, and Lymphatics	4-16

HEART

Key Facts

Macroscopic Anatomy
- Cardiac chamber structure reflects pressure and volume physiology
  - Right atrium (2-6 mmHg) receives systemic venous drainage and provides small atrial "kick" to help fill right ventricle; 2-3 mm wall thickness
  - Right ventricle (15-30 mmHg) pumps blood through pulmonary artery against pulmonary vascular resistance; 4-5 mm wall thickness
  - Left atrium (4-12 mmHg) receives pulmonary venous drainage and provides small atrial "kick" to help fill left ventricle; 2-3 mm wall thickness
  - Left ventricle (100-140 mmHg) pumps blood through aorta against systemic vascular resistance; 13-15 mm wall thickness
- Atrial "sidedness" landmarks
  - Right appendage larger and pyramid-shaped, left is finger-like
  - Right atrial pectinate muscles prominent, left smooth except for appendage
  - Right atrium has coronary sinus ostium, limbus of oval fossa, terminal crest, sinoatrial node, atrioventricular node
- Ventricular "sidedness" landmarks
  - Right septal wall trabecular, left septal wall smooth
  - Tricuspid cordal attachments to right septum; no septal cordal attachments on left
  - Muscle separates tricuspid from pulmonary valves on right; mitral and aortic valves in continuity on left
- Pericardium envelopes and encircles heart
  - Epicardium (visceral pericardium) is a delicate serous layer adhering to heart, whereas the pericardium proper (parietal pericardium) forms a thick fibrous-walled sac surrounding heart
  - Space between epicardium and pericardium contains ~ 30 mL of cushioning fluid

Microscopic Anatomy
- Chamber walls composed of 3 layers
  - Endocardium: Inner single endothelial cell lining with basement membrane and thin layer of fibroelastic connective tissue
  - Myocardium: Middle layer of stratified and interconnected myocytes with associated vessels and stromal cells
  - Epicardium: Outer layer of adipose tissue through which epicardial nerves, arteries, veins, and lymphatics course; bounded by serous epicardial lining
- Interventricular septum contains only myocardium, whereas interatrial septum may contain epicardium separating 2 myocardial layers

Pitfalls/Artifacts
- Contraction bands (in endomyocardial biopsy): These result from compression, stretching, and tearing of myocytes by the bioptome
- Perivascular collagen: Normal amount of dense collagenous tissue surrounds intramyocardial vessels; this is not interstitial fibrosis
- Papillary muscle tip: Dense collagen normally; not fibrosis
- Atrioventricular valve annulus: Dense collagen normally; not fibrosis

Age Variation
- Brown atrophy: Lipofuscin pigment is present in normal heart and increases with age
- Proportion of sarcoplasm to nuclei in infant myocardium is much lower than in adults

Hyperplasia
- Hypertrophy: Increased myocardial mass results from hypertrophy, not hyperplasia
  - Nuclear features: Binucleation, enlargement, hyperchromasia, less ovoid and more rectangular contours (even angulated and bizarre when severe)
  - Myocyte size: Less reliable due to tangential sectioning, variable tissue shrinkage during fixation, and distortion during microtomy

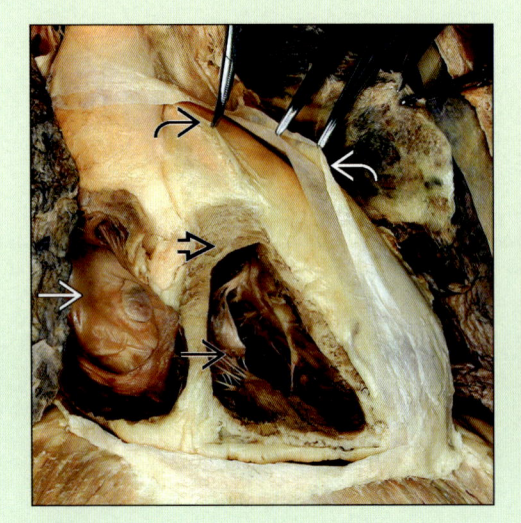

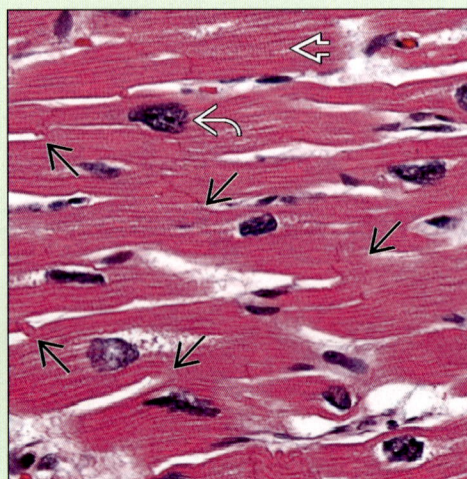

(Left) This view of a cadaver heart illustrates the right atrium ➡, right ventricle ➡, epicardium (visceral pericardium) ➡, parietal pericardium ➡, and myocardium ➡ of the "infundibulum." *(Right)* Cardiomyocytes contain sarcoplasmic cross-striations ➡, centrally placed nuclei ➡, and interconnections between cells ➡ that facilitate cellular electrical "coupling."

HEART

Sarcomere Ultrastructure

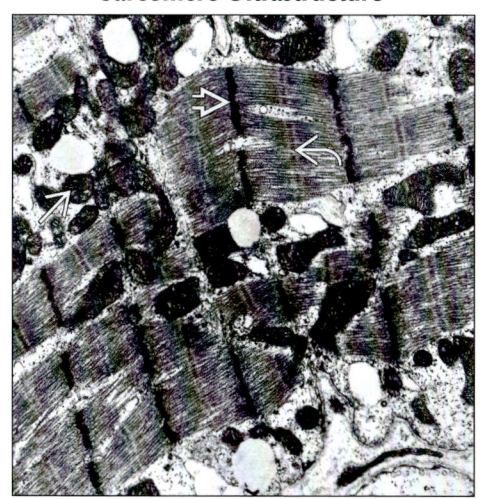

Cardiomyocytes: Cross-Striations

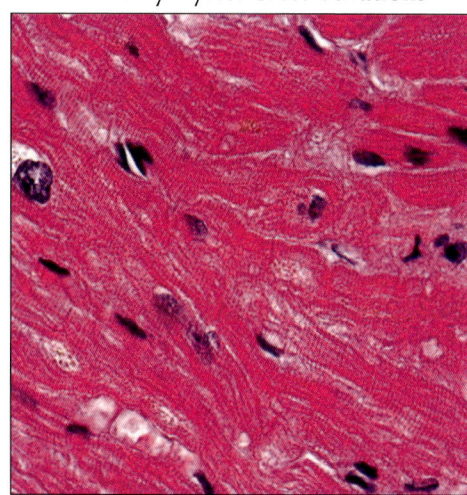

(Left) This EM view (x14,000) shows individual myofilaments within a cardiomyocyte. The Z bands ⇨ anchor the thin actin filaments. M lines ➡ connect thick myosin filaments and represent the center of the A band (between 2 Z lines). Mitochondria ➡ are abundant. *(Right)* Parallel stripes running perpendicular to the long axis of the myocytes are referred to as cross-striations. These result from alignment of hundreds of myofilament Z bands across the width of the cell.

Cardiomyocytes: Intercalated Discs

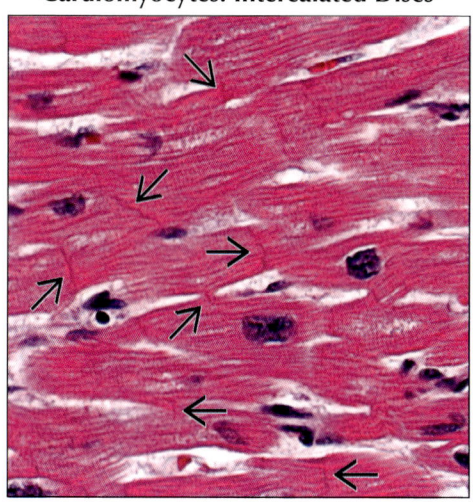

Lipofuscin (Brown Atrophy)

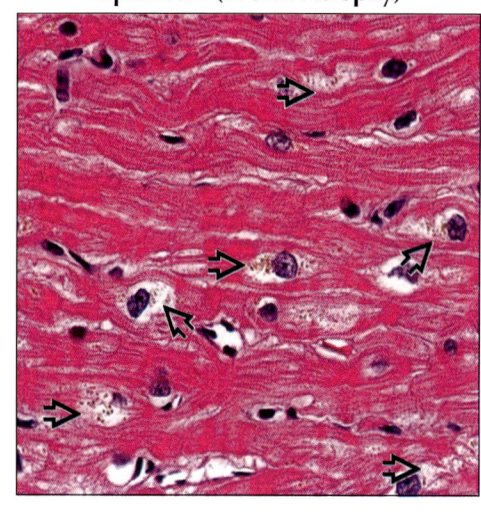

(Left) At the junctions between interconnecting cells, desmosome-rich intercalated discs are seen as dense, irregular eosinophilic lines ➡. *(Right)* Brown atrophy is an age-related phenomenon and consists of the accumulation of granular gold-brown lipofuscin (or lipochrome) pigment around cardiomyocyte nuclei ⇨.

Endocardium

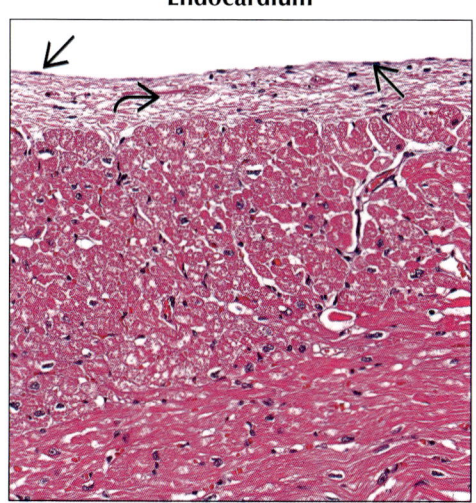

Endocardial Thickening

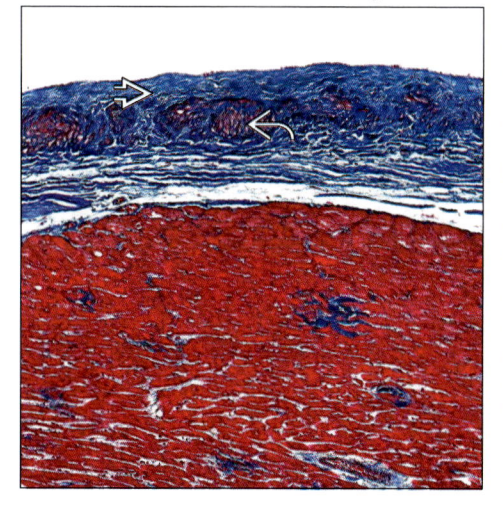

(Left) Ventricular endocardium is comprised of a single layer of endothelial cells ➡ (with flattened inconspicuous nuclei) and varying amounts of subendothelial connective tissue ➡ on the ventricular luminal surface. *(Right)* Thickened endocardium is seen normally in the left atrium and subvalvular portions of the ventricles. There is increased collagen fibrosis ⇨ and elastic tissue. Endocardium also contains a thin smooth muscle layer throughout much of the heart ➡.

HEART

Infant Myocardium

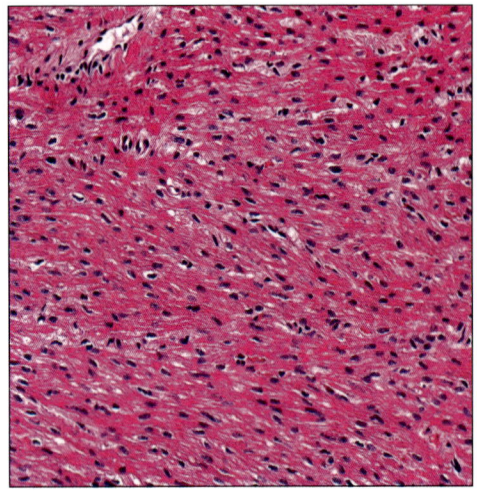

Early Myocyte Hypertrophy

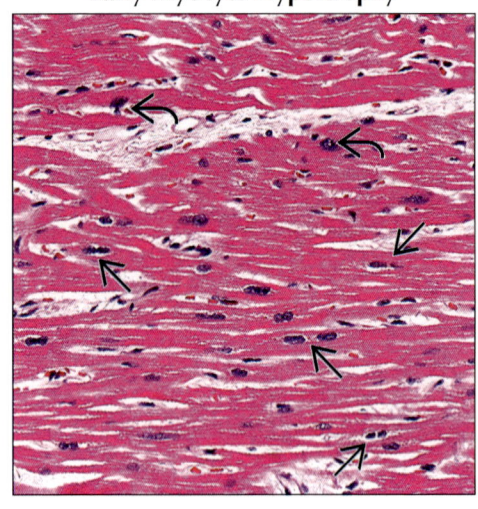

(Left) The proportion of sarcoplasm to nuclei in infant myocardium is much lower than in adults, consistent with the dogma that myocardial growth occurs via hypertrophy and not hyperplasia. **(Right)** This adult myocardium (note the increased sarcoplasm relative to infants) shows early features of (abnormal or pathologic) myocyte hypertrophy, including frequent binucleation of myocytes ⇥ and nuclear darkening and enlargement ⇥.

Severe Myocyte Hypertrophy

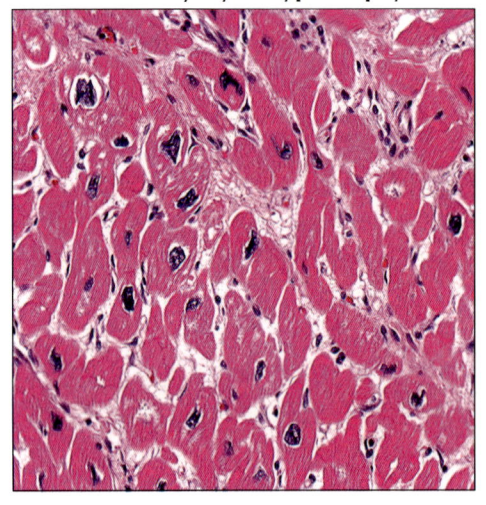

Subendocardial (Ischemic) Vacuolation

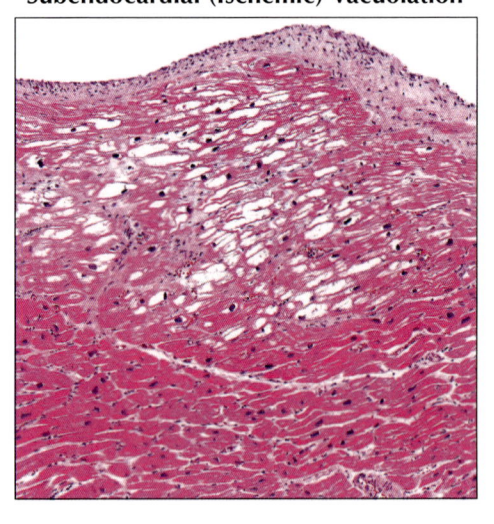

(Left) In severe (abnormal) hypertrophy, the nuclei are dramatically enlarged, hyperchromatic, and irregular. Note the absence of mitoses. Nuclear features are a more reliable measure of hypertrophy than other cell width measurements due to the complex 3-dimensional architecture of cardiomyocytes. **(Right)** Subendocardial myocardium is furthest from coronary blood flow but too deep to receive oxygen and nutrients from luminal blood. In chronic ischemia, starved cells show vacuolation.

Atrial Myocardium

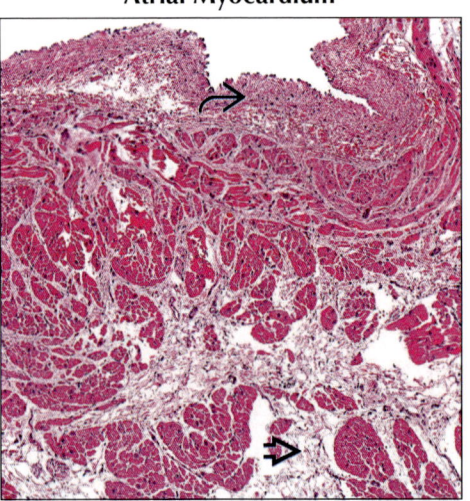

Ventricular Myocardium

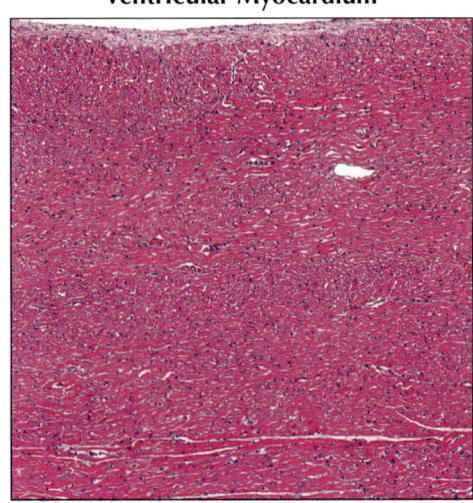

(Left) The atrial walls are thinner than the ventricles, but still contain all 3 tissue layers. The atrial endocardium ⇥ is typically thicker than in the ventricles. The myocardial architecture is also more disorganized and haphazard. Adipose infiltration in the myocardium is also common in the atria ⇥. **(Right)** Aside from being thicker, the ventricular myocardium is also more compact and composed of layers of myocyte "fascicles," successively oriented in alternating directions.

Circulatory System

4

HEART

Papillary Muscle Tip

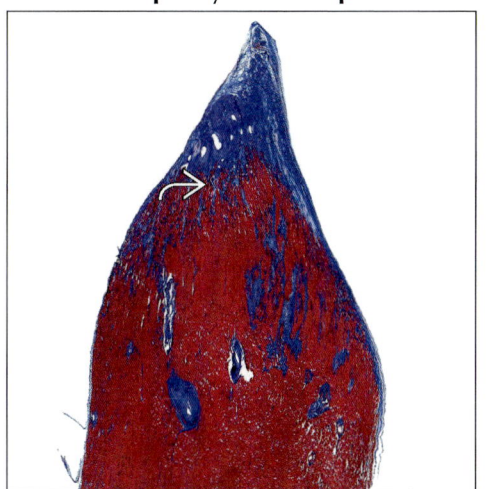

Tricuspid Valve Annulus

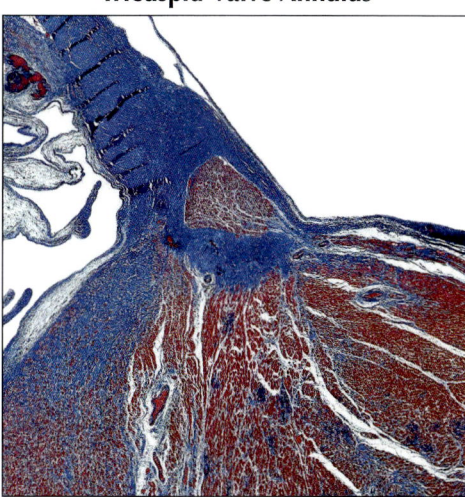

(Left) The tip of a papillary muscle is stained with trichrome to highlight the interdigitation of myocardium and dense collagenous valve apparatus (tendinous cord) tissue ➡. Cross sections through the tips of the papillary muscle may falsely appear to have increased interstitial fibrosis, though this is a normal anatomic phenomenon. *(Right)* Similar to the papillary muscle tip, the dense collagenous interventricular valve annulus also shows some interdigitation with myocardium.

Intramyocardial Vessels

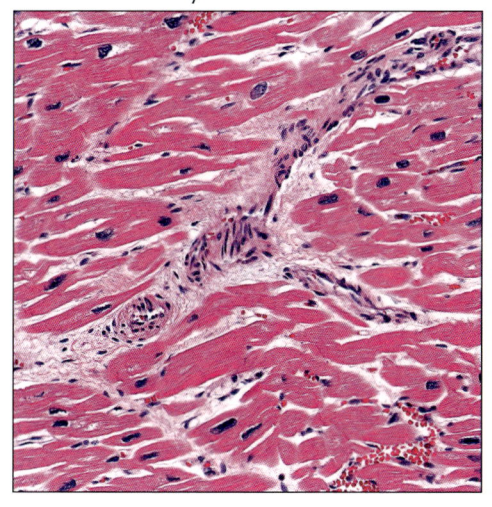

Intramyocardial Vessels

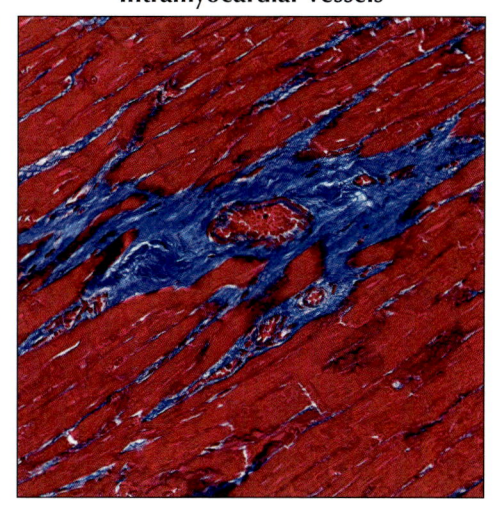

(Left) As penetrating arteries and other intramyocardial vessels course through the myocardium, they are surrounded by a layer of connective tissue. This is normal and should not be confused with pathologic interstitial fibrosis. *(Right)* Trichrome staining highlights the collagenous connective tissue surrounding intramyocardial vessels. Note the absence of collagenous fibrosis between myocytes, where no vessels are seen.

Contraction Band Artifact

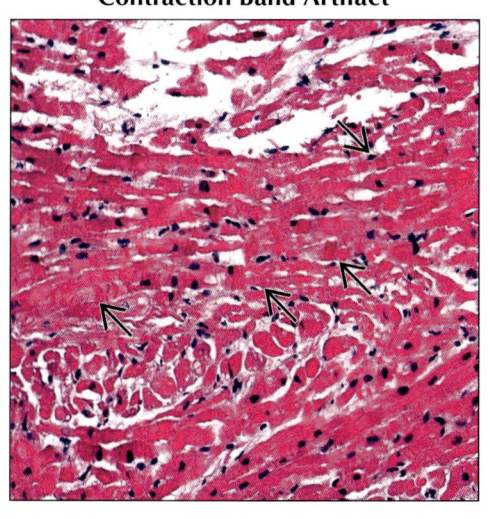

Hydrophilic Polymer Gel Embolus

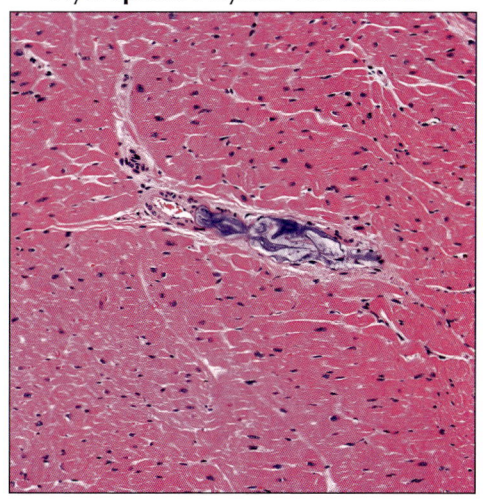

(Left) Contraction bands are thick perpendicular lines ➡ (much thicker than cross-striations or intercalated discs) within myocytes, caused by clumping together of the contractile elements. In full-thickness sections of the heart, these indicate infarction, but in biopsies they do not (rather due to biopsy-related trauma). *(Right)* Hydrophilic polymer coatings are common on endovascular catheters and may embolize to coronary arteries. This is an artifact that is not typically pathologic.

CARDIAC VALVES

Key Facts

Macroscopic Anatomy

- **Semilunar (ventriculoarterial) valves:** Aortic and pulmonary valves; anatomy is similar
- 3 shirt pocket-like cusps or leaflets arranged radially
- Retrograde blood flow from aorta during diastole fills cusp pockets, occluding valve orifice
- Outer "sheath" of these valves varies in composition at different levels
  - Below leaflets (pulmonary): Ventricular septum and right ventricular outflow tract (infundibulum)
  - Below leaflets (aortic): Ventricular septum and anterior mitral leaflet-aortic valve fibrous continuity
  - Behind leaflets: Bulbar or "sinus of Valsalva" portion of aorta or pulmonary artery (and coronary artery ostia in aorta); sinuses are more prominently dilated in aortic valve
  - Above leaflets: Sinotubular junction or supraaortic/pulmonary ridge
- A line of fine fibrosis develops toward top of aortic cusps along line of closure/coaptation; above this line there is often redundant and fenestrated tissue called the "lunula"
- At cusp edge midpoint is a pyramidal focus of fibrosis (nodule of Arantius), from which often emanate fine strands of fibrous tissue (Lambl excrescences)
- **Atrioventricular valves:** Mitral and tricuspid valves; anatomy is similar
  - Each is suspended from a fibrous annulus that separates atria above from ventricle below
  - Each is tethered from below (preventing prolapse into atria during systole) by tendinous cords attached to papillary muscle (outcroppings from ventricular muscle wall)
  - Mitral valve has 2 leaflets (anterior and posterior) supported by 2 papillary muscles (1 at each commissure)
  - Tricuspid valve has 3 leaflets (anterior, posterior, and septal) and 3 papillary muscles

Microscopic Anatomy

- Semilunar and atrioventricular valves share same trilaminar histo-architecture
  - Thickness and proportional contribution of each layer vary
- **Fibrosa:** Dense collagenous layer in continuity with annular connective tissue (and for the semilunar valves, the arterial wall)
  - Bounded on either side by thin layer of elastic fibers (more prominent beneath endothelium)
  - Elastic layers diminish toward free edge of leaflets
  - This layer continues as tendinous cords of atrioventricular valves
- **Spongiosa:** Central layer, composed of loose connective tissue, fibroblasts, and valvular interstitial cells
  - Most prominent near annulus
  - In semilunar valves, atrial myocardium, nerve bundles, and lymphatics may infiltrate spongiosa near annulus
  - This layer also rises to the surface distally in semilunar valves to become "auricularis" layer
- **Ventricularis:** Most elastic fiber-rich layer with multiple layers of elastic tissue
  - Lines ventricular surfaces of both semilunar and atrioventricular valves
  - Also coats tendinous cords

Pitfalls/Artifacts

- Tangential sectioning (when blocking tissue or at embedding)
- Presence of vessels within valve tissue is abnormal, signifies postinflammatory process such as rheumatic valve disease

Age Variation

- Diffuse rubbery thickening, accentuation of noduli Arantii, and mitral annular and sinotubular junction (supravalvular ridge) calcification all occur with aging
- Calcification and fibrosis in the fibrosa in valve sclerosis and expansion of loose connective tissue in spongiosa also occur with aging

(Left) This photo shows the semilunar valves after removal of the great arteries. The pulmonary artery ➡ is anterior and the aorta ➡ posterior with the right coronary ➡ artery branching from the aorta. *(Right)* The atrioventricular valves (tricuspid ➡ and mitral ➡) are shown in this 4-chamber view of the heart. The valves are suspended from annular rings and tethered to papillary muscles ➡ by tendinous cords ➡.

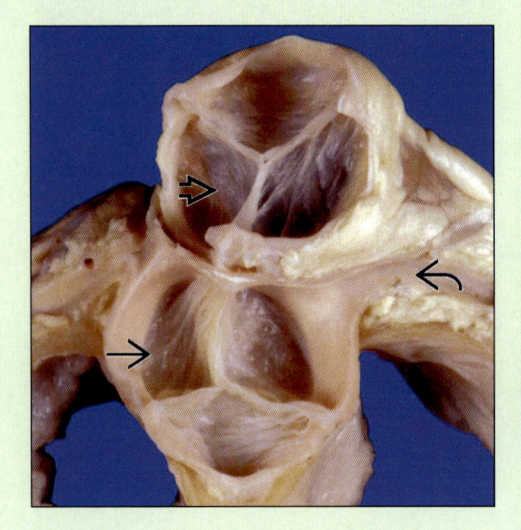

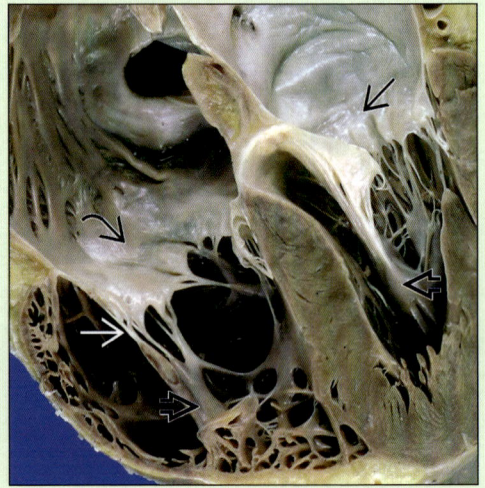

CARDIAC VALVES

Semilunar Valve

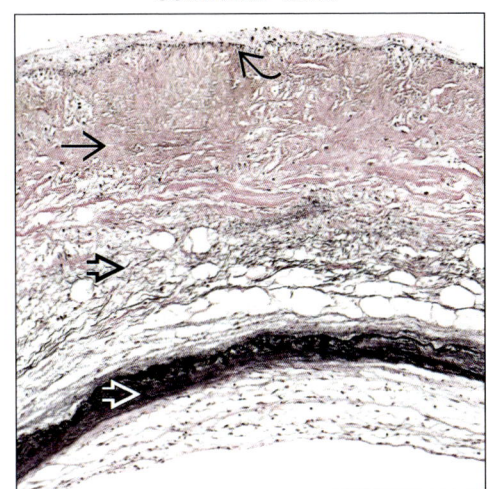

Atrioventricular Valve

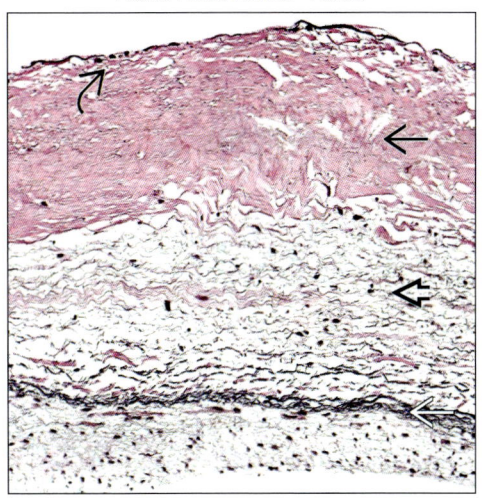

(Left) The 3 distinct valvular layers are the fibrosa ➡, spongiosa ➡, and ventricularis ➡. A fine line of elastic tissue is seen beneath the endocardium overlying the fibrosa layer ➡. The ventricularis layer is the richest in elastic tissue, as shown by the heavy black band on this elastic stain. *(Right)* This photo shows the the 3 distinct valvular layers: Fibrosa ➡, spongiosa ➡, and ventricularis ➡, with the subendocardial elastic layer ➡.

Semilunar Valve (Free Aspect)

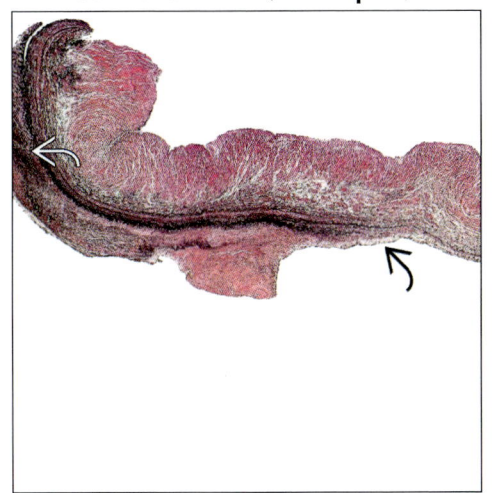

Semilunar Valve (Free Aspect)

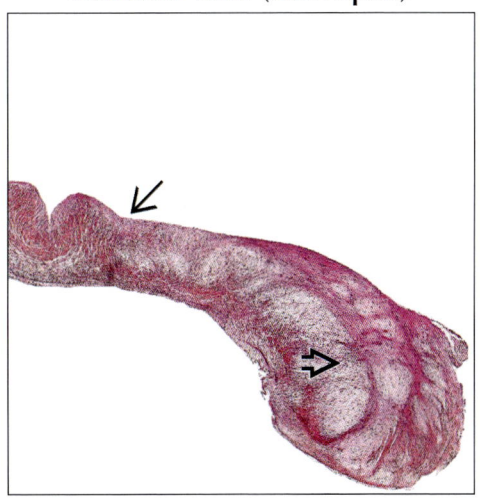

(Left) This photo demonstrates continuity between the aortic valve and the elastic wall of the aortic root ➡, along with the gradual diminution of the ventricularis layer ➡ and fibrosa layer toward the free edge of the cusp. *(Right)* There is gradual diminution of the ventricularis layer and fibrosa layer ➡ with progression toward the free edge of the cusp, shown here. The spongiosa layer expands to become most prominent at the free edge ➡.

Atrioventricular Valve Near Annulus

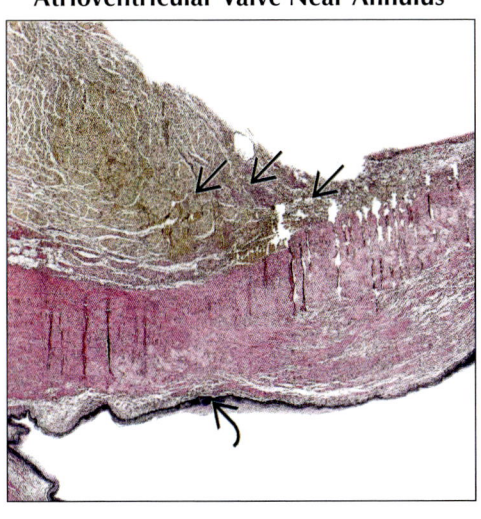

Tendinous Cord

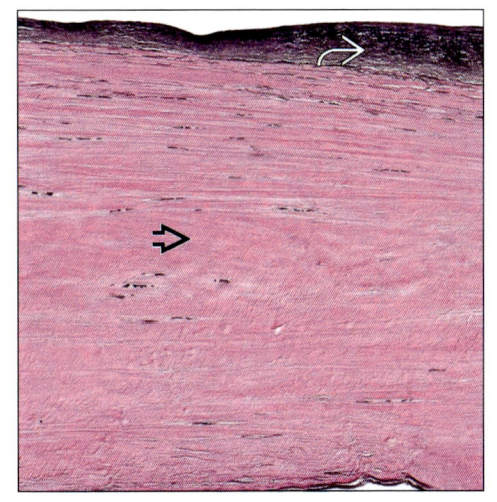

(Left) The myocardium extends (along with lymphatics, fat, and nerves) into the proximal portion of the valve substance ➡. The heavy band of elastic tissue in the ventricularis layer ➡ is also prominent. *(Right)* This section shows a thickened portion of tendinous cord. The core ➡ is dense collagen that is continuous with the valve fibrosa layer. There is a coating of prominent elastic tissue ➡ covering the cords as well.

CARDIAC CONDUCTION SYSTEM

Key Facts

Macroscopic Anatomy
- Sinoatrial (or sinus) node
  - Specialized "pacemaker" myocyte collection in right atrium
  - Subepicardial structure near superior vena cava, overlying the terminal crest (vertical crest on interior wall of right atrium that separates sinus of vena cava from rest of the right atrium)
  - Found at union of smooth-walled "sinus venosus" portion and and trabecular portion of right atrium
  - Supplied by sinus node artery (usually a branch from right coronary)
- Atrioventricular (AV) node
  - Specialized conducting myocytes within tricuspid annulus near atrioventricular (membranous) septum
  - Subendocardial structure found within "Koch triangle," an anatomic area defined by these 3 vertices: (1) Membranous septum, (2) roof of coronary sinus ostium, and (3) tricuspid annulus at a point directly below coronary sinus ostium
  - Supplied by AV nodal artery (usually from posterior descending artery)

Microscopic Anatomy
- Sinoatrial node
  - Compact and polyhedral myocytes surrounded by dense collagenous tissue
  - Sarcoplasm and cross-striations less prominent
  - Sinus nodal artery courses through sinus node
  - Autonomic nerve fibers and ganglia seen in vicinity
- AV node
  - Compact "bulb" of smaller polyhedral myocytes merging with larger stellate to spindled myocytes with vacuolar sarcoplasm toward the His bundle
  - Mesothelial-like cells and cystic structures occasionally intermixed
  - AV nodal artery courses through AV node
  - Connective tissue surrounds node, "insulating" adjacent myocardium
  - Autonomic nerves and lymphatics seen in vicinity
- His bundle and bundle branches
  - Constituent cells mostly smaller than myocardial myocytes and more vacuolated
  - Right bundle branch is smaller and cordlike
  - Left bundle branch is larger and splays out over leftward ventricular septum
- Purkinje cell
  - This term is applied to cells in left bundle branch and distal right bundle branch because they are larger than myocardial myocytes and have more vacuolar cytoplasm
  - As with all conduction system cells, Purkinje cells are myocytes and contain myofibrils by electron microscopy
  - Differ from normal cardiomyocytes by the absence of T tubules and striking abundance of cell:cell junctions

Pitfalls/Artifacts
- Normally occurring smooth muscle bundles in endocardium should not be mistaken for Purkinje cells or conduction system tracts

Age Variation
- Increased ratio of dense collagen to myocytes with increasing age reported by some authors

(Left) This illustration shows the approximate locations of the sinus node ⇨ (subepicardial), atrioventricular node ⇨ (subendocardial), and His bundle ⇨, as well as the bundle branches (subendocardial). *(Right)* The conduction system coordinates each cardiac contraction. Every beat originates in the sinus node and propagates through the atrium to the atrioventricular (AV) node. The AV node, His bundle and bundle branches control contraction of the ventricles.

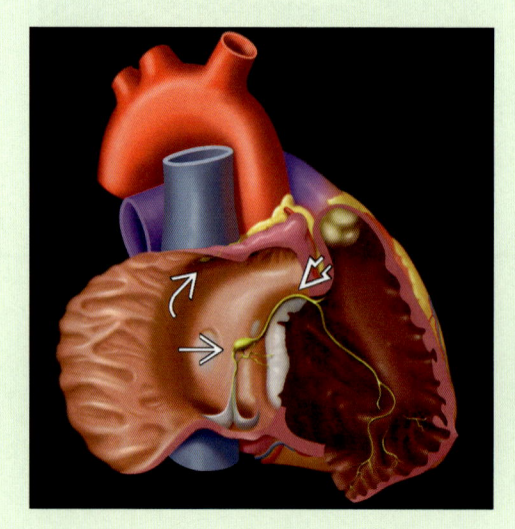

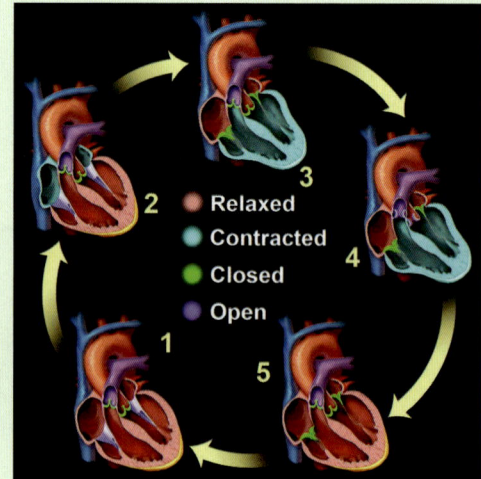

CARDIAC CONDUCTION SYSTEM

Heart, Superior Oblique View

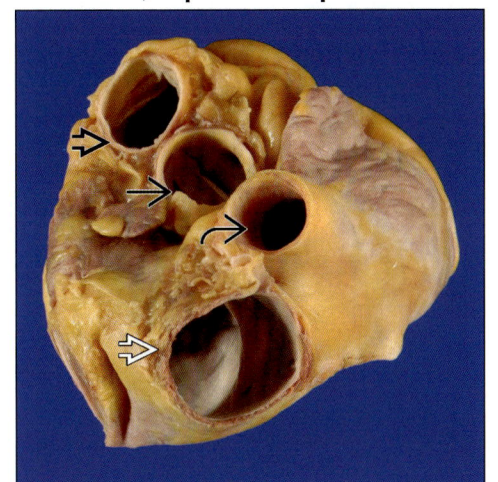

Heart, Superior Oblique View (Sinoatrial Node Block Removed)

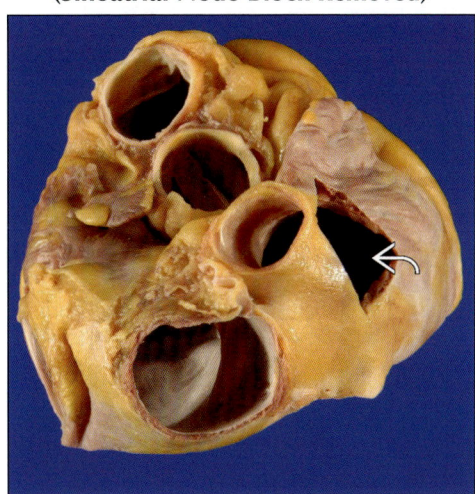

(Left) This heart removed at autopsy illustrates the pulmonary artery ⮕, aorta ⮕, superior vena cava ⮕, and left pulmonary vein confluence ⮕ when viewed from above. *(Right)* A block of tissue ⮕ along the lateral border near the SVC connection, containing the sinus node, has been removed from this heart. Internally, a segment of the terminal crest in the right atrium is removed with this block.

Excised Tissue Block Containing Sinus Node

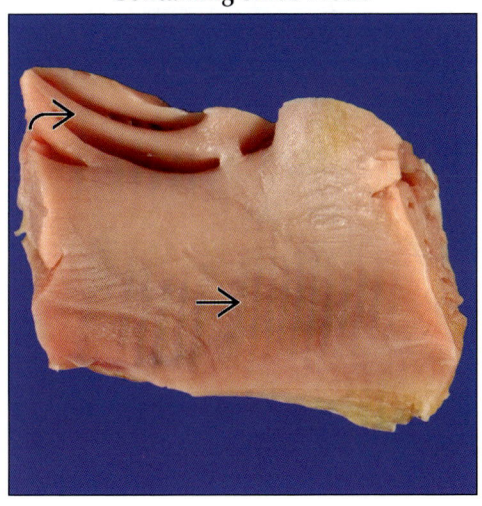

Sinus Node Tissue Block (Cross Sections)

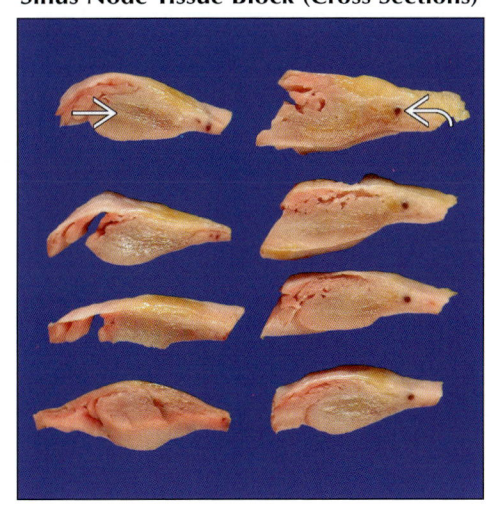

(Left) Viewed from the endocardial aspect, this excised tissue block consists of a portion of terminal crest ⮕ with a few pectinate muscles ⮕ attached. The overlying epicardium (not seen, facing down) is intact. *(Right)* After serial sectioning, the belly of the terminal crest ⮕ is now seen in cross section in each piece. The pinpoint sinus nodal artery ⮕ can also be seen in many of the sections, identifying the locus of the node.

Sinoatrial Node

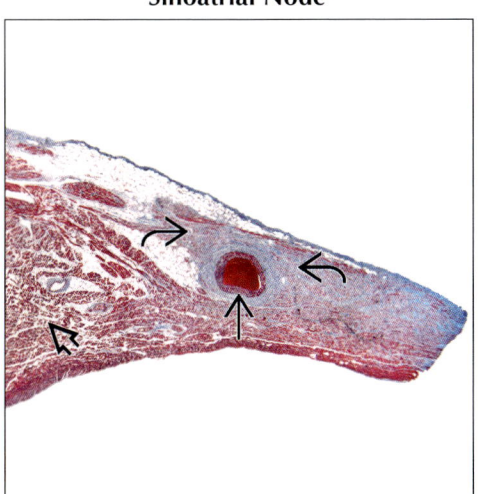

Sinoatrial Node

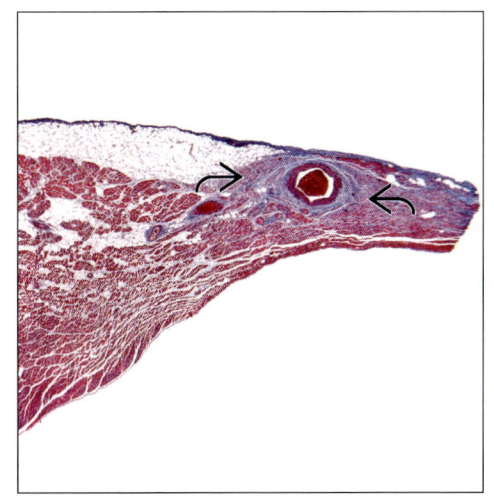

(Left) This trichrome-stained section at low magnification shows the atrial (terminal crest) myocardium ⮕, sinus node artery ⮕, and sinoatrial node itself ⮕, characterized by intermixed dense collagen and small polygonal myocytes. *(Right)* This cross section illustrates the dense connective tissue-rich sinoatrial node tissue ⮕ surrounding the sinus node artery.

CARDIAC CONDUCTION SYSTEM

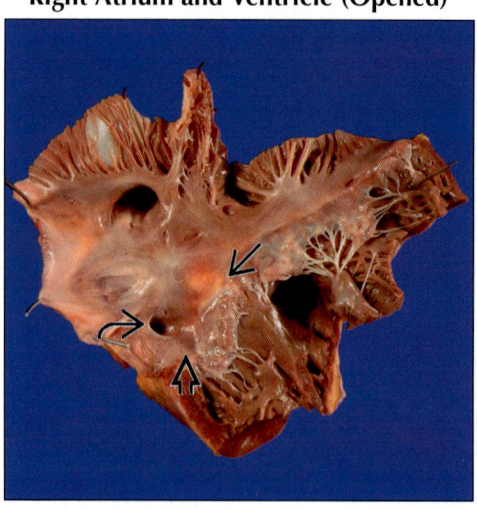

(Left) This trichrome-stained section shows a portion of normal sinoatrial node with accompanying sinus node artery ➡. The nodal myocytes show prominent vacuolization ➡. **(Right)** The right side of the heart has been opened through the tricuspid valve. Koch triangle can be visualized as imaginary lines connecting the roof of the coronary sinus ostium ➡, the tricuspid annulus at a point directly below the coronary sinus ostium ➡, and the membranous septum ➡.

Sinus Node, High Magnification

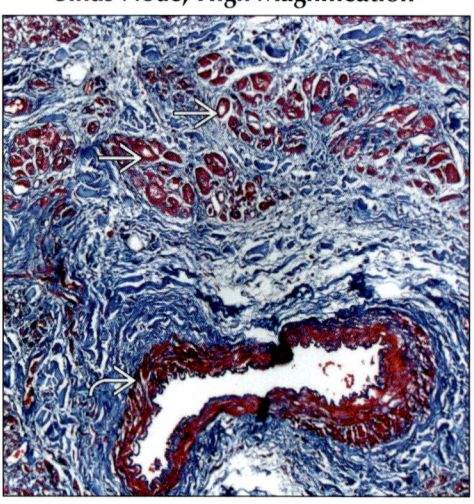

Right Atrium and Ventricle (Opened)

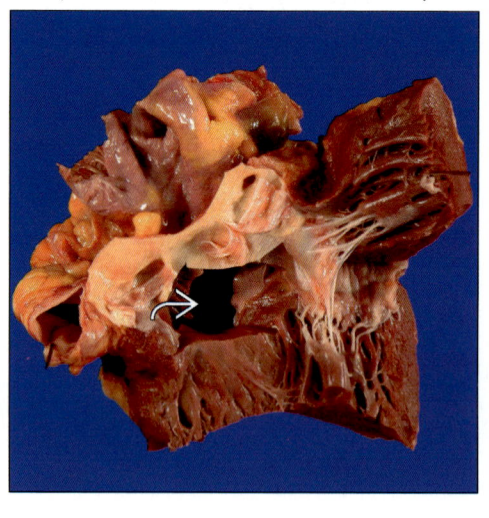

(Left) This view shows the right side of the heart, opened through the tricuspid valve, after the tissue block containing Koch triangle (including the AV node) has been removed ➡. **(Right)** This view demonstrates that the excised tissue block ➡ included the interventricular septum and part of the aortic valve and aorto-mitral fibrous continuity.

Right Atrium and Ventricle, Opened (AV Node Tissue Block Removed)

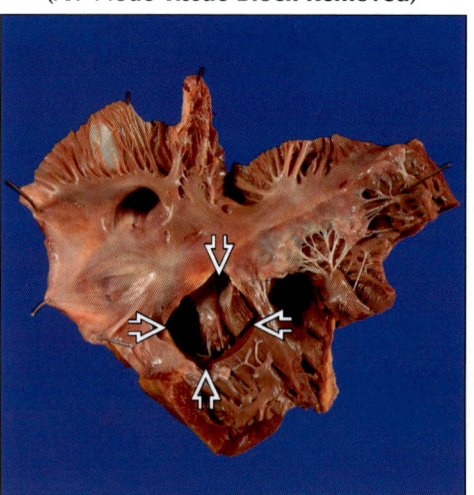

Left Ventricular Outflow Tract, Opened (AV Node Tissue Block Removed)

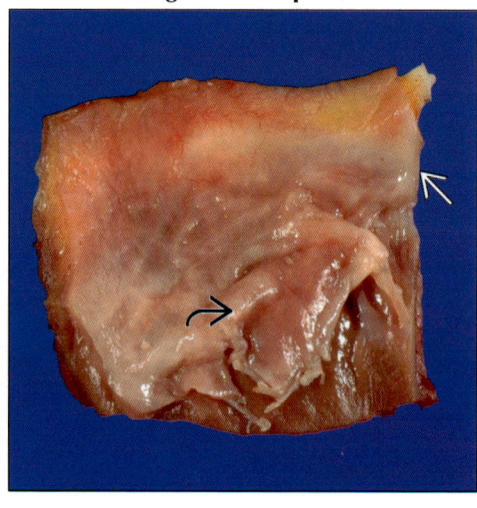

(Left) This view demonstrates that the excised tissue block ➡ also included the portion of anterior mitral valve leaflet that forms the aorto-mitral fibrous continuity. **(Right)** The AV node tissue block is shown with a portion of posterior tricuspid leaflet ➡ that traverses the rightward aspect diagonally. The membranous (atrioventricular) septum is also seen ➡.

Left Atrium and Ventricle, Opened (AV Node Tissue Block Removed)

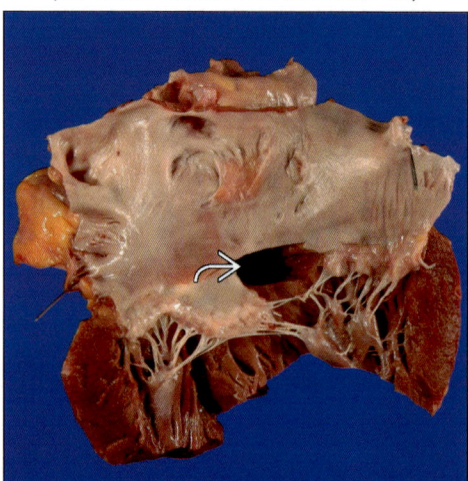

AV Node Tissue Block (Rightward Aspect)

CARDIAC CONDUCTION SYSTEM

AV Node Tissue Block (Leftward Aspect)

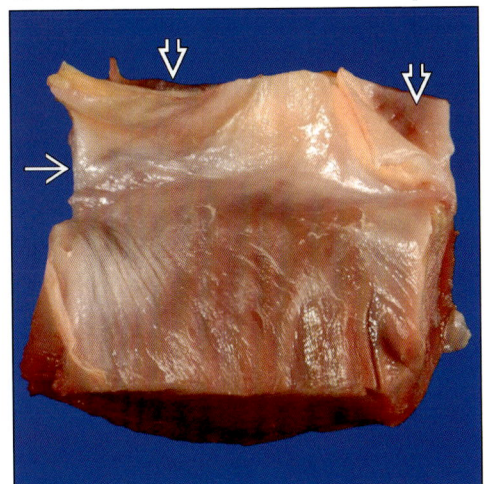

Cross Sections through AV Node Tissue Block

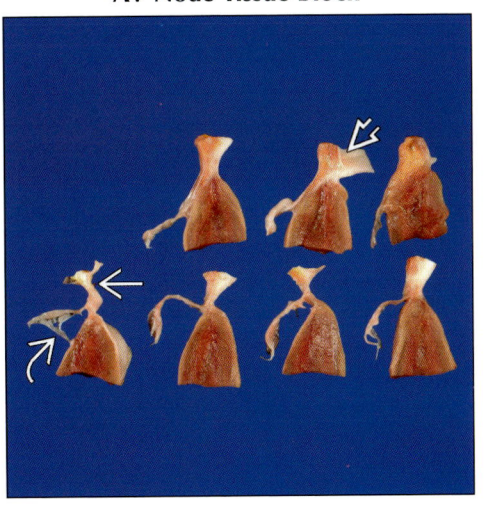

(Left) The left-facing aspect of the AV node tissue block is shown here, with membranous septum ➡ and pockets of 2 aortic valve cusps ➡. *(Right)* Serial cross sections through the excised AV node tissue block illustrate portions of tricuspid valve leaflet ➡, membranous (atrioventricular) septum ➡, and aortic valve cusp ➡.

AV Node: Trichrome

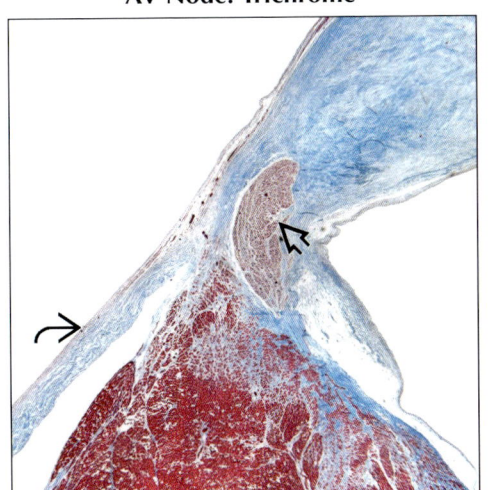

His Bundle and Right Bundle Branch: Trichrome

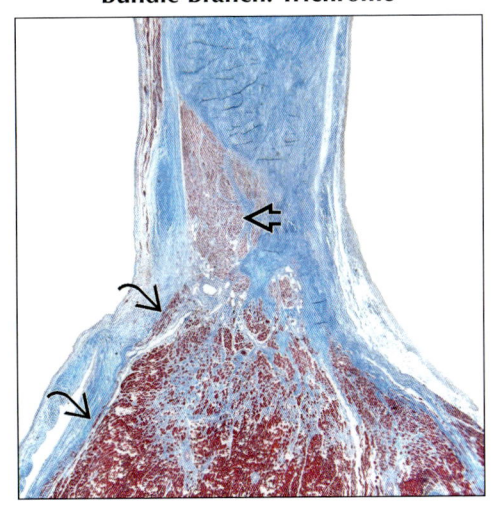

(Left) Intermixed dense collagen and small myocytes comprise the AV node ➡, situated in the annular connective tissue, insulated from the atrial and ventricular myocardium. A portion of tricuspid valve leaflet is also seen ➡. *(Right)* The right bundle branch ➡ consists of a thin, cord-like wisp of conduction system myocytes arising from the main His bundle ➡. Because of its small size, step sections through the paraffin block are typically required to see it well.

Left Bundle Branch: Trichrome

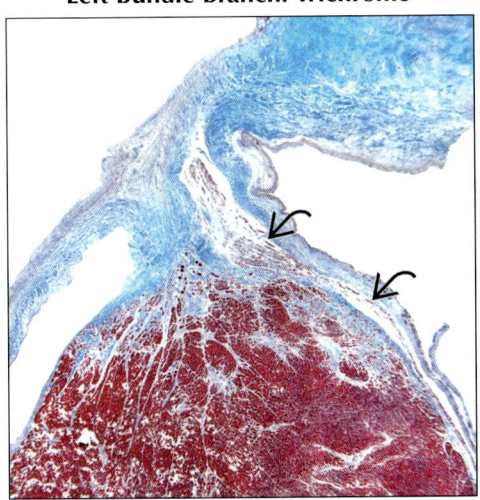

AV Node, High Magnification: Trichrome

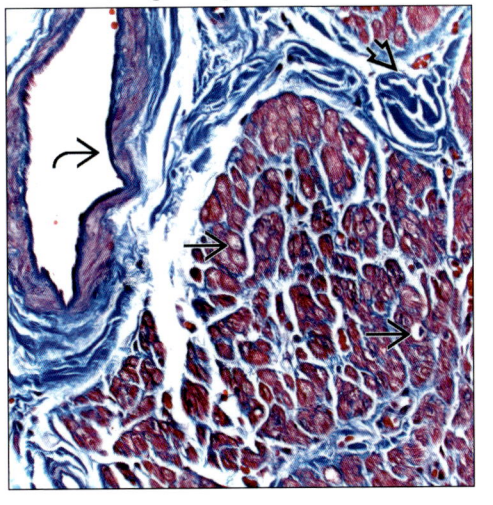

(Left) The left bundle branch ➡ is larger and broadly splays out beneath the left ventricular outflow tract endocardium. The specialized myocytes are smaller than the adjacent normal myocardial myocytes and may also be more vacuolated. *(Right)* This trichrome-stained section shows a portion of the AV node with accompanying AV nodal artery ➡. The conduction system myocytes are compact and show vacuolization of the sarcoplasm ➡. There is also dense collagenous connective tissue in the node ➡.

ARTERIES

Key Facts

Macroscopic Anatomy
- Elastic arteries
  - 1st order branches of aorta (carotid, subclavian, proximal renal, and iliac; also internal mammary arteries)
  - Walls composed of multi-elastic-layer concentric strata
- Muscular arteries
  - Arterial segments in between elastic arteries and arterioles
  - Distinct internal and external elastic lamina
- Arterioles
  - Smooth muscle only, no definite elastic layer

Microscopic Anatomy
- Intimal layer (tunica intima)
  - Single layer of endothelial cells with subendothelial loose connective tissue and smooth muscle cells
- Medial layer (tunical media)
  - Multiple layers of smooth muscle cells with associated elastic tissue
- Adventitial layer (tunica adventitia)
  - Dense connective tissue
- Cerebral arteries, relative to similar caliber arteries outside brain, have
  - No external elastic lamina
  - Very thin adventitia (and Virchow-Robin spaces)
  - Reduced wall thickness:lumen diameter ratio

Pitfalls/Artifacts
- Tangential sectioning of tortuous vessels can result in asymmetric luminal contours and wall thicknesses
- En face sectioning of elastic layers in aortic sections (when not embedded "on edge")

Age Variation
- Intimal thickness increases with age in a manner independent of atherosclerosis
- Mild medial elastic fiber fragmentation in large elastic arteries also can be seen in elderly
- Calcification of internal elastic lamina in muscular arteries (Mönckeberg-type medial calcific sclerosis) is another nonpathologic, age-related phenomenon

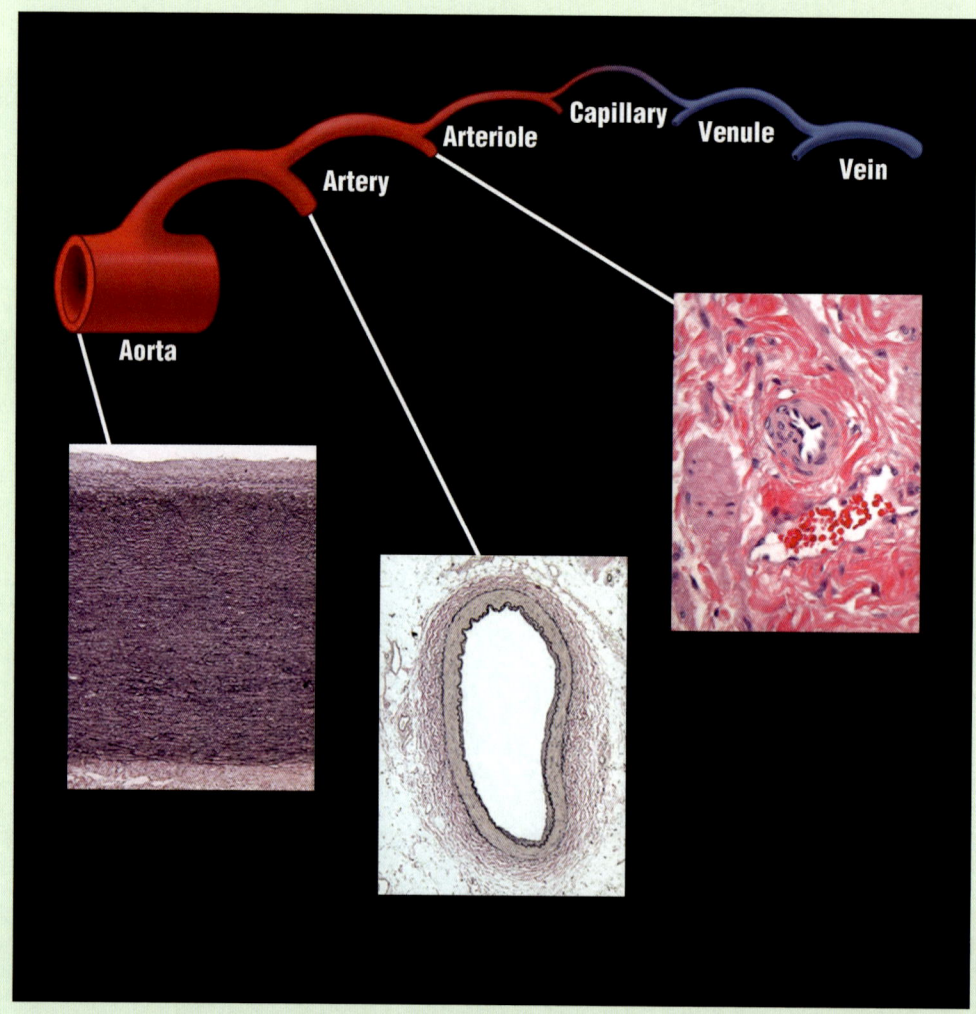

This schematic shows the spectrum of vascular segments from elastic artery to capillaries and back again to the great veins. For each arterial segment, the histologic structure reflects its function. The aorta is rich in elastic tissue, which helps provide recoil to sustain blood flow during diastole. The muscular arteries have some elastic properties but also substantial smooth muscle that contracts and relaxes to alter luminal flow. Arterioles are almost entirely smooth muscle and serve as the main locus of control for peripheral vascular resistance.

ARTERIES

Muscular Artery (Cross Section)

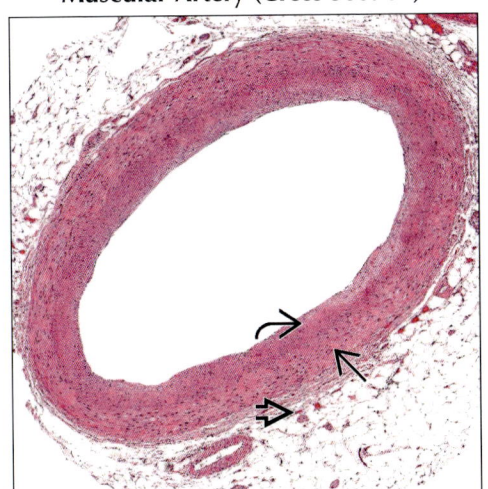

Muscular Artery (Cross Section)

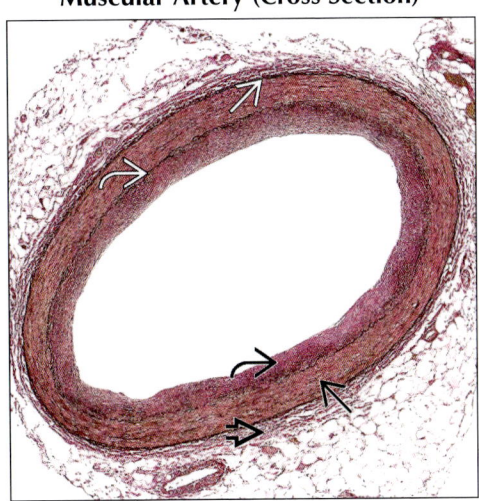

(Left) Photomicrograph of a muscular artery shows the normal configuration and appearance of the intimal ⮕, medial ⮕, and adventitial layers ⮕. *(Right)* Elastic-stained section of muscular artery illustrates the normal configuration and appearance of the intimal ⮕, medial ⮕, and adventitial layers ⮕. The stain also demonstrates the internal ⮕ and external ⮕ elastic laminae.

Muscular Artery (Compressed)

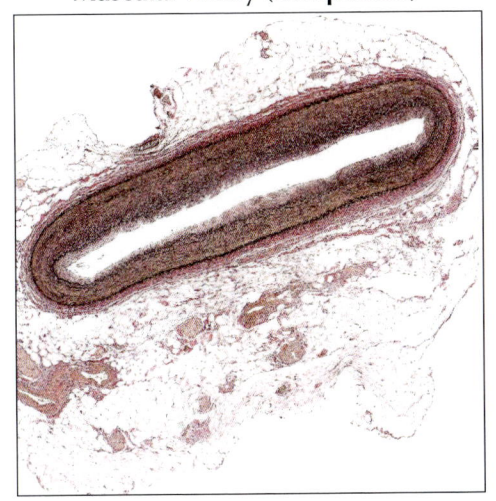

Muscular Artery Branching

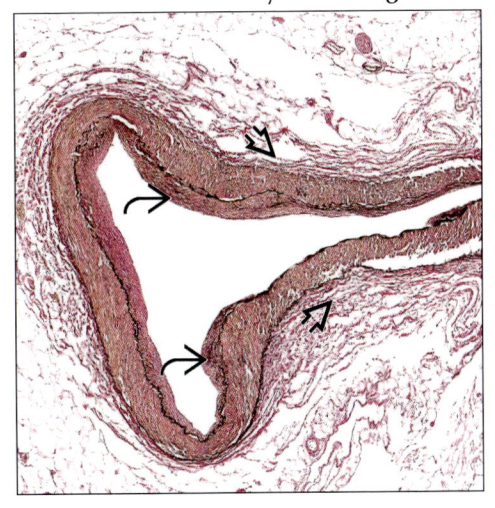

(Left) The lumen of this artery is elongated and narrowed, rather than the usual circular appearance, but this reflects an artifact of compression during tissue fixation. *(Right)* A perpendicular branch ⮕ arises from a muscular artery. Note the difference in caliber between the main artery (cross section) and branch (longitudinal section). Note also that the tissue layers and elastic laminae are continuous from main artery to the branch with thickened intima at the junction ⮕.

Muscular Artery

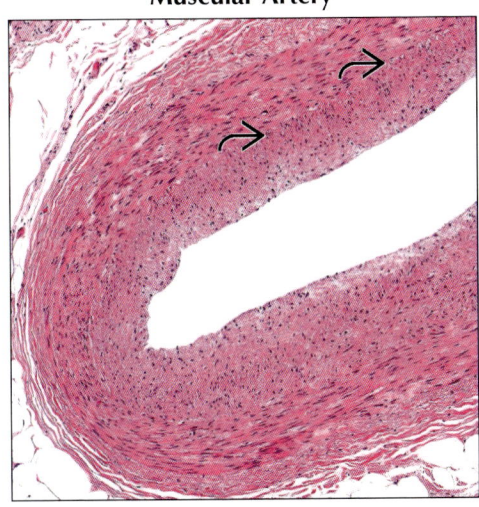

Adventitia and Periadventitial Tissue

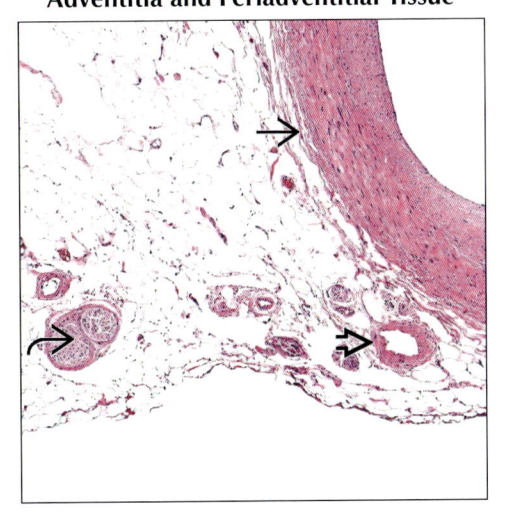

(Left) Photomicrograph of a muscular artery in cross section demonstrates that elastic staining is not always needed to see the wavy, refractile elastic fibers of the internal elastic lamina ⮕. *(Right)* Beyond the adventitia ⮕ there is adipose tissue in which nerve fibers ⮕ and small vessels of the vasa vasorum ⮕ can be found. The vasa vasorum run parallel to the artery but give rise to perpendicular branches that penetrate into the media to supply the smooth muscle cells.

ARTERIES

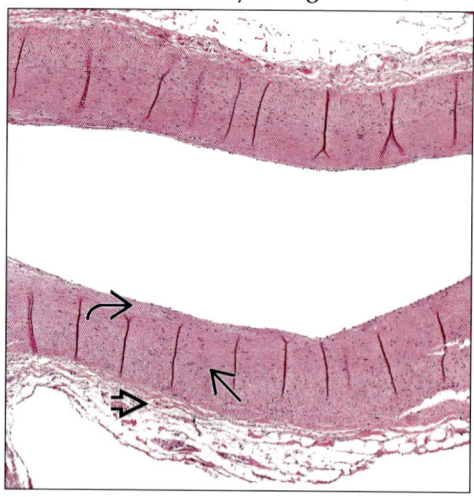

Muscular Artery (Longitudinal)

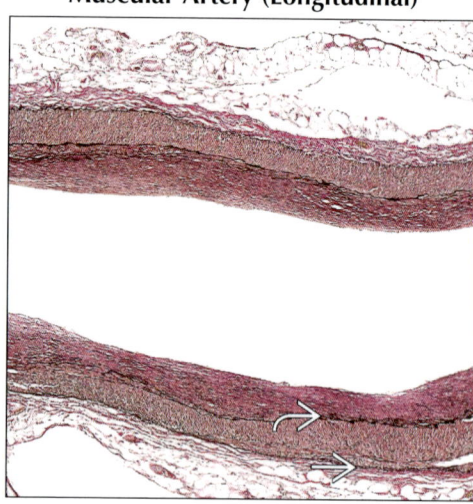

(Left) Longitudinal section of an arterial segment (as opposed to cross section) shows the same tri-layered architecture with intima ⇨, media ⇨, and adventitia ⇨. **(Right)** Elastic stain of a longitudinally sectioned muscular artery demonstrates the internal ⇨ and external elastic ⇨ laminae.

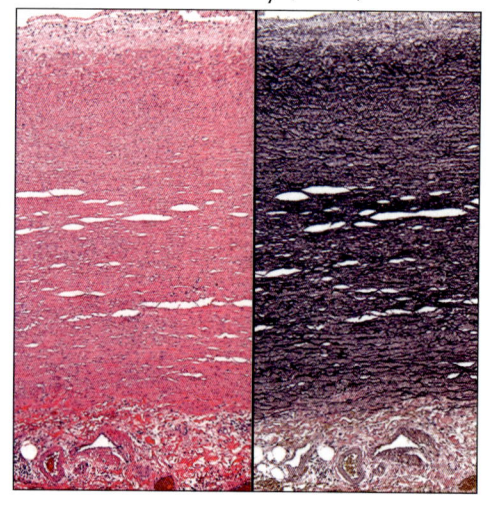

Elastic Artery (Aorta)

(Left) Photograph compares H&E and elastic staining of the aortic wall. Note the relatively thin intimal layer; nearly the entire thickness of the wall is comprised of media with alternating elastic fiber and intervening smooth muscle layers. The adventitia is also prominent with large vasa vasorum readily apparent. **(Right)** Normal aortic wall is composed of multilayered strata of wavy elastic fibers.

Tangential Sectioning Artifact

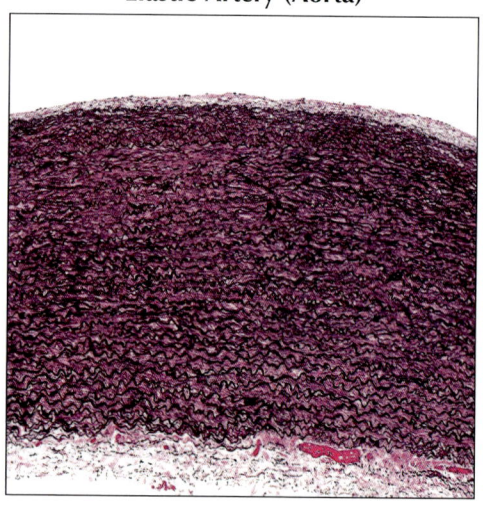

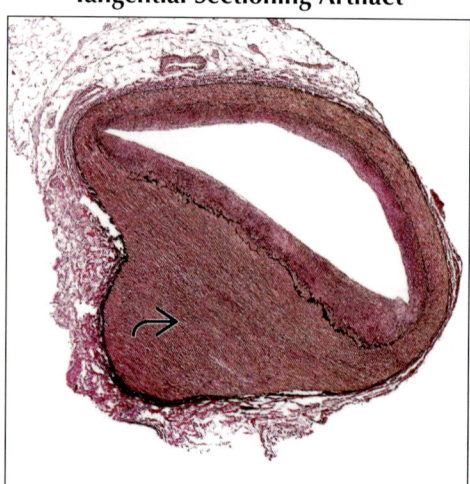

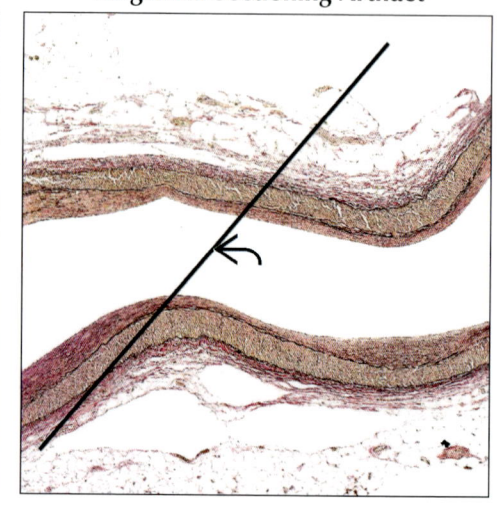

(Left) An asymmetric bulging ⇨ is seen on 1 side of this vessel (otherwise in cross section). Elastic staining shows that this is composed of medial layer. The orientation of the medial smooth muscle is altered relative to the cross-sectional areas (another clue to tangential sectioning). **(Right)** A slightly tortuous segment of muscular artery is shown with a line ⇨ representing a tangential plane that could give rise to an artificial bulge secondary to sectioning artifact.

ARTERIES

Elastic Artery (Internal Mammary Artery)

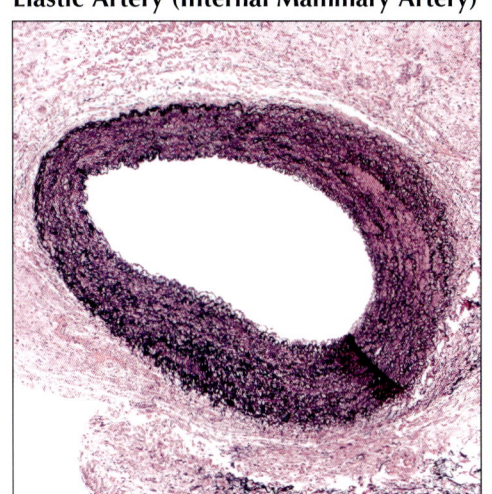

Atherosclerotic Plaque (Longitudinal)

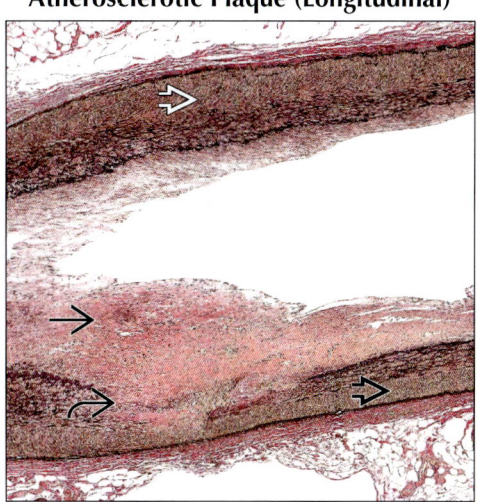

(Left) The internal mammary arteries are unique as the smallest caliber elastic arteries in the arterial tree. These are used as conduits in coronary bypass surgery, so this feature is helpful distinguishing conduit vessels from the native target vessel histologically. *(Right)* This artery contains an atherosclerotic plaque ➡. Note the dissolution of the internal elastic lamina ➡ and atrophy of the media underlying the plaque ➡ (compared to the medial thickness opposite ➡).

Atherosclerotic Plaque (Cross Section)

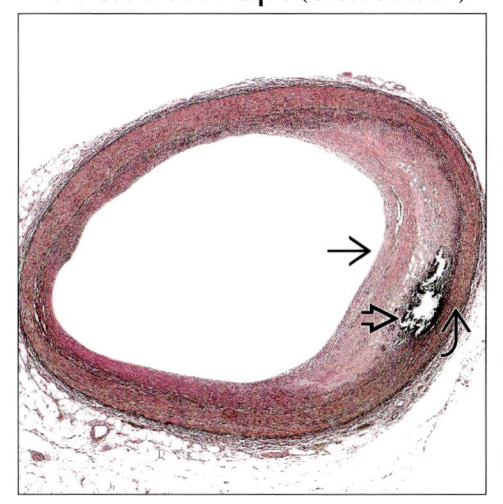

Medial Calcific (Mönckeberg-Type) Sclerosis

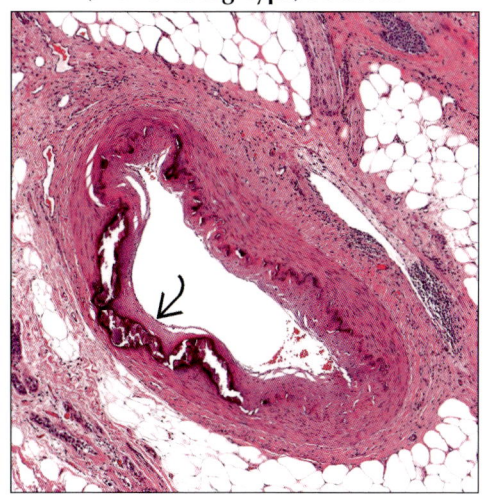

(Left) Elastic staining of this muscular artery shows atherosclerotic plaque ➡ in the intima (inside the internal elastic lamina). Atrophy of the underlying media ➡ and focal calcification ➡ are also seen. *(Right)* Paraffin section of muscular artery shows extensive calcification ➡ centered on the internal elastic lamina. This is largely an age-related phenomenon and of no major clinical significance.

Chronic Medial Dissection

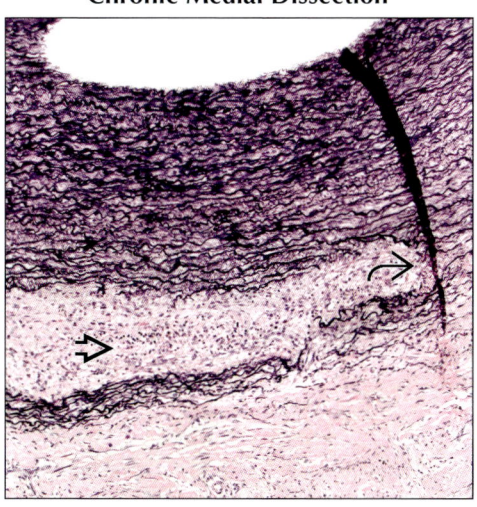

Vasculitis: Disruption of Internal Elastic Lamina

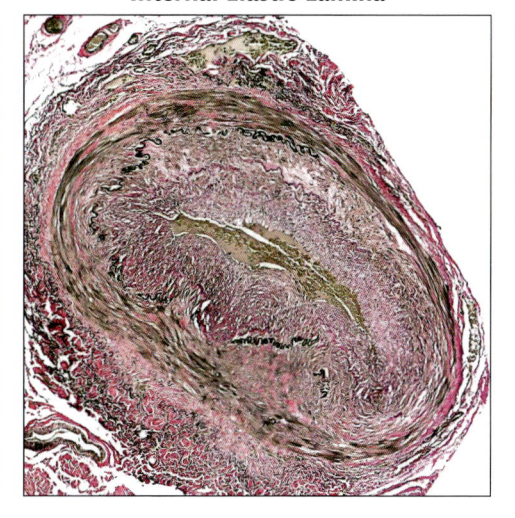

(Left) Photomicrograph shows an elastic artery with chronic medial dissection plane. A new cavity (false lumen) has developed in a dissection plane ➡ within the media, filled with old, organized thrombus ➡. *(Right)* This is a markedly abnormal vessel, showing an important hallmark of inflammatory damage caused by vasculitis. The inflammation causes discrete breaks in the internal elastic lamina, and there is replacement of smooth muscle with collagen and fibroblasts (fibrosis).

CAPILLARIES, VEINS, AND LYMPHATICS

Key Facts

Macroscopic Anatomy
- Veins
  - Thinner wall and larger caliber compared to accompanying arteries
  - Valves cause periodic widening within larger veins
  - Venous circulation is high volume but low flow
- Lymphatics
  - Difficult to see macroscopically
  - Visualization during surgery aided by preoperative ingestion of lipids since chylomicrons are taken up by lymphatics
  - Lymphatic mapping in vivo performed by injecting fluorescent dyes or radioactive isotopes (lymphoscintigraphy)
  - Larger lymphatics may have a "beads on a string" appearance due to lymphatic valves

Microscopic Anatomy, Capillaries
- Lack muscular media
- Lack elastic fibers
- Composed only of endothelial cells with basement membrane and supporting pericyte(s)
- Smallest diameter (~ 5-40 μm) but greatest aggregate surface area in the circulatory system
- Capillary density is proportionate to the metabolic activity of an organ/tissue
- 3 primary types
  - Fenestrated: Pores (60-90 nm) perforating endothelial cytoplasm, forming direct communication to extracellular space (kidney, GI tract, endocrine organs)
  - Continuous: Absent fenestrations; endothelium forms a barrier to extracellular space (muscle, nervous tissue)
  - Sinusoid: Complex 3-dimensional endothelial-lined cavity (liver, spleen, bone marrow)
- Portal system: Capillary bed bound by venous drainage on either end (pituitary, liver)

Microscopic Anatomy, Veins
- Venules
  - Transition from capillaries somewhat arbitrary, based on size
  - Pericytes still present
  - More subendothelial connective tissue than capillaries
  - At most, a single smooth muscle medial layer (often absent)
  - High endothelial venules: Specialized venular segment within lymph nodes; site of leukocyte migration
- Veins
  - Intima: Endothelium and connective tissue; absent internal elastic lamina
  - Media: Variable thickness; greatest in lower extremities, mesentery, uterus, umbilicus, and nearly absent in CNS, retina, medullary bone, penis
  - Adventitia: Most prominent layer; predominantly longitudinally oriented bundles of dense collagen &/or smooth muscle with coarse elastic fibers
  - Valves are present in most veins, composed of paired infoldings from intimal layer

Microscopic Anatomy, Lymphatics
- Lymphatics
  - Smallest lymphatics resemble capillaries, but with larger lumina and less rounded contours
  - Larger lymphatics have thin wisps of muscular media and intimal valves
  - Lack elastic tissue
  - Negligible basement membrane layer
  - Podoplanin (D2-40) and LYVE-1 expressed in lymphatic endothelium

Age Variation
- Phlebosclerosis: Age-related medial and adventitial fibrosis, with less frequent intimal thickening and calcification

(Left) This photomicrograph shows capillaries within organizing granulation tissue. Capillaries consist of endothelial cells ➡ with a basement membrane and supporting pericytes ➡. (Right) This is a small vein. The intimal layer ➡ consists of only endothelium and loose collagen. The media is essentially absent. Longitudinal smooth muscle bundles comprise the adventitia ➡.

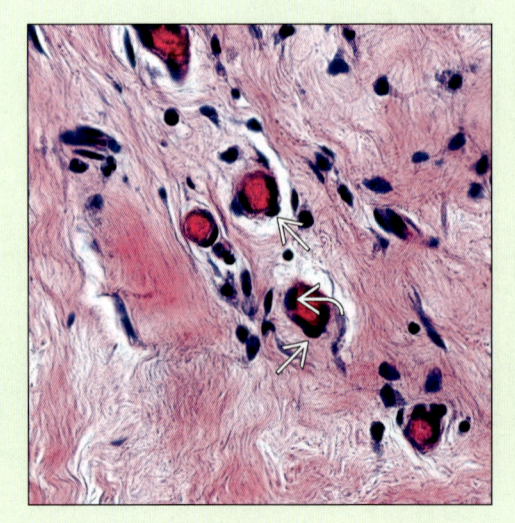

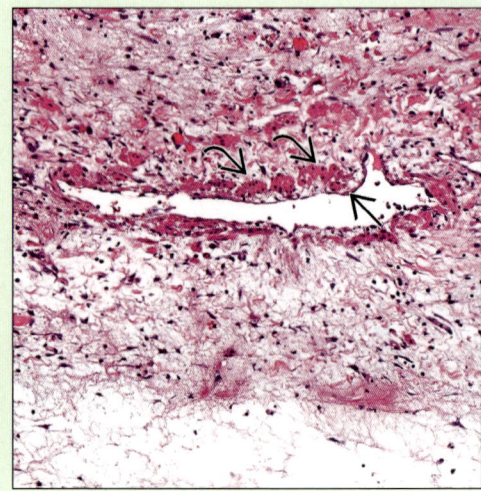

CAPILLARIES, VEINS, AND LYMPHATICS

Medium-Sized Vein in Cross Section

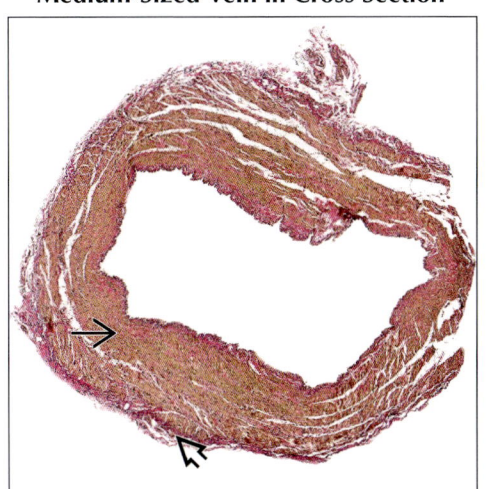

Medium-Sized Vein in Longitudinal Section

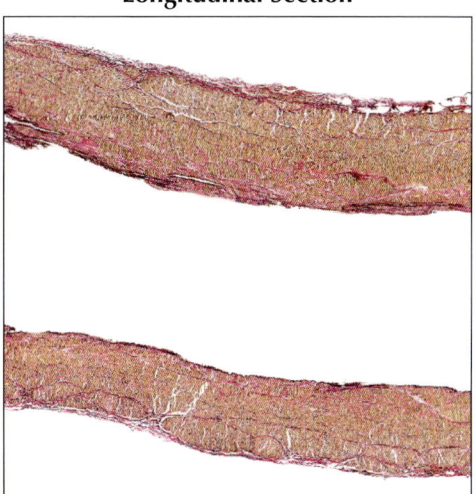

(Left) Veins lack a well-developed internal elastic layer beneath the intima. This small saphenous vein branch has substantial muscular media ⇾. There is abundant adventitial elastic tissue ⇾, but it does not form a discrete lamina. The adventitia is stratified with longitudinal and circumferential bands of smooth muscle and collagen. *(Right)* This longitudinal section of a saphenous vein branch shows that most of the adventitial bundles run parallel to the vessel length.

Organizing Granulation Tissue, Capillaries

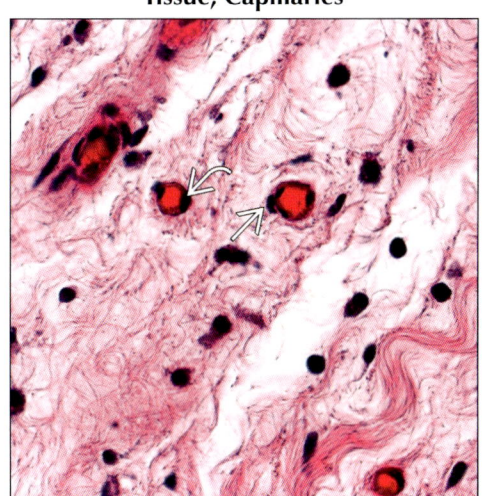

Capillaries, Renal Medulla

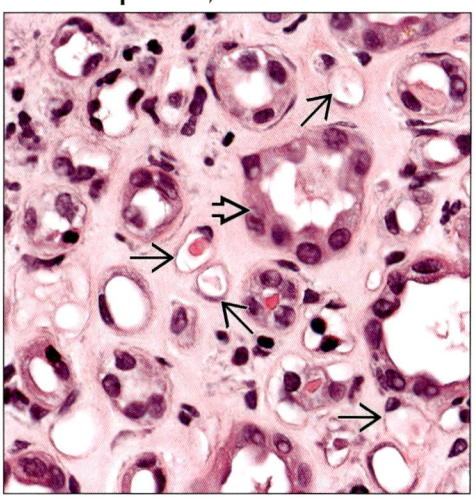

(Left) Capillaries surrounded by a loose connective tissue matrix are a component of the classic wound healing response. By light microscopy, the endothelial cells ⇾ and supporting pericytes are clearly seen ⇾. *(Right)* These capillaries ⇾ are composed of a single endothelial cell circumscribing the lumen. They run alongside renal tubules ⇾ and form part of the vasa recta, running parallel to Henle loops in the renal papillae.

Pulmonary Alveolar Capillaries

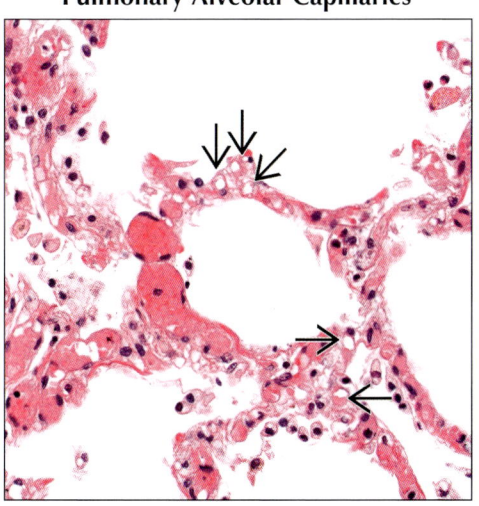

Cerebral Cortical Capillary

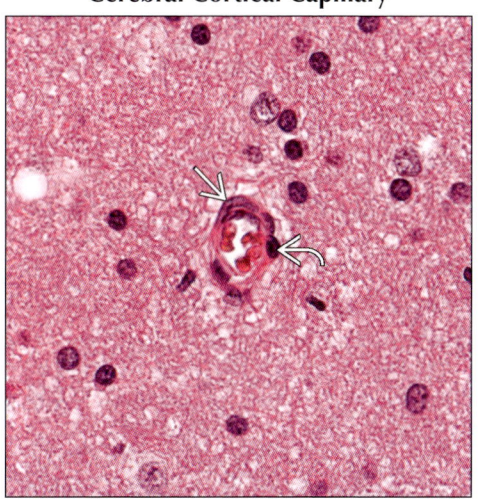

(Left) Contiguous capillaries comprise the bulk of the alveolar septal structure, allowing maximum surface area exposure for gas exchange. Several capillaries with open lumina can be seen in this section ⇾. *(Right)* Continuous-type capillaries account for the blood-brain barrier, which limits solute exchange in CNS circulation. As with other capillaries, endothelial cells ⇾ and supporting pericytes ⇾ are seen by light microscopy.

CAPILLARIES, VEINS, AND LYMPHATICS

Fenestrations in Glomerular Capillaries

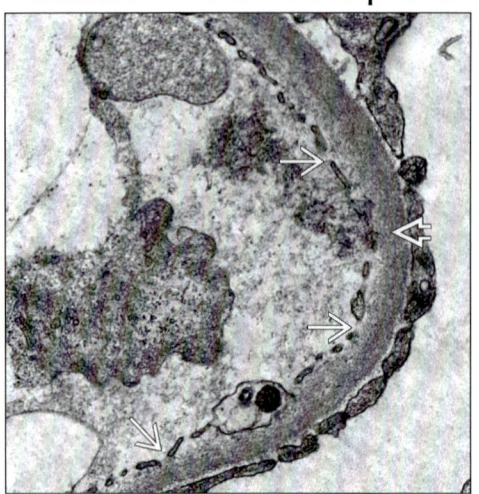

(Left) This electron micrograph shows glomerular capillary fenestrated endothelium. Endothelial cytoplasm forms a discontinuous "dashed" line to the left of the glomerular basement membrane ➡. The clear spaces (pores) ➡ between the cytoplasm allow free communication with the extracellular compartment.

Comparison of Vein, Lymphatic, and Artery

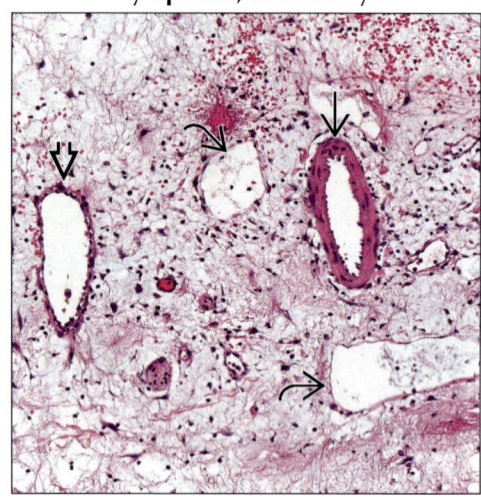

(Right) This photograph of adjacent vein ➡, lymphatics ➡, and artery ➡ in cross section highlights their structural differences.

Medium-Sized Vein and Artery

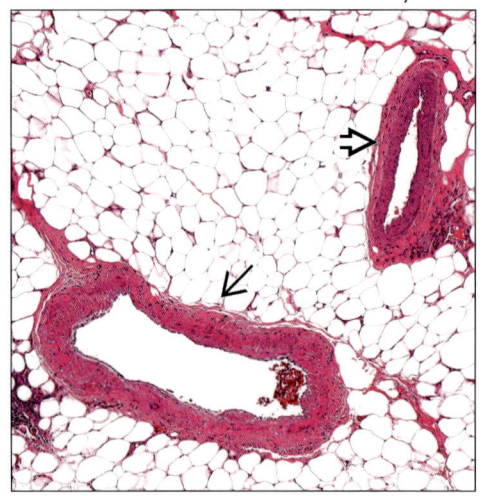

(Left) This section contains a medium-sized vein ➡ and accompanying artery ➡. Veins lack an internal elastic lamina and have thinner, less orderly medial smooth muscle. The vein adventitia is the most prominent layer, and most adventitial bundles are oriented longitudinally.

Small Vein and Muscular Artery

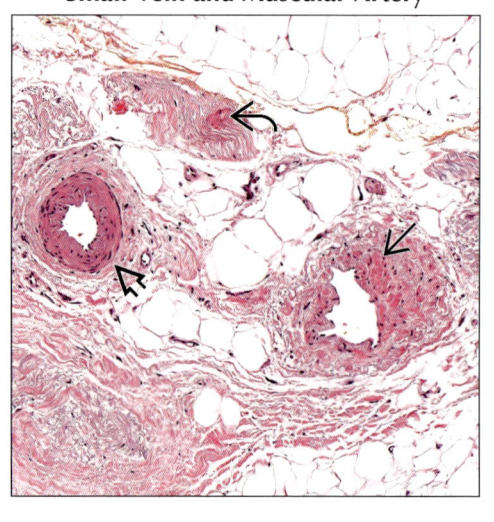

(Right) This vein ➡ has an irregular lumen profile and prominent longitudinal adventitial collagen bundles. An artery is next to it for comparison ➡. A nerve is also seen in this "neurovascular bundle" ➡.

High Endothelial Venule (Longitudinal Section)

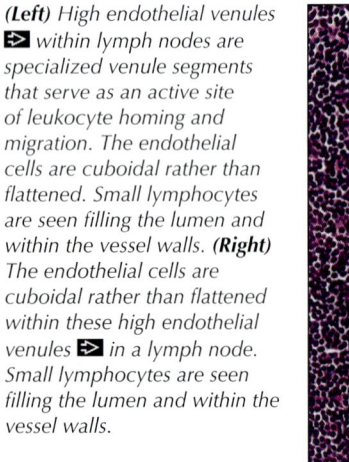

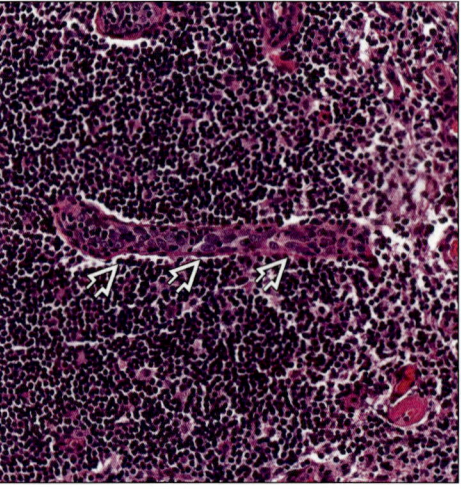

(Left) High endothelial venules ➡ within lymph nodes are specialized venule segments that serve as an active site of leukocyte homing and migration. The endothelial cells are cuboidal rather than flattened. Small lymphocytes are seen filling the lumen and within the vessel walls.

High Endothelial Venules (Cross Section)

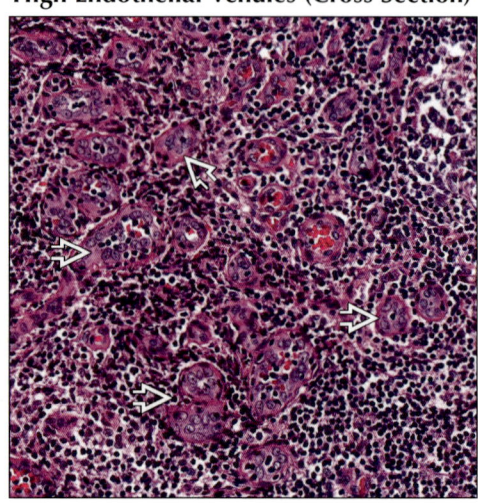

(Right) The endothelial cells are cuboidal rather than flattened within these high endothelial venules ➡ in a lymph node. Small lymphocytes are seen filling the lumen and within the vessel walls.

CAPILLARIES, VEINS, AND LYMPHATICS

Lymphatic Vessels

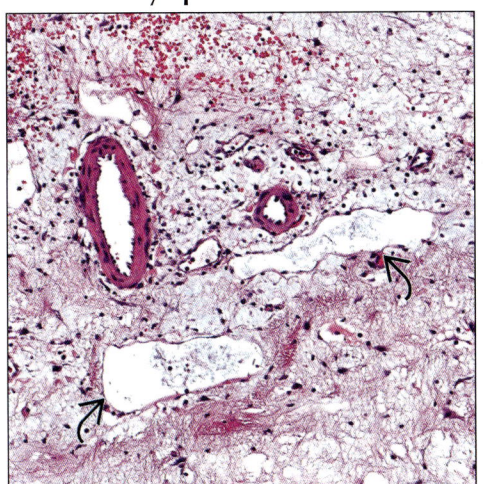

Pulmonary Vein

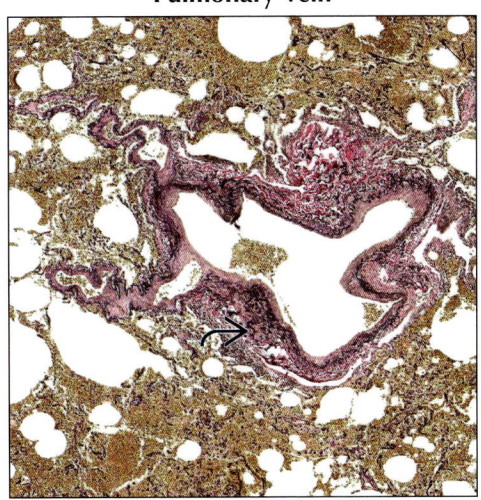

(Left) Two dilated lymphatic vessels ⇨ are seen within organizing granulation tissue. Lymphatics are composed of a single layer of endothelial cells with minimal supporting connective tissue. There is little to no muscular medial wall. They often have irregular luminal contours. *(Right)* Veins in the lung are recognized by the absence of an accompanying airway. No internal elastic lamina is seen. The adventitial elastic fibers ⇨ are coarse and poorly organized.

Pulmonary Venules and Lymphatics

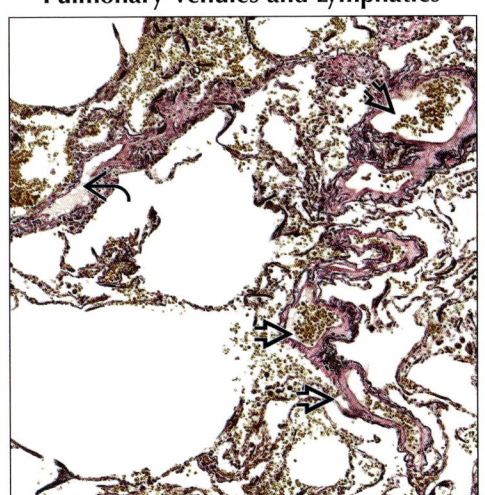

Pulmonary Lymphatics

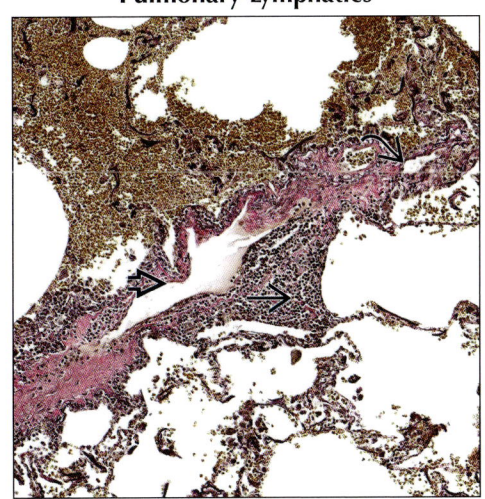

(Left) Venules and lymphatics in the lung travel in the interlobular septa. Venules ⇨ have a better developed elastic adventitia and contain blood. Lymphatics ⇨ show more irregular luminal contours, thinner walls, and no luminal blood cells. *(Right)* This lymphatic channel ⇨ shows complex luminal branching and some associated extranodal lymphoid tissue ⇨. A small vein ⇨ is also present for comparison.

Arteriovenous Malformation

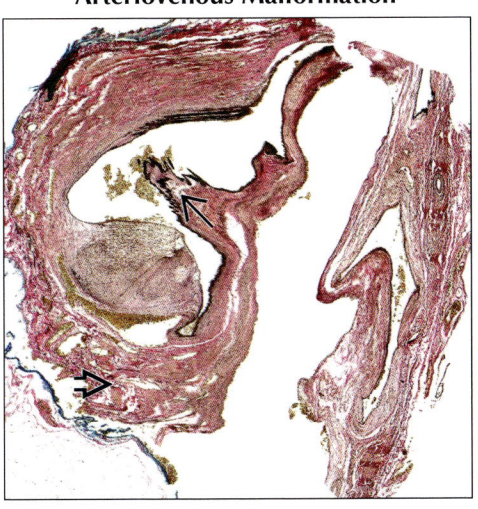

Arteriovenous Malformation

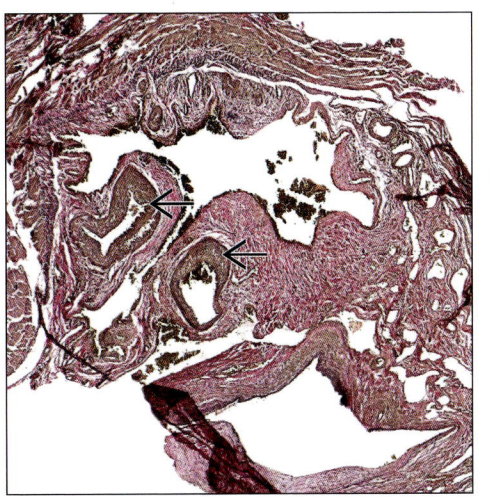

(Left) Hybrid vessel walls with arterial (internal elastic lamina ⇨) and venous (absent internal elastic lamina and prominent adventitial collagen and longitudinal smooth muscle ⇨) features are seen in this AVM. *(Right)* Irregular cavernous lumina and vessel walls showing venous features (absent internal elastic lamina and prominent adventitial bundles) are seen in this AVM. Disproportionately thick-walled vessels are also embedded in the walls of larger vessels ⇨.

SELECTED REFERENCES

HEART

1. Mehta RI et al: Hydrophilic polymer emboli: an under-recognized iatrogenic cause of ischemia and infarct. Mod Pathol. 23(7):921-30, 2010

2. Veinot JP et al: Light microscopy and ultrastructure of the blood vessels and heart. In Silver MB et al: Cardiovascular Pathology. Philadelphia: Churchill Livingstone. 30-53, 2001

3. Billingham ME: Normal heart. In Sternberg SS: Histology for Pathologists. 1st ed. New York: Raven Press. 215-30, 1992

CARDIAC VALVES

1. Schoen FJ: Cardiac valves and valvular pathology: update on function, disease, repair, and replacement. Cardiovasc Pathol. 14(4):189-94, 2005

2. Kitzman DW et al: Age-related changes in the anatomy of the normal human heart. J Gerontol. 45(2):M33-9, 1990

CARDIAC CONDUCTION SYSTEM

1. Anderson RH et al: The anatomy of the cardiac conduction system. Clin Anat. 22(1):99-113, 2009

2. Anderson RH et al: The architecture of the sinus node, the atrioventricular conduction axis, and the internodal atrial myocardium. J Cardiovasc Electrophysiol. 9(11):1233-48, 1998

3. Bharati S et al: The morphology of the AV junction and its significance in catheter ablation. Pacing Clin Electrophysiol. 12(6):879-82, 1989

4. Bharati S et al: Morphology of the sinus and atrioventricular nodes and their innervation. Prog Clin Biol Res. 275:3-14, 1988

ARTERIES

1. Heistad DD et al: Blood flow through vasa vasorum of coronary arteries in atherosclerotic monkeys. Arteriosclerosis. 6(3):326-31, 1986

2. The ageing aorta. Lancet. 2(8469-70):1402-3, 1985

3. Lie JT et al: Spectrum of aging changes in temporal arteries. Its significance, in interpretation of biopsy of temporal artery. Arch Pathol. 90(3):278-85, 1970

CAPILLARIES, VEINS, AND LYMPHATICS

1. Jackson DG: The lymphatics revisited: new perspectives from the hyaluronan receptor LYVE-1. Trends Cardiovasc Med. 13(1):1-7, 2003

2. Harmon JV Jr et al: Venous valves in subclavian and internal jugular veins. Frequency, position, and structure in 100 autopsy cases. Am J Cardiovasc Pathol. 1(1):51-4, 1987

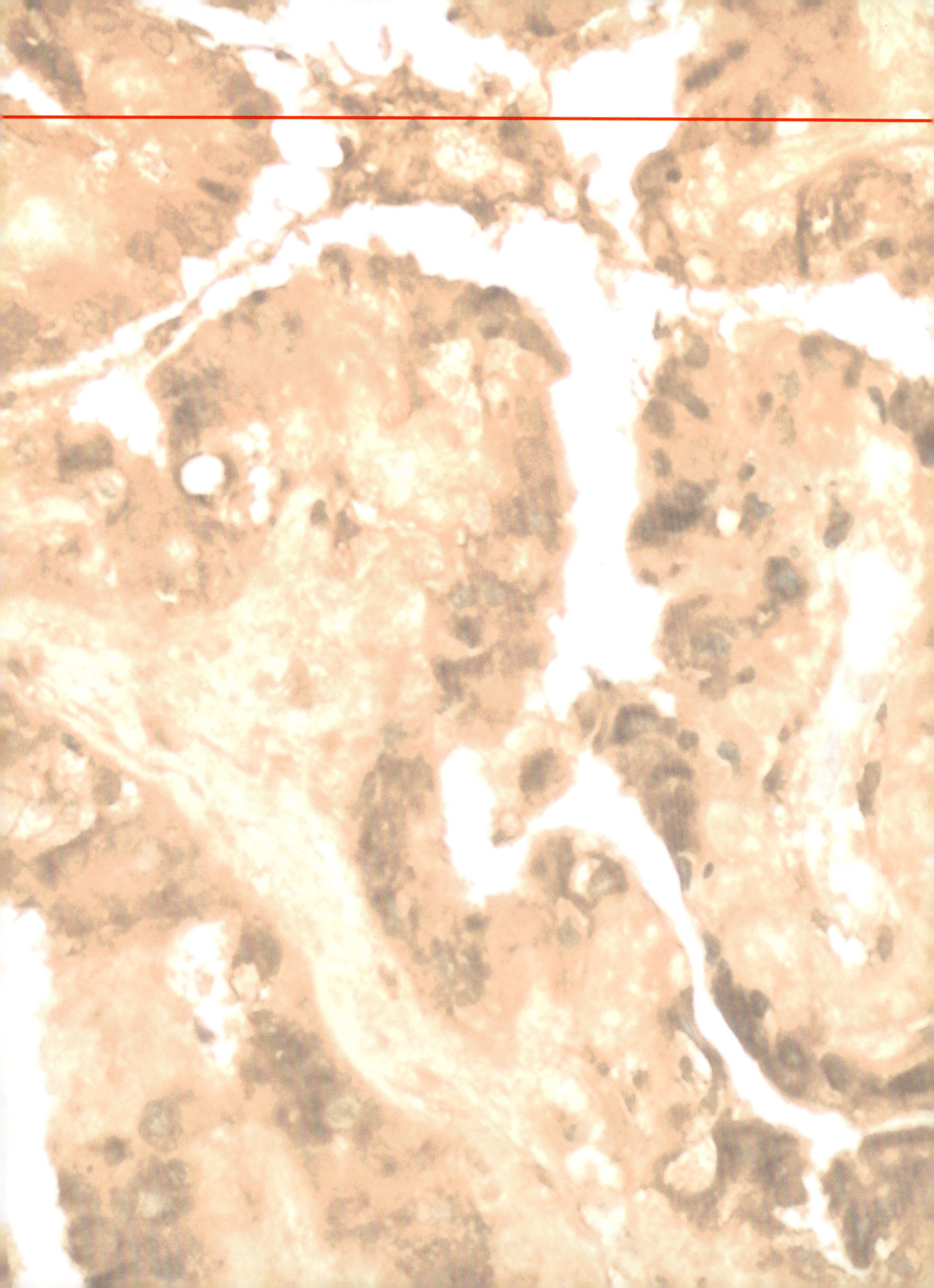

Nervous System

Peripheral Nervous System   5-2

Central Nervous System   5-6

Meninges   5-10

Choroid Plexus   5-12

PERIPHERAL NERVOUS SYSTEM

Key Facts

Macroscopic Anatomy
- Nerve trunks: Glistening grayish-white cords
- 12 cranial nerves and 31 spinal nerves
- Spinal nerves connected to spinal cord via 2 roots: Anterior (efferent/motor), posterior (afferent/sensory)
- Sensory cell bodies: In posterior (dorsal) root ganglion
- Motor cell bodies: SC anterior horn, brainstem nuclei
- Distally spinal nerves divide: Anterior + posterior rami
  - Supplying anterior and posterior parts of the body
  - Anterior rami-supplying limbs form nerve plexuses
  - Upper: Cervical, brachial; lower: Lumbar, sacral

Microscopic Anatomy
- Neuron/ganglion cell: Basic anatomic/functional unit
  - Highly specialized with complex morphology
- Perikaryon (soma): Large, spherical neuron cell body
  - Large euchromatic pale nuclei, prominent nucleoli
- Nissl substance: Basophilic material in cytoplasm
  - Granular endoplasmic reticulum and ribosomes
- Neurofibrils: Silver + neurofilaments, neurotubules
- Dendrites: Multiple branching short processes
  - Receive impulses and conduct to soma
- Axon: Single, slender, long; conducts away from soma
  - Axoplasmic flow and retrograde transport system
- Dense core granules present in nerve terminals

Non-neuronal (Satellite) Cells
- Schwann cells: Neural crest derived; S100 positive
  - Separated from endoneurium by basal lamina
- Perineurial cells: Fibroblast derived; EMA positive
  - Their tight junctions form perineurial barrier
- Endoneurial capillaries from vasa nervorum
  - Endothelium tight junctions (blood-nerve barrier)
- More than a few endoneurial leukocytes is abnormal

Peripheral Nerve Organization
- Peripheral nerve: Bundle of nerve fibers (CNS: Tract)
- Ganglion: Collection of neuron cell bodies, glial cells
  - Relay station during nerve impulse transmission
  - Autonomic or sensory, based on impulse direction
- Nerve fiber: Long process of a neuron (usually axon)
  - Grouped into fascicles by connective tissue sheaths
  - Myelinated (2-18 μm) and unmyelinated (0.2-3 μm)

- Myelin: Lipoprotein complex; insulating sheath
  - Pale, unstained halo around axon on H&E stains
  - Thickness of sheath proportional to axon diameter
- Nodes of Ranvier: Junctions (gaps) in myelination
  - Internodal segment myelinated by 1 Schwann cell
  - Variable number of fibers enveloped (5-20 axons)
  - Internodal distance increases with axon diameter
- Synapse: Specialized membranous contact (neurons)
  - Usually: Axon of 1 to the dendrites of another

Types of Neurons
- Based on axon/dendrite configuration (polarity)
  - Multipolar: Several branching dendrites, 1 axon, polygonal (stellate-pyramidal) soma
  - Unipolar (pseudounipolar): Single T-shaped process branches into axon/dendrites; rare (in ganglia)
  - Bipolar: Single dendrite and single axon at opposite poles of spindle-shaped soma; rare (retina, cochlea)
- Based on axon length (Golgi types)
  - Type I: Extensive dendrites, long axon forms nerve
  - Type II: Short axons; interneurons in CNS pathways
- Based on stimulus direction (motor vs. sensory)
  - Motor: Control effector organs (muscles, glands)
  - Sensory: Receive stimuli from environment

Connective Tissue Sheaths
- Endoneurium: Delicate connective tissue, few cells
  - Surrounds each individual nerve fiber
- Perineurium: Multilayered concentric cells, collagen
  - Encloses each fiber bundle/fascicle
  - Fuses to form sensory endings, motor endplate
  - Blends with pia-arachnoid
- Epineurium: Dense fibrous connective tissue
  - Envelops main nerve trunk (several bundles)
  - Merges with surrounding adipose tissue
  - Continuous with dura mater

Pitfalls/Artifacts
- Crush injury/artifact resembles axonal degeneration
- Electrocautery/thermal artifact may mimic infarction
- Crushed vessels mistaken for healed/fibrotic vasculitis
- Fixation in hyperosmolar solution causes shrinkage
  - Empty space around neurons mistaken for atrophy

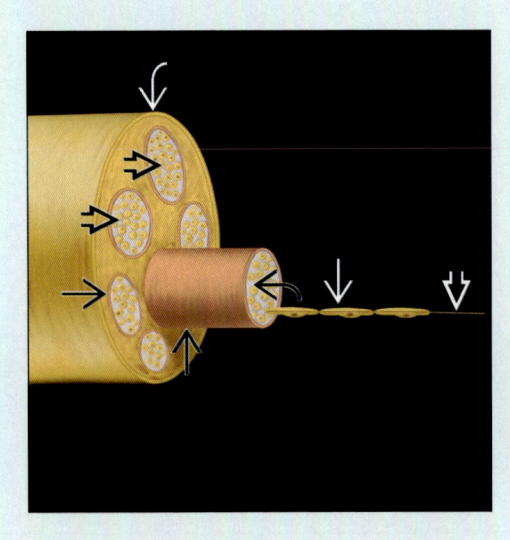

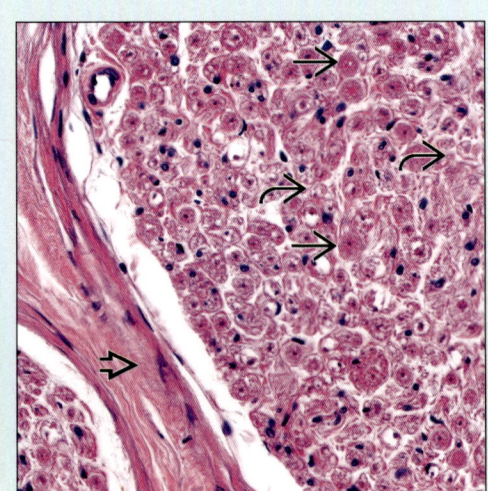

(Left) Each axon ⇨ is surrounded by myelin-producing Schwann cells ⇨ and covered by endoneurium ⇨. Multiple axons are grouped into fascicles ⇨, each covered by perineurium ⇨. Several fascicles together are bound by epineurium ⇨, forming the main nerve trunk. *(Right)* High-power view of peripheral nerve cross section shows individual fibers (axons) ⇨ in parallel arrays, surrounded by endoneurium ⇨ and bundled into fascicles covered by perineurium ⇨. (Courtesy P. Burger, MD.)

PERIPHERAL NERVOUS SYSTEM

Normal Peripheral Nerve

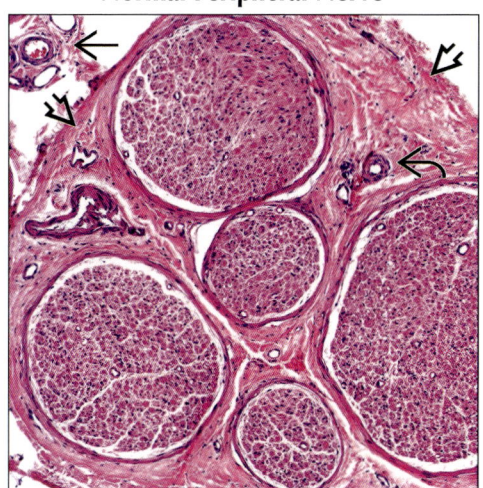

Normal Peripheral Nerve

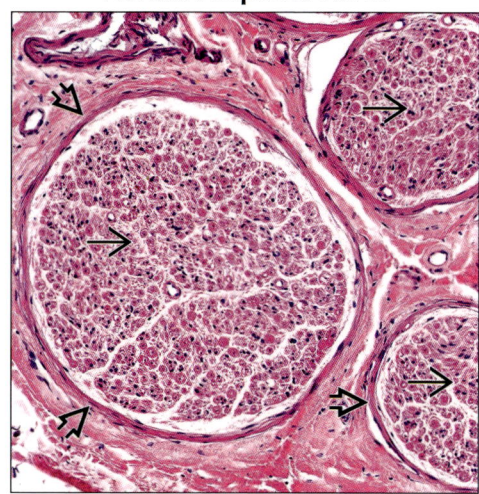

(Left) Each main nerve trunk is enveloped by epineurium ➔, the outer layer of dense fibrous connective tissue that merges with surrounding fibroadipose tissue ➔. Blood vessels ➔ (vasa nervorum) pass through this epineurium to reach the nerves. *(Courtesy P. Burger, MD.)* *(Right)* Peripheral nerves are composed of multiple bundles (or fascicles) ➔, each enclosed by perineurium ➔. *(Courtesy P. Burger, MD.)*

Normal Peripheral Nerve

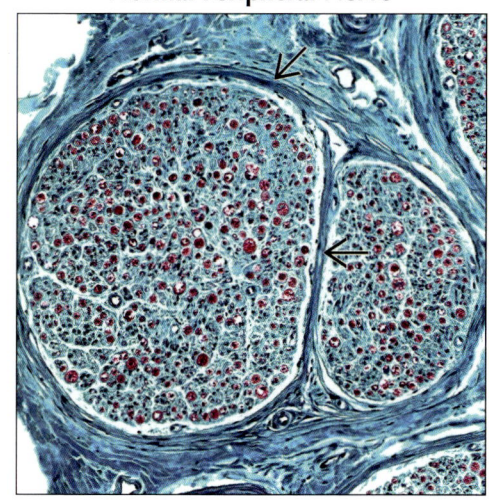

Normal Peripheral Nerve

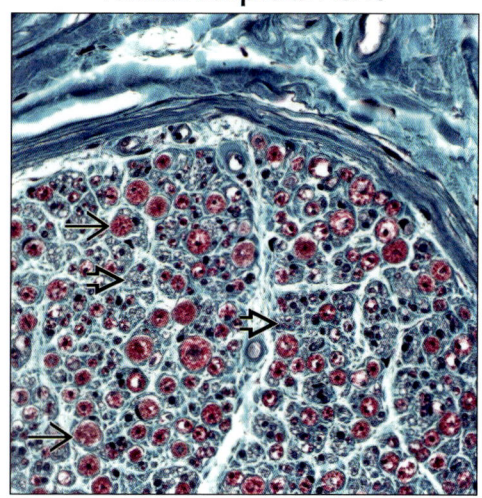

(Left) Peripheral nerve axons are red on trichrome stain and connective tissue is blue-green. Perineurium ➔, composed of multiple concentric layers of flattened cells and collagen, surrounds each bundle/fascicle. *(Courtesy P. Burger, MD.)* *(Right)* The individual nerve fibers stain red ➔ and the endoneurium ➔ is blue-green. Endoneurium is composed of satellite cells and fine connective tissue that extends around and between each individual nerve fiber. *(Courtesy P. Burger, MD.)*

Dorsal Spinal Root (Sensory) Ganglion

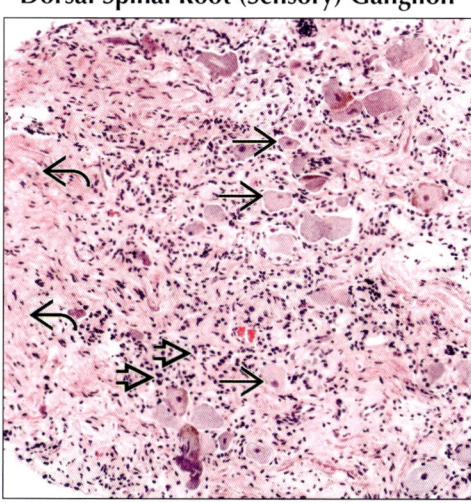

Dorsal Spinal Root (Sensory) Ganglion

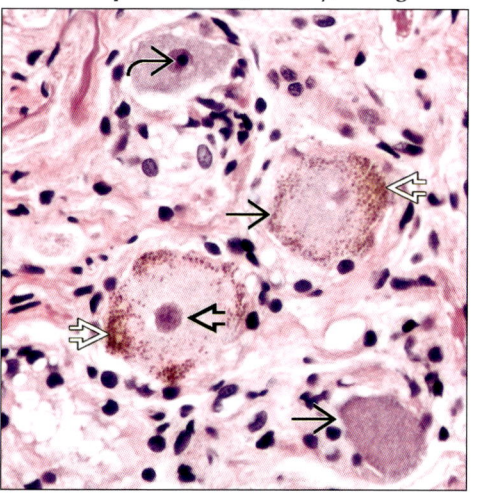

(Left) A section from the dorsal root ganglion (T10 level) shows clusters of neuronal cell bodies ➔. The surrounding smaller, darker nuclei ➔ belong to satellite cells. The longitudinal bundles of nerve fibers ➔ belong to the spinal nerve associated with this ganglion. *(Right)* This high-power view shows large spherical perikarya ➔ with large, pale, centrally located nuclei ➔ and prominent nucleoli ➔. Brown-blue Nissl substance ➔ can be seen in the cytoplasm.

PERIPHERAL NERVOUS SYSTEM

Normal Peripheral Nerve

(Left) The perineurium ⇒ around this single, small nerve fascicle is composed of collagen and spindle-shaped perineurial cells. The empty space ⇒ is due to fixation artifact and should not be mistaken for atrophy. Nuclei of non-neuronal satellite cells ⇒ in the endoneurium mostly belong to Schwann cells. **(Right)** A trichrome-stained section of a nerve fascicle shows axons and myelin sheaths in red ⇒ and the delicate connective tissue of endoneurium in blue ⇒.

Normal Peripheral Nerve

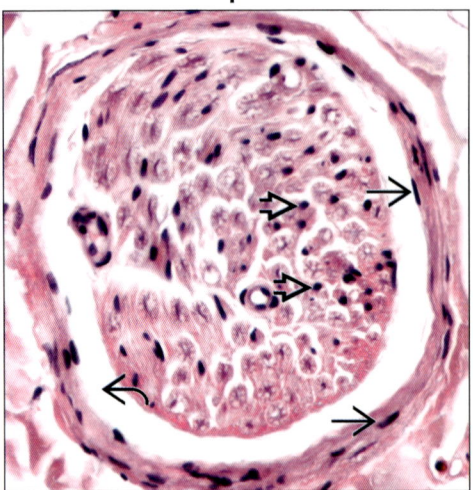

Normal Peripheral Nerve

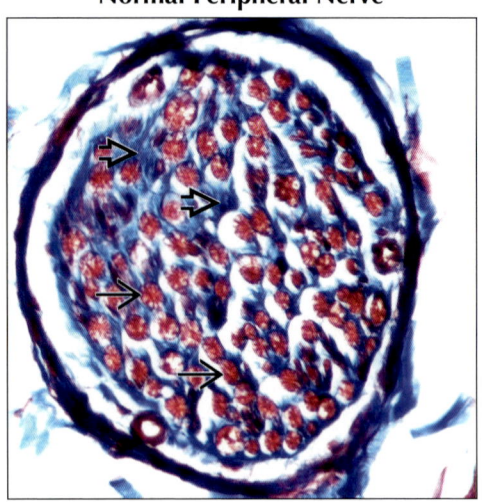

(Left) Immunohistochemical stain for neurofilament protein shows large, myelinated axons ⇒ that are strongly positive. The variable diameters of the staining axons reflect different amounts of myelin surrounding each nerve fiber/axon. Unmyelinated axons are very narrow and difficult to detect. **(Right)** The myelin stains dark blue in this toluidine blue-stained plastic section. A mixture of large- ⇒ and small- ⇒ diameter myelinated nerve fibers can be seen.

Normal Peripheral Nerve

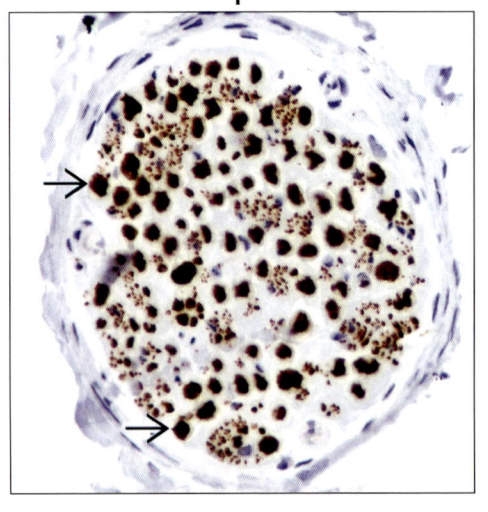

Normal Peripheral Nerve

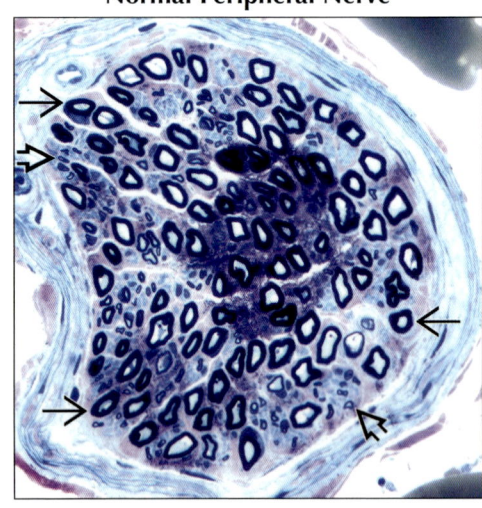

(Left) This Toluidine blue, longitudinal section shows nodes of Ranvier ⇒, seen as gaps in myelination. The internodal segment between is myelinated by a single Schwann cell. (Courtesy B. Scheithauer, MD.) **(Right)** Luxol-fast blue stains myelin ⇒ blue-cyan (seen here around large-diameter axons ⇒, which are stained black with a Bielschowsky stain). Small-diameter axons ⇒ are unmyelinated. This can identify demyelinating/remyelinating processes. (Courtesy B. Scheithauer, MD.)

Normal Peripheral Nerve

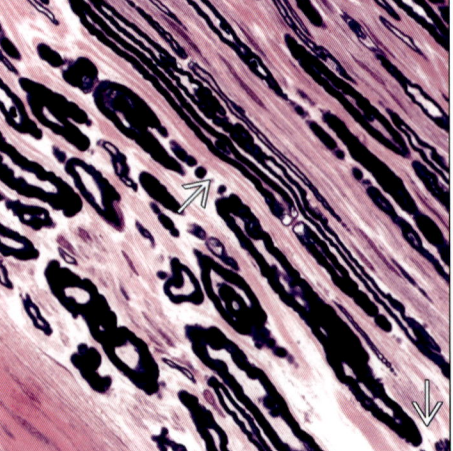

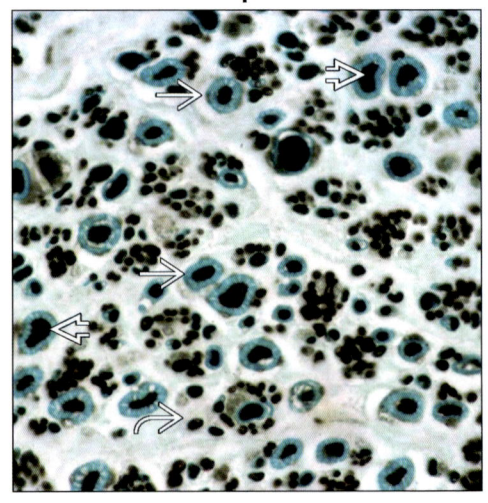

PERIPHERAL NERVOUS SYSTEM

Normal Peripheral Nerve

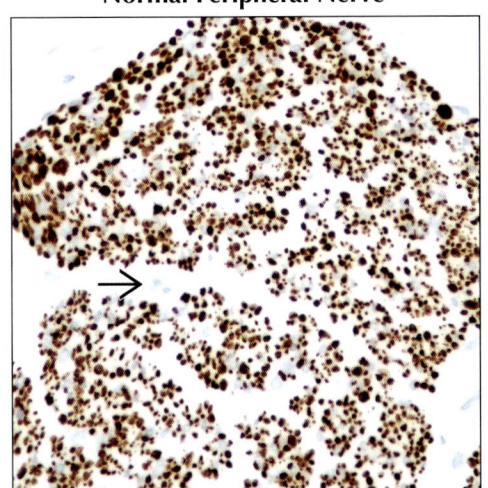

Normal Peripheral Nerve

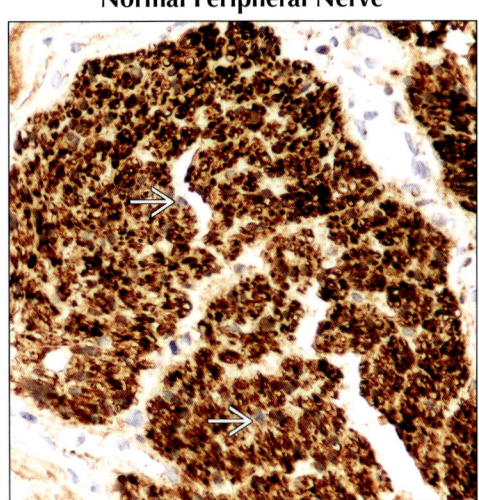

(Left) This medium-power neurofilament protein (NFP) stain shows a cross section of peripheral nerve with strongly positive fascicles of nerve fibers. The space ⇒ between fascicles represents perineurium. **(Right)** S100 protein shows Schwann cells staining strongly positive in the endoneurium, while surrounding nerve fibers ⇒ are negative.

Normal Peripheral Nerve

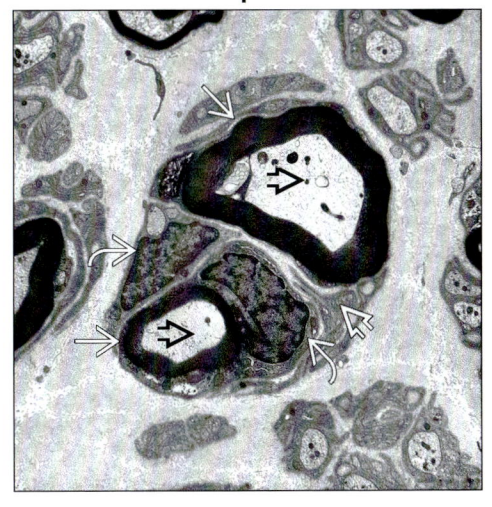

Myenteric Ganglionitis

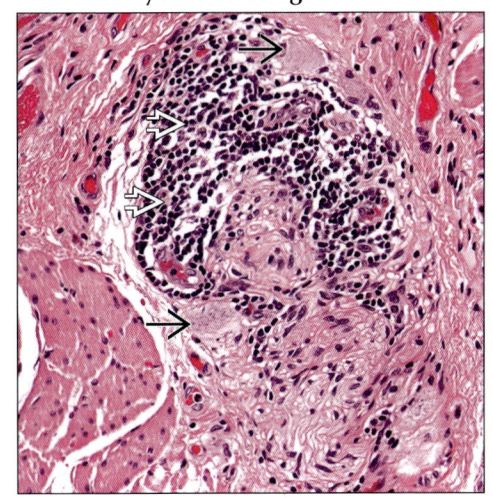

(Left) Axons ⇒ are surrounded by myelin sheaths ⇒ produced by Schwann cells. Schwann cell nuclei ⇒ and cytoplasm ⇒ with abundant endoplasmic reticulum are also seen. (Courtesy P. Boyer, MD, PhD.) **(Right)** This section from the colon wall shows Auerbach (myenteric) plexus, a collection of ganglion cells ⇒ in the enteric nervous system. Increased numbers of lymphocytes ⇒ as seen here are abnormal, but the cause is not always clear.

Peripheral Nerve Tumor

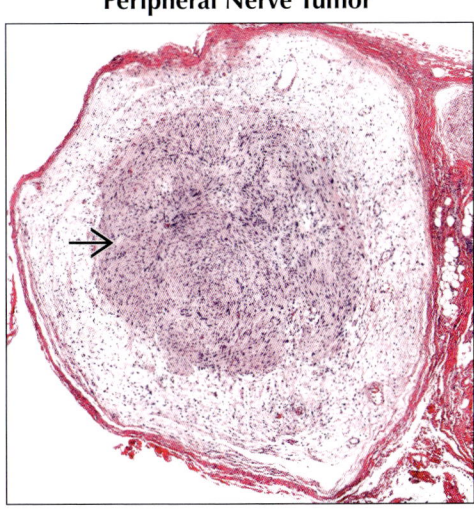

Peripheral Nerve Tumor

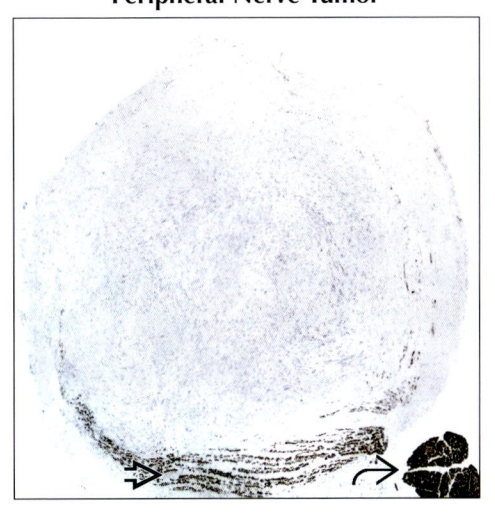

(Left) This cross section from a peripheral nerve shows a Schwannoma ⇒ in the center of the nerve trunk, displacing normal nerve fibers to the periphery. **(Right)** Neurofilament protein (NFP) staining shows a Schwannoma that does not stain, whereas the peripherally displaced normal nerve fibers ⇒ as well as a neighboring nerve ⇒ are both positive.

CENTRAL NERVOUS SYSTEM

Key Facts

Macroscopic Anatomy: Brain
- Supratentorial components (over tentorium cerebelli)
  - Cerebrum: Frontal, parietal, temporal, occipital lobes
  - Cerebral cortex has 6 layers: Molecular, external granular, external pyramidal, internal granular, internal pyramidal, polymorphic/multiform
  - Subcortical white matter: Projection fibers (connect cortex to and from subcortical nuclei), commissural fibers (axons that cross between hemispheres)
  - Fissures/sulci separate gyri/lobes: Sylvian fissure/lateral sulcus (temporal from frontal/parietal), longitudinal cerebral fissure (left/right hemispheres)
  - Deep basal ganglia nuclei (caudate, putamen, globus pallidus); diencephalon (thalamus, hypothalamus)
- Infratentorial components (posterior fossa contents)
  - Cerebellum: Superior, middle, and inferior peduncles
  - Cerebellar cortex has 3 layers (outer hypocellular molecular, central Purkinje cell, inner/deep granular)
  - Brainstem (midbrain, pons, medulla): Cranial nerve motor nuclei, sensory nuclei, and autonomic nuclei
- Ventricular system: Hollow chambers/connections that contain CSF (2 lateral, 3rd, 4th ventricles)

Macroscopic Anatomy: Spinal Cord
- Central, H-shaped gray matter horns
  - Posterior/dorsal: Sensory input (dorsal root ganglia)
  - Anterior/ventral: Motor neurons to spinal nerves
  - Lateral autonomic (intermediolateral cell columns)
- Surrounding white matter fiber bundles (funiculi)
  - Thickest in cervical SC (ascending/descending fibers)
  - Terminus (filum terminale): Mostly meningeal tissue
- Central canal: Ependyma-lined neural tube remnant

Microscopic Anatomy
- Gray matter: Rich in neuronal and glial cell bodies
- Neuropil: Hypocellular, finely fibrillar meshwork of unmyelinated neuronal and astrocytic cell processes
- Nuclei: Circumscribed aggregates of nerve cell bodies
- Glial cells: Structural/metabolic support, protection
- White matter: Compact bundles (tracts, fascicles) of myelinated axons and supporting oligodendrocytes
- CNS lacks connective tissue and lymphoid elements

- **Neuron (nerve cell)**: Anatomical/functional unit
  - Receive, process, store, transmit information/stimuli
  - Mature neurons: Postmitotic; incapable of division
- Cell body (perikaryon): Spherical, ovoid, or angular
  - Size: 5-10 μm (granular) to 50-100 μm (Purkinje cells)
  - Has microtubules, neurofilaments, prominent Golgi
  - Nissl substance: Granular basophilic areas (rough ER)
- Dendrites: Multiple short processes; receive stimuli
- Axon: Single long process; conducts downstream
  - Short (interneurons) to very long (upper motor)
  - Terminal arborization: End boutons form synapses
- Immunoreactivity for NFP, NeuN, synaptophysin
- Pigmented catecholaminergic neurons (substantia nigra, locus coeruleus): Cytoplasmic neuromelanin
- **Macroglia (neuroectoderm-derived)**
- **Astrocytes**: Most common; outnumber neurons 10:1
  - Protoplasmic: Many short processes; in gray matter
  - Fibrous: Few long processes; mostly in white matter
  - Processes toward neurons (metabolic support), subpial/subependymal (blood-brain-CSF barrier)
  - Cytoplasmic intermediate filament protein (GFAP)
  - Round-oval nuclei (10 μm); Even, pale chromatin
- **Oligodendroglia (oligodendrocytes)**
  - Wrap around/myelinate numerous axon internodes
  - Small round nucleus (8 μm), dense chromatin
  - Perinuclear "halo": Artifactual rim of clear cytoplasm
  - Accumulate around neurons ("neuronal satellitosis")
- **Ependyma**: Epithelioid cuboidal/low columnar cells
  - Line ventricular system (form brain-CSF barrier)
  - Pale vesiculated nucleus (8 μm) on abluminal side
  - Ciliated/microvillous border on ventricular side
- **Microglia**: Mesoderm-derived resident macrophages
  - Small elongated cells with short processes, thin rod nuclei (5-10 μm); express phagocytic marker CD68

Age Variation
- Neurons accumulate substances with increasing age
  - Yellow-brown intracytoplasmic lipofuscin
  - Neurofibrillary tangles, plaques, Hirano bodies
  - Marinesco bodies: Bright red intranuclear inclusions
- Astrocytes accumulate corpora amylacea in processes
  - Spherical inclusion bodies of glucose polymers

(Left) Midline sagittal brain section (medial view) shows the frontal ➡, parietal ➡, and occipital ➡ lobes of the cerebral hemispheres, as well as the cerebellum ➡, pons ➡, and medulla ➡. (Courtesy M. Nielsen, MS.) *(Right)* Inferior view shows the 2 cerebellar hemispheres ➡, beginning of spinal cord ➡, pons ➡, and optic chiasm ➡. The longitudinal cerebral fissure ➡ separates left from right cerebral hemispheres, here at the level of frontal lobes ➡. (Courtesy M. Nielsen, MS).

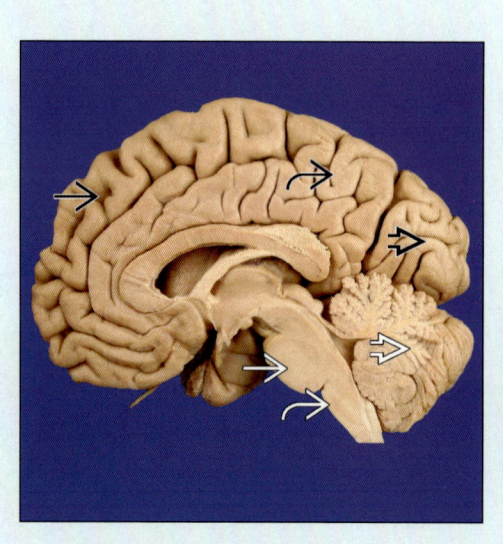

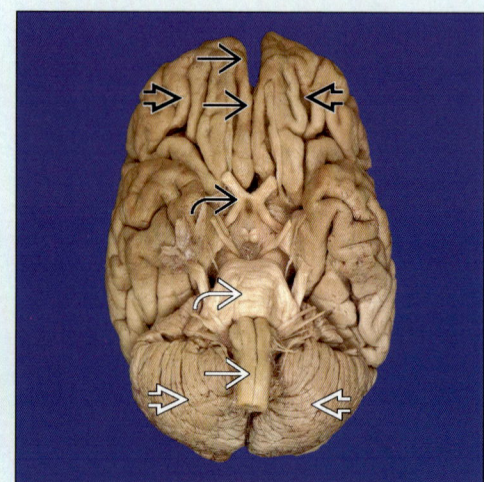

CENTRAL NERVOUS SYSTEM

Coronal Brain Section

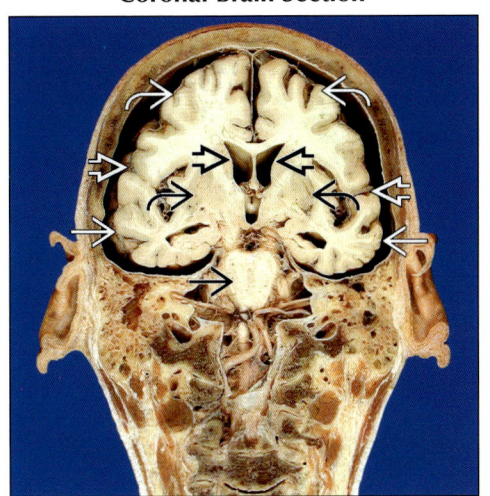

Cerebral Cortex Layers

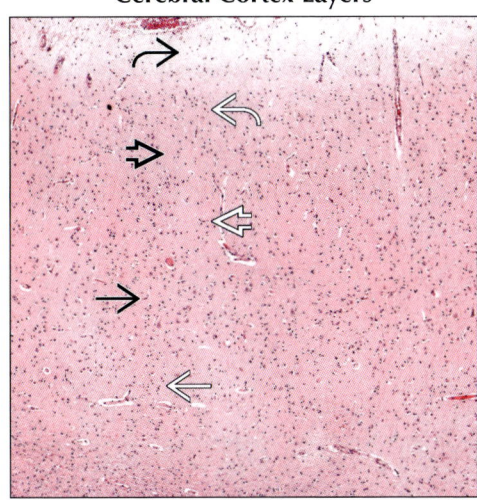

(Left) Anterior view of coronal head section shows the Sylvian fissure or lateral sulcus ➔, separating temporal ➔ from frontal ➔ lobes. Also seen are the paired lateral ventricles ➔, deep nuclei of basal ganglia ➔ and pons ➔. *(Courtesy M. Nielsen, MS.)* *(Right)* This photo shows the 6 layers of the cerebral cortex between the pia mater (top) and subcortical white matter (bottom left): Molecular ➔, external granular ➔, external pyramidal ➔, internal granular ➔, internal pyramidal ➔, and polymorphic or multiform ➔.

Cerebral Cortex Cells

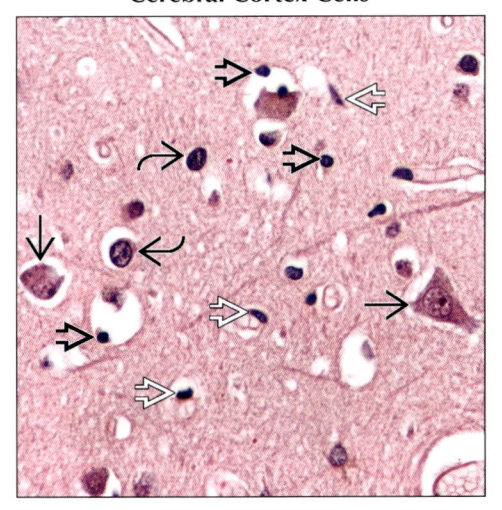

Cerebellar Cortex Layers

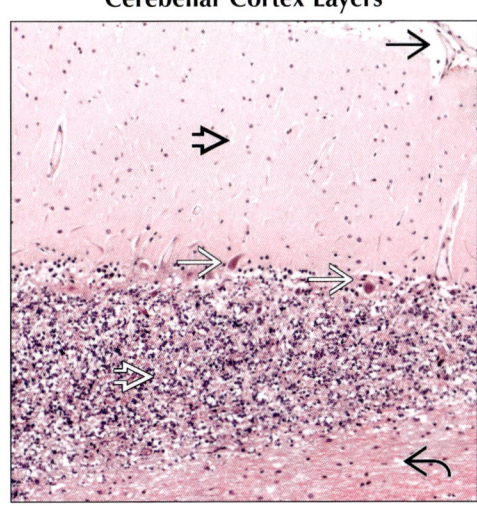

(Left) The cellular components of the cerebral cortex (and all of the CNS) include neurons ➔, astrocytes ➔, oligodendrocytes ➔, and microglia ➔. *(Right)* This view shows the 3 layers of the cerebellar cortex between surface pia mater ➔ and the white matter ➔ of cerebellar medulla: Outer hypocellular molecular layer ➔, middle/central Purkinje cell layer ➔, and inner/deep hypercellular granular cell layer ➔. The small cells of the latter are difficult to recognize histologically as classic neurons.

Purkinje Cell Layer

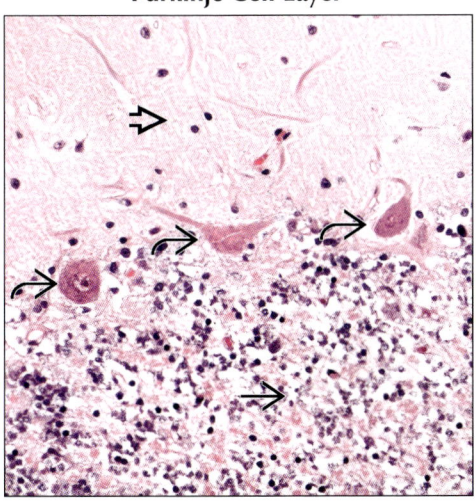

Purkinje Cell

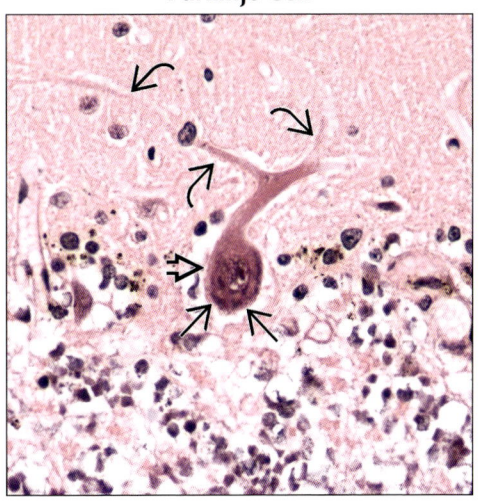

(Left) The intermediate lamina of the cerebellar cortex consists of a single cell layer of Purkinje cells ➔, sitting between the outer, relatively hypocellular molecular layer ➔, and the inner, densely populated granular cell layer ➔. *(Right)* Purkinje cells in the cerebellar cortex are composed of a large (50 μm) nerve cell body (perikaryon) ➔ with a prominent vesicular nucleus, granular basophilic Nissl bodies/substance ➔, and a dendritic arbor ➔ that extends deep into the molecular layer.

CENTRAL NERVOUS SYSTEM

Cervical Spinal Cord

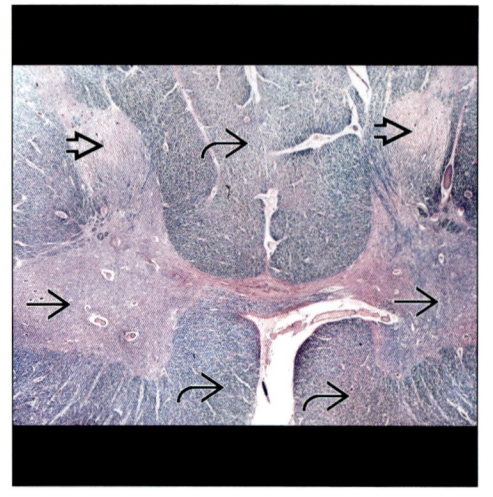

Thoracic Spinal Cord

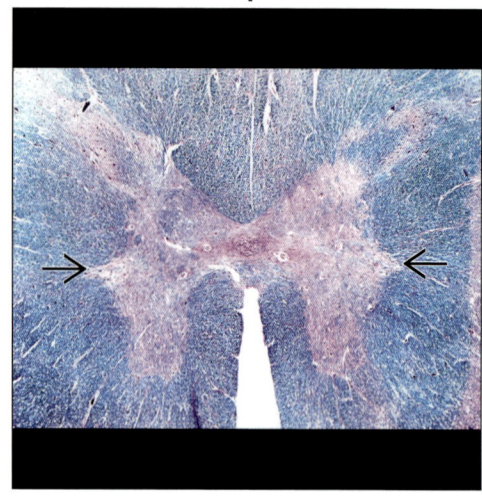

(Left) Cross section of cervical spinal cord shows large anterior/ventral horns ⇨ of gray matter containing motor neurons that innervate upper extremities. Posterior/dorsal horns ⇨ get sensory input from dorsal root ganglia. Funiculi of white matter fibers ⇨ are thickest here (largest number of ascending and descending tracts). **(Right)** Thoracic cord has smaller anterior/posterior horns, but also contains the lateral horns ⇨ of the intermediolateral cell column (sympathetic autonomic) neurons.

Lumbosacral Spinal Cord

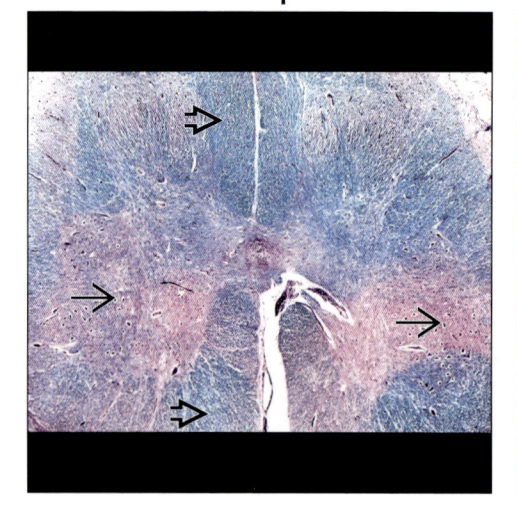

Spinal Cord, Central Canal

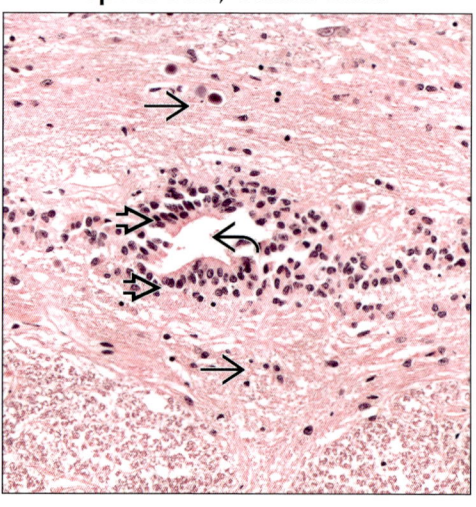

(Left) Lumbosacral spinal cord has very large anterior/ventral gray matter horns ⇨ that house motor neurons supplying the lower extremities. White matter tracts ⇨ are thinner here, as small numbers of ascending tracts have joined. **(Right)** The central canal of the spinal cord is lined (as is the ventricular system) by ciliated cuboidal/columnar ependyma cells ⇨. The lumen ⇨, often obliterated in adults, contains CSF. Surrounding gray matter ⇨ is part of the gray commissure.

Spinal Cord Gray Matter

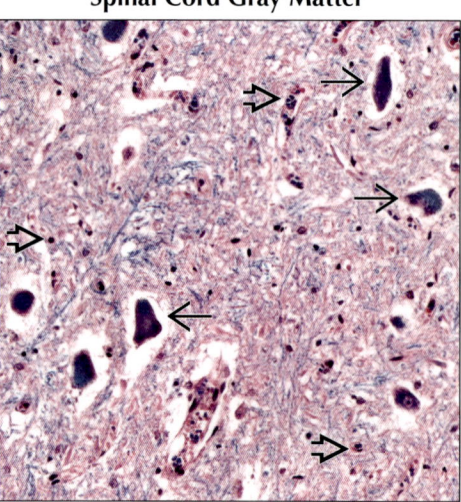

Spinal Cord White Matter

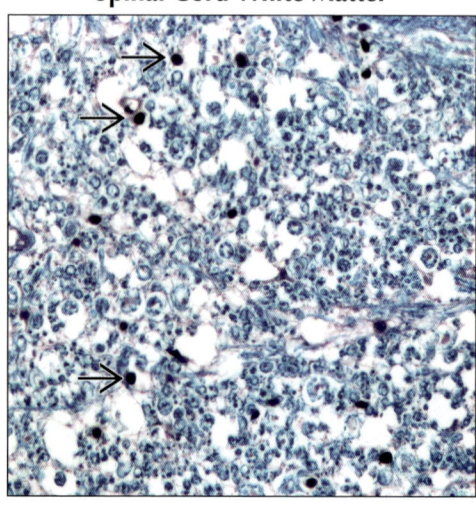

(Left) Spinal cord gray matter contains multiple neuronal cell bodies ⇨ and nuclei of various supporting glial cells ⇨ amid the finely fibrillar background of the neuropil meshwork. The latter is composed of unmyelinated (negative in this Luxol fast blue stain) neuritic and astrocytic cell processes. **(Right)** Luxol fast blue stain highlights the blue myelinated axons of neurons in the white matter of the cord (and CNS), and the small dense round nuclei of oligodendrocytes ⇨ that produce this myelin sheath.

CENTRAL NERVOUS SYSTEM

White Matter Axons

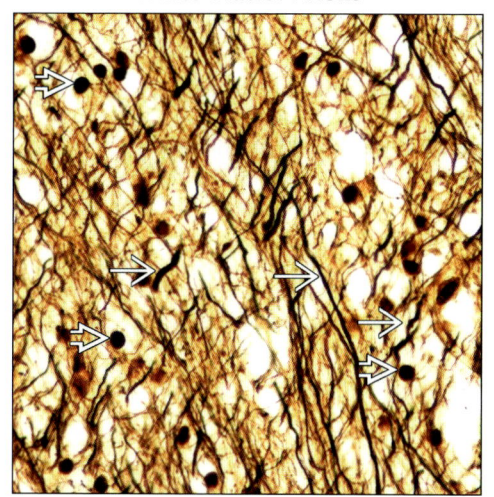

GFAP-Positive Astrocyte

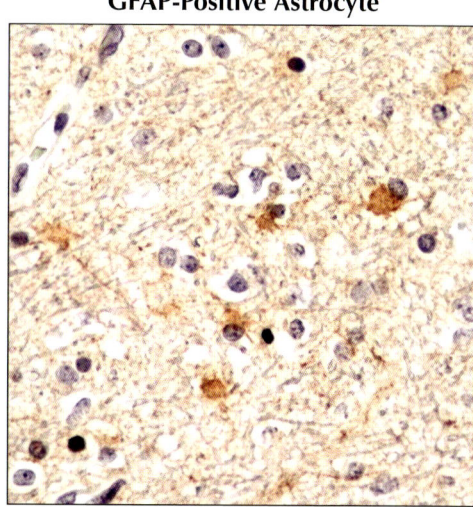

(Left) High-power view of a Bielschowsky silver stain highlights the argyrophilic (silver-positive) long axonal processes ⇨ of neurons in largely uniform white matter, peppered by the nuclei of myelinating oligodendroglia ⇨. *(Right)* High-power view of an immunohistochemical stain for glial fibrillary acidic protein (GFAP) highlights immunoreactive astrocytes with "star-shaped" cytoplasm, round pale nuclei, and multiple processes.

Synaptophysin-Positive Neuron

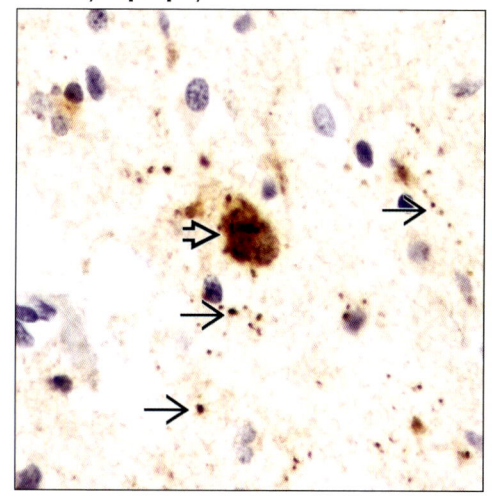

Substantia Nigra Neurons

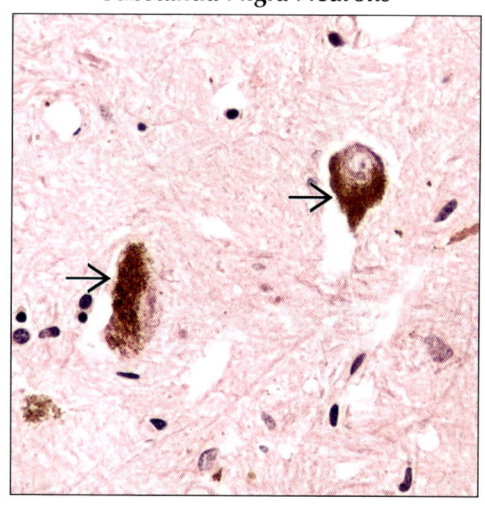

(Left) Synaptophysin is a widely used marker of neuronal differentiation that is found in synaptic vesicles, and thus highlights the nerve cell body ⇨ and proximal dendrites of a large neuron in a punctate pattern. In the background neuropil, diffuse, finely granular staining ⇨ indicates synaptic contacts. *(Right)* Pigmented catecholaminergic neurons of the brainstem (substantia nigra in midbrain, locus coeruleus in the pons) contain neuromelanin, seen as coarse dark brown cytoplasmic granules ⇨.

Lipofuscin Accumulation

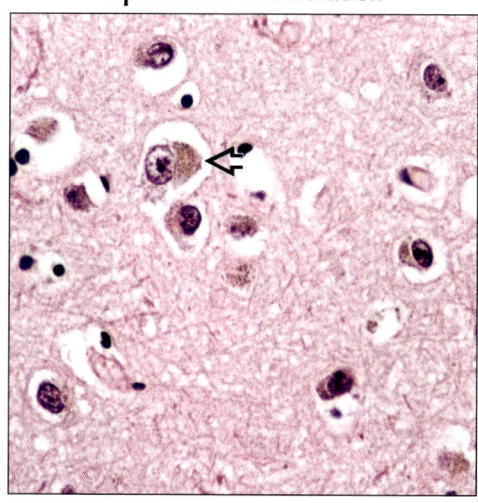

Senile (Neuritic) Plaque

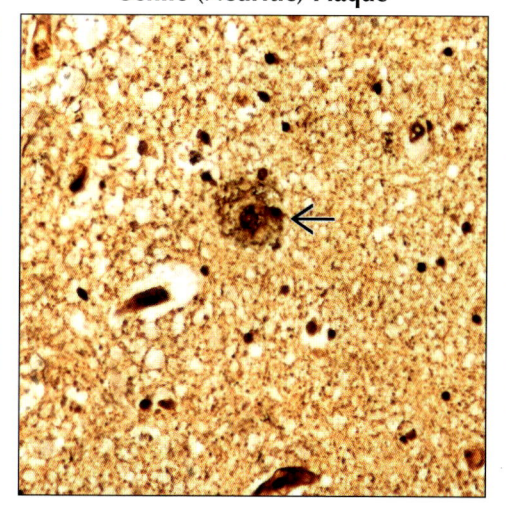

(Left) Lipofuscin ⇨ (lipochrome or "wear and tear" pigment) is a pale, yellow-brown cytoplasmic accumulation seen with age in neurons, and often peripherally displaces nucleus and organelles. *(Right)* Bielschowsky silver stain shows a senile plaque ⇨, seen in the aging brain as an ill-defined round cluster of extracellular granular material (abnormal neurites) that alters the smooth fibrillarity of background neuropil and causes nearby axons to disperse. Mature plaques are visible on H&E and acquire a central eosinophilic core that is positive for amyloid.

MENINGES

Key Facts

Macroscopic Anatomy
- Meninges consist of 3 separate layers of connective tissue membranes that envelop the central nervous system (CNS)
  - Dura mater, arachnoid mater, and pia mater
  - Leptomeninges = arachnoid and pia
- Dura mater (pachymeninx, meninx fibrosa)
  - Tough outermost layer
  - Composed of 2 tightly juxtaposed or fused layers of dense fibrous connective tissue that separate to form dural venous sinuses (major venous channels)
  - Outer (external) layer of dura is adherent to inner skull and functions as periosteum of cranium
  - Inner dura layer joins arachnoid to form infoldings that separate parts of the brain (falx cerebri, falx cerebelli, tentorium cerebelli, diaphragm sellae)
  - Inner dural layer penetrated by arachnoid villi, draining veins
  - Potential spaces: Epidural (between dura and cranium/vertebral canal); subdural (between dura and underlying leptomeninges)
- Arachnoid mater
  - Delicate, thin, continuous, and transparent membrane closely apposed to dura mater above
  - Wispy, web-like connective fibers (arachnoid trabeculae) adjoin arachnoid to underlying pia
  - Subarachnoid space (between pia and arachnoid): Contains CSF, superficial cerebral arteries and veins
  - Subarachnoid cisterns: Enlarged areas of subarachnoid space (e.g., cisterna magna), may contain in addition cranial nerves
- Pia mater
  - Internal delicate membrane covers brain surface, follows contours (gyri and sulci)
  - 2 closely attached layers
  - Outer layer (epipia): Covers CNS surface, coats all penetrating arterioles/venules until they become capillaries
  - Inner layer (intima pia): Closely apposed to peripheral astrocytic end processes (pia-glial limiting membrane)
  - Potential space: Subpial (between pia and underlying brain/spinal cord surface)

Microscopic Anatomy
- Dura mater
  - Elastic and dense collagen fibers arranged in laminae
  - Contains numerous blood vessels
  - Cerebral venous sinuses lined by endothelium
- Arachnoid mater
  - Composed of 2 layers (subdural and inner) of mesothelial cells
  - Compact central layer: Polygonal cells, round nuclei, pale cytoplasm
  - Desmosomes and intercellular tight junctions form barrier
  - Granulations: Small aggregates/clusters near intracranial venous sinuses
- Pia mater
  - Loose connective tissue: Collagen and elastic fibers
  - Thin sheet of flattened mesothelial cells with desmosomes and gap junctions

Pitfalls/Artifacts
- Arachnoiditis ossificans
  - White plaques covering dorsal leptomeninges of spinal cord (thoracic, lumbar, sacral)
  - Composed of laminated and hyalinized fibrous tissue
  - Incidental autopsy finding, no relevant clinical history
  - True mineralization occurs with prior symptomatic inflammation or trauma
- Leptomeningeal melanocytes
  - Normal cellular components of pia and arachnoid
  - Impart a brown discoloration grossly, especially over ventral midbrain

Age Variation
- Dura can fuse with skull in older individuals
- Nonspecific calcifications in dura increase with age
  - Also seen in chronic renal failure
- Arachnoid mater and granulations increase in size, thicken with advancing age due to collagen deposition

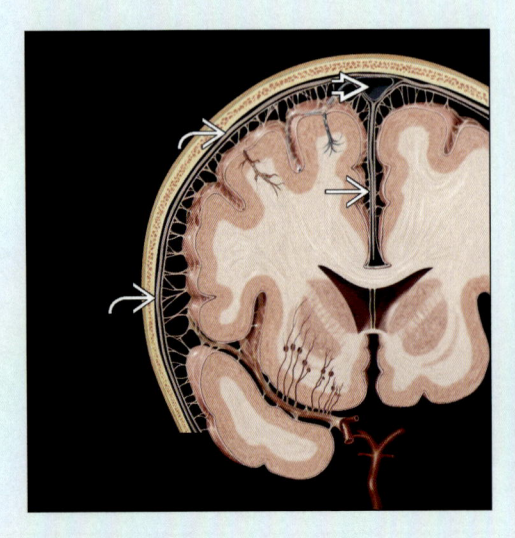

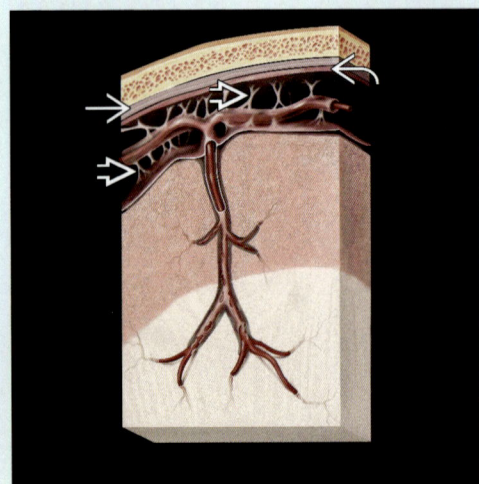

(Left) This coronal view shows the brain and cranial dura mater ⇒. The 2 layers (outer and inner) of the dura mater separate to form the superior sagittal sinus ⇒. The inner dural layer joins the underlying arachnoid to form the falx cerebri ⇒. (Right) The dense fibrous dura mater ⇒ overlies the delicate translucent arachnoid ⇒, which is closely attached to it. Web-like connective tissue fibers ⇒ (arachnoid trabeculae) join the arachnoid to the underlying pia mater.

MENINGES

Dura Mater

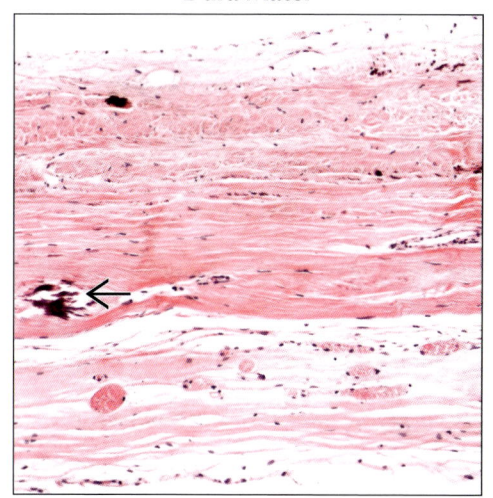

Superior Sagittal Sinus

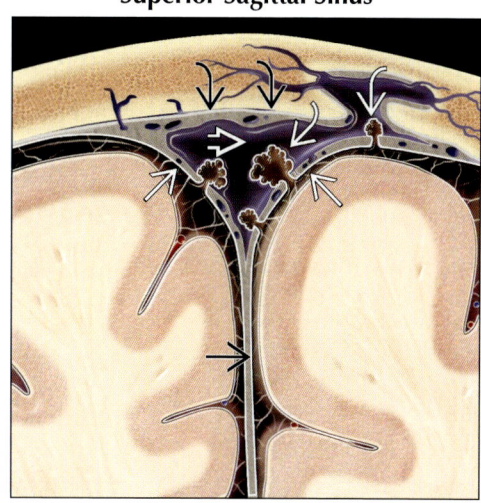

(Left) The dura mater is composed of dense fibrous connective tissue. The outer and inner layers are often fused and difficult to distinguish. Nonspecific calcifications ➔ can be seen, especially with increasing age. (Right) The superior sagittal sinus ➔ is a venous channel formed by the separation of the outer ➔ (periosteal) and inner ➔ (meningeal) dural layers. Arachnoid granulations ➔ are projections of the arachnoid-covered, CSF-containing subarachnoid space into the blood-filled venous sinus.

Arachnoid and Subarachnoid Space

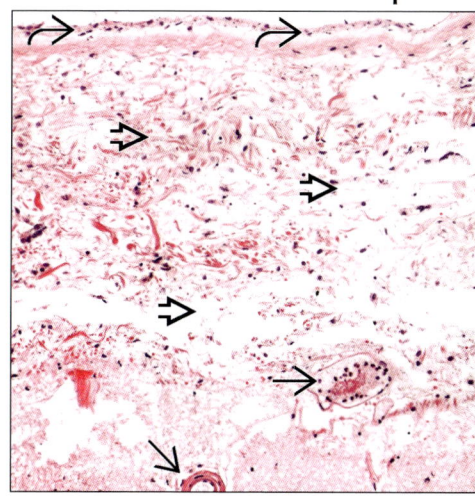

Leptomeninges

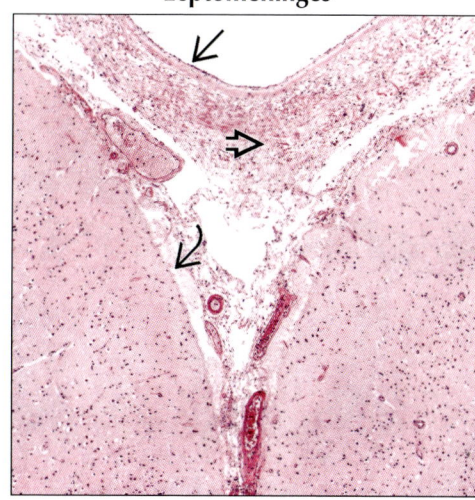

(Left) The subarachnoid space is a potential space found below the arachnoid membrane ➔ and occupied by CSF, superficial cerebral vessels ➔, and arachnoid trabeculae ➔ (connective tissue fibers between arachnoid and underlying pia). (Right) This low-power view illustrates the relationships between the arachnoid ➔ (thin layer of mesothelial cells), subarachnoid space ➔, and pia mater ➔ (delicate membrane covering the brain, adherent to gyri and sulci).

Pia Mater

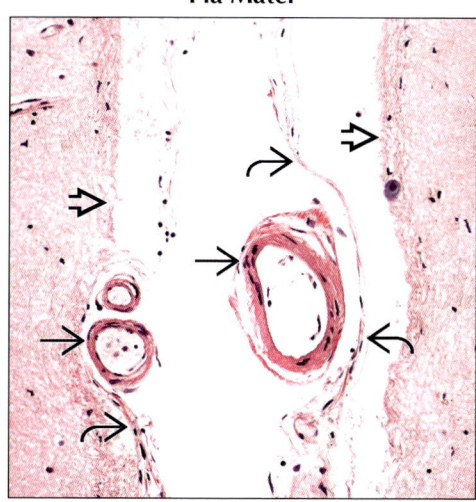

Arachnoid Cyst

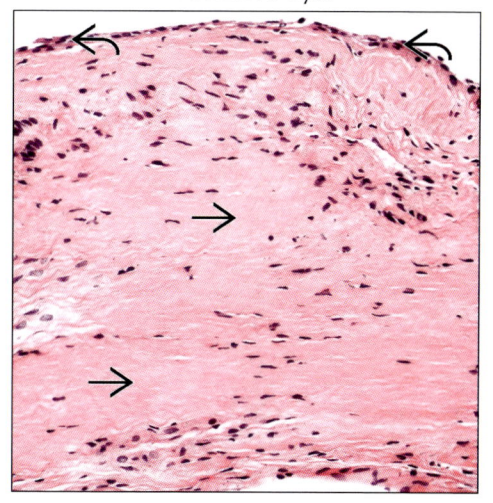

(Left) The pia mater is a delicate membrane ➔ that coats the brain surface ➔ as well as penetrating cerebral vessels ➔. The potential space between the pia mater and CNS surface is called the subpial space. (Right) Arachnoid cysts are usually congenital and asymptomatic. The arachnoid is replaced by dense fibrosis ➔, but the characteristic overlying single cell layer of mesothelium ➔ is still visible.

CHOROID PLEXUS

Key Facts

General Concepts
- Specialized vascular organ in ventricles of CNS
- Site of CSF production by choroid epithelial cells

Locations
- Lateral ventricles: Body, atrium, and temporal horns
- Roof of 3rd and 4th ventricles, foramina of Monro
- Cerebellopontine angle cisterns (subarachnoid)

Microscopic Anatomy
- Invaginated pia mater folds (vascular leptomeninges)
  - Papillary, frond-like processes project into ventricles
  - Loose tissue core of collagen, dilated blood vessels
  - Small nests of meningothelial (arachnoid) cells
- Covered by single layer of cuboidal/low columnar cells
  - Modified ependyma cells: Larger, hobnailed surface
  - Greatly increased surface area due to villi, microvilli
  - Tight intermediate junctions (blood-CSF barrier)

Pitfalls/Artifacts
- Biopsy tissue compression can mimic hypercellularity
  - Misinterpreted as choroid plexus papilloma
  - Normal choroid cells retain hobnail appearance
  - True papilloma is contrast-enhancing mass
- In unusual location or as "floater" by carryover
  - May be misinterpreted as metastatic carcinoma
  - Normal choroid plexus is not cytologically atypical

Age Variation
- Mineral salt deposition in connective tissue cores
  - Seen with increasing age; accounts for radiodensity
- Cytoplasmic vacuoles, cystic xanthomatous change
  - Common incidental finding with increasing age; no pathologic significance
- Choroid plexus cysts
  - Common, often in fetuses; some associated with aneuploidy (trisomy 18, 21)

(Left) This graphic shows the sites of choroid plexus in the brain, including the roof of the 3rd ➡ and 4th ➡ ventricles. *(Right)* This low-power view demonstrates the papillary architecture of the choroid plexus, characterized by frond-like processes of vascular leptomeningeal tissue that project into the ventricular lumen.

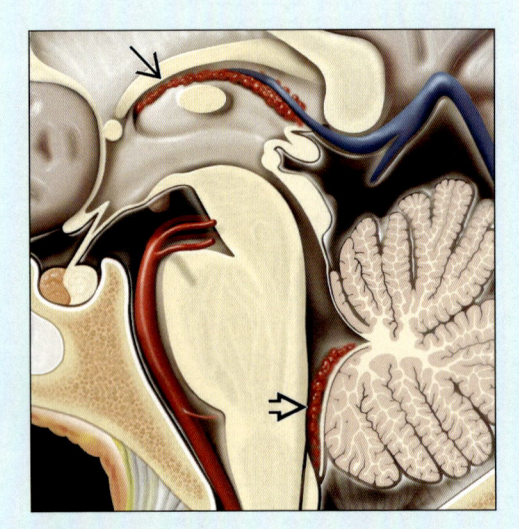

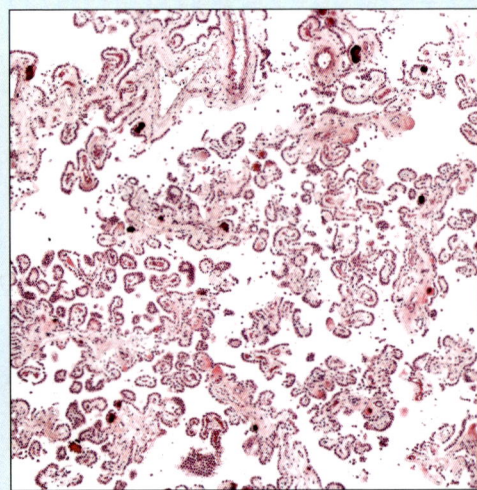

(Left) The cores of loose connective tissue and dilated blood vessels ➡ in the choroid plexus are covered by a single cell layer of modified ependyma cells ➡. *(Right)* This high-power view shows the choroid plexus ➡ and ependyma cells ➡ covering the surface of the ventricle wall ➡. In contrast to the ependyma cells, from which they are derived and with which they are continuous, choroid epithelial cells are larger, with a more "hobnailed" or "tombstone" appearance.

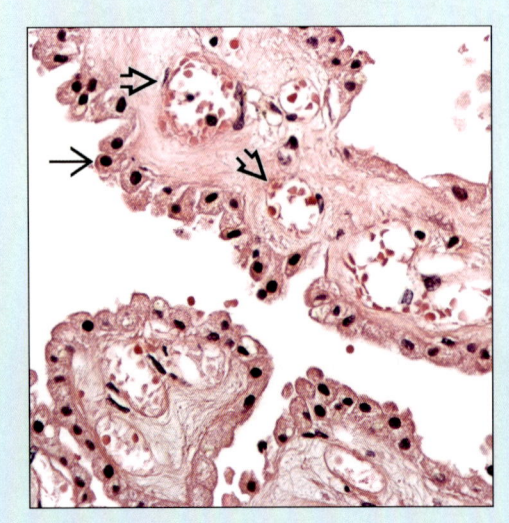

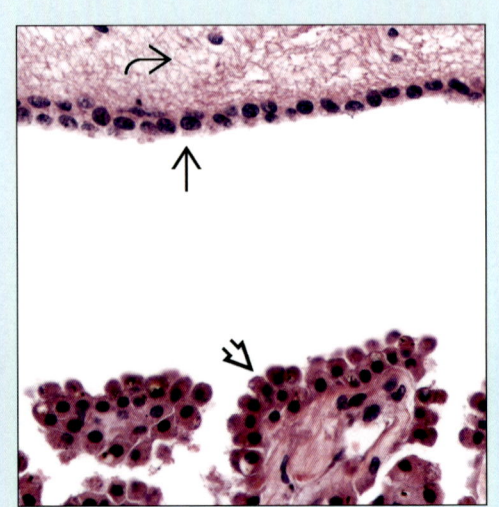

CHOROID PLEXUS

Mineralization

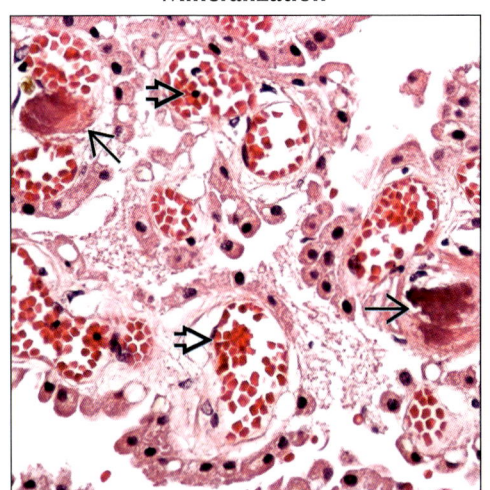

Psammomatous Calcification

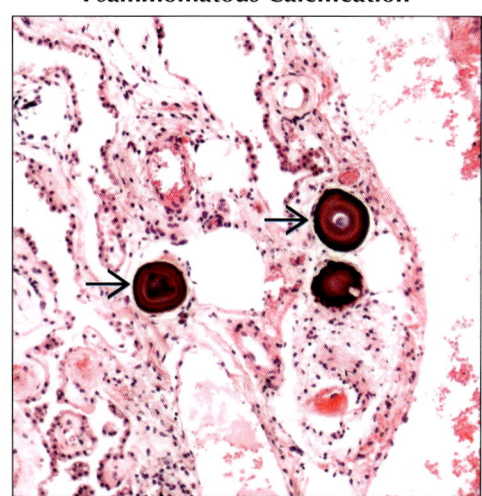

(Left) High-power view of the choroid plexus shows dilated, congested vessels ⇨ and mineral salt deposition ⇨ in connective tissue cores. The latter is more common with increasing age and accounts for radiodensities often observed in the ventricles. *(Right)* The calcifications ⇨ within the connective tissue cores of choroid plexus may assume a laminated, concentric appearance (psammoma bodies).

Choroid Plexus Cyst

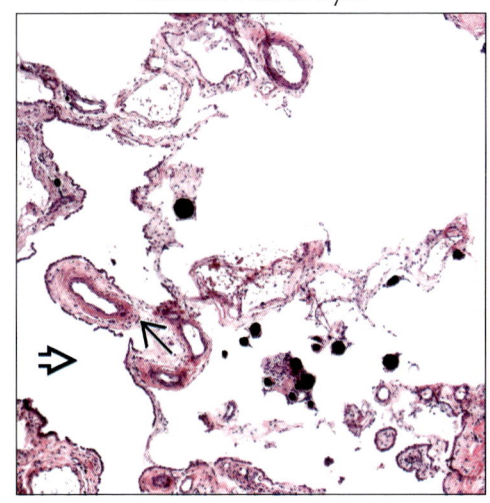

Cystic Xanthomatous Change

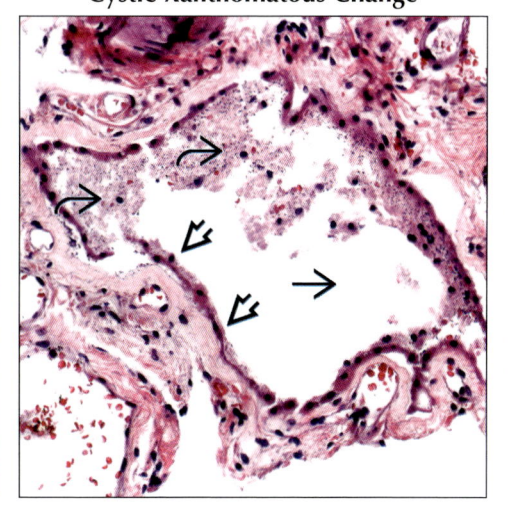

(Left) Choroid plexus cysts are a common benign lesion often seen in fetuses. Vascular connective tissue fronds of choroid plexus ⇨ can be seen surrounding the lumen of the cyst ⇨. *(Right)* This photograph of cystic xanthomatous change shows a cystic lumen ⇨ filled with xanthoma cells (foamy macrophages) ⇨ and surrounded by attenuated choroid epithelial cells ⇨. This is a common incidental finding, seen with older age, but it has no specific pathologic significance.

Choroid Plexus Papilloma

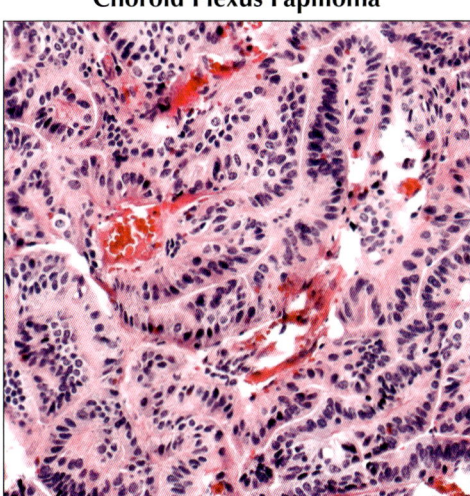

Choroid Plexus Papilloma

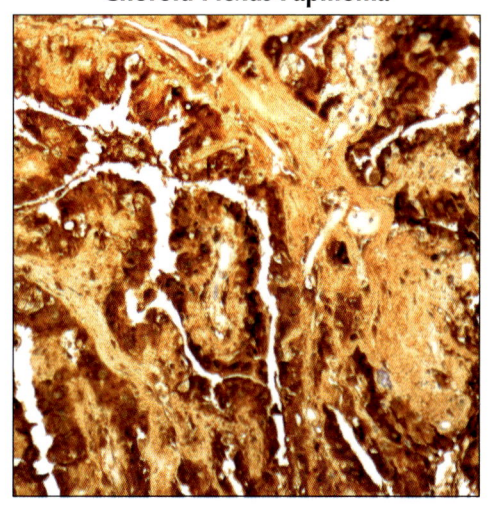

(Left) Choroid plexus papilloma is a benign neoplasm of choroid epithelial cells. Compared to normal choroid plexus, papillomas form a contrast-enhancing mass and are more hypercellular. The crowded cells have a higher nuclear to cytoplasmic ratio and lack the "hobnail" appearance. *(Right)* Choroid plexus cells are immunopositive for prealbumin, as seen here in a choroid plexus papilloma. However, this stain cannot distinguish a papilloma from a normal choroid plexus.

SELECTED REFERENCES

PERIPHERAL NERVOUS SYSTEM

1. Topp KS et al: Peripheral nerve: from the microscopic functional unit of the axon to the biomechanically loaded macroscopic structure. J Hand Ther. 25(2):142-51; quiz 152, 2012

2. Ortiz-Hidalgo C et al: Peripheral nervous system. In Mills SE: Histology for Pathologists. 3rd ed. Philadelphia: Lippincott Williams & Wilkins. 241-71, 2007

3. Smith B: Anatomy and histology of peripheral nerve. In Kimura J: Handbook of Clinical Neurophysiology. Vol. 7. Peripheral Nerve Diseases. Waltham: Elsevier. 3-22, 2006

4. Thomas PK et al: Diseases of the peripheral nerves. In Graham DI et al: Greenfield's Neuropathology. Vol. 2. 6th ed. London: Arnold. 367-94, 1997

5. Junqueira LC et al: Basic Histology. 8th ed. Norwalk: Appleton & Lange. 152-80, 1995

CENTRAL NERVOUS SYSTEM

1. Papura V et al: Glial cells in (patho)physiology. J Neurochem. 121(1):4-27, 2012

2. Tremblay MÈ et al: The role of microglia in the healthy brain. J Neurosci. 31(45):16064-9, 2011

3. Sofroniew MV et al: Astrocytes: biology and pathology. Acta Neuropathol. 119(1):7-35, 2010

4. Fuller N et al: Central nervous system. In Mills S: Histology for Pathologists. 3rd ed. Philadelphia: Lippincott Williams & Wilkins. 273-319, 2007

MENINGES

1. Fuller N et al: Central nervous system. In Mills S: Histology for Pathologists. 3rd ed. Philadelphia: Lippincott Williams & Wilkins. 273-319, 2007

2. Barshes N et al: Anatomy and physiology of the leptomeninges and CSF space. Cancer Treat Res. 125:1-16, 2005

3. Mawera G et al: The function of arachnoid villi/granulations revisited. Cent Afr J Med. 42(9):281-4, 1996

4. Greenberg RW et al: The cranial meninges: anatomic considerations. Semin Ultrasound CT MR. 15(6):454-65, 1994

CHOROID PLEXUS

1. Damkier HH et al: Epithelial pathways in choroid plexus electrolyte transport. Physiology (Bethesda). 25(4):239-49, 2010

2. Fuller N et al: Central nervous system. In Mills S: Histology for Pathologists. 3rd ed. Philadelphia: Lippincott Williams & Wilkins. 273-319, 2007

3. Emerich DF et al: The choroid plexus: function, pathology and therapeutic potential of its transplantation. Expert Opin Biol Ther. 4(8):1191-201, 2004

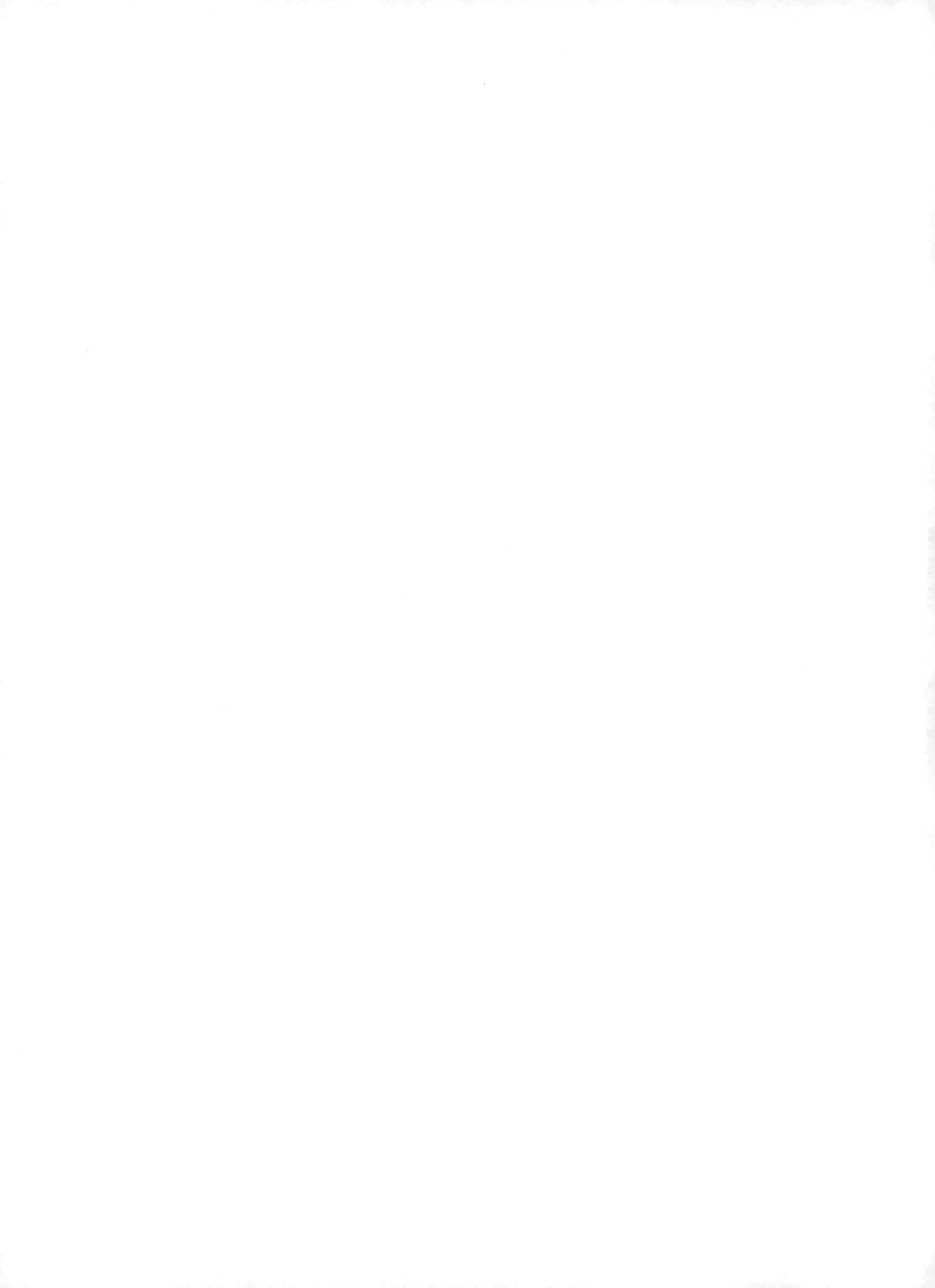

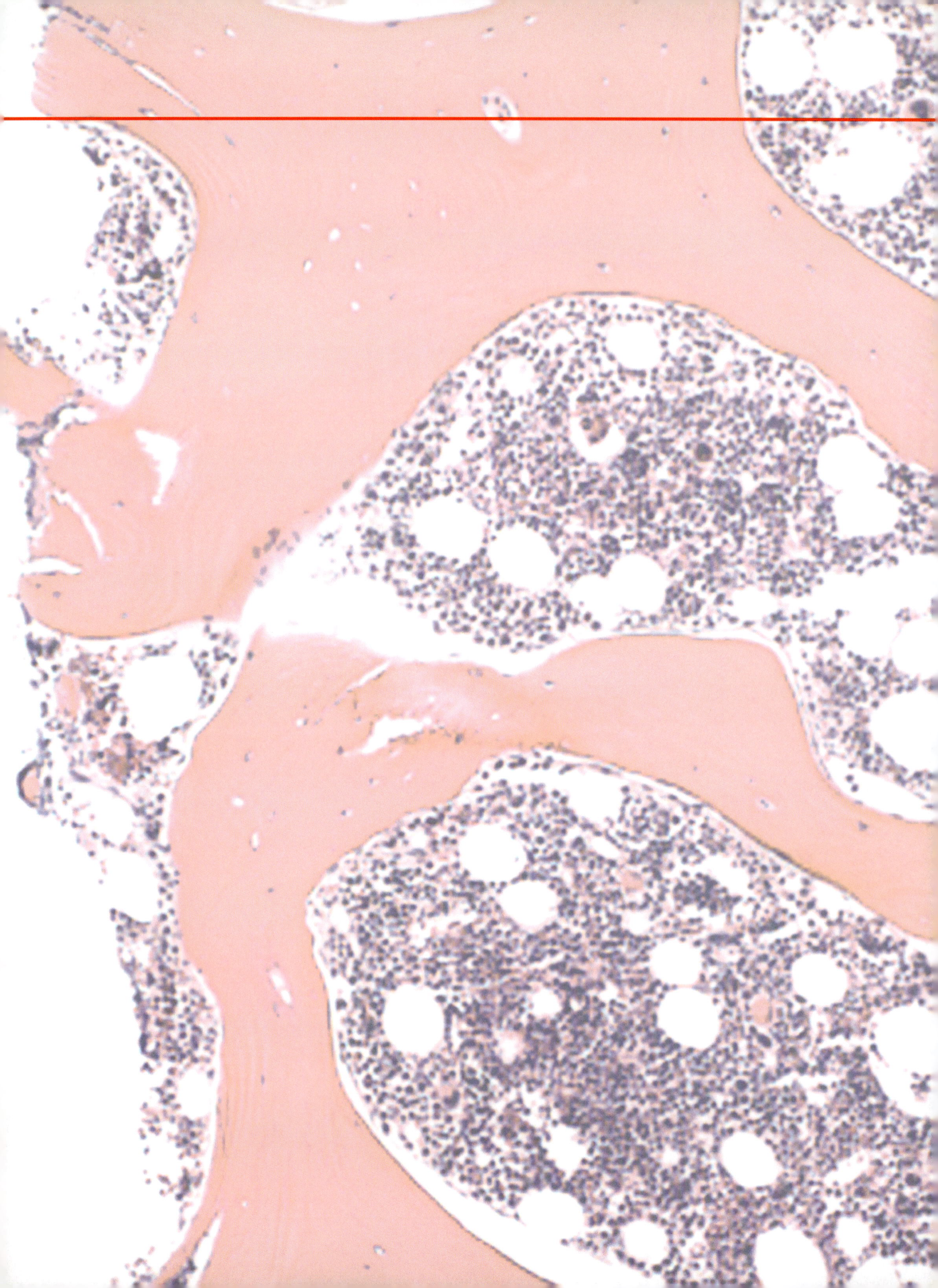

Hematopoietic and Immune Systems

Overview of the Immune System	6-2
Lymph Nodes	6-6
Spleen	6-10
Bone Marrow	6-14
Peripheral Blood	6-22
Thymus	6-26

OVERVIEW OF THE IMMUNE SYSTEM

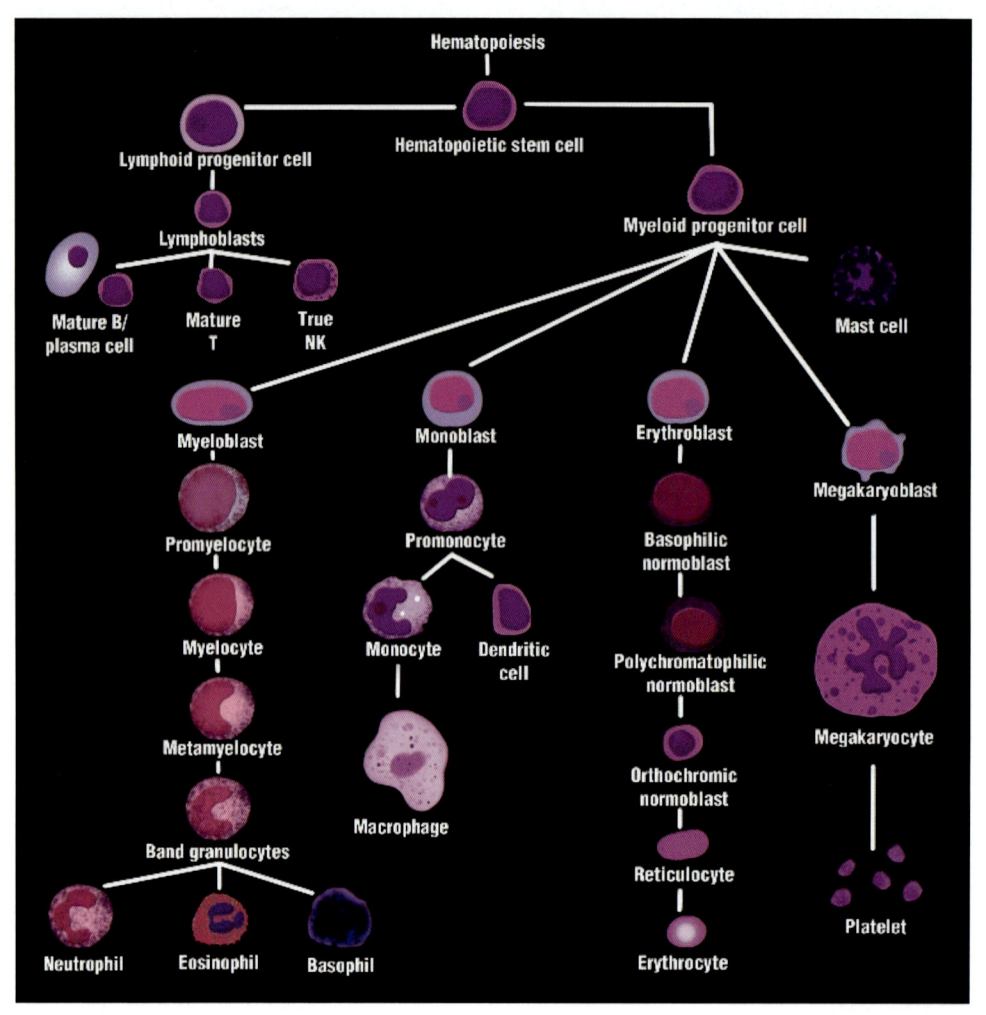

This schematic illustrates general features of lymphoid and myeloid cell derivation from pluripotent stem cells. Both myeloid and lymphoid lineage cells are derived from a common precursor cell. The general maturation stages, from immature to fully differentiated hematopoietic cells, are listed.

TERMINOLOGY

Definitions
- Conceptually divided into innate and adaptive immunity
- **Innate immunity**
  - Rapid and stereotyped response
  - Consists of physical, chemical, and biological barriers
  - Resistance is not acquired through interaction with antigen
    - Recognize foreign carbohydrates on surface of microorganisms
  - Carried out by specialized cells
    - Macrophages/monocytes, neutrophils, dendritic cells, natural killer cells, mast cells, eosinophils, and basophils
  - Main mechanisms include
    - Phagocytosis
    - Release of inflammatory mediators
    - Activation of complement system proteins
    - Synthesis of acute phase proteins, cytokines, and chemokines
  - Present in all individuals
  - Does not change or adapt following contact; nonspecific
- **Adaptive immunity**
  - Induced following contact with foreign antigens
  - Dependent on activation of specialized cells and soluble molecules produced by lymphocytes
    - NK/T, T, and B lymphocytes (TLs and BLs), dendritic cells, or antigen-presenting cells
    - Soluble molecules include antibodies, cytokines, and chemokines
    - Exhibits diversity, memory, and specificity
  - Involves 2 main components
    - Cell-mediated (e.g., cytotoxic TLs)
    - Antibody-mediated (antibody-producing BLs)
  - Specificity and diversity of recognition are key

COMPONENTS OF THE INNATE IMMUNE SYSTEM

Dendritic Cells
- Engulf and present antigens to lymphocytes

OVERVIEW OF THE IMMUNE SYSTEM

- ○ Antigens are presented bound to MHC molecules
- ○ Act as bridge from innate to adaptive immune system
- Originate in bone marrow and migrate to peripheral tissues where they reside (skin, liver, intestine)
  - ○ Migrate to regional lymph nodes upon activation

Neutrophils
- Most abundant leukocytes in peripheral blood
- Constitute 40-60% of circulating leukocytes
- Activated by bacterial products, complement proteins (e.g., C5a), immune complex, chemokines, and cytokines
- Involved in phagocytosis
- Contain primary, secondary, and tertiary granules

Macrophages
- Referred to as monocytes in peripheral blood
- Constitute 3-8% of circulating leukocytes
- Monocytes give rise to macrophages and myeloid dendritic cells in tissues
- Engulf pathogens and cellular debris; efficient phagocytes
  - ○ Process and present antigens via MHC molecules to lymphocytes

Natural Killer Cells
- Originate from common progenitor cells in bone marrow
- Constitute 5-20% of circulating leukocytes
- Important line of nonspecific defense
  - ○ Recognize and lyse virus-infected cells, bacteria, protozoa, and tumor cells
    - ▪ Lysis mediated by perforins and granzymes
    - ▪ Virus-infected cells and tumor cells are susceptible due to their low expression of MHC class I proteins
  - ○ Recruit neutrophils and macrophages
  - ○ Activate dendritic cells and T and B lymphocytes
  - ○ Secrete proinflammatory cytokines

Mast Cells
- Derived from hematopoietic progenitor cells in bone marrow
  - ○ Migrate to peripheral tissues where differentiation and maturation occur
  - ○ Distributed along blood vessels, nerves, and under epithelial surface of skin and mucous membranes
  - ○ Abundant in areas of environmental contact
  - ○ Typically not observed in circulation
- Play key role in acute inflammatory reactions
  - ○ Type I hypersensitivity reactions
- Upon activation, both preformed and newly formed mediators are released
  - ○ Preformed mediators: Vasoactive amines, proteases, heparin, IL-4, TNF-α, and granulocyte-macrophage colony-stimulating factor (GM-CSF)
  - ○ Newly formed mediators: Platelet activating factor, arachidonic acid derivatives, cytokines
  - ○ Release of mediators results in: Inflammatory cell migration, increased vascular permeability, mucus secretion, increased gastrointestinal motility, and bronchoconstriction

Basophils
- Derived from hematopoietic progenitor cells in bone marrow
- Constitute < 1% of circulating leukocytes
- Cytoplasmic granules contain mediators similar to mast cells
- May contribute to immediate hypersensitivity reactions

Eosinophils
- Derived from hematopoietic progenitor cells in bone marrow
- Constitute ≤ 5% of circulating leukocytes
- Found in greater numbers in mucosal regions and in patients with allergies &/or asthma
- Important infection-fighting cells
- Strong antiparasitic action
  - ○ Adhere to parasites and pathogens coated with IgE or IgA
  - ○ Release granular contents upon binding and activation
- Important components in allergic reactions and asthma
- Produce and store various proteolytic granules
- Recruited by adhesion molecules and chemokines

Complement System (CS)
- 3 forms of CS activation: Classical, alternative, and via mannose-binding lectin
  - ○ **Classical activation:** Stimulated by antigen-antibody reactions
  - ○ **Alternative activation:** Stimulated by polysaccharides from yeasts and gram-negative bacteria
  - ○ **Mannose-binding lectin activation:** Stimulated by mannose-containing proteins and carbohydrates on microbes (e.g., viruses and yeasts)
  - ○ Consists of ~ 20 plasma glycoproteins
  - ○ Upon activation, glycoproteins acquire proteolytic activity and activate subsequent components in cascade effect
  - ○ Mediators alter vascular permeability and contribute to inflammatory response
  - ○ End result is formation of membrane attack complex (MAC)
    - ▪ Promotes osmotic lysis and removal of target cell/infectious agent
  - ○ Other anti-infectious functions include
    - ▪ Opsonic action of C3b
    - ▪ Release of soluble C3a and C5a (anaphylatoxins)
    - ▪ Inflammatory infiltrate induced by C5a

Major Histocompatibility Complex
- HLA genes reside within genetic complex referred to as major histocompatibility complex (MHC)
- **Class I MHC proteins**
  - ○ Glycoproteins found on surfaces of nearly all nucleated cells
  - ○ HLA-A, HLA-B, and HLA-C loci encode numerous different proteins that make up MHC class I proteins
- **Class II MHC proteins**
  - ○ Highly polymorphic glycoproteins found on surface of certain cells; macrophages, B cells, dendritic cells of spleen, and Langerhans cells of skin
  - ○ HLA-D loci encode for class II MHC proteins (i.e., DP, DQ, DR)
  - ○ Composed of 2 polypeptides; both encoded by MHC locus
    - ▪ Hypervariable region (provides polymorphism) and constant region (site of CD4 T-cell binding)

OVERVIEW OF THE IMMUNE SYSTEM

- Association of antigen with MHC class proteins allows recognition by T cells
  - CD8-positive cytotoxic T cells recognize antigen complexed with class I MHC
  - CD4-positive helper T cells recognize antigen complexed with class II MHC

COMPONENTS OF THE ADAPTIVE IMMUNE SYSTEM

B Lymphocytes
- Lymphoid progenitors arise from pluripotent stem cells within bone marrow and give rise to BLs
- BLs undergo maturation within bone marrow
  - Pro B cell → pre B cell I → pre B cell II → immature B cell → mature B cell → plasmocyte and memory cell
- Mature BLs migrate to secondary lymphoid organs (e.g., lymph nodes and spleen)
- Immunoglobulins (Igs)
  - Igs consist of 2 heavy chains (α, γ, δ, ε, μ) and 2 light chains (κ, λ)
  - Membrane immunoglobulins (IgM, IgD) recognize antigens
  - During differentiation, changes in constant portion of heavy chain allow for class switching (e.g., IgD or IgM → IgG, IgE, or IgA)

T Lymphocytes
- Lymphoid progenitors arise from pluripotent stem cells within bone marrow and give rise to TLs
- TL differentiation, maturation, and selection take place within thymus
  - Maturation process involves expression of functional T-cell receptor and coreceptors CD4 &/or CD8
  - Positive selection: Selects TLs capable of interacting with MHC I or II; positively selected TLs migrate from thymic cortex towards medulla; TLs that do not interact with MHC I or II undergo apoptosis
  - Negative selection: TLs that have survived positive selection but interact too strongly with "self" peptides are removed by way of apoptosis; process allows for self-tolerance
- TLs recognize processed antigens presented by MHC molecules on surface of antigen-presenting cell
- T-cell receptors
  - Formed by 2 peptide chains of immunoglobulin superfamily
    - Variable and constant regions
  - Undergo recombination process similarly to BL immunoglobulins
  - Formed by α and β chains in 95% of circulating TLs (αβ-TLs)
  - Formed by γ and δ chains in 5% of circulating TLs (γδ-TLs)
- CD4 TLs
  - Recognize antigens presented by class II MHC molecules
  - Responsible for orchestration of other cells involved in immune response
    - Activation of BLs, macrophages, and CD8 TLs
  - T-helper (Th) lymphocytes
    - Subdivided by cytokine production patterns during activation and effector patterns
    - **Th1 lymphocytes**: Produce IFN-γ and IL-2; function in phagocyte activation and opsonizing antibody production
    - **Th2 lymphocytes**: Produce IL-4, IL-5, IL-6, IL-10, and IL-13; function in BL activation, BL differentiation, antibody production, and eosinophil activation
    - **Th17 lymphocytes**: Produce IL-17, IL-22, IL-26, M-CSF, GM-CSF; function in myeloid expansion, chemokine production, and inflammatory cytokine production
- CD8 TLs (cytotoxic TLs)
  - Recognize antigens presented by class I MHC molecules
  - Recognize viral infected and tumor cells
  - Induce apoptosis in target cell via perforins, granzymes, and through expression of FasL receptor (CD95)
- Regulatory TLs
  - Function in immune system regulation and autotolerance
  - Produce immunosuppressive cytokines (e.g., IL-4, IL-10, TGF-β)
  - Express high levels of CD25

Lymphoid Tissues
- Naive (non-antigen-stimulated) BLs and TLs populate lymph nodes, spleen, tonsils, and mucosa-associated lymphoid tissue
- Provide microenvironment for naive BLs and TLs to encounter specific antigen
- Contain antigen-presenting cells that produce necessary cytokines to maintain BLs and TLs
- Communicate with tissues via lymphatics and blood vessels

CLINICAL IMPLICATIONS

MHC and Transplantation
- Success of transplantation requires compatibility of donor and recipient MHC class proteins
- Class II MHC plays the major role
- Severity and rapidity of rejection depend on degree of difference between donor and recipient MHC class proteins
  - **Hyperacute allograft rejection**: Occurs within minutes of engraftment due to large amounts of preformed antibody (e.g., anti-ABO antibodies)
  - **Acute allograft rejection**: Occurs within 11-14 days of engraftment; marked decrease in vascular circulation with increased mononuclear infiltrate and eventual necrosis; T-cell mediated
  - **Chronic allograft rejection**: Occurs months to years following engraftment; thought to be related to incompatibility of minor histocompatibility antigens and immunosuppressive drug side effects; results in atherosclerosis of vasculature
  - Allografts require some degree of immunosuppression
- **Graft versus host reaction**
  - Graft T cells proliferate in irradiated immunocompromised host

OVERVIEW OF THE IMMUNE SYSTEM

Basic Characteristics of Immunoglobulin Classes

Immunoglobulin Class	Structure	Characteristics
IgD	Monomeric	Membrane-bound immunoglobulin; part of naive B-lymphocyte membrane receptor
IgM	Monomeric; pentameric	Monomeric form present on surface of nearly all B lymphocytes; produced early in primary immune response to antigen; pentameric form present in serum; does not cross placenta
IgG	Monomeric	Main immunoglobulin of acquired immunity; has capacity to cross placenta
IgE	Monomeric	Involved in response to allergic and parasitic processes; mediator of immediate hypersensitivity; interaction with basophils and mast cells results in histamine release
IgA	Monomeric and dimeric	Present in gastrointestinal, respiratory, and urogenital tract mucosa; prevents colonization of mucosa by bacteria and viruses

Selection of HLA Disease Associations

HLA Molecule	Disease Association	Comments
HLA-B27	Ankylosing spondylitis (AS)	Found in >95 % of AS patients; absence of HLA-B27 essentially excludes AS.
HLA-DQ2, HLA-DQ8	Celiac disease	
HLA-DRB1*01:03	Ulcerative colitis	
HLA-DRB1*07	Crohn disease	
HLA-DQB1*06:02, HLA-DR2	Narcolepsy	Absence of HLA-DQB1*06:02 tends to exclude narcolepsy
HLA-DQ2, HLA-DQ3	Insulin-dependent diabetes mellitus	No value in routine testing of patients
HLA-DRB1	Rheumatoid arthritis	DRB1*04:01, 04:04, 04:05, and 04:08 are the main susceptibility subtypes

- ○ Graft T cells reject cells with "foreign" MHC class proteins
- ○ May occur in perfectly MHC class I and II matched patients due to differences in minor antigens
- ○ Results in severe organ dysfunction
  - ▪ Common symptoms: Maculopapular rash, diarrhea, hepatosplenomegaly, and jaundice
  - ▪ Reaction can be reduced by treating allograft with antithymocyte globulin or monoclonal antibodies to reduce mature T cells in allograft

MHC and Autoimmune Disease
- Many autoimmune diseases occur in individuals with expression of certain MHC genes (HLA associations)
- Associations have strong negative predictive value but weak positive predictive value (e.g., presence of a certain HLA type/subtype does not predict disease but its absence may be helpful in excluding disease)

LYMPHOID ORGANS

Lymph Node
- Small oval-shaped organ of immune system
- Distributed throughout body
- Linked by lymphatic vessels that drain into left subclavian vein via thoracic duct

Spleen
- Located in upper left quadrant of abdomen
- Largest secondary immune organ in body
- Functions as mechanical filter of old, damaged, or defective red blood cells, reserve of monocytes, and site of active immune response through innate and adaptive immune pathways
- Initiates immune reactions to blood-borne antigens

BONE MARROW

Hematopoiesis
- Contains hematopoietic stem cells, which give rise to 3 types of blood cells
  - ○ Red blood cells (erythrocytes)
  - ○ Leukocytes (lymphocytes and granulocytes)
  - ○ Megakaryocytes/platelets (thrombocytes)

THYMUS

T-Cell Maturation
- Specialized organ of immune system involved in T-cell education, selection, and maturation

LYMPH NODES

Key Facts

Macroscopic Anatomy
- Round or reniform shape
- Normally do not exceed 1 cm in diameter
  - Larger during stimulation (2-3 cm in diameter)
  - Suspect malignancy if diameter > 3 cm
- Tan-pink homogeneous cut surface
- Blood supply
  - Arteries and veins enter and exit at hilus, respectively
- Lymphatics
  - Afferent lymphatics enter in subcapsular sinus
  - Efferent lymphatics exit at hilus

Microscopic Anatomy
- **4 compartments**: Cortical area (follicles), paracortex, medullary region, and sinuses
- **Primary follicle**: Homogeneous nodules of small darkly staining naive inactivated B lymphocytes
- **Secondary follicle**
  - Shows changes associated with antigenic stimulation (e.g., germinal center [GC], polarization, tingible body macrophages)
  - GC composed of centroblasts, centrocytes, small lymphocytes, tingible body macrophages, dendritic reticulum cells, and few small T cells
  - Zonation: Related to direction of antigen processing and process of B-cell maturation from centroblasts to centrocytes: Dark zone = predominantly centroblasts oriented towards center of LN; light zone = predominantly centrocytes, oriented towards periphery
- **Mantle zone**
  - Similar characteristics as primary follicle
  - Small dark staining tightly packed B cells that surround GC
- **Marginal zone**
  - Less compact B cells, more abundant cytoplasm, located along outer layer of mantle zone
- **Paracortex**
  - Interfollicular area composed predominantly of T cells, with post capillary/high endothelial venules, and interdigitating cells (IDC)
  - T cells are mostly small and naive, may become activated and change into larger immunoblasts upon stimulation
  - IDCs involved in antigen presentation, when present in large numbers, impart a mottled appearance
- **Medullary region**
  - Cords of cells: Lymphocytes, plasmacytoid lymphocytes, mature plasma cells, plasmablasts, and rare mast cells
  - Site of plasma cell proliferation, differentiation, and antibody production
  - Cords are separated by medullary sinuses
- **Sinuses**
  - Primarily in medullary region, but do extend up into cortex
  - Subcapsular sinus located directly beneath capsule
  - Carry lymph from afferent lymphatics through lymphoid parenchyma into efferent lymphatics located at LN hilum
  - Lined by thin, pale-staining endothelial cells; acquire a lining of macrophages within hilum
  - Contain macrophages, lymphocytes, plasma cells, immunoblasts, and occasional neutrophils

Anatomic Variation
- Inguinal lymph nodes commonly appear fibrotic; may distort LN architecture
- Paraaortic and parailiac lymph nodes may show sclerotic or hyaline deposits

Pitfalls/Artifacts
- Distinguish Bcl-2 expression in a primary follicle from Bcl-2 expression in follicular lymphoma (FL)
  - Primary follicles will express Bcl-2 and CD5 and will lack distinctive neoplastic cytomorphologic appearance of FL

Hyperplasia
- Enlarged reactive LNs with prominent follicular hyperplasia (FH) more common in younger age groups
  - Considered atypical in elderly and should prompt close evaluation

(Left) This lymph node graphic shows the usual arrangement of cortical-based follicles ⮕. The directional flow of lymph through afferent ⮕ and efferent ⮕ lymphatics is indicated by yellow arrows. (Right) This illustration of a secondary follicle shows many of the key histologic features: Light and dark zonation, tingible body macrophages ⮕, follicular dendritic cells ⮕, mantle zone ⮕, and marginal zone ⮕.

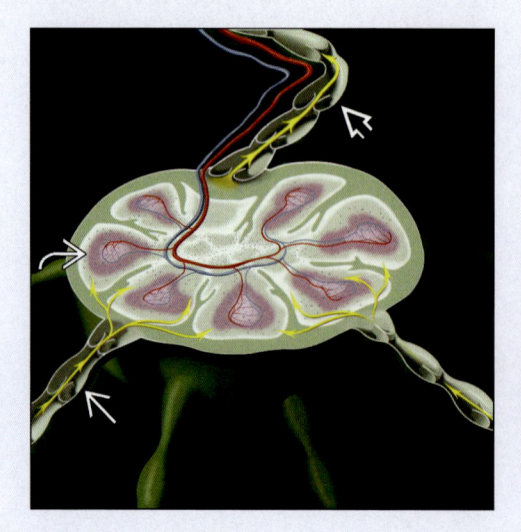

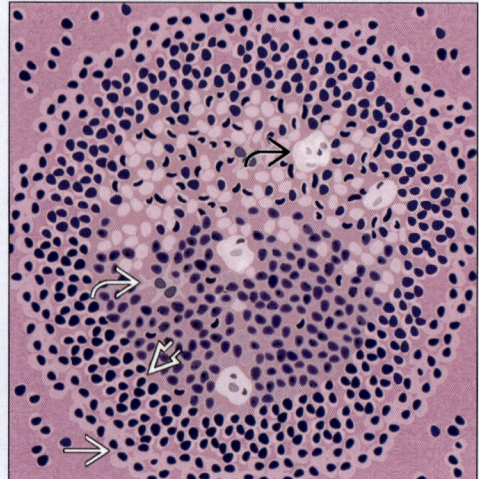

LYMPH NODES

Lymph Node

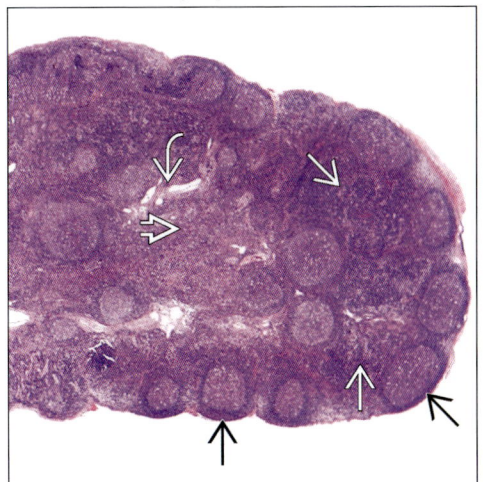

Lymph Node Follicle

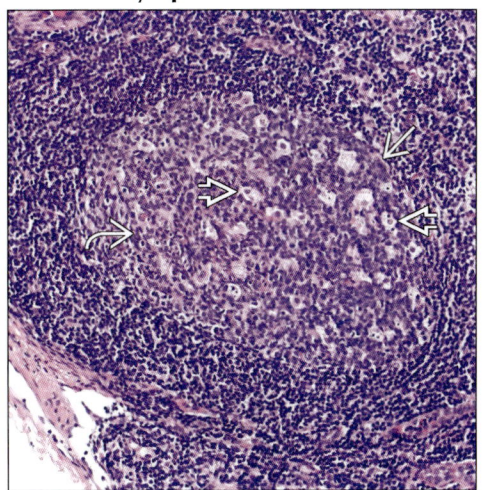

(Left) Cortically based secondary follicles ⇨, paracortex ⇨, medullary region ⇨, and sinuses ⇨ are visualized in this reactive-appearing LN. (Right) Polarization (light ⇨ and dark zones ⇨) and prominent tingible body macrophages ⇨ impart a starry sky pattern in this secondary follicle. The dark zone is composed predominantly of centroblasts that, following antigenic stimulation, mature into centrocytes located primarily within the light zone.

Secondary Follicle

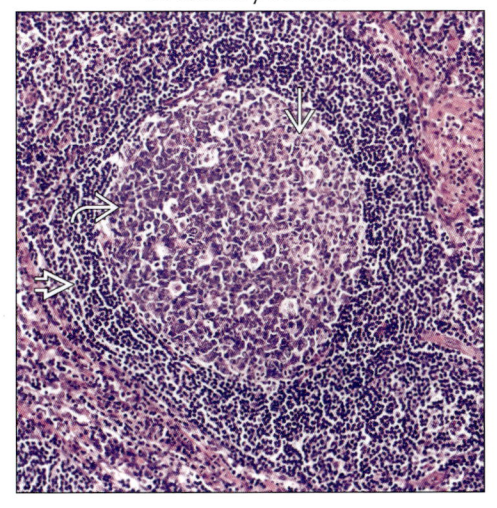

Neoplastic Follicle

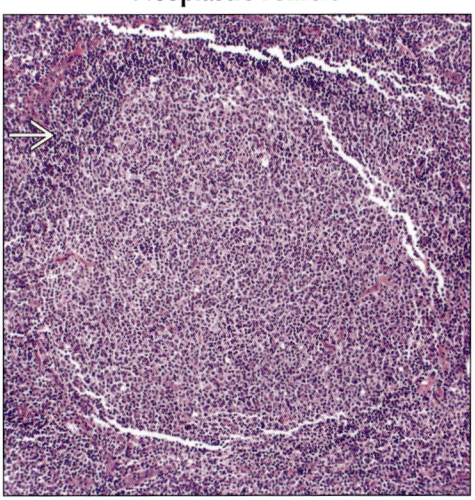

(Left) A secondary follicle with dark and light zonation and a distinct surrounding mantle zone ⇨ is shown. The dark zone ⇨ consists predominantly of immature centroblasts and a few immunoblasts while the light zone ⇨ consists of more mature centrocytes. The surrounding mantle zone consists of naive B cells. (Right) This neoplastic follicle from a follicular lymphoma lacks polarization and tingible body macrophages and has a diminished mantle zone ⇨.

Germinal Center

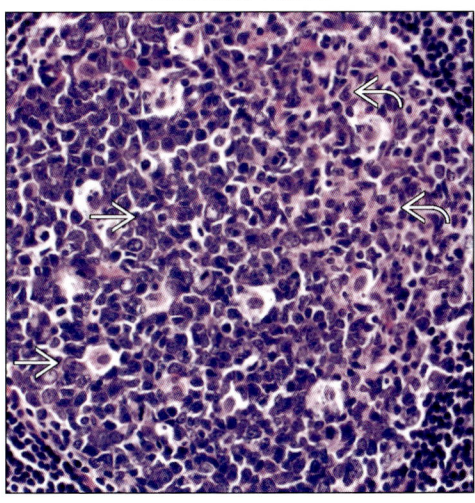

Tingible Body Macrophages

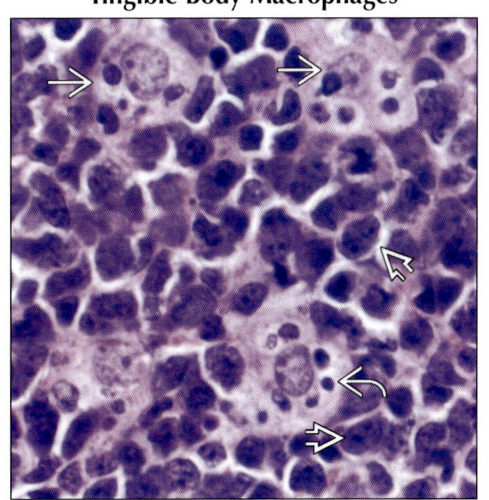

(Left) The predominance of centroblasts ⇨ in the dark zone and centrocytes ⇨ in the light zone of this germinal center is illustrated here at high power. (Right) The dark zone of a germinal center contains several tingible body macrophages, shown here ⇨ at high power. Note the cytoplasmic debris ⇨. This finding is common among antigenically activated secondary follicles. The centroblasts show large oval nuclei that often have multiple nucleoli ⇨.

LYMPH NODES

CD20 Immunostain, Lymph Node

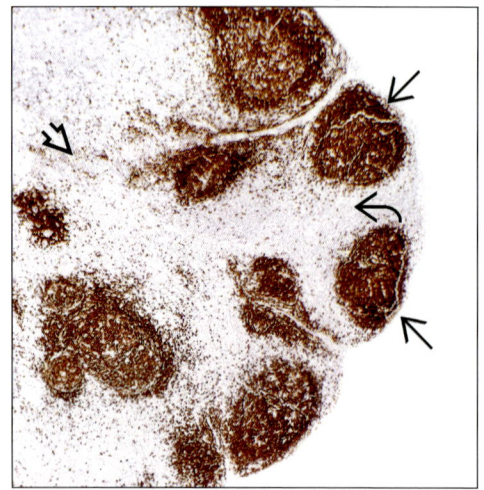

CD20 Immunostain, Follicle

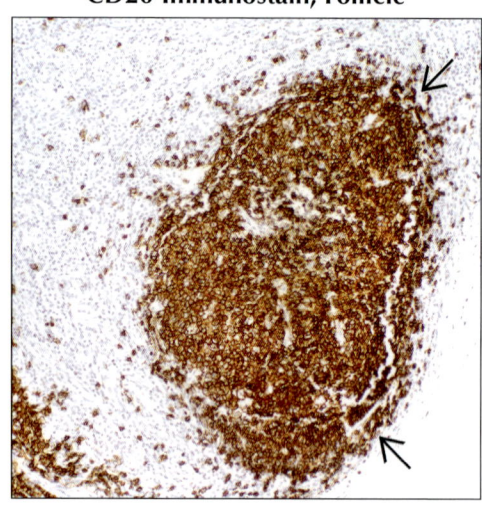

(Left) CD20 immunostaining highlights B cells of the cortical-based follicles ➡ in this lymph node. Note the paucity of CD20(+) B cells in the paracortical ➡ and medullary ➡ regions of the lymph node. *(Right)* Medium-power view shows a cortical-based lymph node follicle ➡ that is composed primarily of CD20(+) B cells.

CD3 Immunostain, Lymph Node

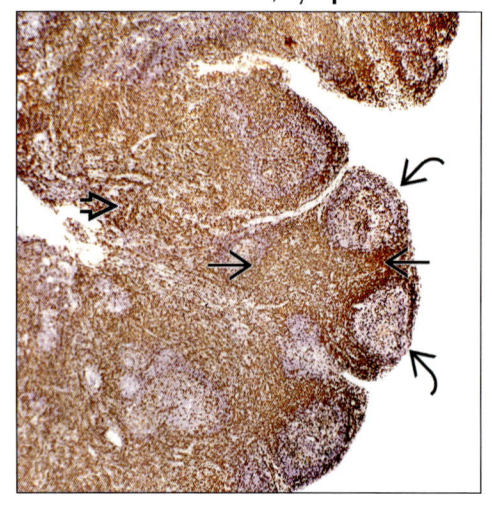

CD3 Immunostain, Follicle

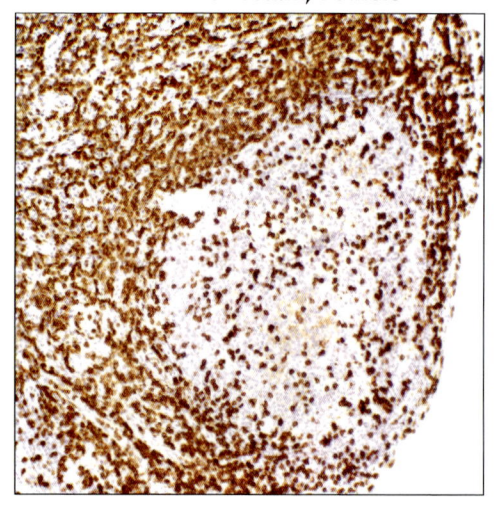

(Left) This CD3 immunostain highlights the general distribution of the CD3(+) T cells within the paracortical ➡ and medullary ➡ regions. Note the few scattered T cells (follicular helper T cells) seen within the B-cell-predominant follicles ➡. *(Right)* CD3 immunostain at medium power highlights the scattered T cells within the germinal center (follicular helper T cells), and the predominance of T cells within the paracortical region.

Bcl-2 Immunostain, Lymph Node

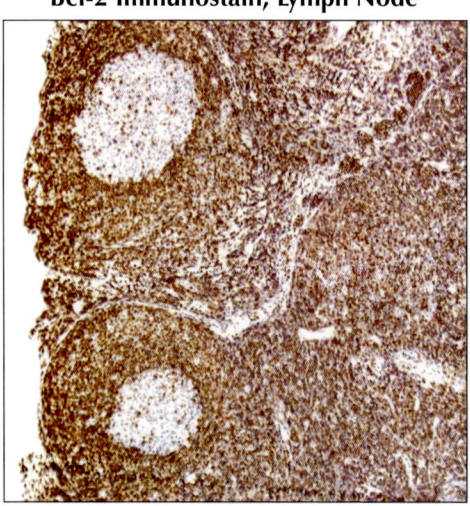

Ki-67 Immunostain, Follicle

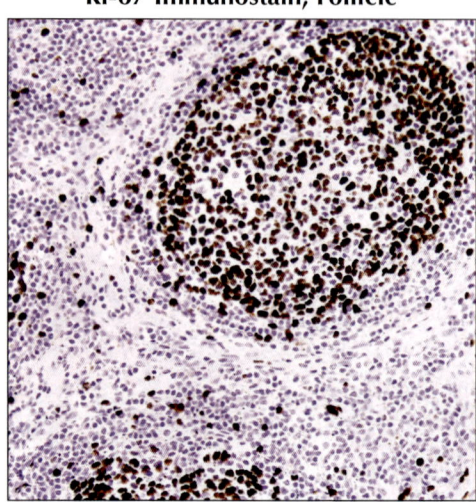

(Left) Bcl-2 immunostaining shows the typical staining pattern of a reactive lymph node: Negative staining in the germinal center and positive staining in all other areas. Bcl-2 has antiapoptotic activity, so the lack of Bcl-2 expression in B cells undergoing antigen-driven selection in the germinal center allows these cells to undergo apoptosis if necessary. *(Right)* Ki-67 immunostaining shows a polarized appearance (dark and light zones), which is typical of a benign reactive follicle.

LYMPH NODES

Lymph Node Subcapsular Sinus

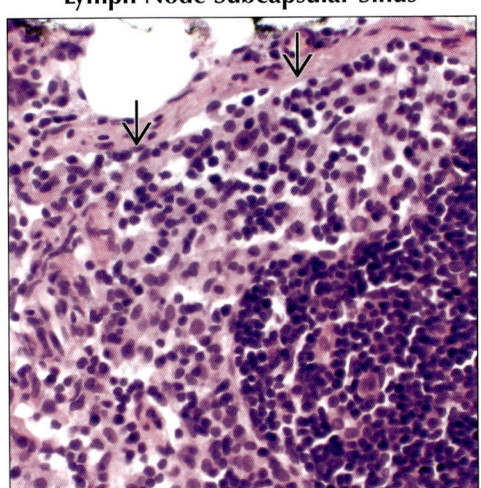

Lymph Node Medullary Region

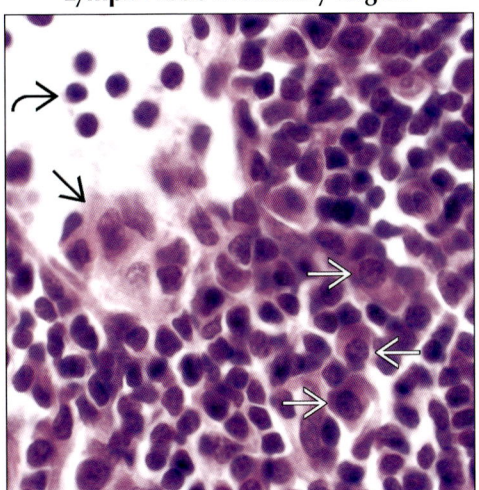

(Left) A dilated subcapsular sinus ➡ with numerous histiocytes (round nuclei, abundant eosinophilic cytoplasm) and scattered small lymphocytes is shown at medium power. *(Right)* A small portion of a medullary cord with mature plasma cells ➡ is shown at high power. Adjacent is a dilated sinus with scattered histiocytes ➡ and small lymphocytes ➡.

Paracortical Hyperplasia

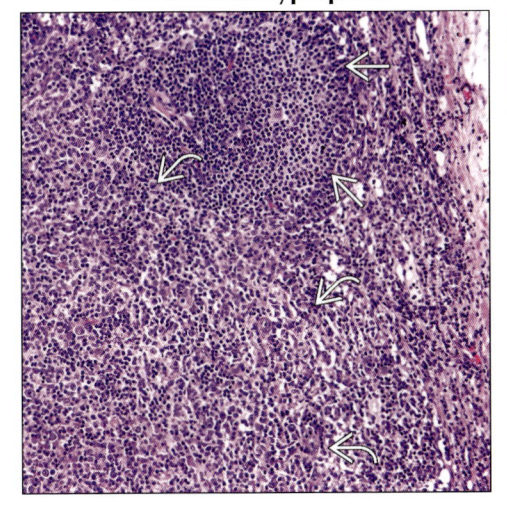

Paracortical Hyperplasia

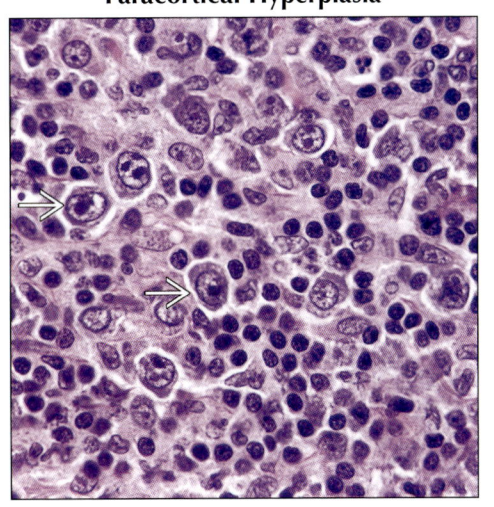

(Left) This reactive lymph node has marked paracortical (interfollicular) ➡ expansion. A residual follicle ➡ is at the top of the field. This feature is commonly associated with viral-mediated lymphadenopathies. *(Right)* A hyperplastic paracortex with a heterogeneous cell population is shown. Note the large immunoblasts ➡ with prominent centrally located nucleoli admixed with small lymphocytes and histiocytes. These features are commonly associated with viral infections.

Thoracic Lymph Node

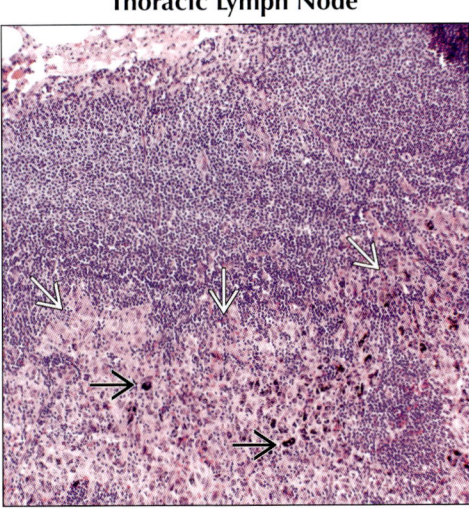

Thoracic Lymph Node

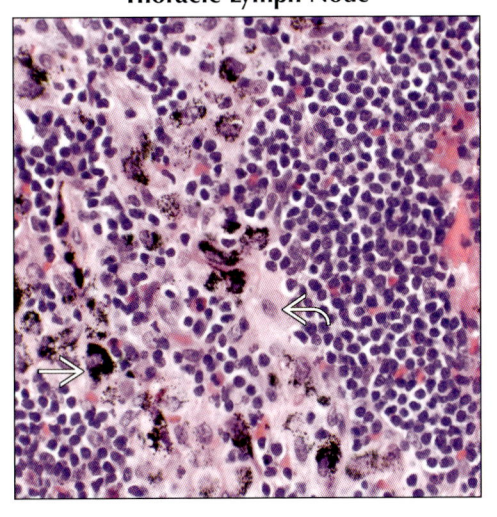

(Left) Thoracic lymph nodes often show abundant anthracotic pigment ➡ that is typically associated with histiocytic infiltrates ➡ and distortion of the usual lymph node architecture as seen above. *(Right)* The abundant anthracotic pigment ➡ and scattered histiocytes ➡ are shown at high power. These features are common among thoracic/pulmonary lymph nodes.

SPLEEN

Key Facts

Macroscopic Anatomy
- Bean-shaped organ covered by smooth capsule
- Blood supply via splenic artery
  - Splenic artery enters at hilus and branches in spleen

Microscopic Anatomy
- **Splenic vasculature**
  - Blood enters spleen via splenic artery, which then branches into trabecular arteries
  - Accompanied by veins and lymphatic vessels, branching trabecular arteries surrounded by dense connective tissue comprise splenic cuff
  - Trabecular arteries emerge from connective tissue and become arterioles of white pulp (central arterioles), which are surrounded by periarteriolar lymphatic sheath (PALS)
  - Central arterioles continue into follicles (follicular arterioles)
  - Follicular arterioles become smaller and terminate in marginal zone or form vascular tuft of capillaries in red pulp
  - Capillaries in red pulp end as sheathed capillaries
  - Sheathed capillaries lack direct communication to sinuses
  - Arteries, arterioles, and capillaries are lined by endothelial cells
  - Sheathed capillaries are lined by concentrically arranged macrophages and reticular fibers that become continuous with reticular network (stroma) of red pulp (cords)
  - Sheathed capillaries in conjunction with cords function as filtering unit of spleen
  - Red cells enter adjacent sinuses via sheathed capillaries and cords
- **Red pulp**
  - Loose reticular network of capillaries, penetrating venous sinuses, and cords
  - Venous sinuses are large leaky vessels lined by discontinuous layer of cuboidal littoral cells; type of endothelial cell that stains with both histiocytic and endothelial markers
  - Splenic cords (cords of Billroth) represent tissue between venous sinuses; contain reticular cells, macrophages, and plasma cells
- **White pulp**
  - Consists of B- and T-cell compartments
  - **Follicles**: B-cell compartments may be seen as primary follicles (unstimulated) or secondary follicles (antigen stimulated with germinal center present); follicles are surrounded by rim of mantle zone cells and outer rim of marginal zone cells
  - **Periarteriolar lymphatic sheath (PALS)**: T-cell compartment that lies adjacent to arterioles; irregular areas composed primarily of CD4(+) T cells
- **Perifollicular zone**
  - Area adjacent to follicles and T-cell compartments
  - Indicated by numerous erythrocytes directly adjacent to lymphoid cells
  - Capillaries and sheathed capillaries are also present in this zone

Pitfalls/Artifacts
- Extremely vulnerable to autolysis
- Additional stains may be helpful to visualize splenic architecture (e.g., reticulin, periodic acid-Schiff)

Age Variation
- White pulp does not contain well-formed follicles until birth
- Maturing hematopoietic precursors are commonly seen in fetal spleen
- Secondary follicles are more common in patients < 20 years of age
- Patients > 20 years of age typically have fewer secondary follicles
- Hyalinization of vessels is common in both old and young patients
- Extramedullary hematopoiesis in adult spleen is associated with pathologic conditions

(Left) The functional filtering unit of the spleen is illustrated. Red cells pass from the sheathed capillaries lined by concentrically arranged macrophages ➔ into the cords ➔ and then into the sinuses ➔. Old &/or abnormal red cells will be removed during this process. (Right) White ➔ and red pulp ➔ are viewed at low power in this section of normal spleen. A thin splenic capsule ➔ with slivers of branching trabeculae ➔ is also noted.

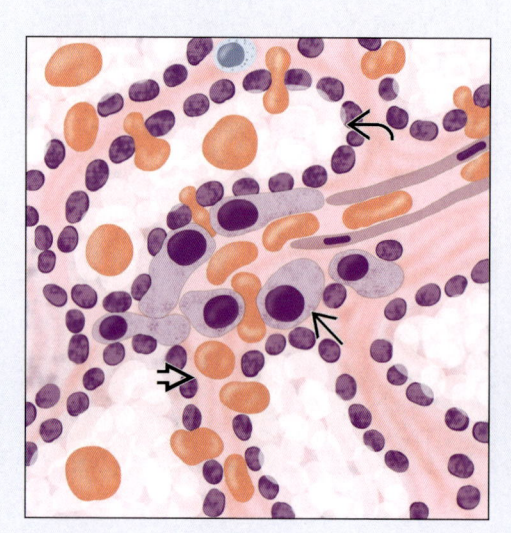

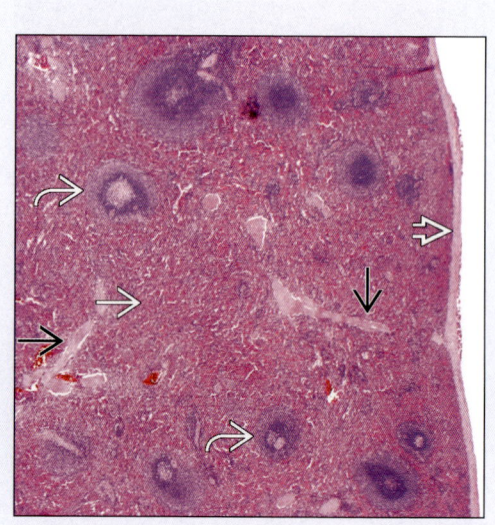

SPLEEN

Spleen: Red and White Pulp

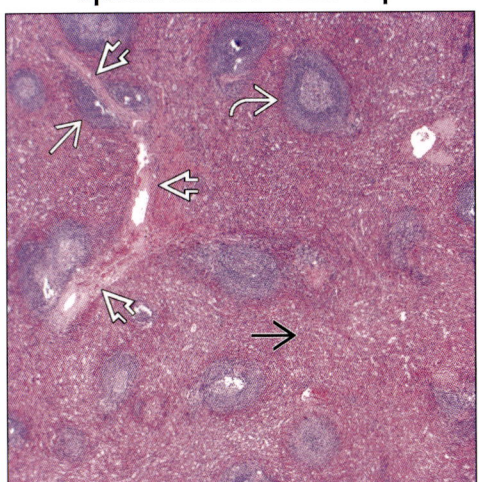

White Pulp: Secondary Follicle

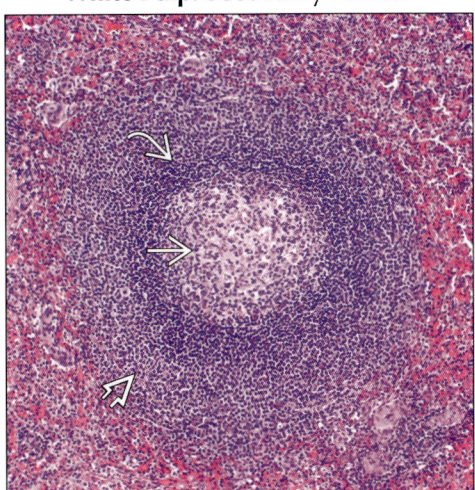

(Left) Nearly all splenic compartments are illustrated in this image: White pulp (B-cell ➡ and T-cell ➡ compartments), red pulp ➡, and splenic cuff ➡. (Right) A B-cell follicle is shown at medium power. The follicle shows features of activation, as noted by the germinal center ➡. Note the surrounding rim of dense small lymphocytes and the less dense and more expanded rim of lymphocytes, which represent the mantle ➡ and marginal ➡ zones, respectively.

White Pulp: Follicle

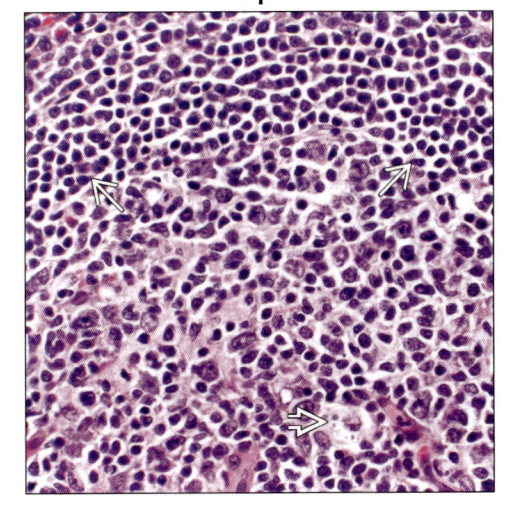

White Pulp: Follicle

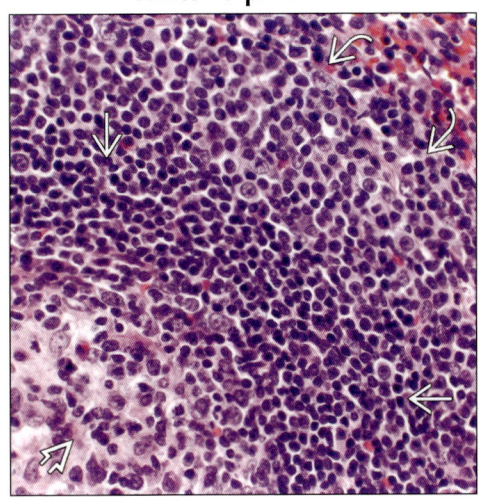

(Left) Splenic follicles show many of the same features as those of lymph nodes. In this secondary (antigen-stimulated) follicle, a tingible body macrophage ➡ is seen within the germinal center, and surrounding mantle zone ➡ is shown. (Right) This high-power view illustrates the mantle zone ➡ (dense rim of small B cells with scant cytoplasm), the outer marginal zone ➡ (less dense rim of B cells with more abundant cytoplasm), and a small section of germinal center ➡.

White Pulp: Follicle and PALS

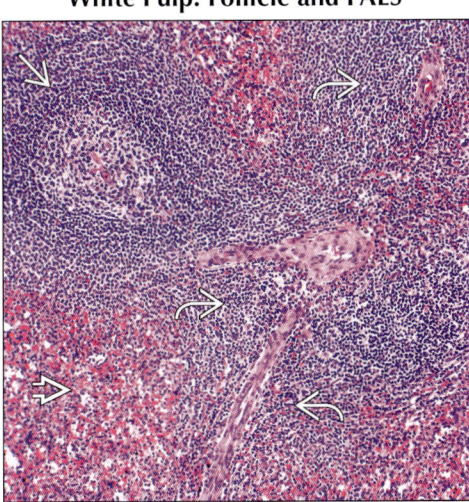

Spleen: Perifollicular Zone

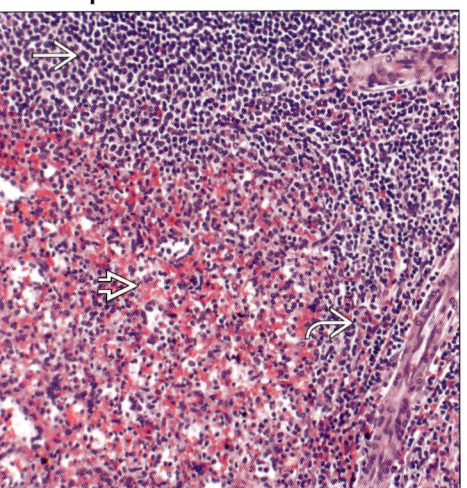

(Left) The T-cell compartment (periarteriolar lymphatic sheath [PALS]) ➡, B-cell compartment (follicle) ➡, and perifollicular zone ➡ are shown. The T-cell and B-cell compartments together make up the white pulp. (Right) The perifollicular zone ➡ lies adjacent to the follicle ➡ and T-cell compartment (periarteriolar lymphatic sheath) ➡ and contains numerous erythrocytes in addition to capillaries and sheathed capillaries (not shown).

SPLEEN

(Left) Red pulp consists of capillaries, venus sinuses, and splenic cords (cords of Billroth). Several follicles along the edges are also present. **(Right)** A branching capillary lined by flattened endothelial cells is shown ➡. In the spleen, arterioles lead to capillaries, which then lead to sheathed capillaries that are lined by concentrically arranged macrophages.

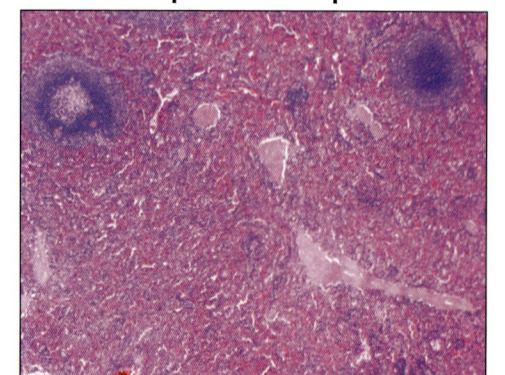

Spleen: Red Pulp

Red Pulp: Splenic Capillary

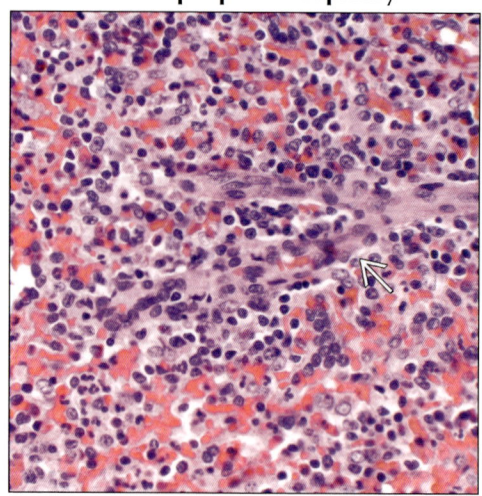

(Left) A splenic capillary lined by flat endothelial cells ➡ precedes the sheathed capillary ➡, which is lined by concentrically arranged macrophages and a network of reticular cells and fibers. **(Right)** Sinuses lined by littoral cells, a type of cuboidal endothelial cell that stains for both endothelial and histiocytic markers, are shown ➡. Several small capillaries are also noted along the bottom. Note the flatter endothelial cells ➡ that line the capillaries.

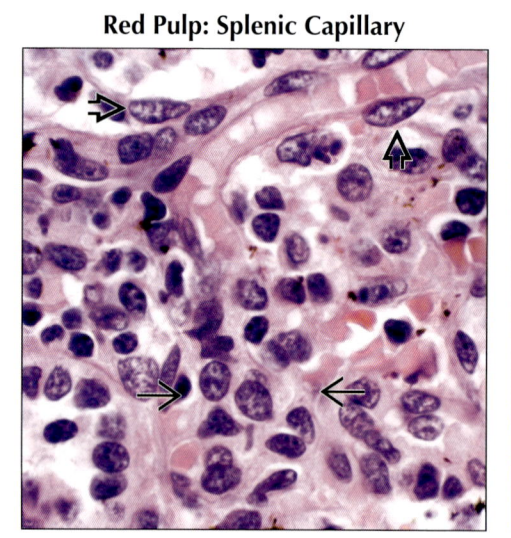

Red Pulp: Splenic Capillary

Red Pulp: Sinuses

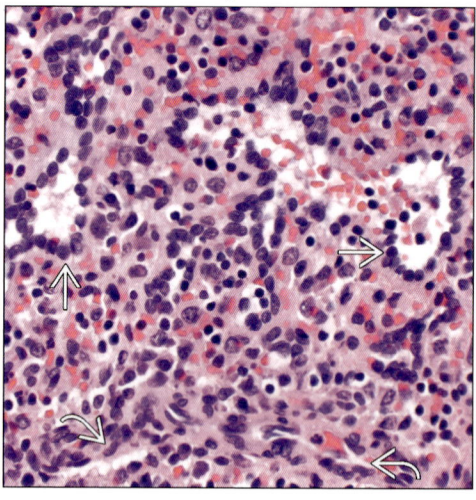

(Left) Capillaries ➡, sheathed capillaries ➡, and a sinus are shown. Note the abundant hemosiderin ➡ in the macrophages that are part of the sheathed capillaries and cords. **(Right)** Splenic cords ➡ that contain macrophages, reticular cells, and plasma cells represent the tissue that lies between the sinuses. Note the individual red cells that are passing from the cords into the sinuses ➡. Old &/or damaged red cells that cannot squeeze through will be removed by the spleen.

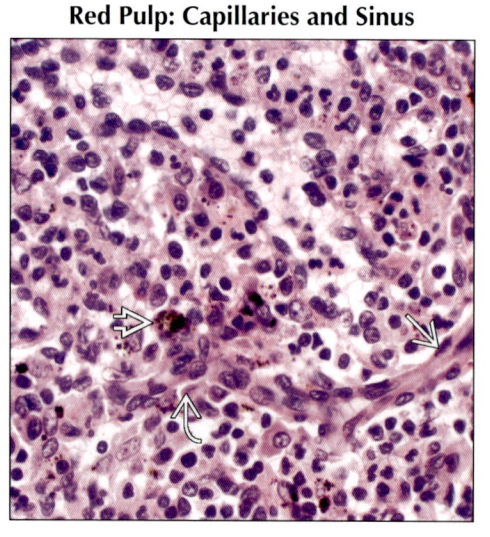

Red Pulp: Capillaries and Sinus

Red Pulp: Cords and Sinuses

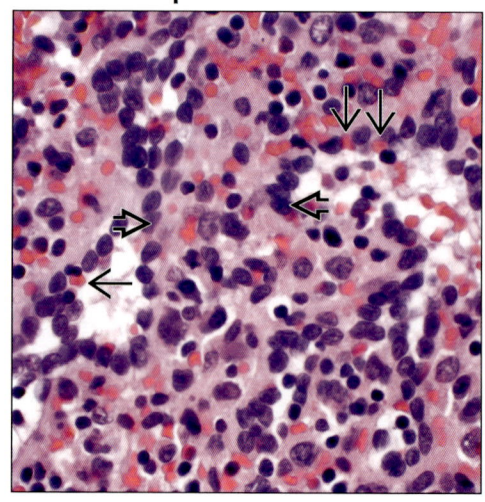

SPLEEN

Splenic Congestion

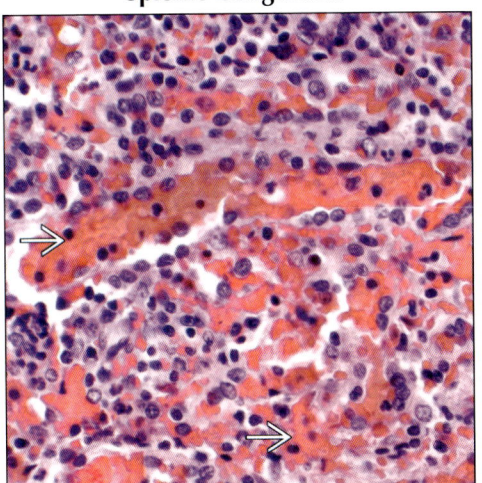

Spleen: CD20 Immunostain

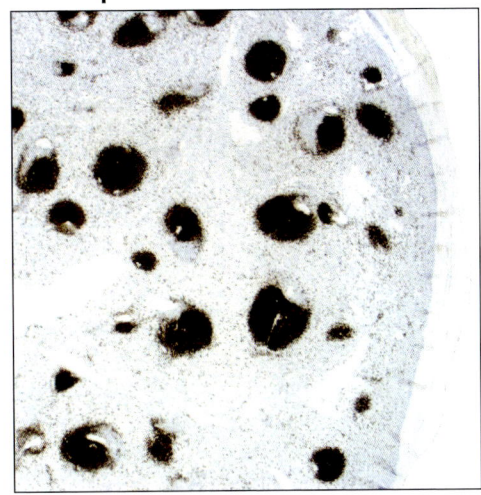

(Left) Sinuses filled with packed red blood cells ⇨ are seen in this image from a congested spleen. *(Right)* Scattered B-cell follicles are highlighted by CD20 in this spleen that has undergone follicular hyperplasia.

Spleen: CD20 Immunostain

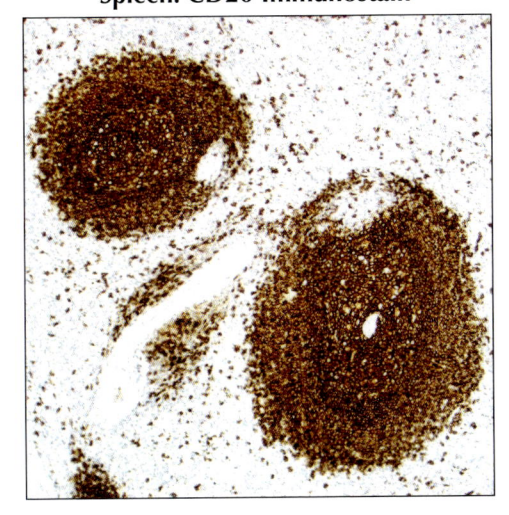

Spleen: CD3 Immunostain

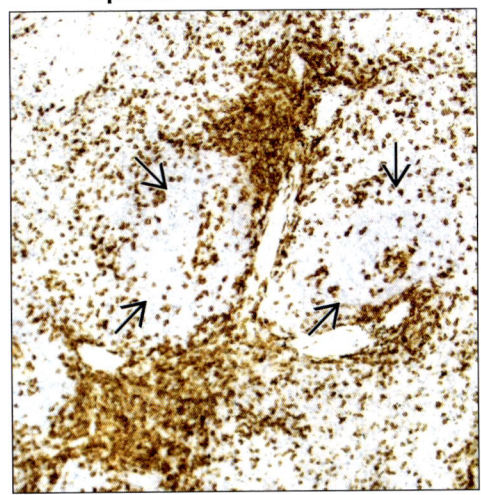

(Left) A CD20 immunostain highlights the B-cell follicles of this spleen. *(Right)* The T-cell compartment (periarteriolar lymphatic sheath) is highlighted by CD3. Note the negative areas of staining ⇨ that represent the B-cell follicles. Together, these 2 compartments make up the white pulp of the spleen.

Spleen: Factor VIII Immunostain

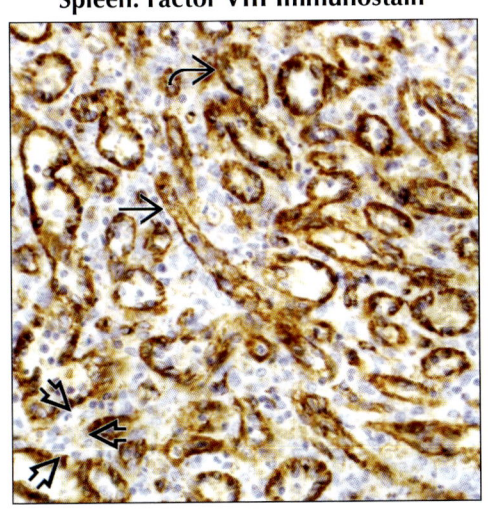

Red Pulp: Reticulin Stain

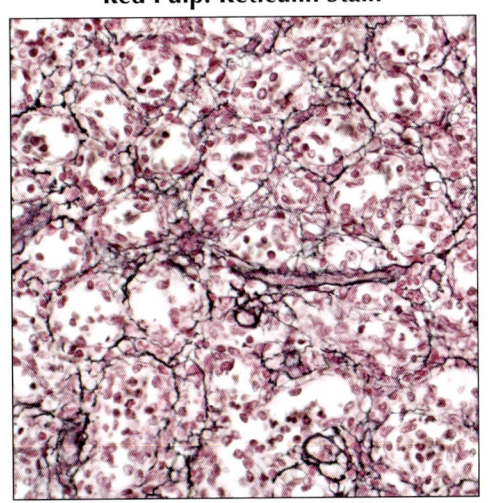

(Left) The splenic sinuses ⇨ and capillaries ⇨ are highlighted by factor VIII. The space between the sinuses represents the splenic cords (cords of Billroth) ⇨. After passing through the cords into the sinuses, the red cells then progress to venules and veins. *(Right)* The reticulin network of the sinuses and capillaries is highlighted. The more discontinuous reticulin network of the sinuses allows for the passage of cells from the cords into the sinuses.

BONE MARROW

Key Facts

Hematopoiesis
- Cell production in bone marrow (BM) is exquisitely regulated; both inducers and suppressors in microenvironment
- Both hematopoietic (HP) and mesenchymal stem cells delineated by functional properties &/or immunophenotype
- Cell types produced by HP stem cells include erythrocytes (RBCs), neutrophils, eosinophils, basophils, monocytes/macrophages/dendritic cells, mast cells, lymphocytes, natural killer cells, osteoclasts, and platelets
- Microenvironment specifies each lineage production site at submicroscopic level
- Mesenchymal stem cells produce fat cells, osteoblasts, vessels, and stromal cells
- Blast is designation for earliest identifiable cell in each HP lineage
- Unique features of HP include endomitosis of megakaryocytic lineage cells and enucleation to create mature RBCs

Macroscopic Anatomy
- Specimens that can be assessed include BM core biopsies, imprint preparations, clot sections, and BM aspirate smears
- Anticoagulated aspirate samples can be used for numerous specialized studies, including flow cytometry, cytogenetics, and molecular assays

Microscopic Anatomy
- Granulopoiesis: Myeloblast to neutrophil maturation process characterized by progressive increase in cytoplasmic granulation essential for cell function
  - Immature granulocytic cells reside adjacent to bony trabeculae and around blood vessels
  - Both enzymatic (cytochemical) stains and immunophenotyping can be used to delineate lineage and stage of maturation of granulocytic cells
- Erythropoiesis: Erythroblast to RBC maturation process characterized by RNA loss, hemoglobin gain, nuclear shrinkage, & ultimate extrusion
  - Erythroid cells form colonies by adhering to central macrophages
  - Erythroid cells are best identified by morphology and immunophenotyping for CD71, glycophorin A, and hemoglobin A
  - Iron in erythroid cells and macrophages can be assessed by Prussian blue staining
- Megakaryopoiesis: Megakaryoblast to platelet maturation process characterized by progressive doubling of DNA without mitosis, creating a very large cell with lobulated nuclei and abundant cytoplasm
  - Megakaryocytes reside adjacent to sinuses to facilitate platelet release directly into circulation by shedding cytoplasm
  - Megakaryocytic cells, especially immature and small forms, can be delineated by immunophenotyping for CD61, CD42b, CD41, and factor VIII
- Fat cells and macrophages are key components of the BM microenvironment
- Macrophages play a role in the regulation of hematopoiesis and in iron storage
- Plasma cells reside adjacent to blood vessels, are generally infrequent
- Mast cells reside within bone marrow particles and can be highlighted by CD117 and tryptase

Pitfalls/Artifacts
- Poor specimen quality is major source of diagnostic problems
- Aspiration of the medullary space is common in core biopsies where aspiration is performed 1st, then biopsy is done close to aspiration site

Age Variation
- There is distinctive age-based variation in cellularity, bone features, number of lymphocytes, lymphoid immunophenotype
  - Both osteoclasts and osteoblasts are seen along bony trabeculae in children and adolescents, reflecting active bone remodeling
  - Overall cellularity declines with age; most pronounced in very elderly patients

(Left) Schematic illustrates likely hematopoietic ➡ and mesenchymal ➡ stem cells, which reside in distinct niches. Osteoblasts ➡ and macrophages ➡ play key roles in hematopoietic regulation. (Right) This graph displays age-related variations in the proportion of erythroid, granulocytic, and lymphoid lineages within bone marrow. Note the age-related variation of erythroid and lymphoid lineage cells, while granulocytic lineage cell levels are fairly stable throughout life.

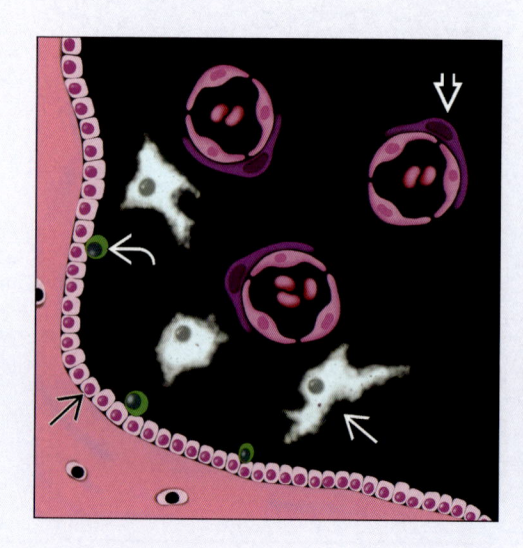

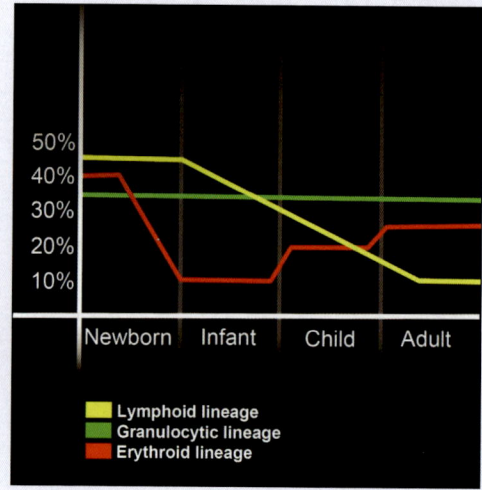

BONE MARROW

Bone Marrow Aspirate

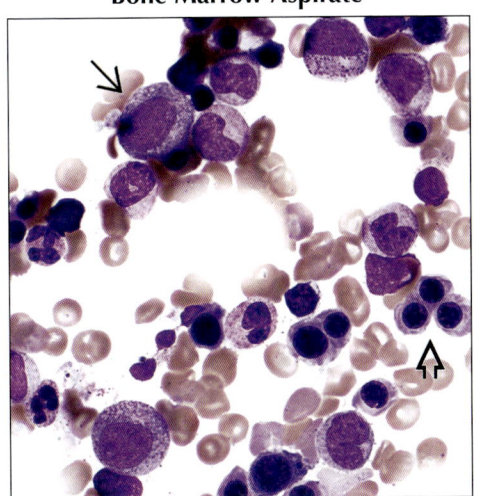

Bone Marrow Aspirate

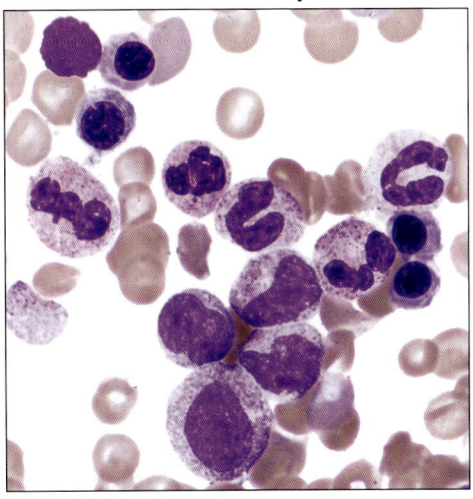

(Left) This bone marrow aspirate smear at intermediate magnification shows an admixture of developing myeloid and erythroid cells. Note that the immature myeloid cells are least numerous ⇨, and the maturing forms predominate with intact nuclear and cytoplasmic maturation. Erythroid cells ⇨ are generally less numerous than granulocytic cells. (Right) The morphologic features of the nuclei and cytoplasm of developing hematopoietic cells are best appreciated at high magnification.

Bone Marrow Clot Section

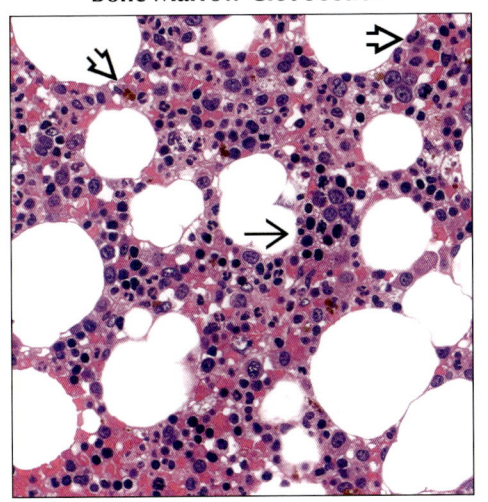

Bone Marrow Core Biopsy

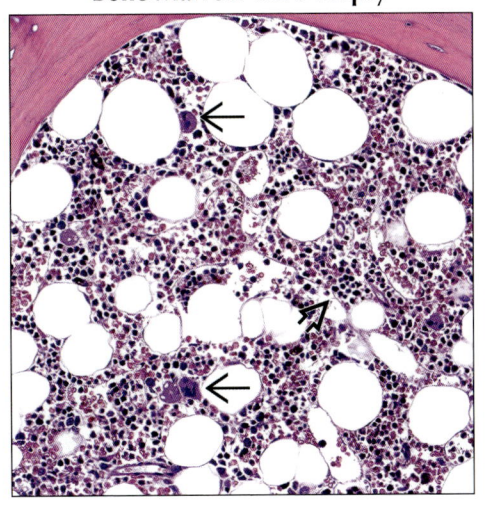

(Left) On clot sections, the overall cellularity can be assessed (70% in this image). In addition, hematopoietic cells, including erythroid colonies, are also evident ⇨. Note hemosiderin in the individually dispersed macrophages ⇨. (Right) On bone marrow core biopsies, bony trabeculae are evaluated in addition to hematopoietic and stromal cells. Bony trabeculae in normal adult patients do not show evidence of remodeling. Note dispersed megakaryocytes ⇨ and erythroid colonies ⇨.

Bone Marrow Clot Section

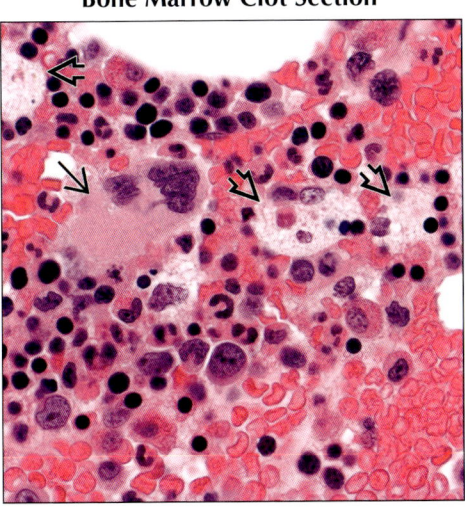

Macrophage, Aspirate Smear

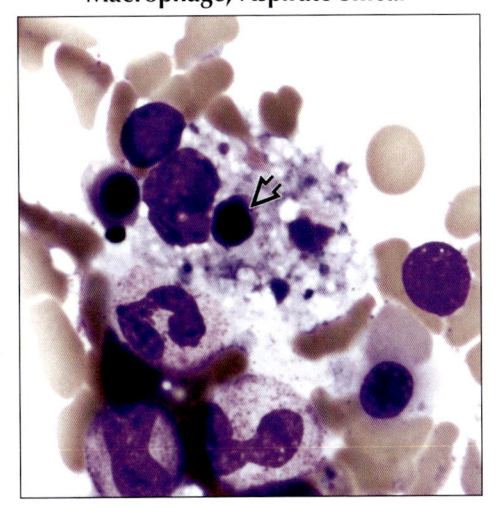

(Left) This bone marrow clot section shows an individual megakaryocyte ⇨ and multiple foamy macrophages ⇨. Macrophages are typically inconspicuous on clot and core biopsy sections. (Right) Macrophages can be assessed on bone marrow aspirate smears and should be evaluated for nuclear features and cytoplasmic contents. Note the ingested nucleus, likely from an erythroid cell ⇨. The adjacent hematopoietic cells are unremarkable.

BONE MARROW

Granulocytic Lineage Cells

(Left) This bone marrow aspirate smear shows numerous maturing granulocytic lineage cells, including promyelocytes ⇨, myelocytes ⇨, metamyelocytes ⇨, band neutrophils ⇨, and a mature segmented neutrophil ⇨.
(Right) Immature granulocytic cells, such as this central promyelocyte ⇨, have basophilic cytoplasm with sparse granules, while myelocytes ⇨ and successive granulocytic lineage cells have eosinophilic cytoplasm due to secondary granules.

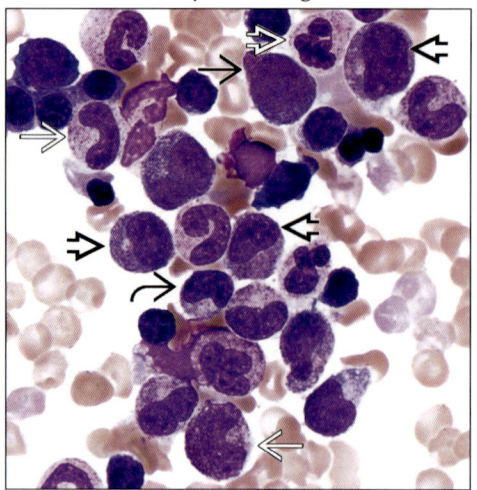

Immature Granulocytic Cells

Maturing Granulocytic Cells

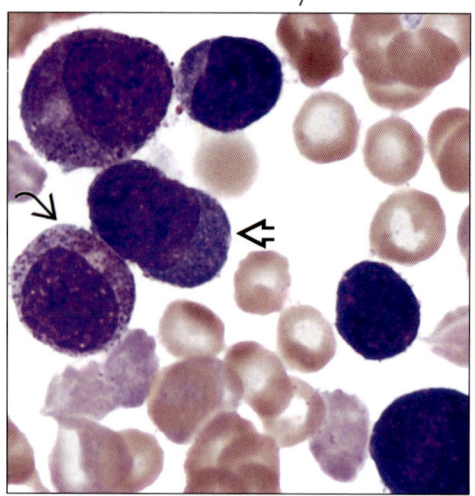

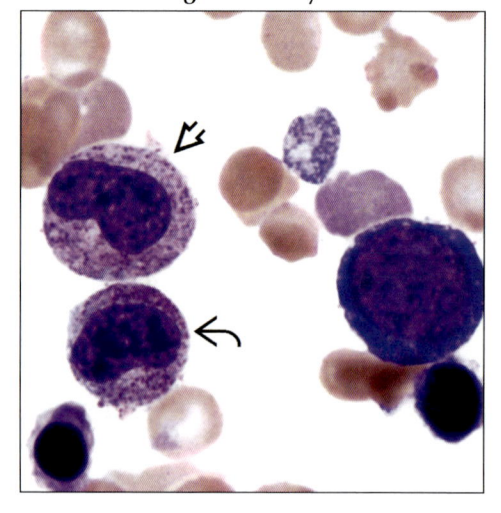

(Left) Nuclear indentation distinguishes a metamyelocyte ⇨ from a myelocyte ⇨, although maturation is a biologic continuum. Note that darker primary granules are more conspicuous in the myelocyte. **(Right)** Band neutrophils ⇨ are distinguished from segmented neutrophils ⇨ by nuclear features. Band neutrophils have uniform C-shaped nuclei without constriction. Terminal maturation is characterized by progressive nuclear lobulation, just beginning in the neutrophil shown here.

Stages of Granulocytic Maturation

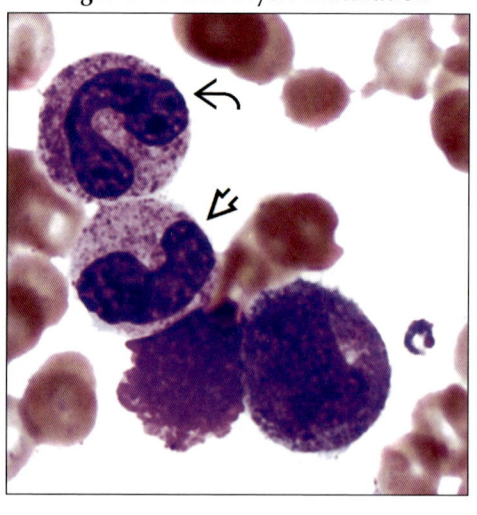

Paratrabecular Granulocytic Precursor Cells

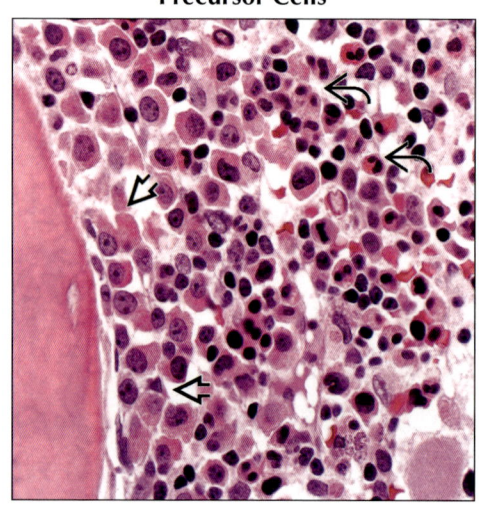

(Left) The normal paratrabecular localization of immature granulocytic lineage cells ⇨ is evident in this high-magnification image of a bone marrow core biopsy. More mature granulocytic lineage cells ⇨ are localized in the central regions of the core biopsy and are thus readily available for release into circulation. **(Right)** The lower edge of this biopsy shows the paratrabecular localization of normal immature granulocytic lineage cells that are highlighted by myeloperoxidase staining ⇨.

Paratrabecular Granulocytic Precursors

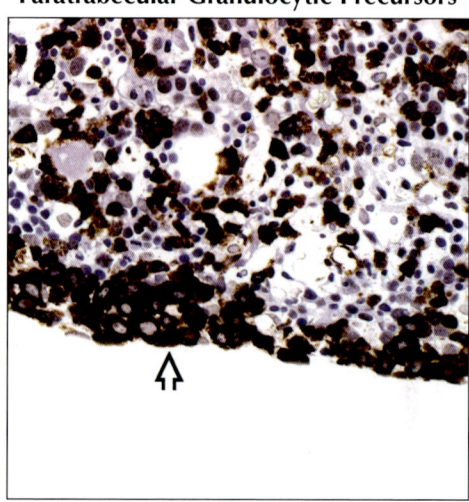

BONE MARROW

Erythroblasts

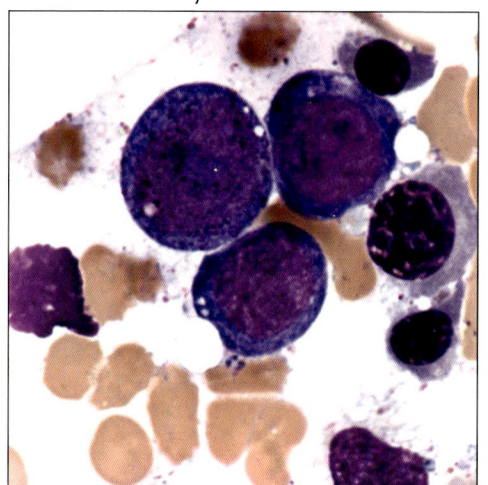

Erythroid Colony

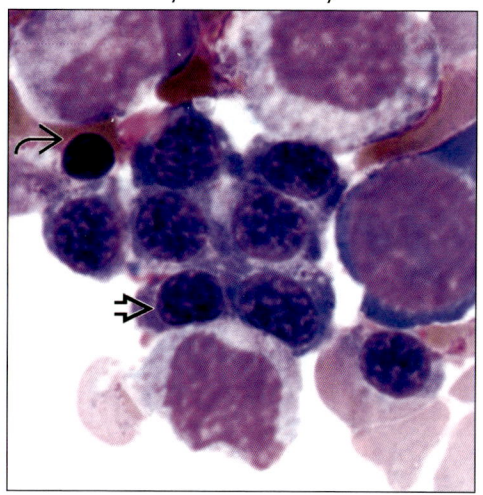

(Left) Erythroblasts (center) are characterized by a high nuclear to cytoplasmic ratio and deeply basophilic cytoplasm. Dramatic nuclear and cytoplasmic changes characterize maturation. (Right) More mature erythroid lineage cells show gray to eosinophilic cytoplasm reflecting hemoglobin production. There is dramatic nuclear shrinkage and pyknosis ⇨ with ultimate extrusion of the pyknotic nucleus ⇨. Erythroid cells tend to aggregate in colonies.

Macrophage With Adherent Erythroids

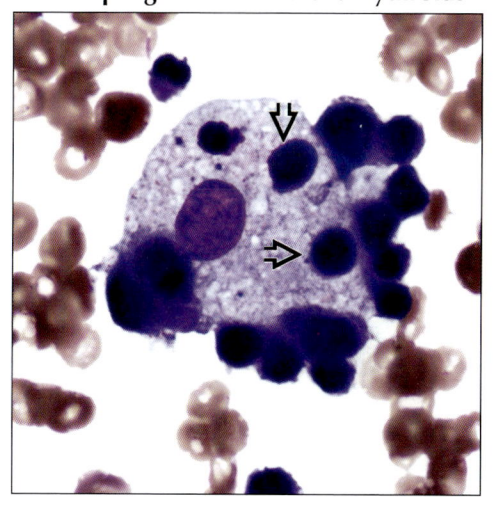

Storage Iron in Macrophage

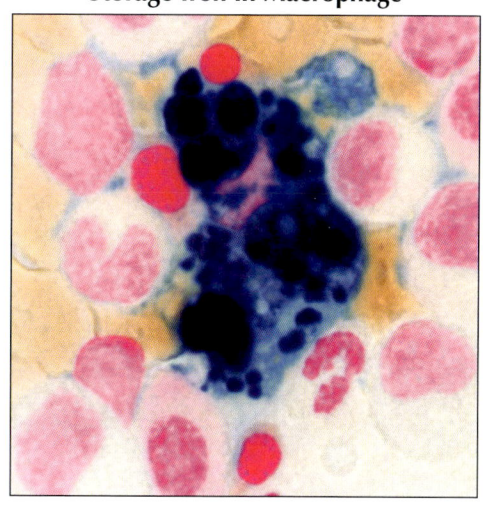

(Left) Erythroid cells selectively attach to macrophages, producing a so-called nurse cell. This adherence is critical for iron homeostasis. The macrophage is also immediately available to ingest extruded pyknotic erythroid cell nuclei ⇨ in the terminal stages of erythrocyte maturation. (Right) This macrophage, seen on an aspirate smear, contains abundant storage iron as seen in this iron stain.

Megakaryocytes

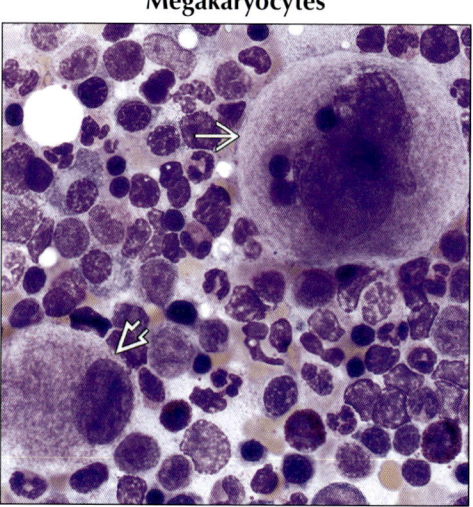

Mature Megakaryocyte

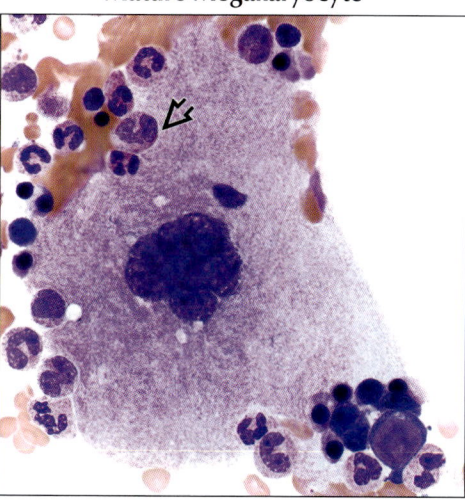

(Left) An immature megakaryocyte with a nonlobate nucleus is evident ⇨ compared to a hyperlobated mature megakaryocyte ⇨. Megakaryocyte maturation is characterized by progressive doubling of DNA without cell division (endomitosis). (Right) This mature megakaryocyte has voluminous amounts of cytoplasm, which will eventually shed off directly into the circulation as platelets. Neutrophils may pass through megakaryocyte cytoplasm ⇨.

BONE MARROW

Fat Cell

Mast Cell

(Left) Adipose (fat) cells are a normal constituent of the bone marrow microenvironment. These cells can have multiple vesicles, especially during regeneration following bone marrow suppression. (Right) Mast cells are an inconspicuous cell in bone marrow aspirate smears, especially within the darkest staining regions of bone marrow particles. The dark purple granules of mast cells obscure the round nucleus.

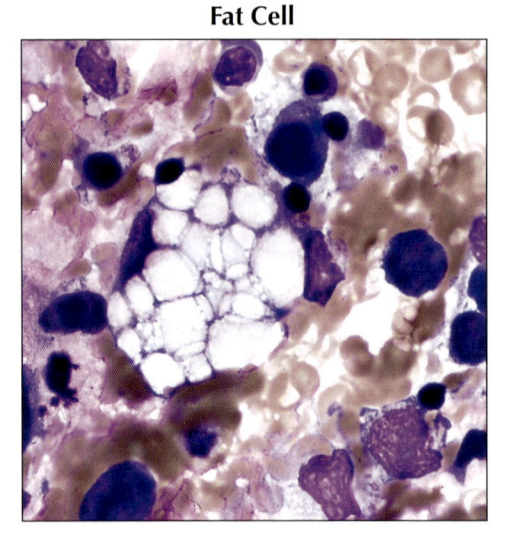

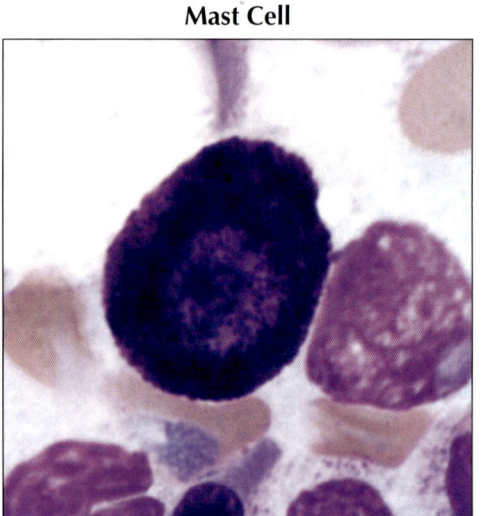

Plasma Cells

Perivascular Plasma Cells

(Left) Plasma cells ➦ are evident on bone marrow aspirate smears and can be identified by their eccentric nuclei and basophilic cytoplasm. A pale paranuclear hof region is evident ➡. Plasma cells may be confused with erythroid precursor cells ➤ because both cell types have deeply basophilic cytoplasm. (Right) Plasma cells are present in a perivascular location on bone marrow core biopsy sections ➡.

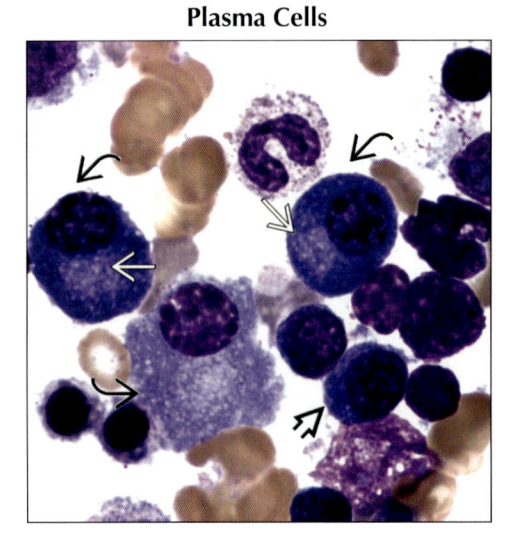

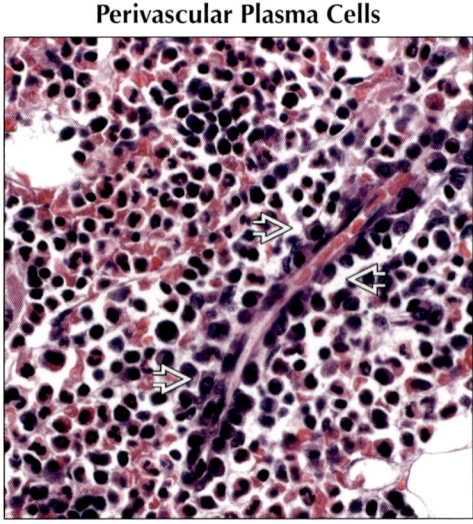

Perivascular Plasma Cells

Binucleate Plasma Cell

(Left) Immunohistochemical staining for CD138 can highlight the number, distribution, and location of plasma cells on bone marrow core biopsy sections. Note that the CD138-positive plasma cells form a collar around small blood vessels. (Right) Binucleated plasma cells ➤ may be seen on bone marrow aspirate smears. Binucleation is not indicative of a neoplastic plasma cell disorder and can be seen in many reactive processes.

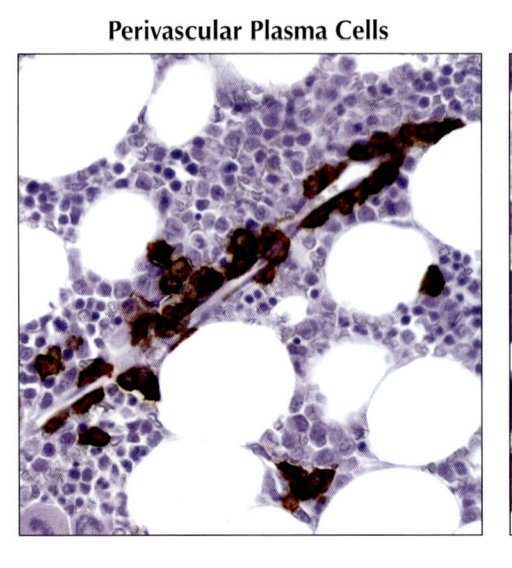

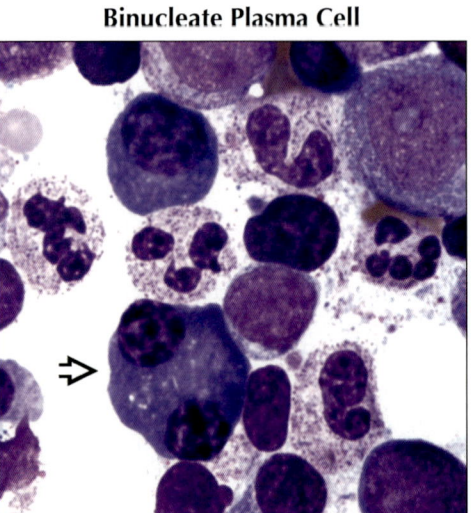

BONE MARROW

Osteoblasts
Osteoblast

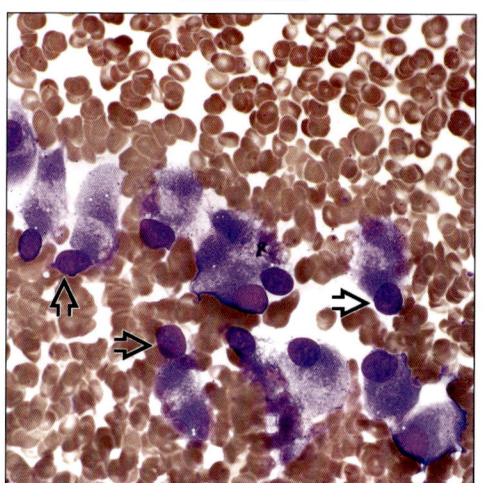

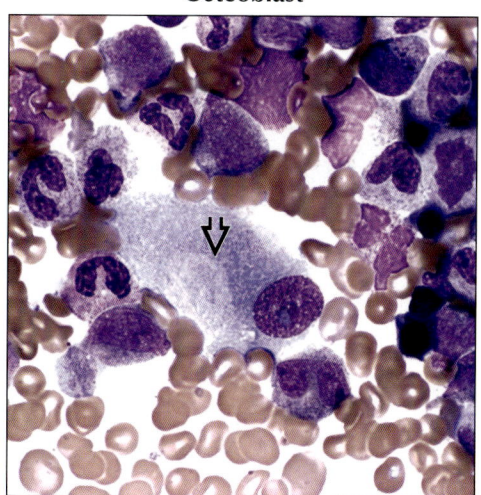

(Left) Osteoblasts are bone-forming cells that can be seen on bone marrow aspirate smears, especially in pediatric patients. They can be numerous in children with physiologic active bone growth and remodeling. Osteoblasts have markedly eccentric nuclei that appear to be separating from the cytoplasm ⇨. *(Right)* On high magnification, an osteoblast is characterized by an eccentric nucleus and a hof (cytoplasmic pale area) which, unlike the plasma cell, is separated from the nucleus ⇨.

Osteoclast
Osteoclast With Bone Sand

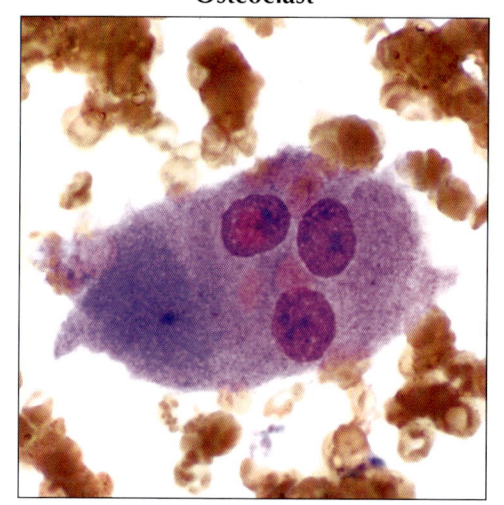

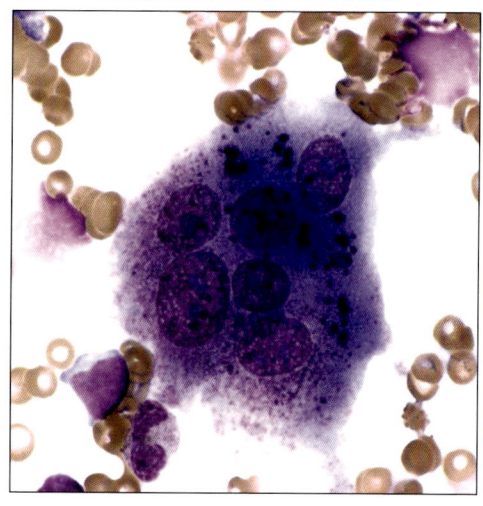

(Left) Osteoclasts can also be seen on bone marrow aspirate specimens in pediatric patients. These cells are characterized by multiple separate nuclei rather than the interconnected lobulation of megakaryocytes. Osteoclasts are hematopoietic stem cell derived and function in bone resorption. *(Right)* More mature osteoclasts may contain coarse cytoplasmic bone sand. Osteoclasts are very large cells that may be confused with either megakaryocytes or multinucleated histiocytes.

Osteoclast in Lacunar Space
Osteoblasts Rimming Bone

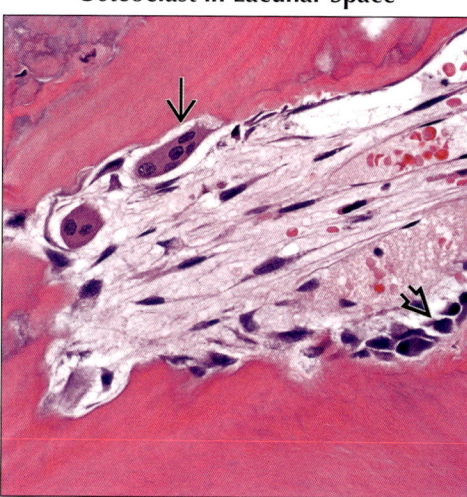

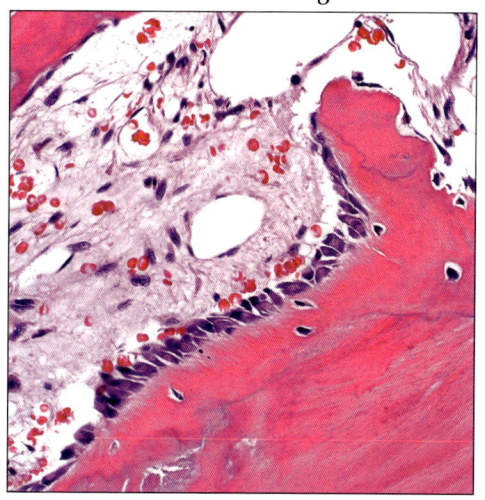

(Left) Bony remodeling is a normal feature in bone marrow core biopsy specimens from children. Osteoclasts reside in lacunar spaces ⇨ whereas osteoblasts rim the bony trabeculae ⇨. Osteoclasts are derived from hematopoietic stem cells, whereas osteoblasts are derived from mesenchymal stem cells. *(Right)* Prominent osteoblast rimming is evident adjacent to the bony trabeculae in this bone marrow core biopsy from a teenager. Osteoblasts are bone-forming cells and are normally present in children and adolescents.

BONE MARROW

Clumping on Aspirate Smear

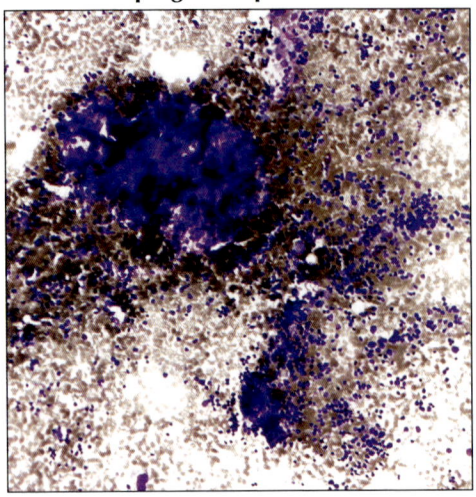

Skin in Core Biopsy Specimen

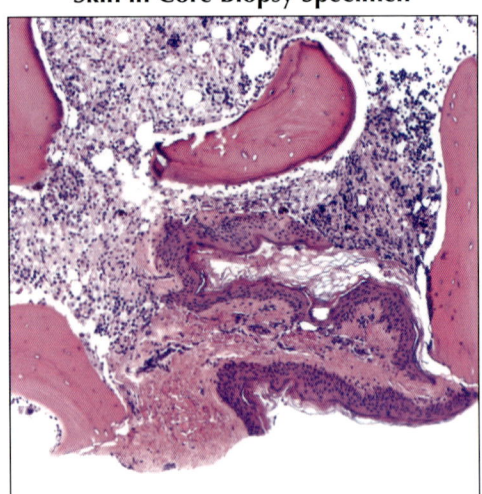

(Left) Prominent clumping is present on this aspirate smear, reflecting early specimen clotting. This phenomenon may greatly skew differential cell counts and distort cytologic assessment. (Right) Skin can sometimes be forced through the trocar needle during the bone marrow core biopsy procedure, as shown in this bone marrow core biopsy section. This has become more common due to concerns regarding scarring of the skin from lancing the entry site prior to inserting the trocar needle.

Aspiration Artifact

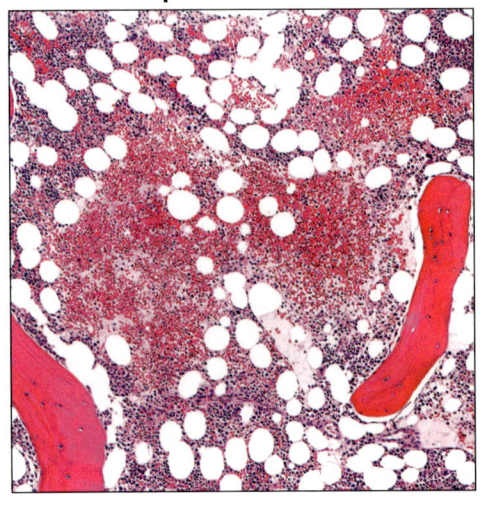

Adequate and Inadequate Core Biopsies

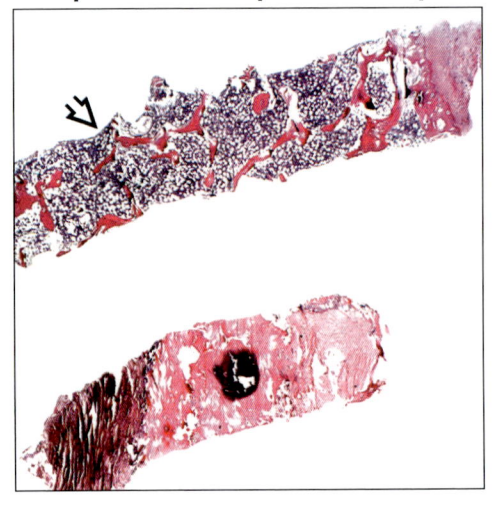

(Left) Partial bone marrow aspiration artifact is evident in the center of this bone marrow core biopsy section, showing an area in the biopsy devoid of marrow. Aspiration artifact is caused by performing the biopsy too close to the prior aspiration site. Aspiration artifact can be avoided by performing the biopsy first. (Right) This composite shows a sizable, intact, technically excellent bone marrow core biopsy ➢ adjacent to an inadequate core biopsy showing crushed bone without hematopoietic cells.

Gelatinous Transformation

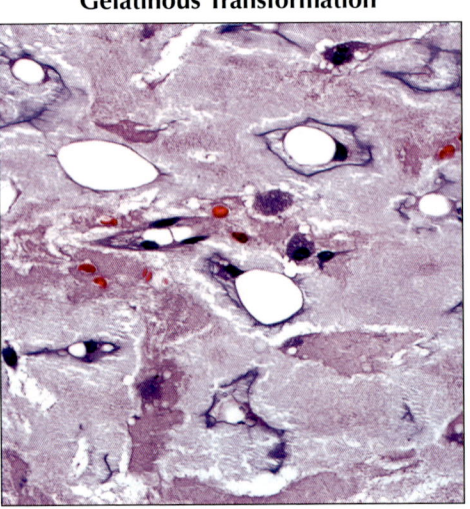

Previous Biopsy Site

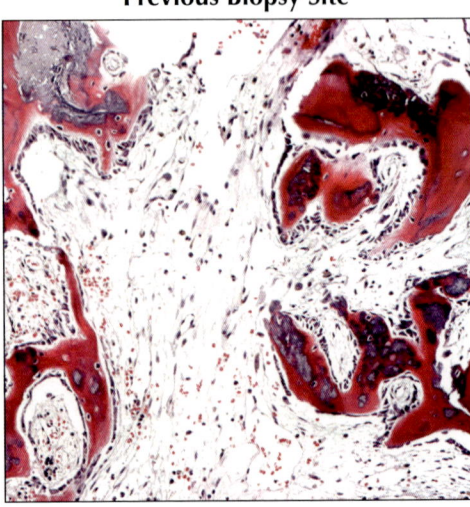

(Left) Gelatinous transformation, a change in the marrow secondary to cachexia, can mimic bone marrow aspirate artifact. RBCs are infrequent in areas of gelatinous transformation whereas numerous RBCs are present with aspiration artifact. (Right) This bone marrow core biopsy section is taken from a previous core biopsy site. Note fibrosis and prominent bone remodeling that reflects the repair process from the previous biopsy.

BONE MARROW

Bone Marrow Aspirate, Newborn

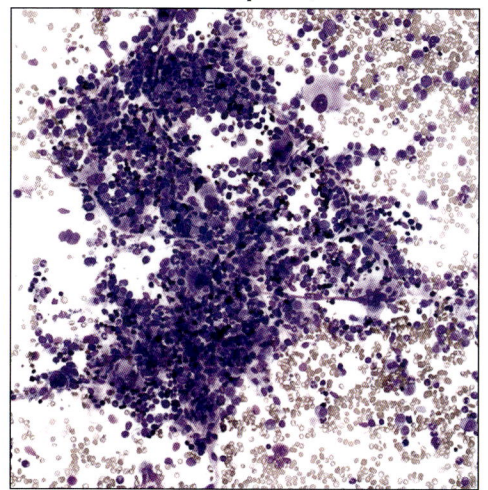

Bone Marrow Core Biopsy, Infant

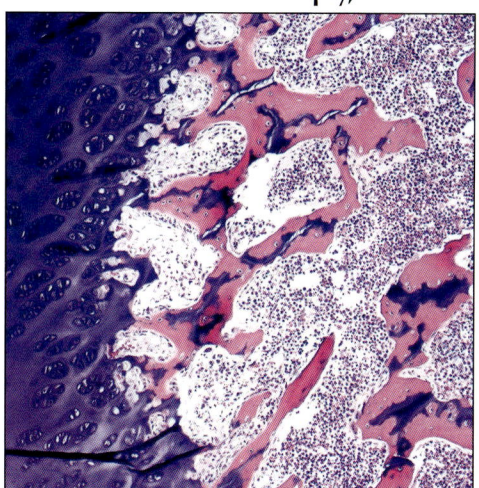

(Left) This bone marrow aspirate smear from a newborn shows approximately 100% cellularity since few, if any, fat cells are present. This high level of cellularity is physiologic in newborns and infants. *(Right)* This bone marrow core biopsy from a 21-month-old infant shows prominent bony remodeling and mineralization, physiologic for patient age. Note that cellularity approaches 100%, also physiologic for age.

Hematogones

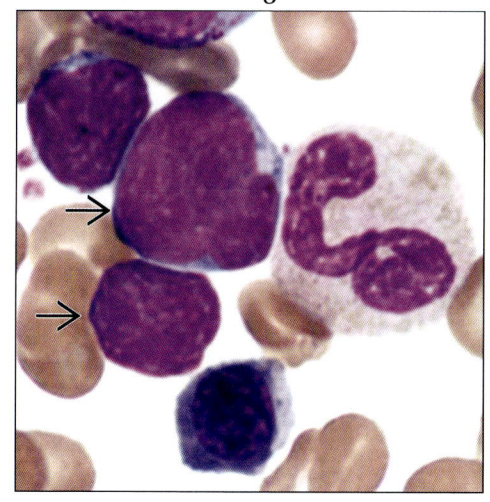

Prominent Hematogones, Young Patient

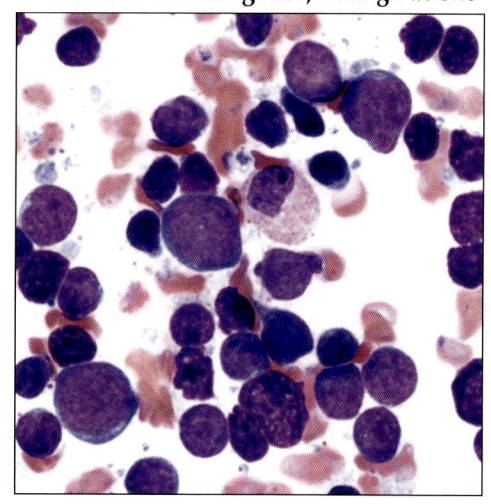

(Left) Hematogones are benign lymphoid precursor cells that show a range in overall cell size. On high magnification, hematogones show dense nuclear chromatin with inconspicuous nucleoli and scant cytoplasm ➔. *(Right)* Lymphoid cells are especially prominent on bone marrow aspirate smears from young patients. These cells often have morphologic features of hematogones (benign lymphoid precursor cells). Specimens with physiologically increased hematogones can be misdiagnosed as leukemia.

Bone Marrow Core, Adolescent Male

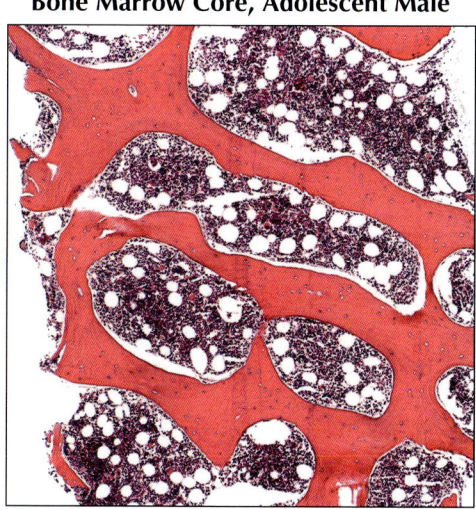

Bone Marrow Core Biopsy, Middle-Aged Woman

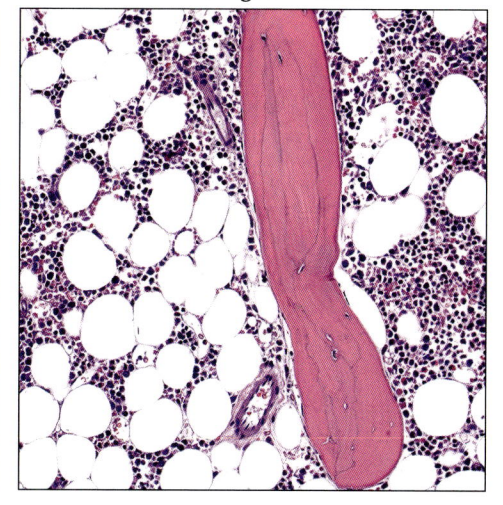

(Left) This bone marrow core biopsy is from a 17-year-old male and shows prominent bone remodeling and thick bony trabeculae, physiologic for age. Note that overall cellularity is about 75%, normal for age. *(Right)* This bone marrow core biopsy from a 52-year-old woman shows approximately 50% fat cells and 50% hematopoietic cells. Increasing amounts of bone marrow fat cells with decreasing hematopoietic cells is typical with aging. Bony trabeculae are also thinner than in younger patients.

PERIPHERAL BLOOD

Key Facts

Macroscopic Anatomy
- Total blood volume varies by body size
- Blood comprises about 7% of total body weight
- Adult blood volume is about 5 liters
- Blood consists of cells (predominantly red blood cells [RBCs]) and plasma
- By centrifugation, blood can be separated into packed RBCs (hematocrit), plasma, and white blood cells (WBCs) (called buffy coat)

Microscopic Anatomy
- All normal circulating cells are bone marrow derived
- Blood is assessed by automated cell counting and morphologic review
- Clinical and laboratory integration is essential
- Numerous RBC parameters are assessed to gauge number, size, shape, hemoglobin content, and uniformity
- WBCs enumerated, differentiated into specific types
- Automated WBC differentials include neutrophils, lymphocytes, monocytes, eosinophils, and basophils
- Absolute WBC counts are more useful than percentages
- In blood, about half of the neutrophils are circulating, and the other half have attached to the endothelium (marginated cells)
- Only the circulating pool of neutrophils is included in the WBC count
- Migration to tissues is key for WBC function
- Platelets are enumerated and sized

Pitfalls/Artifacts
- Automated cell counting may be inaccurate in aged specimens or specimens exposed to high temperatures
- Cryoglobulins, cold agglutinins, and other substances can interfere with automated cell counting
- Large cells and microfilarial worms are selectively pulled to the feather edge and may not be conspicuous in the region of the slide where morphology assessed
- Poor stain quality may interfere with cell identification and morphologic assessment
- Platelet clumping and satellitism cause spurious platelet counts
- Degranulated basophils may be misidentified
- Lymphocytes in neonates and young children may have immature nuclear features
- Normal ranges for RBC parameters/absolute neutrophil counts are lower in individuals of African ancestry

Age Variation
- Highly specific age- and sex-related normal ranges have been established
- Residence at high altitude impacts normal ranges for RBC parameters
- Term neonates exhibit higher RBC parameters with nucleated RBCs and higher WBCs than other ages
- Blood features in preterm neonates include lower RBC count, higher MCV, and more nucleated (N)RBCs compared to term infants
- Blood smear review of a normal neonate shows polychromasia, macrocytosis, NRBCs, and left shift
- WBC count is typically above 15,000 per mm^3 in term neonates due to high numbers of neutrophils
- WBC count declines rapidly after birth, due to neutrophil reductions; RBC parameters gradually decline; NRBCs absent after 1st week
- By about 2 weeks of age, lymphocytes predominate; this finding persists throughout early childhood
- After puberty, RBC parameters are higher in males than females
- Normal ranges for RBC parameters in the advanced elderly are not clear cut, especially the definition of anemia

Hyperplasia
- Expansions in neutrophils, lymphocytes, eosinophils, monocytes, and platelets may occur in a variety of reactive conditions
- The cause of these reactive conditions can usually be determined by clinical correlation
- A significant absolute basophilia is uncommon in reactive conditions and is generally linked to clonal myeloid neoplasms

---

(Left) By automated cell counting techniques, cells pass single file through an aperture and are counted, sized, and interrogated. These 2 graphs illustrate the size profile (i.e., mean corpuscular volume ➤) of normal RBCs. The 2 most prominent peaks on the WBC histogram illustrate lymphocytes ➤ and granulocytes ➤. (Right) Based on size and cytoplasmic granularity, differential counts are performed. Lymphocytes ➤ are small and agranular, whereas neutrophils are larger and granular ➤.

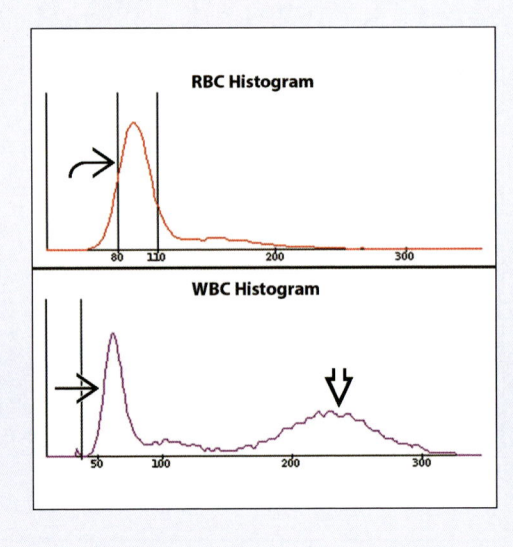

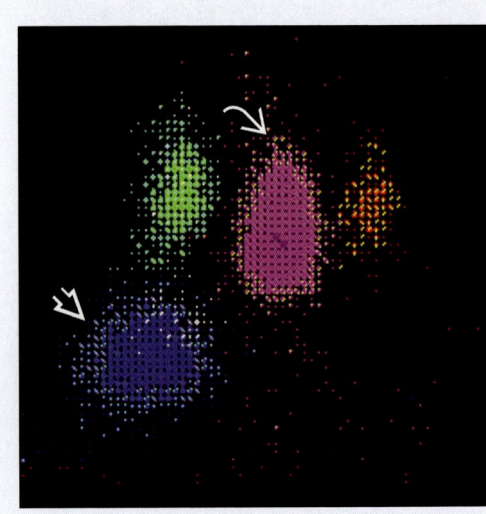

PERIPHERAL BLOOD

Normal Blood (Adult)

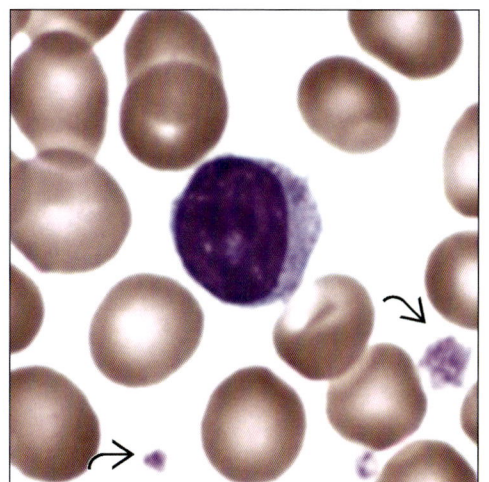

Normal White Blood Cells

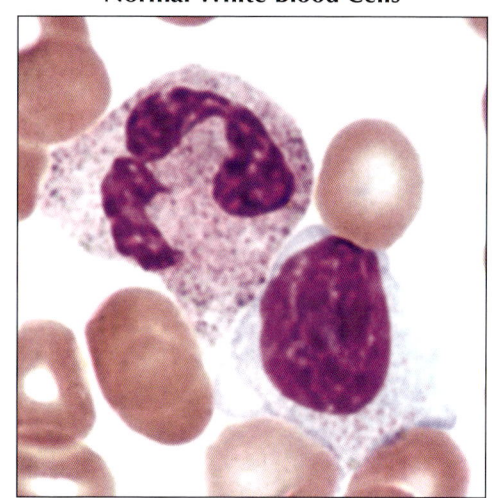

(Left) This peripheral blood smear from a normal adult female shows uniform erythrocytes with a normal central pallor, normal platelets, and a nonactivated lymphocyte. There is some variation in platelet size ➚, but all platelets are well granulated. *(Right)* A normal neutrophil and a large granular lymphocyte are evident at high magnification on this blood smear from an adult. Large granular lymphocytes are present in low numbers in blood; cells with this morphology are either NK cells or cytotoxic/suppressor T cells.

Neutrophil

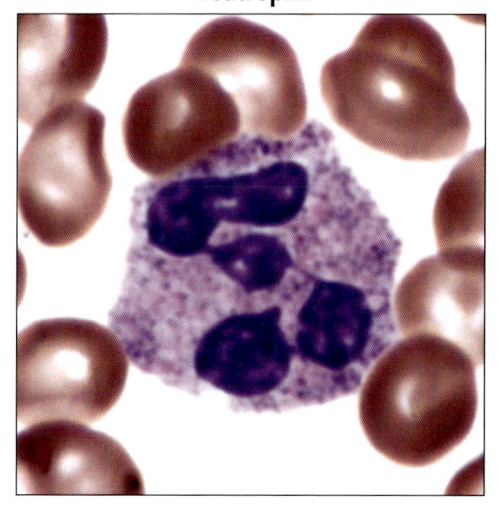

Monocyte

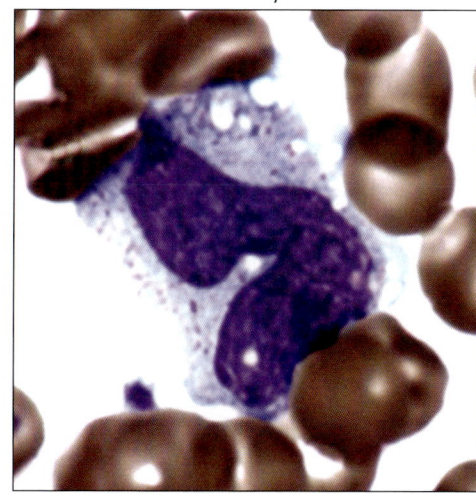

(Left) Normal neutrophil nuclear segmentation and normal granulation of the cytoplasm are evident in this circulating neutrophil. Neutrophils typically have 3-5 nuclear lobes with a thin strand of chromatin connecting these lobes. The cytoplasm has a pinkish tint from secondary granules. *(Right)* A monocyte is characterized by large size, blue-gray cytoplasm with occasional granules and vacuoles, and a somewhat folded nucleus. The nuclear chromatin has a "hills and valleys" appearance.

Eosinophil

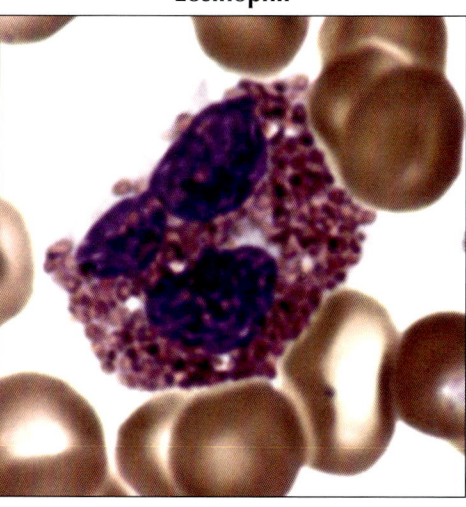

Basophil

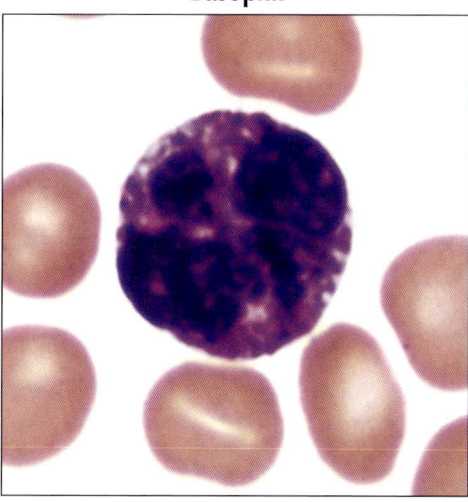

(Left) Eosinophils are recognized by the distinctive eosinophilic, refractile appearance of the secondary granules as shown on the blood smear. Eosinophils typically have 2 nuclear lobes, but sometimes 3, as illustrated here. *(Right)* Basophils are the least numerous WBC in the blood. The secondary granules of basophils are dark and coarse. These granules often overlie the nucleus, which typically shows 3-4 nuclear lobes. Note the adjacent normal RBCs.

PERIPHERAL BLOCD

Clumped Platelets

(Left) Platelet clumping is a common artifact in peripheral blood and may interfere with accurate platelet counts. Manual scanning for platelet clumps is recommended on blood smears when thrombocytopenia is detected by automated counting.

Platelet Satellitism

(Right) Platelet satellitism is an artifactual phenomenon in which platelets adhere to neutrophils. A spuriously low platelet count can result from satellitism. Repeat testing utilizing a different anticoagulant is recommended.

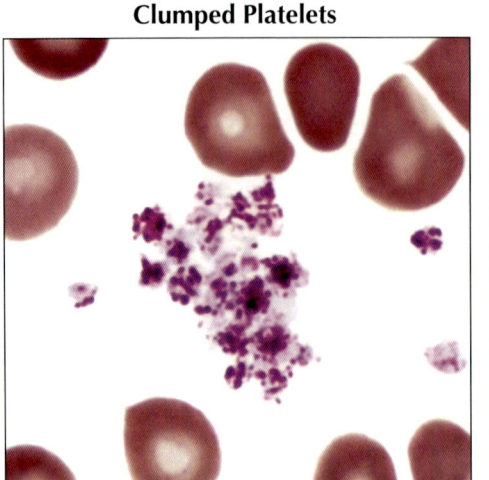

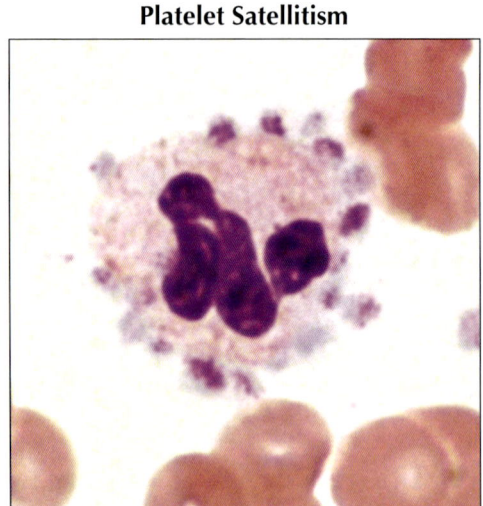

Cryoglobulin

(Left) The extracellular amorphous blue globules shown here are cryoglobulin. They can precipitate in peripheral blood, interfering with automated cell counting.

Agglutination

(Right) Erythrocyte agglutination is common in patients with a cold agglutinin. Agglutination often results with cooling of the specimen during transport after phlebotomy. Warming the specimen eliminates the agglutination so that accurate automated cell counts can occur. Note the clumps of erythrocytes in this photograph.

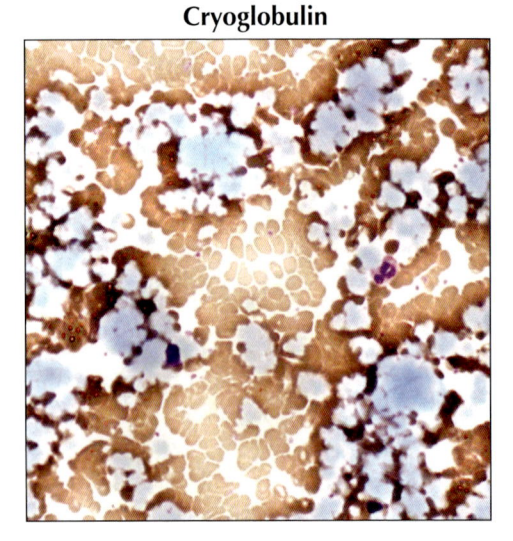

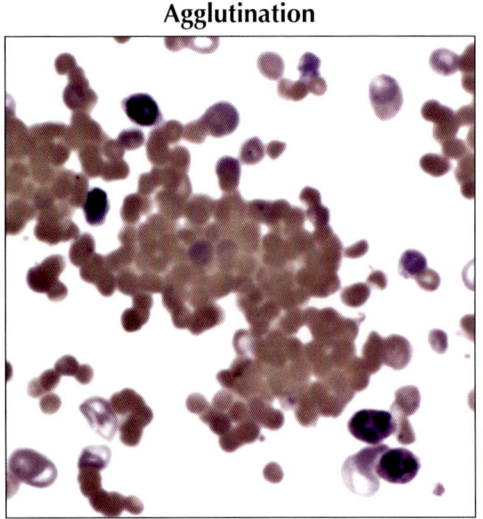

Partial Degranulation of a Basophil

(Left) This photo compares a partially degranulated basophil (lower right) with a normal neutrophil (upper left). Note that basophil granules still overlie the nucleus. Note the broken neutrophil ▷, a so-called basket cell.

Toxic Neutrophils

(Right) Toxic neutrophils, as illustrated here, can mimic basophils because of the prominent basophilic granulation that characterizes an activated neutrophil. This appearance is due to staining changes in the activated secondary granules.

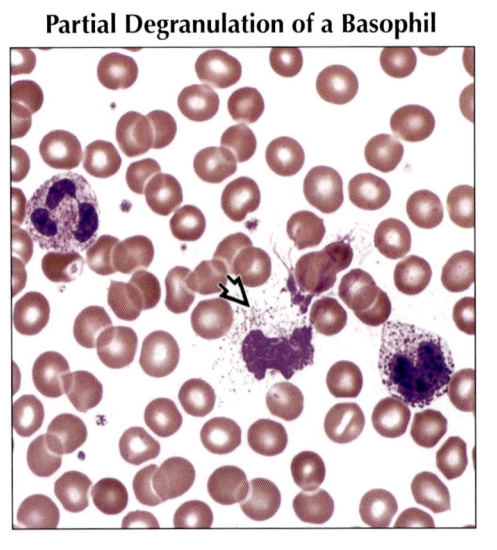

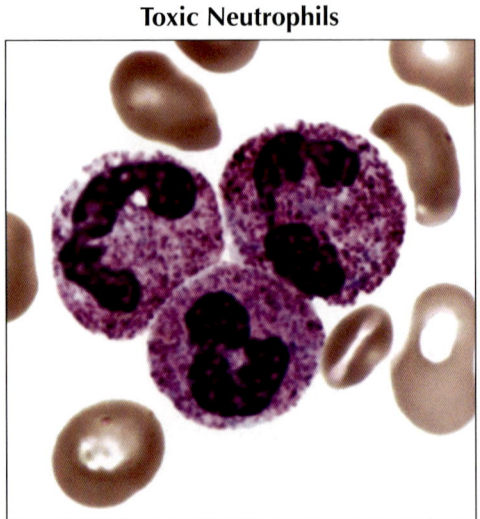

PERIPHERAL BLOOD

Newborn Blood

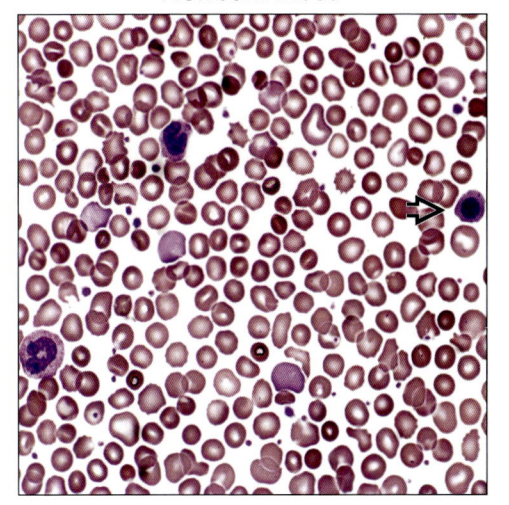

Normal Term Newborn

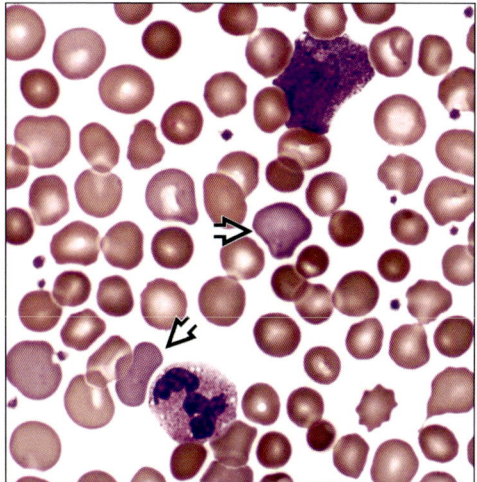

(Left) This blood smear from a term newborn shows a high number of erythrocytes and many reticulocytes, which is physiologic for this age. A leukocytosis with left shift is also physiologic for age, as are nucleated red blood cells ⊵. The leukocytosis, polychromasia, and NRBCs should all decline shortly after birth in healthy babies. *(Right)* Features that are physiologic in the newborn period are illustrated in this peripheral blood smear, including prominent polychromasia ⊵, left shift, and leukocytosis.

Normal Immature Lymphocyte in an Infant

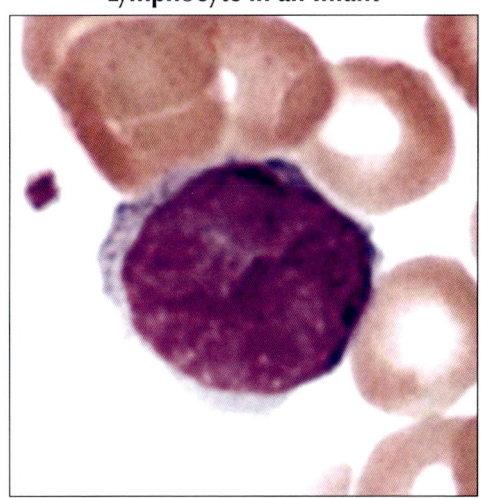

Normal Lymphocyte Spectrum in an Infant

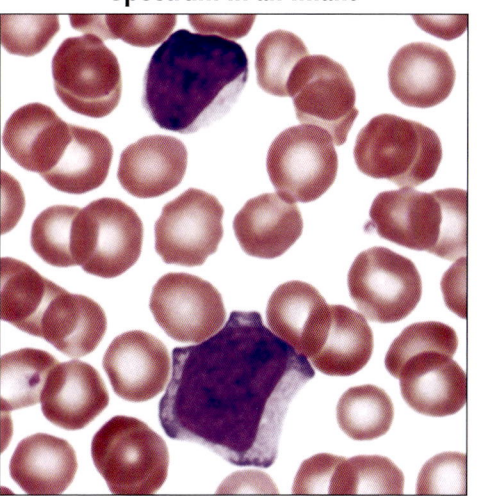

(Left) Immature lymphocytes are physiologic in infants and young children, even though they are reminiscent of lymphoblasts. These cells have dispersed chromatin and scant cytoplasm. Hematopoietic parameters are normal, a finding useful in the distinction from leukemia. *(Right)* This peripheral blood smear is from a 4-month-old infant. It shows a more normal-appearing lymphocyte (top) in conjunction with a larger lymphocyte that exhibits some nuclear immaturity. The size and nuclear features are physiologic for this age.

Normal Blood, 4-Month-Old Infant

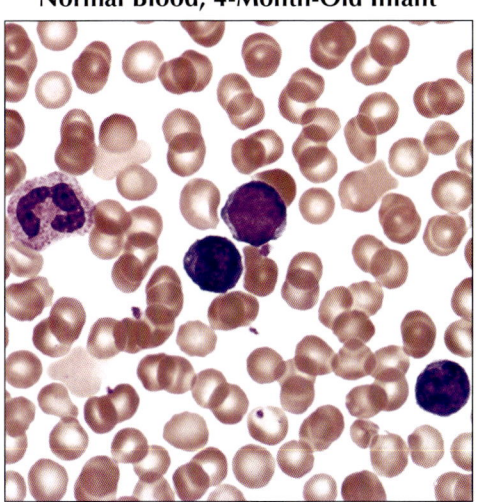

Feather Edge

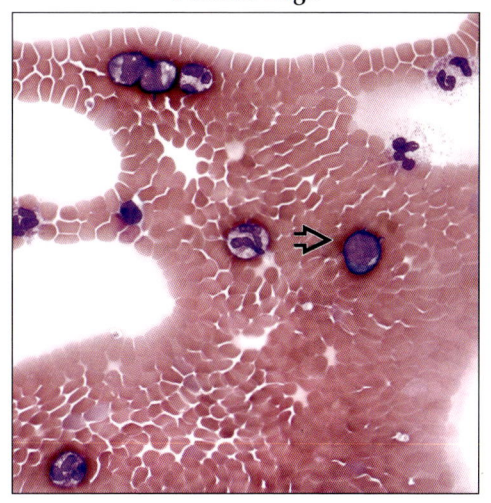

(Left) This blood smear from a 4-month-old boy shows a predominance of lymphoid cells (absolute lymphocyte count of 10.8×10^9/L), which is physiologic for age. *(Right)* It is important to scan the feather edge of a smear during manual morphologic review to detect cells and even microfilarial worms that have been "dragged" to this portion of the blood smear. Larger cells such as this immunoblast ⊵ are often pulled to the feather edge in the preparation of blood smears as well.

THYMUS

Key Facts

Macroscopic Anatomy
- Located in anterosuperior mediastinum
- Lobulated midline organ responsible for T lymphocyte development
  - Lobules have 2 compartments: An outer cortex and an inner medulla

Microscopic Anatomy
- Outer fibrous capsule
- Cortex contains numerous T lymphocytes and sparse epithelial cells
- Medulla contains larger proportion of epithelial cells to lymphocytes
- Hassall corpuscles found in medulla

Pitfalls/Artifacts
- Atrophied thymic remnants can mimic a neuroendocrine proliferation
- Regional brown fat can be misinterpreted as a hibernoma or liposarcoma

Age Variation
- Size and weight of thymus increase from birth to puberty
- Prepubertal thymus is overtly cellular with a prominent dual epithelial/lymphocyte population
- After puberty, thymus begins to atrophy (physiologic involution) and is progressively replaced by mature adipose tissue
- Adult thymus shows significantly decreased cellularity, epithelial cell atrophy, a paucity of lymphocytes, and mature fat infiltration

Hyperplasia
- True thymic hyperplasia is increase in size of thymus
- Lymphoid hyperplasia is due to influx of reactive B cells, such as in myasthenia gravis

(Left) The pediatric thymus is markedly compartmentalized, with lobules of lymphoepithelial tissue separated by wispy fibrous interstitium ➡. Hassall corpuscles can often be seen at low magnification ➡.

(Right) Within each lobule are 2 compartments: A dark outer cortex ➡ and a pale inner medulla ➡. This disparity in color is due to the presence of significantly more lymphocytes in the cortex than in the medulla.

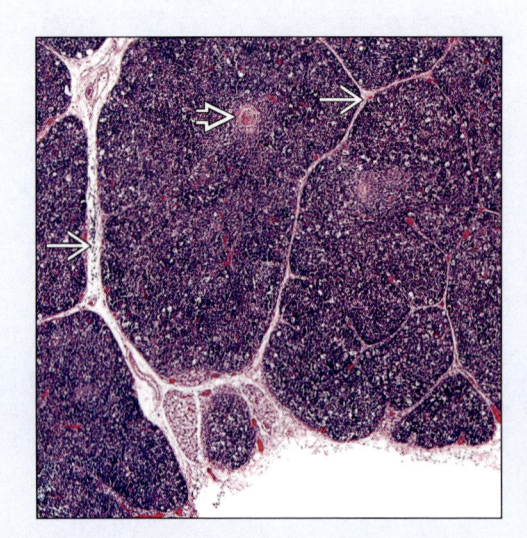

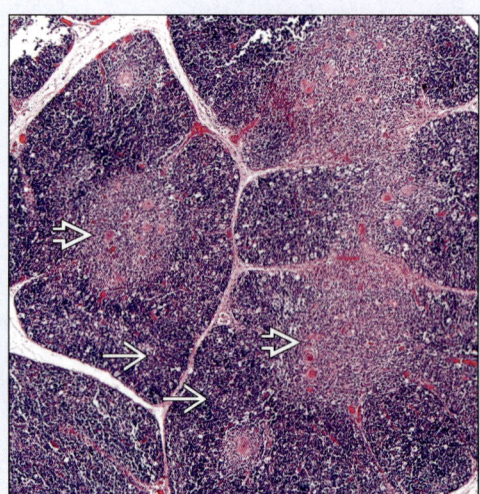

(Left) There is usually a connective tissue capsule at the periphery of the thymus ➡. This capsule varies in size from thin and wispy to thick and fibrous. It is contiguous with the fibrous interstitium between the thymic lobules.

(Right) The cortex ➡ is composed predominantly of immature T lymphocytes and a few epithelial cells, giving it a darker appearance than the adjacent medulla ➡. The pink squamoid Hassall corpuscles are easily visible against the background of lymphocytes ➡.

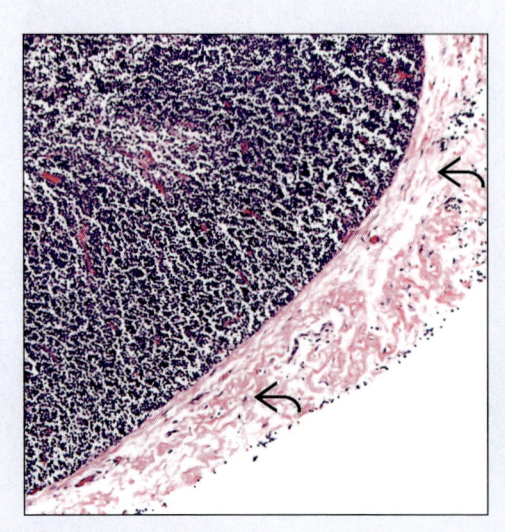

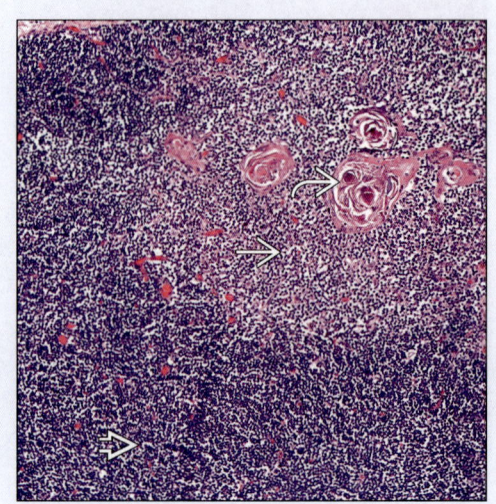

THYMUS

Thymic Cortex

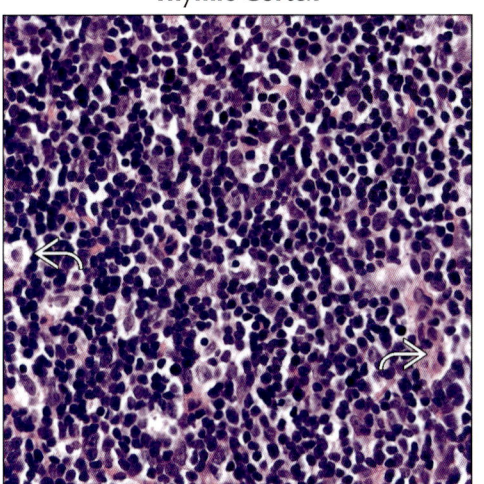

Thymic Medulla

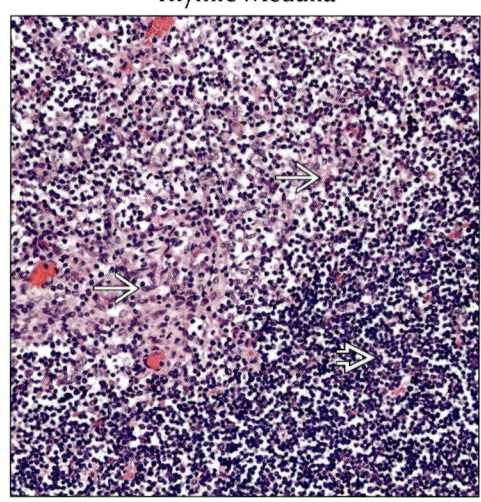

(**Left**) The immature T lymphocytes found in the thymic cortex have very little cytoplasm and are closely packed. The larger thymic epithelial cells are interspersed between the lymphocytes and can be identified by their more abundant cytoplasm ➡. (**Right**) Compared to the cortex, the thymic medulla contains a much larger population of pink, thymic epithelial cells ➡ and a smaller proportion of dark T lymphocytes ➡.

Hassall Corpuscles

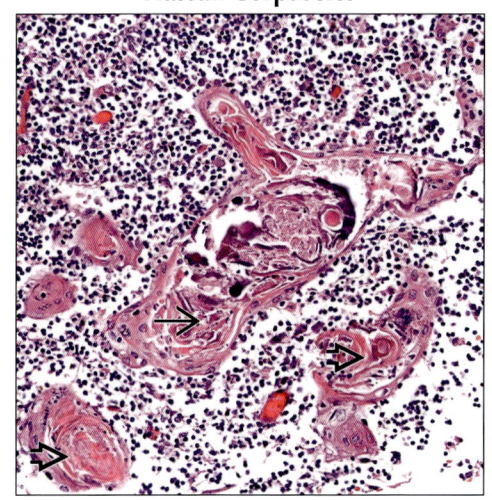

Physiologic Involution

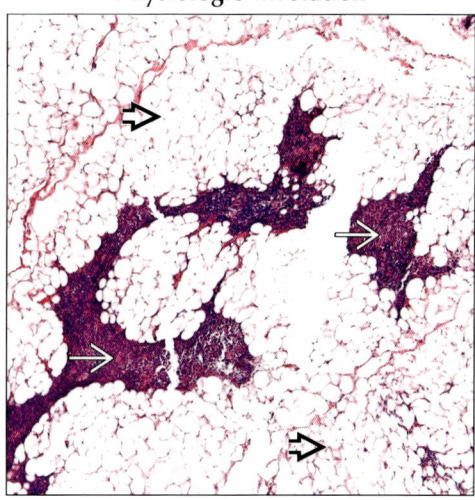

(**Left**) Hassall corpuscles are composed of keratinized epithelial cells arranged in concentrically oriented nests ➡, which often contain keratin debris ➡. These unique structures are easily seen in the medulla even at low magnification and are very useful in identifying thymic tissue. (**Right**) After puberty, the thymus begins the process of physiologic involution, or atrophy, during which the thymic lymphoepithelial tissue ➡ is gradually replaced by mature fat. ➡.

Atrophic Epithelial Elements

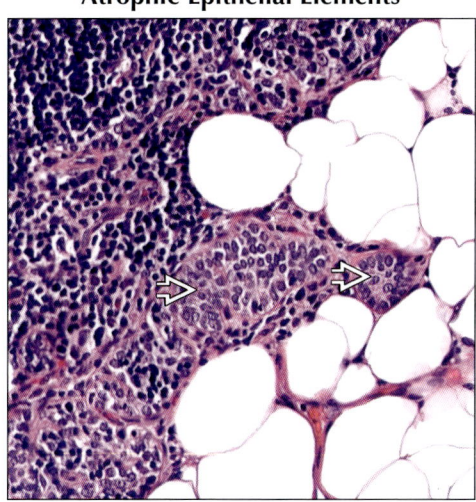

Brown Fat

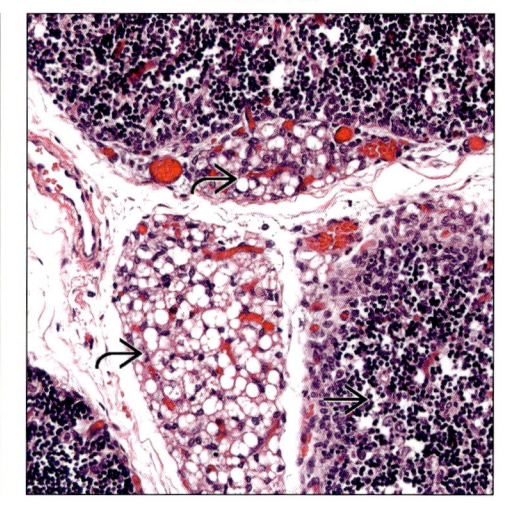

(**Left**) During the process of involution, thymic atrophy can result in small nests or aggregates of atrophied epithelial cells ➡ that are reminiscent of neuroendocrine proliferations, such as a carcinoid tumor. (**Right**) In the pediatric population, the mediastinum contains a prominent component of brown fat ➡. It is not unusual to see nests or sheets of these multivacuolated, often pink granular cells adjacent to the thymic lobules ➡.

SELECTED REFERENCES

OVERVIEW OF THE IMMUNE SYSTEM

1. Murphy SP et al: Innate immunity in transplant tolerance and rejection. Immunol Rev. 241(1):39-48, 2011
2. Chaplin DD: Overview of the immune response. J Allergy Clin Immunol. 125(2 Suppl 2):S3-23, 2010
3. Cruvinel Wde M et al: Immune system - part I. Fundamentals of innate immunity with emphasis on molecular and cellular mechanisms of inflammatory response. Rev Bras Reumatol. 50(4):434-61, 2010
4. Mesquita Júnior D et al: Immune system - part II: basis of the immunological response mediated by T and B lymphocytes. Rev Bras Reumatol. 50(5):552-80, 2010
5. Waldner H: The role of innate immune responses in autoimmune disease development. Autoimmun Rev. 8(5):400-4, 2009
6. Alam R et al: 3. Lymphocytes. J Allergy Clin Immunol. 111(2 Suppl):S476-85, 2003
7. Parkin J et al: An overview of the immune system. Lancet. 357(9270):1777-89, 2001
8. Alam R: A brief review of the immune system. Prim Care. 25(4):727-38, 1998

LYMPH NODES

1. Buettner M et al: Lymph node dissection-- understanding the immunological function of lymph nodes. Clin Exp Immunol. 169(3):205-12, 2012
2. Natkunam Y: The biology of the germinal center. Hematology Am Soc Hematol Educ Program. 1:210-5, 2007
3. Wolniak KL et al: The germinal center response. Crit Rev Immunol. 24(1):39-65, 2004

SPLEEN

1. Cesta MF: Normal structure, function, and histology of the spleen. Toxicol Pathol. 34(5):455-65, 2006
2. Mebius RE et al: Structure and function of the spleen. Nat Rev Immunol. 5(8):606-16, 2005
3. Scothorne RJ: The spleen: structure and function. Histopathology. 9(6):663-9, 1985

BONE MARROW

1. Kostyak JC et al: Calcium- and integrin-binding protein 1 regulates megakaryocyte ploidy, adhesion, and migration. Blood. 119(3):838-46, 2012
2. Bianco P: Bone and the hematopoietic niche: a tale of two stem cells. Blood. 117(20):5281-8, 2011
3. Hattangadi SM et al: From stem cell to red cell: regulation of erythropoiesis at multiple levels by multiple proteins, RNAs, and chromatin modifications. Blood. 118(24):6258-68, 2011
4. Ottersbach K et al: Ontogeny of haematopoiesis: recent advances and open questions. Br J Haematol. 148(3):343-55, 2010
5. Lee SH et al: ICSH guidelines for the standardization of bone marrow specimens and reports. Int J Lab Hematol. 30(5):349-64, 2008
6. Metcalf D: Hematopoietic cytokines. Blood. 111(2):485-91, 2008
7. Cotelingam JD: Bone marrow biopsy: interpretive guidelines for the surgical pathologist. Adv Anat Pathol. 10(1):8-26, 2003

PERIPHERAL BLOOD

1. Jaso J et al: A synoptic reporting system for peripheral blood smear interpretation. Am J Clin Pathol. 135(3):358-64, 2011
2. Proytcheva MA: Issues in neonatal cellular analysis. Am J Clin Pathol. 131(4):560-73, 2009
3. Buttarello M et al: Automated blood cell counts: state of the art. Am J Clin Pathol. 130(1):104-16, 2008
4. Robins EB et al: Hematologic reference values for African American children and adolescents. Am J Hematol. 82(7):611-4, 2007
5. Wakeman L et al: Robust, routine haematology reference ranges for healthy adults. Int J Lab Hematol. 29(4):279-83, 2007
6. Cheng CK et al: Complete blood count reference interval diagrams derived from NHANES III: stratification by age, sex, and race. Lab Hematol. 10(1):42-53, 2004

THYMUS

1. Kendall MD: Functional anatomy of the thymic microenvironment. J Anat. 177:1-29, 1991
2. Schulof RS et al: Thymic physiology and biochemistry. Adv Clin Chem. 26:203-92, 1987
3. Kendall MD et al: Heterogeneity of the human thymus epithelial microenvironment at the ultrastructural level. Adv Exp Med Biol. 186:289-97, 1985

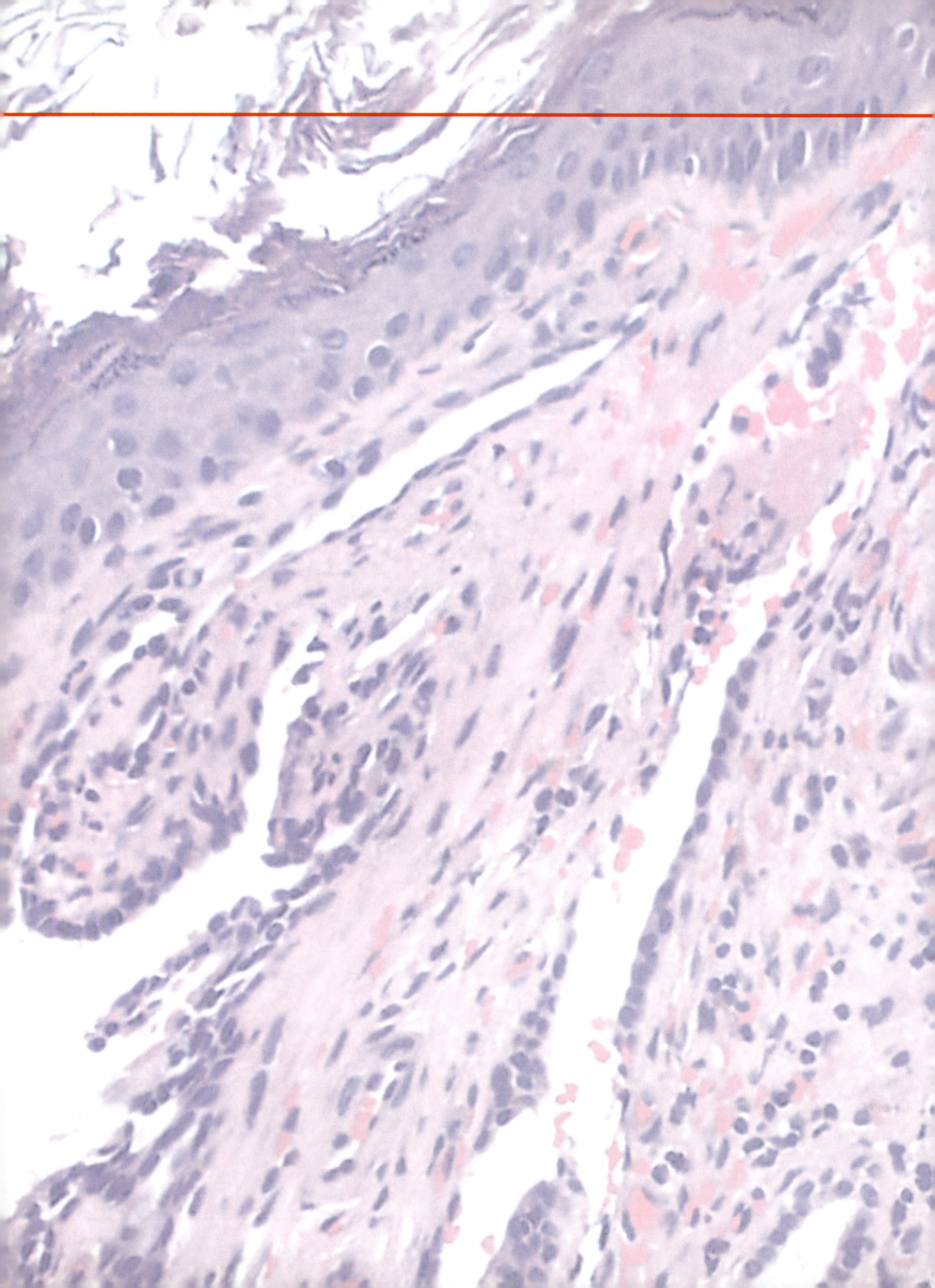

Head and Neck

Eye and Ocular Adnexa	7-2
Oral Mucosae	7-12
Gingivae	7-14
Minor Salivary Glands	7-16
Teeth	7-18
Tongue	7-22
Tonsils/Adenoids	7-26
Ear	7-30
Nose and Paranasal Sinuses	7-34
Pharynx	7-38
Larynx	7-40
Major Salivary Glands	7-44

EYE AND OCULAR ADNEXA

Key Facts

Macroscopic Anatomy
- Eyelid: Skin and conjunctival covering of eye
- Cornea: Transparent outermost structure that refracts incoming light
- Iris: Membranous diaphragm with a central opening (pupil)
- Lens: Biconvex crystalline structure that focuses light on retina
- Vitreous: Gel-like material filling posterior cavity
- Sclera: White, tough outer covering of globe
- Retina: Complex organization of nerve cells and processes that translate light into electrical impulses to the brain via the optic nerve
- Optic nerve: Cranial nerve conveying signals from the retina to the brain
- Orbital soft tissue: Supportive fat, muscle, and collagen

Microscopic Anatomy
- Schlemm canal: Drainage channel for aqueous
- Schwalbe ring: The termination of Descemet membrane
- Ciliary body: Supports lens via zonular fibers
- Choroid: Vascular layer between sclera and retina
- Lacrimal glands: Serous glands that produce tears
- Meibomian gland: Sebaceous glands in tarsus
- Glands of Moll: Eyelash follicle glands composed of apocrine cells
- Glands of Zeis: Sebaceous glands that empty into the eyelash follicle

Age Variation
- Focal thickening of peripheral Descemet membrane (Hassall-Henle warts)
- Thickening and hyalinization of the pars plicata and ciliary processes

(Left) This graphic illustrates the globe in a sagittal section. The globe is supported by muscle ⇨ and adipose tissue ⇨. *(Right)* In this sagittal section, the cornea ⇨, iris ⇨, lens ⇨, vitreous body ⇨, and ciliary body ⇨ can be identified. The anterior chamber is the space between the anterior iris and posterior cornea and the posterior chamber is comprised of the space between the vitreous and the posterior aspect of the iris. (Courtesy H. Brown, MD.)

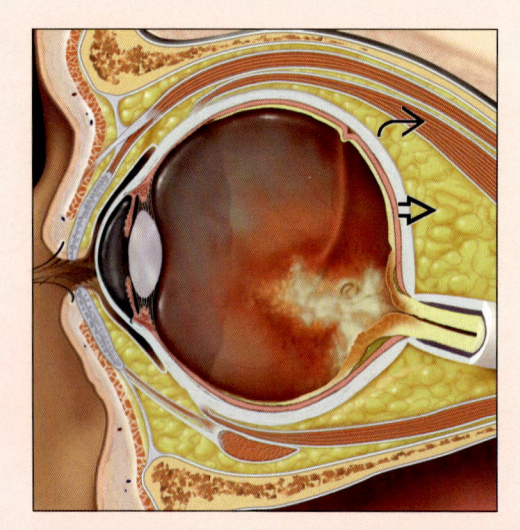

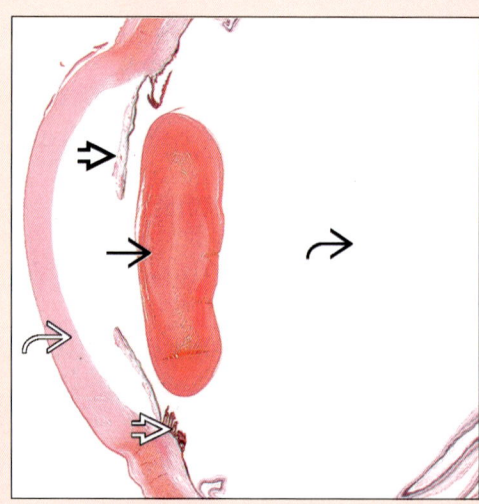

(Left) In this low-power field of the posterior globe, the head of the optic nerve ⇨, the retina ⇨, choroid ⇨, and the sclera ⇨ can be identified. (Courtesy H. Brown, MD.) *(Right)* The anterior chamber of the globe is situated between the posterior cornea ⇨ and the anterior iris ⇨. At low power, the lens is composed of eosinophilic material ⇨. The iris sphincter constricts and dilates to adjust the amount of light that the lens is allowed to focus on the retina. (Courtesy H. Brown, MD.)

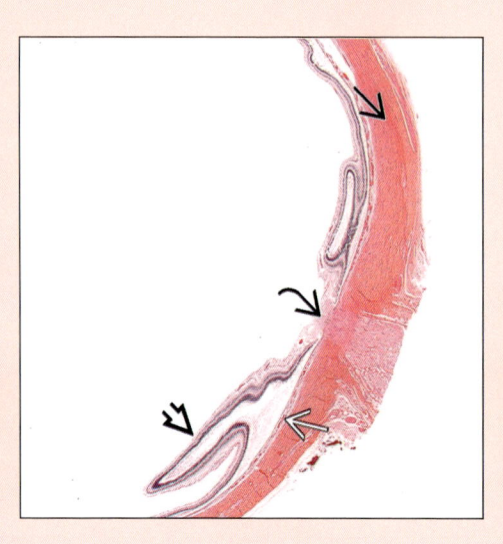

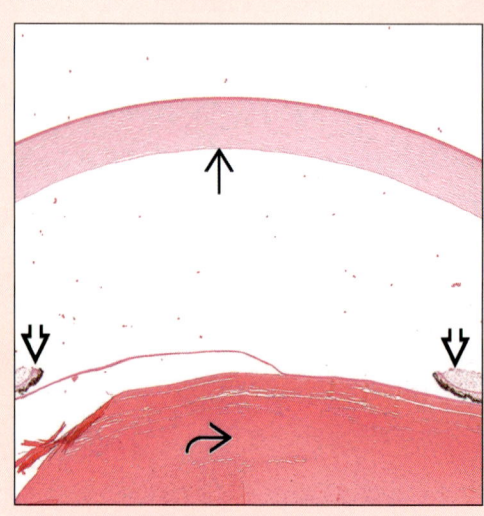

EYE AND OCULAR ADNEXA

Cornea: Stratified Squamous Epithelium

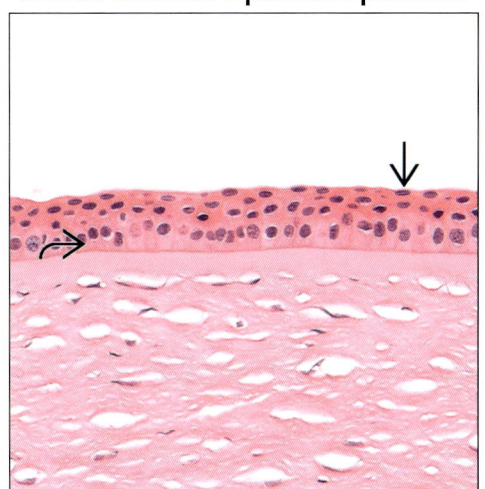

Cornea: Basal Lamina

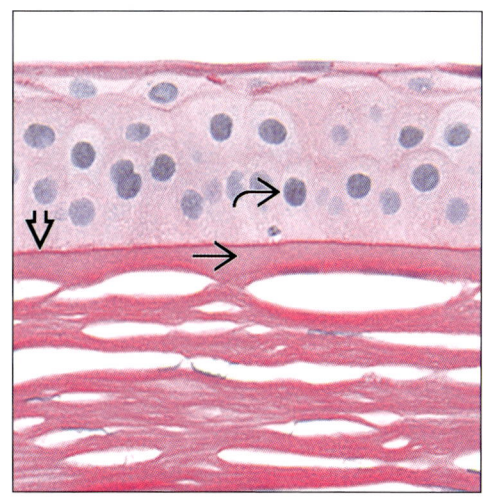

(Left) Corneal epithelium is a nonkeratinizing, stratified, squamous epithelium with nuclei present in all layers. The basal layer ➡ of the epithelium is composed of larger, more columnar cells, and as the cells rise to the corneal surface, they become flattened ➡. (Courtesy H. Brown, MD.) *(Right)* The corneal epithelium ➡ rests upon a thin basal lamina, stained bright pink in this periodic acid-Schiff preparation ➡. The acellular band beneath the basal lamina is the Bowman layer ➡. (Courtesy H. Brown, MD.)

Cornea: Stroma

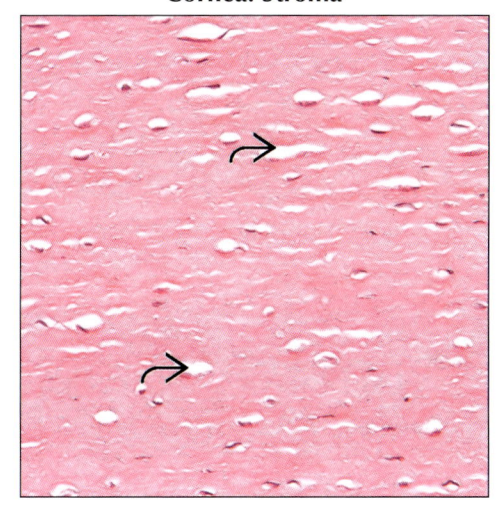

Cornea: Descemet Membrane

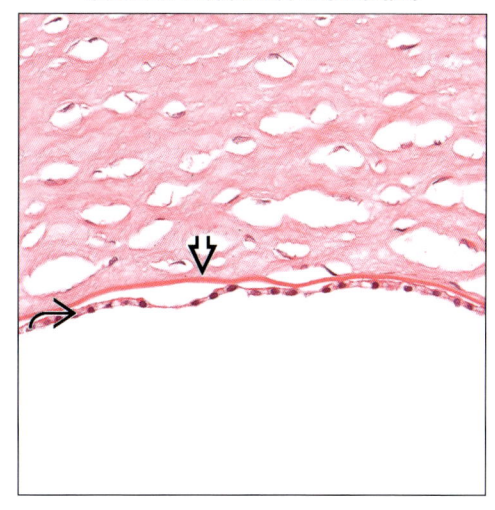

(Left) The corneal stroma is composed of regularly spaced collagen fibers embedded in an extracellular matrix. Of note, no blood vessels or lymphatics are present in the corneal stroma. The cleft-like spaces ➡ are secondary to tissue fixation/processing. (Courtesy H. Brown, MD.) *(Right)* The posterior cornea is lined by a single layer of cuboidal "endothelium" ➡ (a misnomer as it does not line a vessel). The Descemet membrane ➡ is the basement membrane of the "endothelium." (Courtesy H. Brown, MD.)

Cornea: Descemet Membrane

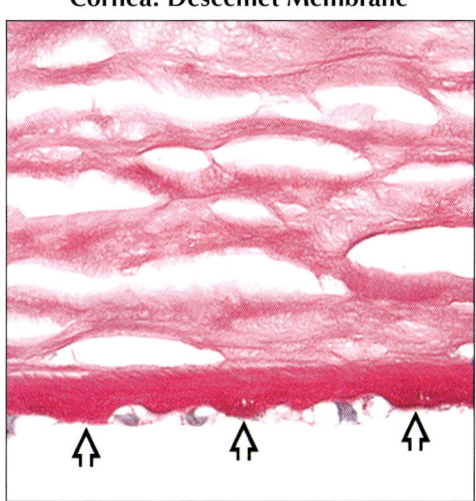

Corneoscleral Limbus

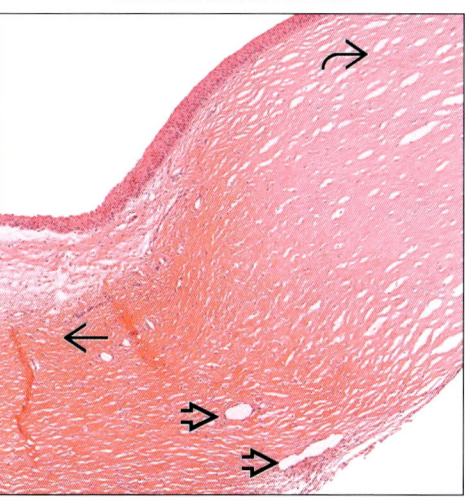

(Left) Normal, age-related changes are seen in the Descemet membrane consisting of focal thickenings ➡ (Hassall-Henle Warts), that appear to alternate with the posterior "endothelium." (Courtesy H. Brown, MD.) *(Right)* The junction of the cornea ➡ and the sclera ➡ is known as the corneoscleral limbus, seen here. The corneoscleral limbus is an important surgical landmark and posteriorly contains several structures ➡ that are vital to the flow of aqueous fluid. (Courtesy H. Brown, MD.)

EYE AND OCULAR ADNEXA

Corneoscleral Limbus

Sclera: Episclera

(Left) The corneal stroma ⇨ and iris ⇨ can be seen forming the anterior chamber angle ⇨. The canal of Schlemm ⇨ is anterior to the iris. As the corneal stroma blends into the sclera, delicate blood vessels (absent in the corneal stroma) can be identified ⇨. (Courtesy H. Brown, MD.) (Right) The episclera composes the outermost layer of the sclera and contains more numerous blood vessels ⇨ admixed with collagen and fibroblasts ⇨. (Courtesy H. Brown, MD.)

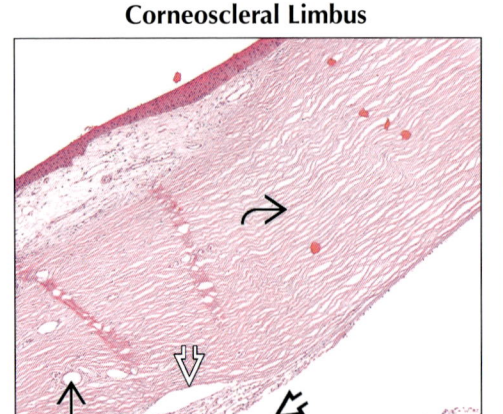

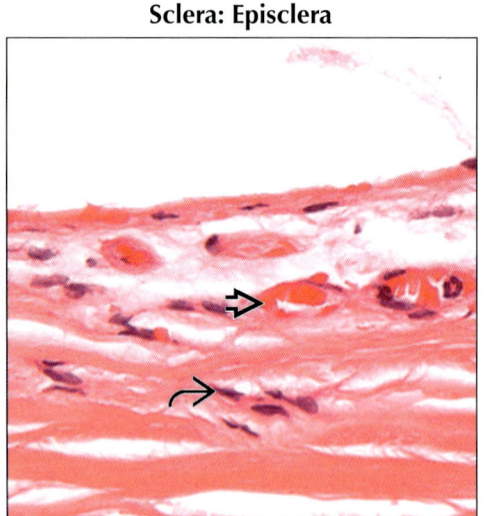

Sclera: Stroma

Sclera: Lamina Fusca

(Left) The middle portion, and the bulk of the sclera, is the scleral stroma. The stroma is composed of varying sizes of collagen fibers admixed with elastic fibers. Within the stroma, rare fibroblasts ⇨ and blood vessels ⇨ may be identified. (Courtesy H. Brown, MD.) (Right) The lamina fusca, seen here under the scleral stroma ⇨, composes the innermost layer of the sclera. The lamina fusca is composed of melanocytes ⇨, collagen, and fibroblasts ⇨. (Courtesy H. Brown, MD.)

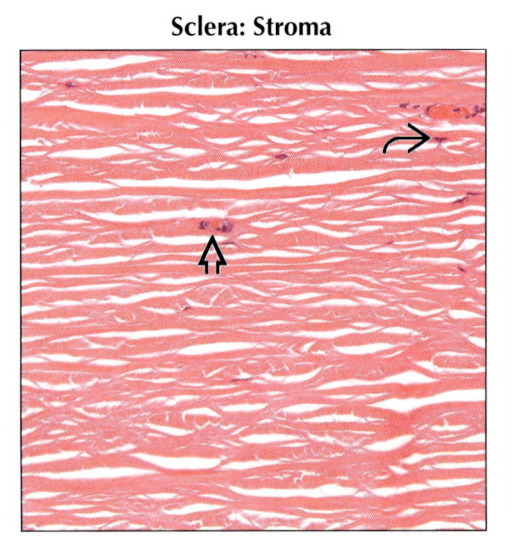

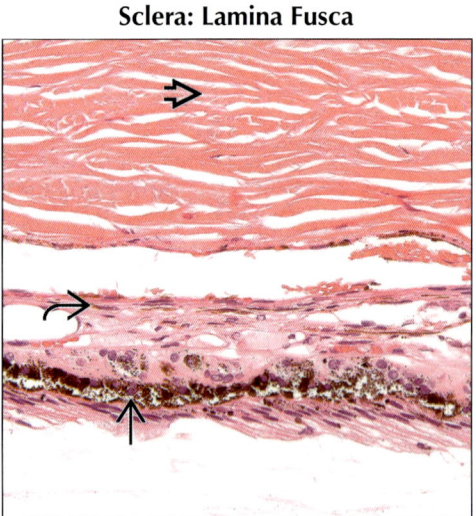

Sclera: Vessels

Canal of Schlemm

(Left) Blood vessels ⇨ and fibroblasts ⇨ are present within the sclera. The episclera ⇨ is located at the top of the image. (Courtesy H. Brown, MD.) (Right) Aqueous fluid from the anterior chamber circulates through the trabecular meshwork ⇨ and drains into the canal of Schlemm ⇨. From there, it flows into the episcleral venous plexus via aqueous veins. Blockage of the aqueous flow at any of these points may lead to increased intraocular pressure and glaucoma. (Courtesy H. Brown, MD.)

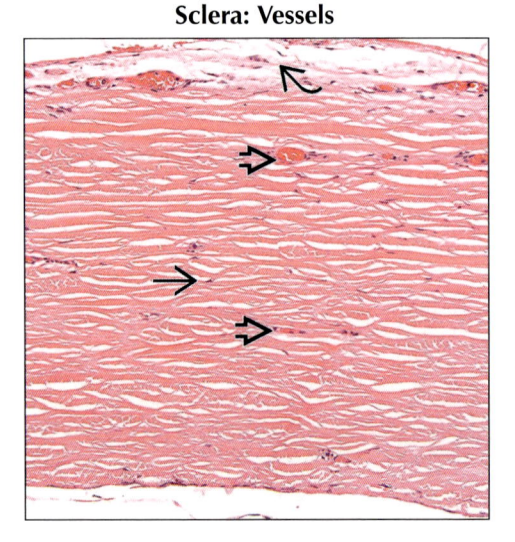

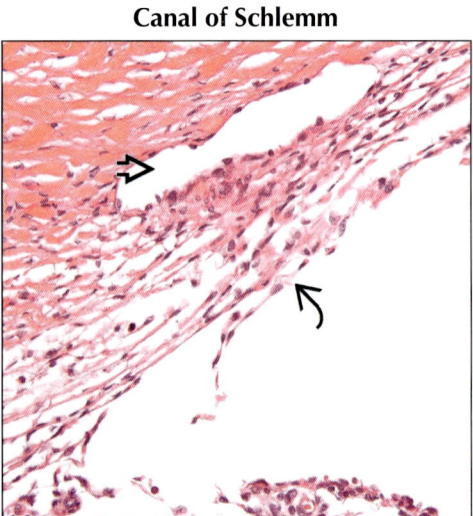

EYE AND OCULAR ADNEXA

Schwalbe Ring

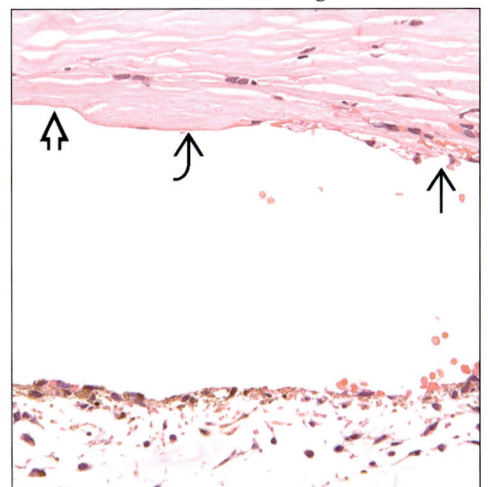

Conjunctiva: Palpebral Conjunctiva

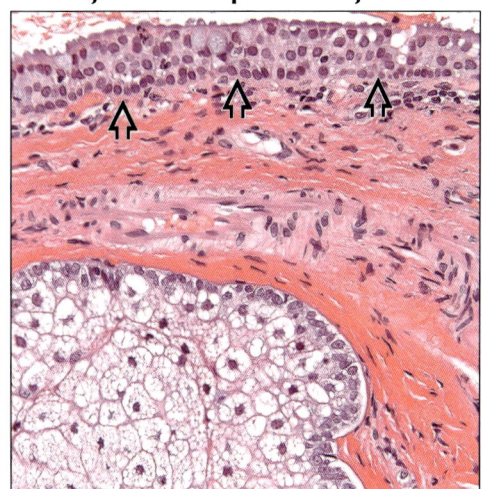

(Left) Schwalbe ring identifies the termination ➔ of Descemet membrane ▷ peripherally. The trabecular meshwork ➔ begins immediately beyond the Schwalbe ring. (Courtesy H. Brown, MD.) *(Right)* The conjunctiva ▷ is the thin, transparent lining relatively covering the inner surface of the eyelid (palpebral conjunctiva) and reflected onto the anterior surface of the globe (bulbar conjunctiva). Its function is to allow the eyelid to slide smoothly over the globe. (Courtesy H. Brown, MD.)

Conjunctiva: Lymphoid Aggregates

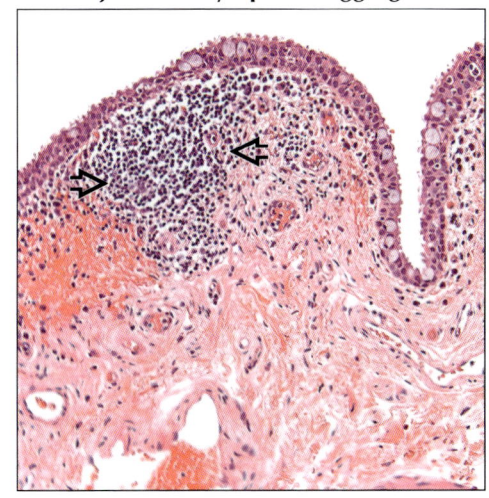

Conjunctiva: Bulbar

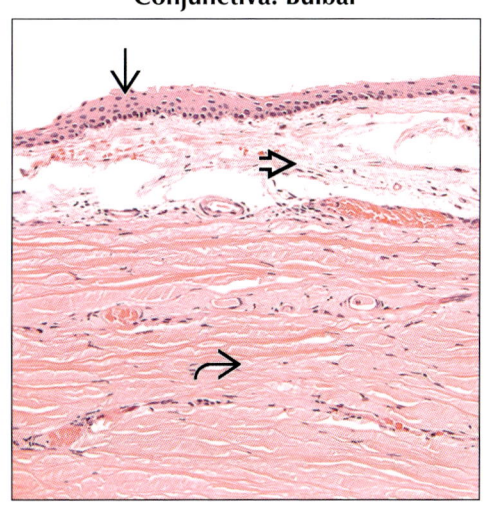

(Left) Occasional aggregates of lymphocytes ▷ may be identified within the conjunctiva. Lymphoid aggregates tend to be more common in the area of the superior and inferior fornices. They are not a sign of chronic infection. (Courtesy H. Brown, MD.) *(Right)* The portion of the conjunctiva overlying the sclera ➔ is known as the bulbar conjunctiva ➔. The bulbar conjunctival stroma is composed of loose connective tissue ▷. (Courtesy H. Brown, MD.)

Conjunctiva: Superior and Inferior Fornix Openings

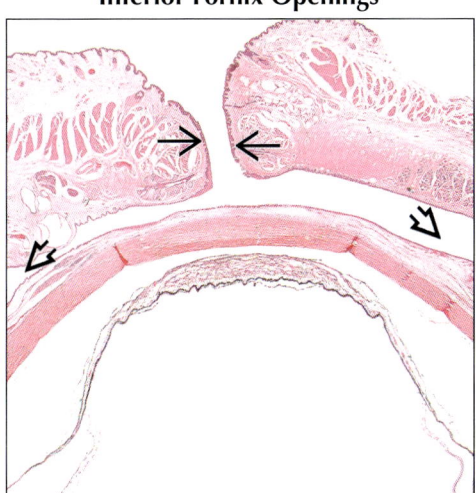

Conjunctiva: Fornix

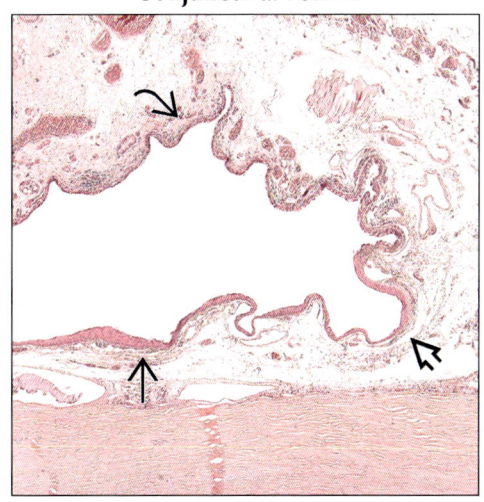

(Left) The conjunctiva terminates anteriorly at the beginning of the squamous lining of the eyelids ➔. The junction of the palpebral conjunctiva and the bulbar conjunctiva occurs in the superior and inferior fornix, the openings of which can be seen here ▷. (Courtesy H. Brown, MD.) *(Right)* The palpebral conjunctiva ➔ and the bulbar conjunctiva ➔ meet in the fornix ▷. It is in this region that lymphoid aggregates and abundant epithelial goblet cells can be identified. (Courtesy H. Brown, MD.)

EYE AND OCULAR ADNEXA

Conjunctiva: Goblet Cells

Iris

(Left) Goblet cells ⇨ are seen in the forniceal conjunctiva. Goblet cells are large mucin-containing cells with grey-blue cytoplasm and basal nuclei. This mucin helps to lubricate the eyelid and conjunctiva. (Courtesy H. Brown, MD.)

(Right) The iris ⇨ can be seen in the middle of this photo. The origin of the iris (iris root ⇨) is from the anterior ciliary face ⇨. Smooth muscle fibers in the iris cause the pupil to constrict and dilate, regulating the amount of light entering the lens. (Courtesy H. Brown, MD.)

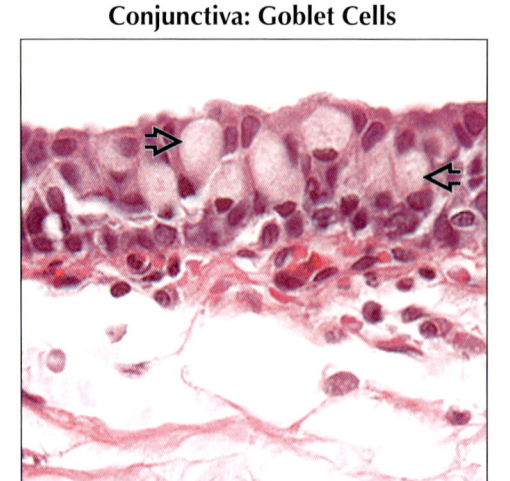

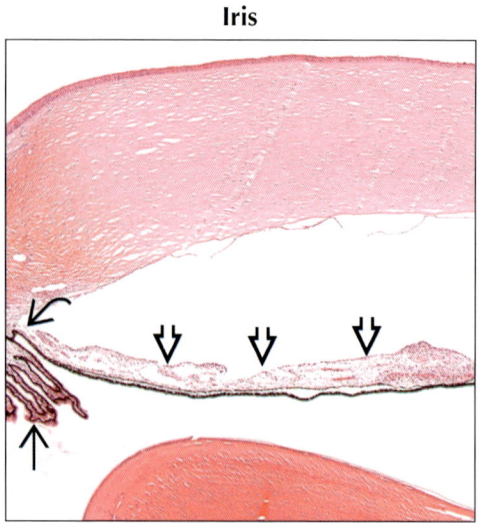

Iris: Stroma

Lens and Ciliary Body

(Left) The iris is composed of connective tissue, smooth muscle ⇨, blood vessels ⇨, nerve cells, and melanocytes. The number of stromal melanocytes determines the color of the iris. The anterior surface lacks an epithelial lining, while the posterior epithelial lining is heavily pigmented ⇨. (Courtesy H. Brown, MD.) (Right) This gross photo of the anterior half of the eye is taken from behind and shows the lens ⇨, surrounding ciliary body ⇨, and retina ⇨. (Courtesy H. Brown, MD.)

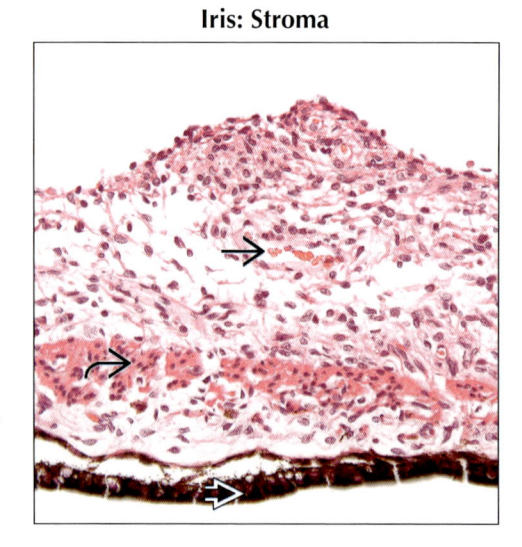

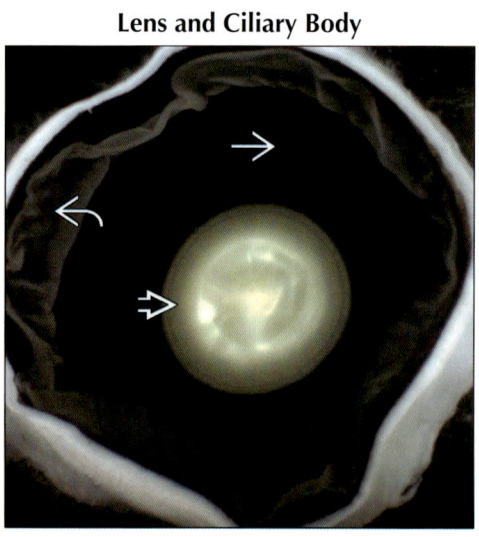

Lens and Ciliary Body

Ciliary Body: Epithelium

(Left) Higher magnification shows the 2 zones of the ciliary body: The pars plicata ⇨ (ridged ciliary processes) and the pars plana, which is more peripheral and flat ⇨. (Courtesy H. Brown, MD.) (Right) The epithelium that lines the ciliary body is composed of 2 distinct layers. The innermost layer ⇨ is nonpigmented and abuts the posterior chamber, while the outer layer is pigmented ⇨ and adjacent to the ciliary body stroma ⇨. (Courtesy H. Brown, MD.)

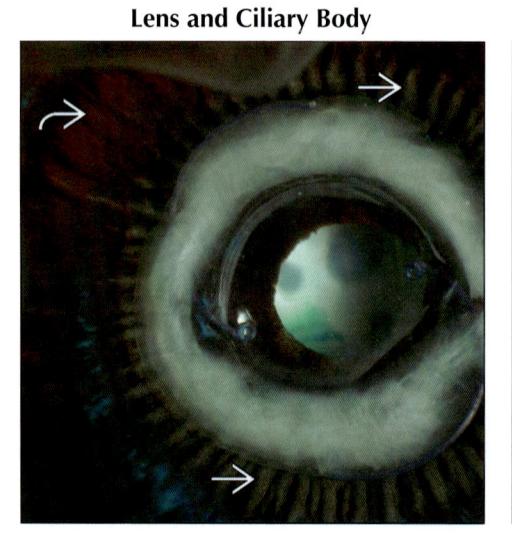

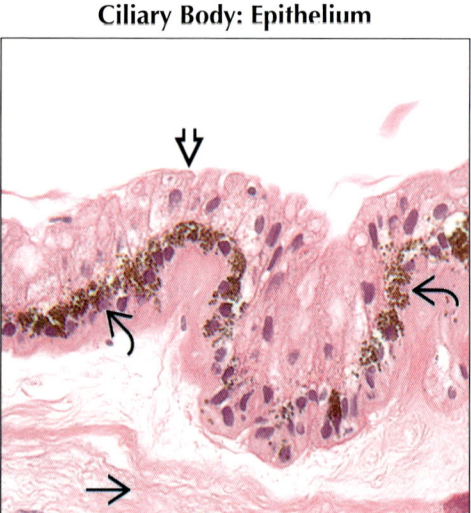

EYE AND OCULAR ADNEXA

Ciliary Body: Zonular Fibers

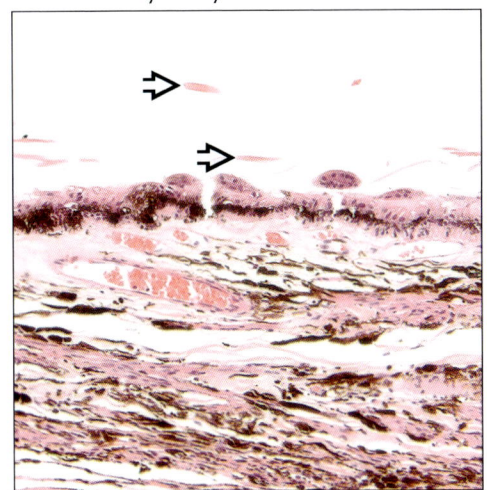

Ciliary Body: Pars Plicata

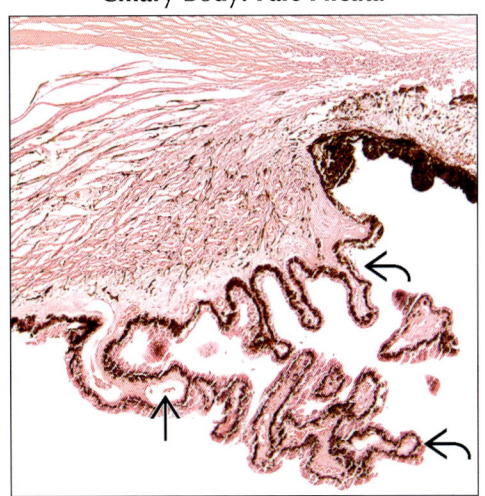

(Left) Thin, acellular, eosinophilic zonular fibers ⇨ may be identified extending from the pars plana of the ciliary body to the lens equator. The zonular fibers anchor the lens to the ciliary body, and decreases in zonular tension allow alteration in lens curvature. (Courtesy H. Brown, MD.) (Right) The fold-like pars plicata can be seen here ⇨. The fibrovascular cores of the pars plicata ⇨ produce the aqueous humor. (Courtesy H. Brown, MD.)

Ciliary Body: Pars Plicata Aging Changes

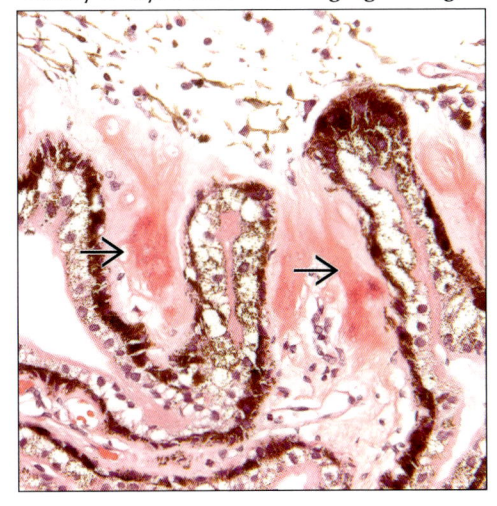

Ciliary Body: Smooth Muscle

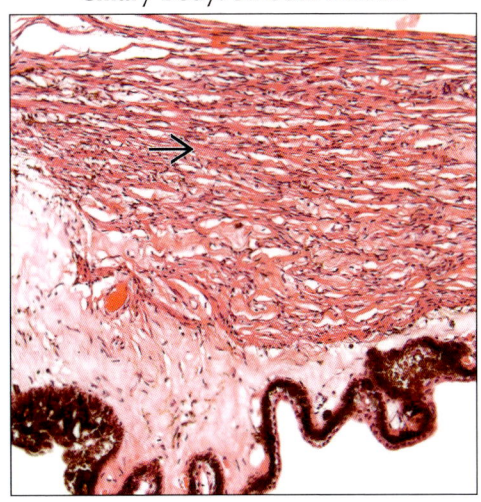

(Left) The amount of stroma present in the pars plicata increases with age. In this section, the stroma is thickened and hyalinized ⇨. (Courtesy H. Brown, MD.) (Right) The ciliary muscle (smooth muscle) ⇨ forms the bulk of the ciliary body. Although histologically difficult to distinguish, 3 layers of muscle (inner circular, middle oblique, and outer longitudinal) are present. Contraction relaxes the zonular fibers and allows the lens to change shape. (Courtesy H. Brown, MD.)

Ciliary Body: Pigment Within Smooth Muscle

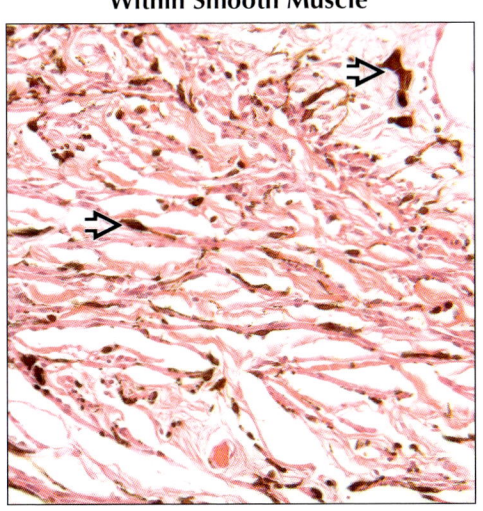

Choroid

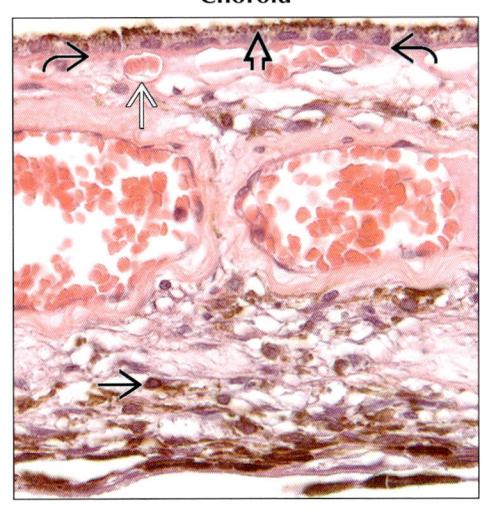

(Left) Interspersed within the smooth muscle of the ciliary body, numerous pigmented melanocytes ⇨ may be identified. (Courtesy H. Brown, MD.) (Right) The choroid begins posterior to the ciliary body and terminates at the optic nerve, lying between the retina and the sclera. The choroid is composed of vessels with interspersed melanocytes ⇨ and fibroblasts. Bruch membrane ⇨ is the basement membrane for both the choriocapillaris ⇨ and pigmented retinal epithelium ⇨. (Courtesy H. Brown, MD.)

EYE AND OCULAR ADNEXA

Retina: Ora Serrata

(Left) The ora serrata ⇨ is the anterior termination of the retina. The neurosensory retina ⇨ is contiguous with the nonpigmented ciliary epithelium ⇨. (Courtesy H. Brown, MD.) **(Right)** The 10 retinal layers: (1) internal limiting membrane, (2) nerve fiber layer, (3) ganglion cell layer, (4) inner plexiform layer, (5) inner nuclear layer, (6) outer plexiform layer, (7) outer nuclear layer, (8) external limiting membrane, (9) rods and cones, and (10) retinal pigment epithelium. (Courtesy H. Brown, MD.)

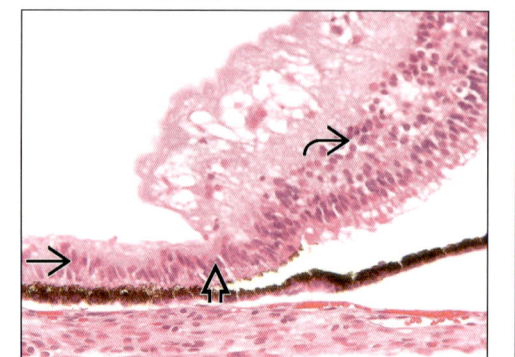

Retina: Multilayered Epithelium

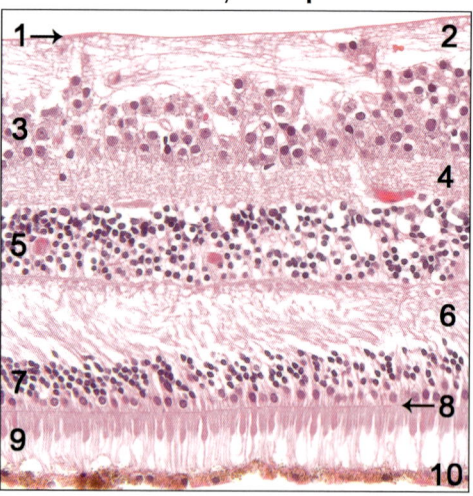

Retina: Macula

(Left) Grossly, the macula lutea appears as a yellow spot within the retina. The macula is a region of the retina that can be identified histologically when the ganglion cell layer is > 1 cell thick, as seen here ⇨. (Courtesy H. Brown, MD.) **(Right)** Away from the macula, the ganglion cell layer thins. This image of peripheral retina shows only rare ganglion cells ⇨. (Courtesy H. Brown, MD.)

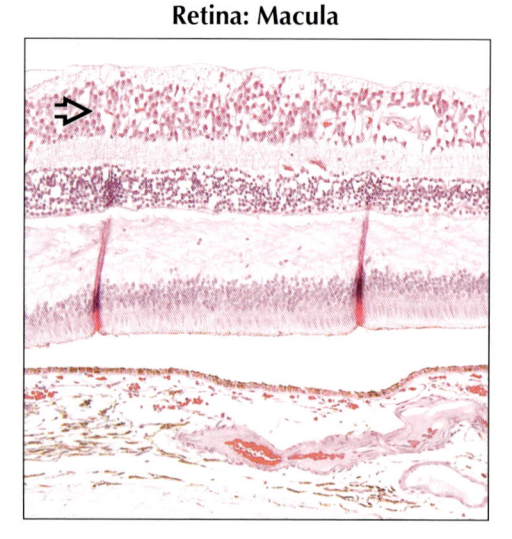

Retina: Nonmacular

Optic Nerve: Head

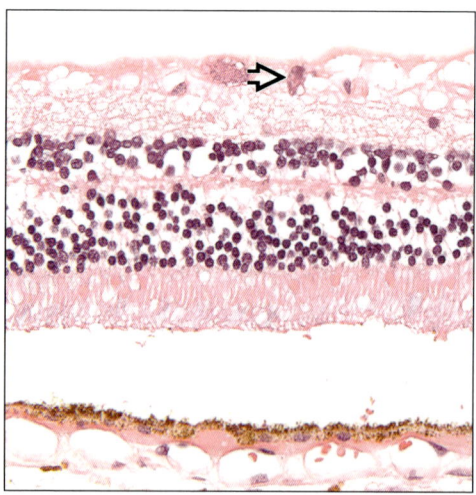

(Left) The optic nerve ⇨ exits the posterior aspect of the globe. Note the absence of nuclear layers of the retina overlying the most anterior aspect of the optic nerve ⇨, leading to the presence of a physiological "blind spot." (Courtesy H. Brown, MD.) **(Right)** A cross section of the optic nerve shows the nerve ⇨ centrally, surrounded by a thin pia mater, arachnoid ⇨, and the much thicker dura mater ⇨. (Courtesy H. Brown, MD.)

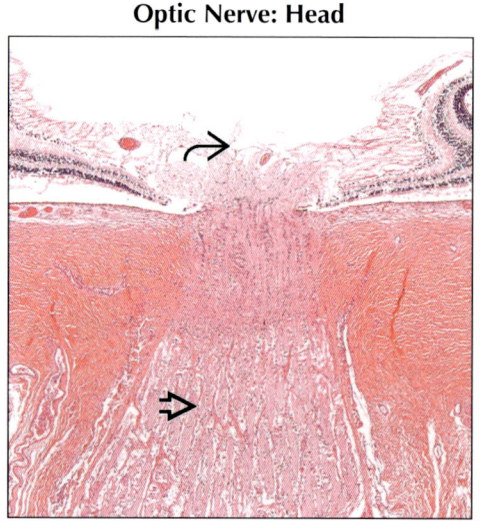

Optic Nerve

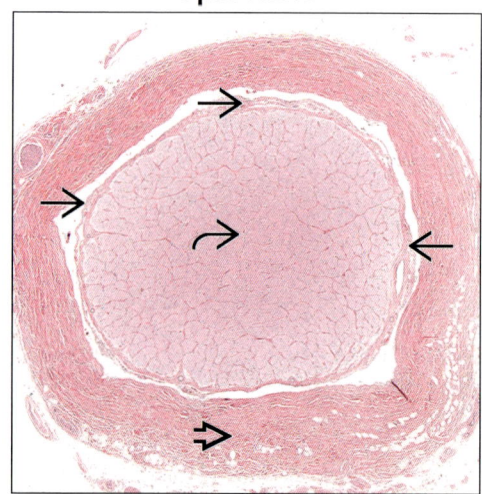

EYE AND OCULAR ADNEXA

Optic Nerve

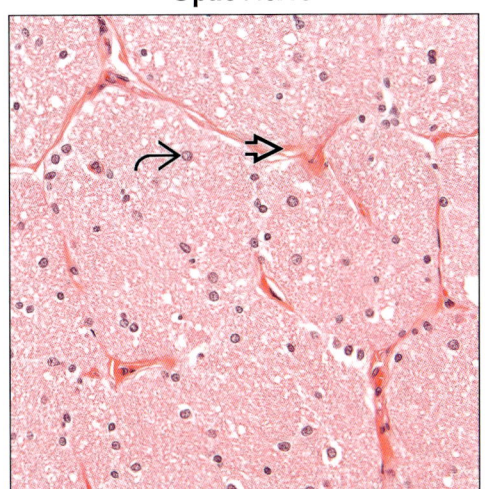

Optic Nerve: Central Artery and Vein

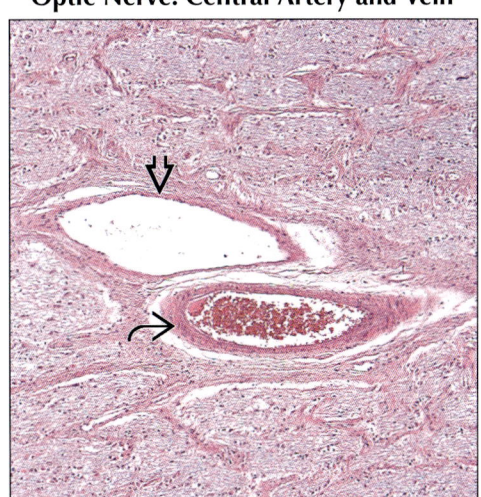

(Left) High-power examination of the central portion of the optic nerve reveals glial cells ⇨ and nerve bundles, divided into fascicles by delicate fibrovascular septa ⇨. (Courtesy H. Brown, MD.) *(Right)* This high-power cross section shows the central artery ⇨ and vein ⇨. These structures can be identified in the middle of the optic nerve in its most anterior aspect (extending to the head of the nerve), entering and exiting the nerve 1-1.5 cm posterior to the globe. (Courtesy H. Brown, MD.)

Lens

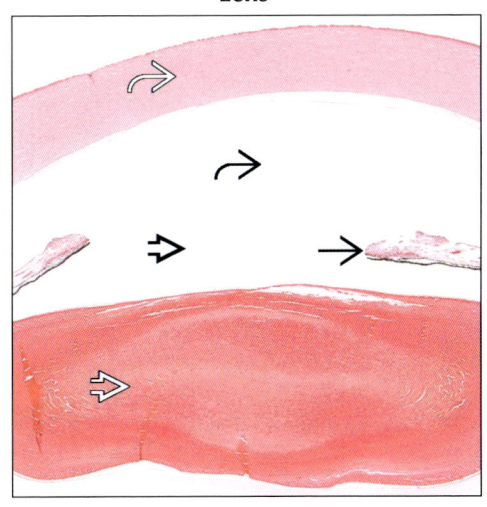

Lens: Equator

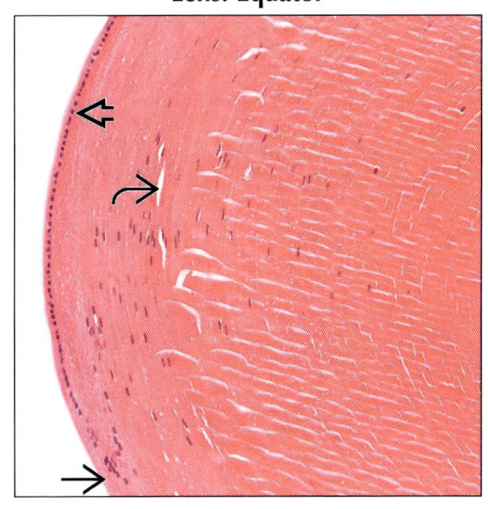

(Left) This low-magnification image of the anterior globe illustrates the lens ⇨ lying posterior to the iris ⇨, anterior chamber ⇨, and cornea ⇨. The pupil consists of the opening within the center of the iris ⇨. (Courtesy H. Brown, MD.) *(Right)* The equator of the lens is located peripherally. In this area, the monolayer lens epithelium lining the anterior lens ⇨ elongates to form lens fibers ⇨. Small clefts in the lens stroma ⇨ are secondary to specimen processing. (Courtesy H. Brown, MD.)

Lens: Anterior

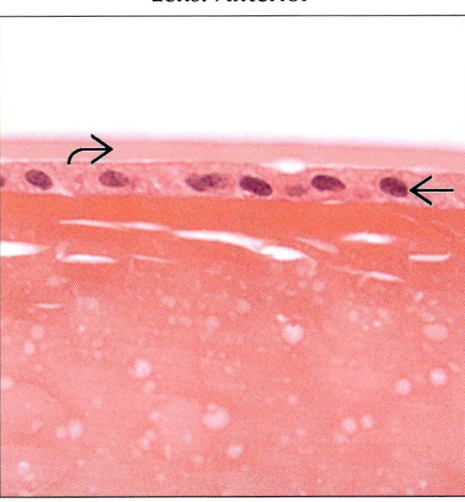

Lens: Posterior

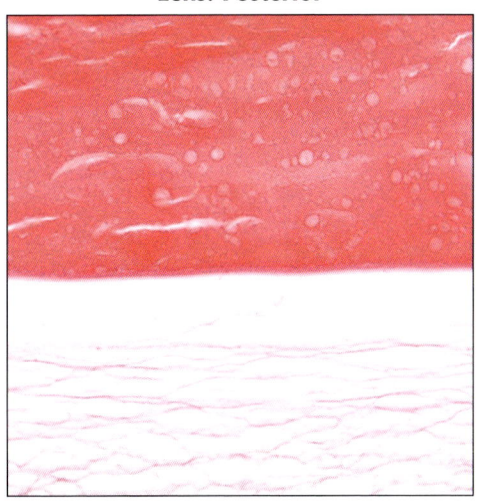

(Left) A thin carbohydrate-rich lens capsule ⇨ encircles the lens, and the equator is the site of attachment for the zonular fibers that connect the lens to the ciliary body. The lens capsule is the basement membrane of the cuboidal epithelial cells ⇨. (Courtesy H. Brown, MD.) *(Right)* The posterior aspect of the lens lacks an epithelial layer. Since only anterior epithelium is present postnatally, the anterior capsule thickens with age while the posterior does not. (Courtesy H. Brown, MD.)

EYE AND OCULAR ADNEXA

Lens and Ciliary Body

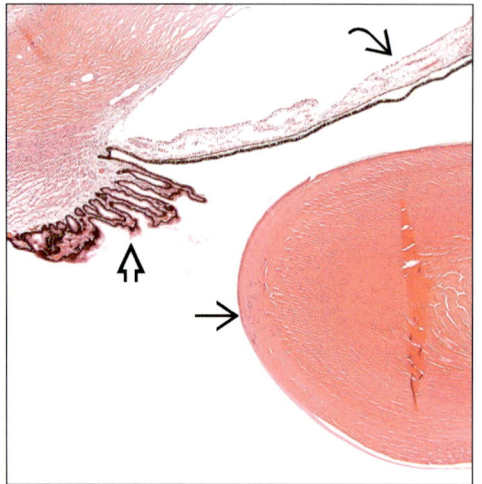

Vitreous

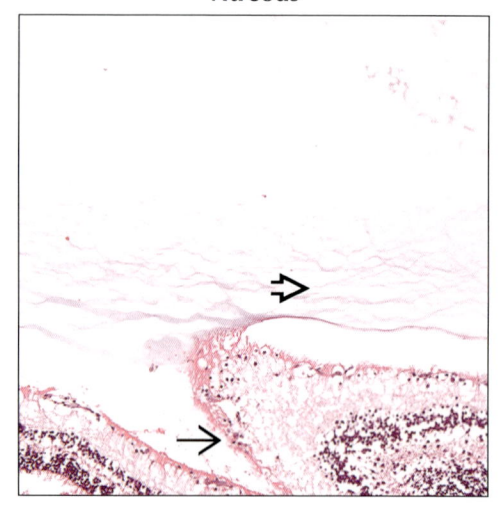

(Left) The equator of the lens ⇨ is in close approximation to the ciliary body ⇨ and held in place by zonular fibers (invisible at this magnification). The iris can be seen anterior to the lens ⇨. (Courtesy H. Brown, MD.)
(Right) The nearly acellular, transparent vitreous ⇨ fills the area posterior to the lens, extending circumferentially to the multilayered retinal epithelium ⇨. The vitreous is a gel-like substance principally composed of water and hyaluronic acid. (Courtesy H. Brown, MD.)

Eyelid

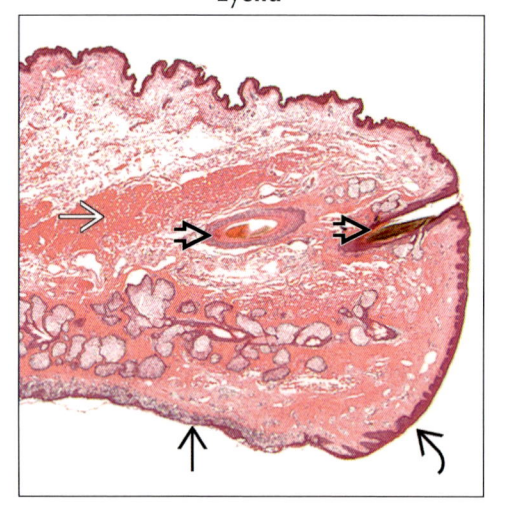

Eyelid: Meibomian Glands

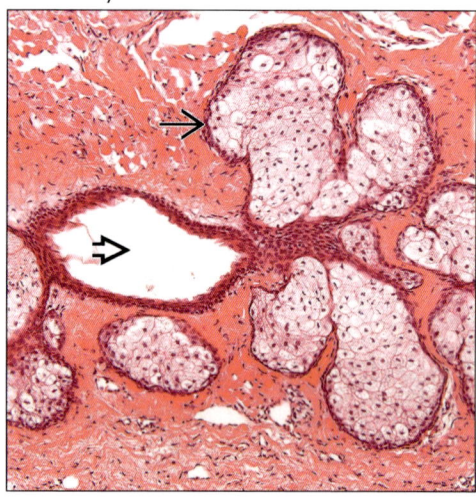

(Left) This section of the eyelid demonstrates the palpebral conjunctiva ⇨ merging with epidermis of the anterior eyelid ⇨. The eyelid contains many structures, including orbicularis muscle ⇨, glands, and the cilia (eyelashes) ⇨. (Courtesy H. Brown, MD.)
(Right) One of the most abundant types of glands is the sebaceous meibomian glands ⇨ that are found in the tarsus in the posterior portion of the eyelid. Here, acini of meibomian glands are seen in association with a central duct ⇨. (Courtesy H. Brown, MD.)

Eyelid: Glands of Moll and Zeis

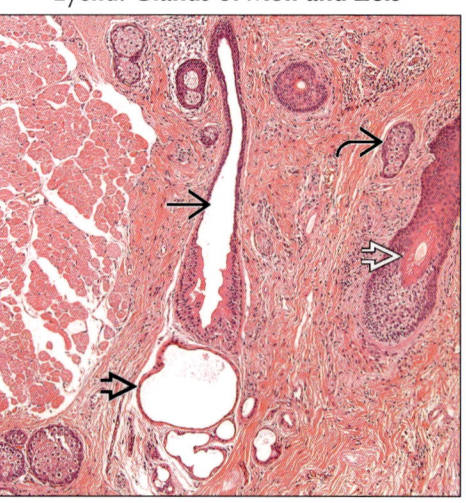

Eyelid: Accessory Lacrimal Glands

(Left) The glands of Moll ⇨ are apocrine glands that drain via a duct ⇨ into the hair follicles that make up the eyelashes. The glands of Zeis ⇨ are sebaceous glands that may be found in the same area and drain into the hair follicle ⇨ as well. (Courtesy H. Brown, MD.) (Right) Accessory lacrimal glands ⇨ may be identified within the most superior and inferior portions of the eyelids at the bases of the tarsal plates ⇨, and in the superior and inferior fornices of the conjunctiva. (Courtesy H. Brown, MD.)

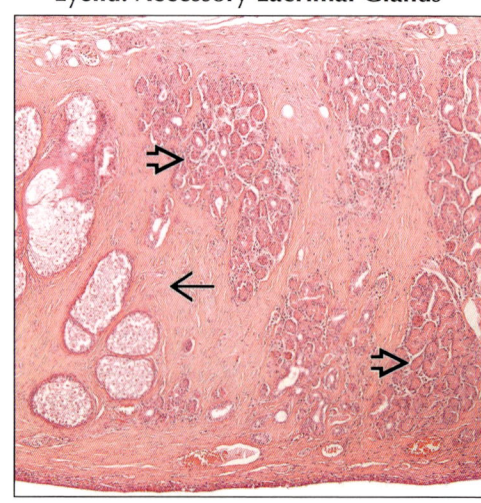

EYE AND OCULAR ADNEXA

Eyelid: Tarsus

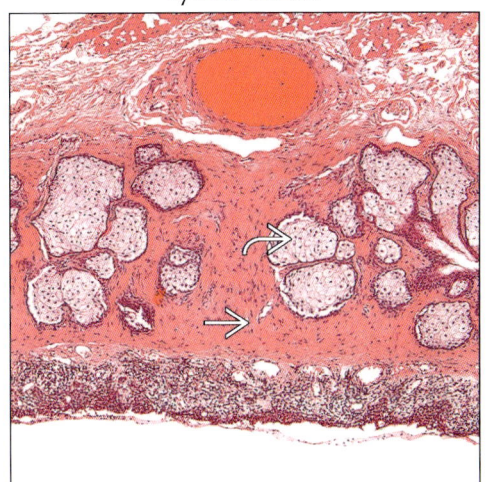

Lacrimal Glands & Duct

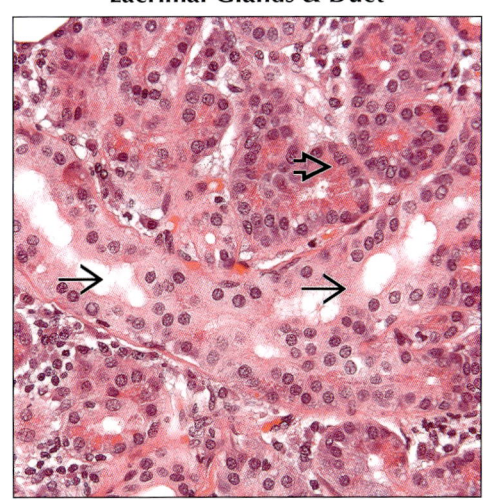

(Left) The tarsus (or tarsal plate) is composed of dense collagen ➔ and is present in the posterior aspect of the eyelid. It contains the meibomian glands ➔. (Courtesy H. Brown, MD.) (Right) The lacrimal glands are composed of serous-type cells ➔ that drain into a central duct ➔. The glands are found within the superior lateral orbit. (Courtesy H. Brown, MD.)

Eyelid: Punctum Canaliculus

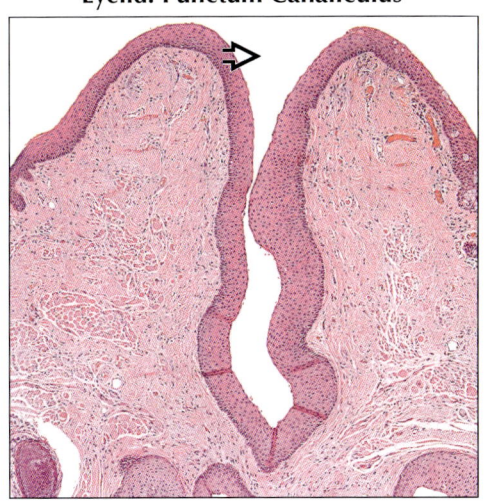

Lacrimal Canaliculus

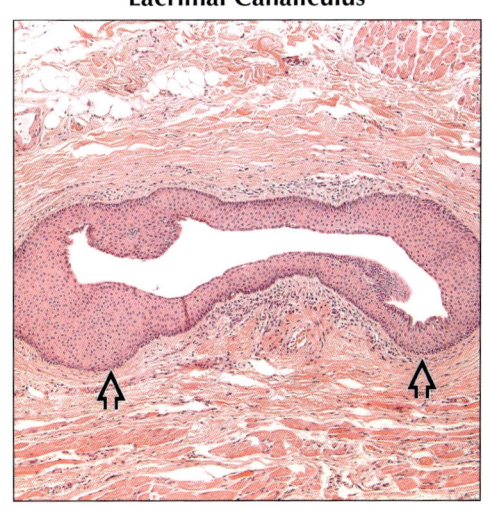

(Left) Tears drain from the lacrimal ducts into the fornices of the conjunctiva and lubricate the anterior globe surface. The tears drain into the punctum canaliculus (opening ➔), which is situated in the medial aspect of each eyelid. (Courtesy H. Brown, MD.) (Right) Tears drain from the punctum canaliculus into the lacrimal canaliculi ➔. The paired canaliculi (1 superior and 1 inferior) are located in the medial portion of each eye. The lining is composed of stratified nonkeratinizing squamous epithelium. (Courtesy H. Brown, MD.)

Lacrimal Sac

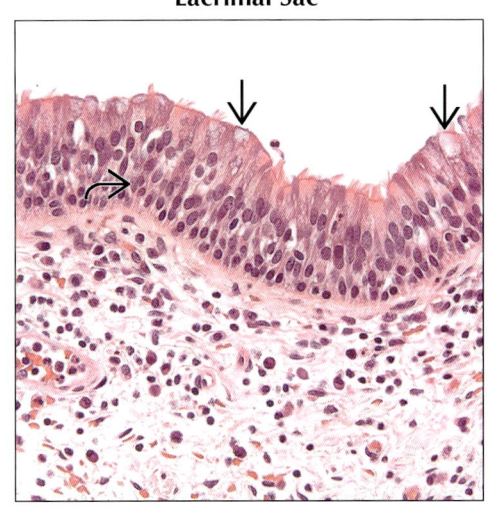

Orbital Soft Tissue

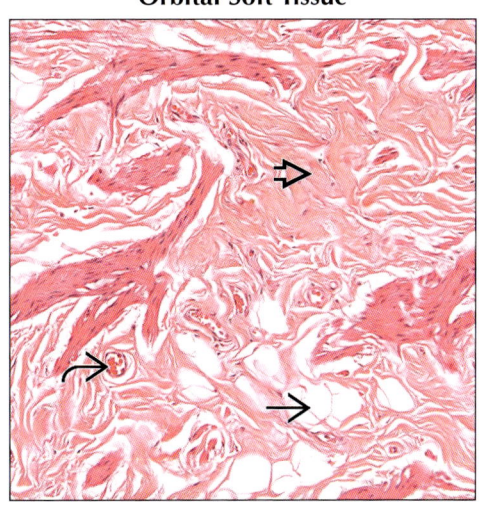

(Left) From the lacrimal canaliculi, the tears drain into the lacrimal sacs, where they collect and drain via the nasolacrimal duct into the sinuses. The lining of the nasolacrimal duct consists of a pseudostratified, ciliated, columnar epithelium ➔ with occasional goblet cells ➔. (Courtesy H. Brown, MD.) (Right) The orbital soft tissue is composed of mature adipose tissue ➔ and supporting collagenous tissue ➔. Small blood vessels are also present ➔. (Courtesy H. Brown, MD.)

ORAL MUCOSAE

Key Facts

Macroscopic Anatomy
- Pink, red, or brown in color
- Moist
- Smooth surface
- Lack appendages seen in skin

Microscopic Anatomy
- Epithelium
  - Stratified squamous type
  - Orthokeratinized in areas exposed to high friction, like palate
  - Nonkeratinized in most other areas of oral cavity
  - Parakeratinized as mucosa transitions to skin on lip
  - Rete ridges are present
  - Pigmentation: Melanin (endogenous) or foreign (exogenous)
  - Nonkeratinocytes: Melanocytes, Langerhans cells, Merkel cells, and lymphocytes
- Lamina propria
  - Composed of dense connective tissue
  - Sebaceous glands (called Fordyce granules) are commonly found in lip and buccal mucosa
  - Inflammatory cells variably present
- Submucosa
  - Dense when overlying bone/periosteum
  - Loose when overlying muscle
  - Contains blood vessels, nerves
  - Minor salivary glands and ducts are present

Age Variation
- Epithelium usually becomes thinner and more fragile with aging
- Fordyce granules increase

(Left) The oral cavity is lined with oral mucosae. This protective lining transitions from skin to mucosae at the lips and is continuous with the mucosae of the digestive system. Their protective functions are essential, and the mucosae are also a first-line defense against microorganisms and infection. The extent of the oral mucosae is designated as blue. (Right) Oral mucosae (blue) are involved in secretion as well as sensations such as touch, temperature, and taste on the tongue.

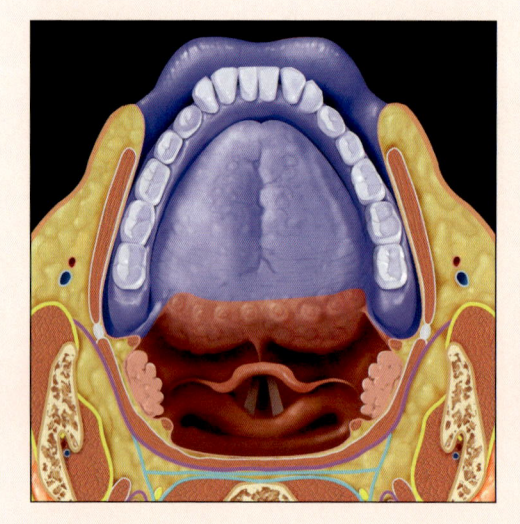

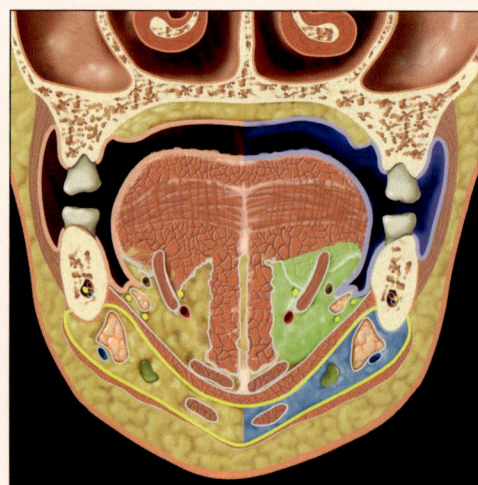

(Left) A low-power view of oral mucosae shows the normal components: Epithelium ➡ with its distinctive rete ridges is easily discernible from the underlying lamina propria ➡. The distinction between the lamina propria and submucosa is not always as easy to recognize. The submucosa may contain fat, glandular tissue, nerves, and blood vessels. (Right) This drawing shows the 3 layers of oral mucosae: Epithelium ➡, lamina propria ➡, and the submucosa ➡.

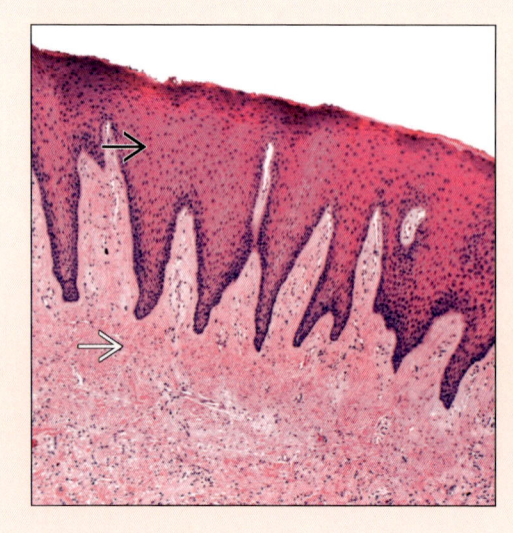

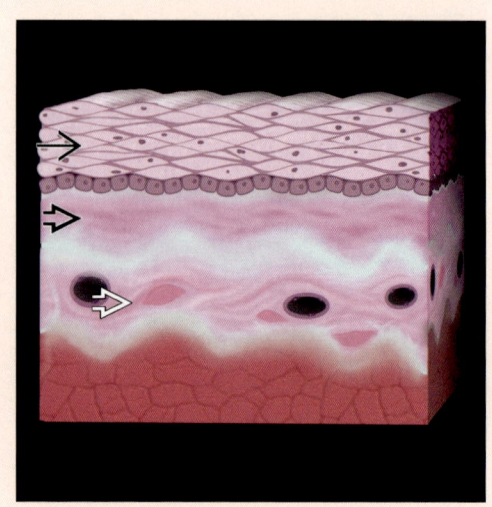

ORAL MUCOSAE

Epithelium

Epithelium

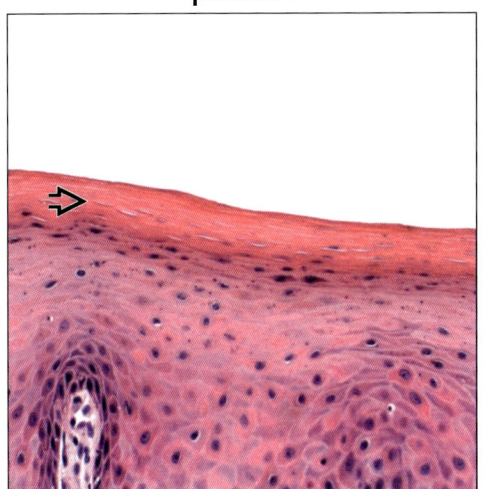

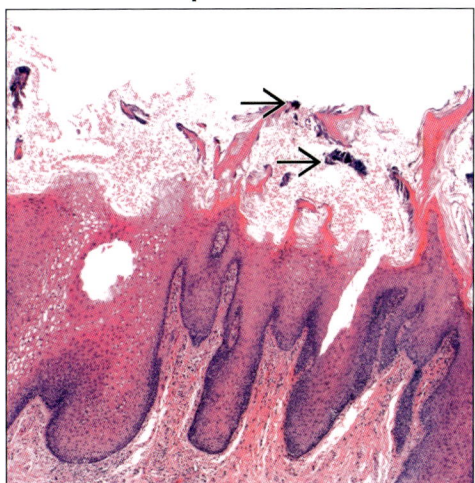

(Left) The keratinization of oral epithelium varies with location and the relative amount of friction to which the tissue is exposed during normal eating or other habits. This image shows epithelium from the palate, surfaced by orthokeratin, flat eosinophilic cells with no nuclei ➡. (Right) This image shows an example of hyperorthokeratotic epithelium seen on the tongue. This appearance is the result of exposure to strong mechanical forces. Note the adherent bacterial colonies ➡.

Epithelium

Epithelium

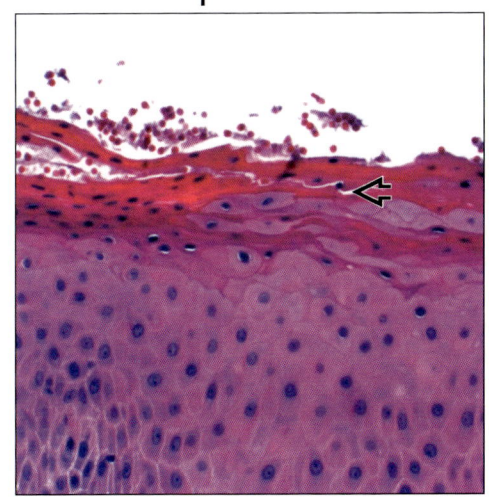

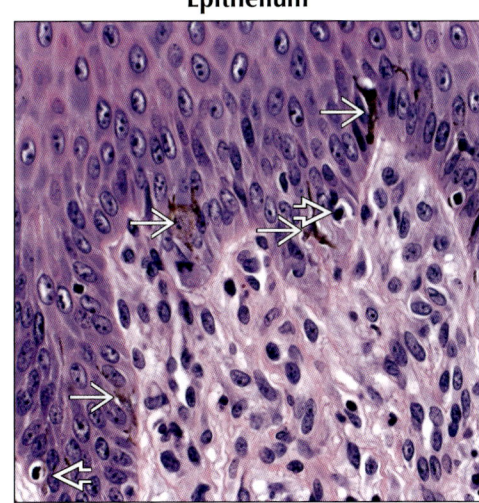

(Left) Areas with increased friction or areas like the epithelium near the lips may show areas of parakeratinization, characterized by flat eosinophilic cells with retained pyknotic nuclei ➡. (Right) The color of mucosae varies among individuals, much like the color of skin. This image shows deposition of melanin ➡ along the basal layer of epithelium. The number of melanocytes ➡ found in the epithelium is generally consistent from one person to the next, despite color variation.

Lamina Propria

Submucosa

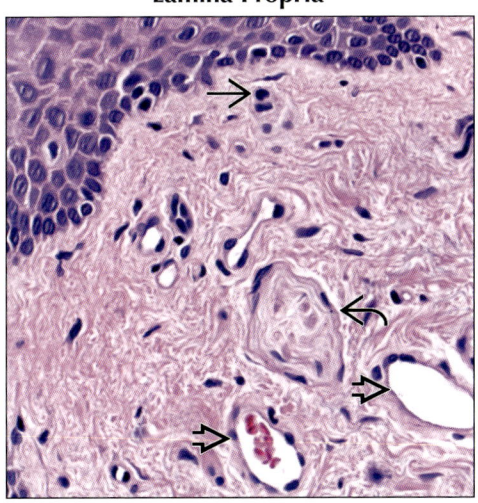

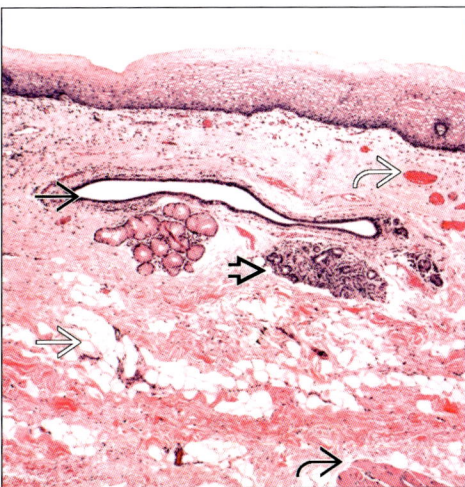

(Left) This image shows a low-power view of the lamina propria and submucosa. Lymphocytes ➡ are a normal finding in the lamina propria. Small blood vessels ➡ and nerve twigs ➡ are found slightly deeper. (Right) This image shows blood vessels ➡, a relatively large salivary gland duct ➡ and a minor salivary gland ➡ within the submucosa. Deep to these structures, adipose tissue ➡ and muscle ➡ are seen.

GINGIVAE

Key Facts

Macroscopic Anatomy
- Gingivae: Mucosae that cover the alveolar ridge, most closely associated with the teeth (masticatory mucosae)
  - Moist and pink, red, or brown with fine stippling
  - Attached gingiva: Adherent to associated bone
  - Free gingiva: Tissue that forms a cuff around the cervix (neck) of the tooth
  - Gingival crevice: Space between free gingiva and tooth, extends from tip of free gingiva (papilla) to the cementoenamel junction (CEJ) of the tooth

Microscopic Anatomy
- Epithelium
  - Stratified squamous; parakeratinization or orthokeratinization may be present, thins in gingival crevice
  - Rete ridges: Long and sometimes narrow to provide strength for tissues exposed to shearing forces of chewing
  - Melanin pigmentation varies with population
  - Nonkeratinocytes: Melanocytes, Langerhans cells, Merkel cells, and lymphocytes
- Lamina propria
  - Composed of dense connective tissue collagen fibers
  - Sebaceous glands (Fordyce granules) are seen, but less frequently than in other oral mucosal sites
  - Inflammatory cells variably present
  - Capillaries
  - Small nerve twigs
  - Odontogenic epithelial rests
- Mucoperiosteum
  - Provides a firm and direct attachment to underlying periosteum of bone of maxilla and mandible
  - No submucosal layer in gingiva

Age Variation
- Epithelium becomes thinner and more fragile with age
- Prevalence of gingivitis approaches 100% with increased age
  - Other local factors are associated: Crowding, dental caries, mouth breathing, and iatrogenic causes

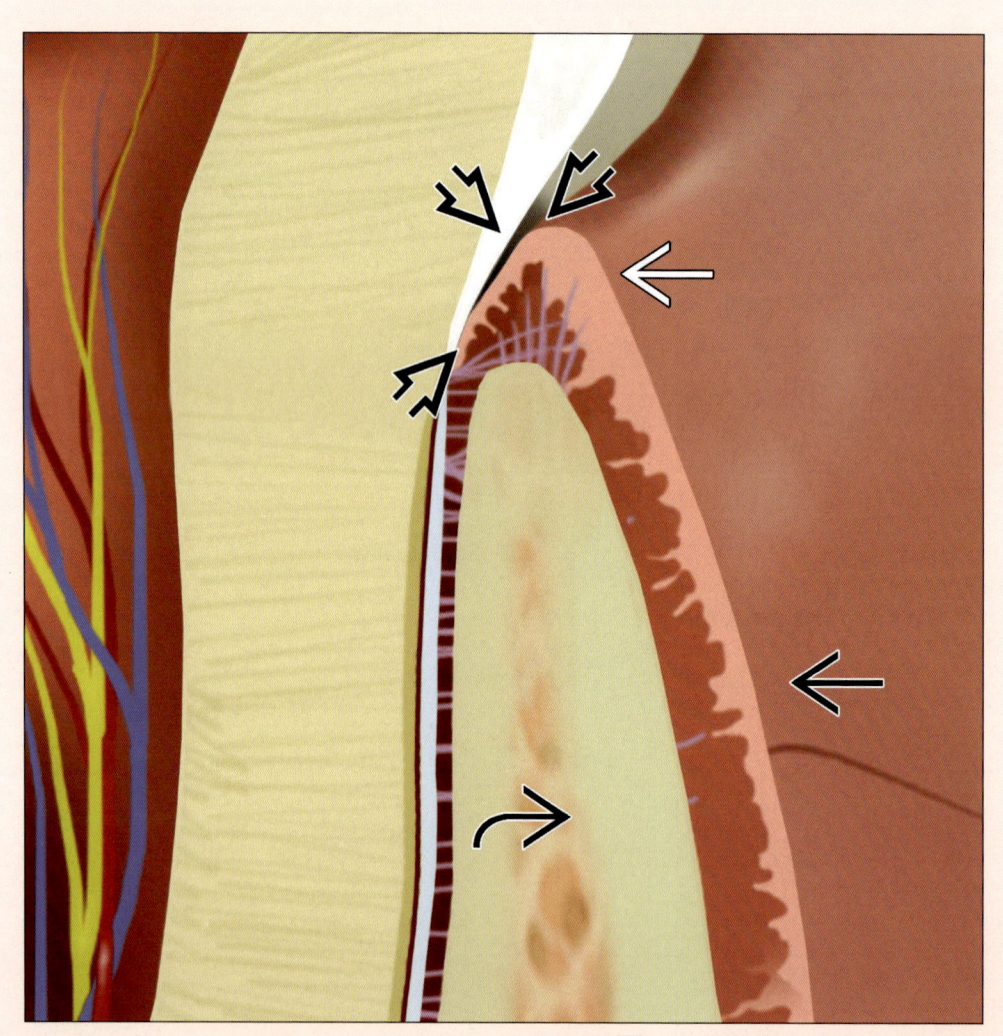

This graphic shows the relationship of the gingivae to the tooth and the alveolar bone ➡. The gingiva intimately associated with the bone is referred to as the attached gingiva ➡, while the gingiva that forms a cuff around the tooth is designated as the free gingiva ➡. The space, or potential space, that is created from the tip of the free gingiva to the attachment of the gingiva to the tooth, at the cementoenamel junction (CEJ), is called the gingival crevice ➡. This space is an excellent environment for pathogens, and the presence of an inflammatory infiltrate is not uncommon. This space is also also the area generally targeted during dental cleanings.

GINGIVAE

Gingivae: Gross

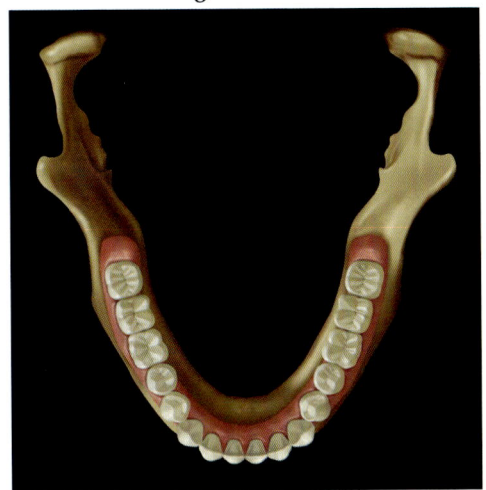

Gingivae: Gross

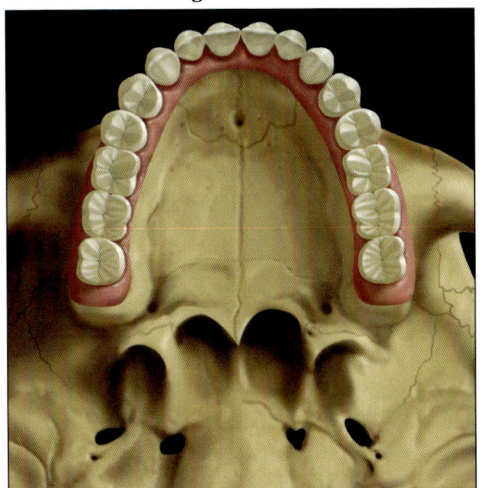

(Left) The attached gingiva provides a protective layer for the underlying bone (mandible in this image). Macroscopically, this tissue is firm and immobile with a pink stippled surface. *(Right)* The forces involved in biting and chewing food expose the gingivae to mechanical forces, such as compression and shearing. Additionally, the tissues are exposed to numerous microorganisms found in the normal oral flora. The gingivae help provide a barrier to infection.

Gingivae: Epithelium

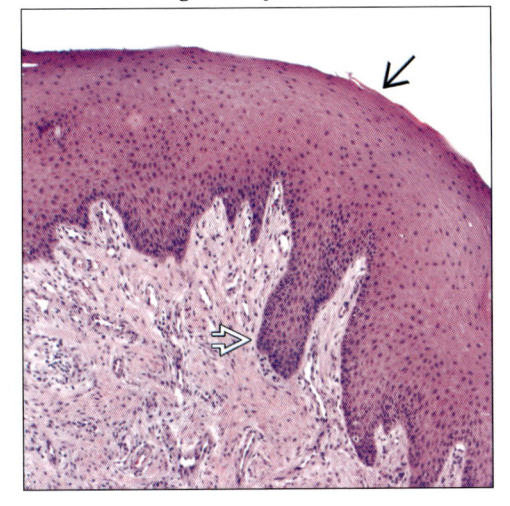

Gingivae: Epithelium

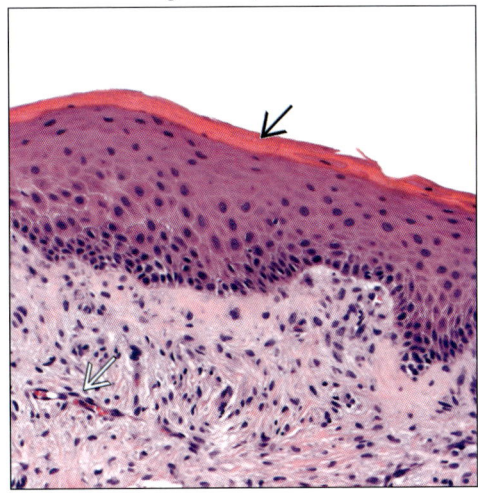

(Left) A hematoxylin and eosin stained tissue shows a section of gingiva. The epithelium in this particular location has a parakeratinized surface ➡. The rete ridges are long, and in some areas, narrow ➡. *(Right)* This section of gingiva shows fewer rete ridges and has an orthokeratinized surface ➡. The underlying lamina propria contains small capillary loops ➡. Sparse inflammatory cells and nerve twigs are sometimes seen in the lamina propria.

Melanin Pigment

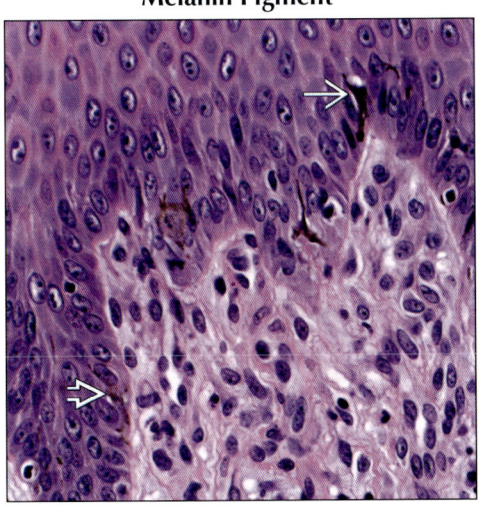

Odontogenic Epithelial Rests

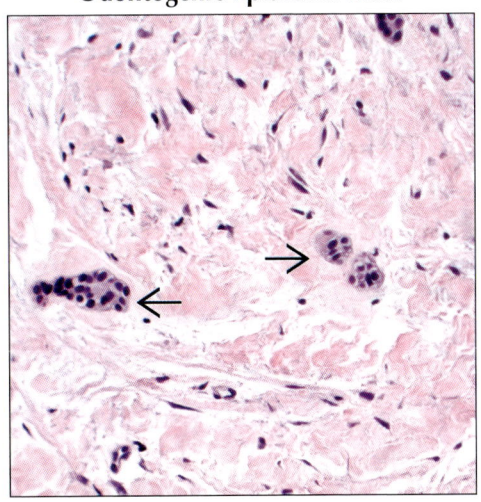

(Left) The pigmentation of gingivae within a population may vary as much as skin color; however, there tends to be a relationship between amount of pigmentation seen in the skin and the gingivae. The melanin pigmentation seen here ➡ is produced by melanocytes ➡. Melanocytes lack desmosomes and may have visible dendritic processes that extend between the cells of the epithelium. *(Right)* Odontogenic epithelial rests ➡ can be seen, especially in the posterior areas of gingiva.

MINOR SALIVARY GLANDS

Key Facts

Macroscopic Anatomy
- 500-1,000 lobules of minor salivary glands
  - Buccal mucosa, lips, floor of mouth, tonsillar pillars, hard and soft palate
  - Tongue: Blandin and Nunn glands and von Ebner glands

Microscopic Anatomy
- Minor glands are either primarily mucous, primarily serous, or a mixture of both
- Acini are rounded collections of mucous or serous cells surrounding a central lumen
- Mucous cells
  - Large polygonal shape with pale, basophilic, mucin-filled cytoplasm
  - Dense, basaloid nuclei flattened against basement membrane
- Serous cells
  - Polygonal shape; cytoplasm has dense, strongly staining eosinophilic secretory granules
  - Round, more open nuclei found in central or basal 1/3 of cell
  - In glands where mucous cells predominate, serous cells may form serous demilunes, or collections of serous cells surrounding terminal part of mucous acini
- Myoepithelial cells
  - May rarely be seen as spindled cells associated with acini
- Ducts
  - Intercalated ducts: Small in size, lined by low cuboidal cells with scant cytoplasm and round nuclei
  - Striated ducts: Larger, lined by columnar and eosinophilic cells with uniform round nuclei
  - Excretory: Largest, lined by pseudostratified columnar epithelium

(Left) This low-power view of seromucous minor salivary glands ➡ shows the unencapsulated relationship the glands has with the surrounding tissue. These glands, from the buccal mucosa, are intimately associated with the nearby connective and adipose tissue. Small excretory ➡ ducts are seen between lobules. (Right) This high-power image of a seromucous gland shows the distinct mucous cells ➡ filled with basophilic mucin, and associated serous, granular demilunes ➡.

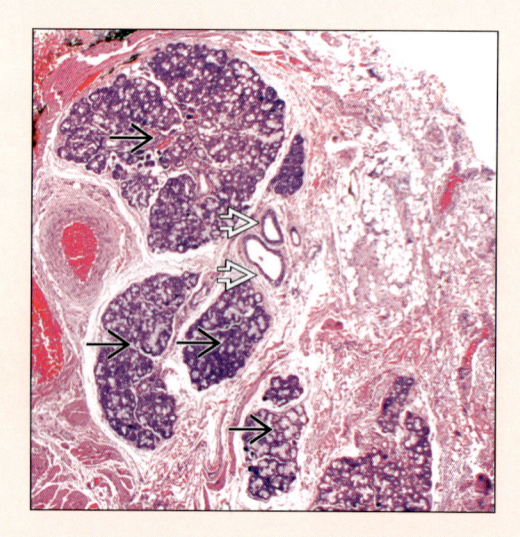

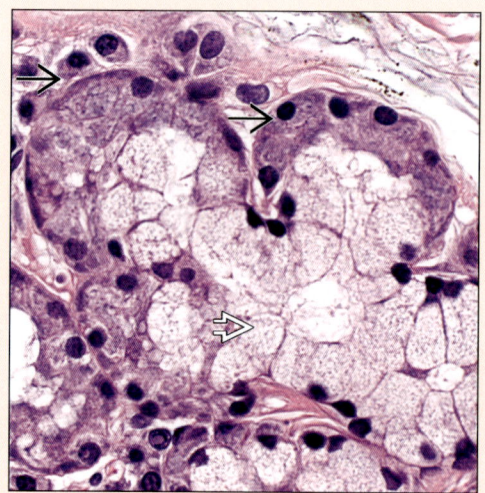

(Left) A medium-power image of a seromucous minor salivary gland shows several seromucous units with mucous acini ➡ capped by serous demilunes ➡. Secretions are collected from the secretory units by ducts. Note the striated duct ➡ lined by columnar cells with round uniform nuclei. (Right) A low-power image shows the von Ebner minor salivary glands. These glands are found in association with the circumvallate papillae found on the posterior dorsal tongue.

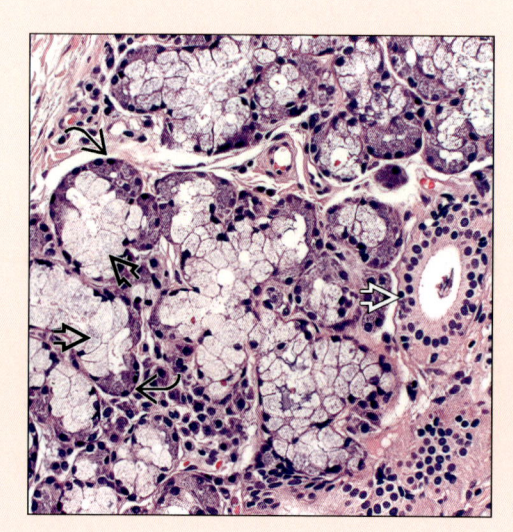

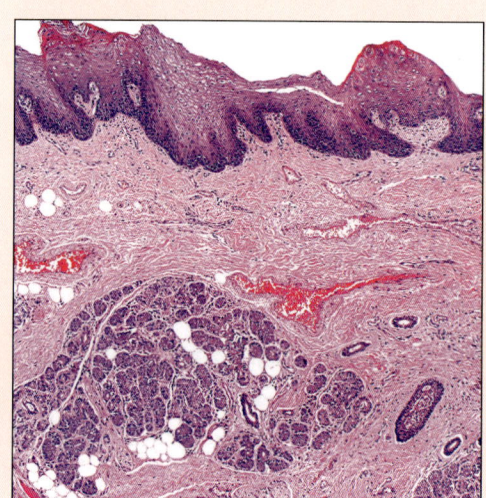

MINOR SALIVARY GLANDS

von Ebner Glands

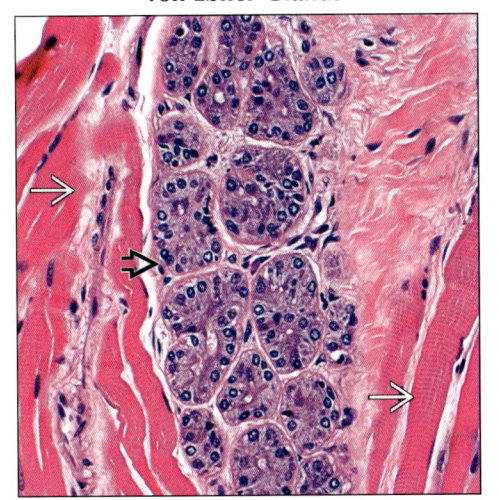

Excretory Duct

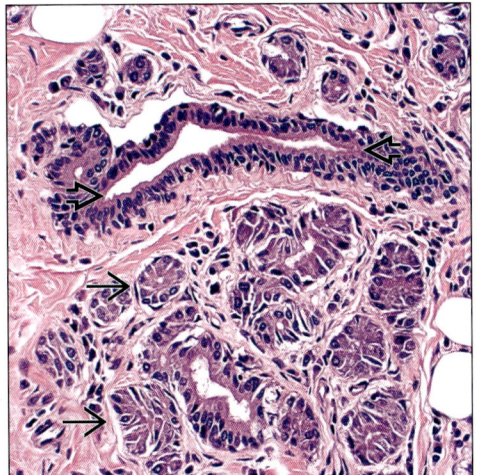

(Left) An image of the serous von Ebner glands ➡ shows the close association to the surrounding skeletal muscle ➡. When minor salivary glands develop neoplasms, this intimate association can make determining invasion difficult. (Right) H&E image shows serous acini ➡ with an adjacent excretory duct ➡, usually shorter than those in major glands. This type of duct is lined by pseudostratified columnar epithelium, supported by surrounding fibrous connective tissue.

Blandin and Nunn Glands

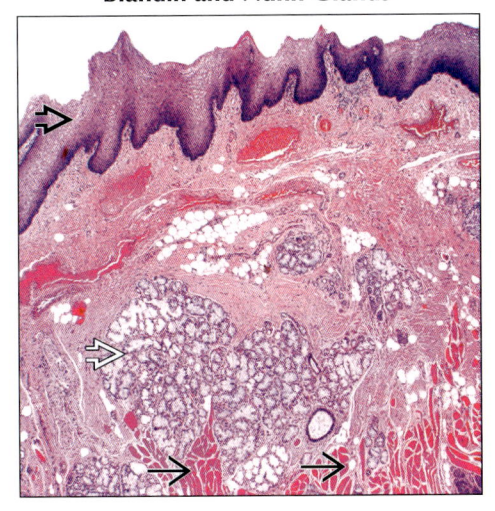

Blandin and Nunn Glands

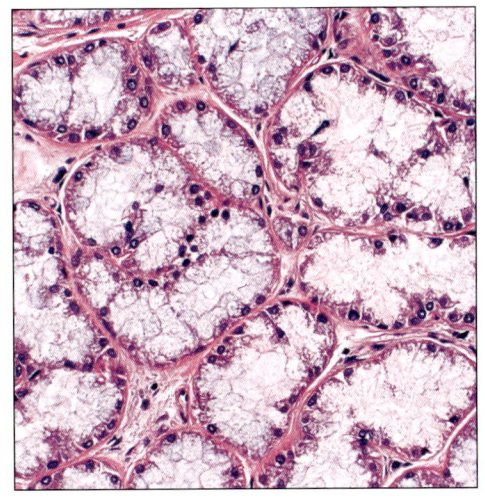

(Left) Low-power image shows the minor salivary glands found in the anterior tongue, called the Blandin and Nunn glands. Note the overlying mucosal epithelium ➡, hyperkeratotic in this case. These unencapsulated glands ➡ are closely associated with the muscle ➡ of the tongue. (Right) This high-power view shows the Blandin and Nunn glands. This type of gland consists of entirely mucous acini, with each acinus surrounded by thin connective tissue septae.

Mucous Acinus and Intercalated Duct

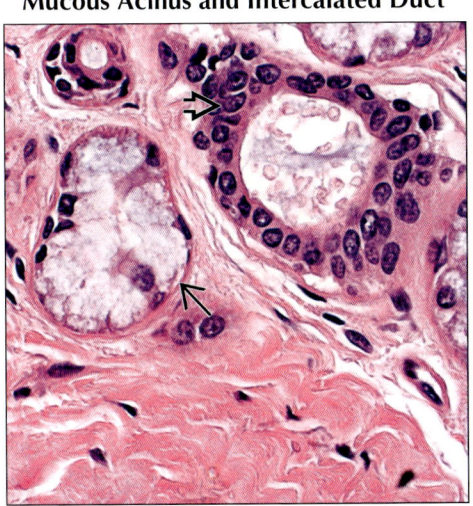

Mucous Cells

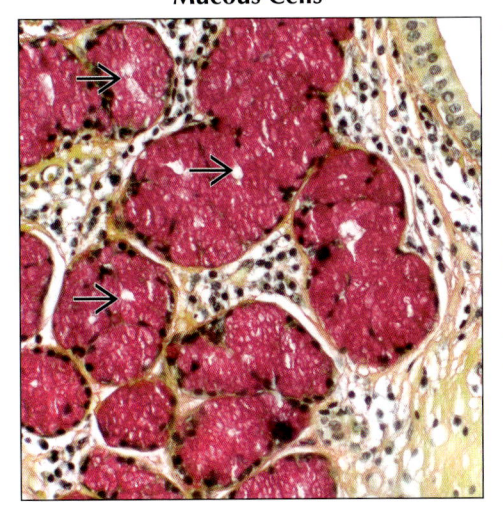

(Left) High-power image shows a mucous acinus ➡ adjacent to an intercalated duct ➡. The small size of this type of duct makes them very inconspicuous in routine H&E slides. Intercalated ducts are lined by cuboidal, eosinophilic cells with centrally placed nuclei. (Right) A high-power image of a mucicarmine stain highlights mucous cells. The intense pink staining assists in locating the small central lumina of the mucous acini ➡.

TEETH

Key Facts

Macroscopic Anatomy
- Crown
  - The part of tooth easily seen clinically
  - Surfaced by hard, brittle, translucent enamel supported by underlying dentin
  - Pulp forms central chamber of tooth that supplies nutrition and contains nerve supply
- Root
  - Anchors tooth to alveolar bone
  - Root number varies depending on tooth
  - Apical foramen is opening through which blood and nerve supply enter and exit tooth

Microscopic Anatomy
- Enamel
  - Acellular, highly mineralized, 96% inorganic material made up of hydroxyapatite crystals
  - Crystals are aligned to create rods
  - Immature enamel has a basophilic, fish scale appearance on H&E sections
- Dentin
  - 70% mineralized tissue
  - Eosinophilic, closely packed tubules
  - Odontoblasts are responsible for production of dentin, and their processes occupy tubules
  - Reparative dentin deposited at site of injury shows distorted tubular pattern
- Pulp
  - Loose connective tissue that resembles primitive mesenchyme
  - Odontoblasts line pulp chamber
  - Stellate fibroblasts
  - Small blood vessels
- Periodontal ligament (PDL)
  - Thin fibrous attachment between root and surrounding bone
  - Permits slight movement of teeth
  - Seldom preserved or seen on routine processing
- Cementum
  - Mineralized organic material that resembles bone
  - Cementocytes are responsible for production of cementum and occupy its lacunae
  - Location where enamel and cementum meet (or sometimes overlap) is referred to as cementoenamel junction (CEJ)

Pitfalls/Artifacts
- Teeth need to be decalcified for routine H&E slides
  - Mature enamel is lost to processing
- Often, teeth that are submitted are surgically sectioned, losing normal anatomy/histology

Age Variation
- Primary (deciduous)
  - 20 teeth: Smaller in size, erupt between 6-30 months of age
  - 8 incisors
  - 4 canines
  - 8 molars
- Secondary (permanent)
  - 32 teeth: Larger in size, erupt starting at ~ 6 years of age
  - 8 incisors
  - 4 canines
  - 8 premolars
  - 12 molars
- Changes found in both primary and secondary teeth
  - Hyperdontia (supernumerary teeth)
  - Hypodontia
  - Dentin continues to be laid down with age, reducing or obliterating the size of dentin tubules and shrinking the pulp chamber
  - Attrition: Loss of tooth structure due to tooth-to-tooth contact
  - Abrasion: Loss of tooth structure due to tooth-to-non-tooth contact (i.e., contact with tooth brush)
  - Erosion: Loss of tooth structure due to chemical process
  - Caries: Loss of tooth structure due to bacterial decay
  - Teeth generally darken with age
  - Dental restorations may alter or replace normal histology
  - Teeth may be lost due to disease or trauma

(Left) This graphic shows the mandibular permanent teeth: Incisors ➔, canines ➔, premolars ➔, and molars ➔. The teeth occupy approximately 1/5 of the surface area of the mouth. (Right) This graphic shows the maxillary permanent teeth: Incisors ➔, canines ➔, premolars ➔, and molars ➔. The maxillary and mandibular teeth work together for proper eating and speech.

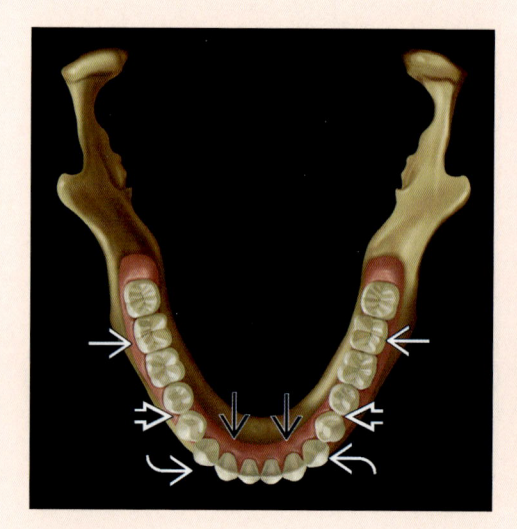

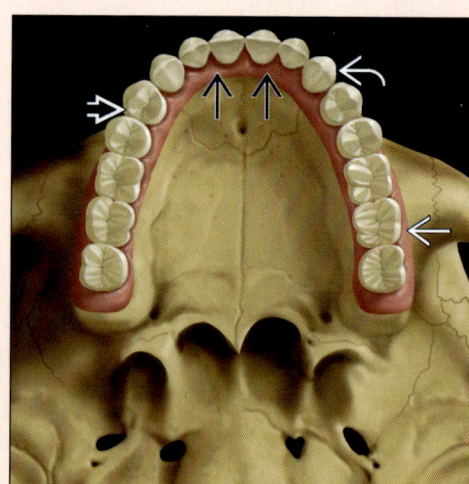

TEETH

Normal Full Dentition: Child

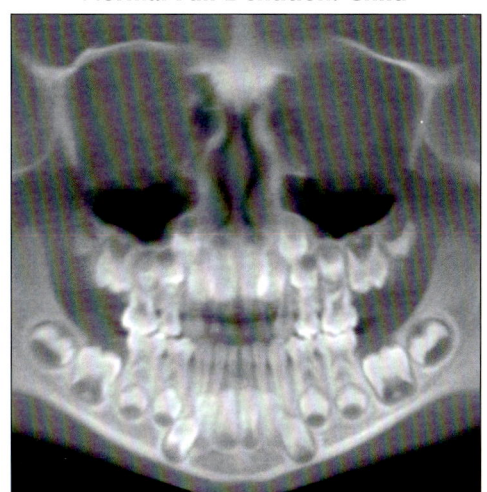

Normal Full Dentition: Young Adult

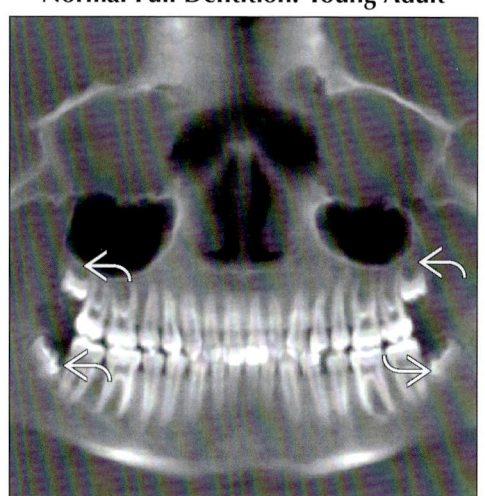

(Left) This image shows the normal full dentition of a child, likely around 5 years of age. All primary teeth are erupted, and the developing permanent teeth can be seen within the jaws. *(Right)* This image shows the normal full dentition of a young adult. Note that the 3rd molars are yet unerupted ➡. The eruption of the 1st permanent teeth begins around the age of 6 years, with the 1st molars, and generally ends in the early 20s with the eruption of the 3rd molars.

Tooth: Major Components

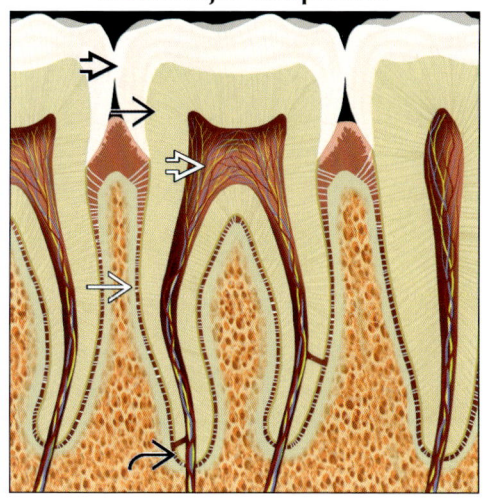

Tooth: Radiographic Image

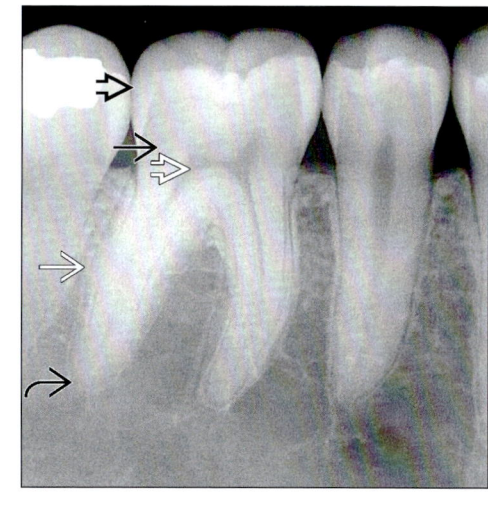

(Left) This graphic shows the major components of a tooth. Enamel ➡ surfaces the crown and is supported by underlying dentin ➡. The pulp ➡ is found centrally and communicates with surrounding bone via the foremen at the apex ➡. The periodontal ligament (PDL) ➡ is in close association with the root. *(Right)* In this radiographic image, the components of the tooth are readily seen: Enamel ➡, dentin ➡, pulp ➡, apex of the tooth ➡, and PDL ➡.

Cusp of Canine Tooth

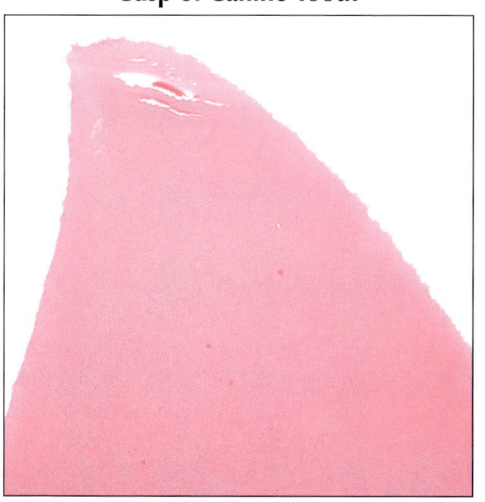

Enamel Matrix

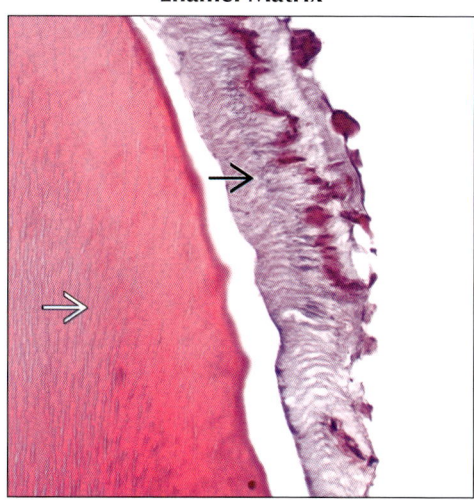

(Left) This image shows the cusp of a canine tooth. Due the the demineralization process required for routine H&E preparations, no enamel is present. Enamel is an inorganic material made up primarily of hydroxyapatite crystallites. *(Right)* Enamel matrix ➡, or immature enamel, is less mineralized and can be seen on routine H&E. Mature teeth do not have enamel matrix; however, this specimen is from an odontoma. Note the underlying dentin ➡.

TEETH

Root of Tooth: Apex

Pulp Chamber

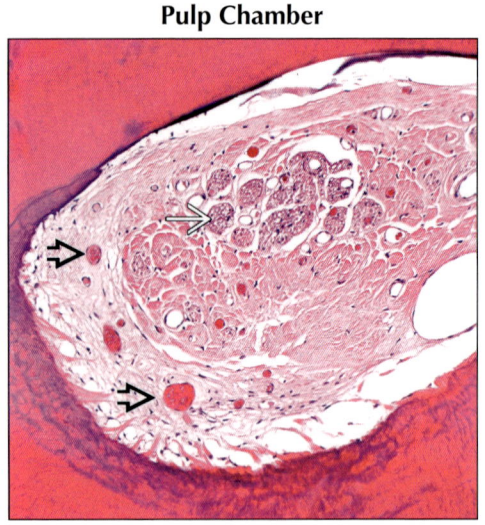

(Left) This image shows the root of the tooth near the apex ➡. The apex of the root is the area where the main foremen is seen; however, smaller accessory foramina may be found anywhere on the root surface. (Right) This image shows a cross section of the pulp chamber as it narrows toward the foramen. The foramen allows for entry and exit of vessels ➡ and nerves ➡. Infection of the pulp may create swelling, resulting in the disruption of the blood supply and tooth death.

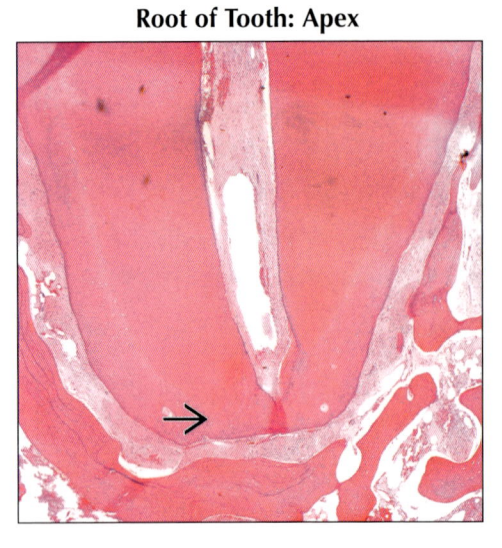

Dentin-Pulp Complex

Pulp

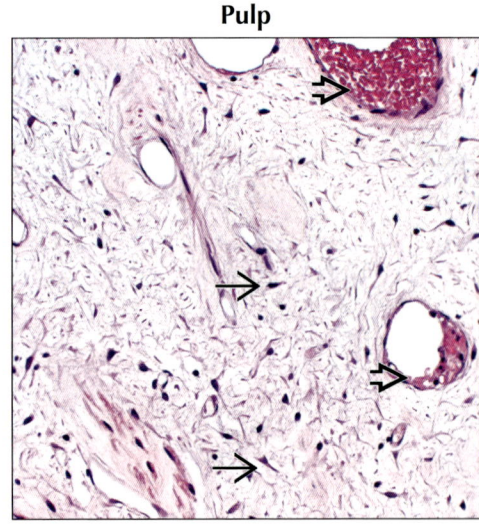

(Left) This high-power image shows the dentin-pulp complex. The odontoblasts ➡ form a single layer along the periphery of the pulp and have processes that extend into the tubules. It is the presence of these cells and their processes that makes dentin a sensitive tissue, unlike enamel. (Right) This high-power view of the pulp shows its loose matrix, which is made up of fibroblasts ➡, collagen, and ground substance. Note the presence of small vessels ➡ with red blood cells.

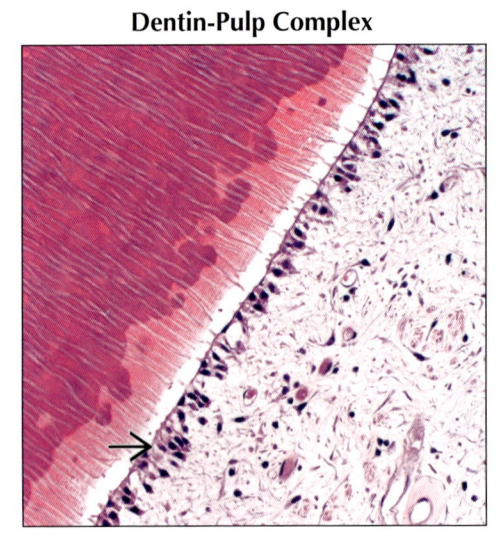

Periodontal Ligament

Periodontal Ligament

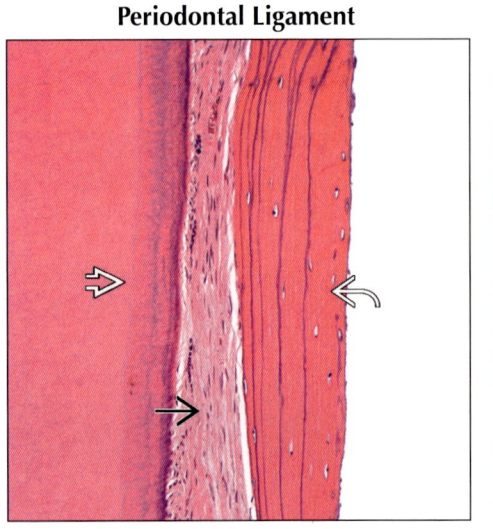

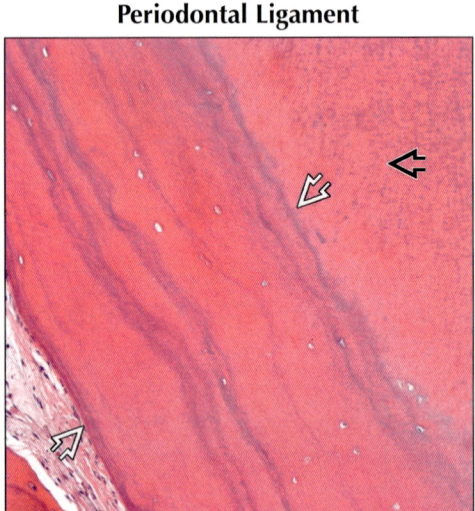

(Left) The periodontal ligament (PDL) ➡ provides attachment between the tooth root ➡ and the surrounding alveolar bone ➡. The PDL is made up of fibrous connective tissue that allows for slight movement during normal eating and biting. It is also the PDL that allows for the correction of malocclusion by orthodontic movements. (Right) This high-power view shows the relationship of the tooth to the PDL. Note the transition of dentin ➡ into cementum ➡.

TEETH

Dentin

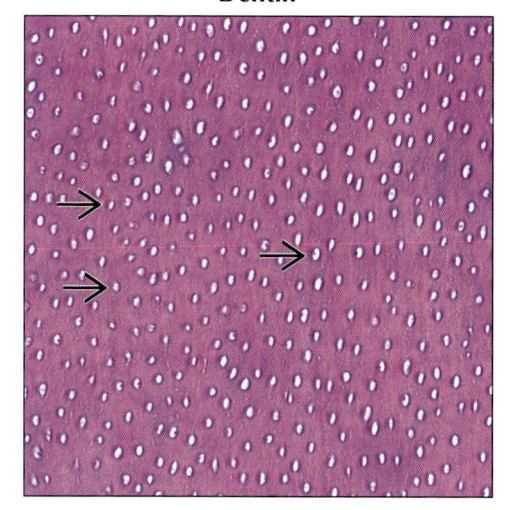

Dentin

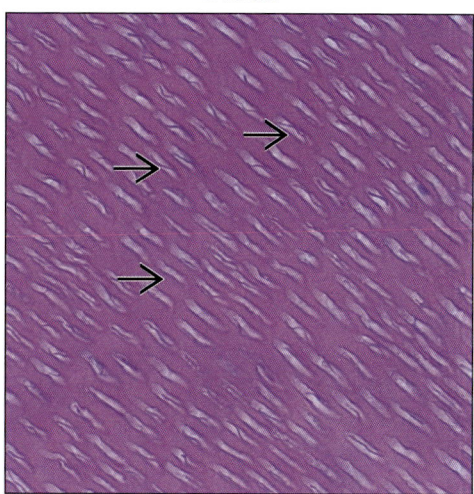

(Left) This high-power cross section of demineralized dentin shows characteristic small tubules ➡. *(Right)* A high-power longitudinal section of dentin shows the slight curvature of the tubules ➡. These tubules are filled with fluid and odontoblast processes. The tubules, however, make the dentin vulnerable to invasion of bacteria, which may result in dental caries. Severe infection may result in the infection of the pulp in addition to decay of tooth structure.

Reparative Dentin

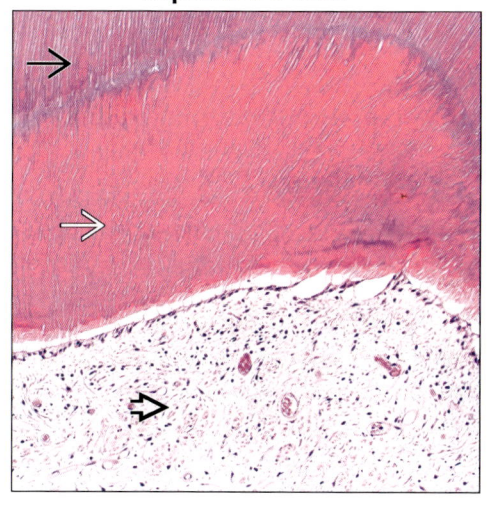

Enamel Matrix

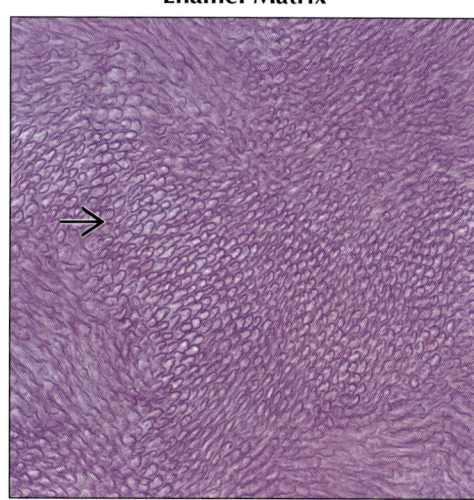

(Left) Insult to the tooth due to caries or mechanical trauma results in the deposition of reparative dentin ➡, seen here adjacent to normal dentin ➡. Reparative dentin has fewer and more irregular tubules; this may be due to the fact that it is likely rapidly laid down in an attempt to protect the pulp ➡. *(Right)* A high-power view shows a classic, basophilic fish scale appearance ➡ of enamel matrix. Mature enamel, unlike matrix, is destroyed by routine tissue processing.

Enamel Matrix

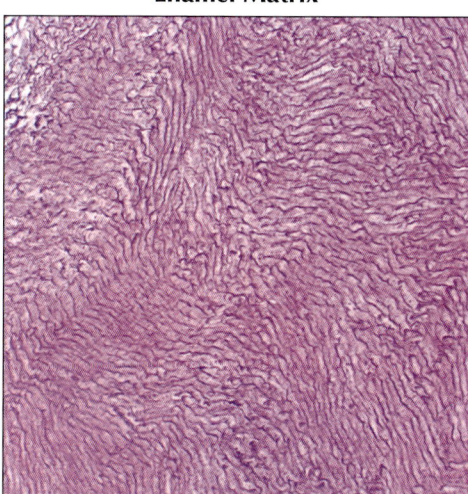

Graphic of SEM Image of Enamel

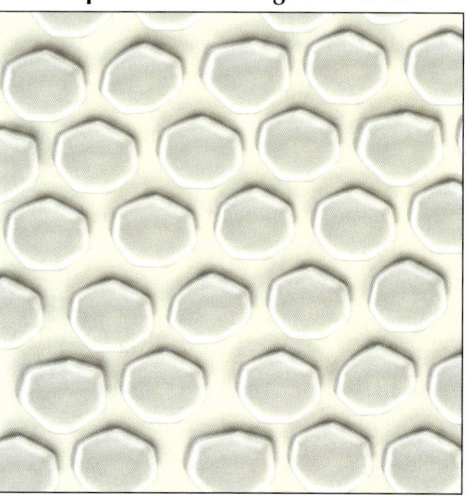

(Left) This photograph illustrates enamel matrix. Mature enamel is 96% inorganic and acellular. Unlike dentin, it is nonvital and not sensitive when affected by caries or trauma. Enamel cannot be regenerated or replaced and is, unfortunately, vulnerable to demineralization by acids in the environment because it is so highly mineralized. *(Right)* This illustration depicts a scanning electron microscope (SEM) image of enamel. SEM images are primarily used for research purposes.

TONGUE

Key Facts

Macroscopic Anatomy
- Anterior 2/3 (mobile tongue) and posterior 1/3 (fixed tongue) separated by sulcus terminalis
- Mobile tongue has dorsal and ventral surfaces
  - Dorsal surface covered by various types of papillae
  - Ventral surface smooth, lacks papillae
- Majority of tongue parenchyma consists of striated muscle

Microscopic Anatomy
- Epithelium is modified stratified squamous mucosa with various types of papillae
  - Ventral surface lined by thin, nonkeratinizing, stratified squamous epithelium with blunt rete pegs
- Filiform papillae: Most numerous; line majority of dorsal tongue
  - 2-3 mm long, conical shaped, and curved slightly posteriorly
  - Arranged in vague rows parallel to sulcus terminalis
  - Heavily keratinized and often have oral flora bacterial colonization
- Fungiform papillae: Less common, scattered throughout tongue
  - 0.5-1 mm wide, dome shaped, rise higher than filiform papillae
  - Thin, nonkeratinized epithelium with underlying vascular stroma (appear red-pink in situ)
  - May contain rare taste buds
- Foliate papillae: Only found in lateral tongue posteriorly
  - Parallel ridges lined by nonkeratinized stratified squamous mucosa
  - Rudimentary in humans, with only rare taste buds
- Circumvallate papillae: Arranged in V-shaped (6-14 papillae) orientation anterior to sulcus terminalis
  - 2-3 mm wide, dome shaped, surrounded by a small circular furrow where most taste buds reside
  - Serous (von Ebner) glands secrete into the furrow base and serve to rinse out furrow contents
  - Peripheral to furrow and papilla is a circular mucosal elevation (the vallum) that may have taste buds
- Taste buds: Sensory taste receptors that communicate with the surface via gustatory pore
  - Oval shaped, comprised of 3 cell types: Gustatory (taste), supporting (sustentacular), and basal (regenerative)
  - Gustatory (taste) cells are crescent shaped, simple epithelial cells with pale cytoplasm innervated by nonmyelinated nerves
  - Nonmyelinated nerve fibers communicate with myelinated fibers in papillae connective tissue core, forming subgemmal nerve plexus
  - Besides papillae, taste buds can be seen in glossopalatine arch, soft palate, lingual epiglottis, and posterior pharynx
- Majority of tongue parenchyma comprised of interlacing striated muscle (intrinsic) bundles arranged horizontally, vertically, and longitudinally
  - Orientation ensures high mobility to enhance mastication, phonation, swallowing, etc.
  - Varying amounts of mature adipose tissue located between skeletal muscle bundles
  - Extrinsic muscles also present; have origin outside of tongue proper
  - Richly vascular with numerous anastomoses and rich nerve supply
- Small amount of loose connective tissue located between epithelial surface and underlying muscle
- Mucous minor salivary gland lobules present in muscle in posterior portion of mobile tongue
- Serous minor salivary glands (von Ebner glands) present only underlying circumvallate papillae

Pitfalls/Artifacts
- Salivary gland tissue may be intimately associated with nerves, mimicking perineural invasion
- Neural tissue in connective tissue cores of papillae may be confused with neuromas
- Ectopic tonsil tissue can mimic neoplasms or inflammatory processes

---

(Left) The posterior border of the mobile tongue consists of a V-shaped row of circumvallate papillae ➢. The dorsal tongue has numerous filiform papillae ➡ and scattered fungiform papillae ➡. *(Right)* The linear foliate papillae ➡ are found on the posterior lateral tongue. Note the numerous filiform papillae ➡ on the dorsal tongue. The ventral tongue ➡ is smooth, lacking papillae.

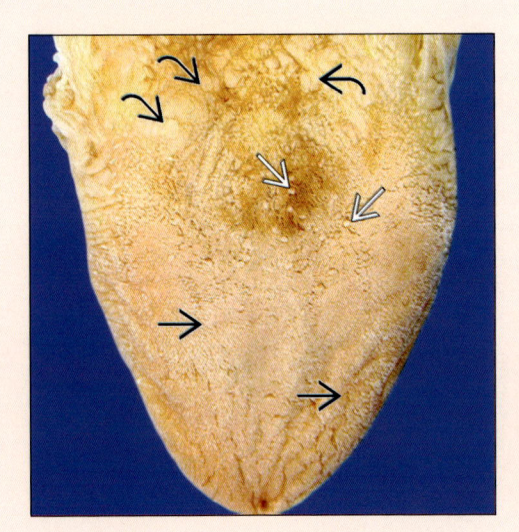

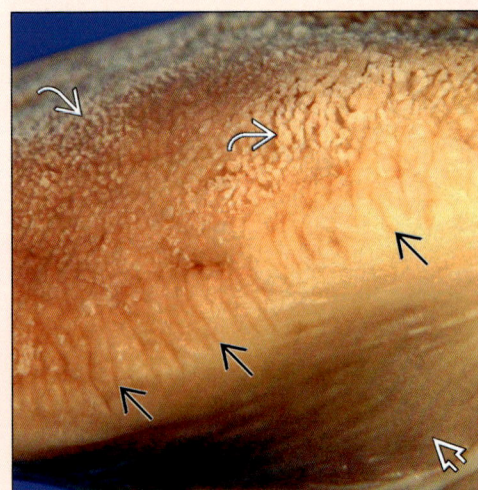

TONGUE

Tongue Parenchyma

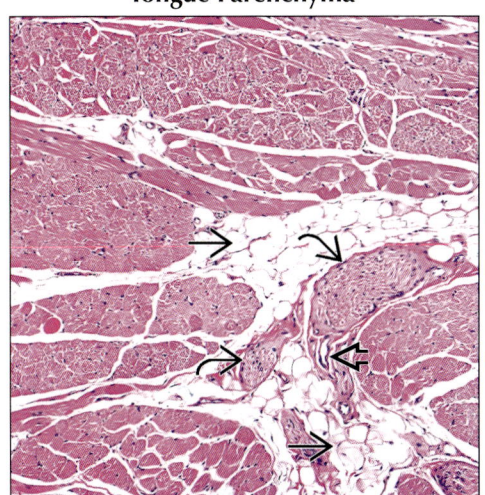

Tongue Muscle

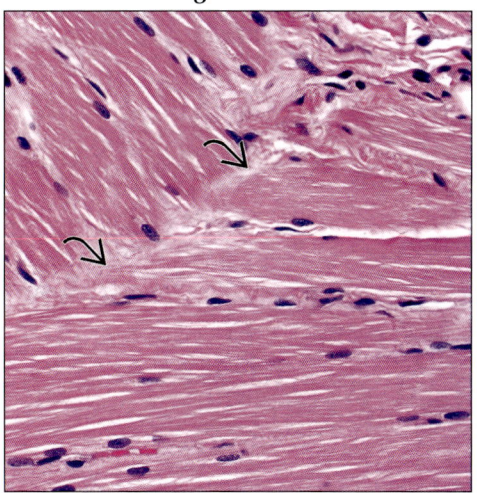

(Left) The bulk of the tongue parenchyma consists of muscle bundles arranged in a 3-dimensional configuration to allow for maximal mobility and functionality. Varying amounts of mature adipose tissue ➔ are associated with the muscle bundles. The tongue is richly innervated ➔ and contains many blood vessels ➔, replete with vascular anastomoses. (Right) Interlacing striated muscle bundles ➔ allow for such essential functions as mastication, phonation, swallowing, etc.

Filiform Papillae

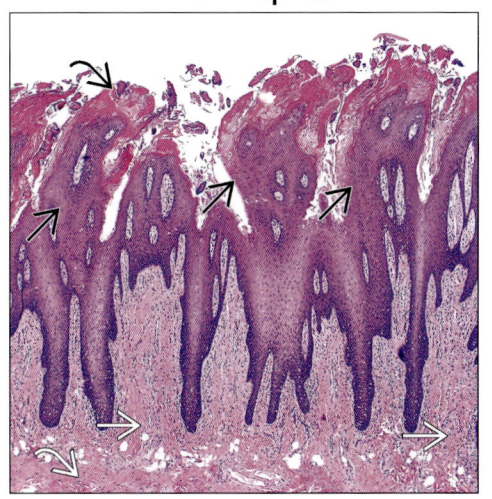

Filiform Papillae

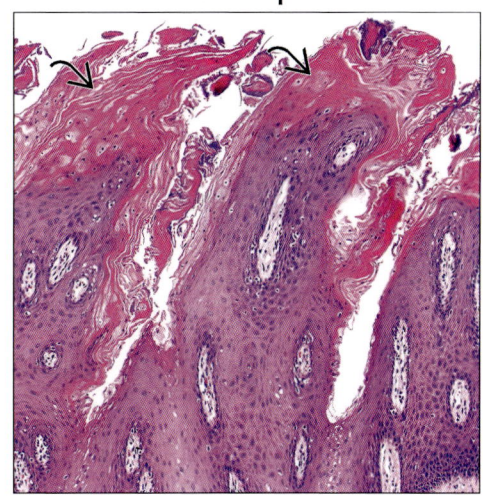

(Left) The dorsal tongue surface is carpeted with conical-shaped, 2-3 mm long, filiform papillae ➔. In contrast to other papillae, the filiform papillae are heavily keratinized ➔, especially on the tips. Throughout the tongue, only a small amount of loose connective tissue ➔ separates the mucosa from the underlying striated tongue muscle ➔. (Right) The tips of the filiform papillae are heavily keratinized ➔. The filiform papillae generally lack taste buds.

Bacterial Colonization of Filiform Papilla

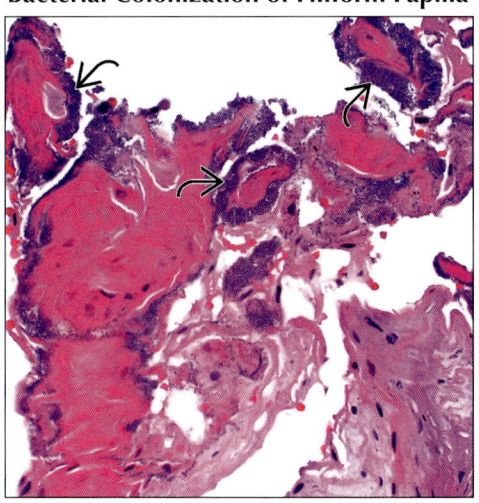

Fungiform Papilla

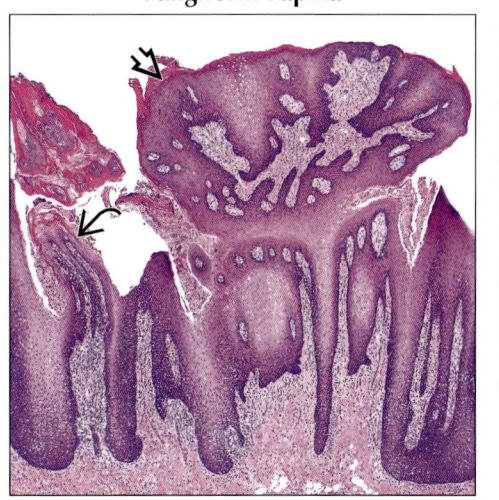

(Left) Bacterial colonization by oral flora bacteria ➔ can be seen to varying degrees in the keratin of filiform papillae. With extensive bacterial colonization, the tongue can appear brown-black macroscopically. (Right) Fungiform papillae ➔ are the second most numerous papillae and are irregularly distributed throughout the tongue between the numerous filiform papillae ➔. These are 0.5-1 mm wide, dome shaped, and slightly taller than the filiform papillae.

TONGUE

Fungiform Papilla

(Left) Fungiform papillae have a thin epithelial surface with limited parakeratinization ⇨ and underlying stroma rich in small blood vessels ⇨, making them look red or pink grossly. The connective tissue stroma has small nerves that innervate the rare taste buds found in some fungiform papillae. **(Right)** Unlike in some mammals, foliate papillae ⇨ are rudimentary in humans. Note the small amount of loose connective tissue separating the mucosa from the striated muscle ⇨.

Foliate Papilla

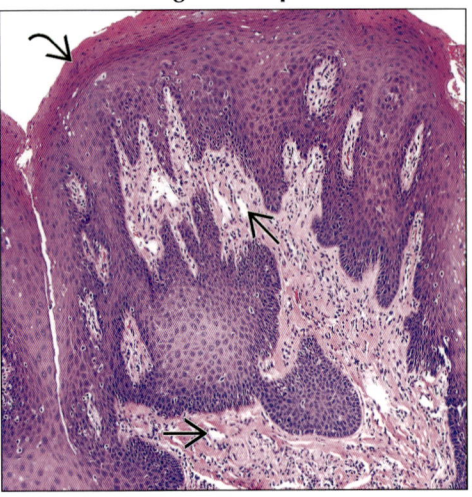

Foliate Papilla

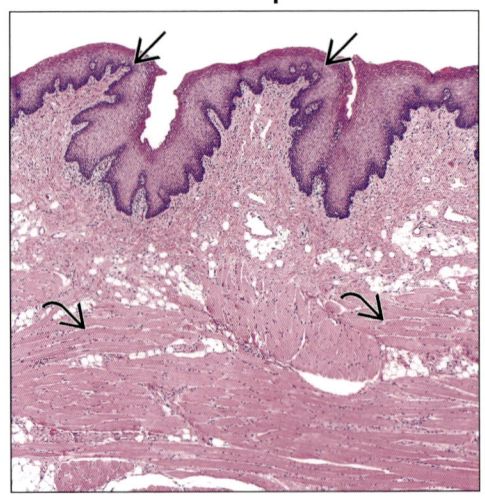

(Left) Foliate papillae can have rare taste buds and are lined by a thin stratified squamous epithelium with minimal parakeratinization ⇨. The connective tissue stroma contains many small blood vessels and nerves. **(Right)** The dome-shaped circumvallate papillae ⇨ are surrounded by a circumferential furrow ⇨ and a circular mucosal ridge (vallum ⇨) lateral to that. von Ebner serous glands ⇨ empty into the base of the furrow ⇨ and are thought to flush out its contents.

Circumvallate Papilla

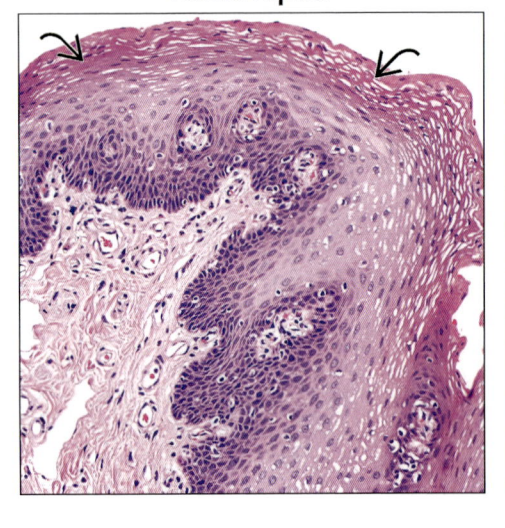

Circumvallate Papilla

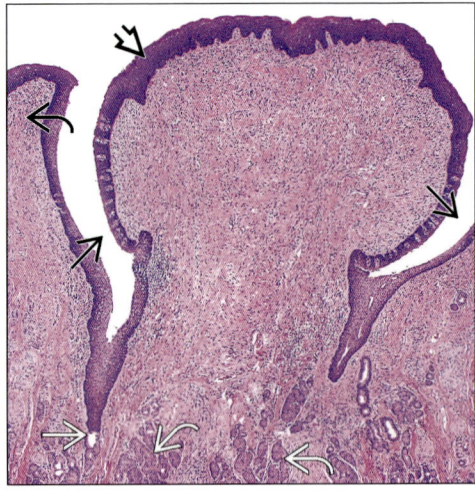

(Left) Circumvallate papillae have a connective tissue core rich in haphazardly arranged small nerves ⇨ that innervate the numerous intraepithelial taste buds ⇨. Taste buds can also be seen in the vallum ⇨. Papillae nerve tissue can be mistaken for neuromas. **(Right)** Taste buds are oval, clear-staining structures ⇨ comprised of crescent-shaped taste, supporting, and basal cells. A taste pore ⇨ transmits tastes via receptors on microvilli to the underlying neurites ⇨.

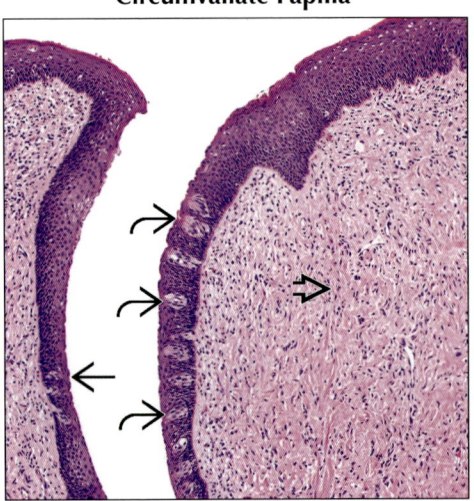

Taste Buds

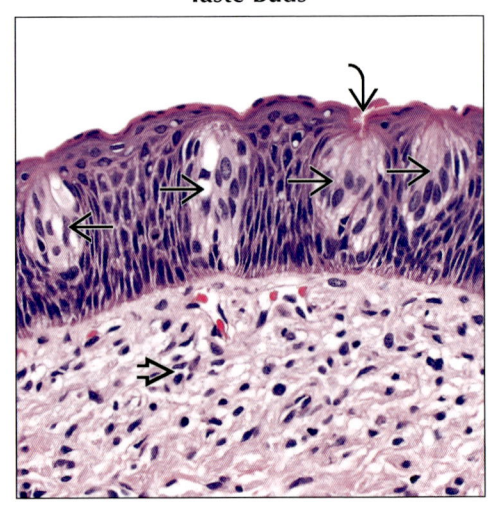

TONGUE

Mucous Glands

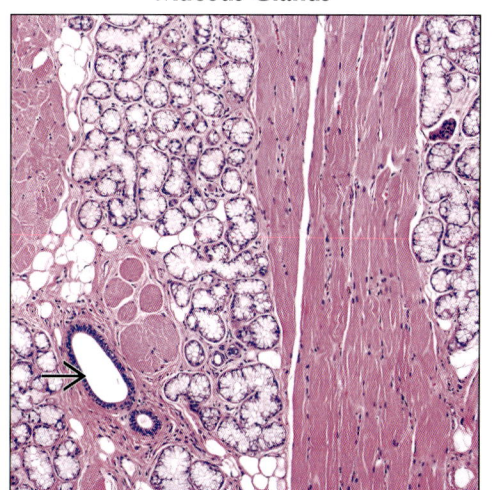

von Ebner Glands

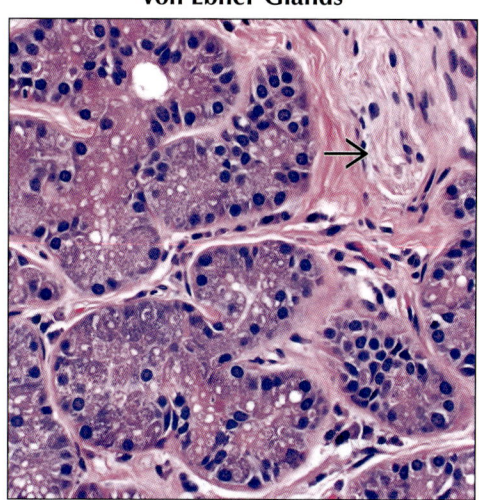

(Left) Salivary gland tissue is present in the posterior portion of the tongue and these consist mostly of mucous gland lobules embedded in striated muscle. The lobules have a central salivary duct ⇥ that drains to the ventral tongue. (Right) von Ebner glands are serous glands located only below the circumvallate papillae. Their ducts drain into the furrows to flush out its contents. Both serous and mucous glands in the tongue are intimately associated with nerves ⇥.

Squamous Metaplasia

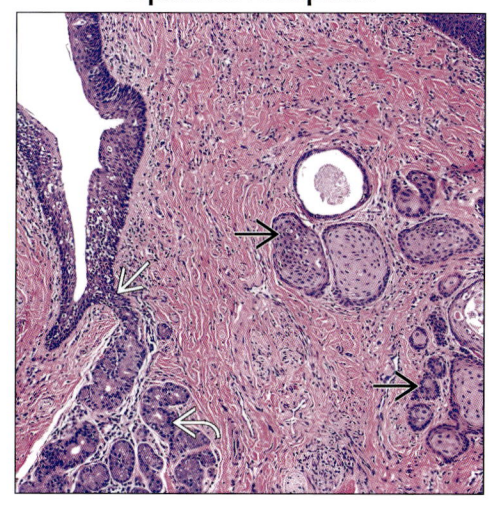

Ectopic Tonsil

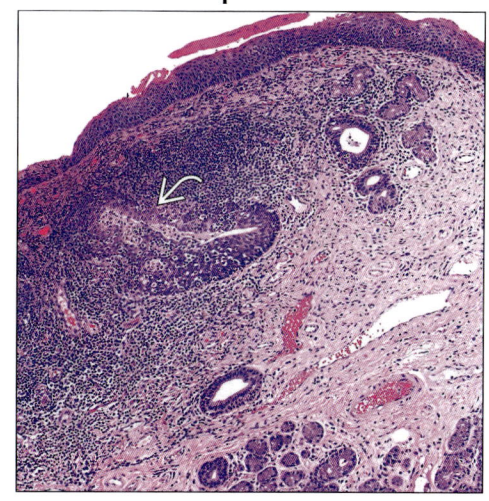

(Left) Serous von Ebner glands ⇥ drain into the furrow ⇥ separating the circumvallate papillae from the adjacent furrow. This is thought to flush out the furrow contents in order to allow for new tastes to be better discriminated. Squamous metaplasia of the salivary gland ducts ⇥ can mimic squamous cell carcinoma on biopsy or at frozen section. (Right) Ectopic tonsil tissue ⇥ can be seen anterior to the sulcus terminalis and can mimic neoplasms or lesions clinically.

Ventral Tongue

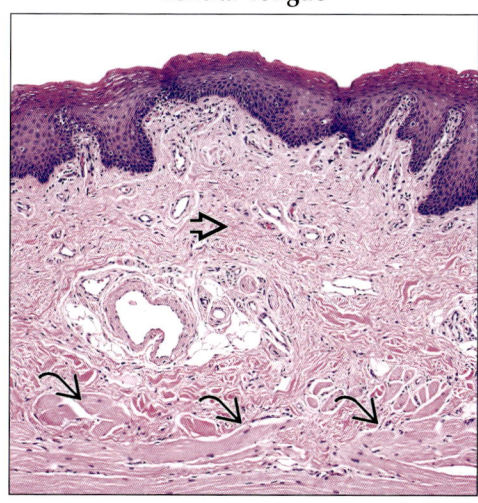

Ventral Tongue

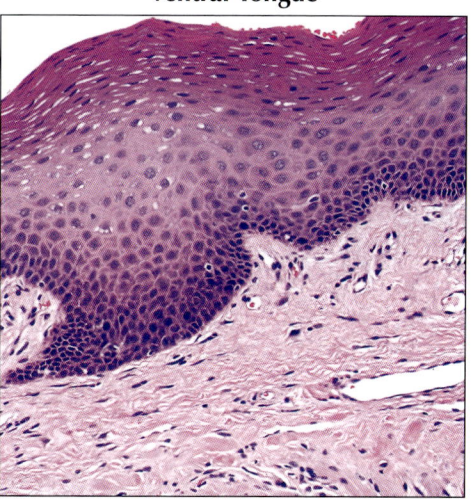

(Left) The ventral tongue lacks papillae, giving it a smooth, glistening appearance macroscopically. Note the small amount of loose connective tissue ⇥ separating the mucosa from the tongue muscle ⇥. (Right) The ventral tongue is lined by a thin, nonkeratinizing, stratified squamous mucosa that lacks the papillae seen throughout the dorsal tongue.

TONSILS/ADENOIDS

Key Facts

Macroscopic Anatomy
- Lymphoid aggregates covered by epithelium that form the majority of Waldeyer ring
  - 3 major tonsils: Palatine, lingual, and pharyngeal
- Palatine tonsil (a.k.a. faucial tonsil, tonsil)
  - Paired tonsils located in lateral oropharynx between palatoglossal (anterior pillar) and palatopharyngeal (posterior pillar) arches
  - Surface is smooth with 15-20 invaginations (crypts) into the tonsil parenchyma
  - Yellow (sulfur) granules often seen within crypts and may be calcified (tonsilloliths)
- Lingual tonsil (a.k.a. base of tongue)
  - Covers surface of posterior 1/3 of tongue (fixed tongue) between sulcus terminalis and valleculae
  - Separated into halves by glossoepiglottic ligament
  - Consists of mucosa-covered nodules with surface invaginations into the tonsil parenchyma (crypts)
- Pharyngeal tonsil (a.k.a. tonsil of Luschka, adenoid)
  - Pyramid-shaped, mucosa-covered nodular tissue located in superior midline of nasopharynx
  - Unlike other tonsils, do not have crypts, but have have elongated folds of the surface mucosa
  - When enlarged clinically, referred to as adenoids (Greek *aden* = gland) because they appear "glandular"

Microscopic Anatomy
- Palatine tonsils
  - Surface is nonkeratinizing stratified squamous epithelium
  - Crypts represent extension of surface mucosa into underlying lymphoid stroma; most are simple, but may be branched, and they extend to the connective tissue pseudocapsule
  - Crypt epithelium contains intraepithelial lymphocytes (both B and T cells) and plasma cells, resulting in distortion of normal architecture with a reticulated appearance (lymphoepithelium)
  - Most crypt epithelial cells have a basaloid appearance with a thin layer of differentiated keratinocytes at the surface
  - Sulfur granules consisting of aggregates of *Actinomyces* and other nonpathogenic oral flora are common in the crypt lumen
  - Deep crypts often contain desquamated keratin debris mixed with oral bacteria and inflammatory cells
  - Lymphoid tissue is comprised of B-cell-rich follicles, many with germinal centers and T-cell-rich interfollicular zones
  - Reactive follicles polarize toward antigenic exposure similar to lymph nodes; unlike lymph nodes, there is no capsule, trabeculae, or sinuses
  - Small mucous salivary glands are present in the connective tissue peripheral to the tonsil; ducts typically drain to the surface
  - Small islands of elastic cartilage can be present in adjacent connective tissue
- Lingual tonsils
  - Histologically very similar to palatine tonsils
  - Crypts are shorter than those in the palatine tonsils
  - Sulfur granules less common than in palatine tonsils
  - Mucous minor salivary glands present, underlying lymphoid tissue
- Pharyngeal tonsil
  - No crypts, but elongated mucosal folds containing lymphoid tissue
  - Surface mucosa is respiratory-type epithelium with variably present foci of squamous epithelium
  - Deep portions of the epithelial folds contain intraepithelial lymphocytes (lymphoepithelium) similar to tonsillar crypts
  - Lymphoid component similar to other tonsils
  - Seromucous minor salivary glands present adjacent to tonsillar tissue; not usually sampled during adenoidectomy

Pitfalls/Artifacts
- Deep crypts may be mistaken for invasive squamous cell carcinoma, especially on frozen section

Age Variation
- Tonsils largest in childhood, progressively atrophy following puberty

(Left) The mucosal surface of the palatine tonsil is mainly smooth ➔, with approximately 15-20 surface invaginations ➔. Tonsils are largest in childhood and gradually atrophy by adulthood. **(Right)** The cut surface shows that the surface invaginations correspond to crypts ➔ that extend deeply into the lymphoid stroma, close to the underlying compressed connective tissue pseudocapsule ➔.

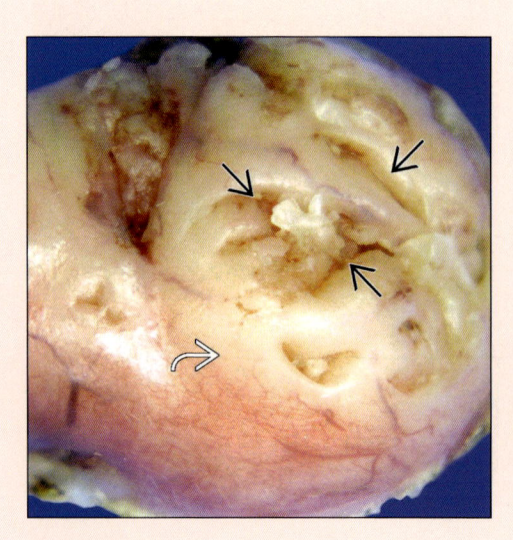

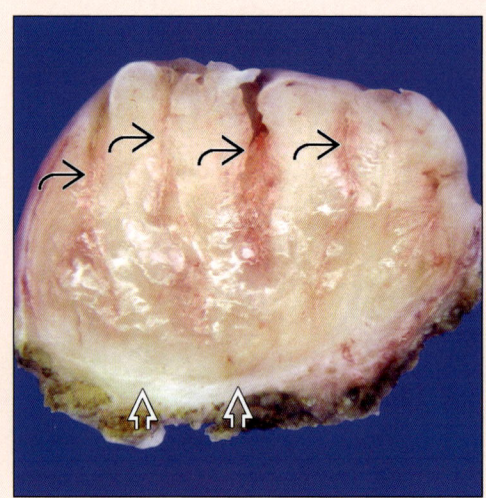

TONSILS/ADENOIDS

Palatine Tonsil

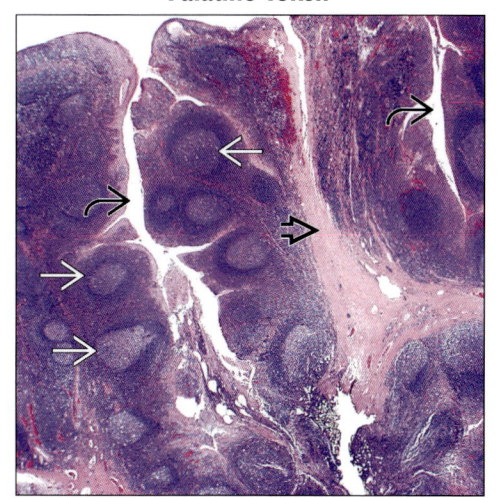

Palatine Tonsil

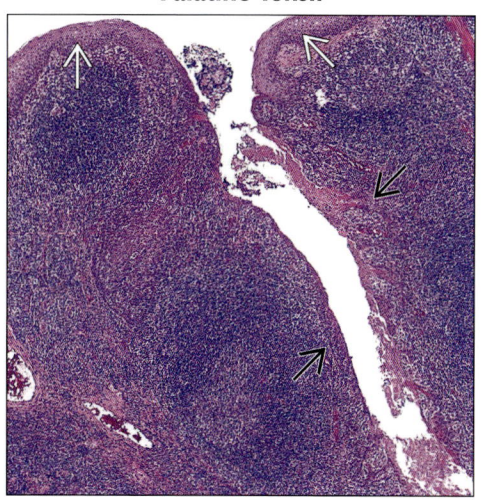

(Left) Tonsillar crypts ➡ represent invaginations of the surface mucosa into the lymphoid stroma. Unlike lymph nodes, tonsils lack capsules, sinuses, and trabeculae, but do have connective tissue bands that extend to the surface ➡. The stroma is mainly comprised of lymphoid aggregates ➡ and interfollicular small lymphocytes. *(Right)* The surface epithelium is nonkeratinizing stratified squamous mucosa ➡, which becomes a specialized lymphoepithelium in the crypt zones ➡.

Tonsillar Crypts: Palatine Tonsil

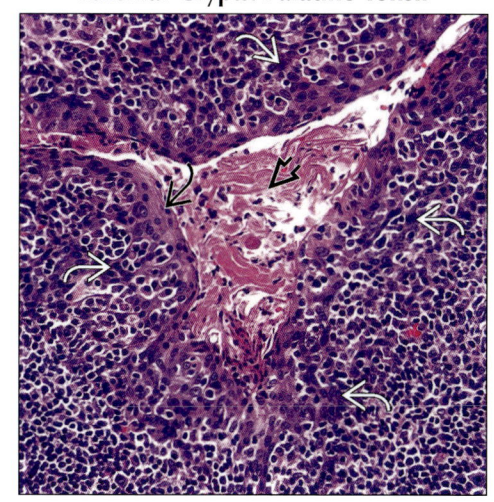

Lymphoepithelium

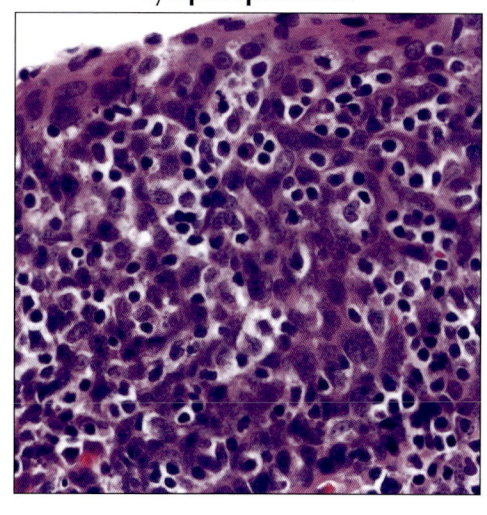

(Left) Crypt epithelium is distorted by infiltrating lymphocytes and plasma cells, which impart a reticular appearance. The squamous cells are predominantly basaloid ➡. The surface has a thin layer of differentiated keratinocytes ➡. Although nonkeratinizing, desquamated squamous cells often accumulate within the crypts ➡. *(Right)* The lymphoepithelium consists of basaloid keratinocytes with infiltrating lymphocytes and plasma cells, imparting a reticulated appearance.

CD3 Immunohistochemistry

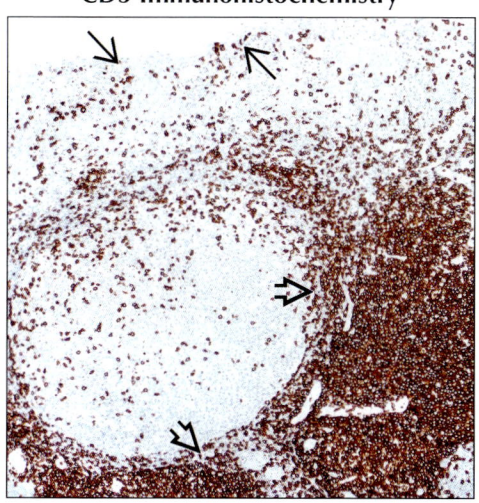

CD20 Immunohistochemistry

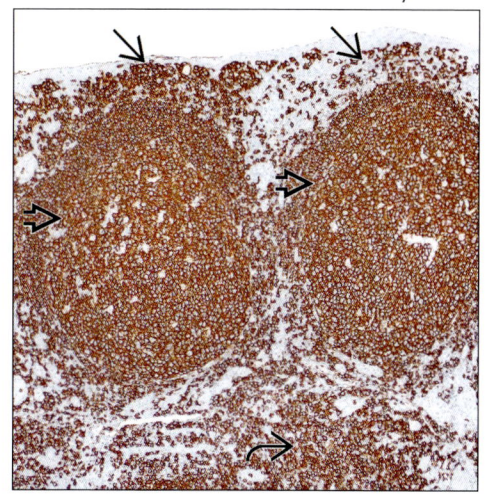

(Left) CD3 immunohistochemical staining highlights interfollicular T-cell-rich zones ➡ in normal tonsil. Note the presence of scattered T cells within the lymphoepithelium ➡. *(Right)* CD20 immunohistochemical staining highlights B-cell-rich follicles ➡ in normal tonsil. Many B cells are also present in the T-cell-rich interfollicular zones ➡. Note the presence of more abundant B cells within the lymphoepithelium ➡.

TONSILS/ADENOIDS

Sulfur Granules

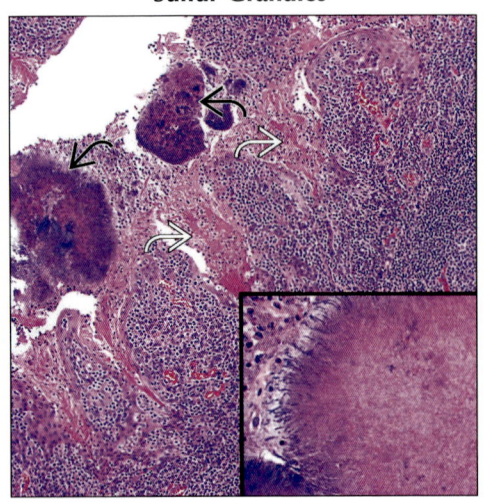

Mucous Glands: Palatine Tonsil

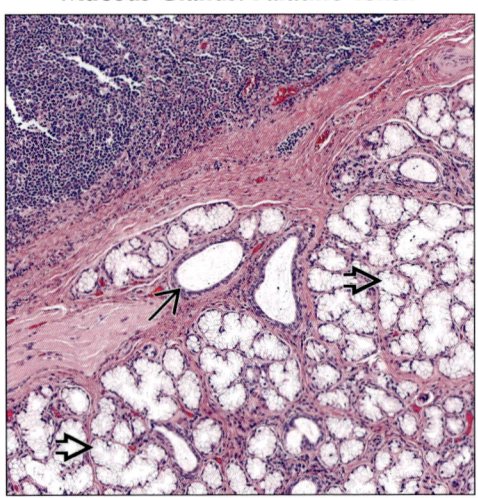

(Left) Tonsil crypts are blind-ending and typically accumulate luminal debris, such as desquamated keratin ➔ and aggregates of oral bacteria ➔. This likely contributes to the development of chronic tonsillitis clinically. The inset demonstrates a sulfur granule composed of numerous actinomycotic organisms mixed with other oral flora. *(Right)* The connective tissue pseudocapsule contains scattered small mucous glands ➔ with ducts ➔ draining to the surface.

Ectopic Cartilage

Lingual Tonsil

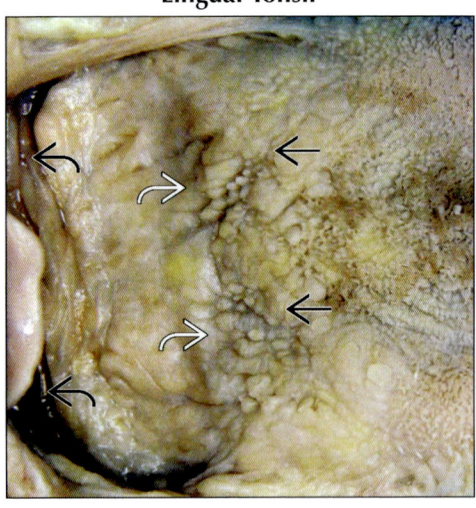

(Left) Small nodules of ectopic cartilage ➔ may be seen in the tonsillar connective tissue pseudocapsule. These are often associated with mucous glands and likely represent 2nd branchial cleft developmental abnormalities. *(Right)* The lingual tonsil (base of tongue) consists of irregular nodular tissue ➔ corresponding to mucosa-covered lymphoid tissue with surface invaginations. It is located posterior to the sulcus terminalis ➔ and anterior to the valleculae ➔.

Lingual Tonsil

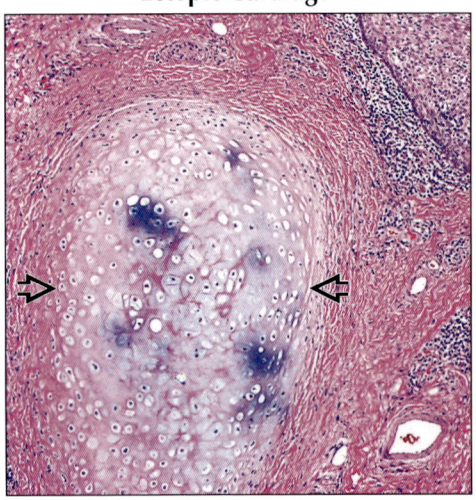

Lingual Tonsil

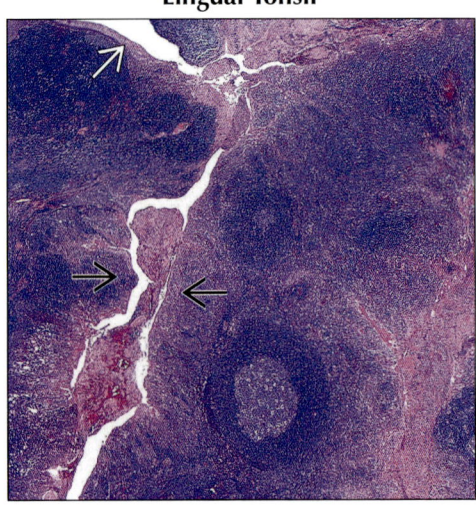

(Left) Similar to the palatine tonsils, lingual tonsillar crypts ➔ represent invaginations of the surface mucosa into the lymphoid stroma. They are shorter than those seen in the palatine tonsil and often extend downward to underlying skeletal muscle and salivary glands ➔. *(Right)* The surface epithelium is nonkeratinizing stratified squamous mucosa ➔, which becomes a specialized lymphoepithelium in the crypt zones ➔.

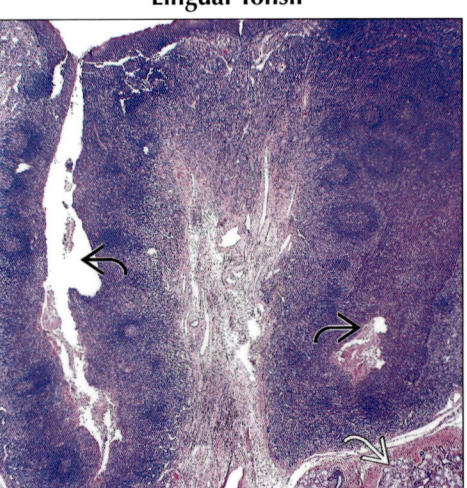

TONSILS/ADENOIDS

Lymphoepithelium: Lingual Tonsil

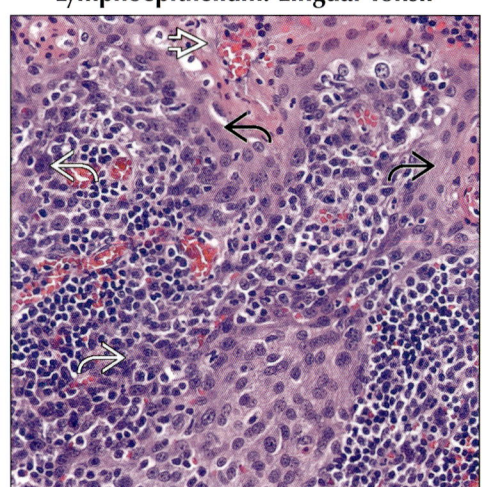

Mucous Glands: Lingual Tonsil

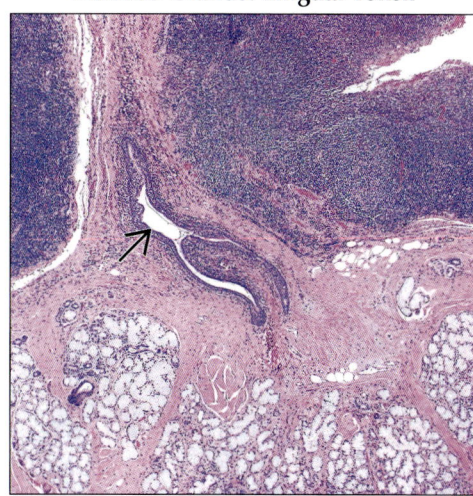

(Left) The lingual tonsil crypt epithelium is similar to that of the palatine tonsil. Basaloid keratinocytes ➡ are infiltrated by lymphocytes and plasma cells, which distort the mucosa. The surface has a thin layer of differentiated keratinocytes ➡. Desquamated keratin debris can accumulate in the lumen ➡. *(Right)* Identical to the palatine tonsils, scattered small, pure mucous glands with ducts ➡ draining to the surface are seen in the connective tissue pseudocapsule.

Pharyngeal Tonsil

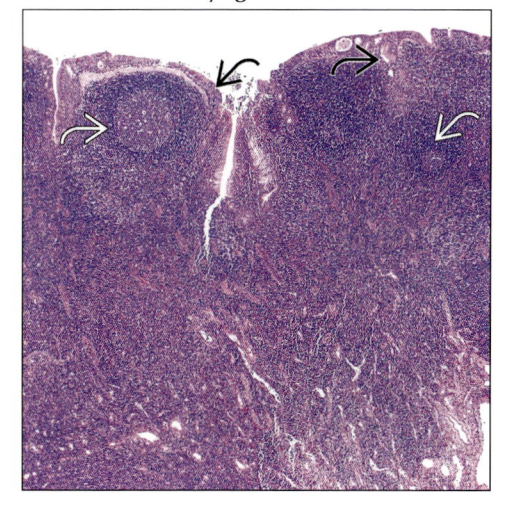

Pharyngeal Tonsil Folds

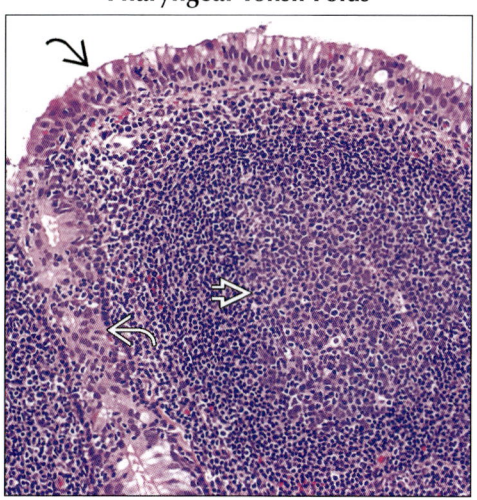

(Left) Unlike other tonsils, the pharyngeal tonsil does not have true crypts, but instead has variably elongated mucosal folds ➡ that contain lymphoid tissue composed of follicles ➡ and interfollicular lymphocytes. *(Right)* Primary lymphoid follicles and germinal centers ➡ are intimately associated with the nasopharyngeal surface mucosa ➡ and mucosal folds ➡. Intraepithelial lymphocytes are present, similar to other tonsils.

Pharyngeal Tonsil Epithelium

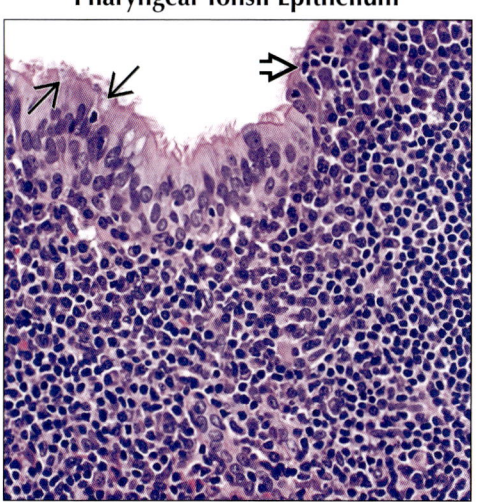

Deep Pharyngeal Tonsil Folds

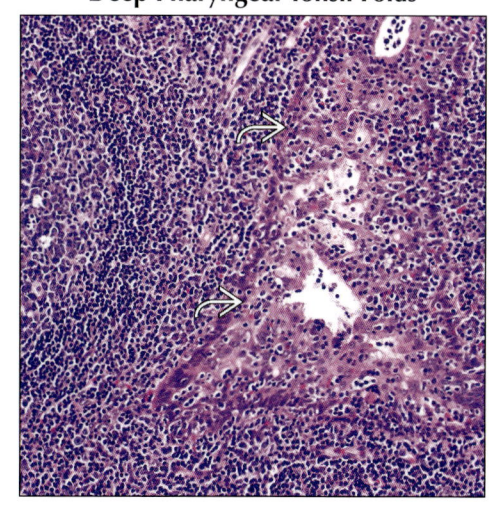

(Left) Unlike other tonsils, the mucosa of the pharyngeal tonsil is a ciliated, pseudostratified, columnar epithelium with scattered goblet cells ➡, identical to respiratory-type epithelium. Note areas of intraepithelial lymphocytes and plasma cells ➡. *(Right)* At the deeper aspects of the mucosal folds, the epithelium contains more intraepithelial lymphocytes and plasma cells, resulting in a characteristic lymphoepithelium ➡ similar to other tonsils.

EAR

Key Facts

Macroscopic Anatomy
- Composed of 3 regions: External ear, middle ear, and inner ear
- External ear is composed of the auricle (pinna), external auditory canal, and outer surface of tympanic membrane
  - Main function is sound conduction
- Middle ear is composed of the tympanic cavity, inner surface of tympanic membrane, ossicles, mastoid air cells, and internal auditory canal (eustachian tube)
  - Main function is sound conduction for auditory portion of inner ear
- Inner ear is comprised of the membranous labyrinth embedded within the medial petrous temporal bone (osseous labyrinth) and consists of the cochlea, semicircular canals, vestibule (saccule and utricle), and endolymphatic sac organ
  - Main functions are sensory reception for hearing and balance

Microscopic Anatomy
- External ear
  - Auricle is a modified skin structure with a cartilaginous skeleton and contains normal skin adnexal structures
  - Outer 1/3 of external auditory canal is supported by cartilage that is continuous with the auricular elastic cartilage and has modified apocrine glands (ceruminous glands) instead of eccrine glands
  - Inner 2/3 of external auditory canal lined by epidermis typically devoid of adnexal structures/glands and supported by portions of the temporal bone instead of cartilage
  - Tympanic membrane is covered by epidermis externally and nonsquamous cuboidal epithelium internally with a connective tissue framework
- Middle ear
  - Tympanic cavity is lined by modified respiratory epithelium consisting of a single layer of cuboidal epithelium; no glands or squamous epithelium present under normal circumstances but may have patches of ciliated columnar epithelium
  - Ossicles are composed of compact lamellar bone; incudomallear and incudostapedial joints are diarthroses with synovial lining
  - Mastoid air cells are lined by flat cuboidal modified respiratory epithelium adherent to underlying periosteum
  - Proximal 1/3 of internal auditory canal is intraosseous, while distal 2/3 is surrounded by hyaline cartilage
  - Internal auditory canal is lined by ciliated columnar epithelium; goblet cells and seromucous glands can be seen mainly in cartilaginous component
  - Lymphoid aggregates (tubal tonsil) can be seen in internal auditory canal, especially in children
- Inner ear
  - Semicircular canal, utricle, and saccule are lined by specialized epithelia with specialized sensory hair cells (rarely, if ever, seen in a surgical specimen)
  - Endolymphatic sac organ lined by low cuboidal to columnar epithelium, which may have papillary structures in sac portion
  - Cochlea is a highly specialized, complex sensory organ that is rarely, if ever, seen in a surgical specimen

Pitfalls/Artifacts
- Chronic otitis media can result in glandular "metaplasia," mimicking gland-forming neoplasms (primarily the so-called middle ear adenoma or carcinoid tumor)
- Squamous metaplasia in middle ear cavity is always abnormal and likely results from migration of external auditory canal epithelium into middle ear via defects in tympanic membrane
  - This can lead to destructive keratin-producing tumors known as cholesteatomas
- Chronic injury to tympanic membrane, usually from chronic otitis media, can lead to sclerosis and secondary dystrophic calcification known as tympanosclerosis

(Left) The external ear auricular cartilaginous framework ⇨ is in continuity with the external auditory canal at the concha. The outer 1/3 is supported by cartilage ⇨, and the inner 2/3 is supported by bone ⇨. (Right) The outer 1/3 of the external auditory canal is lined by squamous epithelium with numerous associated hair follicles, sebaceous glands ⇨, and modified apocrine sweat glands ⇨ known as ceruminous glands.

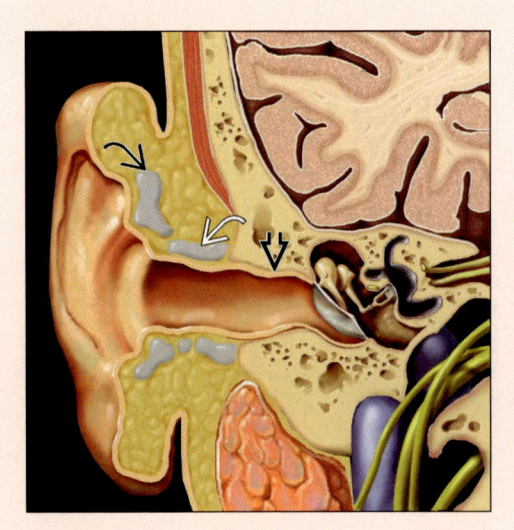

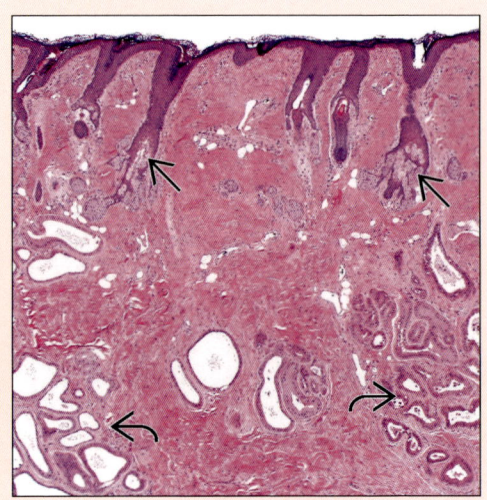

EAR

External Auditory Canal

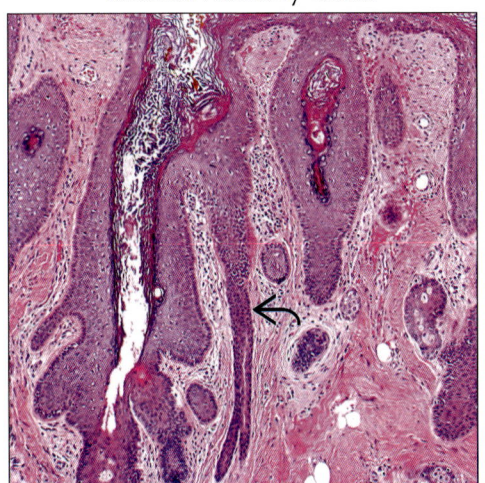

Ceruminous Glands

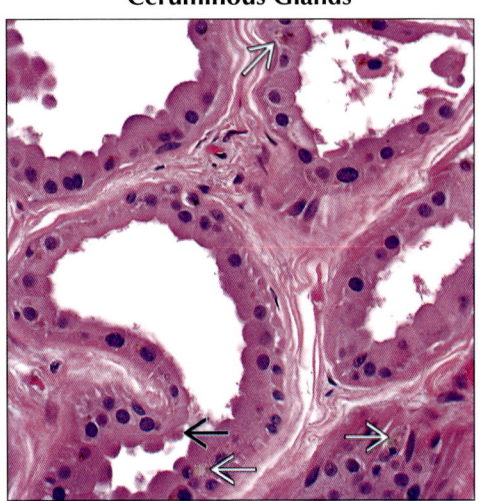

(Left) Cutaneous adnexal structures are numerous in the outer 1/3 of the canal, but are typically absent in the inner 2/3, which is lined by epithelium adherent to bone. Ceruminous gland ducts ➔ may drain to the surface or empty into the pilosebaceous unit as shown here. (Right) Ceruminous glands are modified apocrine glands characterized by cells with abundant granular eosinophilic cytoplasm, apical snouts ➔, apocrine-type secretion, and yellow cytoplasmic granules ➔.

Auricular Cartilage

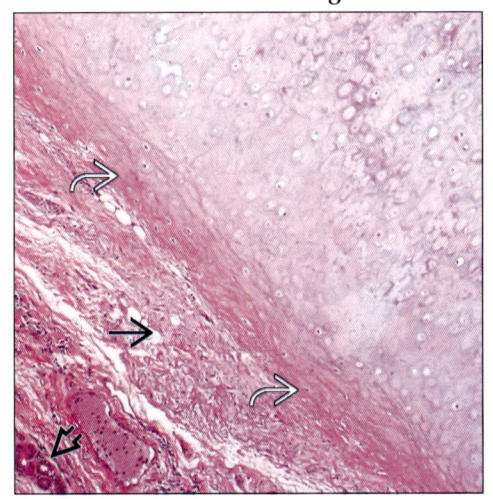

Ear Lobule

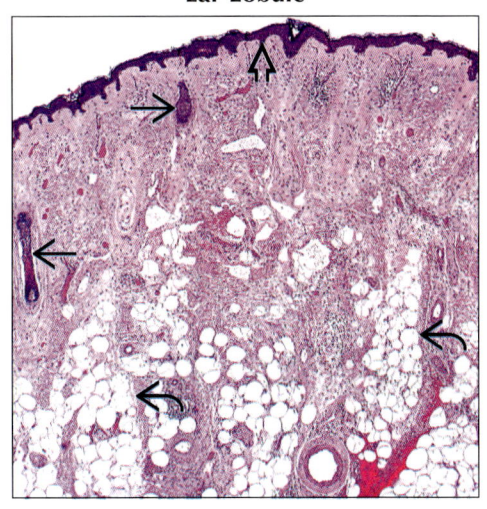

(Left) The auricular and external auditory canal cartilages are elastic-type cartilages. The cartilage is separated from the cutaneous adnexal structures and ceruminous glands ➔ by loose connective tissue ➔ and a thin perichondrium ➔. (Right) The ear lobule is similar to the rest of the auricle; it is lined by squamous epithelium ➔ with adnexal structures ➔. In contrast, no cartilage framework is present, but the stroma does contain abundant mature adipose tissue ➔.

Tympanic Membrane

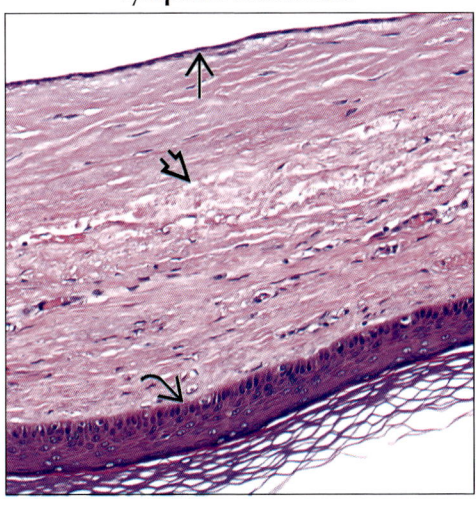

Tympanosclerosis

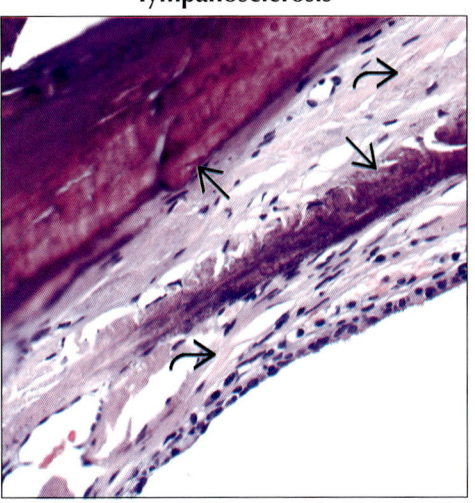

(Left) The tympanic membrane consists of a thin connective tissue plate ➔ lined externally by squamous epithelium ➔ devoid of adnexal structures, and internally by modified respiratory epithelium ➔. This tympanic membrane shows thickened, sclerotic connective tissue stroma due to chronic irritation. (Right) Chronic injury to the tympanic membrane can result in subepithelial sclerosis ➔ with secondary dystrophic calcification ➔, known as tympanosclerosis.

EAR

Middle Ear

(Left) The tympanic cavity ⇨ contains the 3 ossicles ➔ (malleus, incus, and stapes from lateral to medial) and is delimited laterally by the the tympanic membrane ➔. The tympanic cavity is in continuity with the internal auditory canal ➔, which extends to the lateral nasopharynx. (Right) Tympanic cavity epithelium typically consists of flattened respiratory-type epithelium ⇨ lacking underlying glands. Here it is seen adjacent to a paraganglioma ⇨.

Tympanic Cavity

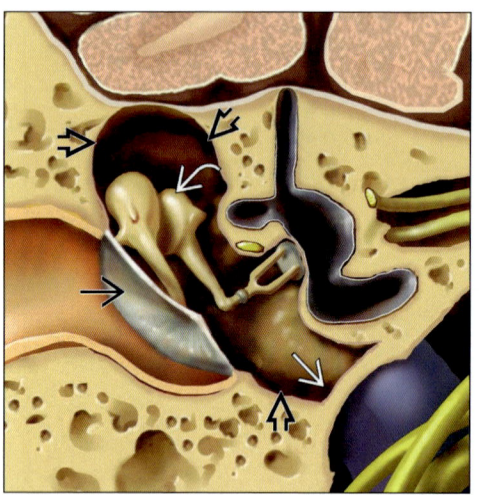

Tympanic Cavity

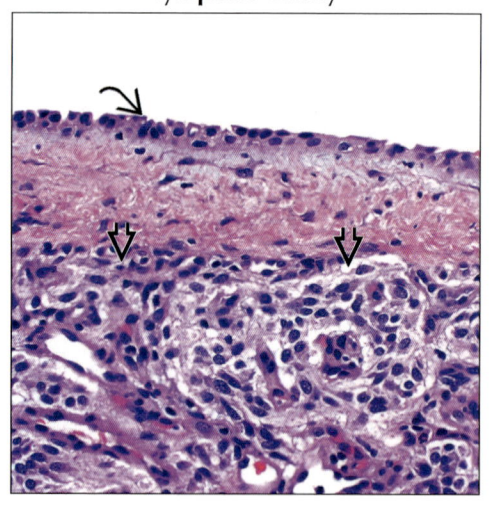

(Left) While normally lined by cuboidal respiratory-type epithelium, patches of columnar respiratory epithelium complete with cilia ➔ are present to varying degrees lining this jugulotympanic paraganglioma ⇨. (Right) Squamous epithelium is not present under normal circumstances in the middle ear. Its presence indicates a cholesteatoma ➔ as seen here. These are often associated with chronic inflammation ➔ and glandular metaplasia ➔, indicating chronic otitis.

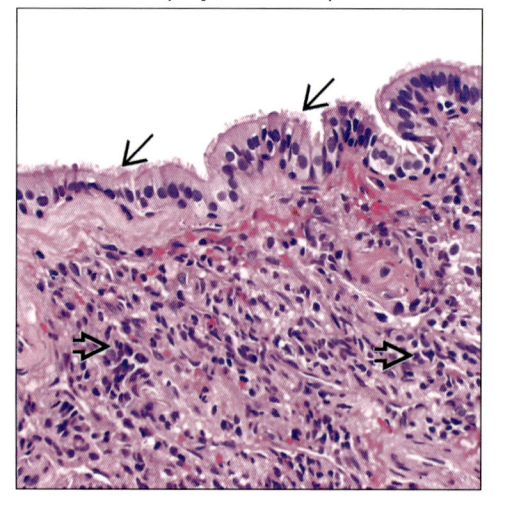

Cholesteatoma and Chronic Otitis Media

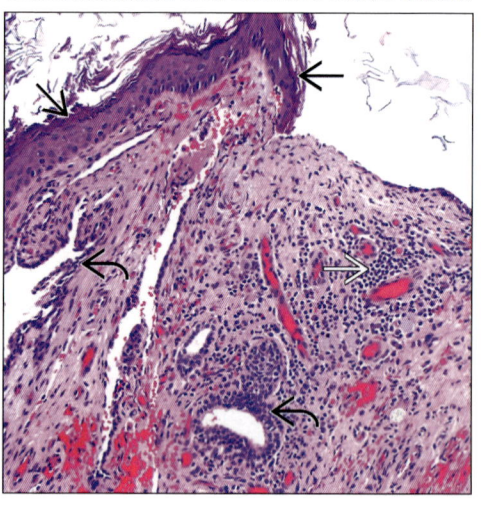

Middle Ear Ossicle (Incus)

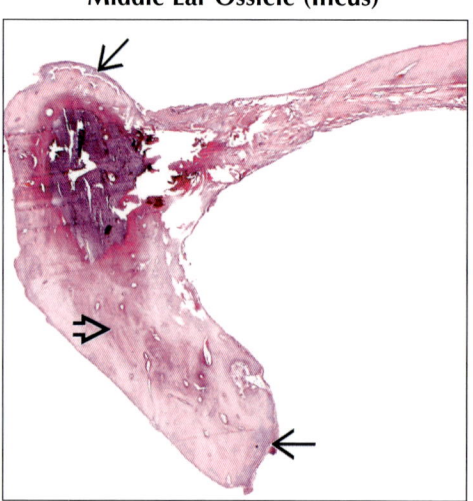

(Left) The ossicles arise from membranous ossification and consist of compact lamellar bone ⇨. Islands of persistent cartilage ➔ can be seen at the ends of most of the ossicles. (Right) The ossicles predominantly consist of compact lamellar bone ➔ with osteocytes ⇨ set within lacunae as well as varying numbers of haversian systems. Islands of cartilage ⇨ can be seen at the periphery of most ossicles.

Ossicles

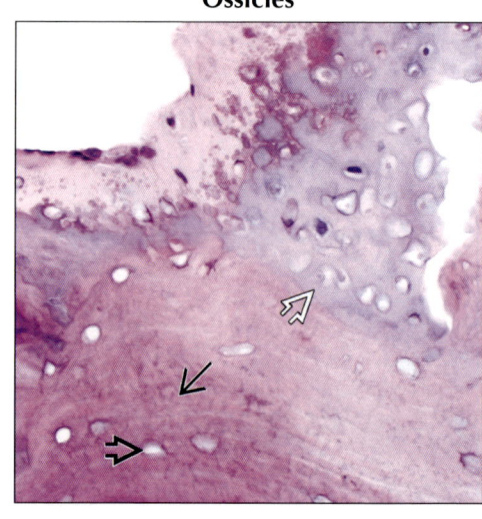

EAR

Ossicles

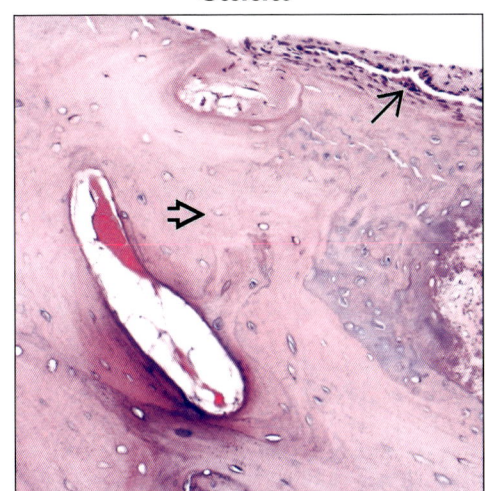

Mastoid Air Cells

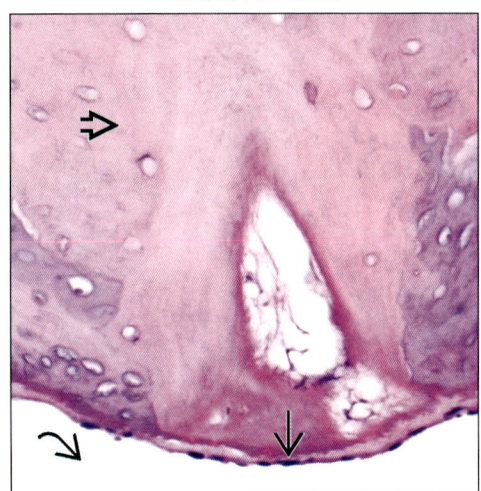

(Left) This section from a stapes bone demonstrates compact lamellar bone ⇨. Tympanic cavity epithelium ⇨ typically lines the periosteal surface of the ossicles. The epithelium is identical to the tympanic cavity epithelium except that the presence of cilia is uncommon. **(Right)** Mastoid air cells consist of air-filled cystic spaces ⇨ within the dense compact lamellar temporal bone ⇨. The lining is identical to the tympanic cavity and is tightly adherent to bone ⇨.

Internal Auditory Canal

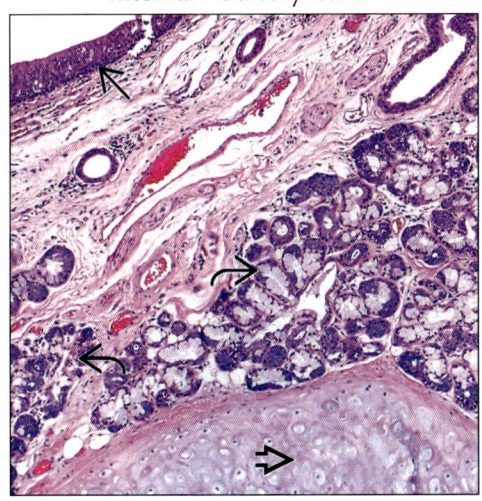

Internal Auditory Canal

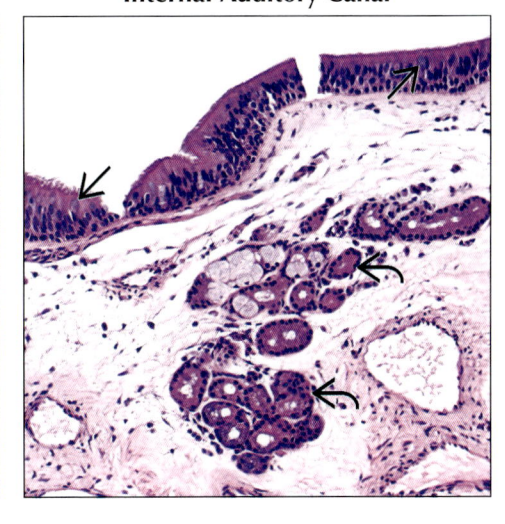

(Left) The internal auditory canal is lined by respiratory-type epithelium ⇨. It is present within bone proximally, but a hyaline cartilage tube ⇨ supports it distally. Submucosal seromucous glands ⇨ are present in the distal 2/3 (cartilaginous portion). **(Right)** The internal auditory canal is lined by respiratory-type epithelium, but goblet cells ⇨ and seromucous glands ⇨ can be seen, primarily in the distal 2/3. Lymphoid aggregates (tubal tonsil) may be seen as well.

Endolymphatic Sac

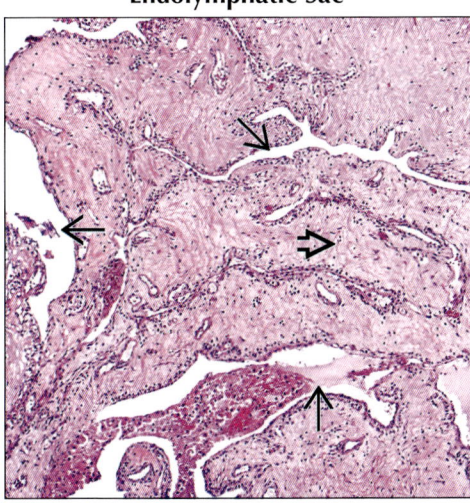

Endolymphatic Sac

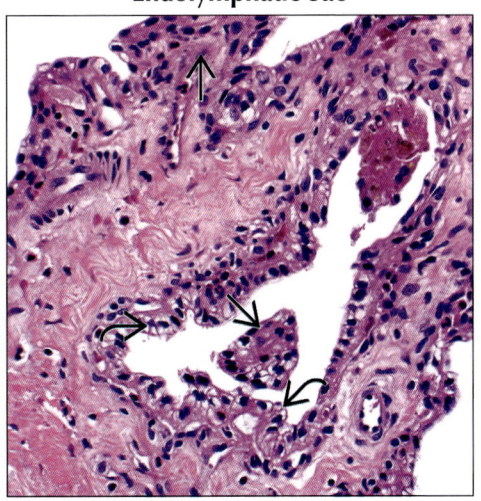

(Left) While not typically seen as a surgical specimen, portions of the endolymphatic sac can be seen in tumor resection specimens. These appear as epithelial-lined cystic spaces ⇨ embedded within loose connective tissue ⇨ or bone. **(Right)** The endolymphatic sac is lined by flat cuboidal to columnar epithelium and may have small papillae ⇨. The cells have small central nuclei and clear to pale eosinophilic cytoplasm ⇨, and rest on a loose vascular connective tissue stroma.

NOSE AND PARANASAL SINUSES

Key Facts

Macroscopic Anatomy
- Paired nasal cavities extend anteriorly from nares (nostrils) and posteriorly to choanae and are separated by nasal septum
  - Consist of 3 distinct regions: Vestibule, respiratory, and olfactory
- Vestibule communicates with external environment and contains hairs that act as coarse filter
- Respiratory region is the most voluminous portion of nasal cavity
  - Medial wall is constituted by nasal septum, which is smooth
  - Lateral wall contains 3 coiled bony projections called turbinates, which increase surface area and induce turbulence to inhaled air
  - Floor is smooth and sits on hard palate and anterior maxilla
- Olfactory region occupies majority of roof of nose and extends medially onto superior nasal septum and laterally onto superior portion of superior turbinate
- Paired air-filled paranasal sinuses include maxillary, frontal, ethmoid, and sphenoid sinuses
  - They communicate with, and are directly connected to, the nasal cavity via several ostia

Microscopic Anatomy
- External nose is covered by epidermis with high concentration of sebaceous glands and fine hairs
- Vestibule consists of epidermis that is continuous with surface skin and contains sebaceous glands, sweat glands, and coarse hairs
- Majority of nasal cavity is lined by ciliated pseudostratified columnar respiratory epithelium
  - Epithelium is ectodermally derived and is referred to as Schneiderian membrane
  - There is short transition of nonciliated columnar or transitional epithelium between vestibule and ciliated epithelium
  - 3 cell types are identifiable: Basal cells, goblet cells, and ciliated columnar cells
- Lamina propria contains numerous seromucous glands, which drain to surface via small ducts
- Scattered melanocytes are present in surface mucosa, glands, and lamina propria
- Turbinates are lined by same Schneiderian membrane but contain more prominent, specialized vascular component
  - Vessels form dense network of variably sized spaces resembling erectile tissue
  - Vessels have thick muscular walls and contract and dilate to regulate temperature and secretions
  - Osseous core consists of thin plates of lamellar bone with intraosseous vessels
- Nasal septum is composed of hyaline cartilage anteriorly, with remainder being plates of lamellar bone
  - Focal collection of ectatic thin-walled vessels can be seen on anterior cartilaginous portion (known as Kiesselbach area or Little area)
- Olfactory mucosa is specialized sensory epithelium lined by ciliated pseudostratified columnar epithelium
  - 3 cell types are identifiable: Basal cells, ciliated columnar supporting/sustentacular cells, and olfactory neural cells
  - No goblet cells are present in olfactory region
  - Sustentacular cells may have lipofuscin pigment in older individuals
  - Olfactory neural cells are bipolar spindle cells with olfactory sense receptor cilia present on surface and axons at basal surface
  - Olfactory neural cells collect in lamina propria to form myelinated nerves that traverse cribriform plate to join olfactory nerve
  - Specialized serous secretory glands (glands of Bowman) are present in lamina propria and empty to surface via small ducts
- Sinuses are lined by Schneiderian membrane, but it is thinner, less vascular, and contains fewer seromucous glands

(Left) This coronal CT scan illustrates the nasal cavity with inferior ➡ and middle turbinates ➡ and paranasal sinuses ➡. The cribriform plate ➡ forms the roof, and the floor ➡ sits on the hard palate. (Right) The nasal vestibule ➡ communicates with the environment and contains coarse hairs. The lateral nasal wall contains superior ➡, middle ➡, and inferior ➡ turbinates. (Courtesy M. Nielsen, MS.)

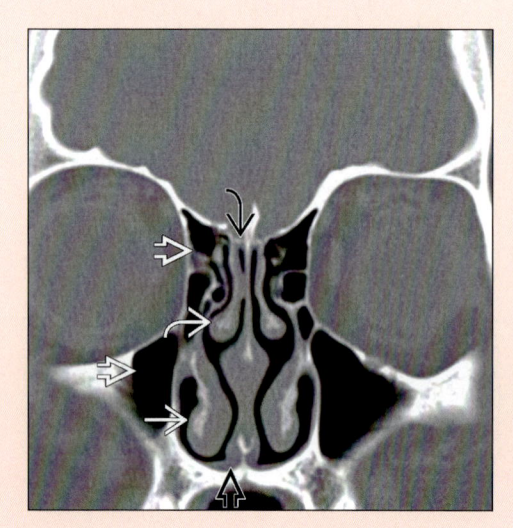

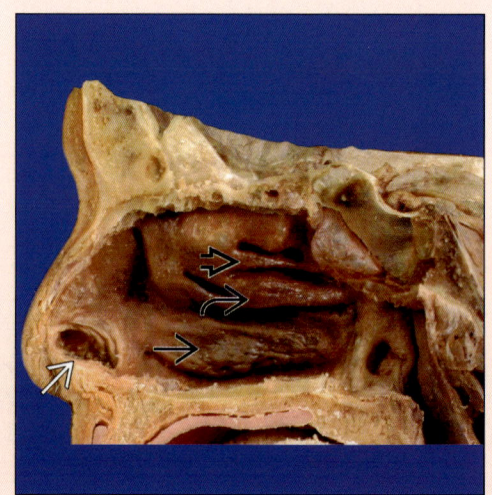

NOSE AND PARANASAL SINUSES

Turbinate

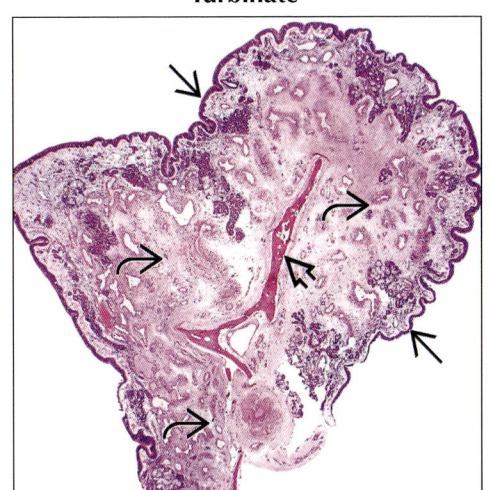

Turbinate Lamina Propria

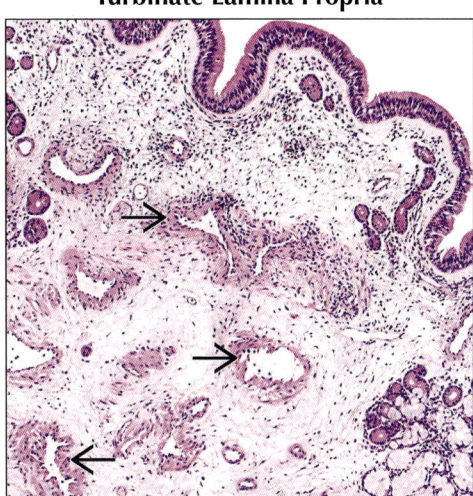

(Left) This cross section of a middle turbinate shows the delicate, curved bone core ➡ surrounded by thick lamina propria ➡, rich in variably sized vessels and covered by Schneiderian mucosa ➡. (Right) The lamina propria of the nasal mucosa, especially the turbinates and inferior septum, contains a network of variably sized venous sinuses with thick muscular walls ➡. These sinuses can rapidly constrict/dilate in response to various stimuli and histologically resemble erectile tissue.

Schneiderian Mucosa

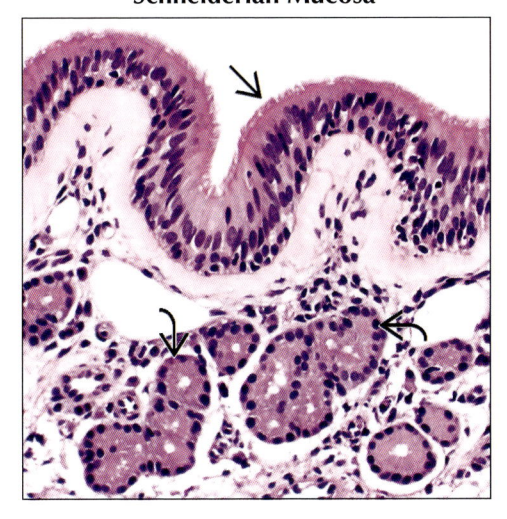

Distal Turbinate

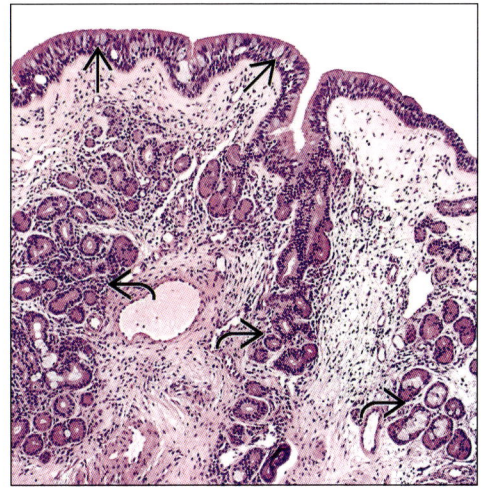

(Left) Similar to the rest of the respiratory region, the turbinates are lined by ciliated pseudostratified columnar epithelium ➡ with scattered mucous (goblet) cells. Varying numbers of seromucous glands ➡ are present in the lamina propria and drain directly to the surface via small ducts. (Right) There are regional differences in turbinate histology. The most distal region, which directly confronts inhaled air, is relatively rich in mucous cells ➡ and salivary glands ➡.

Proximal Turbinate

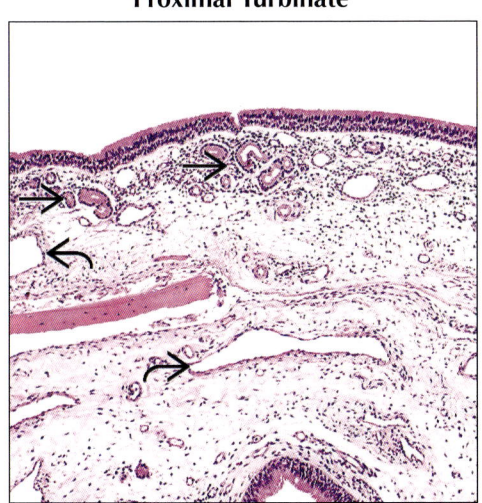

Turbinate Bone

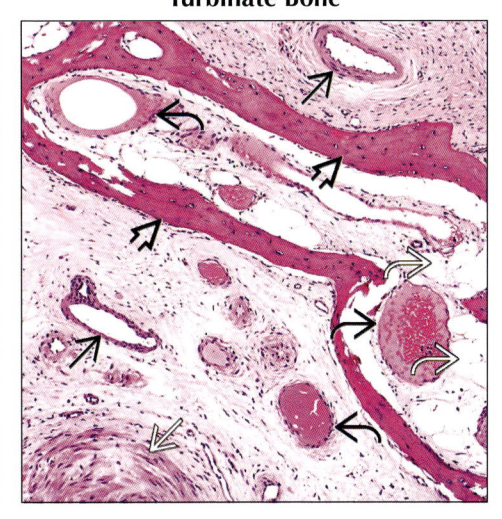

(Left) The turbinate stalk has a thinner lamina propria with fewer vessels ➡ and salivary glands ➡. The epithelium has fewer mucous cells as well. (Right) Turbinate bone is composed of thin trabeculae of mature lamellar bone ➡. Similar to the lamina propria, there are numerous muscular veins ➡, dilated vessels ➡, and arteries ➡ that may mimic vascular neoplasms or malformations. Although there may be adipose tissue ➡, no hematopoietic elements are present.

NOSE AND PARANASAL SINUSES

(Left) The nasal vestibule is lined by skin with stratified squamous epithelium ⇨ containing all layers of normal epidermis. There are numerous hairs ⇨ with associated sebaceous glands ⇨. The coarse hairs and secretions act to trap inhaled particulate matter. **(Right)** The transition from vestibule to respiratory mucosa is gradual, with thinning of the epidermis ⇨, loss of pilosebaceous units, and increased venous vasculature ⇨ with occasional salivary glands and ducts ⇨.

Nasal Vestibule

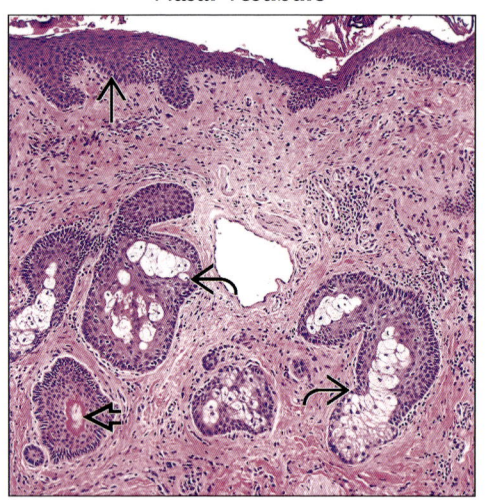

Vestibule: Respiratory Transition

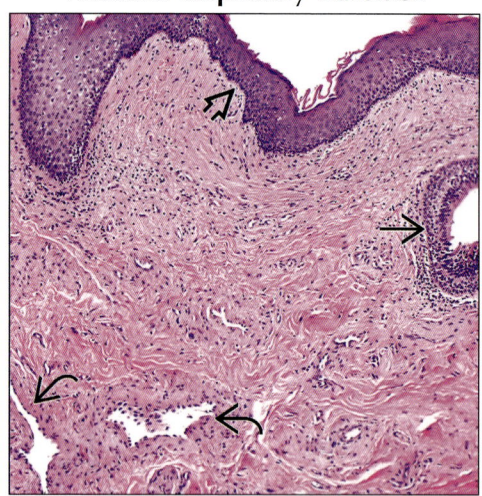

(Left) Similar to the turbinates, the remainder of the respiratory portion of the nasal cavity is lined by ciliated pseudostratified columnar epithelium ⇨ with numerous seromucous minor salivary glands ⇨. The lamina propria also contains numerous venous sinuses ⇨ that warm inhaled air. **(Right)** Mucoserous glands ⇨ drain to the surface via small excretory ducts ⇨. The Schneiderian epithelium is pseudostratified and columnar, containing cilia and scattered mucous (goblet) cells ⇨.

Respiratory Region

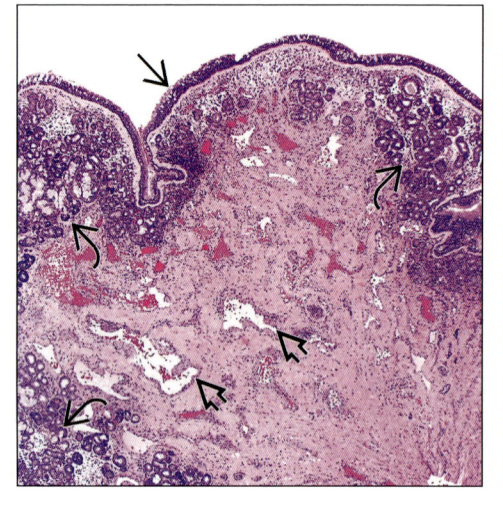

Respiratory Region

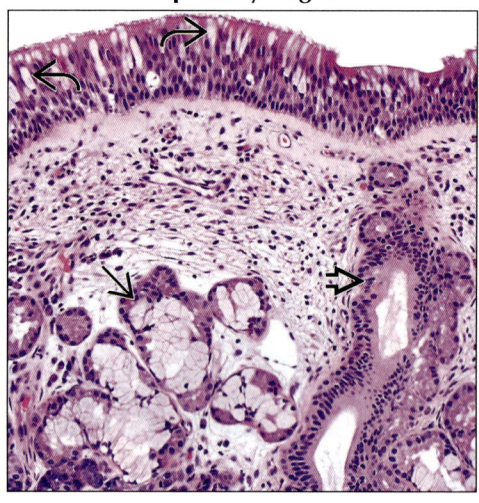

(Left) The nasal septum consists of a plate of hyaline cartilage associated with 4 smaller bony plates ⇨ fused with fibrous sutures ⇨. **(Right)** Olfactory mucosa is a modified ciliated pseudostratified columnar mucosa ⇨ with specialized intraepithelial olfactory nerve cells. These neurons fuse to form olfactory nerve bundles ⇨ in the lamina propria. Specialized olfactory glands (Bowman glands) ⇨ are also present in the lamina propria and are unique to olfactory mucosa.

Septal Cartilage

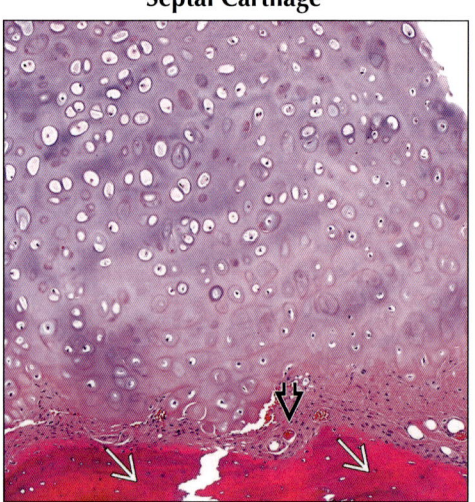

Olfactory Region

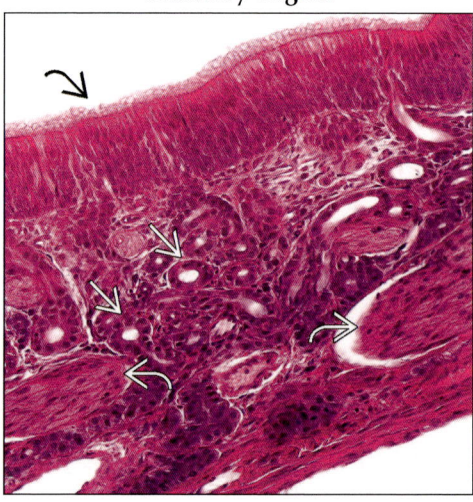

NOSE AND PARANASAL SINUSES

Olfactory Epithelium

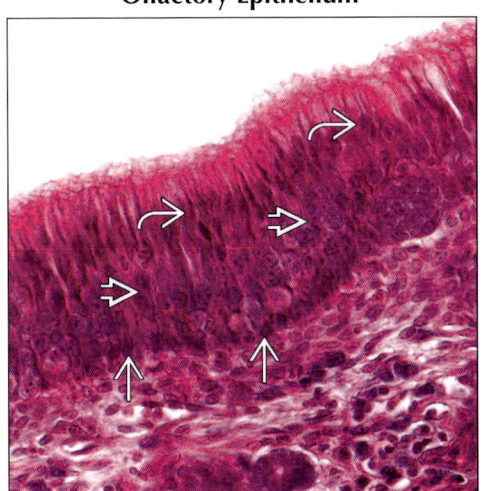

Glands of Bowman

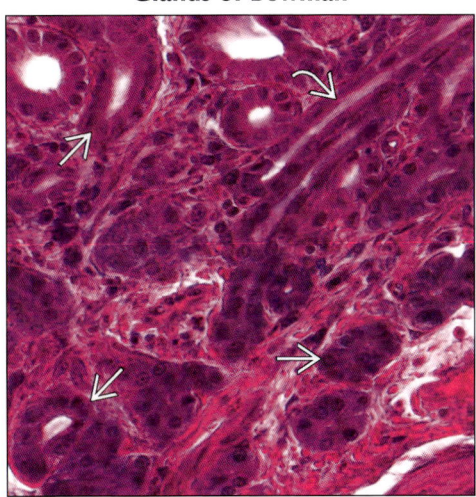

(Left) Olfactory epithelium contains bipolar olfactory nerve cells with nuclei ➡ stratified between the more uniform superficial nuclei of the ciliated columnar supporting (sustentacular) cells ➡ and the progenitor basal cells ➡. No mucous cells are present in the olfactory mucosa. *(Right)* Olfactory glands ➡ are unique to the olfactory region. They are tubulovillous serous glands that may have lipofuscin pigment in the cytoplasm. They drain into a small central duct ➡.

Secretory Duct

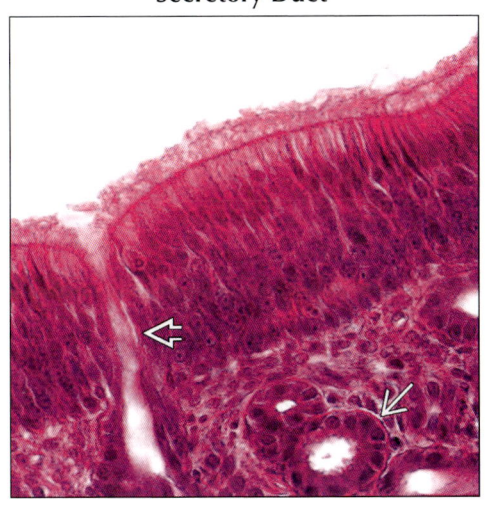

Paranasal Sinus Ostia

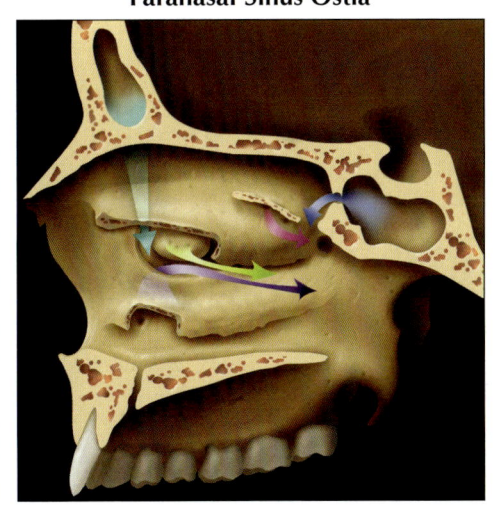

(Left) Olfactory glands ➡ drain secretions directly to the surface via short ducts ➡. The secretions are thought to trap and dissolve odoriferous substances, allowing new substances to be recognized. *(Right)* The paranasal sinuses are air-filled spaces in the bones adjacent to the nasal cavity and are named after the bones in which they are situated. They communicate with the nose via small openings (ostia) as follows: Blue = sphenoid; pink and green = ethmoid; aqua = frontal; purple = maxillary.

Paranasal Sinus

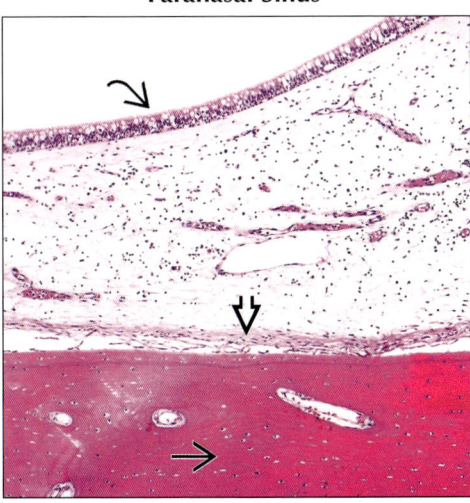

Paranasal Sinus

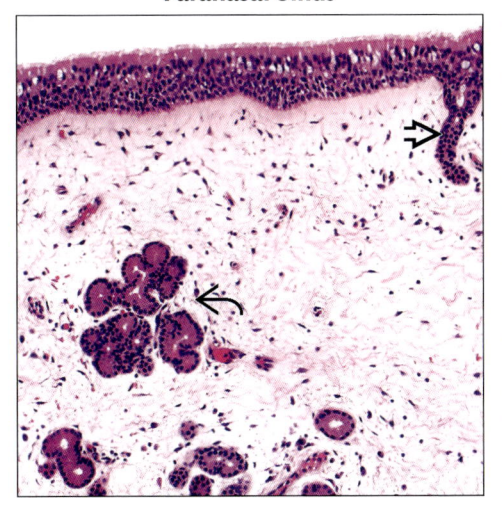

(Left) The paranasal sinuses are lined with ciliated pseudostratified (Schneiderian) mucosa with mucous cells ➡, which is in continuity with the nasal mucosa via ostia. The mucosa is thinner and attaches to the periosteum ➡ of the various sinus bones ➡. *(Right)* In contrast to nasal mucosa, seromucous glands ➡ are less numerous and more randomly distributed. These drain to the surface via small ducts ➡. Also, the stroma does not contain a prominent vascular component.

PHARYNX

Key Facts

Macroscopic Anatomy
- 3 functionally and anatomically distinct subsites
- Nasopharynx extends from choanae to superior (nasal) soft palate border
  - Includes pharyngeal tonsils and posterolateral walls (with eustachian tube openings)
- Oropharynx extends from superior soft palate border to hyoid bone/valleculae
  - Includes palatine tonsils, tonsillar pillars, base of tongue, soft palate, uvula, and posterolateral walls
- Hypopharynx extends from hyoid bone/valleculae to inferior cricoid cartilage border
  - Includes pyriform sinuses, postcricoid region, and posterolateral walls

Microscopic Anatomy
- Nasopharynx lined by both ciliated respiratory-type epithelium and stratified squamous epithelium
  - Pharyngeal tonsil consists of surface invaginations extending into lymphoid stroma
  - Scattered, less prominent lymphoid aggregates can be seen in the non-tonsil mucosa
  - Mixed seromucous minor salivary glands are present in submucosa
- Oropharynx lined by stratified squamous epithelium
  - Palatine tonsils and lingual tonsil (base of tongue) consist of lymphoepithelial crypts extending into lymphoid stroma
  - Pure mucous and scattered mixed minor salivary glands are present in submucosa
- Hypopharynx lined by stratified squamous epithelium
  - Pure mucous and scattered mixed minor salivary glands are present in submucosa
- No muscularis mucosa in any of the subsites

(Left) The nasopharynx extends from the choanae ➡ to the superior soft palate ➡. The oropharynx extends from the superior soft palate to the valleculae ➡. The hypopharynx extends from the valleculae to the inferior cricoid cartilage ➡ and includes the pyriform sinuses ➡. *(Right)* The pharyngeal tonsil (adenoid) is lined by ciliated respiratory-type epithelium ➡ with elongated mucosal folds ➡ extending into lymphoid tissue composed of follicles ➡ and interfollicular lymphocytes.

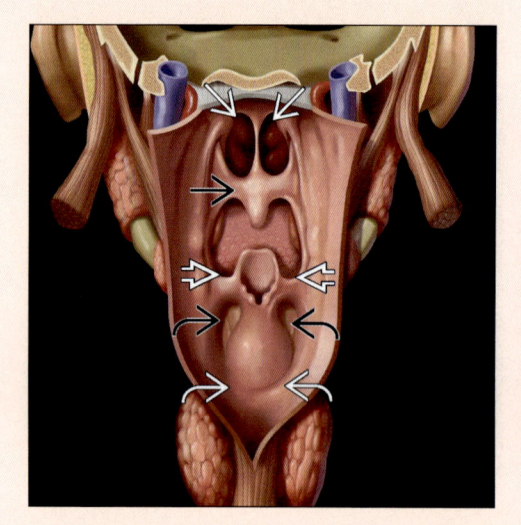

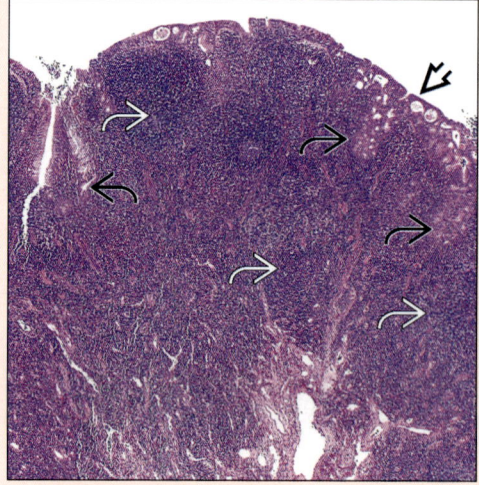

(Left) The nasopharynx is lined by both ciliated respiratory-type epithelium and stratified squamous epithelium. The pharyngeal tonsil, roof, and anterior regions are lined by respiratory-type epithelium ➡. Numerous submucosal mixed seromucous minor salivary glands are present ➡. *(Right)* Scattered submucosal (non-tonsillar) lymphoid aggregates ➡ are present throughout the nasopharynx. The overlying mucosa consists of stratified squamous epithelium ➡ alternating with respiratory-type epithelium ➡.

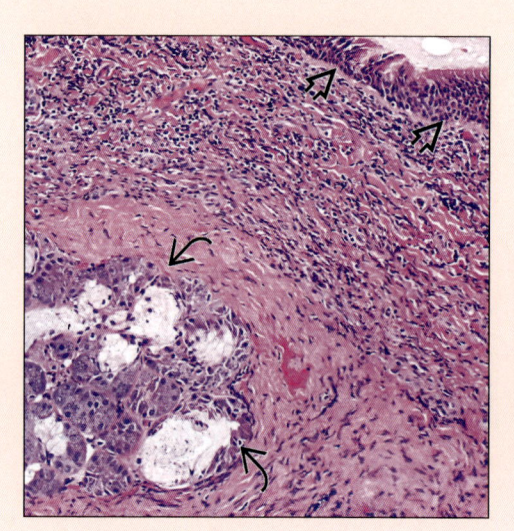

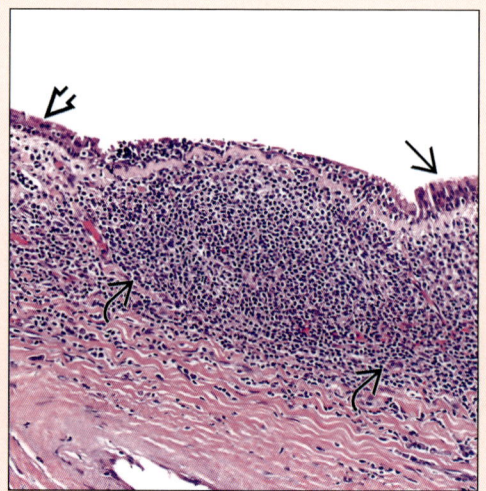

PHARYNX

Thornwaldt Duct Cyst

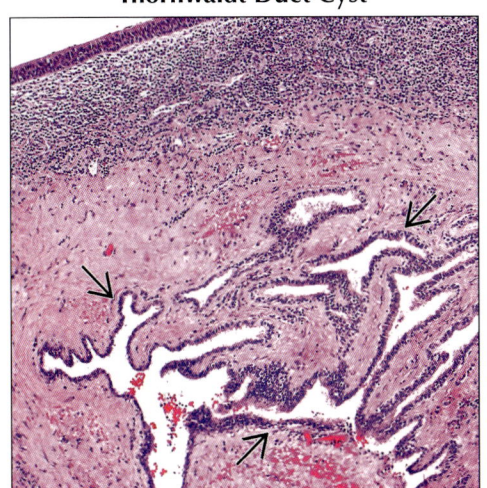

Oropharyngeal Mucosa

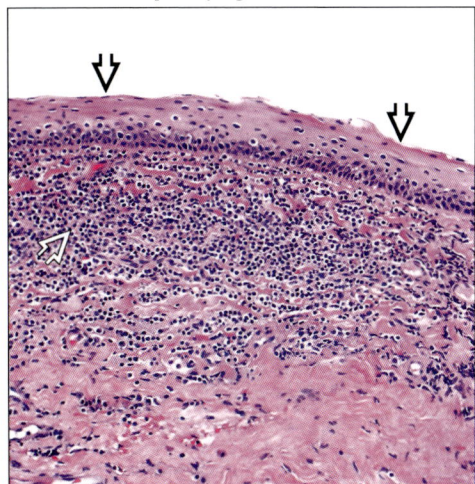

(Left) The developing notochord is in close proximity to the nasopharynx roof. Submucosal notochord remnants can persist and lead to developmental cysts, such as this Thornwaldt duct cyst ⇨. Microscopic remnants of Rathke pouch are also present in the nasopharynx roof of most individuals. (Right) The oropharynx is lined purely by nonkeratinizing stratified squamous epithelium ⇨. Scattered submucosal (non-tonsillar) lymphoid aggregates ⇨ are present throughout the oropharynx.

Tonsil

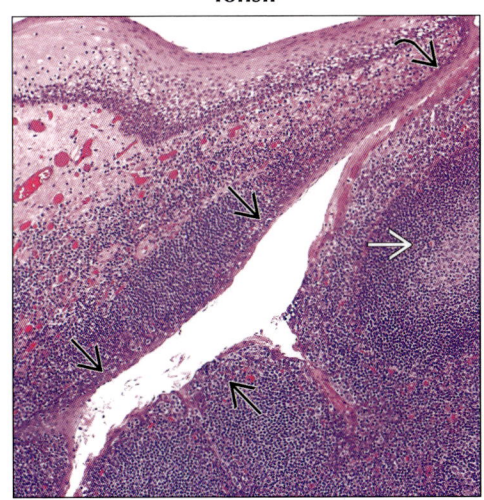

Uvula

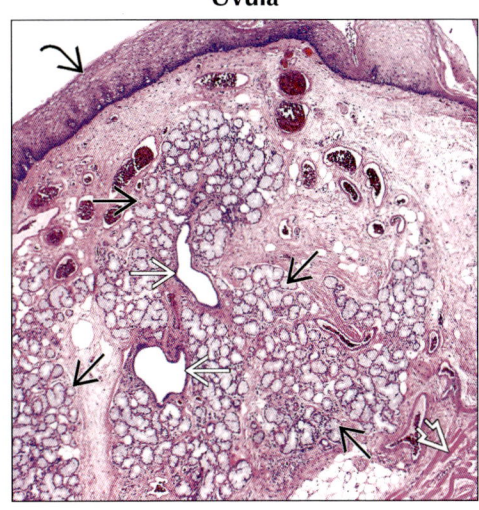

(Left) Palatine and lingual tonsil crypts represent invaginations of the surface squamous epithelium ⇨ into the lymphoid stroma, which becomes a specialized lymphoepithelium ⇨. The stroma is mainly composed of lymphoid aggregates ⇨ and interfollicular small lymphocytes. (Right) The uvula is lined by stratified squamous epithelium ⇨ and contains numerous mucous salivary gland lobules ⇨ with ducts ⇨. Thin bundles of skeletal muscle ⇨ are present in the uvula stroma.

Hypopharynx

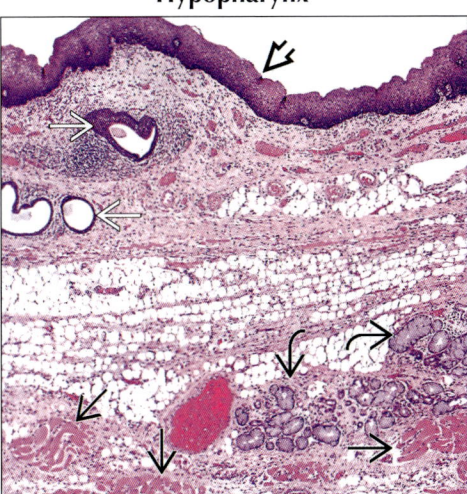

Hypopharynx

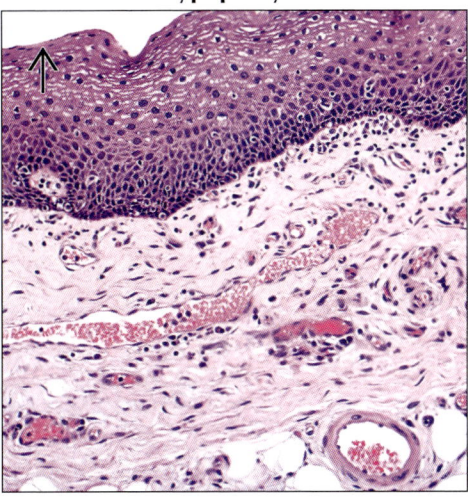

(Left) Similar to the oropharynx, the hypopharynx is lined entirely by nonkeratinizing stratified squamous epithelium ⇨. Scattered, predominantly mucous, minor salivary gland lobules ⇨ are present in the submucosa with ducts ⇨ draining to the surface. Pharyngeal constrictor skeletal muscle ⇨ is present below the submucosa. (Right) Although the surface typically consists of nonkeratinizing squamous mucosa ⇨, exposure to irritants such as tobacco smoke can result in surface keratosis.

LARYNX

Key Facts

Macroscopic Anatomy

- Extends from the epiglottic tip superiorly to the inferior border of cricoid cartilage inferiorly
  - Main functions are phonation and preventing aspiration of ingested or inhaled particles
- Composed of cartilaginous framework supported by ligaments as well as intrinsic and extrinsic muscles
  - Main cartilages are epiglottic, thyroid, cricoid, and arytenoid cartilages
- Covered by mucosa
- Composed of 3 regions: Supraglottis, glottis, and subglottis
  - Supraglottis extends from epiglottis to superior portion of true vocal cords and includes epiglottis, aryepiglottic folds, false vocal cords, and ventricles; embryologically derived from 3rd and 4th branchial arches
  - Glottis extends from superior portion of true vocal cords inferiorly for 1 cm and includes true vocal cords (folds), anterior commissure, and posterior commissure; embryologically derived from 6th branchial arch
  - Subglottis extends from inferior glottis to inferior border of cricoid cartilage; embryologically derived from 6th branchial arch
- Anterior commissure tendon (Broyles ligament) is where the vocal cord elastic tissue attaches to thyroid cartilage
  - Represents "weak" point where carcinomas can spread beyond larynx
- Pre-epiglottic space: Adipose and loose connective tissue anterior to epiglottis
- Paraglottic space: Adipose and loose connective tissue deep to true and false vocal cords
  - Bounded by cricovocal membrane, thyroid cartilage, quadrangular membrane, and pyriform sinus

Microscopic Anatomy

- Lined by both ciliated columnar epithelium with mucous (goblet) cells and nonkeratinized stratified squamous epithelium
  - Majority of supraglottic and glottic larynx are covered by squamous epithelium with occasional patches of ciliated columnar epithelium in supraglottis
  - Superior portion of supraglottic larynx is always squamous whereas lower half is more likely to have patches of ciliated columnar epithelium
  - Ventricles and subglottis are always lined by ciliated columnar epithelium
- Submucosal seromucous glands are present throughout, with exception of true vocal cords
- Submucosa of true vocal cords is loose connective tissue without lymphatics or salivary glands and is known as Reinke space
  - True vocal cords have band of elastic tissue (vocal ligament), which sits adjacent to vocalis (skeletal) muscle
- Epiglottis is elastic cartilage and has varying numbers of fenestrations whereas remaining laryngeal cartilages are hyaline cartilages
  - Epiglottic fenestrations and anterior commissure are weak points where laryngeal carcinomas can spread beyond larynx

Age Variation

- At birth, larynx is lined entirely by ciliated pseudostratified respiratory mucosa; with age, it is gradually replaced by nonkeratinizing stratified squamous mucosa except for ventricle, subglottis, and rare microscopic patches in supraglottis
- Thyroid and cricoid cartilages ossify to varying degrees with age but are ossified in most adults
  - Ossification begins in 2nd-3rd decade; occurs earlier in men
- Oncocytic metaplasia of seromucous gland ducts is common over age 50

Metaplasia

- Patients who smoke have less ciliated columnar mucosa secondary to squamous metaplasia
- Chondroid metaplasia of vocal cord ligament is not uncommon (1-2% of autopsy larynges); may be seen in diagnostic biopsies as well as laryngectomies

(Left) The glottis contains the true vocal cords ➡, which are just below the ventricles ➡. The supraglottis is also composed of the epiglottis ➡, false vocal cords ➡, and aryepiglottic folds ➡. (Right) The vocal cord ligaments ➡ as well as their attachment at the anterior commissure ➡ can be seen in this graphic. The paraglottic space ➡ is between the thyroid cartilage and vocal cords.

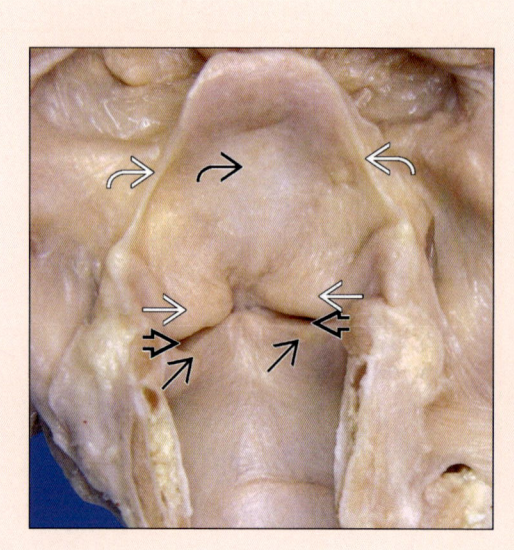

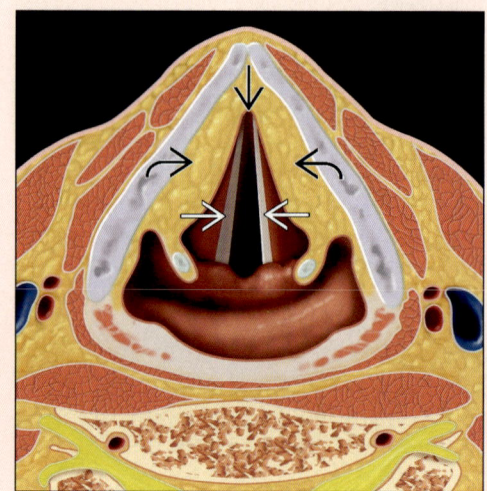

LARYNX

Laryngeal Cartilages (Anterior)

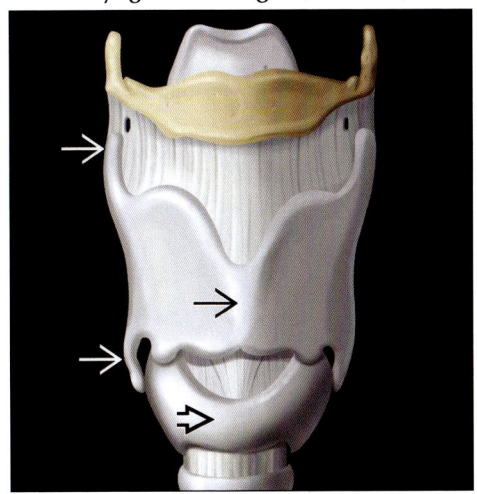

Laryngeal Cartilages (Posterior)

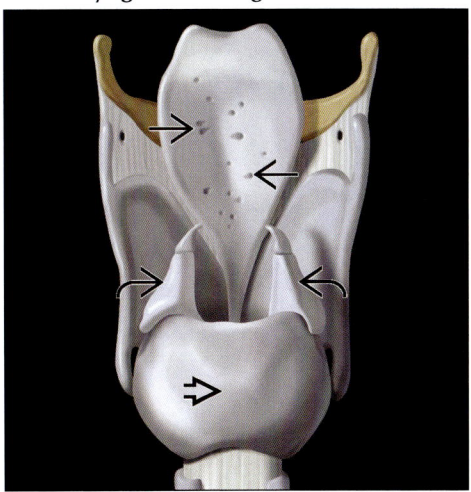

(Left) The main laryngeal cartilages are the epiglottic, thyroid, and cricoid cartilages. The thyroid cartilage is broad anteriorly but does not form a complete ring. There are superior and inferior horns ➡ and a notch just above the laryngeal prominence ➡ ("Adam's apple"). The cricoid cartilage ➡ forms a complete ring, being narrower anteriorly. *(Right)* The epiglottis has small holes (fenestrations) ➡, and the arytenoids ➡ sit on the posterior cricoid cartilage ➡.

Epiglottis

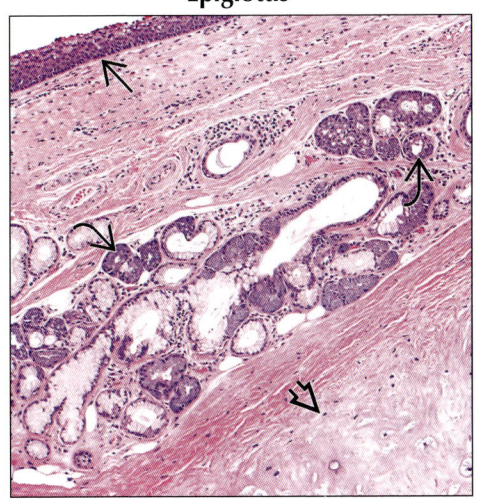

Epiglottic Fenestrations

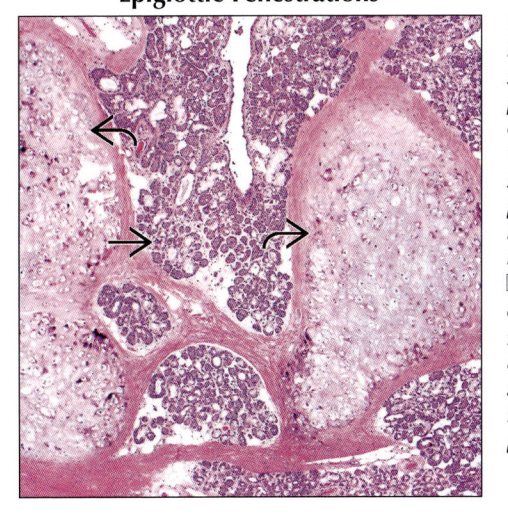

(Left) The epiglottis in adults is typically lined by stratified squamous epithelium ➡, but patches of ciliated columnar epithelium may be present as well. Numerous submucosal seromucous glands ➡ are present in the supraglottic larynx and typically are situated near the epiglottic cartilage ➡. *(Right)* The epiglottis is elastic cartilage ➡ and has fenestrations ➡, which usually contain seromucous glands, and may serve as a conduit for carcinomas to enter the preepiglottic space.

Aryepiglottic Fold

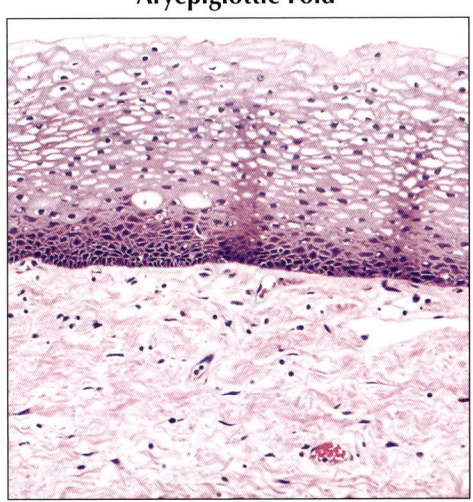

Arytenoid Cartilage

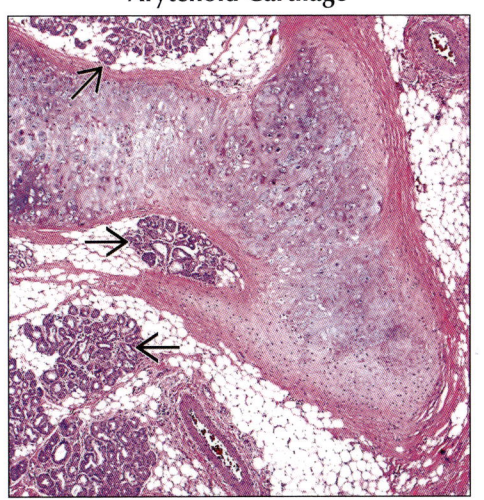

(Left) The aryepiglottic folds are part of the supraglottic larynx and extend from the epiglottis to the arytenoid cartilages. They are usually lined by stratified squamous epithelium without keratinization and have less numerous minor salivary glands in the subepithelial stroma. They represent one of the mucosal margins in laryngectomy specimens. *(Right)* The arytenoid cartilages are small hyaline cartilages associated with mucoserous glands ➡ and are important in phonation.

LARYNX

Vocal Cords

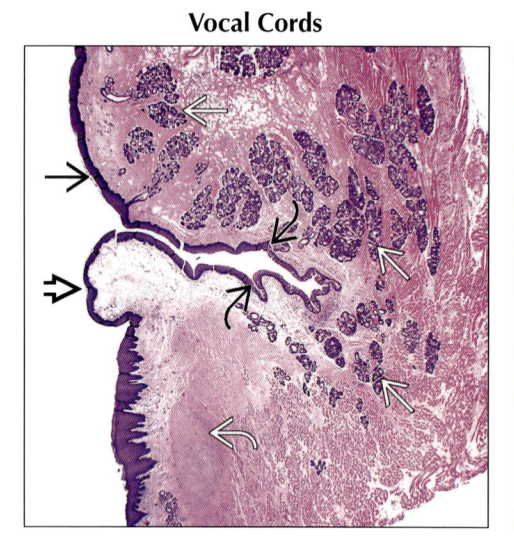

Ventricle and Saccule

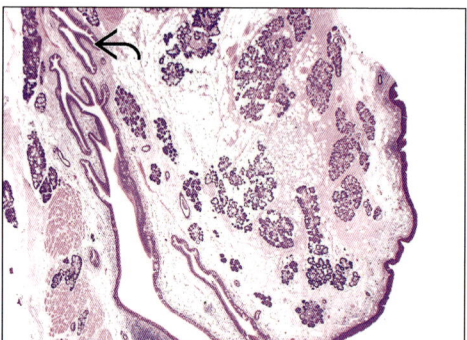

(Left) The true vocal cord ⇨ with vocalis ligament ⇨ is lined by squamous epithelium and is devoid of mucoserous glands. The false vocal cord ⇨ is lined by squamous or respiratory epithelium and has mucoserous glands ⇨. The ventricle ⇨ is lined by respiratory epithelium and also contains mucoserous glands. (Right) The anterior portion of the ventricle ⇨ contains the saccule ⇨, a segment that extends caudally and can result in cystic dilation if obstructed.

Reinke Space

True Vocal Cord

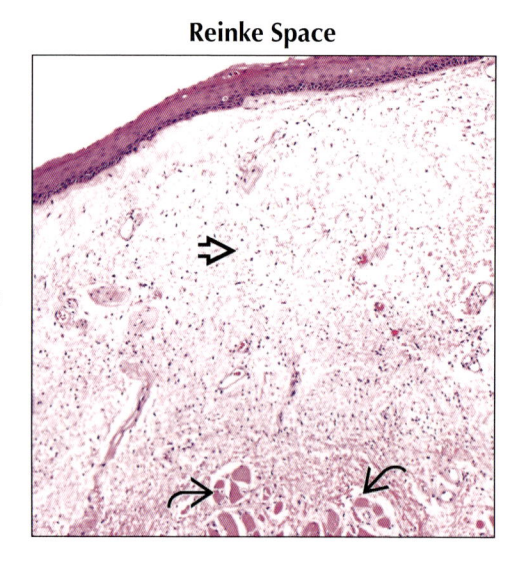

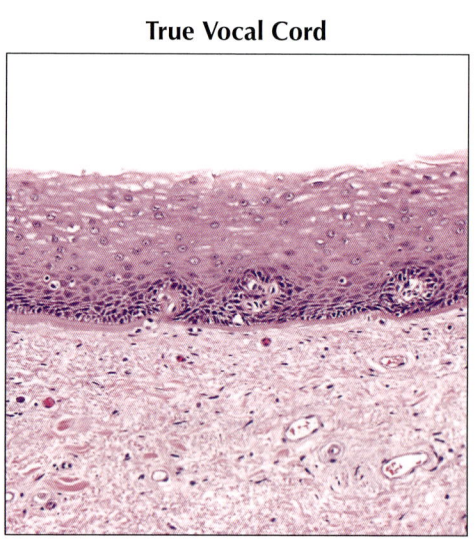

(Left) True vocal cords contain the vocalis muscle ⇨. The lamina propria ⇨ between the vocalis muscle and surface epithelium (Reinke space) contains relatively few capillaries and lacks lymphatic channels. This explains the better prognosis of low-stage glottic carcinomas and the etiology of vocal cord nodules. (Right) The true vocal cords are lined by nonkeratinizing squamous epithelium, approximately 5-20 cells thick. Voice abuse and irritant exposure can lead to keratosis.

Vocal Cord Ligament

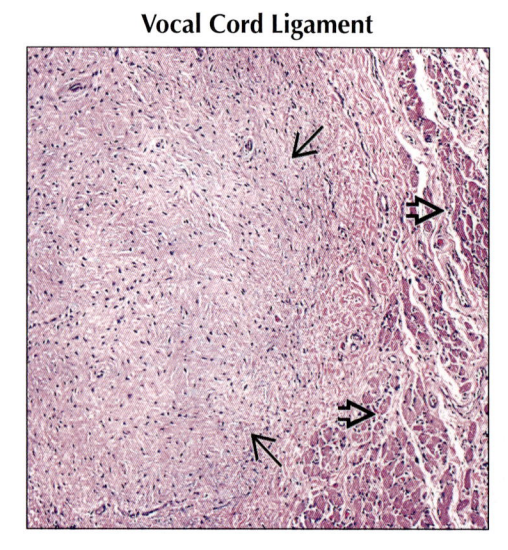

Cartilaginous Metaplasia of Vocal Cord Ligament

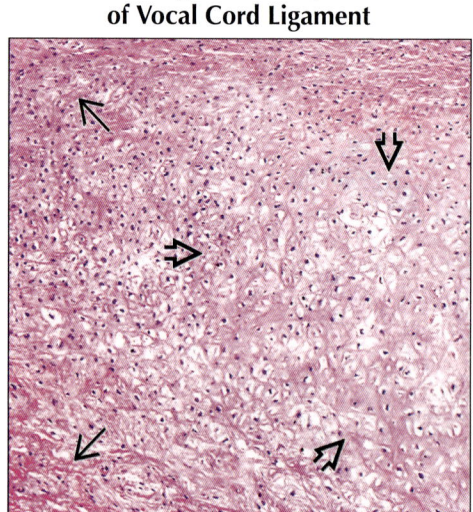

(Left) The vocalis muscle ⇨ consists of a band of connective tissue rich in elastic fibers and often can be seen adjacent to the vocal ligament ⇨. (Right) Chondroid metaplasia ⇨ of the larynx is not uncommon and usually occurs in the posterior 2/3 of the vocal cord ligament ⇨. In contrast to true cartilage, the periphery is not sharply demarcated, and elastic fibers can be seen extending into the metaplastic focus. Chondroid metaplasia can be seen in other parts of the larynx as well.

LARYNX

Lymphoid Aggregate

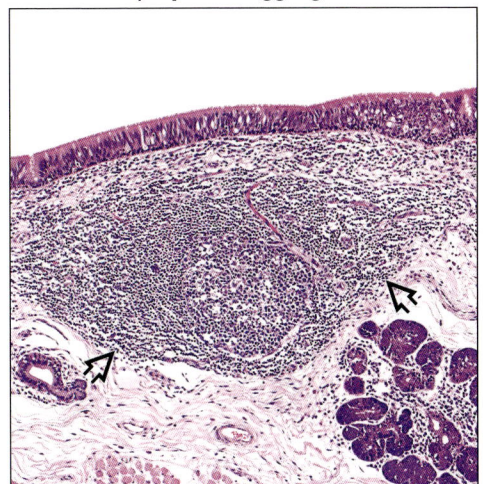

Saccule

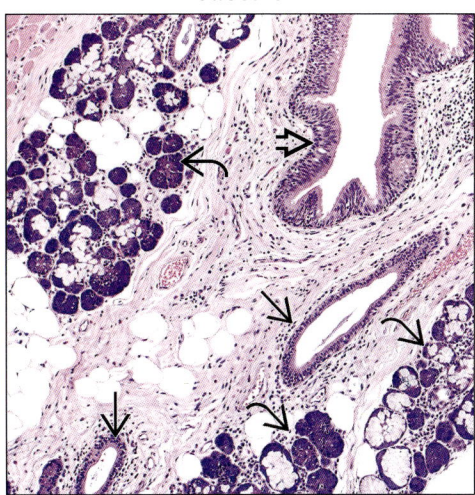

(Left) Lymphoid aggregates ⇨ can be seen in the larynx but are uncommon. When present, they are typically seen in the supraglottic larynx. (Right) The laryngeal saccules represent caudal extensions of the ventricles and are normal. They are lined by respiratory epithelium ⇨ and contain numerous mucoserous glands ⇨ that drain to the mucosal surface via small ducts ⇨. Both the saccule and the ducts can become obstructed, leading to saccular and ductal cysts, respectively.

Saccular Cyst

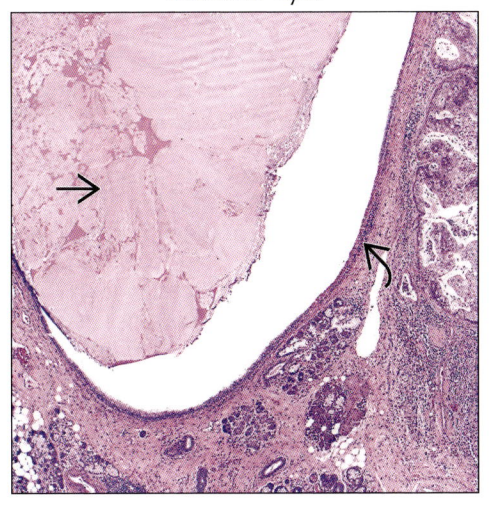

Thyroid Cartilage

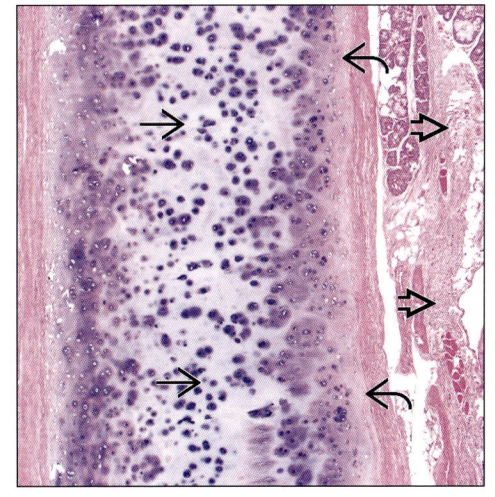

(Left) Saccular cysts represent cystic dilation of the laryngeal saccule; they present in the supraglottis and histologically are respiratory epithelium-lined cysts ⇨ containing mucin ⇨. They usually result from obstruction by invasive squamous cell carcinomas. (Right) In contrast to the epiglottis, most of the other laryngeal cartilages are composed of hyaline cartilage ⇨ with an adjacent perichondrium ⇨. The paraglottic space ⇨ can be seen adjacent to this thyroid cartilage.

Ossification of Thyroid Cartilage

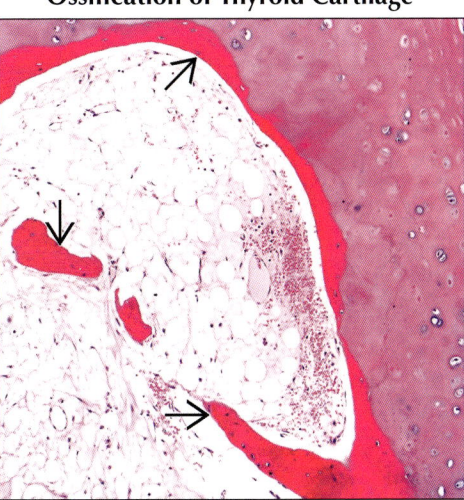

Subglottis

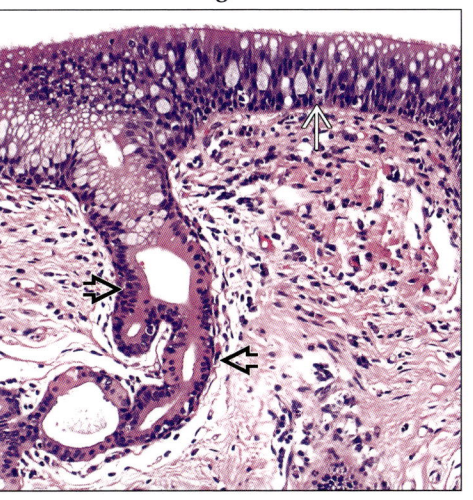

(Left) The thyroid and cricoid cartilages of most adult larynges undergo extensive ossification ⇨ by adulthood. This is an important oncologic point, as nonossified cartilage is typically an excellent barrier to invasion by carcinomas. Once ossified, it is easier for carcinomas to breach the laryngeal cartilages and subsequently spread beyond the larynx. (Right) The subglottis is lined by respiratory mucosa ⇨ with mucoserous glands that drain to the surface via small ducts ⇨.

MAJOR SALIVARY GLANDS

Key Facts

Macroscopic Anatomy

- Major salivary glands include paired parotid, submandibular (submaxillary), and sublingual glands
  - Surrounded by delicate fibrous capsule with intraglandular septae dividing them into lobules
- Parotid glands (15-30 g) are the largest, are located subcutaneously anterior to ear, and are divided by facial nerve into superficial and deep lobes
  - Superficial lobe is larger, flat, and quadrangular whereas deep lobe is wedge-shaped and extends into parapharyngeal space
  - Main (Stensen) duct (~ 7 cm) traverses through masseter and buccinator muscles and drains to oral cavity opposite 2nd maxillary molar
  - Only gland with intraparenchymal lymph nodes
- Submandibular glands (~ 10 g) are located in deep posterior floor of mouth behind mandible
  - Main (Wharton) duct (~ 5 cm) traverses floor of mouth and drains to oral cavity at sublingual caruncle, just lateral to frenulum
- Sublingual glands (2-4 g) are located in anterior floor of mouth behind mandible
  - Main (Bartholin) duct drains into submandibular duct near its termination
  - Numerous small (Rivinus) ducts drain directly to floor of mouth along plica sublingualis

Microscopic Anatomy

- Salivary functional unit (viz., salivon) consists of acinus and draining duct system
- Acini can be serous, mucous, or mixed, and composition can be used to distinguish major salivary glands
  - Parotid is purely serous, submandibular is mixed with serous predominance, and sublingual is mixed with mucous predominance
  - Serous acini are spherical with pyramid-shaped cells containing large basophilic zymogen granules
  - Mucous acini are more tubular with round cells containing sialomucin granules
  - Mixed acini consist of mucous acini with crescent-shaped caps of serous cells (serous demilunes)
- Acinar lumina drain into branching duct system that modifies saliva and delivers it to oral cavity
- Intercalated ducts are intralobular and are located between acini and striated ducts
  - Lined by single layer of cuboidal cells
  - Longest in parotid, shorter in submandibular, and very short in sublingual gland
- Striated ducts are intralobular and deliver saliva to larger excretory ducts
  - Lined by columnar cells with eosinophilic cytoplasm and parallel striations at basal aspect
  - Striations represent basal membrane invaginations with numerous mitochondria and play role in modifying saliva
  - Longest in submandibular, shorter in parotid, and very short in sublingual gland
- Interlobular and main excretory ducts are located in interlobular septae and outside gland, respectively
  - Lined by pseudostratified columnar epithelium with rare goblet cells; become stratified and squamous near their termination in oral cavity
- Contractile myoepithelial cells are flat cells with numerous cytoplasmic processes (basket cells) that aid in propagating secretions
  - Present between epithelial cells and basal lamina in acini, intercalated ducts, and proximal striated ducts
- Noncontractile basal cells are present in striated and excretory ducts
- Parotid parenchyma contains abundant mature adipose tissue; submandibular gland has less
  - Large branches of facial nerve are seen in parotid interlobular septae
- Rare sebaceous cells or lobules can be seen in many parotid gland and some submandibular ducts

Pitfalls/Artifacts

- Intranodal epithelial inclusions may mimic metastases

Age Variation

- Atrophy and oncocytic metaplasia are more common with age

(Left) Branches of the facial nerve ➡ artificially divide the quadrangular superficial parotid lobe from the deep lobe. The main duct ➡ drains into the oral cavity opposite the 2nd maxillary molar. *(Right)* The deep parotid lobe ➡ is wedge-shaped and extends into the parapharyngeal space. Note the intraparotid lymph nodes ➡ and the facial nerve branch ➡ separating the deep lobe from the superficial lobe.

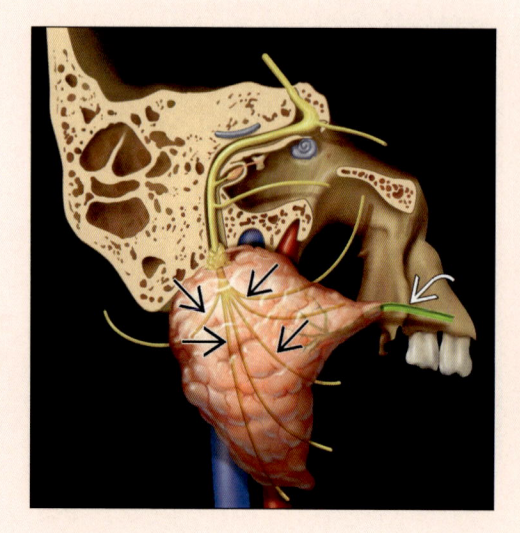

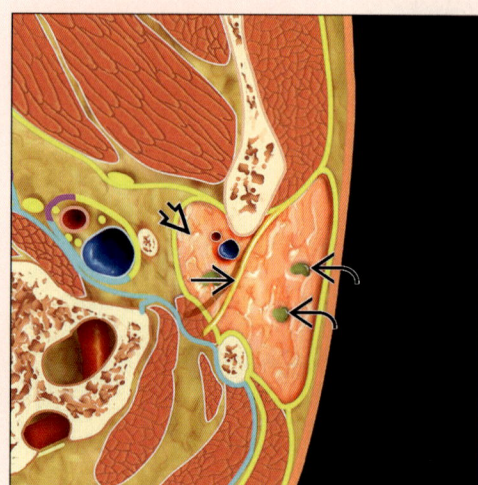

MAJOR SALIVARY GLANDS

Submandibular and Sublingual Glands

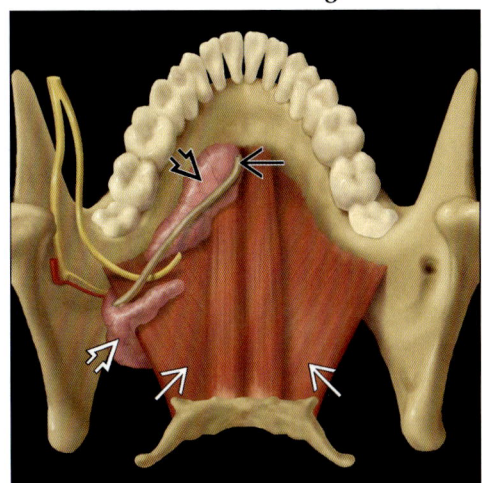

Parotid Lobules

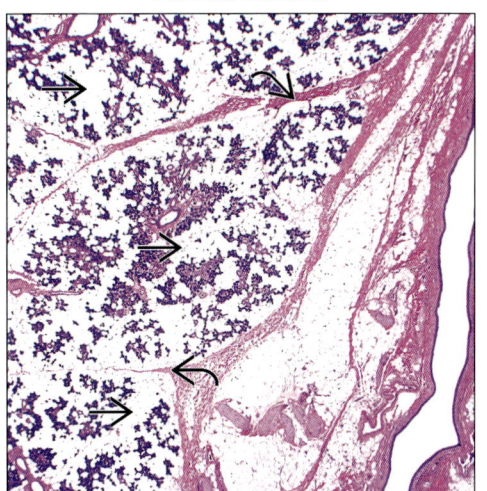

(Left) Submandibular glands ➭ sit below the mylohyoid muscles ➭. A small portion extends above the muscle, and the main duct ➭ extends medially to drain into the oral cavity at the sublingual caruncle. The sublingual gland ➭ is above the muscle, and its main duct drains into the submandibular duct. (Right) Fibrous septae ➭ extend from the capsule to divide the parotid into indistinct lobules. This parotid, from an older individual, contains abundant adipose tissue ➭.

Parotid Excretory Ducts

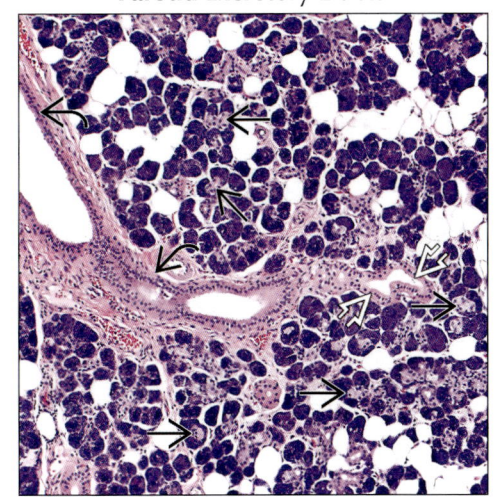

Parotid Acini

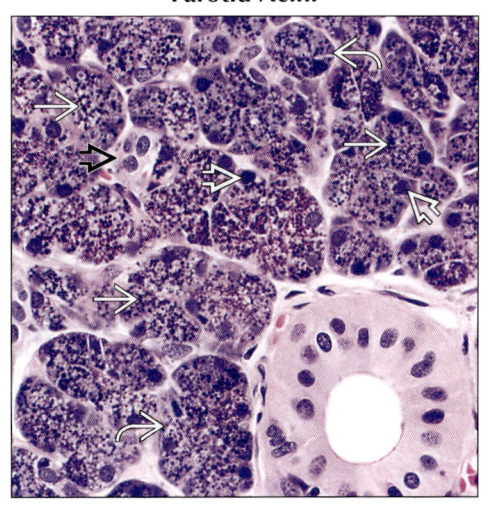

(Left) Intercalated ducts ➭ receive secretions from acini and are easily recognizable in parotid glands. They deliver secretions to intralobular striated ducts ➭, which drain to progressively larger intralobar ➭ and interlobar excretory ducts. (Right) Serous acini ➭ are spherical and drain into intercalated ducts ➭. The secretory cells are pyramidal with basal nuclei ➭ and cytoplasm containing numerous coarse, basophilic secretory (zymogen) granules ➭.

Parotid Intercalated Ducts

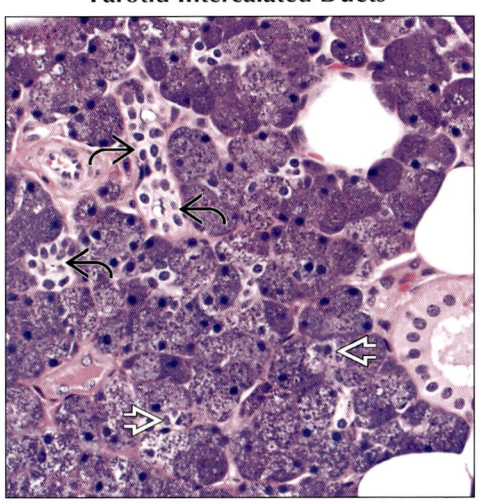

Parotid Striated Duct

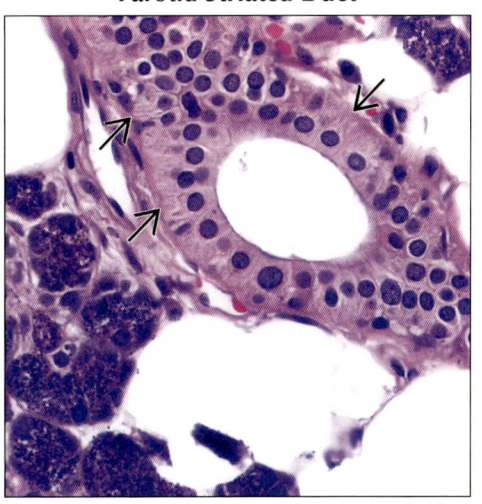

(Left) Intercalated ducts ➭ are lined by simple cuboidal epithelium with pale cytoplasm. Some intercalated duct cells may contain residual zymogen granules ➭. (Right) Striated ducts are simple columnar intralobular ducts that consist of cells with abundant eosinophilic cytoplasm and round central nuclei. Invaginations of the basal cell membrane ➭ account for the striations seen in histologic sections. The cells have numerous mitochondria, which cause the cytoplasmic eosinophilia.

MAJOR SALIVARY GLANDS

Myoepithelial Cells

Intraparotid Lymph Node

(Left) Contractile myoepithelial cells are difficult to discern on H&E but can be appreciated using immunohistochemistry (calponin). They are located around acini ⇨ and intercalated ducts ⇨ and focally in some proximal striated ducts ⇨. (Right) Late embryologic encapsulation accounts for the 5-20 intraparotid lymph nodes that represent 1st-echelon drainage for malignancies of the face, scalp, and ear. They often contain salivary gland inclusions ⇨, which may mimic metastases.

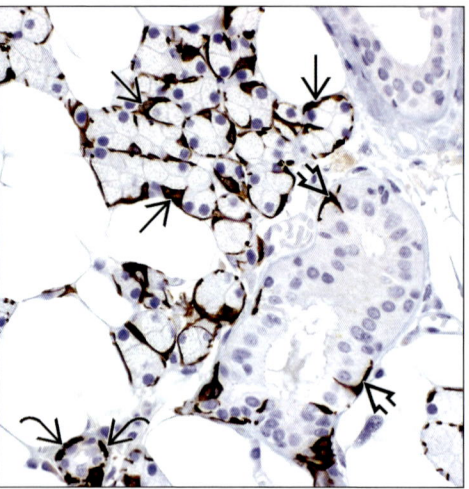

Periparotid Lymph Node

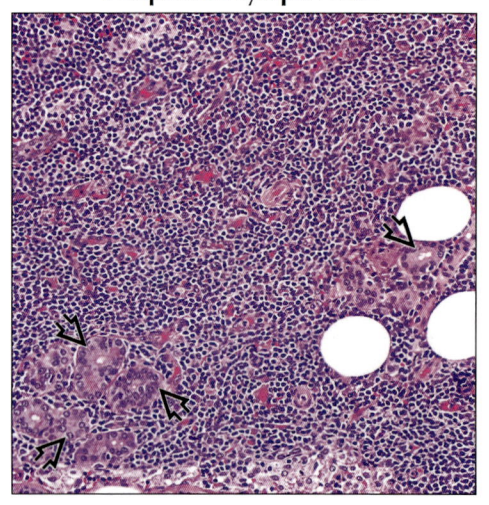

Parotid Atrophy

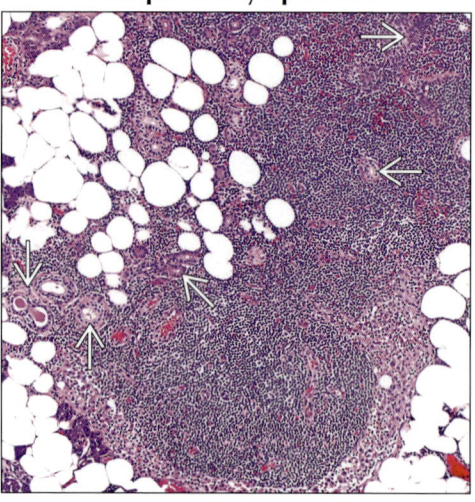

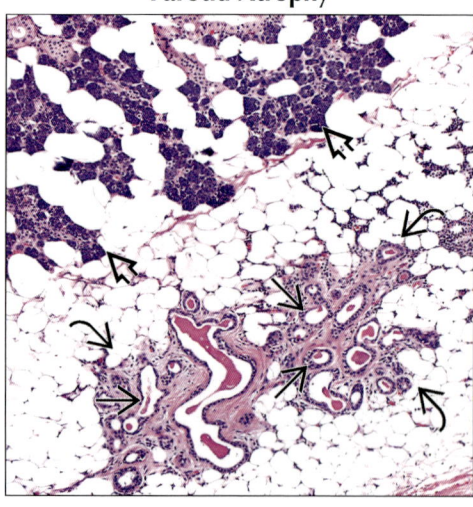

(Left) Similar to intraparotid lymph nodes, periparotid lymph nodes also may contain salivary gland inclusions ⇨, likely due to late embryologic encapsulation as well. These may mimic metastatic disease and can also be a source of extraparotid salivary gland neoplasms. (Right) Focal areas of atrophy ⇨ are common in excised parotid glands ⇨. These result from excretory duct obstruction and may mimic neoplasms. Acini are lost, and only ducts with periductal fibrosis ⇨ persist.

Main Parotid (Stensen) Duct

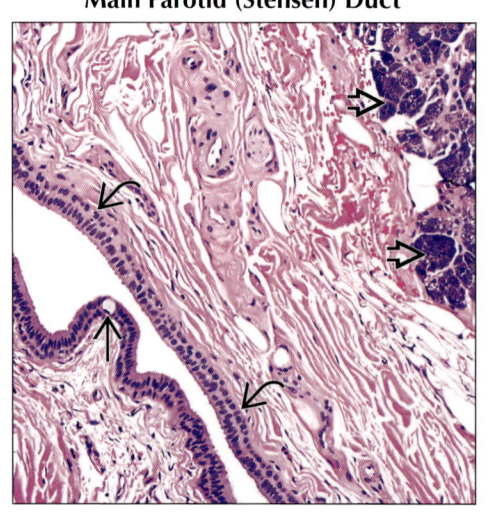

Sebaceous Glands

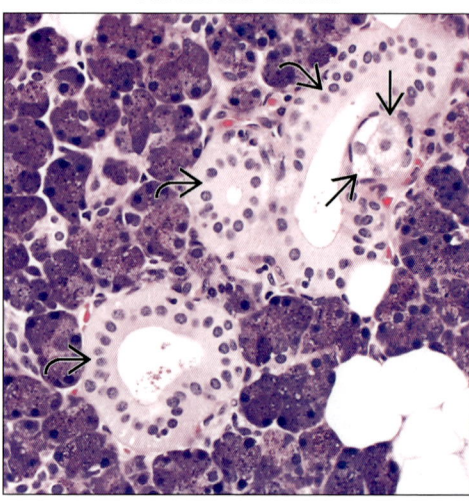

(Left) The main parotid ducts ⇨ traverse connective tissue and muscle to reach their termination in the buccal mucosae. They are lined by pseudostratified or stratified columnar epithelium and may contain goblet cells ⇨ and cilia. Accessory parotid tissue ⇨ can be seen in about 20-50% of people. (Right) Focal sebaceous cells ⇨ or lobules are not uncommon in parotid gland duct epithelium ⇨. They can be seen in the majority of parotid glands with careful examination.

MAJOR SALIVARY GLANDS

Parotid Gland Oncocytic Metaplasia

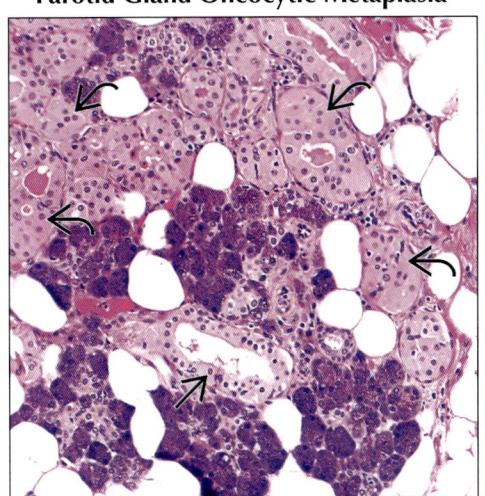

Submandibular Gland

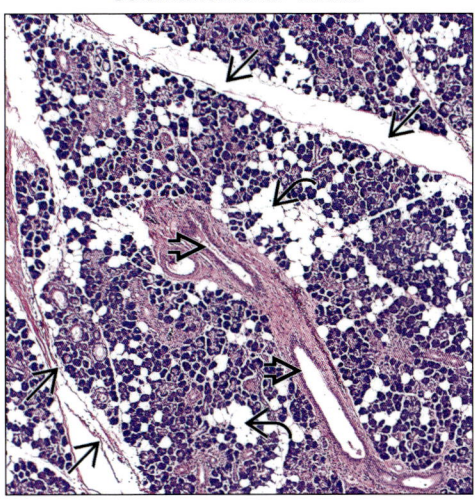

(Left) Oncocytes ➶ are metaplastic cells with granular eosinophilic cytoplasm containing numerous irregular mitochondria. They are often seen in the parotid glands of those > 50 years of age but are less common in submandibular glands. They resemble striated duct cells ➶ superficially. *(Right)* Lobulation ➶ is more pronounced in submandibular glands, and there is less intraparenchymal adipose tissue ➶ than in parotid glands. A central intralobular excretory duct ⮞ is present.

Submandibular Ducts

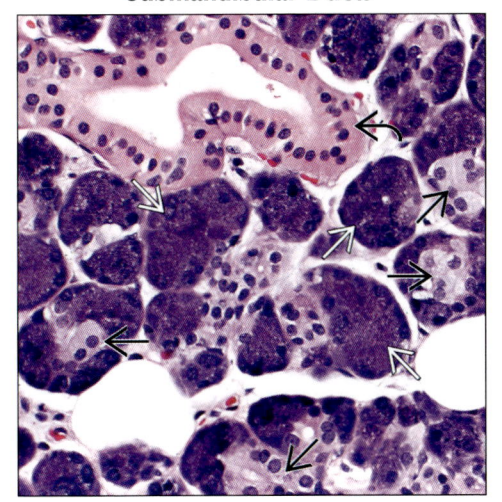

Serous Demilunes

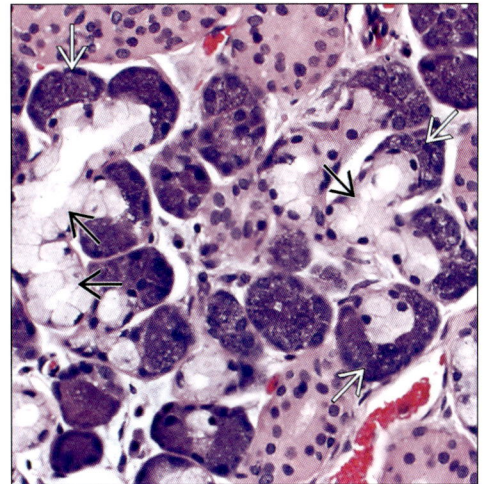

(Left) The submandibular gland is a mixed gland predominantly composed of serous acini ➶ but also containing a minor mucous acinar component. Striated ducts ➶ are longest in the submandibular gland and are easily recognizable. Intercalated ducts ➶ are shorter than in the parotid gland but are easily seen. *(Right)* Serous demilunes consist of tubular mucous acini ➶ capped by a crescent-shaped collection of serous cells ➶. These have been shown to be an artifact of fixation.

Sublingual Gland

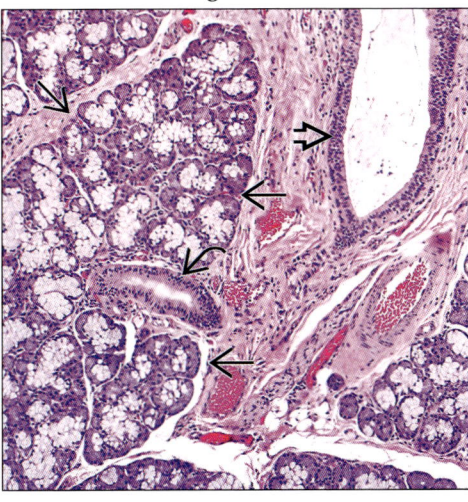

Sublingual Acini

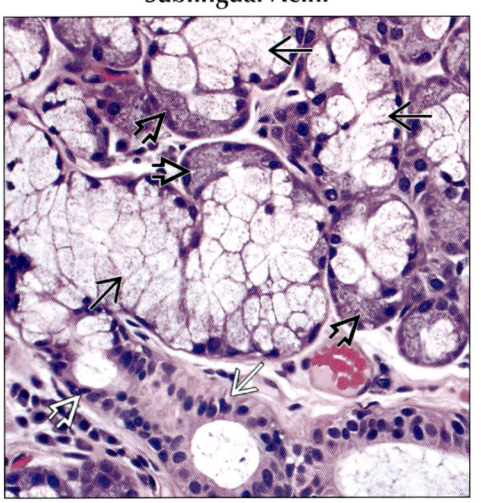

(Left) The sublingual gland is arranged into lobules ➶ but lacks adipose tissue, unlike the other major salivary glands. Intralobular excretory ducts ➶ empty into large interlobular ducts ⮞, which are lined by a pseudostratified columnar epithelium. *(Right)* The sublingual gland is mixed, with a predominance of tubular mucous acini ➶, many of which are capped by serous acini ⮞. They have very short intercalated ducts ⮞ that communicate with short striated ducts ➶.

SELECTED REFERENCES

EYE AND OCULAR ADNEXA

1. Knowles DM et al: Lymphoid hyperplasia and malignant lymphoma occurring in the ocular adnexa (orbit, conjunctiva, and eyelids): a prospective multiparametric analysis of 108 cases during 1977 to 1987. Hum Pathol. 21(9):959-73, 1990
2. Koornneef L: New insights in the human orbital connective tissue. Result of a new anatomical approach. Arch Ophthalmol. 95(7):1269-73, 1977
3. Straatsma BR: Typical and reticular degenerative retinoschisis. Ber Zusammenkunft Dtsch Ophthalmol Ges. 74:123-30, 1977
4. Tripathi RC: Aqueous outflow pathway in normal and glaucomatous eyes. Br J Ophthalmol. 56(3):157-74, 1972
5. Cogan DG et al: Focal senile translucency of the sclera. Arch Ophthalmol. 62:604-10, 1959

ORAL MUCOSAE

1. Ten Cate AR: Oral Histology: Development, Structure, and Function. 3rd ed. St. Louis: Mosby, 1989
2. Wheater PR: Functional Histology. 2nd ed. Edinburgh: Churchill Livingstone. 191-9, 1987

GINGIVAE

1. Neville B et al: Oral and Maxillofacial Pathology. 3rd ed. St. Louis: Saunders, 2009

MINOR SALIVARY GLANDS

1. Ellis G, et al: Tumors of the Salivary Glands. AFIP Atlas of Tumor Pathology Series 4, Fascicle 9. American Registry of Pathology, 2008
2. Wheater PR: Functional Histology. 2nd ed. Edinburgh: Churchill Livingstone. 191-9, 1987

TEETH

1. Neville B et al: Oral and Maxillofacial Pathology. 3rd ed. St. Louis: Saunders, 2009
2. Ten Cate AR: Oral Histology: Development, Structure, and Function. 3rd ed. St. Louis: Mosby, 1989
3. Wheater PR: Functional Histology. 2nd ed. Edinburgh: Churchill Livingstone. 191-9, 1987

TONGUE

1. Oakley B: Neuronal-epithelial interactions in mammalian gustatory epithelium. Ciba Found Symp. 160:277-87; discussion 287-93, 1991
2. Delay RJ et al: Ultrastructure of mouse vallate taste buds: II. Cell types and cell lineage. J Comp Neurol. 253(2):242-52, 1986
3. Farbman AI et al: Structure of taste buds in foliate papillae of the rhesus monkey, Macaca mulatta. Am J Anat. 172(1):41-56, 1985

TONSILS/ADENOIDS

1. Kapoor N et al: Cartilagenous choristoma of palatine tonsil--a case report. Indian J Pathol Microbiol. 46(4):654-5, 2003
2. Nave H et al: Morphology and immunology of the human palatine tonsil. Anat Embryol (Berl). 204(5):367-73, 2001

EAR

1. Lo WW et al: The endolymphatic duct and sac. AJNR Am J Neuroradiol. 18(5):881-7, 1997
2. Michaels L et al: Development of the stratified squamous epithelium of the human tympanic membrane and external canal: the origin of auditory epithelial migration. Am J Anat. 184(4):334-44, 1989
3. Sophian LH et al: Anatomy and histology of the external ear in relation to the histogenesis of external otitis. Laryngoscope. 64(9):772-84, 1954

NOSE AND PARANASAL SINUSES

1. Naessen R: The identification and topographical localisation of the olfactory epithelium in man and other mammals. Acta Otolaryngol. 70(1):51-7, 1970
2. Schneider RA: The sense of smell in man--its physiologic basis. N Engl J Med. 277(6):299-303, 1967

PHARYNX

1. Nicolai P et al: Nasopharyngeal cysts. Report of seven cases with review of the literature. Arch Otolaryngol Head Neck Surg. 115(7):860-4, 1989
2. Ali MY: Histology of the human nasopharyngeal mucosa. J Anat. 99(Pt 3):657-72, 1965

LARYNX

1. Dang-Tran KD et al: Thyroid cartilage ossification and multislice computed tomography examination: a useful tool for age assessment? J Forensic Sci. 55(3):677-83, 2010
2. Stell PM et al: Morphology of the human larynx. III. the supraglottis. Clin Otolaryngol Allied Sci. 6(6):389-93, 1981
3. Hill MJ et al: Chondromatous metaplasia in the human larynx. Histopathology. 4(2):205-14, 1980
4. Stell PM et al: Morphology of the human larynx. II. The subglottis. Clin Otolaryngol Allied Sci. 5(6):389-95, 1980
5. Stell PM et al: Morphometry of the epithelial lining of the human larynx. I. The glottis. Clin Otolaryngol Allied Sci. 3(1):13-20, 1978

SELECTED REFERENCES

6. Nassar VH et al: Topography of the laryngeal mucous glands. Arch Otolaryngol. 94(6):490-8, 1971

MAJOR SALIVARY GLANDS

1. Foschini MP et al: Differential expression of myoepithelial markers in salivary, sweat and mammary glands. Int J Surg Pathol. 8(1):29-37, 2000
2. Toh H et al: Incidence and histology of human accessory parotid glands. Anat Rec. 236(3):586-90, 1993
3. Young JA et al: Morphology and physiology of salivary myoepithelial cells. Int Rev Physiol. 12:105-25, 1977

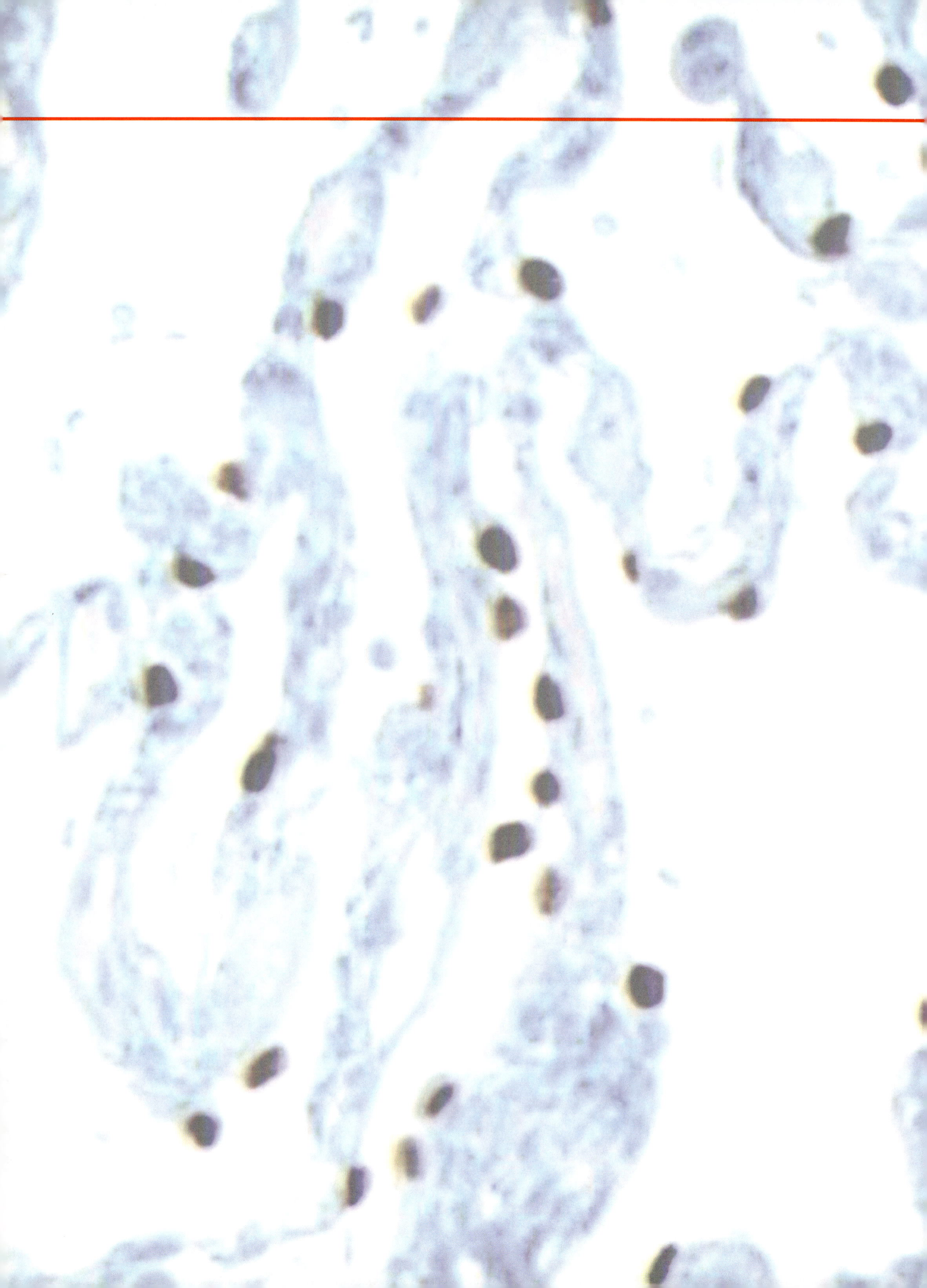

Respiratory System

Trachea 8-2

Lung 8-4

Mesothelium 8-10

TRACHEA

Key Facts

Macroscopic Anatomy
- Tubular structure extending from cricoid cartilage to carina, where it branches into the 2 mainstem bronchi
- Runs directly anterior to esophagus
- Protected anteriorly by C-shaped rings of cartilage
- Posterior aspect is devoid of cartilage and contains trachealis muscle and connective tissue

Microscopic Anatomy
- 4 main layers (superficial to deep)
  - Mucosa: Respiratory epithelium, basement membrane, lamina propria
  - Submucosa: Seromucous glands, vessels, nerves
  - Cartilaginous rings: Hyaline cartilage
  - Adventitia: Loose connective tissue sheath
- Seromucous glands connect to luminal surface of trachea via ducts lined by cuboidal epithelium
- Respiratory epithelium is composed of pseudostratified ciliated columnar epithelium
  - Goblet cells are common
- Smooth muscle (trachealis muscle) is present in posterior trachea
- Seromucous glands are more numerous in posterior trachea

Pitfalls/Artifacts
- Cartilaginous rings can appear highly cellular
- Numerous seromucous glands in posterior trachea can mimic neoplasm

Metaplasia
- Squamous metaplasia: Associated with smoking, chronic irritation
- Oncocytic metaplasia

(Left) This image shows the surface epithelium ⇨, underlying lamina propria, submucosal seromucous glands ⇨, and cartilage ring of the trachea ⇨. The outer adventitia is not shown. (Right) The trachea is lined by a pseudostratified columnar epithelium containing numerous apical cilia ⇨ and scattered goblet cells ⇨. This epithelium is also referred to as "respiratory-type epithelium." The pink basement membrane ⇨ separates the epithelium from the underlying lamina propria.

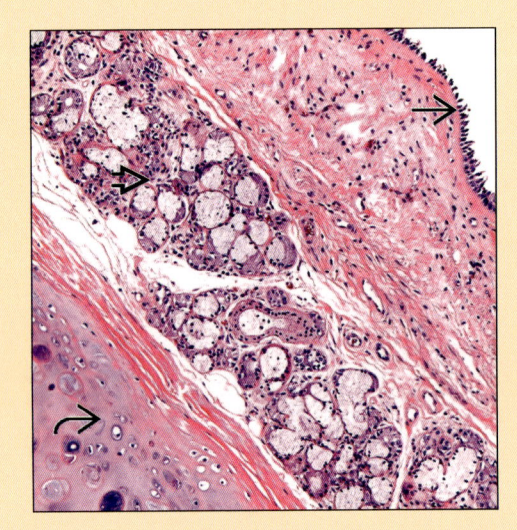

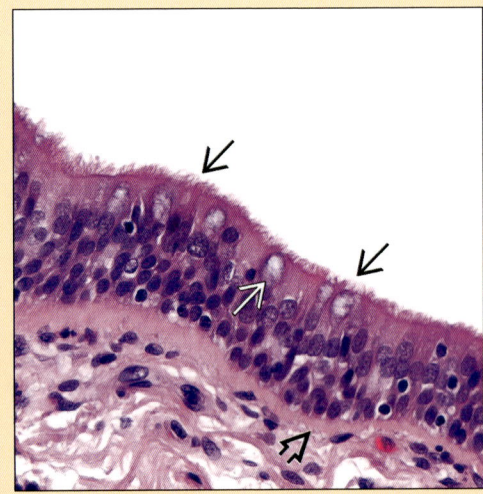

(Left) In the setting of chronic irritation (such as from smoking or other chemicals), it is not unusual for the columnar epithelium to transition into a stratified squamous epithelium (squamous metaplasia). Compared to columnar cells, squamous cells ⇨ are very eosinophilic, round to flat, and lack cytoplasmic mucin. (Right) The lamina propria is a layer of loose connective tissue that contains nerves ⇨, vessels ⇨, and ducts ⇨ that connect the submucosal glands to the luminal surface.

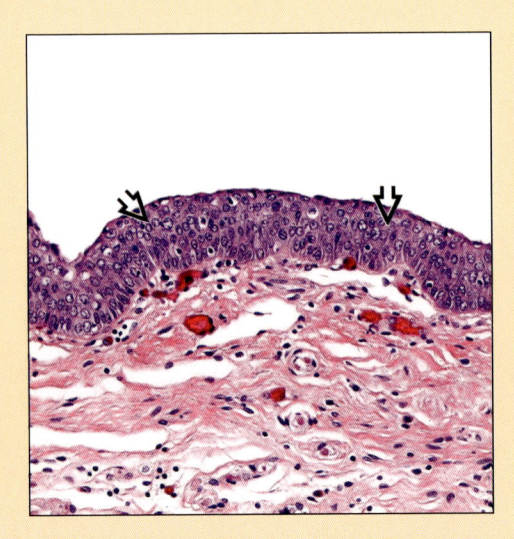

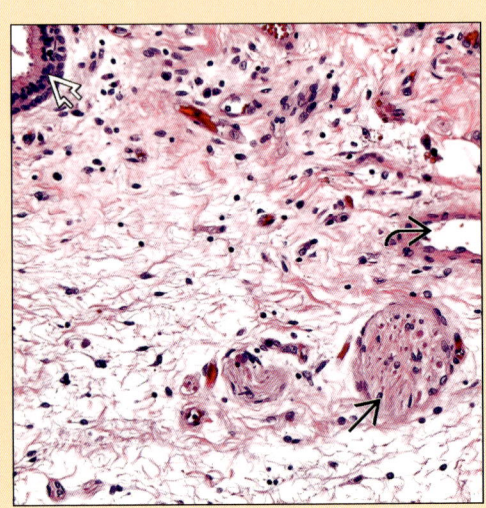

TRACHEA

Seromucous Glands and Ducts

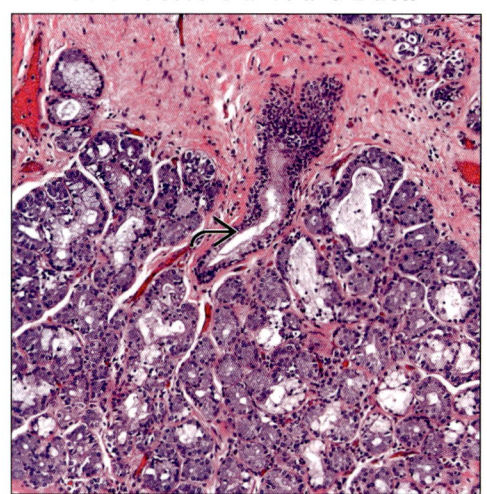

Seromucous Glands

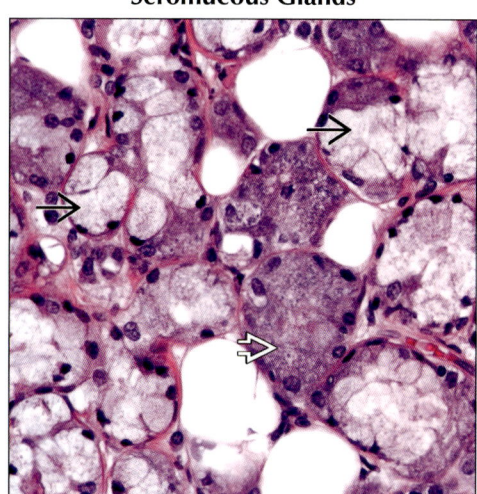

(Left) The submucosal glands of the trachea are very similar to those found in the normal salivary gland. The glands are arranged in lobules, and each lobule is associated with a duct ➡ that conveys the glandular secretions to the luminal surface. *(Right)* Within a lobule, each acinus (cluster of cells) is composed of a variable mixture of serous cells and mucous cells ➡. The serous cells ➡ are usually easily identified by their basophilic, granular cytoplasm.

Squamous Metaplasia

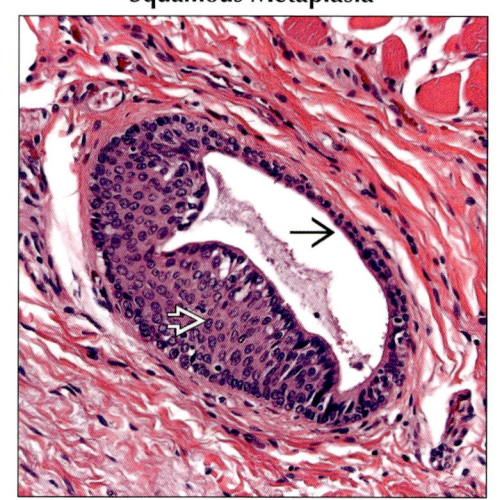

Cartilage Ring

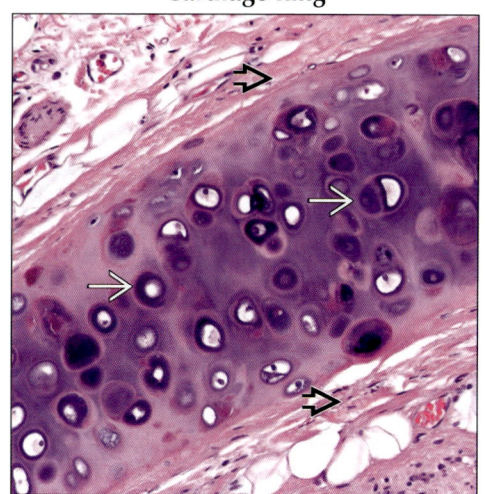

(Left) Similar to the columnar surface epithelium, the epithelial lining (flat cuboidal ➡) of the glandular ducts will occasionally show features of squamous metaplasia ➡, particularly in the setting of chronic irritation. *(Right)* The cartilage rings that protect the trachea anteriorly are found immediately deep to the submucosa. Each demonstrates a fibrous perichondrium ➡ and contains numerous chondrocytes ➡.

Hyaline Cartilage

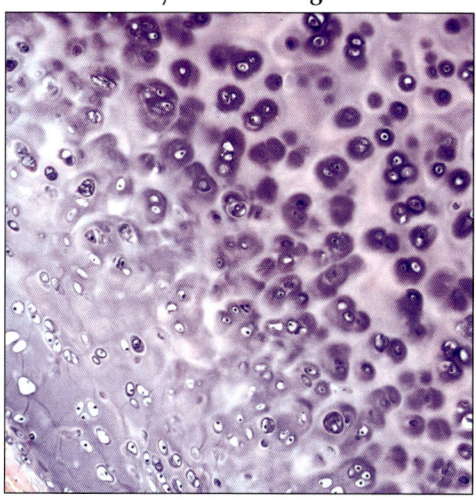

Adventitia

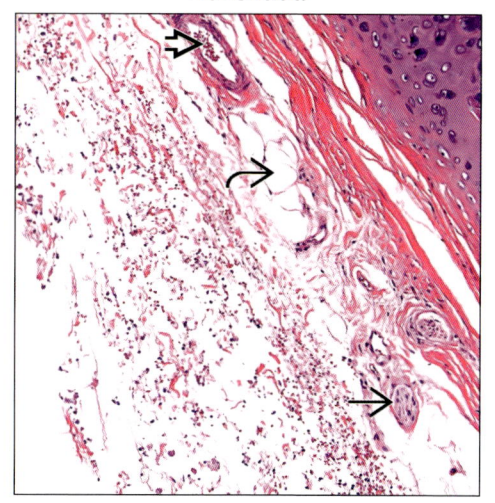

(Left) The cartilage rings are composed of hyaline cartilage, which is the most common type of cartilage in the body. On routine H&E stain, this hyaline cartilage can appear blue, purple, or even pink. *(Right)* The adventitia is loose connective tissue that invests the external surface of the trachea. Similar to the submucosa, it contains fibroblasts, nerve twigs ➡, adipose tissue ➡, and small vessels ➡. There is no mesothelial lining.

LUNG

Key Facts

Macroscopic Anatomy
- Airways
  - Bronchi (> 1 cm in diameter) connect trachea to bronchioles within hilum of lung
  - Bronchioles (usually < 1 cm in diameter) with extensive distal dichotomous branching
  - Terminal bronchioles connect proximal bronchioles with respiratory bronchioles
  - Respiratory bronchioles are connected directly to alveolar ducts, alveolar sacs, and alveoli
  - Alveoli: Sites of gas exchange
- Right lung
  - 3 lobes: Upper, middle, and lower
  - Each lobe divided into 10 bronchopulmonary segments (lobules)
- Left Lung
  - 2 lobes: Upper and lower
  - Presence of lingula (no true middle lobe)
  - Each lobe divided into 9 bronchopulmonary segments (lobules)
- Vasculature
  - Pulmonary arteries provide deoxygenated venous blood from systemic circulation to alveoli for oxygenation
  - Pulmonary veins transport oxygenated blood from alveoli to systemic circulation
  - Bronchial arteries provide oxygenated systemic blood to parenchyma of lung and visceral pleura
  - Bronchial veins remove deoxygenated blood from parenchyma of lung and visceral pleura
- Pleura
  - Visceral pleura invests periphery of each lobe of both lungs
  - Parietal pleura lines inner chest wall
- Lymphatics
  - Rich lymphatic network drains toward hilum

Microscopic Anatomy
- Airways
  - Ciliated pseudocolumnar epithelium with goblet cells
  - Submucosal seromucous glands
  - Smooth muscle present in walls of airways
  - Bronchi have protective anterior cartilaginous rings
  - Lobar and terminal bronchioles lack cartilaginous rings
  - Respiratory bronchioles and alveolar structures are not lined by pseudocolumnar epithelium
- Parenchyma
  - Bronchopulmonary segments contain a central lobar bronchiole and are delineated from adjacent segments by interlobular septae
  - Alveolar tissue is composed of type 1 pneumocytes, type 2 pneumocytes, and alveolar capillaries
  - Alveolar macrophages remove alveolar debris
- Vasculature
  - Lobar bronchioles are paired with pulmonary arteries and contain bronchial arteries in their walls
  - Pulmonary vein branches are in interlobular septae and are not paired with arteries or lobar bronchi
  - Lymphatic channels can be found adjacent to lobar arterioles as well as interlobular septal venules
  - In general, arteries contain a double (inner & outer) elastic lamina, & veins contain a single outer lamina
- Pleura
  - Composed of connective tissue and elastic fibers and lined by mesothelium

Pitfalls/Artifacts
- Pigmented macrophages in smokers
- Crush artifact
- Insufficient inflation prior to tissue processing
- Hemorrhage related to a surgical procedure
- Peribronchial metaplasia
- Foreign body reaction
- Bone marrow emboli
- Megakaryocytes
- Carbon pigment (anthracosis)
- Corpora amylacea
- Meningothelial nodules
- Calcification
- Metaplastic ossification

Age Variation
- Bronchial cartilage may calcify with increased age

(Left) Akin to the trachea, a bronchus is composed of surface epithelium ➡ with underlying seromucous glands (for lubrication) ➡ and C-shaped rings of hyaline cartilage (for structural support) ➡. *(Right)* The bronchi and bronchioles also contain a thin layer of smooth muscle ➡ that allows for bronchoconstriction. An artery ➡ can also be identified in this field.

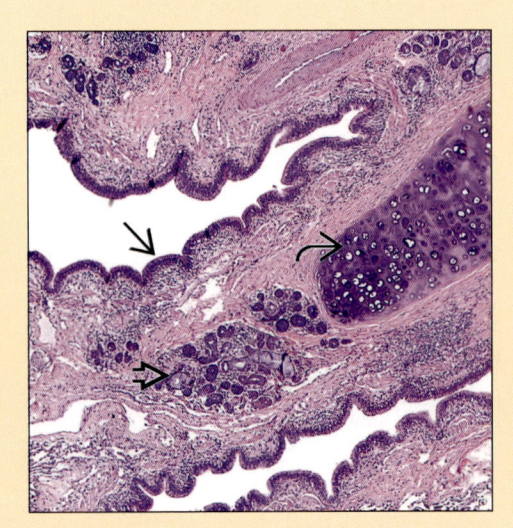

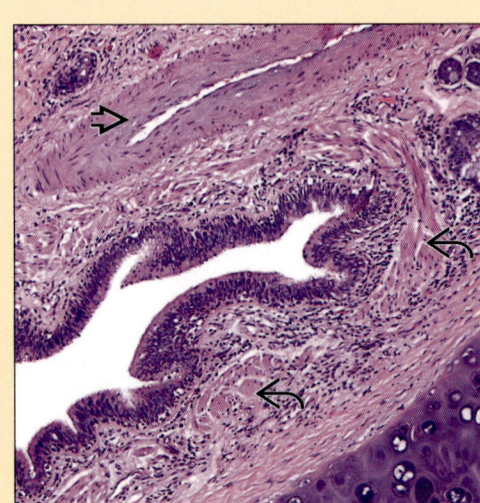

LUNG

Main Bronchi

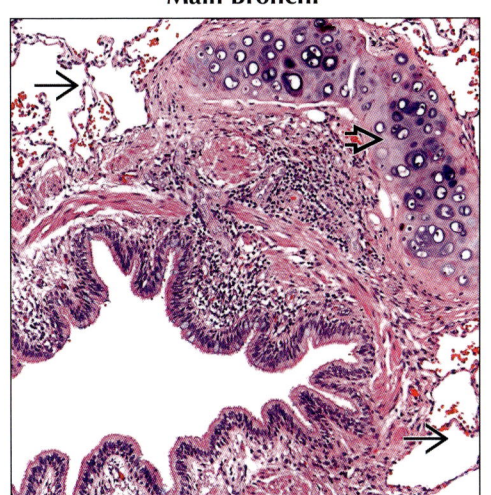

Lobar Bronchioles

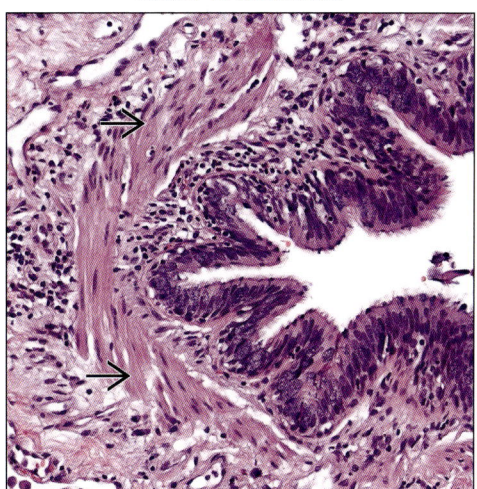

(Left) This image shows a main bronchus as it enters the lung parenchyma (note surrounding alveoli ➔). It also serves to demonstrate how the protective cartilaginous rings ➔ are not completely circumferential and only protect the anterior aspect of the large airways.
(Right) Unlike the large main bronchi, the lobar bronchi do not contain cartilaginous rings. They do, however, contain a ring of smooth muscle ➔ that helps constrict the airway for protective purposes.

Ciliated Pseudostratified Columnar Epithelium

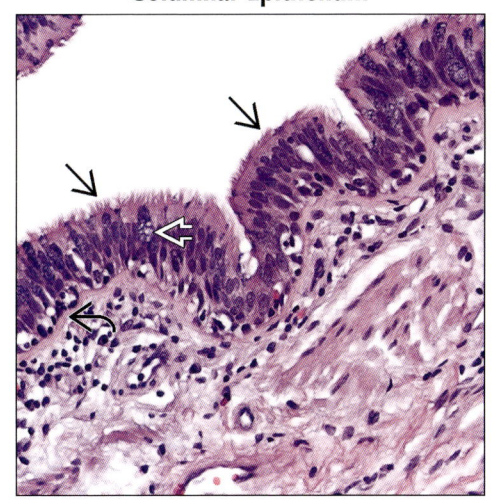

Asthma

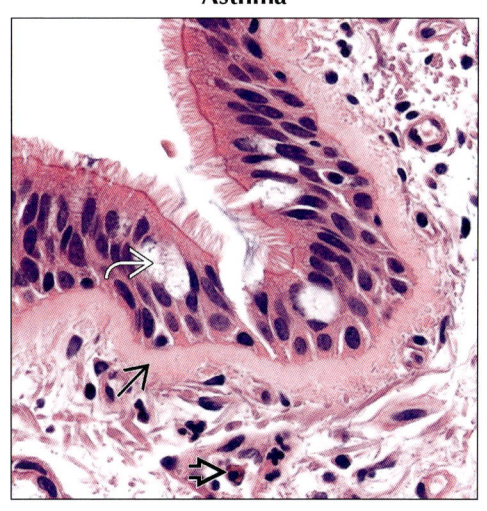

(Left) The respiratory lining is composed of pseudostratified columnar epithelium with prominent apical cilia ➔ and goblet cells ➔. This epithelium rests on a thin, pink basement membrane ➔, which separates the epithelium from the underlying lamina propria.
(Right) In patients with asthma, the basement membrane ➔ is often markedly thickened. Other changes include increased numbers of goblet cells ➔ as well as stromal eosinophils ➔.

Lobar Bronchioles and Arteries

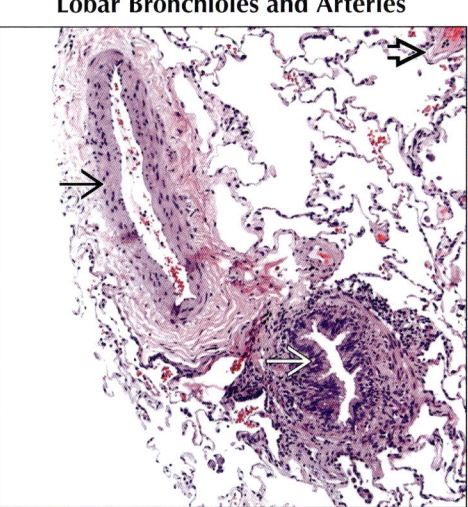

Vasculature

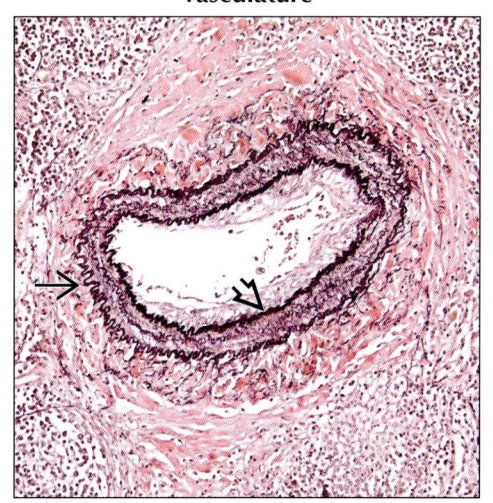

(Left) Lobar bronchioles ➔ are paired with an adjacent pulmonary arteriole ➔. These medium-sized vessels further ramify within the lung parenchyma and show up as small isolated vessels ➔ unaccompanied by an airway. It can be difficult to tell a small venule from an arteriole. (Right) Both arteries and veins contain elastic lamina within their walls; however, the larger arteries show both inner ➔ and outer ➔ lamina, as highlighted in black by an elastin stain.

LUNG

Interlobular Septae

(Left) The interlobular septae ⇨ are composed of loose connective tissue and define the anatomic boundary between lobules. Pulmonary veins ⇨ and lymphatic channels course within these septae. **(Right)** Respiratory bronchioles transfer air into elongated alveolar ducts ⇨, which are in direct communication with multiple alveoli ⇨. Note that in the the normal lung, the alveolar walls ⇨ are very thin and form a relatively intact mesh-like network.

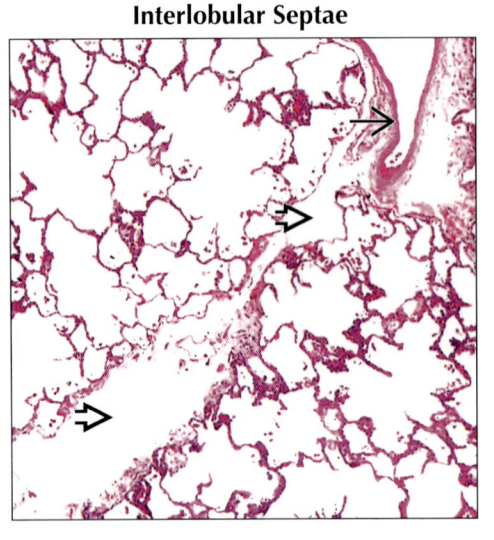

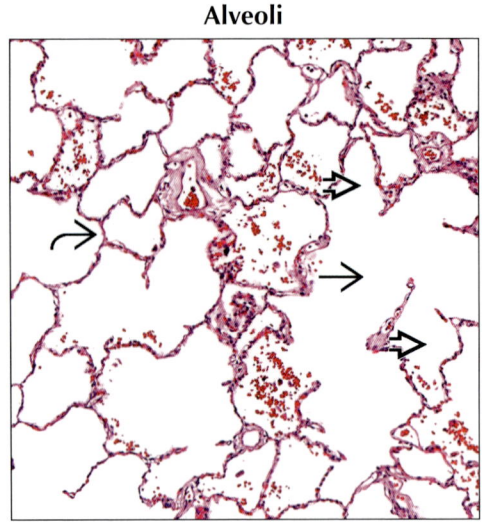

Alveoli

Alveolar Epithelium

(Left) Alveolar epithelium is composed of capillaries (identified by their lumina ⇨) and type 1 and type 2 pneumocytes, which can be difficult to see on routine H&E stain. Tiny alveolar macrophages ⇨ are not uncommon. **(Right)** Even at very high magnification, it can be difficult to identify pneumocytes and distinguish them from endothelial cells. Capillaries, however, are usually easily identified by their open lumina ⇨. Note the single alveolar macrophage ⇨.

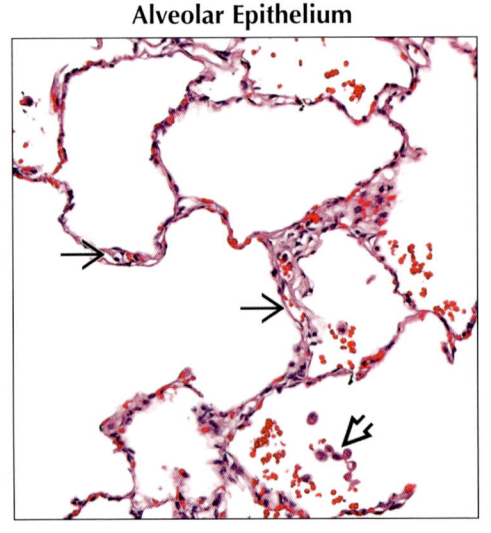

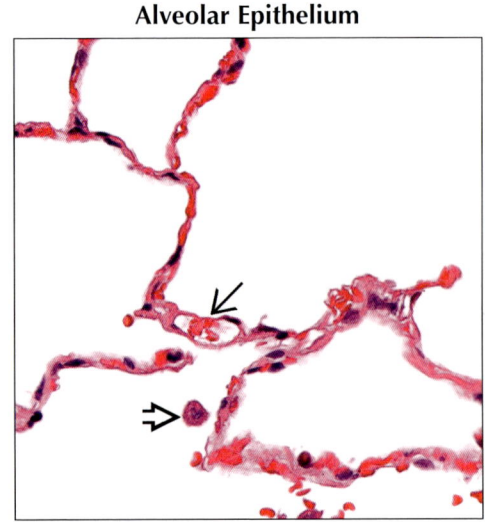

Alveolar Epithelium

Pneumocytes

(Left) Using immunohistochemistry, a thyroid transcription factor-1 (TTF-1) stain highlights the nuclei ⇨ of the alveolar pneumocytes. The endothelial cells of the capillaries ⇨ and the alveolar macrophages ⇨ do not stain. **(Right)** Although alveolar macrophages are typically scant in normal lung, they can be increased ⇨ in patients who smoke. Under these circumstances, they often form large aggregates that fill the alveoli. Sometimes they can appear multinucleated.

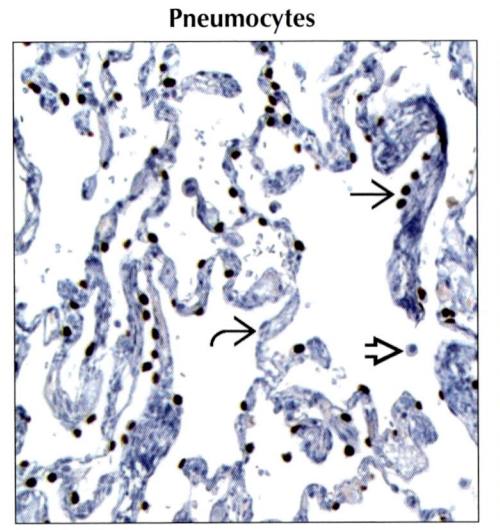

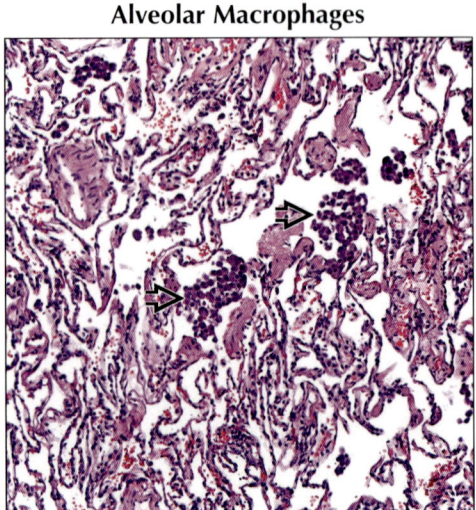

Alveolar Macrophages

LUNG

Pigmented Macrophages

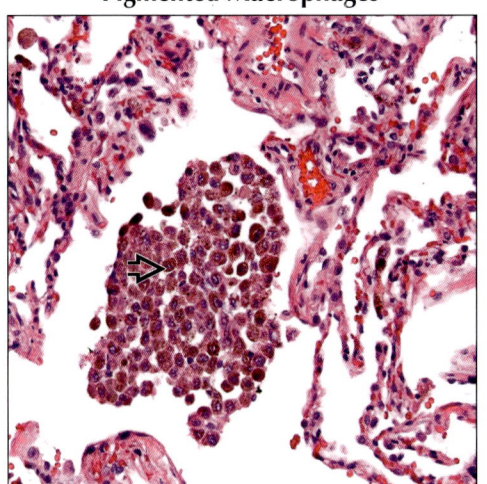

Bronchial-Associated Lymphoid Tissue (BALT)

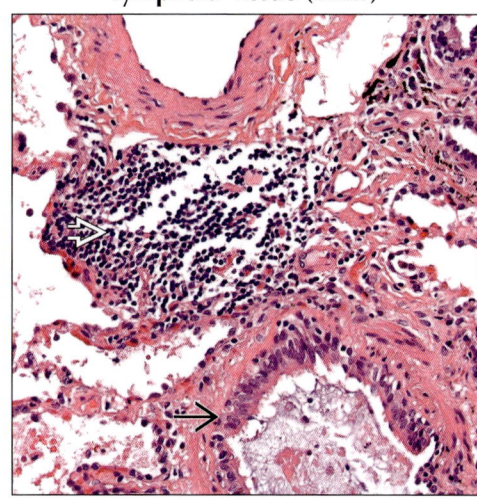

(Left) In smokers, the aggregates of macrophages often show a fine, light brown pigmentation ➡. In contrast, iron (hemosiderin) pigment, such as that seen in true alveolar hemorrhage, is bright golden-brown and chunky. **(Right)** Similar to the gastrointestinal tract, the lung has small aggregates of lymphoid tissue ➡, known as BALT, associated with the bronchioles ➡. They can be enlarged in infectious or inflammatory states and sometimes contain reactive germinal centers.

BALT Crush Artifact

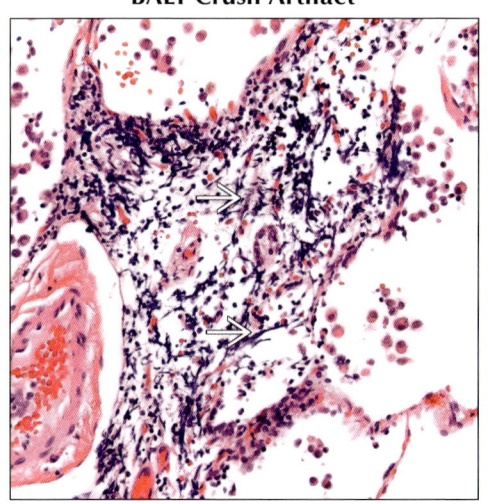

Visceral Pleura

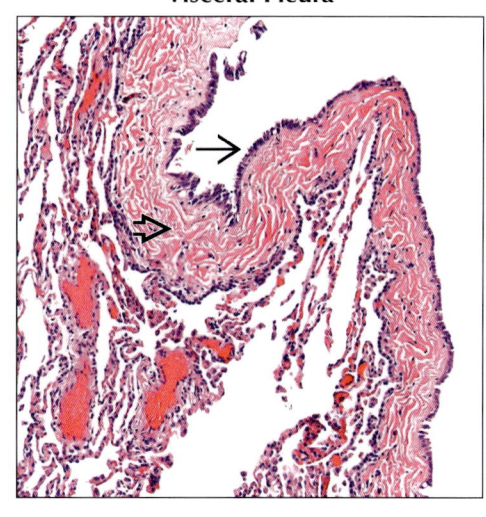

(Left) Lymphocytes are somewhat fragile and are easily crushed during a biopsy procedure. This can give them a spindled (elongated) ➡ appearance that may be mistaken for a neoplasm or fungus. **(Right)** The periphery of each lobe is invested in a rind of fibroconnective tissue and elastin, called the visceral pleura ➡. The external surface is lined by a thin layer of mesothelial cells ➡; however, this lining is not always entirely visible in routine histologic sections.

Peripheral Emphysematous Changes

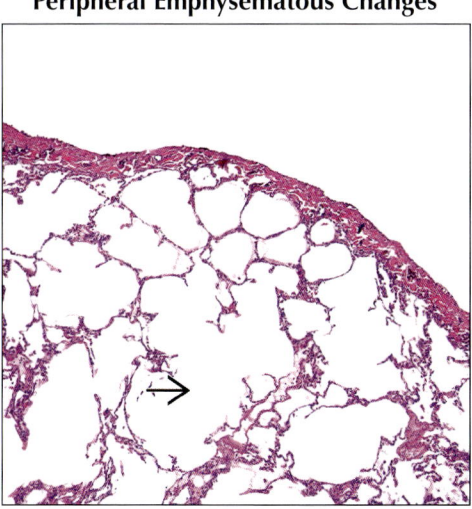

Atelectasis

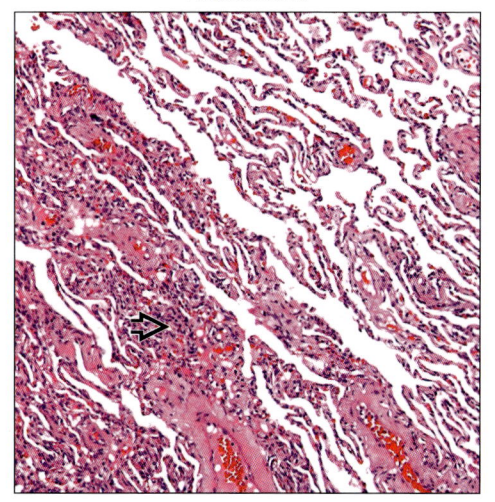

(Left) A common finding in smokers is emphysema, which is characterized by alveolar wall destruction and gives the impression of enlarging alveolar spaces ➡. It is most common at the periphery. **(Right)** Atelectasis is a collapse ➡ of the lung parenchyma. It can be real or artifactual, but it is most commonly due to insufficient inflation of the lung specimen prior to fixation. This impression of increased cellularity can lead to the mistaken notion of fibrotic lung disease.

LUNG

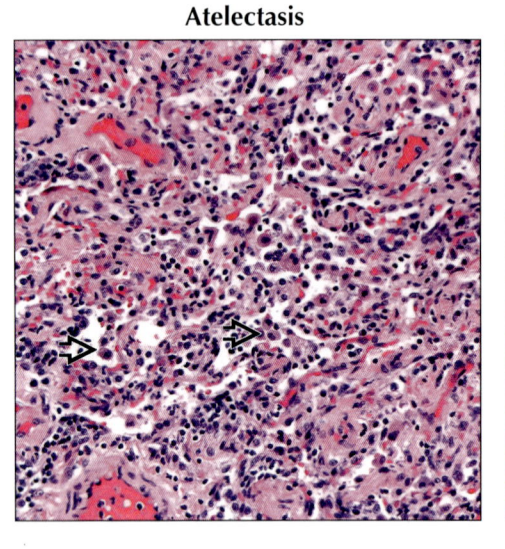

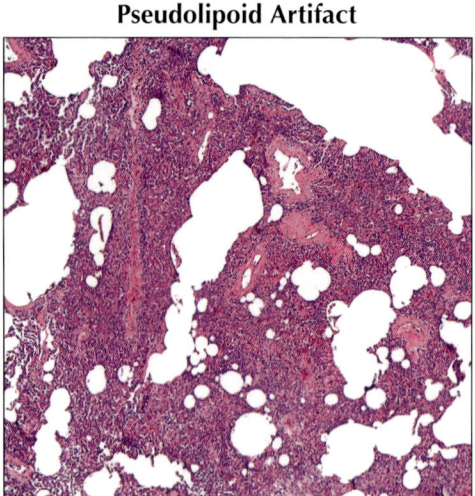

Atelectasis

Pseudolipoid Artifact

(Left) Even when artifactual atelectasis is significant, the normal lung architecture, although compressed, can often still be appreciated. Note the macrophages in the alveoli ➡. (Right) Compression of a lung specimen may lead to the artifactual formation of large, round spaces resembling fat within the tissue. Unlike in cases of lipid aspiration, this artifact shows an absence of multinucleated giant cells around the spaces.

Artifactual Hemorrhage

Peribronchiolar Metaplasia

(Left) Blood ➡ is often seen if the lung is injured during the biopsy/resection process. Unlike true hemorrhage, artifactual (procedure-related) bleeding is patchy and usually does not cross interlobular septae ➡.
(Right) Peribronchiolar metaplasia is due to chronic bronchiolar irritation, such as with cigarette smoking. It is characterized by metaplastic cuboidal cells ➡ that replace the normally flat alveolar epithelium that is immediately adjacent to bronchioles ➡.

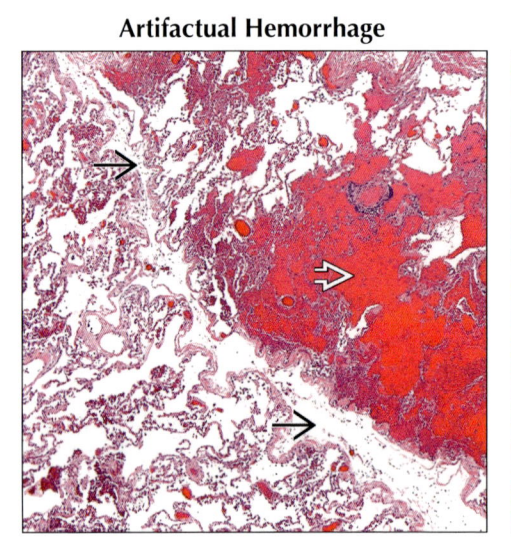

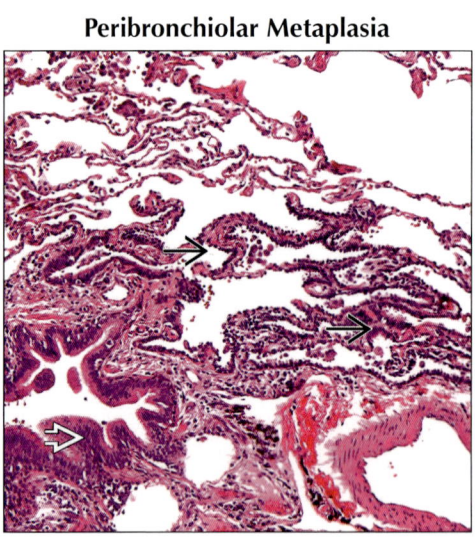

Focal Foreign Body Giant Cell Reaction

Bone Marrow Embolus

(Left) Focal foreign body giant cells ➡ can occasionally be seen reacting to aspirated food particles or talc and other substances. Depending on its composition, a particle ➡ may appear crystalline and glassy unless polarized light is utilized. (Right) It is not uncommon to identify bone marrow tissue ➡ within a pulmonary blood vessel ➡. This finding is common at autopsy and suggests prior bone manipulation (e.g., chest compressions).

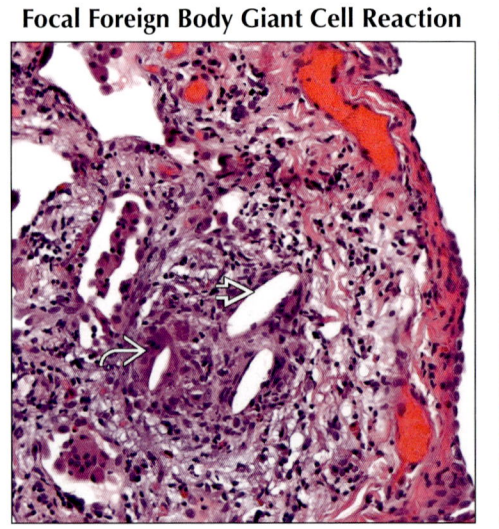

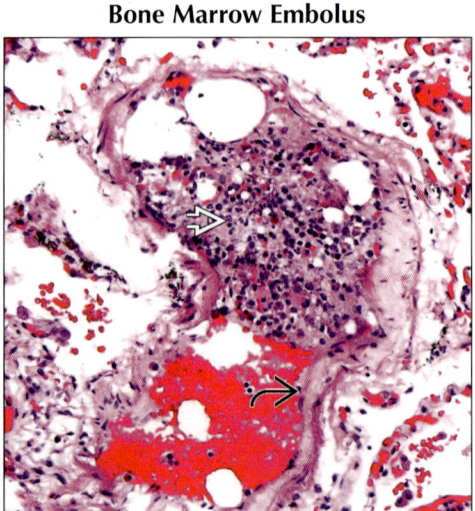

LUNG

Megakaryocytes

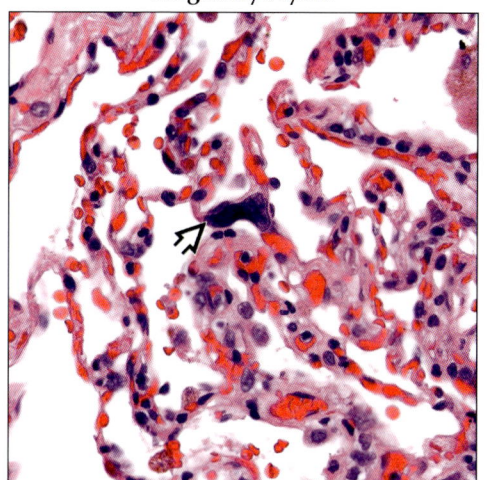

Anthracosis

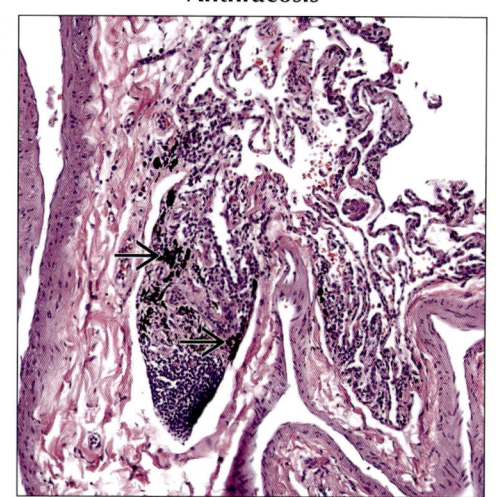

(Left) Megakaryocytes ⊳ within alveolar capillary spaces can be an incidental finding. They are typically large, dark, elongated, and irregularly shaped. They should not be confused with neoplastic cells. *(Right)* A very common finding in lung specimens is the presence of dark carbon (anthracotic) pigment ⊳ within the lung parenchyma, histiocytes, and lymph node sinuses. It is usually most prominent in smokers but can be seen in any city dweller.

Corpora Amylacea

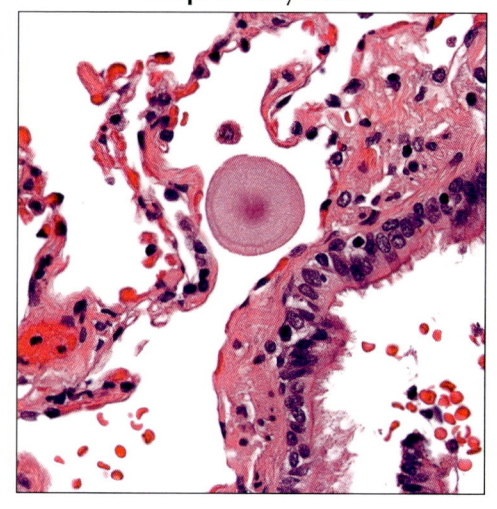

Calcification

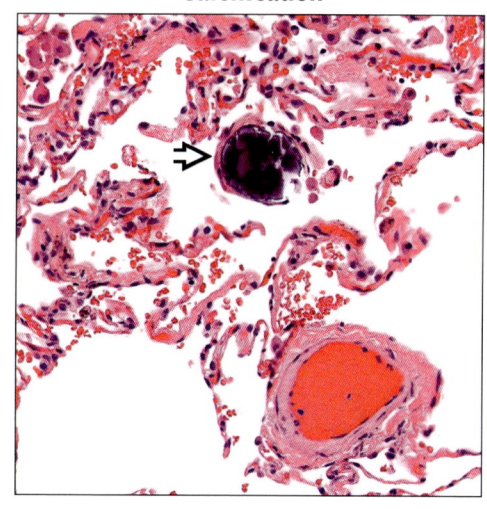

(Left) Similar to what is seen in the prostate, corpora amylacea in the lung are concentrically lamellated pink structures occasionally found within alveoli, particularly in older adults. Their etiology is unclear, and they have no clinical significance. *(Right)* Foci of calcification ⊳ can be seen in pathologic conditions or with increasing age, and may or may not be a significant finding. They are commonly associated with old hyalinized granulomas.

Meningothelial Nodule

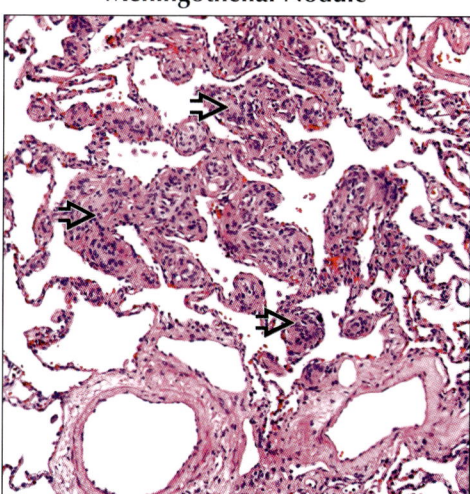

Metaplastic Ossification

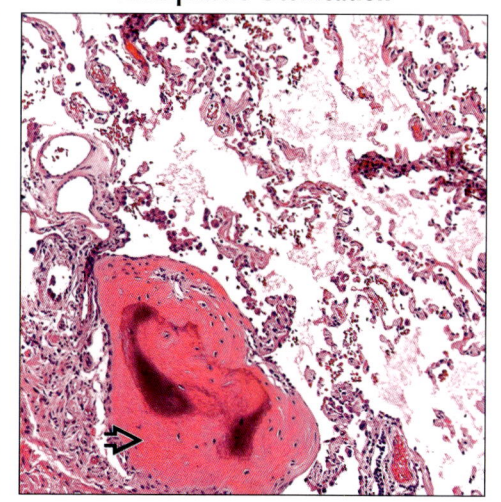

(Left) Meningothelial nodules ⊳ are small, whorled proliferations most often seen in a subpleural distribution. They are often found incidentally and demonstrate histologic and immunophenotypic features of meningeal cells. *(Right)* Mature bone formation ⊳ can rarely be seen in alveoli, particularly in sites of prior inflammation or lung injury, and it can be focal or patchy in distribution. It is also occasionally seen associated with diffuse interstitial (fibrosing) lung disease.

MESOTHELIUM

Key Facts

Macroscopic Anatomy
- Mesothelium lines pleural (chest), pericardial, and peritoneal (abdominal) cavities
- Visceral mesothelium invests regional organs (lungs, intestines) and omental fat
- Parietal mesothelium lines outer surface of cavity
- Abdominal mesentery is where parietal and visceral mesothelial layers meet

Microscopic Anatomy
- Composed of thin layer of cuboidal mesothelial cells overlying submesothelial connective tissue
- Normal mesothelial cells are small, with well-defined cell borders, a single central nucleus with homogeneous chromatin, and no nucleolus
- Reactive mesothelial cells are larger and more conspicuous, with enlarged nuclei and prominent central nucleoli; may show multinucleation; may form papillary structures (hyperplasia)
- In reactive conditions, submesothelium is often thickened and more cellular
- Immunophenotype
  - Positive: Calretinin, cytokeratin AE1/AE3, CK 5/6, WT1, D2-40, HBME-1, thrombomodulin
  - Negative: MOC-31, BER-EP4, B72.3, CEA, CD15

Pitfalls/Artifacts
- Mesothelium is easily denuded and may not be visible
- Odd cuts can lead to misplaced aggregates of mesothelial cells within underlying fat or fibrous tissue
- Mesothelial cells and submesothelial fibroblasts express epithelial antigens (e.g., keratins), which may lead to confusion with carcinoma or mesothelioma

(Left) This image of pleura shows a single layer of normal, nonreactive mesothelial cells ➡. They appear as small cuboidal or flat cells with eosinophilic cytoplasm and indistinct nuclear features. At times, they are difficult to identify in histologic sections and may appear to be absent. *(Right)* This image shows cuboidal mesothelial cells ➡. These cells are easier to identify than flat mesothelial cells but still show a similar bland cytomorphology.

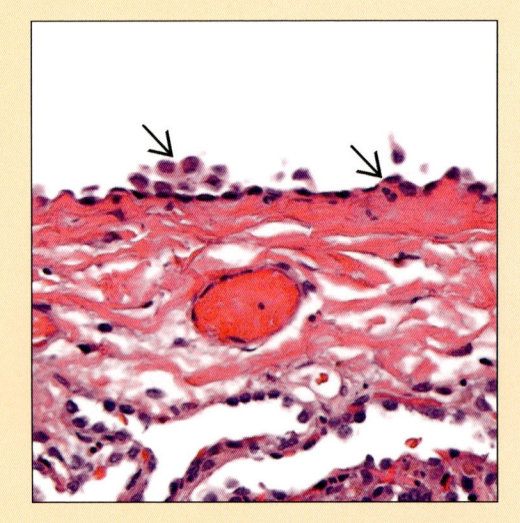

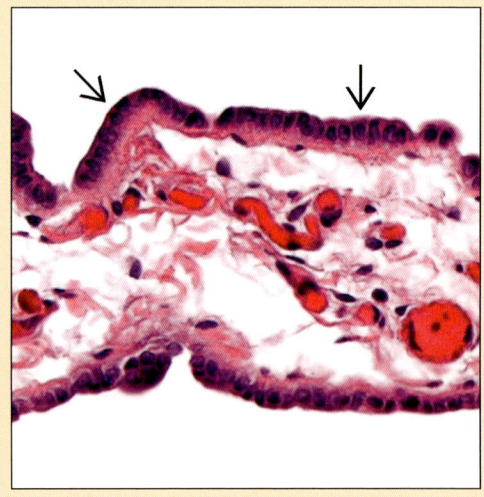

(Left) Reactive mesothelial cells may slough off and appear as nests or sheets of eosinophilic epithelioid cells. They are not cytologically malignant, however, which helps distinguish them from an epithelial malignancy (carcinoma) or mesothelioma. *(Right)* A distinctive feature of reactive mesothelial cells is an open chromatin pattern with 1 to a few small but prominent basophilic nucleoli ➡. This image also shows the characteristic "hobnailing" ➡ or "tombstoning" of these cells.

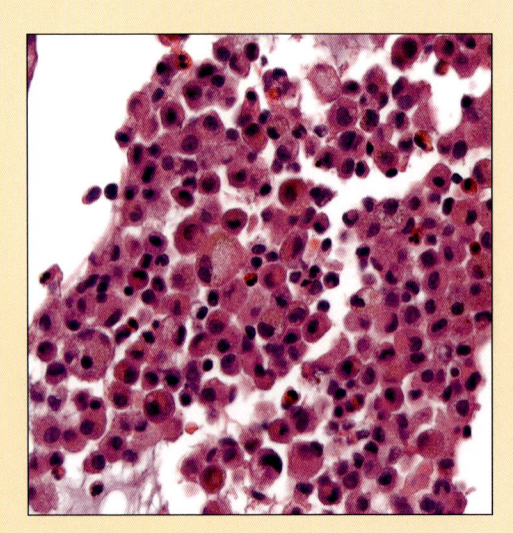

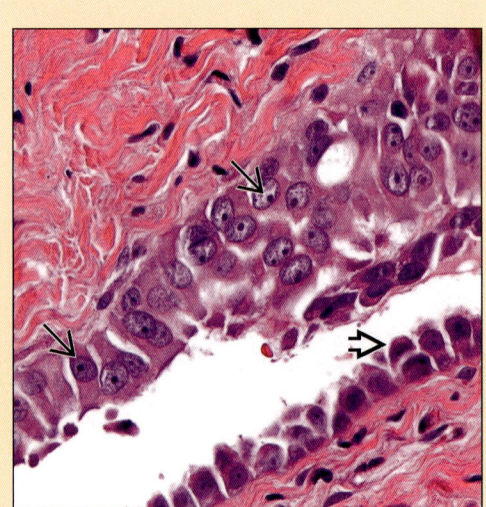

MESOTHELIUM

Mesothelial "Window"

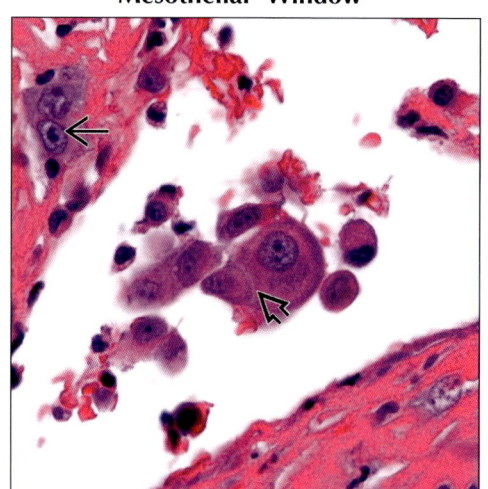

Reactive Mesothelial Cells

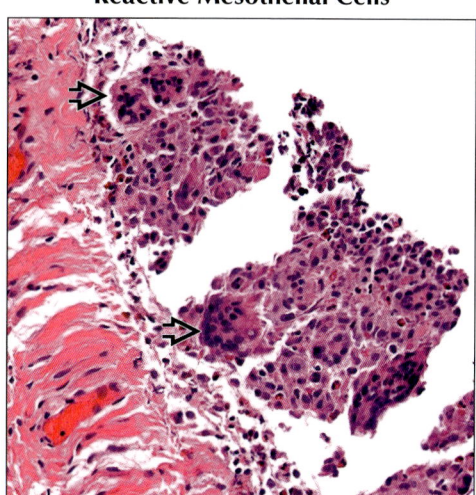

(Left) A unique finding in reactive mesothelial cells is the mesothelial "window," which is a thin, pale zone ⇨ that forms between neighboring cells. Note the prominent reactive nucleoli ⇨. *(Right)* Occasionally, reactive mesothelial cells will show a marked increase in the number of nuclei ⇨, leading to confusion with the multinucleated giant cells of granulomatous infections or foreign body giant cell reactions.

Reactive Papillary Hyperplasia

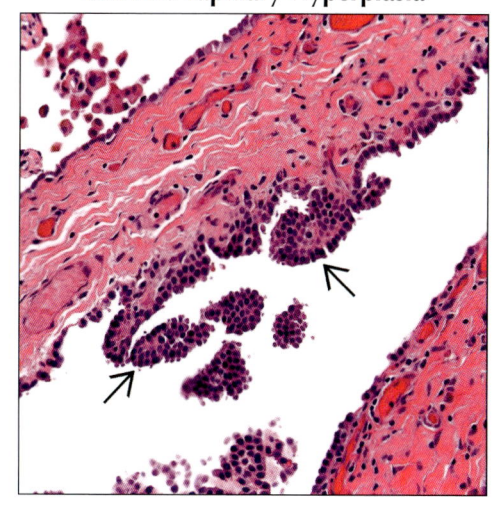

Reactive Papillary Hyperplasia

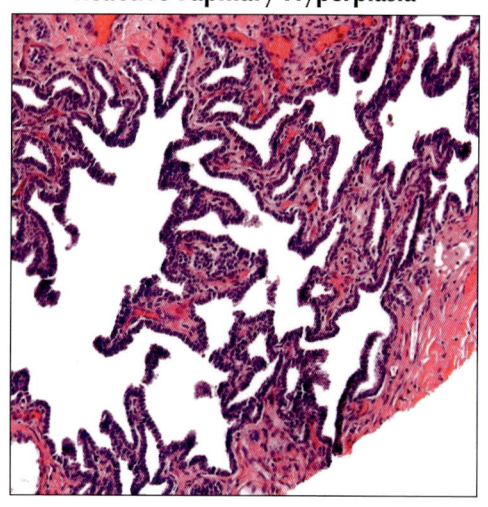

(Left) Reactive mesothelial cells can also form small papillary structures ⇨ that project out into the pleural, pericardial, or peritoneal space. When these changes are diffuse, distinction from a well-differentiated papillary mesothelioma can be very difficult. *(Right)* Reactive papillary mesothelial hyperplasia can be further complicated by tangential sectioning, which can provide the illusion of an infiltrative neoplastic process.

Submesothelial Fibroblasts

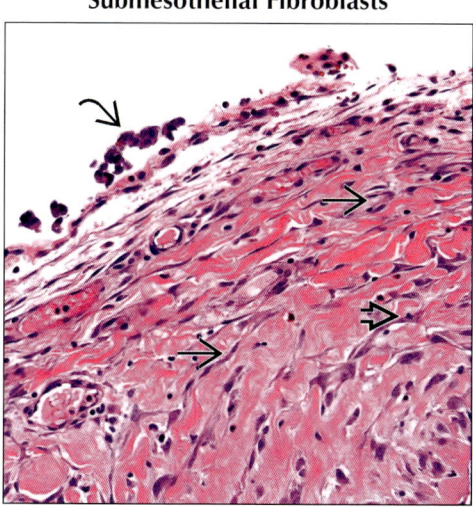

Submesothelial Fibroblasts

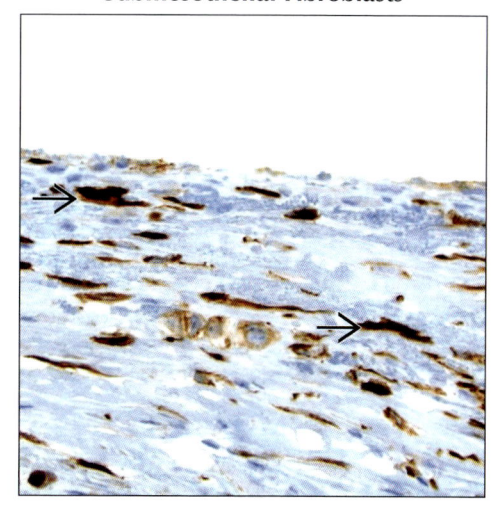

(Left) Submesothelial fibroblasts ⇨ exist in the connective tissue underlying the mesothelium ⇨ and are generally inconspicuous. However, they are more easily identified in reactive conditions, and their cytoplasm becomes more eosinophilic and stellate (angulated) ⇨. *(Right)* Similar to mesothelial cells, submesothelial fibroblasts ⇨ commonly express epithelial antigens by immunohistochemistry, particularly cytokeratin (brown chromogen utilized).

SELECTED REFERENCES

TRACHEA

1. Gail DB et al: Cells of the lung: biology and clinical implications. Am Rev Respir Dis. 127(3):366-87, 1983

2. Breeze RG et al: The cells of the pulmonary airways. Am Rev Respir Dis. 116(4):705-77, 1977

3. Boyden EA: Development of the pulmonary airways. Minn Med. 54(11):894-7, 1971

LUNG

1. Castranova V et al: The alveolar type II epithelial cell: a multifunctional pneumocyte. Toxicol Appl Pharmacol. 93(3):472-83, 1988

2. Gail DB et al: Cells of the lung: biology and clinical implications. Am Rev Respir Dis. 127(3):366-87, 1983

3. Bienenstock J: Gut and bronchus associated lymphoid tissue: an overview. Adv Exp Med Biol. 149:471-7, 1982

4. Kuhn C III: Ultrastructure and cellular function in the distal lung. Monogr Pathol. 19:1-20, 1978

MESOTHELIUM

1. Lee A et al: Mesothelial hyperplasia with reactive atypia: diagnostic pitfalls and role of immunohistochemical studies: a case report. Diagn Cytopathol. 22(2):113-6, 2000

2. Albertine KH et al: The structure of the parietal pleura and its relationship to pleural liquid dynamics in sheep. Anat Rec. 208(3):401-9, 1984

3. Albertine KH et al: Structure, blood supply, and lymphatic vessels of the sheep's visceral pleura. Am J Anat. 165(3):277-94, 1982

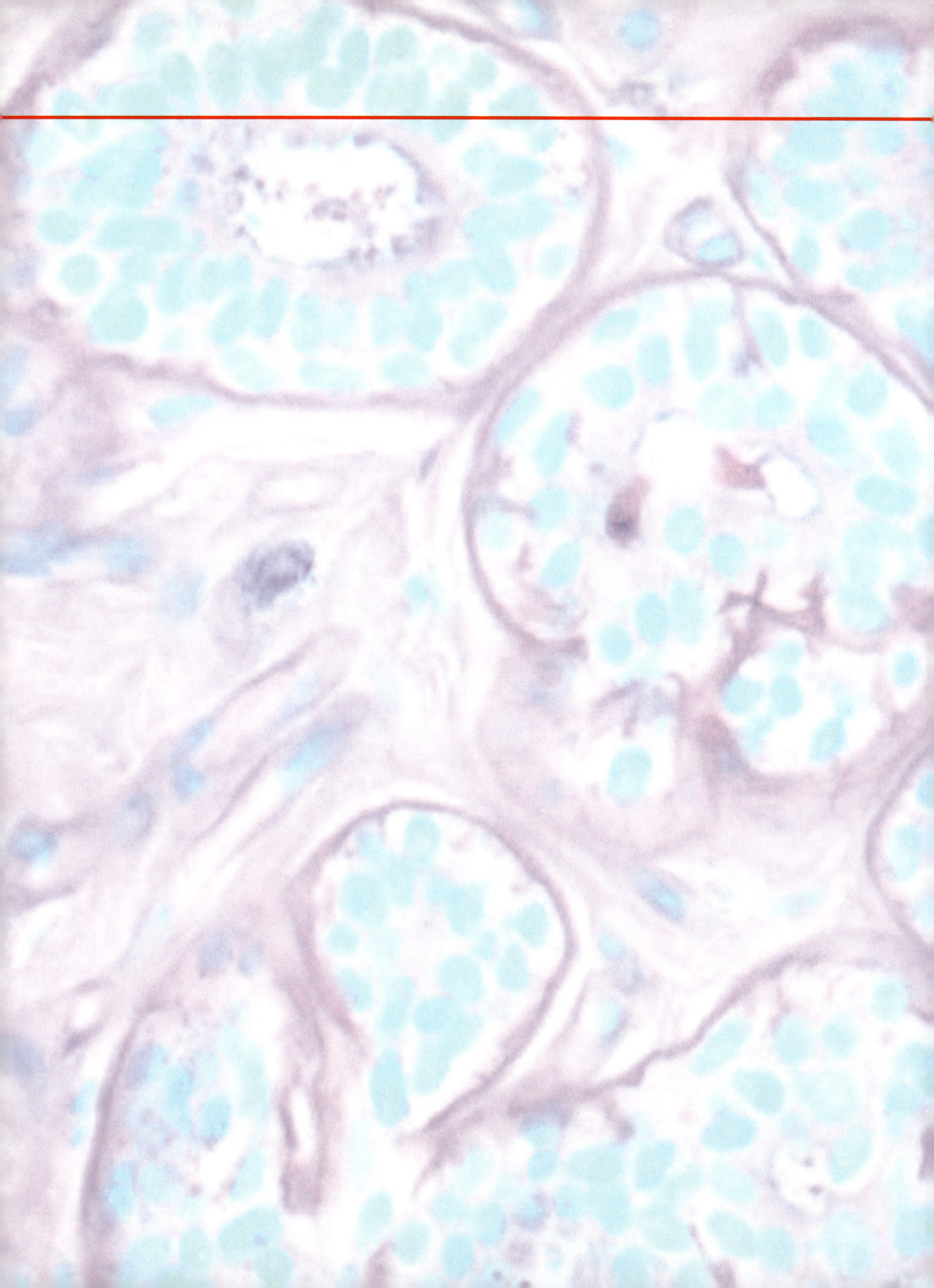

Breast

Breast   9-2

BREAST

Key Facts

Macroscopic Anatomy
- Adult female breast
  - Modified specialized cutaneous glandular structure
  - Located in superficial fascia of anterior chest wall overlying pectoralis major and minor muscles
- Distinctive conical protuberance extending from 2nd to 6th rib in midclavicular line
  - Breast tissue spreads from lateral edge of sternum to anterior axillary line and often extends into axilla
  - Suspensory (Cooper) ligaments are fascial attachments from skin to chest wall
  - Provide support and allow for mobility
- Nipple projects from anterior surface, positioned slightly medial and inferior to center of breast
  - Consists of dense fibrous tissue and smooth muscle bundles covered by hyperpigmented skin
  - Smooth muscle makes the nipple "erectile" and assists with milk expression
  - Milk secretion occurs through 10-15 major duct orifices opening onto nipple surface
- Breast parenchyma consists of branching duct system
  - 15-20 lobes radiate from the nipple, bound together by interlobular connective tissue
  - Ducts are continuous with terminal ductal lobular units (TDLU), responsible for milk production
  - TDLUs are embedded in specialized, hormonally responsive intralobular stroma
  - Glandular tissue is admixed with varying amounts of adipose tissue, responsible for variability in breast size

Physiologic Function
- Secretes milk for nourishment and immunologic protection of the young during postpartum lactation
  - Target organ for a variety of hormones that regulate development and physiologic function
  - Hormonal and growth factor effects result in ongoing lifelong changes in response to menarche, pregnancy, lactation, and menopause
  - These cyclical changes over the life cycle result in a broad range of what might be considered normal breast histology
  - Some histologic patterns seen in specimens submitted for pathologic examination represent variants of physiologic changes

Embryologic/Fetal Development
- Milk lines appear as 2 thickened ventral bands of ectoderm during 5th week of gestation
  - Initially extend from axilla to groin
  - Most of the milk line regresses except for segment in thoracic-pectoral region, forming mammary ridge
  - Rarely, supernumerary nipples &/or ectopic breast tissue can develop in other areas along milk line
  - May enlarge and produce milk during lactation
- Breast tissue development begins with mesenchymal stromal differentiation
  - Induces down growth of overlying epithelium, forming 15-20 epithelial strips
  - Placental hormones initiate canalization of epithelium, increasing mammary tissue

Microscopic Anatomy
- Epidermis of nipple has thick keratin layer
  - Protects against trauma and drying from nursing
  - Lactiferous duct is lined by squamous epithelium where the duct traverses epidermis of nipple
  - Lining cells transition to columnar epithelium distal to lactiferous sinus
- Breast epithelium is composed of a simple bilayer of cells lining entire mammary duct/lobular system
  - Inner luminal cells are required for milk production
  - Outer myoepithelial cells assist with milk ejection
  - Stem cells that give rise to both cell types are present but require special techniques for recognition

Age Variation
- Histology of breast tissue undergoes substantial change during period from early adolescence to menopause
- Estrogen mediates development of ductal tissue; progesterone facilitates TDLU development; prolactin regulates milk production

(Left) The adult female breast is located on the anterior chest wall, overlying the pectoralis muscles ➡. The nipple-areolar complex ➡ is located slightly inferior to center, and connects the overlying skin to the mammary parenchyma ➡. *(Right)* The major breast structures are the nipple-areolar complex ➡, the large duct system ➡, and the terminal duct lobular units ➡. Glandular breast tissue is supported by connective tissue (interlobular and intralobular stroma, and adipose tissue ➡).

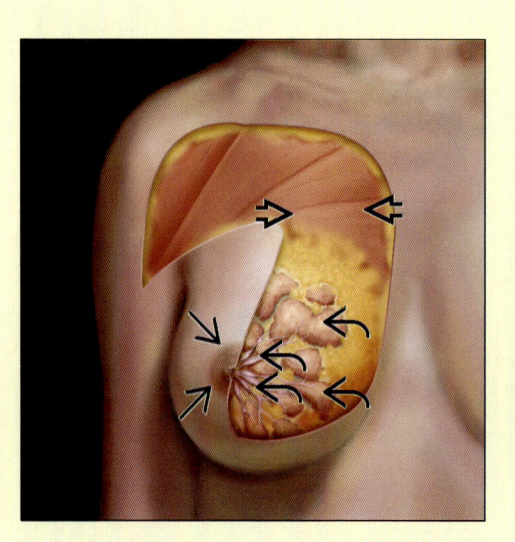

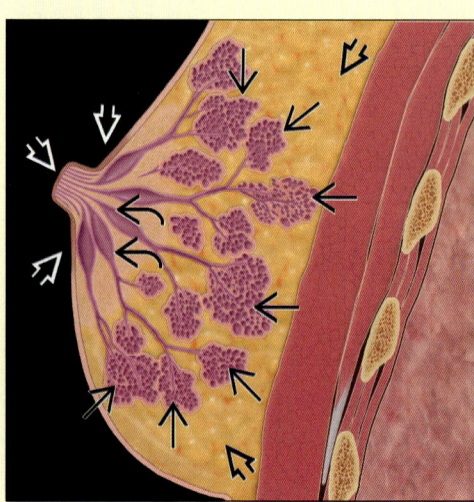

BREAST

Nipple/Areolar Complex

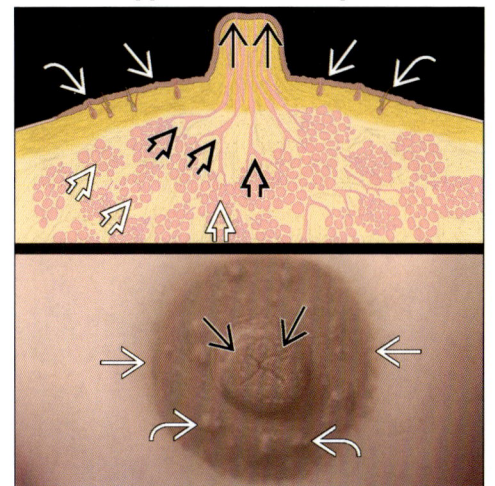

Prophylactic Subcutaneous Mastectomy

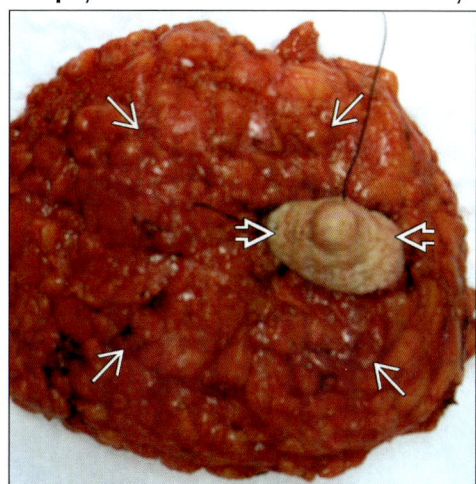

(Left) The nipple-areolar complex is covered by a pigmented squamous epithelium ⇒ and contains sebaceous glands (Montgomery tubercles ⇒). During lactation, milk is produced in the lobules ⇒ and is transported via ducts ⇒ that lead to the nipple orifices ⇒. *(Right)* A mastectomy may be performed to reduce risk of subsequent cancer in some high-risk patients. In this case, the nipple ⇒ and breast tissue were removed, sparing the skin. The anterior breast tissue ⇒ corresponds to the skin flap margins.

Nipple, Gross Evaluation

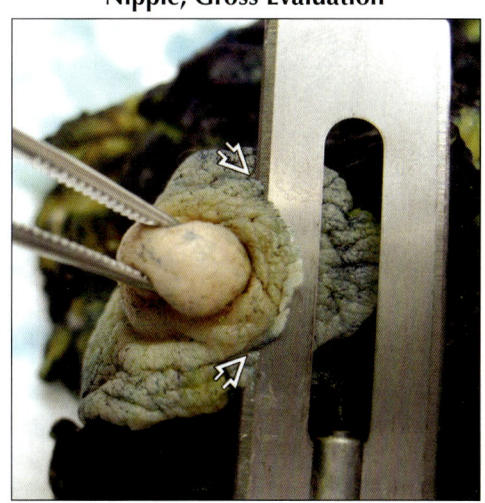

Nipple, Gross Evaluation

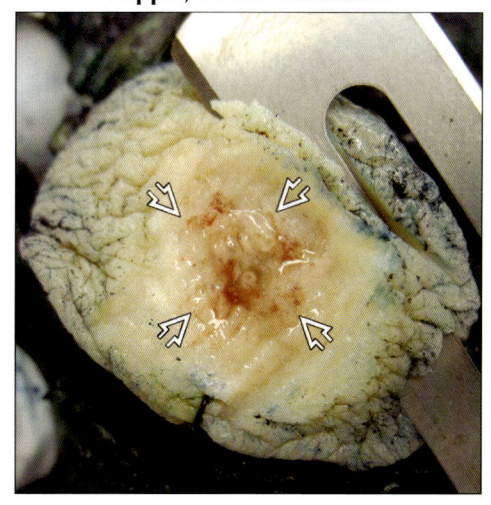

(Left) Microscopic examination of the nipple is important to exclude nipple or skin involvement by disease. The nipple is first removed by carefully cutting across the base ⇒, parallel to the skin surface. *(Right)* After the nipple has been removed, an en face section of the nipple can be taken for microscopic examination of the base of the nipple ⇒. This tissue will show cross sections of the major ducts and lactiferous sinuses as they extend to the nipple surface.

Nipple, Gross Evaluation

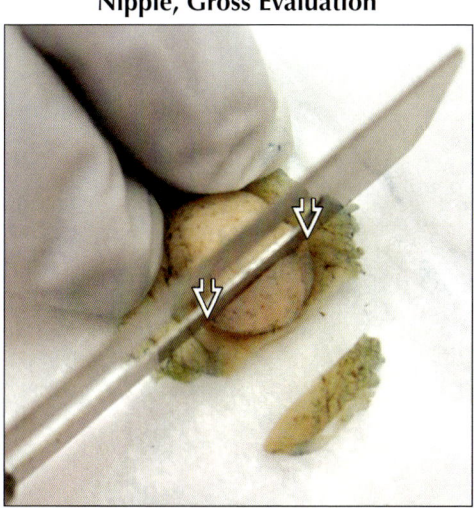

Nipple, Sections for Microscopy

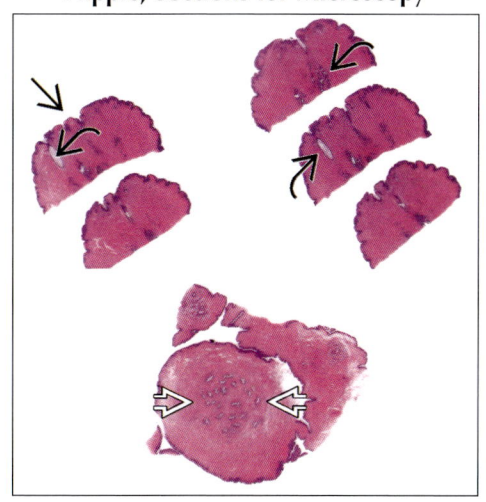

(Left) Perpendicular sections ⇒ of the nipple allow for examination of the overlying nipple epidermis and the lactiferous ducts as they extend to the nipple orifice. *(Right)* Microscopic examination of perpendicular sections of the nipple show the epidermis ⇒ and the major lactiferous ducts ⇒. Microscopic examination of the base of the nipple shows the lactiferous sinuses ⇒.

BREAST

Nipple and Lactiferous Duct

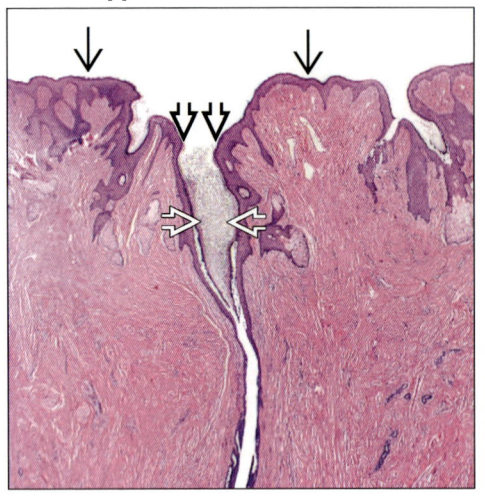

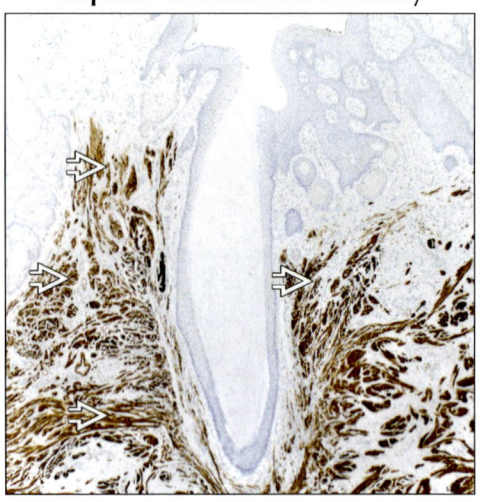

(Left) Squamous epithelium ⇨ covers the nipple and areola. The orifices of the lactiferous ducts are also squamous lined where the duct traverses the epidermis ⇨. Keratin plugs ⇨ may be present in the nipple orifices in the non-lactating breast. **(Right)** Lactiferous ducts in the nipple are surrounded by bundles of smooth muscle ⇨, which are embedded in a collagenous and elastic stroma. Longitudinal muscle bundles along the lactiferous ducts are responsible for nipple erection.

Calponin Immunohistochemistry

Squamous/Columnar Junction

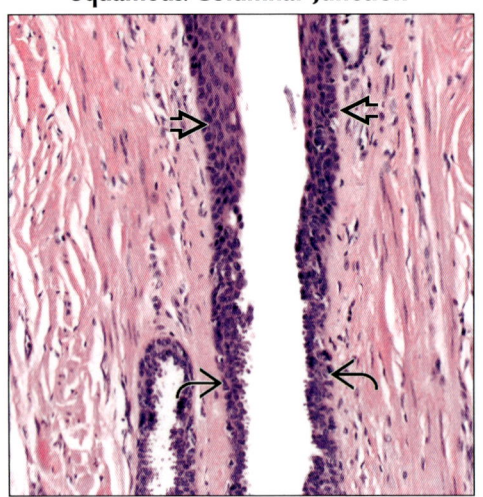

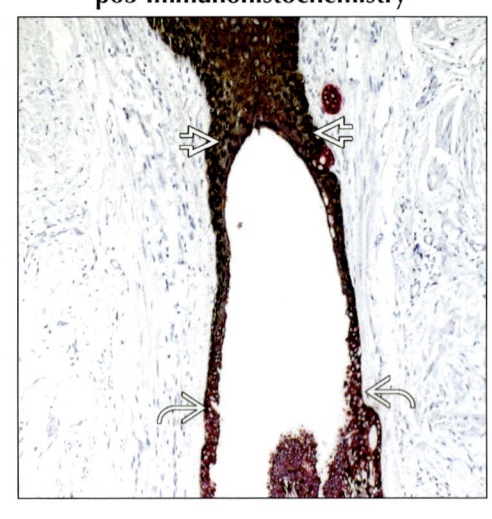

(Left) The squamous epithelium of the epidermis ⇨ dips into the nipple orifice for 1-3 mm, where it joins the columnar epithelium ⇨ to form an abrupt squamo-columnar junction distal to the lactiferous sinus. **(Right)** Immunohistochemistry can be used to highlight the different cell types seen in the squamo-columnar junction of the lactiferous ducts. Cytokeratin 7 stains the luminal cells ⇨ (red chromogen), while CK5/6 and p63 stain the squamous epithelium ⇨ (brown chromogen).

Cytokeratin 7 and CK5/6 With p63 Immunohistochemistry

Lactiferous Sinuses

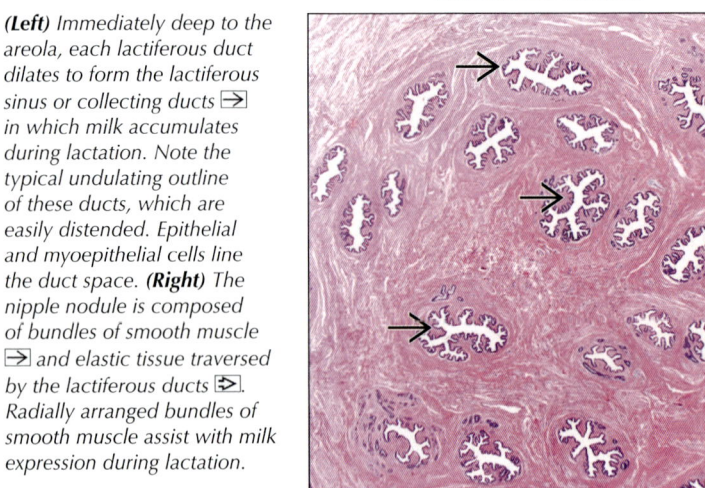

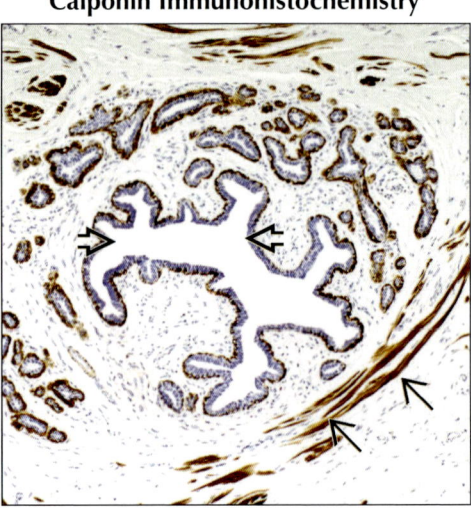

(Left) Immediately deep to the areola, each lactiferous duct dilates to form the lactiferous sinus or collecting ducts ⇨ in which milk accumulates during lactation. Note the typical undulating outline of these ducts, which are easily distended. Epithelial and myoepithelial cells line the duct space. **(Right)** The nipple nodule is composed of bundles of smooth muscle ⇨ and elastic tissue traversed by the lactiferous ducts ⇨. Radially arranged bundles of smooth muscle assist with milk expression during lactation.

Calponin Immunohistochemistry

BREAST

Mammary Duct System

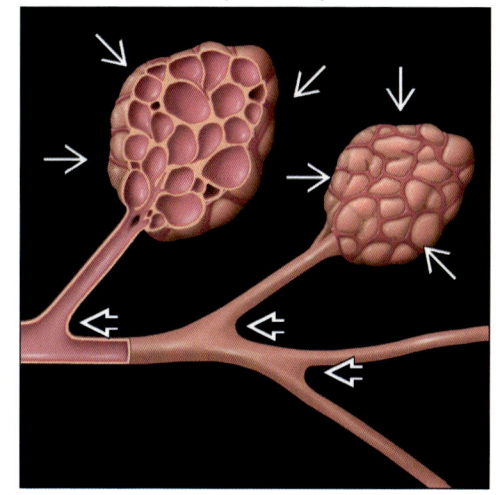

TDLU

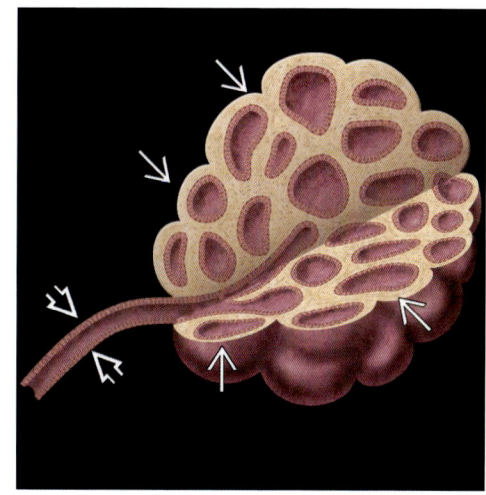

(Left) The epithelial components of the breast consist of a branching system of large and intermediate interlobular ducts ➡ that connect the structural and functional units of the breast (TDLUs ➡) to the nipple. *(Right)* The terminal ductules ➡ end in lobular/glandular units called the TDLUs ➡. Lobule formation from the terminal ducts is apparent within 1 to 2 years after the onset of the menses. Thereafter, glandular development is variable. Full differentiation of the mammary gland is attained during pregnancy.

Interlobular Mammary Ducts

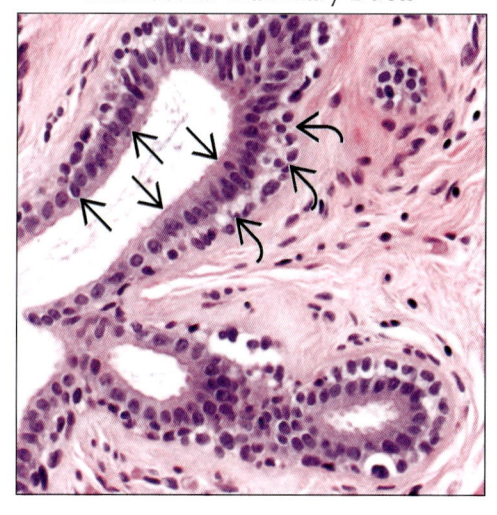

TDLU

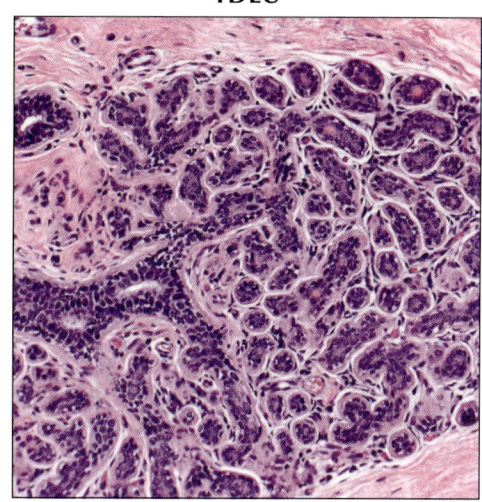

(Left) The mammary ductal/lobular system is composed of a bilayer of cells, extending from the major lactiferous duct to the TDLUs. The luminal cells form a columnar layer ➡ in the interlobular ducts and are surrounded by a layer of myoepithelial cells ➡. *(Right)* The normal histology of the lobules is not constant in the mature female breast because of changes associated with fluctuations in hormonal levels (during menstrual cycle, pregnancy, lactation, and menopause).

Cytokeratin 7 and CK5/6 With p63 Immunohistochemistry

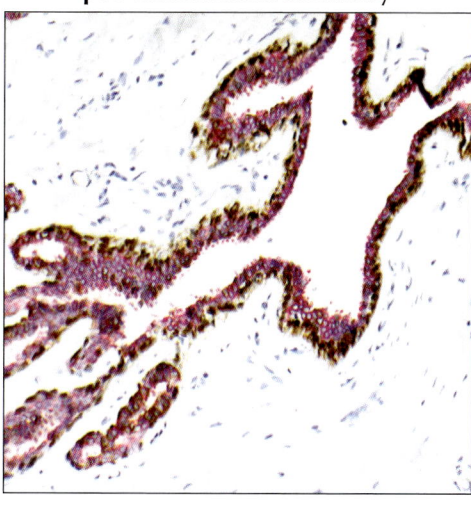

Cytokeratin 7 and CK5/6 With p63 Immunohistochemistry

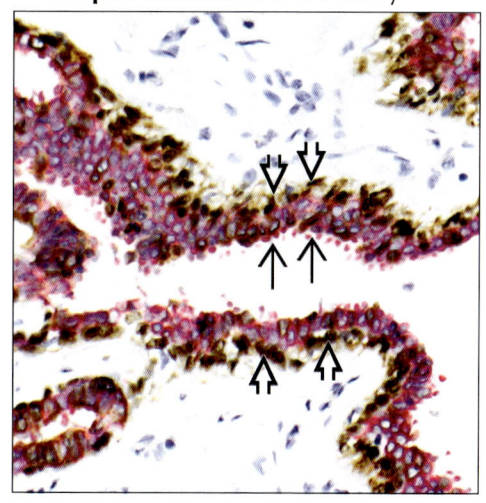

(Left) Luminal and myoepithelial cells differentially express low and high molecular weight cytokeratins, respectively. Luminal cells express low molecular weight luminal cytokeratins (CK 7, red chromogen). Myoepithelial cells express high molecular weight basal cytokeratins (CK 5/14/17) and other distinguishing markers such as p63 (brown chromogen). *(Right)* High-power photo shows luminal cells expressing low molecular weight CK 7 ➡ and myoepithelial cells expressing p63 ➡.

BREAST

TDLU

(Left) TDLUs have an architectural organization similar to a tree if the trunk and branches were hollow. The terminal duct ("trunk") ➔ opens into the acini ("branches") ➔ of the lobule. This "lobulocentric" organization is a key microscopic feature in recognizing normal breast structure. **(Right)** There are 2 types of epithelial cells. Luminal cells express keratins 7, 8, and 18 (red cytoplasmic chromogen ➔). Myoepithelial cells express p63 ➔ (brown nuclear chromogen).

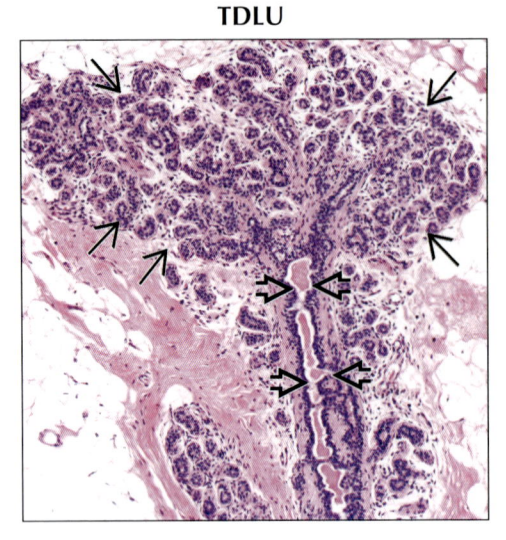

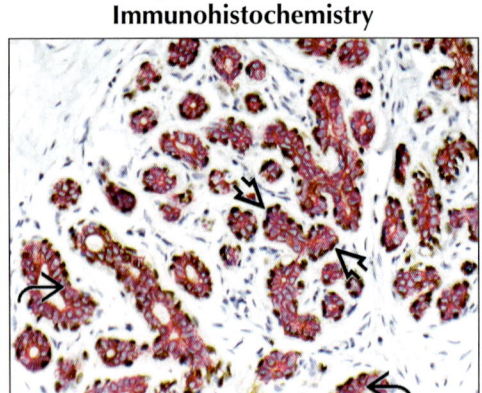

Cytokeratin 7/p63 Immunohistochemistry

Estrogen Receptor Immunohistochemistry

(Left) Not all luminal cells express ER ➔. The content of ER and PR in the normal luminal cells varies with the degree of lobular development, in parallel with cell proliferation. **(Right)** Proliferation is an important part of the growth and development of breast tissue. Scattered Ki-67(+) cells (a marker of proliferation ➔) can be found in the normal TDLU; however, these cells are negative for ER. Different populations of luminal cells within the breast may interact in a paracrine fashion.

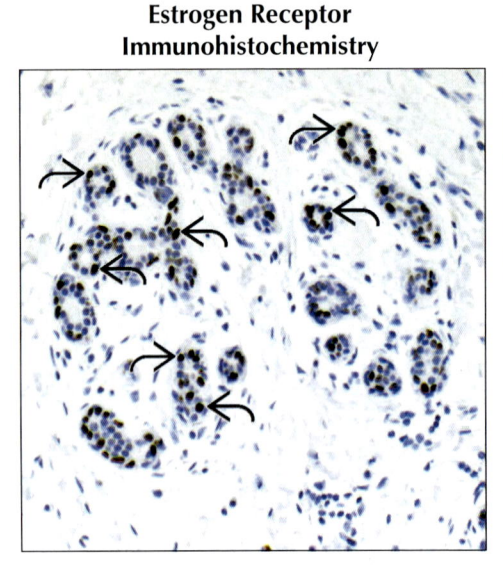

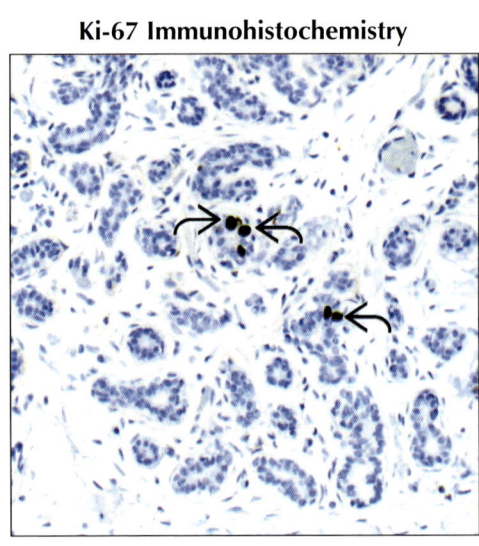

Ki-67 Immunohistochemistry

TDLU

(Left) The basement membrane surrounding the ducts and lobules contains type IV collagen and laminin and appears as a bright pink layer on Alcian blue/PAS staining ➔. This basement membrane is contiguous with that of the large ducts and skin. **(Right)** The TDLU has a specialized intralobular stroma enveloping the acini and consisting of CD34(+) stromal fibroblasts ➔ and capillaries. Lesions arising from this stroma (fibroadenomas and phyllodes tumors) are biphasic.

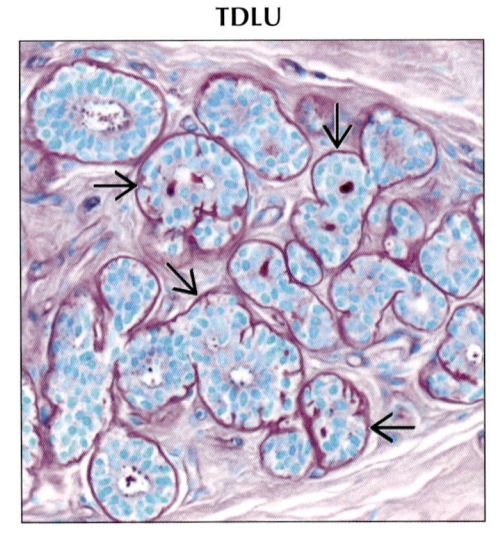

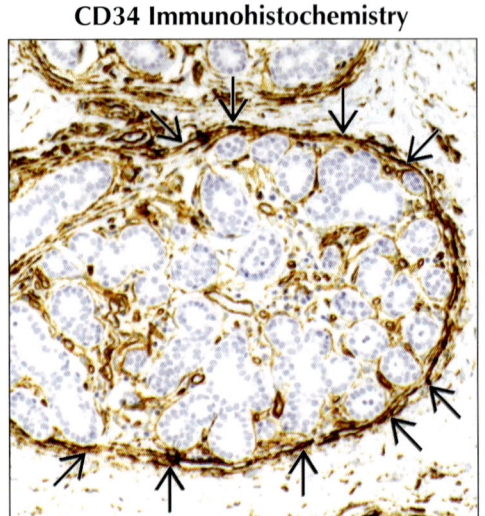

CD34 Immunohistochemistry

BREAST

Pregnancy and Lactation

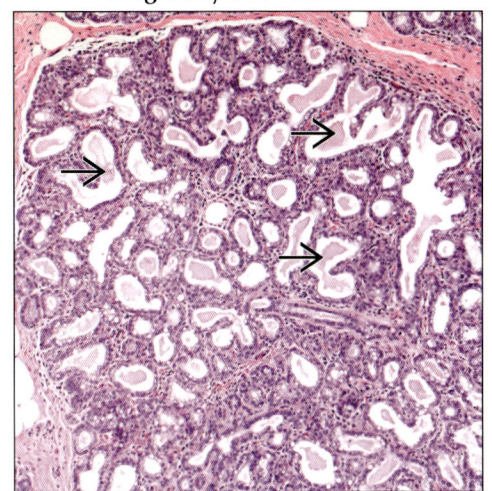

Pregnancy and Lactation

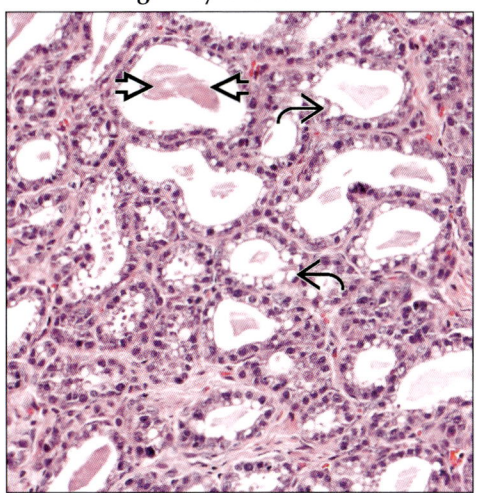

(Left) During early pregnancy, epithelial cells rapidly proliferate, with expansion of both the size and number of lobules due to the influence of placental hormones. The lobular acini dilate and undergo secretory changes in preparation for lactation ➡. *(Right)* The luminal cells of the TDLU become vacuolated ➡ and show nuclear enlargement with prominent nucleoli during pregnancy and lactation. The acinar lumina become progressively dilated and distended by the accumulation of secretory material or colostrum ➡.

Pregnancy and Lactation

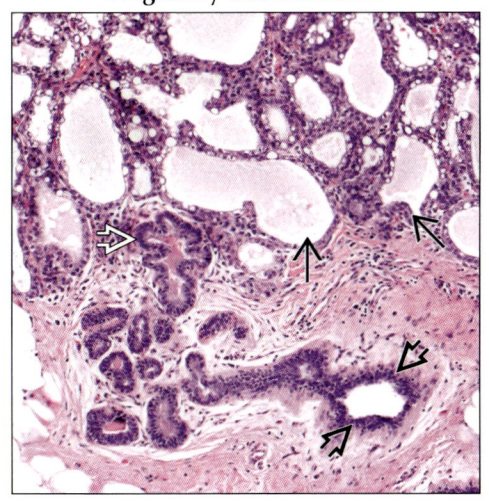

Post-Lactation Involution

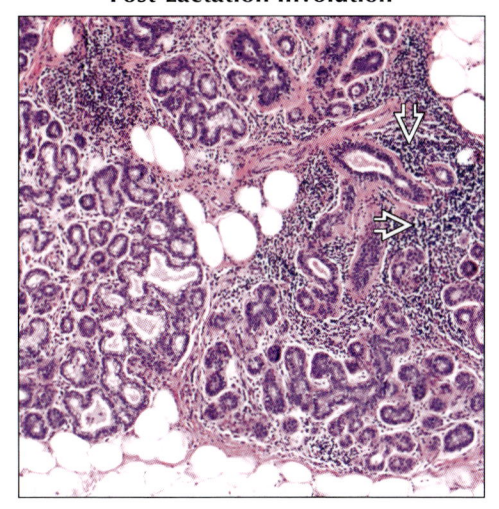

(Left) The large duct system ➡ in lactational breast can be distinguished from the TDLUs ➡ because secretory changes only occur in the TDLUs. There is an abrupt transition from the terminal duct ➡ to the TDLU. *(Right)* The postlactational breast requires both lactogenic hormone deprivation and local signals to undergo glandular involution. A prominent lymphocytic infiltrate surrounds the lobules ➡. The lobules do not regress to their pre-pregnancy state but maintain a more differentiated lobular organization.

Menopause

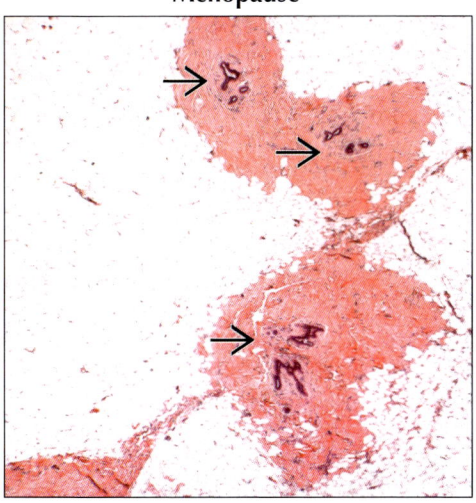

Menopause

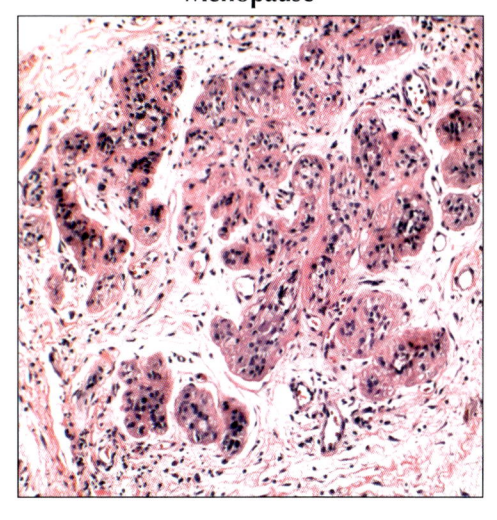

(Left) The breast undergoes involution following menopause and a greater percentage of the breast consists of stroma and fatty tissue. During involution, the lobules and the specialized lobular stroma begin to disappear, leaving only small terminal ducts ➡. The interlobular stroma becomes more fatty, making the breast more radiolucent. *(Right)* In an atrophic lobule, myoepithelial cells and basement membranes become more prominent and luminal cells regress. The myoepithelial cells sometimes appear spindled in shape.

SELECTED REFERENCES

BREAST

1. Russo J et al: Pattern of distribution of cells positive for estrogen receptor alpha and progesterone receptor in relation to proliferating cells in the mammary gland. Breast Cancer Res Treat. 53(3):217-27, 1999

2. Russo J et al: Influence of age and parity on the development of the human breast. Breast Cancer Res Treat. 23(3):211-8, 1992

3. Hultborn KA et al: The lymph drainage from the breast to the axillary and parasternal lymph nodes, studied with the aid of colloidal Au198. Acta radiol. 43(1):52-64, 1955

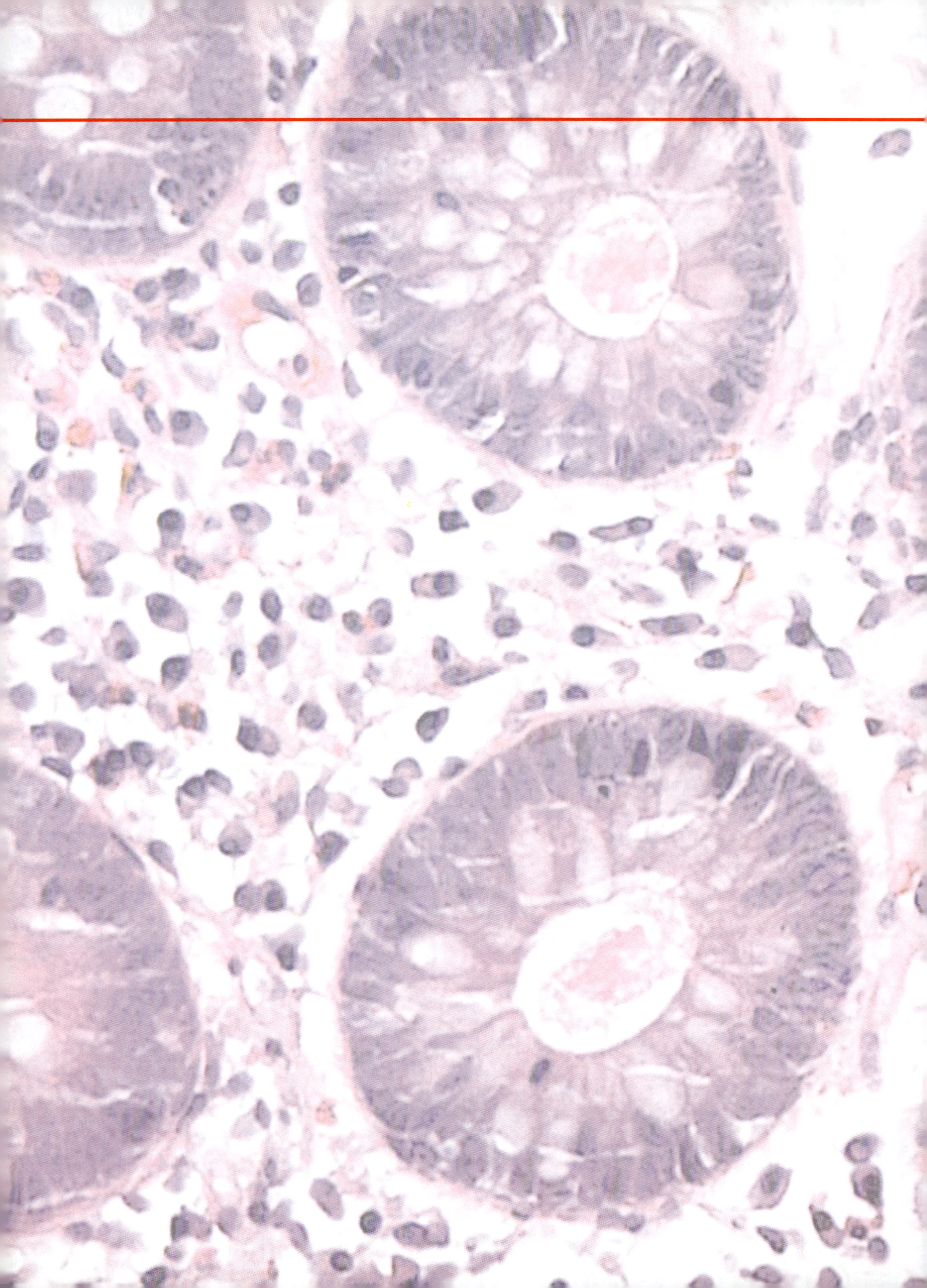

Tubular Gut and Peritoneum

Esophagus	10-2
Stomach	10-8
Small Intestine	10-14
Large Intestine	10-18
Appendix	10-24
Anus and Anal Canal	10-28
Peritoneal Membranes	10-32

ESOPHAGUS

Key Facts

Macroscopic Anatomy
- Muscular tube approximately 25 cm in length
  - Prominent longitudinal folds when not insufflated
  - Z-line: Macroscopically defines the gastroesophageal junction

Microscopic Anatomy
- Epithelium: Stratified squamous with few scattered intraepithelial lymphocytes and Langerhans cells
- Lamina propria: Located under epithelium and above muscularis mucosa; contains blood vessels, inflammatory cells, and mucous glands
  - A minority of people have melanocytes at the epithelial-stromal junction
- Muscularis mucosae: Thin, longitudinal bands of smooth muscle that demarcate the mucosa from the submucosa
- Submucosa: Loose connective tissue containing blood vessels, lymphatics, nerve fibers, and mucous (salivary-type) glands
- Muscularis propria: Thick smooth muscle bundles (inner circular and outer longitudinal layers)
- Adventitia: Most of the esophagus is lined by loose connective fascial sheath; lacks true serosa for most of its length
- Squamocolumnar junction: Transition from stratified squamous epithelium to glandular epithelium
  - Glandular epithelium at junction may be a mix of mucous and oxyntic glands, or exclusively mucous glands

Pitfalls/Artifacts
- Glycogenic acanthosis can mimic candidiasis macroscopically
- Contamination by normal oral flora (bacteria and yeast) can mimic true infection
- Heterotopic tissue (e.g., gastric and sebaceous) can mimic neoplasms macroscopically

Metaplasia
- Intestinal metaplasia (Barrett esophagus)
- Pancreatic acinar metaplasia common; no clinical significance

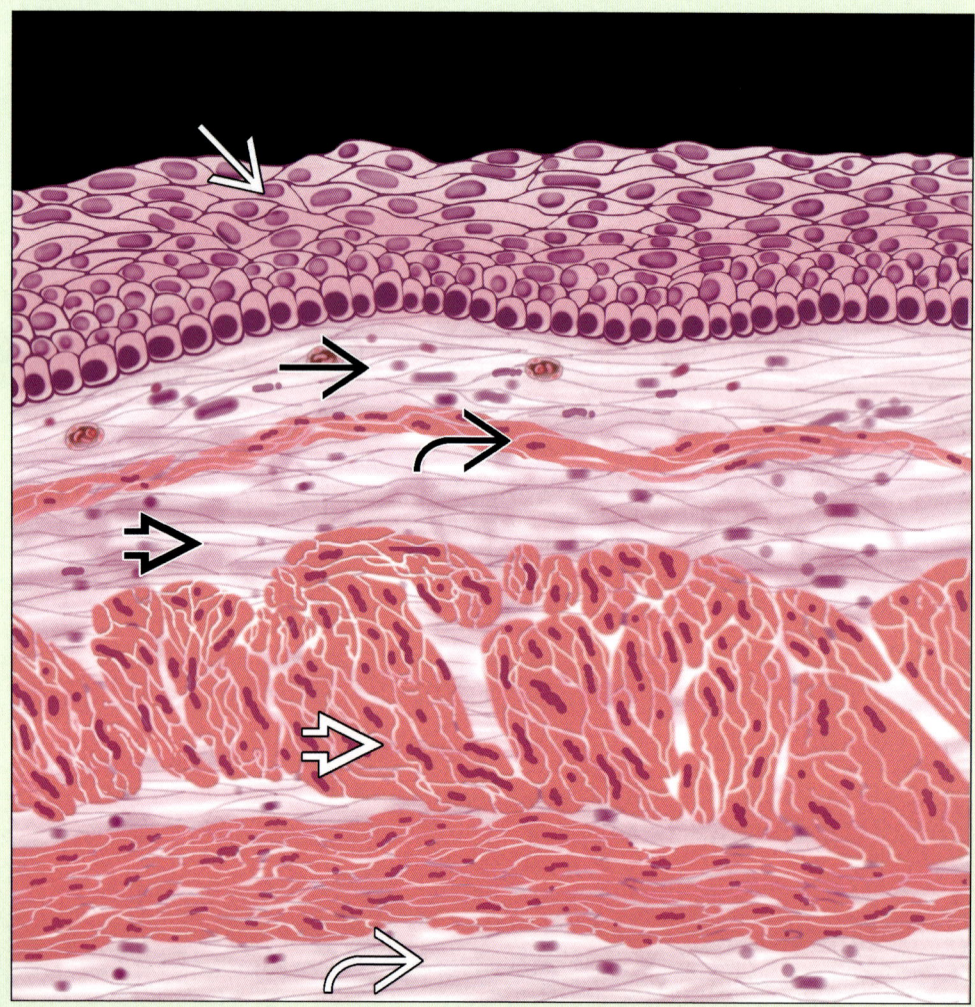

From superficial (luminal) to deep, the anatomical layers of the esophagus are: Stratified squamous epithelium ➡, lamina propria ➡, muscularis mucosa ➡, submucosa ➡, muscularis propria (includes inner circular/circumferential layer and outer longitudinal layer) ➡, and the adventitial connective tissue ➡.

ESOPHAGUS

Squamous Epithelium

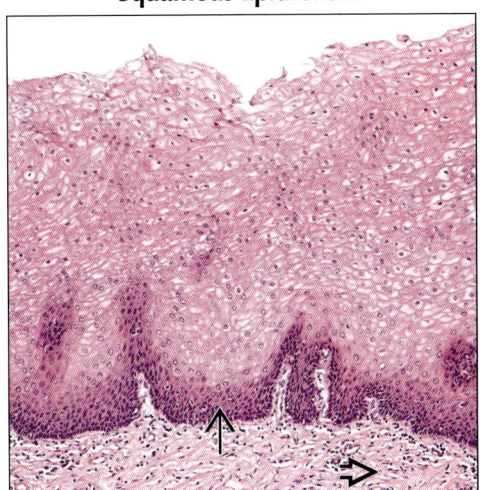

Squamous Epithelium

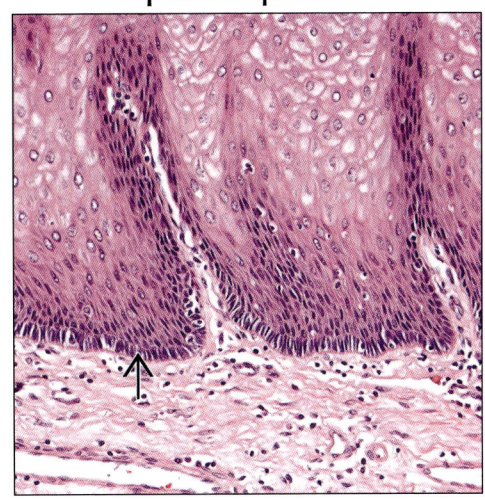

(**Left**) The esophagus is lined by nonkeratinized stratified squamous epithelium. The basal cell layer ⇨ contains actively proliferating basal cells that give rise to the squamous cells above them, which mature further as they progress toward the surface where they are ultimately sloughed off. This renewal process continues indefinitely. Note the underlying lamina propria ⇨. (**Right**) The basal cell layer ⇨ is readily identified due to its higher nuclear density.

Squamous Epithelium

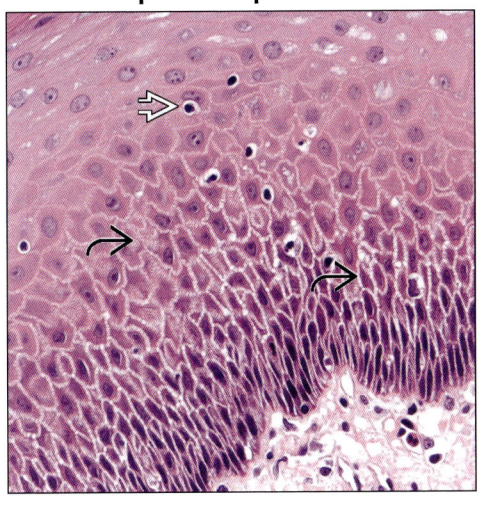

Squamous Epithelium

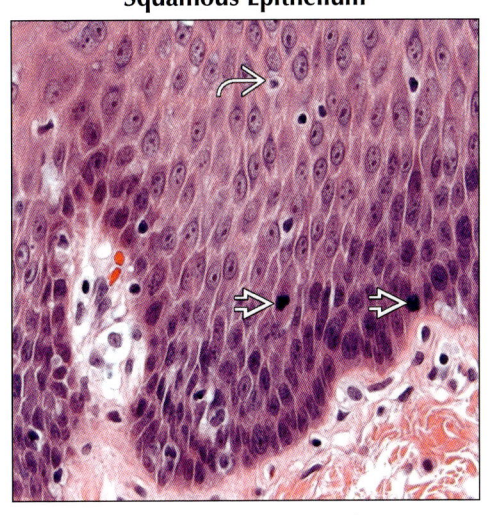

(**Left**) In various reactive conditions (e.g., reflux), the basal half of the epithelium often displays prominent intercellular edema, which highlights the desmosomes ⇨ connecting the squamous cells. Scattered intraepithelial lymphocytes ⇨ are common normally, especially in the basal area. (**Right**) Since it is a site of active proliferation, mitotic figures ⇨ can often be identified in the normal basal layer. They are larger than the intraepithelial lymphocytes ⇨.

Squamous Epithelium, Reactive

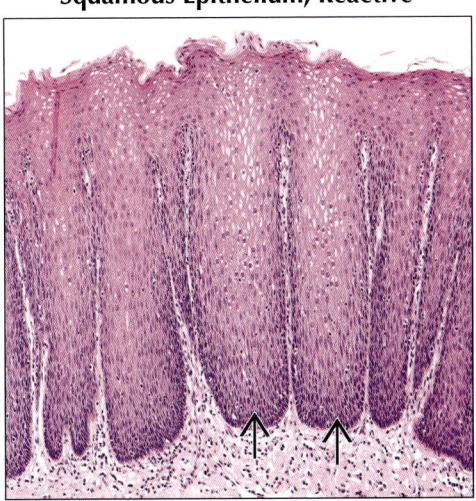

Heterotopia

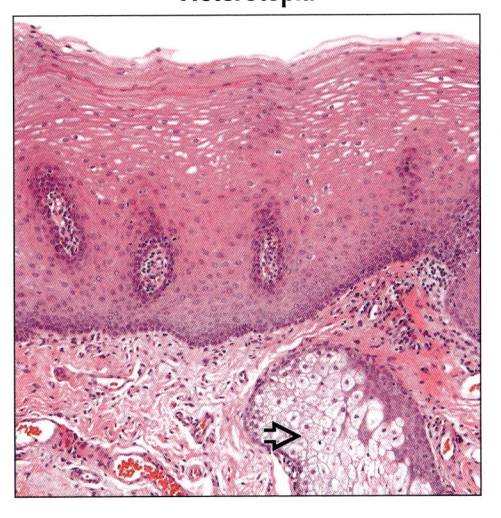

(**Left**) In reactive conditions, elongation of the tongue-like epithelial rete pegs is common ⇨. Compare the significant elongation in this case of reflux to images of the normal esophagus. (**Right**) On occasion, normal mucosal tissue not typically found in the esophagus (such as gastric or sebaceous tissue ⇨) will appear as small nodules in the proximal esophagus. This is considered a normal variant finding (ectopic/heterotopic) and is not neoplastic.

ESOPHAGUS

Glycogenic Acanthosis

(Left) All maturing squamous cells contain some intracytoplasmic glycogen (which gives them a clear appearance), but occasionally the glycogen is prominent ⇨ and grossly nodular, known as glycogenic acanthosis. This is a normal variant, but can mimic candidiasis grossly. (Right) A PAS stain highlights the intracytoplasmic glycogen in glycogenic acanthosis.

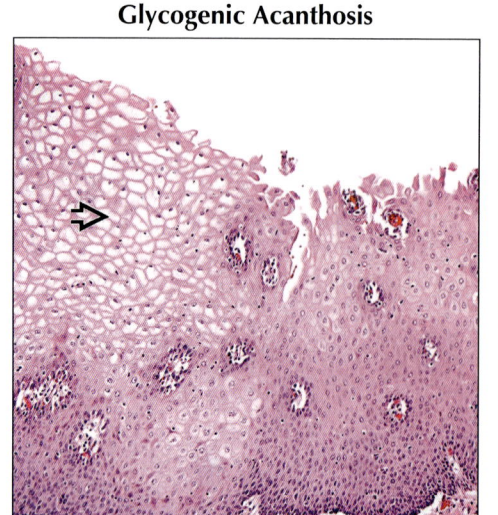

Food Matter / Oral Flora

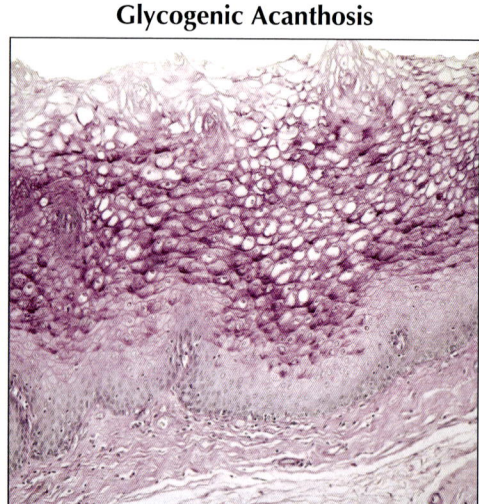

(Left) Food matter is an incidental finding, particularly near esophageal strictures. Meat products appear as red striated skeletal muscle. Accompanying blue clusters of bacteria are often present ⇨. (Right) In addition to bacteria, the oral cavity normally contains fungi (e.g., Candida). These organisms ⇨ are frequently swept up with denuded oral epithelial cells or food and swallowed, and can appear in esophageal biopsies. This should not be mistaken for true infection.

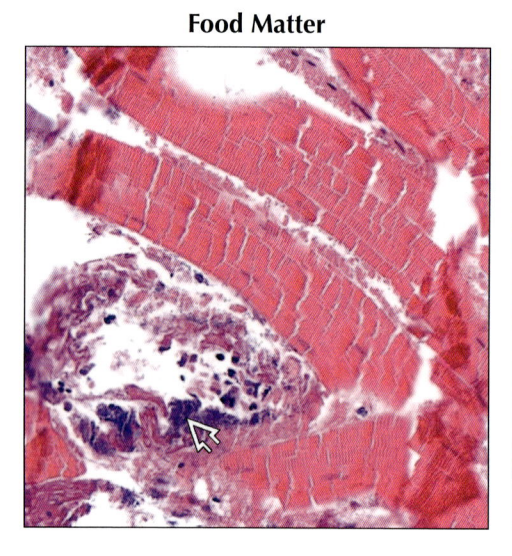

Lamina Propria / Muscularis Mucosa and Submucosa

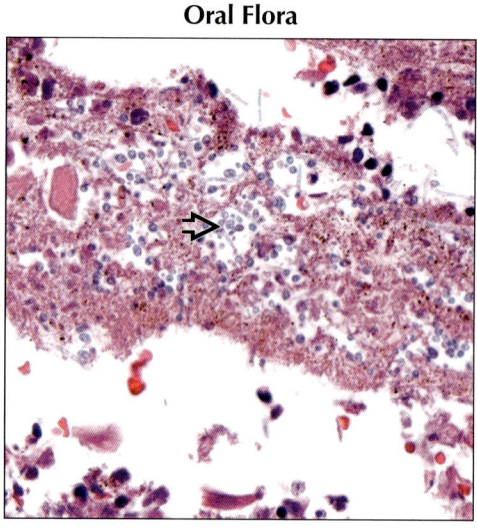

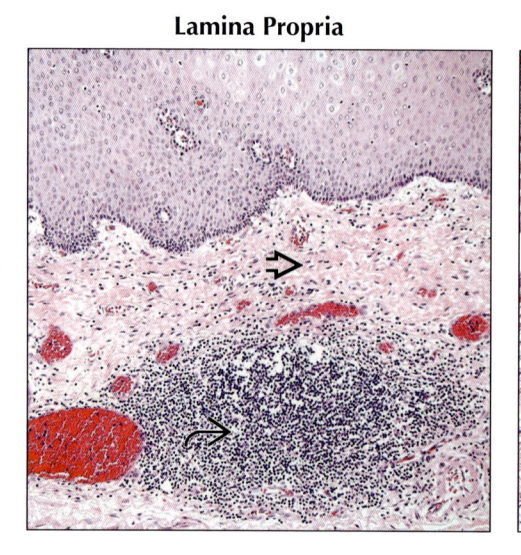

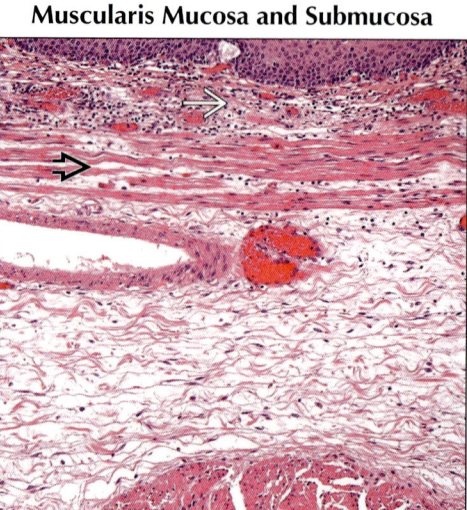

(Left) The lamina propria ⇨ is directly underneath the epithelium. It contains connective tissue with vessels and nerves. Occasional benign lymphoid aggregates ⇨ are seen as well. (Right) The muscularis mucosa ⇨ is typically a thin layer of smooth muscle that demarcates the overlying mucosa from the underlying submucosa. It lies directly under the lamina propria ⇨.

ESOPHAGUS

Muscularis Mucosa

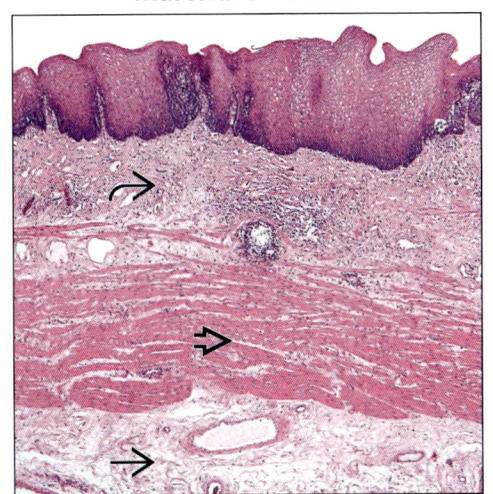

Submucosa

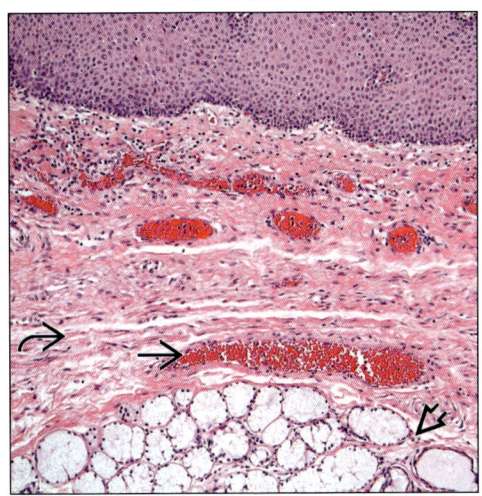

(Left) The muscularis mucosa ⇨ is thicker in the distal esophagus and in some diseases (e.g., Barrett esophagus), sometimes leading to confusion with the muscularis propria. The lamina propria ⇨ and submucosa ⇨ can help orient the tissue. (Right) The submucosa contains loose connective tissue, blood vessels ⇨, lymphatics, inflammatory cells, and submucosal mucous glands ⇨. Note that the muscularis mucosa ⇨ is very thin and difficult to identify in this image.

Submucosal Glands

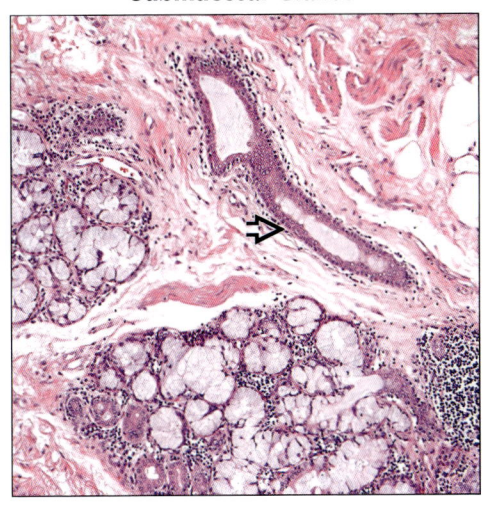

Submucosal Glands

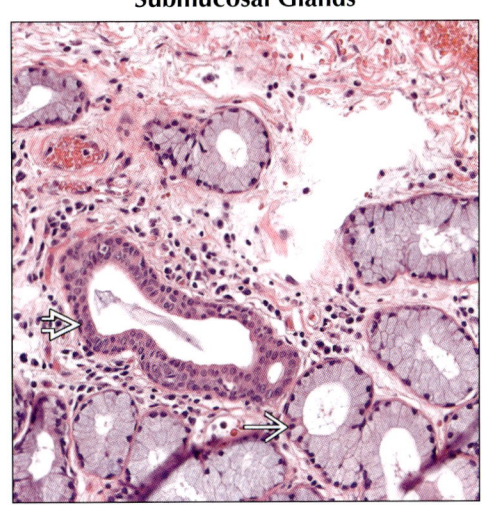

(Left) Submucosal glands are lobular mucous glands associated with a simple duct ⇨. The ducts deliver gland secretions to the surface for lubrication and protection. (Right) Individual acinar units of the submucosal glands, like those in the salivary gland, consist of mucous cells ⇨ arranged radially around a central lumen. The lumen connects to the duct, which is lined by a double layer of cuboidal cells ⇨. A mild lymphoid infiltrate associated with the duct is common.

Muscularis Propria

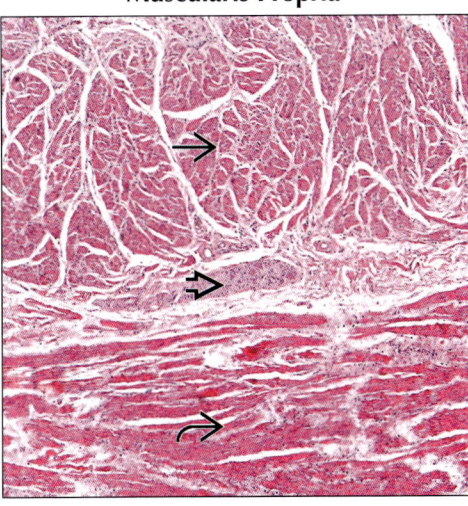

Muscularis Propria

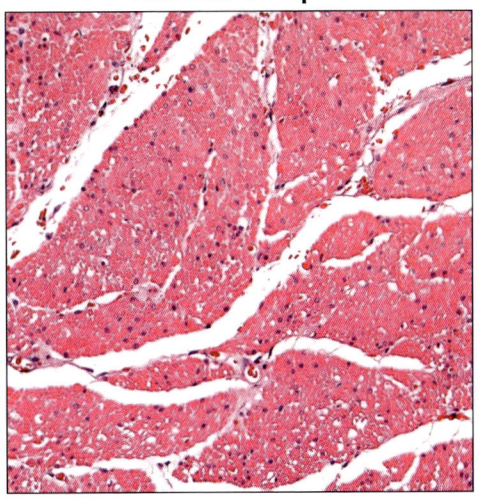

(Left) The muscular propria is divided into an inner circumferential layer ⇨ and outer longitudinal layer ⇨. In between lies the myenteric neural plexus ⇨. (Right) The inner circular (circumferential) layer is composed of smooth muscle that encircles the tubular esophagus. As a result of this orientation, the muscle fibers are often cut in cross section and appear as lobular bundles rather than long fascicles.

ESOPHAGUS

Muscularis Propria

Myenteric Plexus

(Left) In contrast to the inner layer, the outer (longitudinal) layer of the muscularis propria is oriented to run along the length of the esophagus. This creates a streaming fascicular pattern to the smooth muscle cells. (Right) The myenteric neural plexus (also known as Auerbach plexus) is composed of a network of nerve fibers that run the length of the gastrointestinal tract. These nerve fibers branch out to innervate both layers of the muscularis propria.

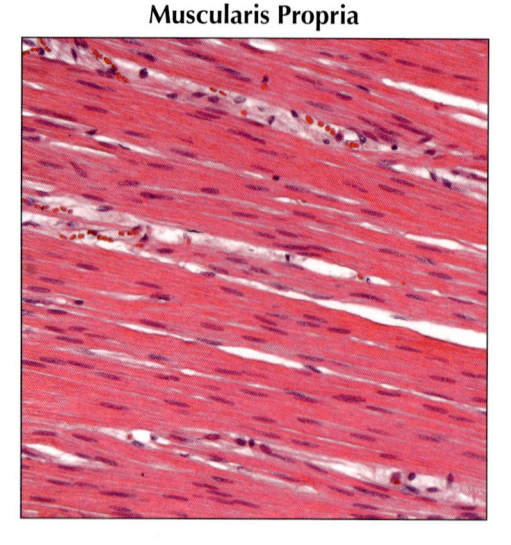

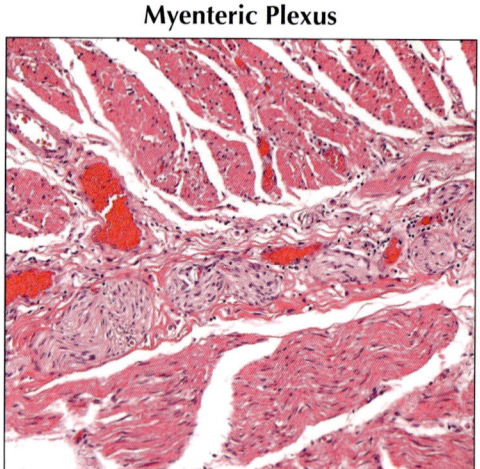

Interstitial Cells of Cajal (ICC)

Myenteric Plexus

(Left) ICCs regulate motility in the gastrointestinal tract and vary in number depending on the site. They are difficult to identify on routine stain, but C-Kit immunostain highlights them ⇨. Note that the smooth muscle cells ⇨ of the muscularis propria in the background do not stain. (Right) Ganglion cells, either individually or in clusters, are present within the network of neural fibers. They are large, round to polygonal cells ⇨ that are present in varying numbers.

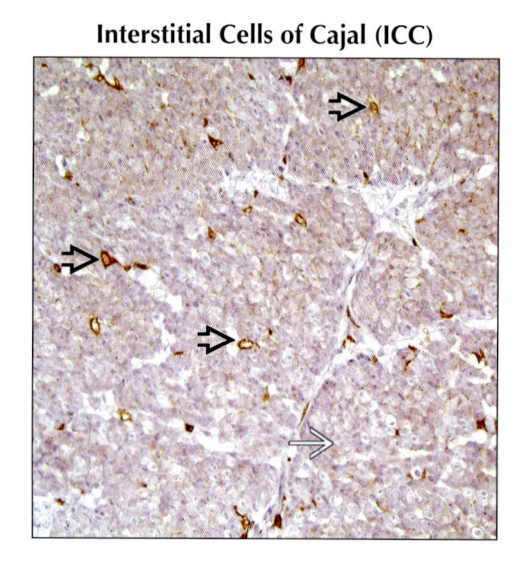

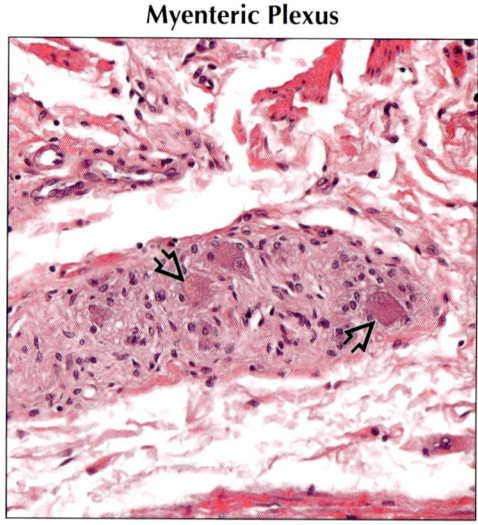

Ganglion Cells

Adventitia

(Left) Ganglion cells have basophilic (blue) cytoplasm with large nuclei and prominent nucleoli. (Right) Beneath the muscularis propria ⇨, the adventitia of the esophagus is a loose connective tissue fascia that forms a sheath around most of the esophagus. It contains fibroblasts, adipose tissue, and neurovascular elements. The majority of the esophagus lacks an outer mesothelial lining.

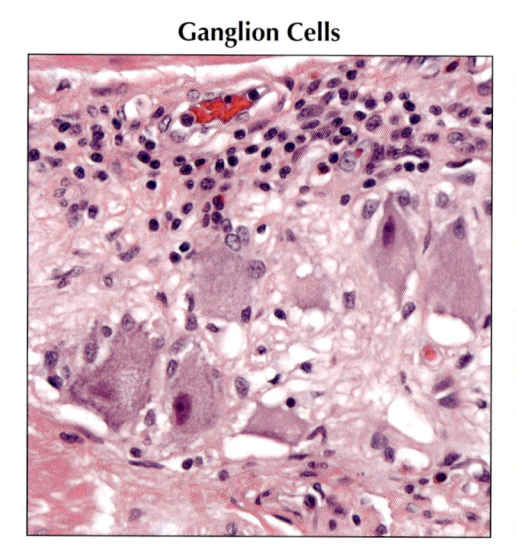

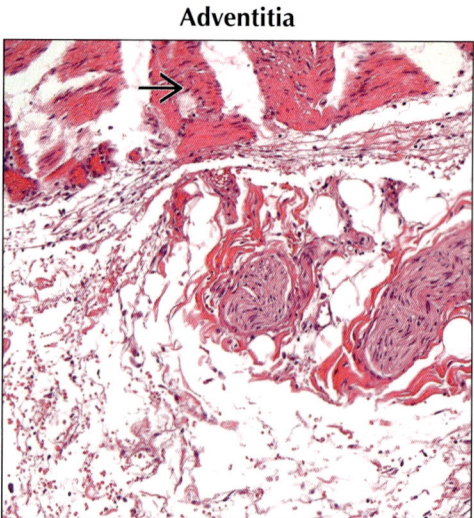

ESOPHAGUS

Squamocolumnar Junction

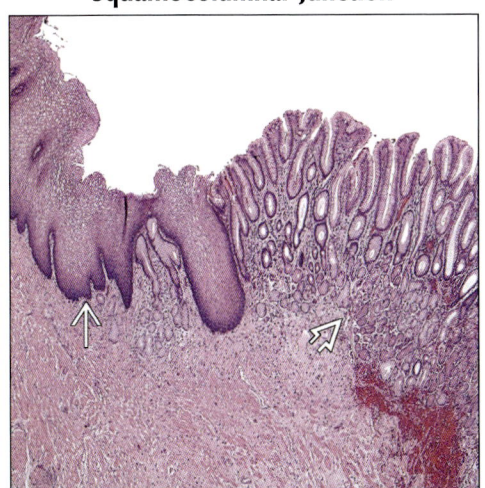

Squamocolumnar Junction

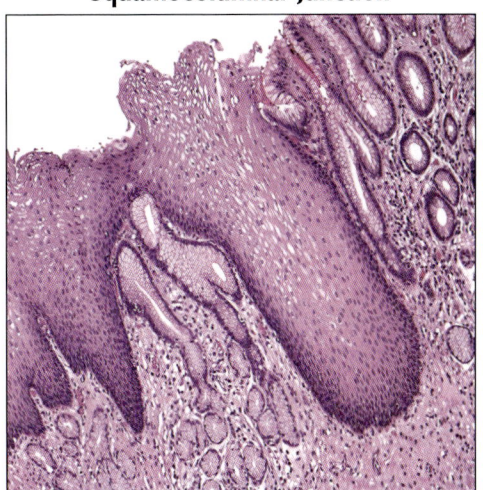

(Left) This photomicrograph illustrates the squamocolumnar junction, or the transition from squamous epithelium ➡ to gastric glandular epithelium ➡. (Right) The gastroesophageal junction, also known as the squamocolumnar junction, is a gradual transition from the stratified squamous epithelium of the esophagus to simple columnar epithelium of the stomach. Due to the gradual change, it is not uncommon to see glandular epithelium admixed with squamous epithelium.

Squamocolumnar Junction

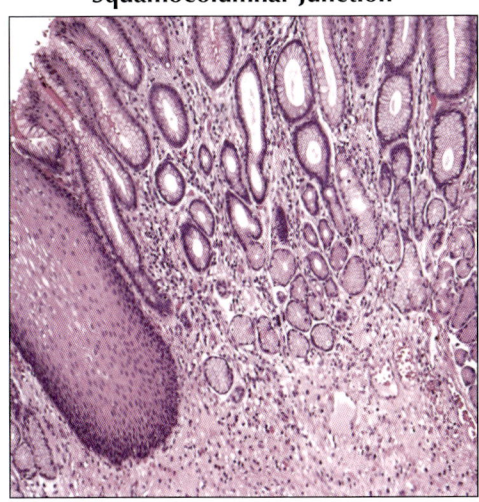

Pancreatic Acinar Metaplasia

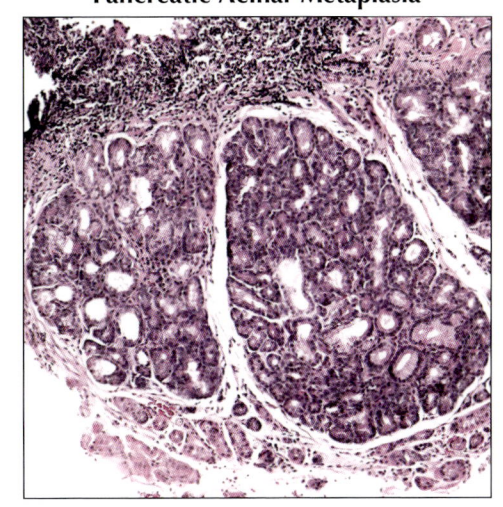

(Left) The glandular epithelium at the squamocolumnar junction may be a mix of oxyntic and mucous glands, or consist primarily of mucous glands. (Right) Small aggregates of pancreatic acinar-type glands are found in up to 5% of biopsies of the GE junction, usually in the deeper part of the mucosa. This finding is known as pancreatic acinar metaplasia, and the origin (true metaplasia vs. heterotopia) is unknown. It has no known clinical significance.

Pancreatic Acinar Metaplasia

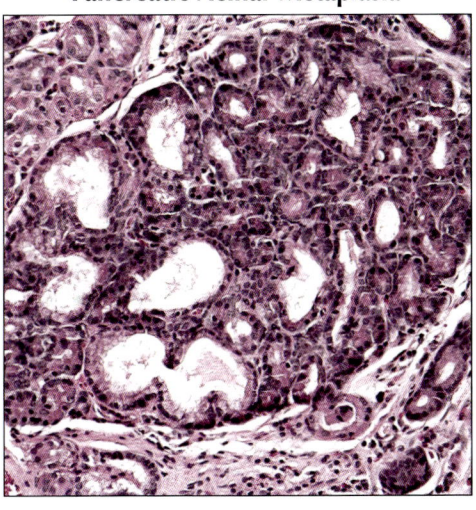

Intestinal Metaplasia

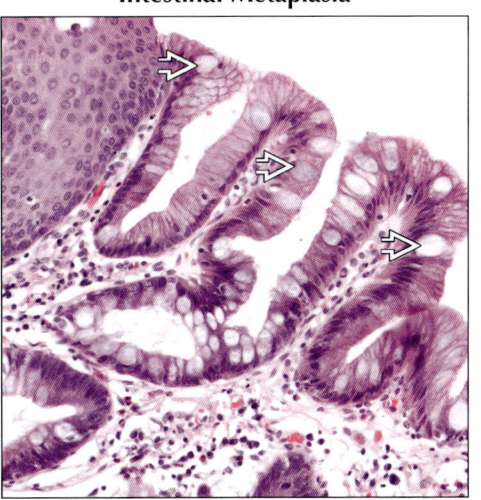

(Left) Pancreatic acinar metaplasia is characterized by groups of pancreatic acinar-like cells in a lobular configuration. Like normal pancreatic acini, many of the cells have supranuclear granular eosinophilic cytoplasm and subnuclear basophilic cytoplasm. (Right) Intestinal metaplasia is characterized by large, barrel-shaped goblet cells ➡ within the epithelium (like those seen in the bowel). This finding is known as Barrett esophagus.

STOMACH

Key Facts

Macroscopic Anatomy
- Sac-like, J-shaped organ in central left upper abdomen
  - Can accommodate up to 1.5 L of food and gastric juice in normal adults
  - Lined by rugae or prominent folds
  - Mucosal surface is finely granular or nodular; nodules are known as areae gastricae
- Cardia: Uppermost portion where esophagus joins stomach
  - Extends 1-2 cm or less
  - Immediately distal to lower esophageal sphincter musculature
- Body: Extends distally from cardia to angularis (bend in lesser curvature near pylorus)
  - Greater curvature on left, inferolateral margin
  - Lesser curvature on right, superomedial margin
  - Angularis roughly divides body from antrum
- Fundus: Cephalad part of the body that forms bulge on upper left of stomach
- Antrum: Distal to angularis; terminates in pylorus
  - Pylorus overlies pyloric sphincter, which is dividing line between stomach and duodenum
- External surface almost entirely covered by peritoneum
  - Greater curvature attached to omentum and mesentery of transverse colon
  - Lesser curvature attached to liver by gastrohepatic ligament

Microscopic Anatomy
- Epithelium consists of mucosa, lamina propria, muscularis mucosa at base
- Types of mucosa do not exactly correlate with gross anatomic divisions
- Mucosa has 2 compartments: Superficial pit (or foveolar) and deep glands
  - Surface/pit epithelium is same throughout stomach
  - Gland type differs with region
  - Cardiac and antral/pyloric glands are mucinous
  - Body and fundus glands contain specialized chief and parietal cells (oxyntic mucosa)
  - Transitional zones can share features of both types of mucosae
- Lamina propria
  - Scant fibromuscular stroma between glands
  - Contains arterioles, venules, and lymphatics
  - Scattered mononuclear cells are normal
- Muscularis mucosa
  - Thin double layer of smooth muscle that separates mucosa from submucosa
- Endocrine cells are present throughout mucosa, but type differs with region
- Submucosa
  - Loose connective tissue containing vessels, lymphatics, nerves, ganglion cells
- Muscularis propria
  - 3 muscle layers: Inner oblique, middle circular, and outer longitudinal
- Subserosa/serosa
  - Thin covering of collagen and single layer of flat mesothelium
  - Present except where stomach is attached to omentum, mesocolon, and ligaments

Pitfalls/Artifacts
- Detached glandular cells can mimic signet ring cells
  - Most often seen in cases of gastritis
- Hypertrophic muscularis mucosa can be seen in numerous inflammatory and neoplastic conditions
  - Do not mistake for muscularis propria
- Proton pump therapy may cause vacuolization, hypertrophy, dilated lumina in oxyntic glands

Age Variation
- Antral/body transitional mucosa extends more proximally with age

Metaplasia
- Intestinal and pyloric-type metaplasia may be seen in a variety of inflammatory conditions

(Left) The anatomic regions of the stomach include the cardia (blue), the fundus (green), the body (yellow), and the pylorus (purple). The duodenum is red and the esophagus is orange in this graphic. (Right) The deeper layer of the mucosa consists of coiled glands ▶ that empty into the bases of the pits. The glands differ in both structure and function in the various regions of the stomach; however, the types of mucosa do not exactly correlate with the gross anatomic division of the stomach.

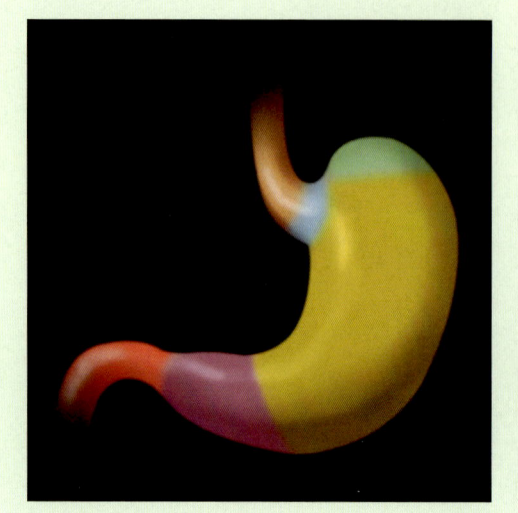

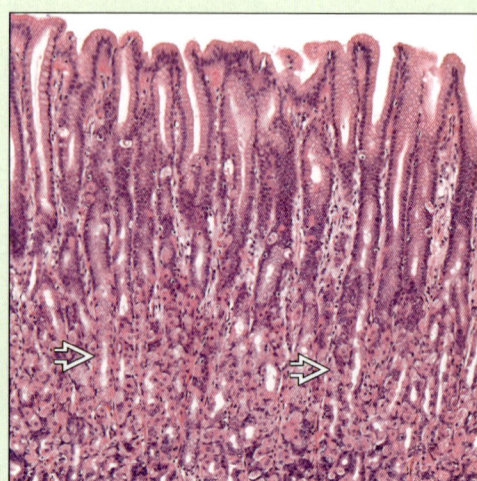

STOMACH

Pits

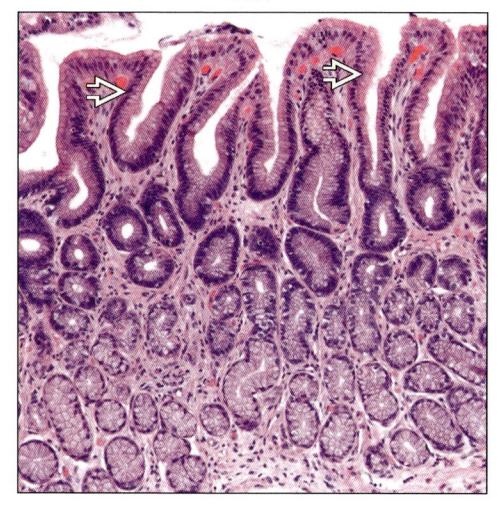

Pit/Surface Epithelium

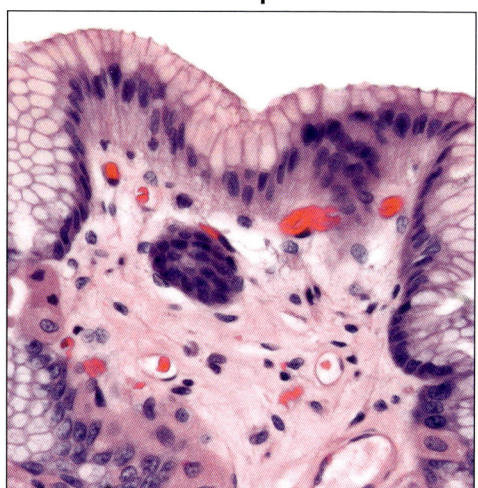

(Left) The superficial gastric mucosa consists of pits ➤ or foveolae, which are invaginations of the surface epithelium. The pits are a conduit to the lumen for glandular secretions. The depth of the pits varies from short in the body (1/4 of total mucosal thickness) to longer in the cardia and antrum (approximately half of total thickness). *(Right)* The surface/pit epithelium is mucinous and tall columnar throughout the stomach, regardless of region. Nuclei are small and basally located.

Pit/Surface Epithelium

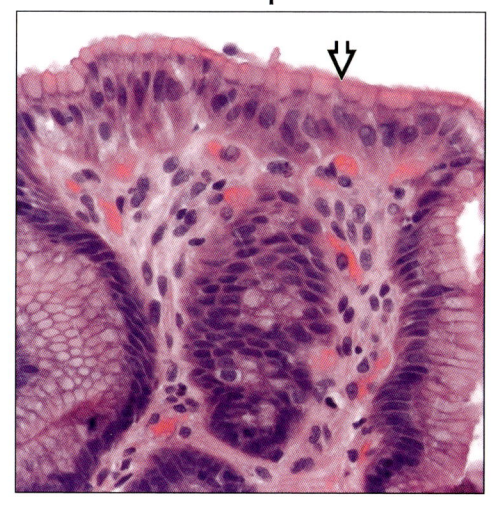

Mucous Neck Cells

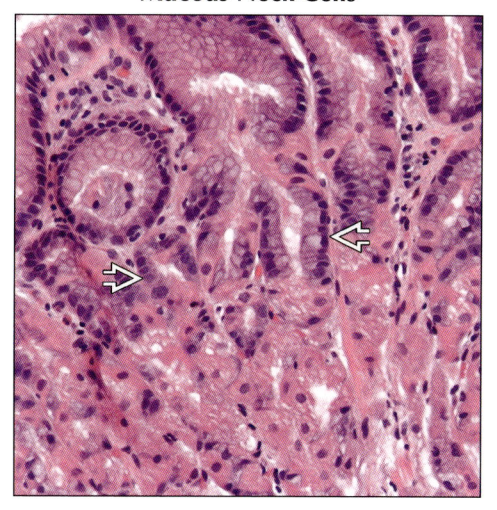

(Left) The surface/pit epithelium often appears to have pale pink apical mucin vacuoles ➤ that contain neutral mucins. *(Right)* The area between the pits and the glands is the neck. Mucous neck cells are mucinous, and the nuclei of the neck region may be slightly larger than those in the pits or the glands ➤. Mucous neck cells are believed to be the proliferative zone for the gastric mucosa.

Endocrine Cells

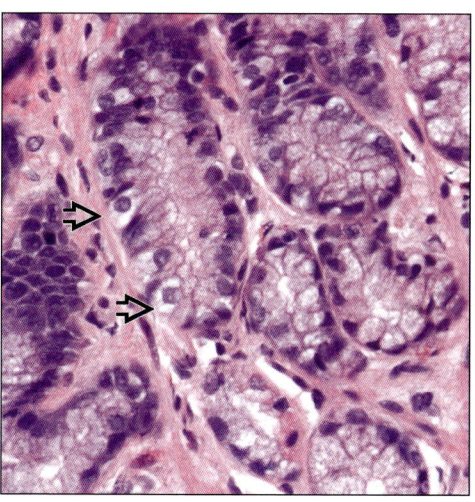

Endocrine Cells

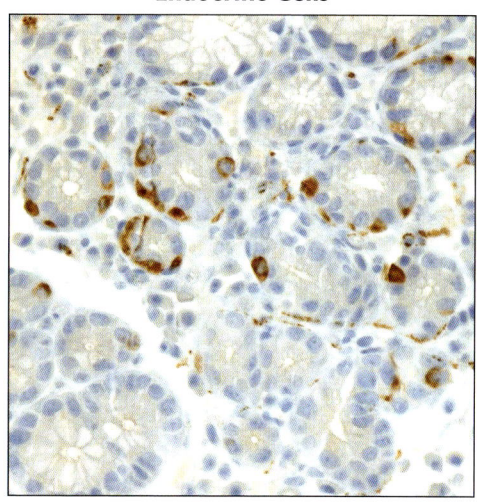

(Left) The type of endocrine cell differs with the region of the stomach. In the antrum, the pale, ovoid cells with gray cytoplasm are the gastrin-producing or G cells ➤. The body contains ECL cells, which produce histamine, in the lower 1/3 of the mucosa near the chief cells. *(Right)* Endocrine cells are present throughout the gastric mucosa but may be difficult to appreciate on H&E. This CD56 stain highlights neuroendocrine cells within the glands.

STOMACH

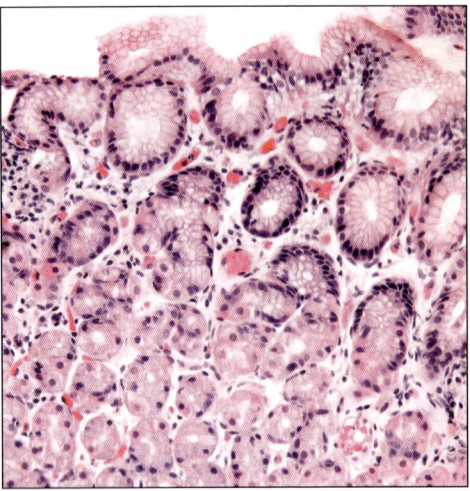

Lamina Propria

(Left) The lamina propria consists of relatively sparse stroma, which normally contains scattered macrophages, lymphocytes, mast cells, and plasma cells. Lamina propria is more abundant in the superficial mucosa between the foveolae. *(Right)* The lamina propria is composed of smooth muscle and loose collagen, and it contains arterioles and venules. In the normal stomach, the lymphatics are present in the lamina propria at the base of the mucosa, not at the surface.

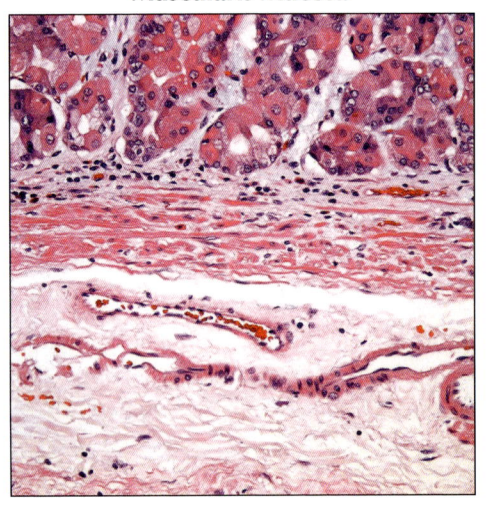

Muscularis Mucosa

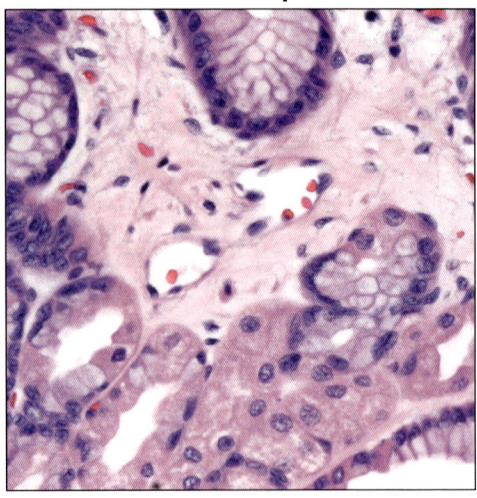

(Left) The muscularis mucosa consists of a thin double layer of smooth muscle that defines the base of the mucosa and separates it from the submucosa. Muscle fibers can occasionally extend into the base of the mucosa. *(Right)* The muscularis mucosa becomes hypertrophic in a wide variety of reactive and neoplastic processes. A hypertrophic muscularis mucosa should not be confused with muscularis propria.

Cardia / Cardia and Antrum

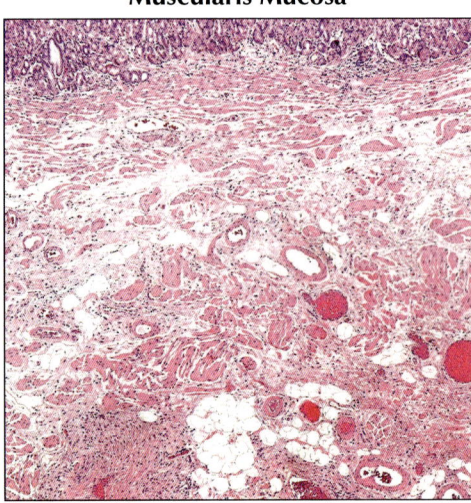

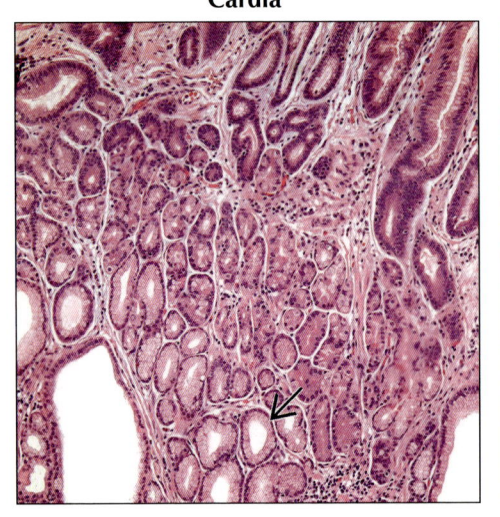

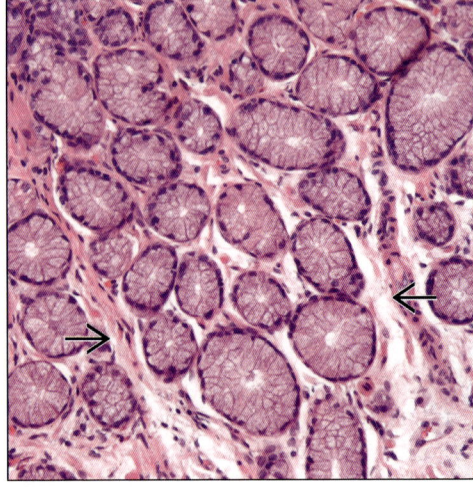

(Left) Cardiac glands are mucinous and loosely aggregated ➡. Occasional cystic glands are normal. The mucosa at the GE junction may be mixed mucinous and oxyntic, as seen here, entirely mucinous, or rarely, entirely oxyntic. *(Right)* The cardia and antrum typically have more stroma than the fundus and body. The mucinous glands of the cardia and antrum may be separated into loose clusters by fine strands of collagen and smooth muscle ➡.

STOMACH

Oxyntic Mucosa

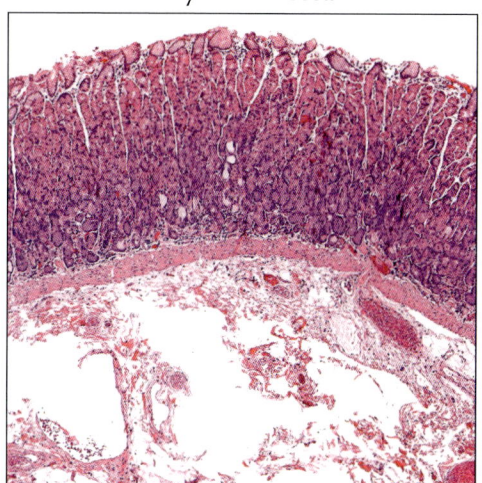

Oxyntic Mucosa

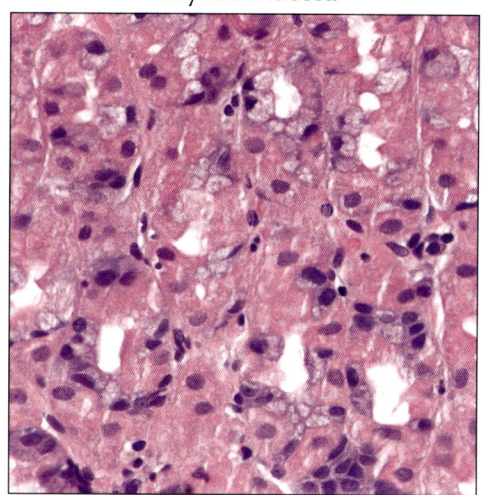

(Left) The fundus and body contain the specialized oxyntic glands. These glands consist of parietal cells, which produce acid, and chief cells, which produce digestive enzymes. The glands in the oxyntic mucosa are tightly packed and straight rather than coiled. **(Right)** Parietal cells are pink, with centrally placed nuclei. Parietal cells secrete acid and intrinsic factor.

Oxyntic Mucosa

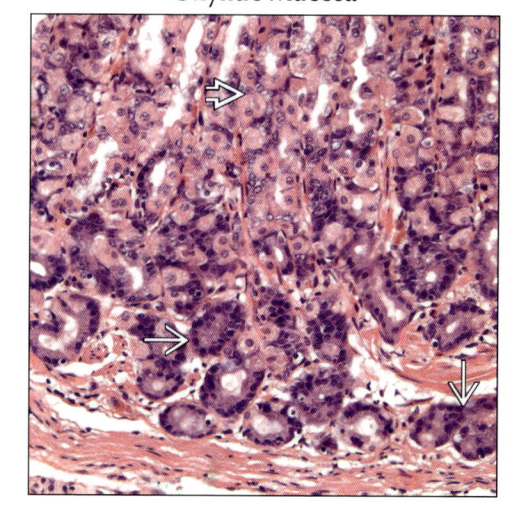

Antrum

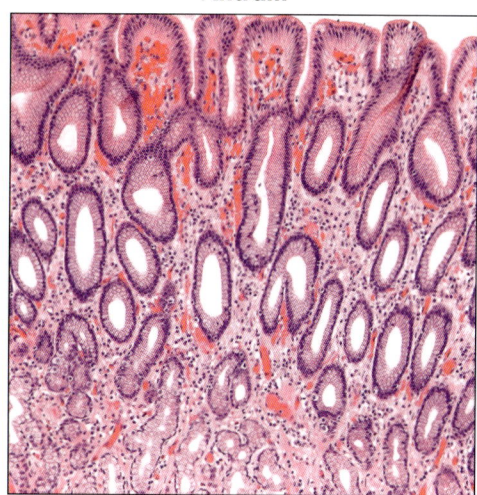

(Left) Parietal cells ➡ are more prominent in the upper part of the mucosa, whereas the darker purple chief cells ➡ are more prominent at the base. Chief cells are cuboidal to columnar with basally located nuclei, and they secrete digestive enzymes such as pepsinogen. **(Right)** The antral and pyloric mucosa is similar to the cardiac mucosa, consisting of mucinous glands with abundant stroma.

Antrum

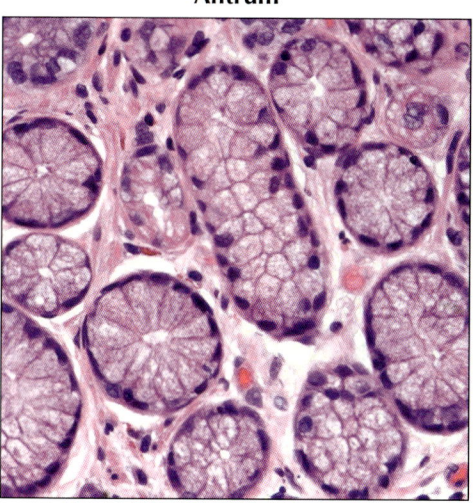

Transitional Mucosa

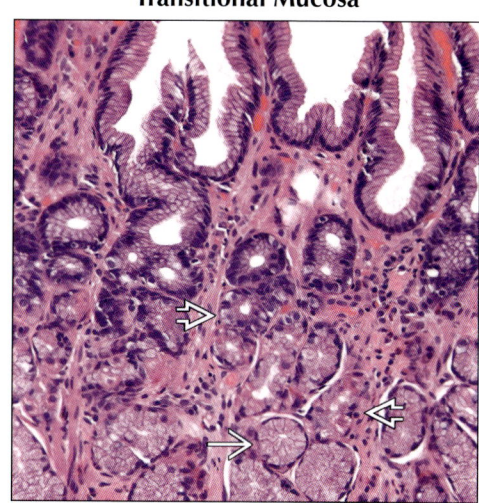

(Left) The mucinous antral glands have bubbly cytoplasm resembling Brunner glands, and small basally located nuclei. **(Right)** Transitional mucosa, such as that at the interface between the body and antrum, may contain both oxyntic ➡ and mucinous ➡ glands. This particular transition migrates proximally with age.

STOMACH

Submucosa
Submucosa

(Left) The submucosa lies beneath the muscularis mucosa and consists of loose connective tissue admixed with smooth muscle and variable amounts of adipose tissue. It contains vessels, lymphatics, nerves, ganglion cells, and scattered mononuclear cells as well.
(Right) The amount of submucosal adipose tissue can be quite prominent in some individuals, as seen here. Note the submucosal vessels ⇨.

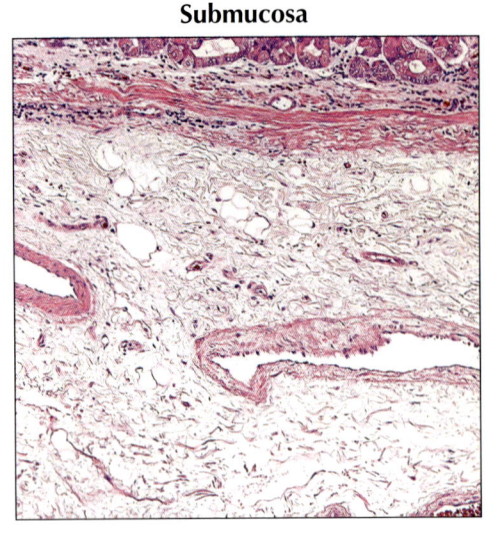

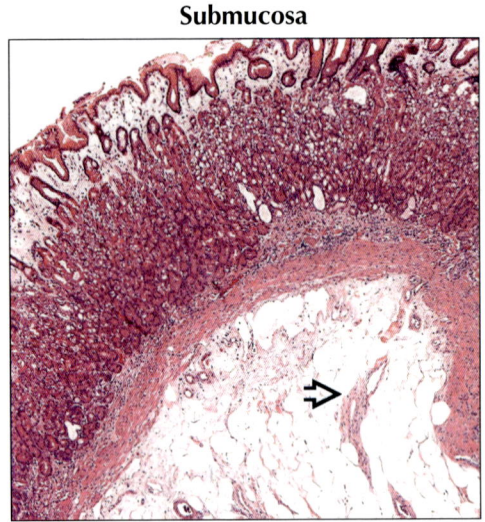

Submucosa
Muscularis Propria

(Left) The nerves and ganglion cells ⇨, known as Meissner plexus, are present within the gastric submucosa.
(Right) Unlike the rest of the tubular gut, the gastric muscularis propria consists of 3 muscle layers: Inner oblique, middle circular, and outer longitudinal.

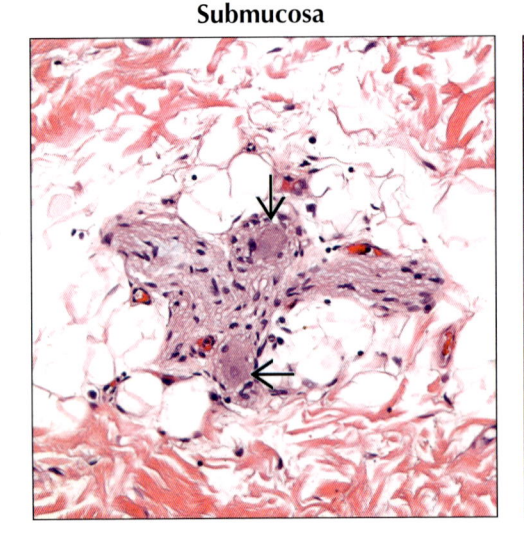

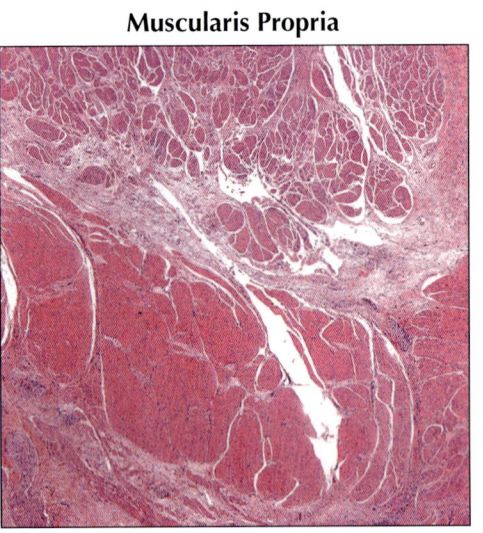

Auerbach Plexus
Subserosa

(Left) The nerves and ganglion cells ⇨ of Auerbach plexus are present between the outer 2 layers of the muscularis propria. **(Right)** The subserosa consists of thin layer of collagen that is present on the external surface of the stomach except where it is attached to the omentum, mesocolon, and ligaments. The subserosa is covered by a single layer of flat mesothelium ⇨, the serosa proper, which is part of the visceral peritoneum.

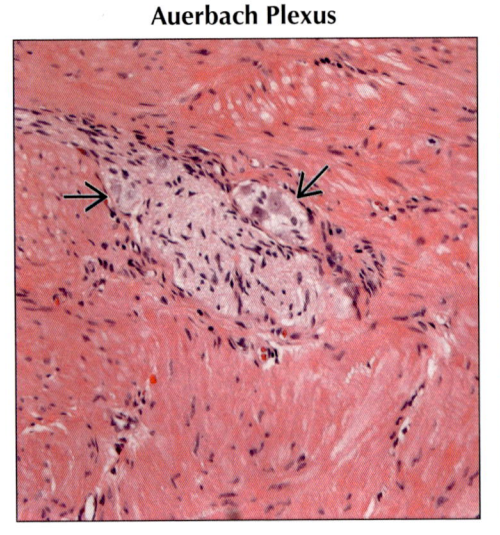

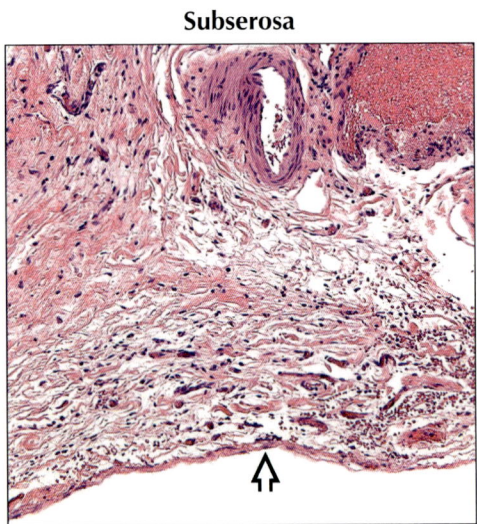

STOMACH

Lymphoid Tissue

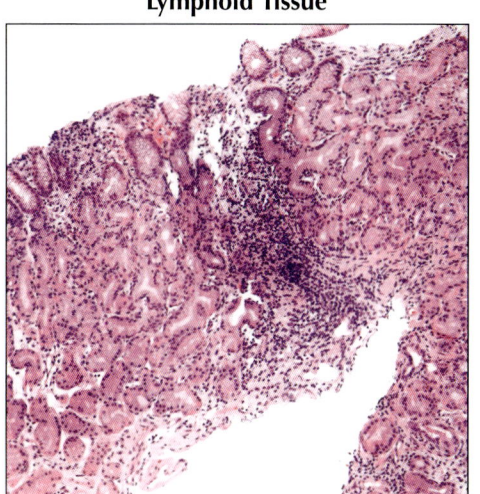

Proton Pump Inhibitor Effect

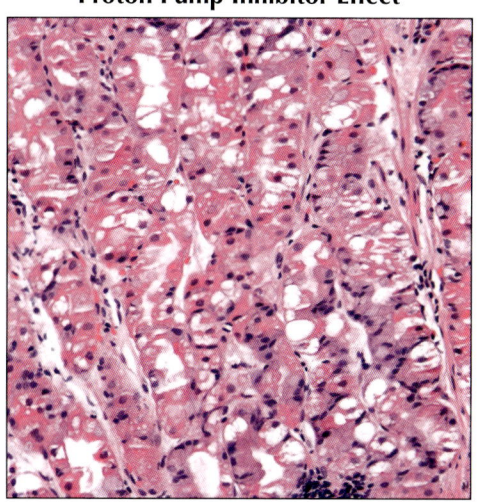

(Left) Whether or not lymphoid tissue is normally present in the gastric stomach is a subject of controversy. However, small lymphoid aggregates are often seen in otherwise normal gastric biopsies. This does not constitute a diagnosis of chronic gastritis. (Right) PPI use can cause numerous changes in parietal cells including cytoplasmic vacuolization, increased glandular tortuosity, dilated glandular lumens, and protrusion of cytoplasm into the gland lumens creating a tufted, irregular appearance.

Pylorus

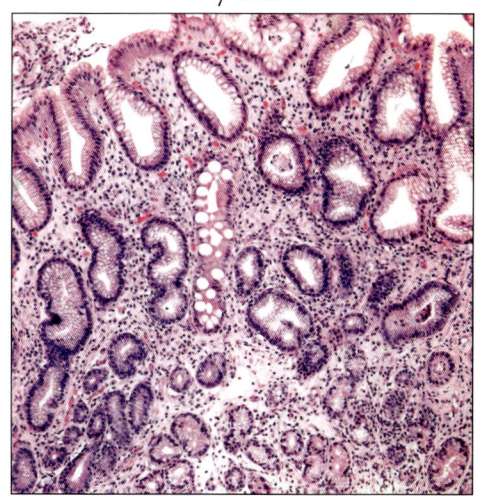

Metaplasia

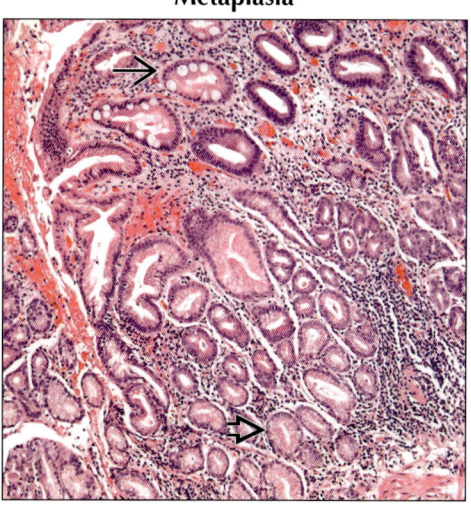

(Left) Foci of goblet cells are normally found in the transition between antral and duodenal mucosa, and their presence in this location does not mean that the patient has intestinal metaplasia. (Right) Both intestinal ⇾ and pyloric ⇾ metaplasia are seen in this fundic biopsy of chronic atrophic gastritis. The intestinal and pyloric glands have replaced the oxyntic mucosa.

Pseudo-Signet Ring Cells

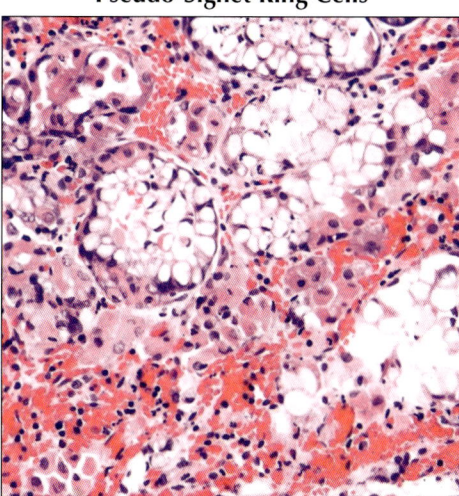

Heterotopic Pancreas

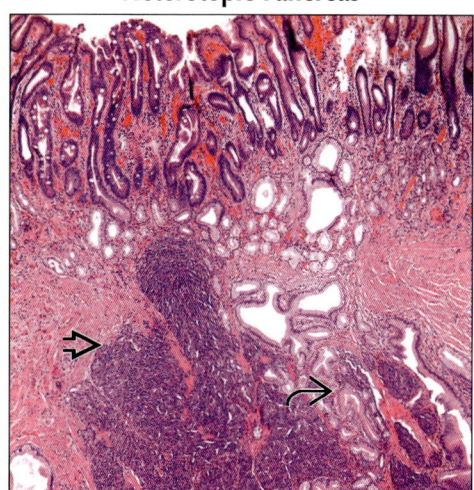

(Left) Detached clusters of signet ring-like cells can be seen in a number of inflammatory conditions. These detached clusters should not be mistaken for true signet ring cell carcinoma. (Right) Heterotopic pancreatic tissue is commonly found within the stomach. This example shows pancreatic acinar ⇾ and ductal ⇾ tissue at the distal antrum/pylorus.

SMALL INTESTINE

Key Facts

Macroscopic Anatomy
- Coiled tubular organ extending from pylorus of stomach to ileocecal valve
  - Average length in adults is 6-7 m
  - Primary function is absorption of nutrients
  - Plicae circulares: Mucosa-covered folds running perpendicular to long axis of small bowel that increase mucosal surface area; permanent folds with submucosal cores
- Duodenum: Most proximal portion; extends from pylorus to duodenojejunal flexure and forms C shape around pancreas
- Jejunum: Middle portion, primarily lies within upper abdomen; no distinct anatomic transition to ileum
- Ileum: Most distal portion, primarily lies within lower abdomen and pelvis

Microscopic Anatomy
- Mucosa: Epithelium, lamina propria, muscularis mucosa
  - 2 compartments: Villi and crypts
  - Normal villous to crypt ratio is 3:1-5:1
  - Epithelium is single layer composed of multiple cell types
  - Delicate basement membrane separates epithelium from lamina propria
- Villous compartment
  - Absorptive cells, goblet cells, endocrine cells
  - Intraepithelial lymphocytes (1 per 4-5 epithelial cells) normal
- Crypt compartment (crypts of Lieberkühn)
  - Crypts are depressions of surface epithelium
  - Absorptive cells, goblet cells, endocrine cells, Paneth cells
  - Mitoses are frequent (1-12 per crypt)
  - Scattered intraepithelial lymphocytes normal
- Lamina propria
  - Forms cores of villi
  - Numerous white blood cells are normally present, including plasma cells, lymphocytes, mast cells, eosinophils, histiocytes
  - Contain vessels and central blind-ending lymphatic channel or lacteal
- Submucosa: Loose connective tissue that contains inflammatory cells, adipose tissue, vessels, lymphatics, nerves, ganglion cells (Meissner plexus)
- Muscularis propria
  - 2 layers: Outer longitudinal and inner circular
  - Muscles partitioned into bundles by thin strands of connective tissue
  - Auerbach plexus lies between layers, as do interstitial cells of Cajal
- Serosa: Mesothelial-lined thin layer of connective tissue external to muscularis propria; contains vessels, lymphatics, and nerves
- Features specific to duodenum
  - More mononuclear cells than distal small bowel
  - Submucosal Brunner glands
  - Villi shorter than in jejunum and ileum
- Features specific to jejunum
  - Taller villi with club-shaped tips
  - No Brunner glands or Peyer patches
- Features specific to ileum
  - Ileocecal valve and rest of submucosa may have very prominent fat
  - Ileum has the most goblet cells
  - Peyer patches

Pitfalls/Artifacts
- Villi may be artifactually shortened by underlying nodules of Brunner glands or lymphoid aggregates
- Persons from tropics may have shorter, broader villi, but villus to crypt ratio is maintained
- Tangentially sectioned tissue may result in artifactual villous blunting
- Picric acid-based fixatives wash out Paneth cell granules, leaving only clear vacuoles
- Refractile brown-black granular pigment of unknown origin often seen in macrophages in Peyer patches in adults

Age Variation
- Peyer patches increase until puberty and regress with age but are present throughout life

---

(Left) Small bowel mucosa consists of the villi and crypt compartments. The villi are long slender projections covered by epithelium; the lamina propria forms the cores of the villi. The crypts ➡ lie between and beneath the villi. Villi cover the entire luminal surface of the small bowel to enhance the surface area. *(Right)* Peyer patches may be very prominent in children, and visible to the naked eye as white nodules ➡. (Courtesy G. Gray, MD.)

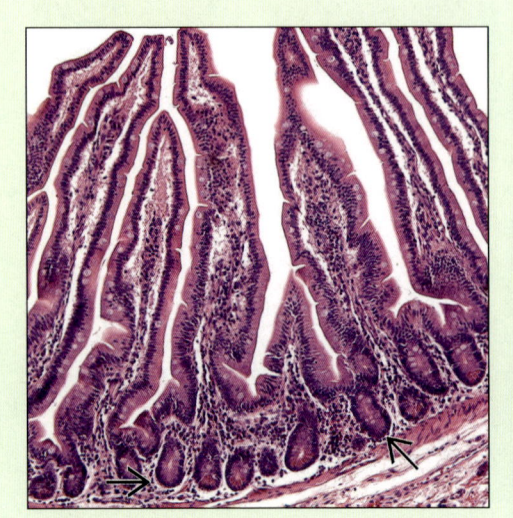

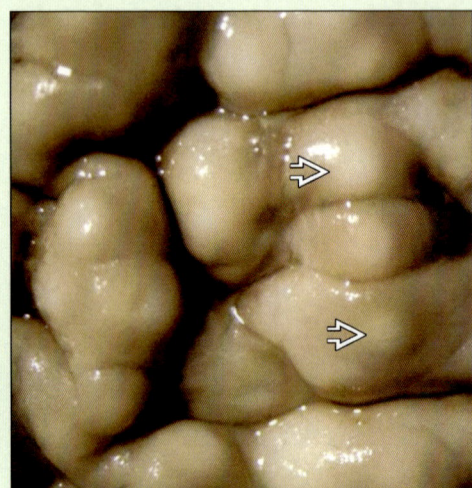

SMALL INTESTINE

Mucosa

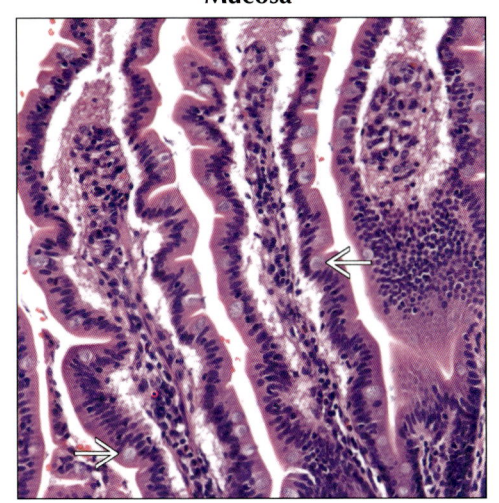

Brush Border

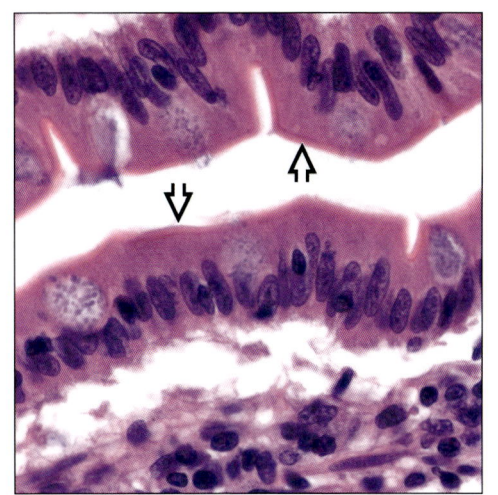

(Left) The absorptive cells are simple columnar cells with round to oval, basally located nuclei and eosinophilic cytoplasm. Goblet cells ➡ are interspersed among the absorptive cells. These barrel-shaped cells with characteristic mucin droplets secrete mucin. *(Right)* The brush border ➡ of the small bowel epithelium is composed of microvilli (best seen on electron microscopy) and the glycocalyx. This complex increases the surface area of the small bowel and houses important digestive enzymes.

Crypts

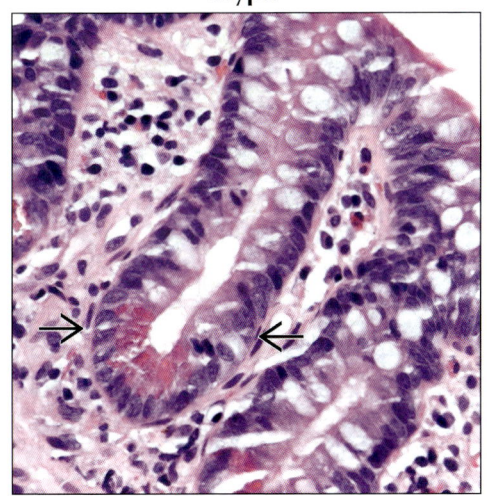

Paneth Cells

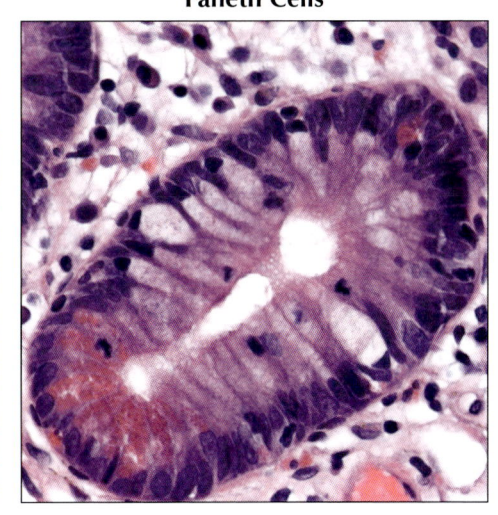

(Left) The epithelium rests on a delicate basement membrane ➡ separating it from the lamina propria. Crypts contain Paneth cells, goblet cells, absorptive cells, neuroendocrine cells, and occasional intraepithelial lymphocytes. Crypts are the regenerative compartment of the mucosa and thus contain mitoses. *(Right)* Paneth cells, present throughout the small bowel, are pyramidal cells with their apices toward the lumina of the crypts. The supranuclear eosinophilic granules contain numerous enzymes, the exact function of which is unknown.

Intraepithelial Lymphocytes

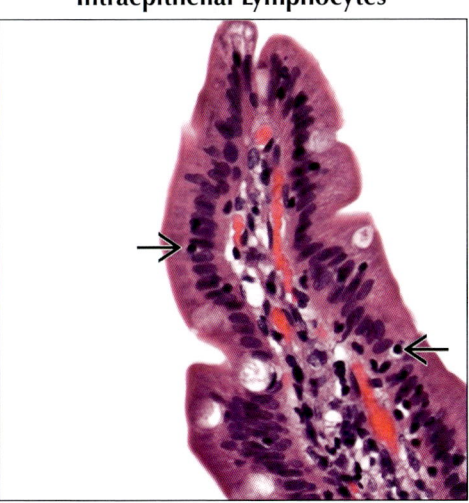

Lacteals

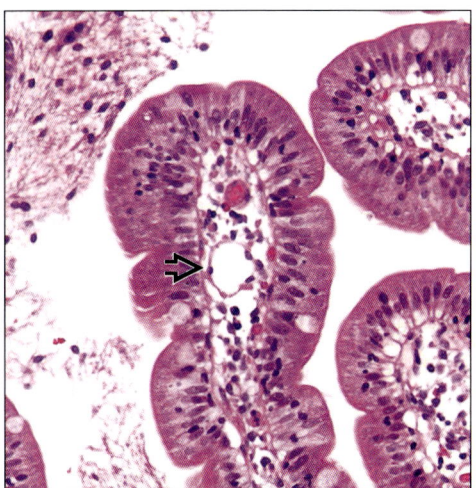

(Left) Intraepithelial lymphocytes ➡ are normally present in the small bowel and are usually located right above the basement membrane of the epithelium. Approximately 1 lymphocyte per 4-5 epithelial cells is considered normal. In the duodenum, the lymphocytes often extend along the sides of the villi and spare the tips. *(Right)* Villi contain a central blind-ending lacteal or lymphatic channel ➡.

SMALL INTESTINE

Lamina Propria

Endocrine Cells

(Left) The lamina propria normally contains plasma cells, lymphocytes, mast cells, histiocytes, and scattered eosinophils. Neutrophils are not a normal component of the inflammatory milieu. *(Right)* Many endocrine cells in the small bowel are pyramid shaped and have small dark pink or red granules. In contrast to Paneth cells ⇨, which have supranuclear granules, endocrine cells have subnuclear granules ⇨.

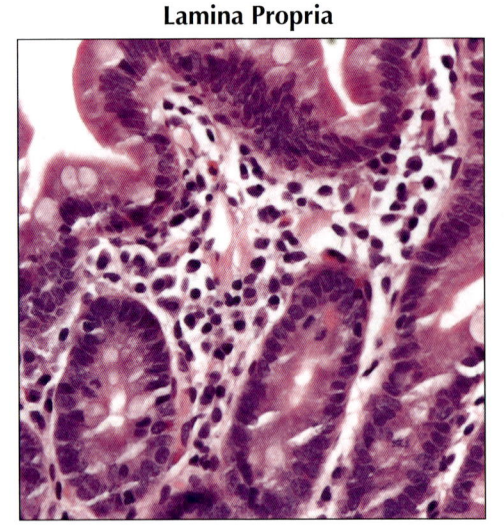

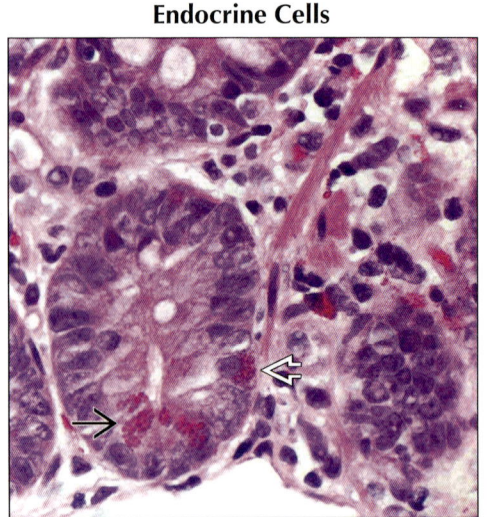

Muscularis Mucosa

Submucosa

(Left) The muscularis mucosa ⇨ is a thin layer of muscle that separates the mucosa, above, from the underlying submucosa. It anchors the mucosa and provides structural support. *(Right)* The submucosa consists of loose connective tissue and contains nerves, vessels, lymphatics, and fat. Meissner plexus is also present ⇨.

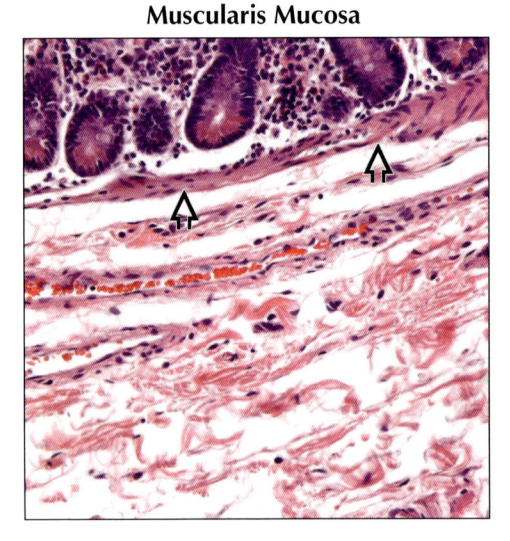

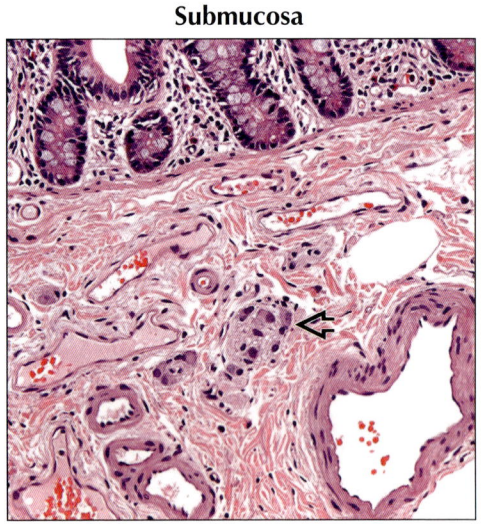

Brunner Glands

Jejunum

(Left) Brunner glands ⇨ are a feature of the duodenum. These tubuloalveolar glands are primarily in the submucosa but may extend into the mucosa, as seen here. They contain cuboidal/columnar cells with small basal nuclei and pale cytoplasm. *(Right)* The jejunal villi are tall and slender but may have broader or club-shaped tips. The jejunum lacks both Brunner glands and Peyer patches.

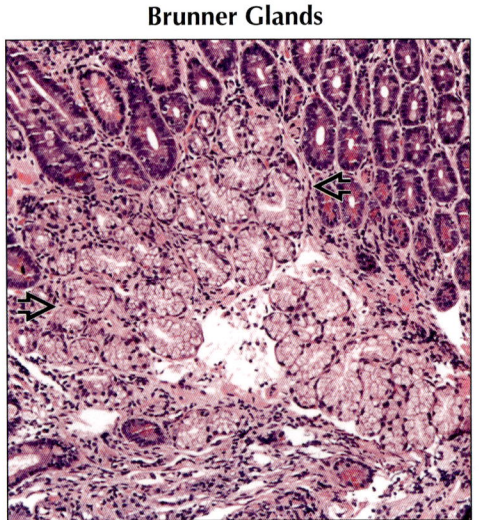

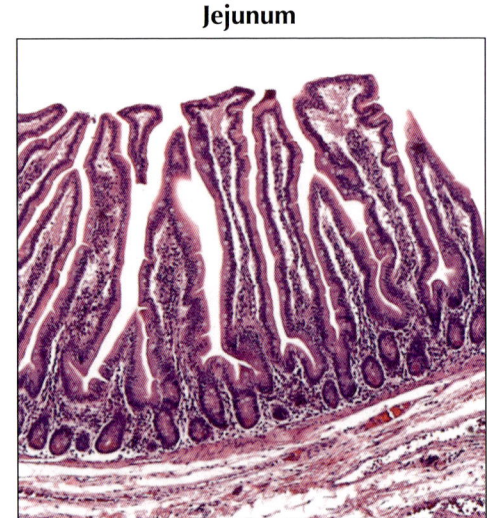

SMALL INTESTINE

Ileum

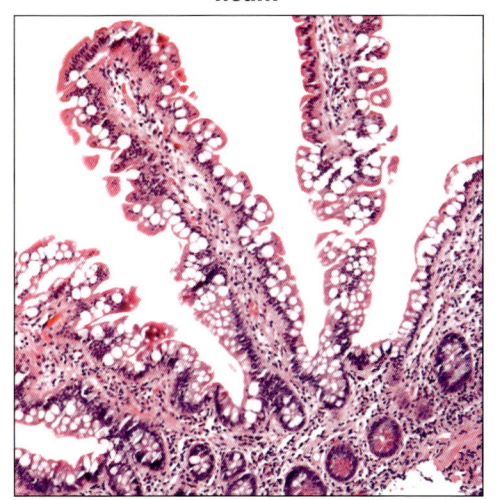

Peyer Patches

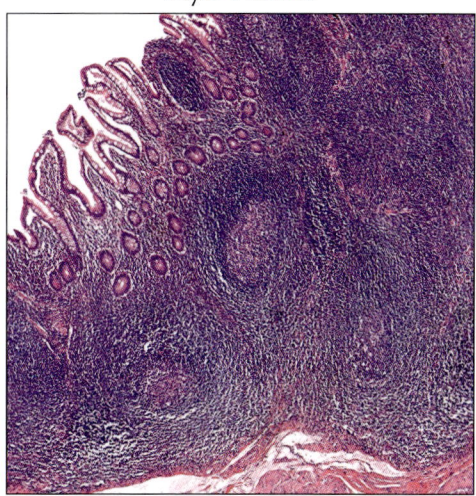

(**Left**) The ileum contains more goblet cells than the more proximal small bowel. (**Right**) Peyer patches are large aggregates of lymphoid tissue that are unique to the ileum. They involve both the mucosa and submucosa, and usually have germinal centers. The overlying follicle-associated epithelium lacks goblet cells. Lymphoid aggregates may be found anywhere in the small bowel, however.

Ileocecal Valve

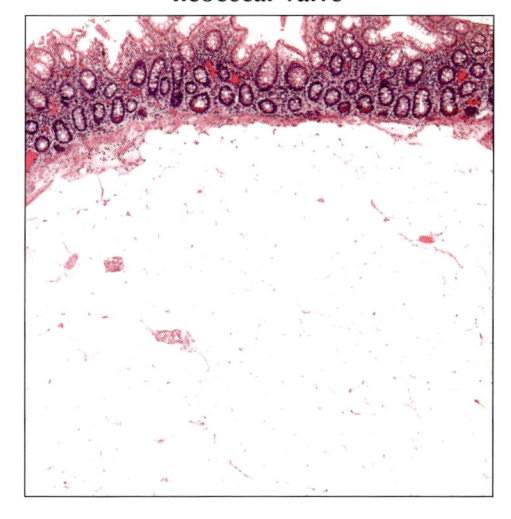

Auerbach Plexus

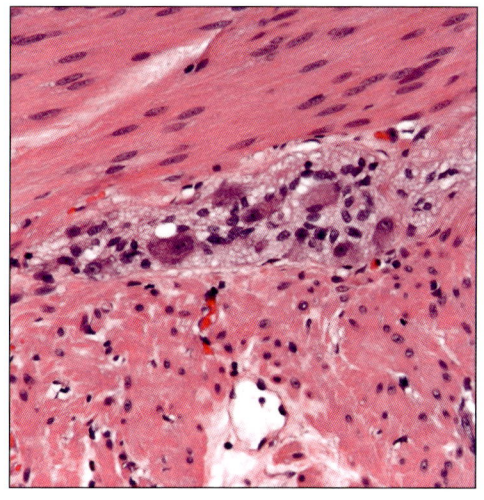

(**Left**) The ileocecal valve, as well as the ileocecal area in general, may contain remarkable amounts of adipose tissue that may even form a mass. (**Right**) The Auerbach plexus lies between the 2 layers of the muscularis propria and contains both nerves and ganglion cells.

Muscularis Propria

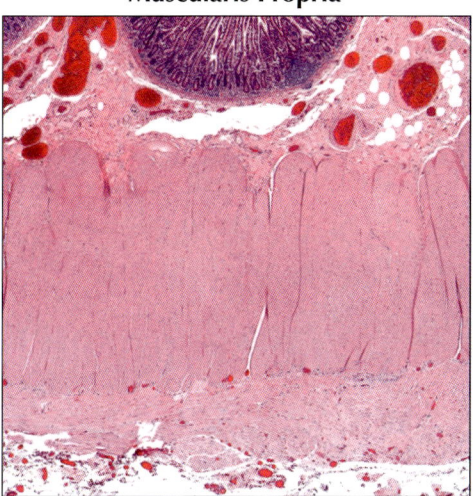

Artifactual Villous Blunting

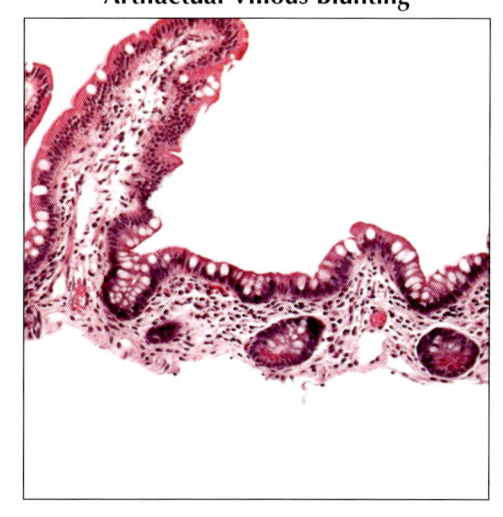

(**Left**) The muscularis propria consists of 2 layers: The outer longitudinal layer and the inner circular layer. (**Right**) When the mucosa is stripped off of the muscularis mucosa during a biopsy procedure, the tissue spreads laterally due to the loss of structural support, and the normal villous architecture may be lost. Note, however, that there is no abnormal intraepithelial lymphocytosis.

LARGE INTESTINE

Key Facts

Macroscopic Anatomy
- Right colon
  - Ileocecal valve, cecum, ascending colon, hepatic flexure, and proximal transverse colon
- Left colon
  - Distal transverse colon, splenic flexure, descending colon, sigmoid colon, rectum
- Ascending, descending, sigmoid, and rectum are retroperitoneal and have no peritoneal serosal lining
  - Important for pathologic staging of malignancies

Microscopic Anatomy
- Mucosa
  - Simple columnar epithelium with apical microvilli and numerous goblet cells
  - Basement membrane
  - Lamina propria
  - Muscularis mucosa
- Submucosa
- Muscularis propria
- Serosa

Pitfalls/Artifacts
- Tangential sectioning
- Pseudolipomatosis
- Tissue cauterization
- Intraepithelial lymphocytes/neutrophils overlying lymphoid aggregates
- Hyperplastic mucosal changes
- Rectal foamy histiocytes (muciphages)
- Melanosis coli
- Bifid crypts
- Biopsy-related trauma
- Vegetable matter

Metaplasia
- Paneth cell metaplasia in left colon

(Left) This image shows the layers of the colon including the mucosa ⇨, submucosa, and muscularis propria. The serosa (not pictured) is external to the muscularis propria. *(Right)* The crypts have a "rack of test tubes" configuration when viewed longitudinally. They are relatively evenly distributed and extend from the luminal surface down to the muscularis mucosa ⇨. They generally do not show branching or distortion.

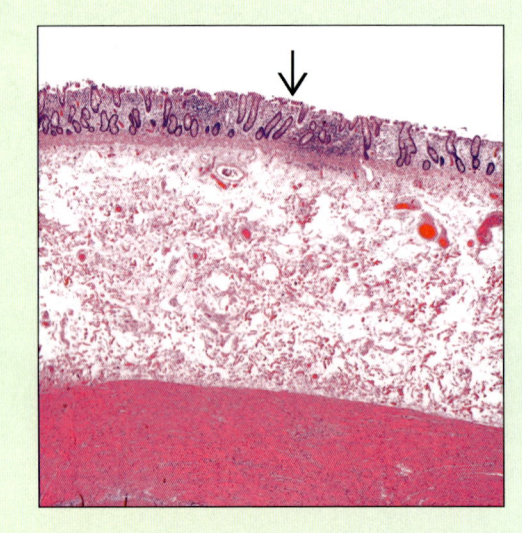

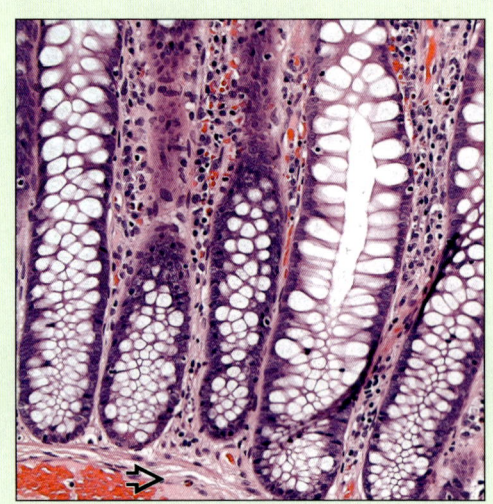

(Left) When viewed from the top down, the colon appears to be a "sea of glands" with regularly spaced crypts. The intervening lamina propria is normally filled with a mixed chronic inflammatory infiltrate. For this reason, a diagnosis of "chronic inflammation" in the colon is inappropriate. *(Right)* The mixed inflammatory infiltrate of the lamina propria includes lymphocytes, plasma cells, and eosinophils ⇨. Scattered normal mitotic figures ⇨ are not an uncommon finding in the crypt epithelium.

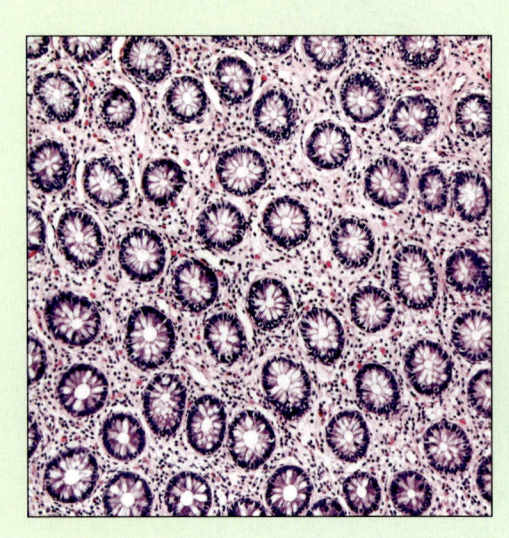

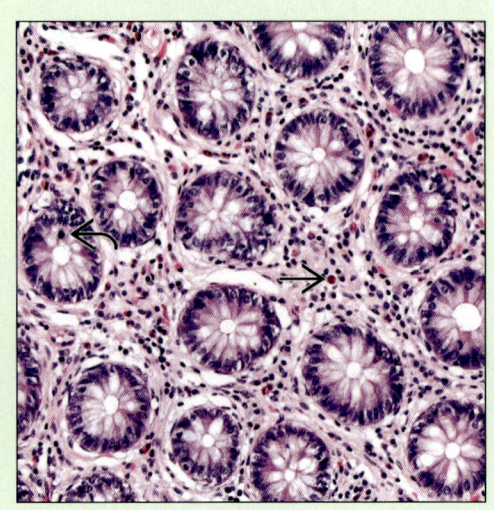

LARGE INTESTINE

Mucosa

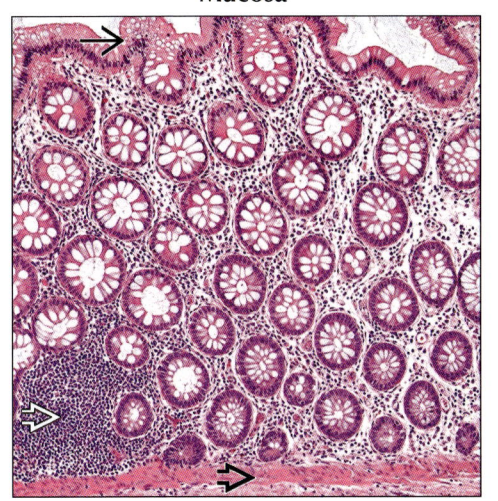

Columnar Epithelium

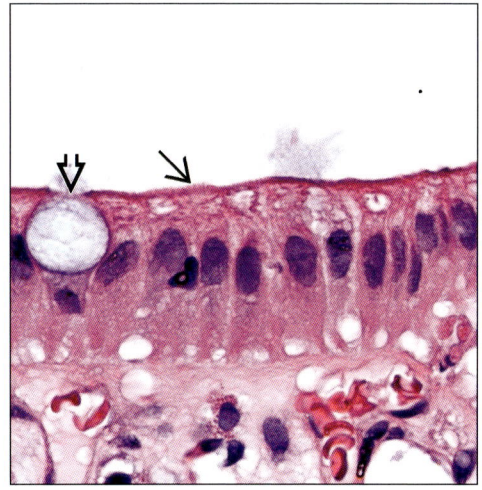

(Left) The mucosa of the large intestine extends from the luminal epithelium at the surface ⇨ down to the muscularis mucosa ⇨. The crypts may appear round instead of tube-like if tissue is oriented obliquely. Note the mucosa-associated lymphoid tissue (MALT) ⇨. *(Right)* The simple columnar epithelium of the colon has a fine brush border containing innumerable microvilli ⇨. Interspersed goblet cells ⇨ are responsible for secreting mucin.

Paneth Cells

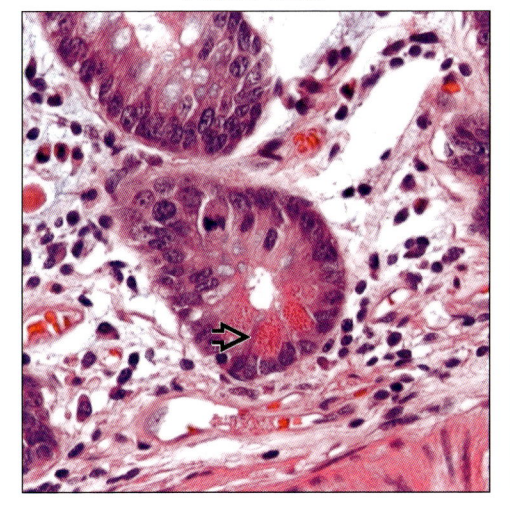

Endocrine Cells

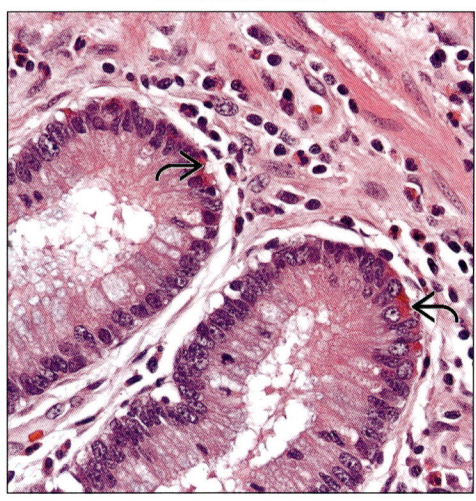

(Left) On the right side of the colon (proximal to the mid-transverse colon), specialized immune cells with prominent pink/red granules (Paneth cells) ⇨ are common. Distal to the mid-transverse colon, Paneth cells are metaplastic and indicate chronic injury. *(Right)* Endocrine cells can also be seen scattered throughout the colon and are identified by their small, basally located red granules ⇨. Unlike Paneth cells, these granules do not face the lumen of the crypt.

Mucosa-Associated Lymphoid Tissue (MALT)

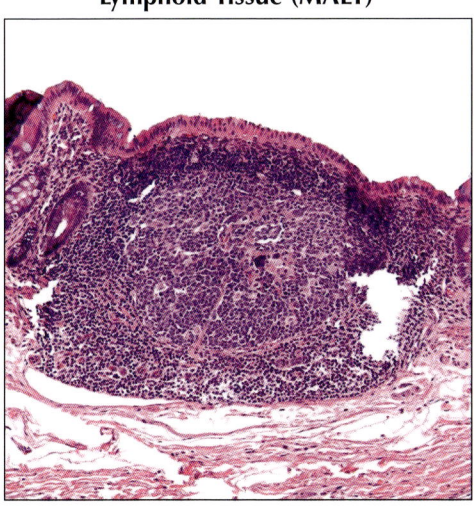

Reactive MALT

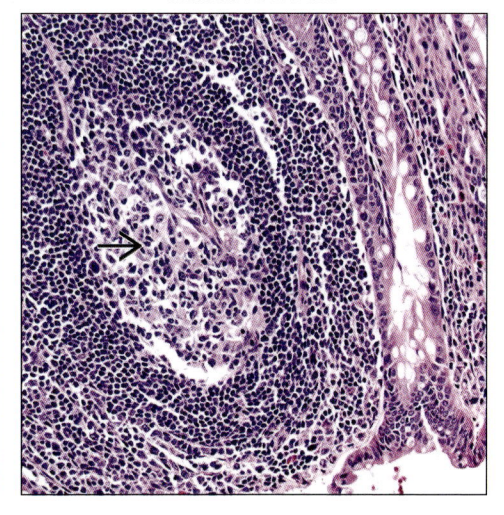

(Left) Mucosa-associated lymphoid tissue, or MALT, is common throughout the colon and represents the colonic component of the immune system. These aggregates function similar to the tonsils or lymph nodes, are composed mostly of T cells, and vary widely in size from small to very large. *(Right)* Some aggregates show a central, reactive germinal center ⇨ that is composed of B cells. These can be seen in any reactive, infectious, or inflammatory condition in the colon.

LARGE INTESTINE

Submucosa

Submucosa

(Left) As is seen in other segments of the gastrointestinal tract, the colonic submucosa contains blood vessels ➔, nerves and ganglion plexi, fibrocollagenous stroma, and downward extensions of the MALT ➔. *(Right)* Sometimes the submucosal tissue is more loose and edematous than dense and fibrous, and the collagen takes on a shredded and splayed appearance. This image also shows 2 nerve twigs ➔ and a blood vessel ➔.

Muscularis Propria

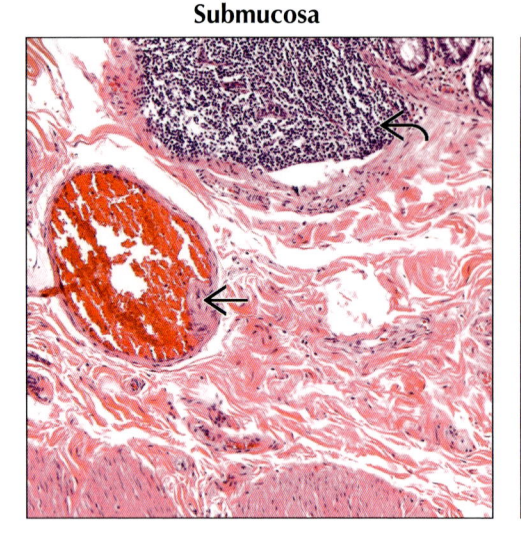

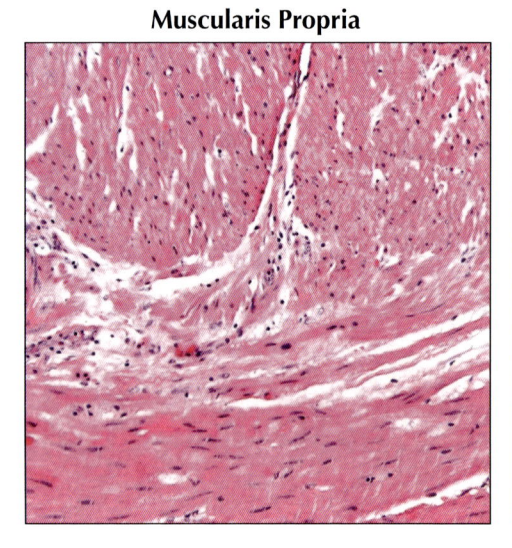

Myenteric Plexus With Ganglion Cells

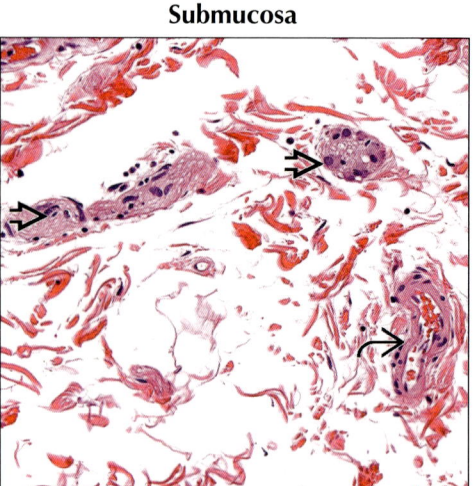

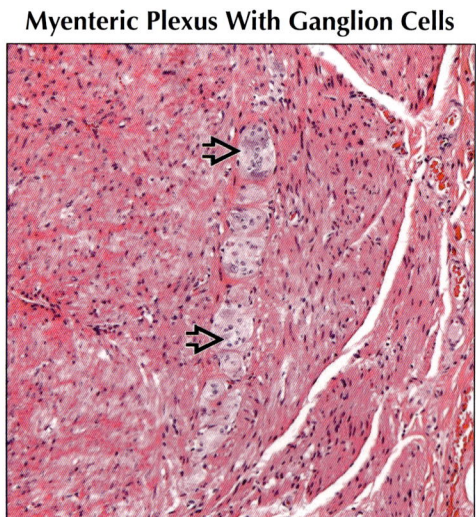

(Left) The muscularis propria is composed of 2 layers of mature smooth muscle: An inner circular layer and an outer longitudinal layer. The longitudinal layer runs the length of the colon (parallel), and the circular layer encircles the colon. *(Right)* In between the 2 layers of the muscularis propria lies the myenteric (Auerbach) nerve plexus ➔, which contains both nerves and ganglion cells and helps coordinate muscular contractions. Outer layer forms 3 thick longitudinal bands; taeniae coli.

Serosa

Lymph Node

(Left) The serosa contains fat, vessels, collagen, fibroblasts, and chronic inflammatory cells. Intraperitoneal segments of colon are lined by mesothelium (not shown). Retroperitoneal segments of large bowel lack a true peritoneal lining; this is important to know for cancer staging purposes. *(Right)* Lymph nodes are commonly found within serosal fat. They are distinguished from lymphoid aggregates by the presence of a pink outer capsule ➔ and subcapsular sinuses ➔.

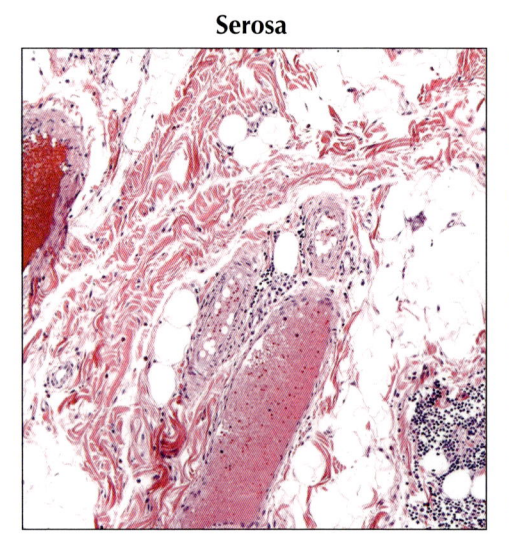

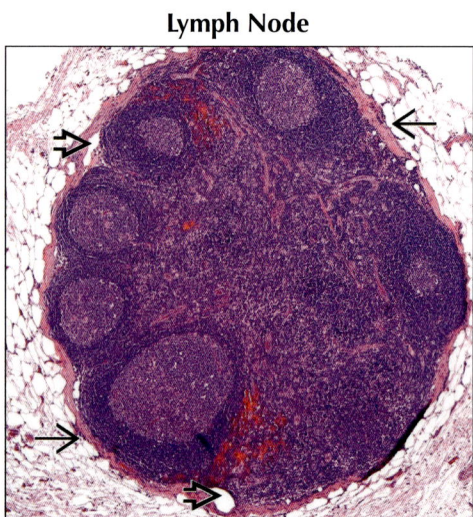

LARGE INTESTINE

Tangential Sectioning

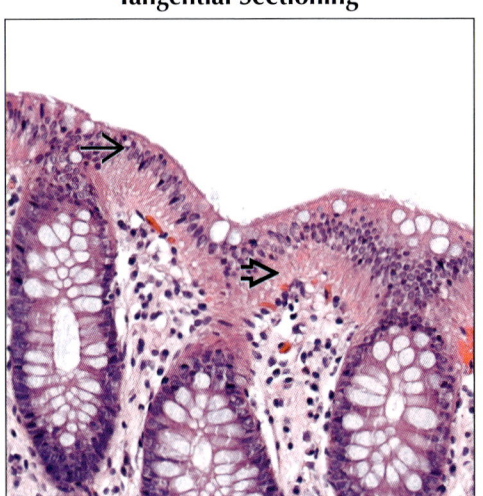

Pseudolipomatosis

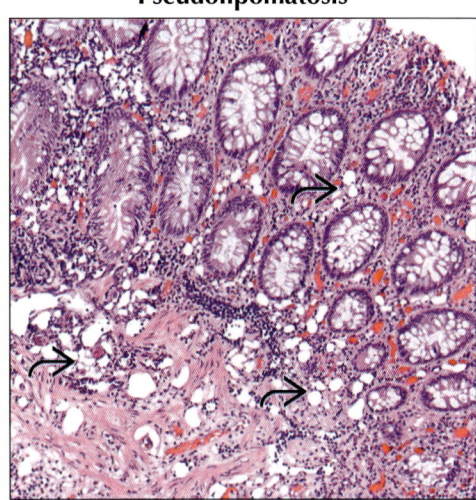

(Left) A common finding in colon biopsies is artificial thickening of the epithelium ⇒ and underlying basement membrane ⇒ due to oblique or tangential sectioning of the tissue. This artifact can generate the impression of nuclear stratification, such as that seen in dysplasia, or a thickened subepithelial collagen band, such as that as seen in collagenous colitis. (Right) Mild endoscope trauma can lead to air ⇒ entering the lamina propria and submucosa, an artifact known as pseudolipomatosis.

Pneumatosis

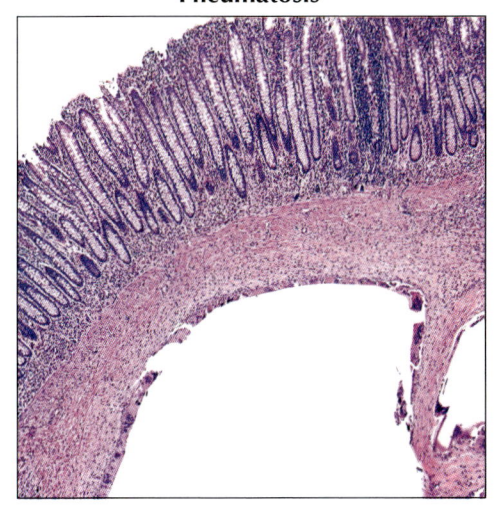

Pneumatosis

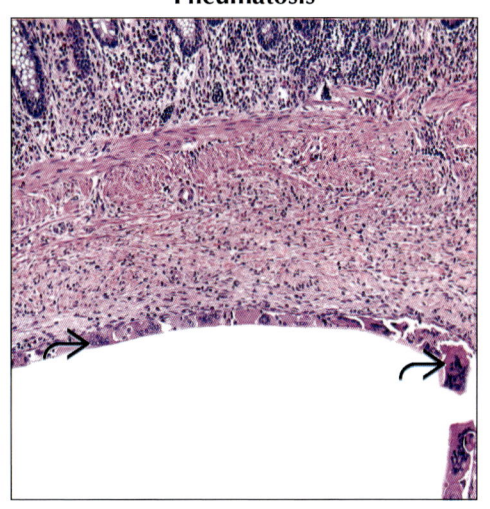

(Left) Pneumatosis is caused by gas entering the submucosa or subserosa of the bowel and is related to various etiologies, including infection and mechanical trauma. Compared to pseudolipomatosis, pneumatosis can be seen endoscopically and is not an artifact. (Right) A higher magnification of pneumatosis shows the characteristic finding of foreign body multinucleated giant cells ⇒ rimming the space filled with gas. This finding is not seen in artifactual pseudolipomatosis.

Tissue Cauterization

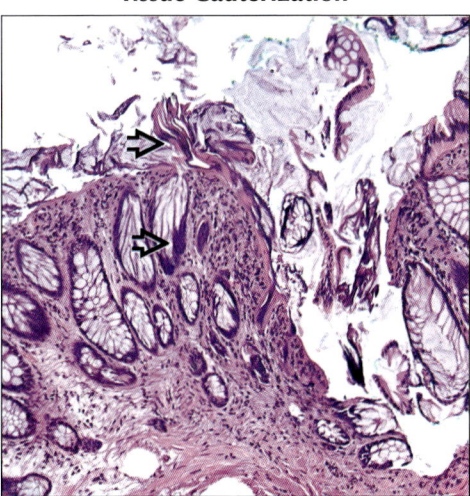

Intraepithelial Lymphocytes

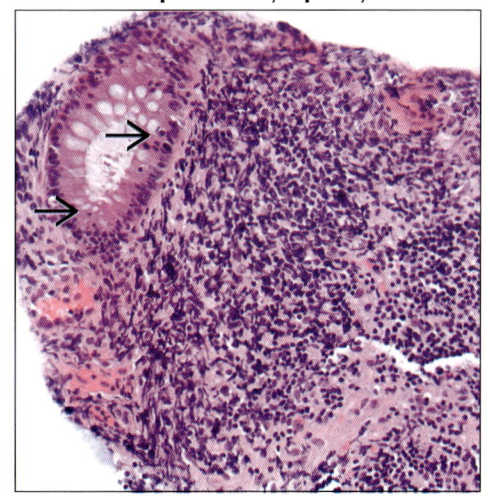

(Left) If the endoscopist uses cautery when collecting tissue, it is very common to see at least some degree of tissue cautery or burning, which gives all affected cells and their nuclei a markedly "stretched out" appearance ⇒. (Right) The epithelium overlying a lymphoid aggregate (MALT) usually shows an increased number of intraepithelial lymphocytes ⇒. This normal finding can lead to a misdiagnosis of lymphocytic colitis, particularly if lymphoid aggregates are numerous.

LARGE INTESTINE

Intraepithelial Lymphocytes

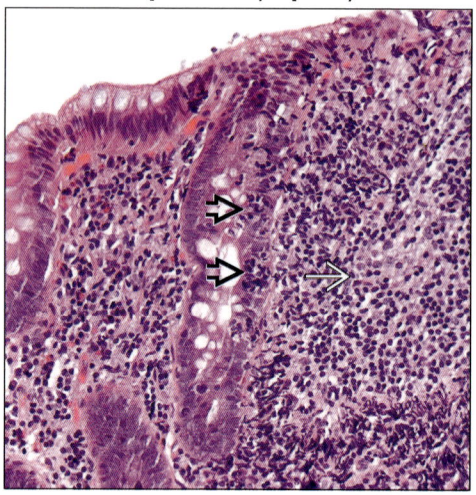

Luminal Debris

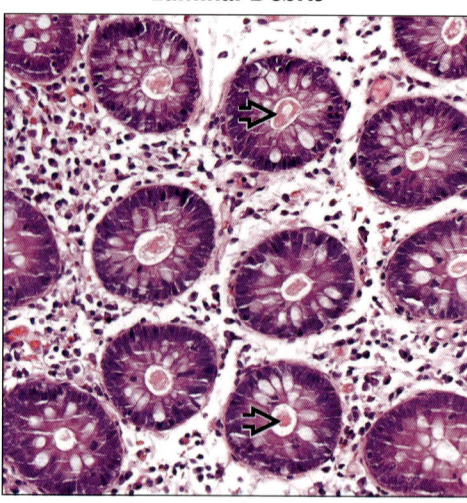

(Left) This image shows a substantial increase in intraepithelial lymphocytes ⇨ adjacent to a reactive lymphoid aggregate ➡. Occasionally intraepithelial neutrophils can also be seen next to lymphoid aggregates as well (not shown). (Right) Biologic matter (such as vegetable matter), admixed with gland secretions, can be seen within the crypt lumina as pink fluffy or chunky material ⇨ and is of no particular significance. It should not be confused with parasitic organisms.

Hyperplastic Mucosal Changes

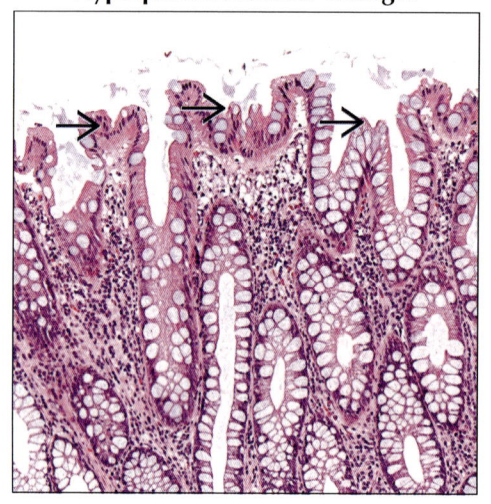

Rectal Histiocytes (Muciphages)

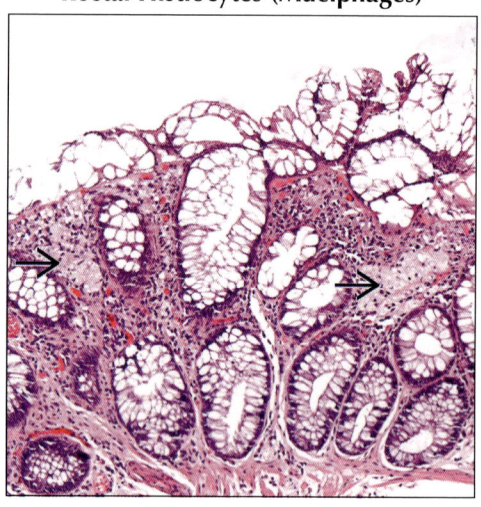

(Left) Hyperplastic mucosal changes are typically seen within the context of mucosal irritation/friction, such as exposure to the fecal stream. It is identified as splitting or branching of the luminal surface epithelium ⇨. Note how there is no distortion at the base of the crypts, which is often a more significant finding. (Right) In the rectum, it is common to find aggregates ➡ of benign foamy histiocytes, known as muciphages. These aggregates vary in size.

Muciphages

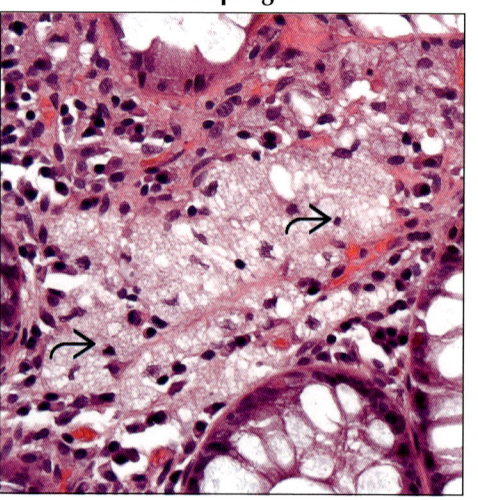

Melanosis Coli

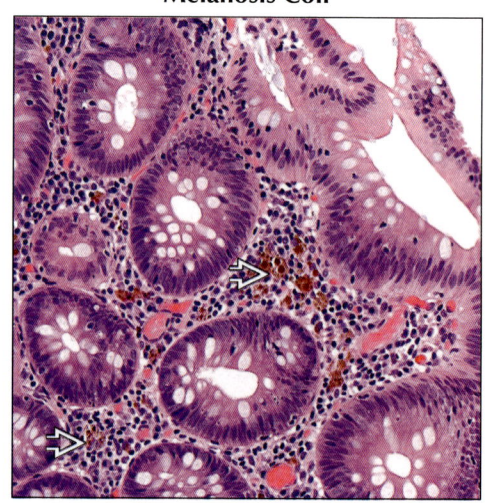

(Left) At high magnification, the muciphages show abundant foamy blue-white cytoplasm and small, dark nuclei ⇨. The lack of nuclear atypia is an important feature and helps distinguish them from the signet ring cells present in some variants of adenocarcinoma. (Right) Melanosis coli is seen as brown/black pigmented macrophages ⇨ predominantly within the colonic mucosa. It is a common finding in patients with chronic laxative usage.

LARGE INTESTINE

Melanosis Coli

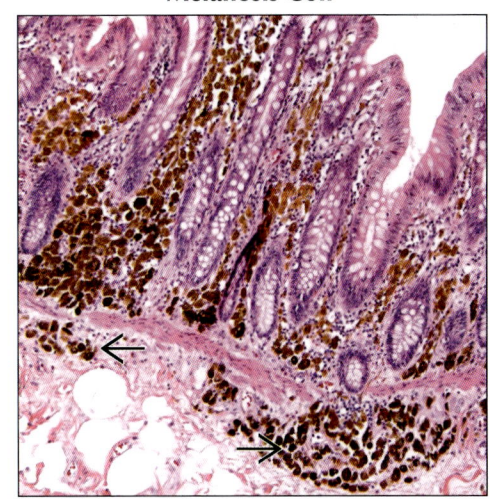

Bifid Crypt

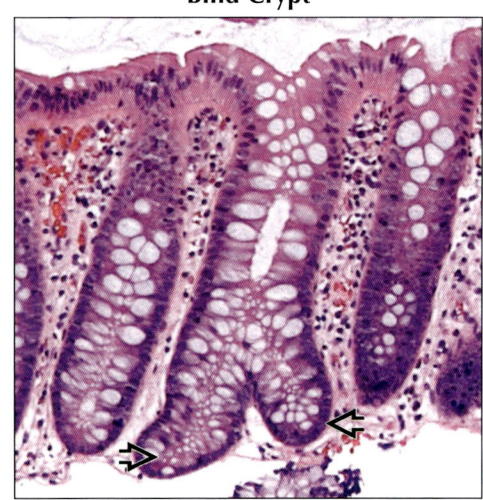

(Left) In some examples of melanosis coli, the pigmented macrophages are very prominent and even extend into the submucosa ⇨. If extensive, this finding may lead to consideration of malignant melanoma. **(Right)** A bifid crypt is a normal variant of a colonic crypt in which the basal aspect demonstrates a fork-like split appearance ⇨. This finding should not be confused with true architectural distortion seen within the context of chronic colitis and inflammatory bowel disease.

Artifactual Mucosal Hemorrhage

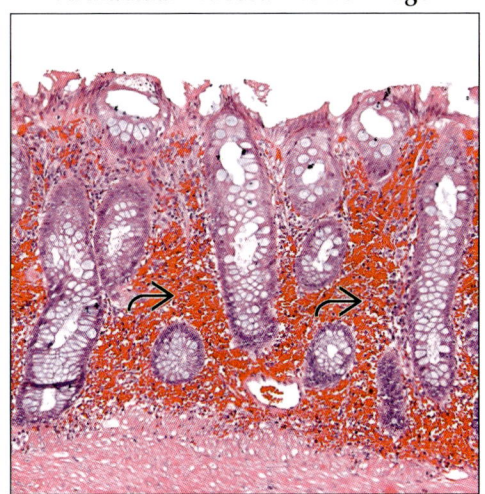

Artifactual Epithelial Telescoping

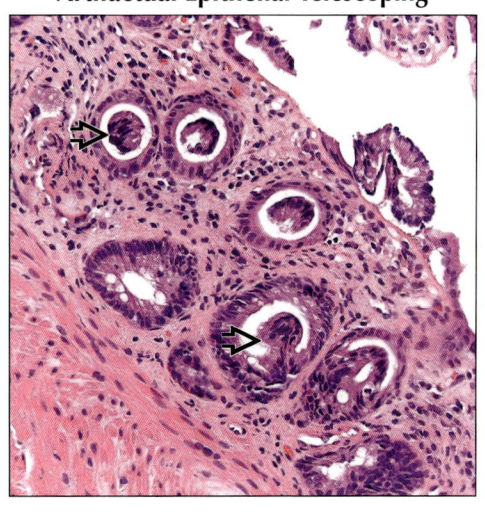

(Left) Nonpathologic hemorrhage ⇨ localized within the lamina propria can be seen as a result of trauma related to the surgical or biopsy procedure or to bowel prep. It is often patchy and confined to the mucosa, but without hemosiderin-laden macrophages (a feature of chronic hemorrhage). **(Right)** As a consequence of aggressive biopsy techniques and tissue compression, colonic crypts can "telescope" within themselves ⇨ and mimic the appearance of an intraluminal organism.

Endoscope Trauma

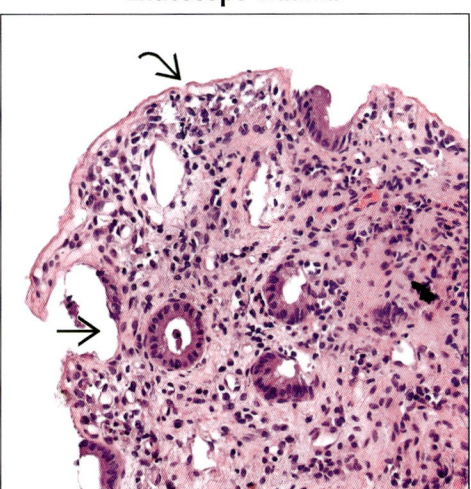

Vegetable Material

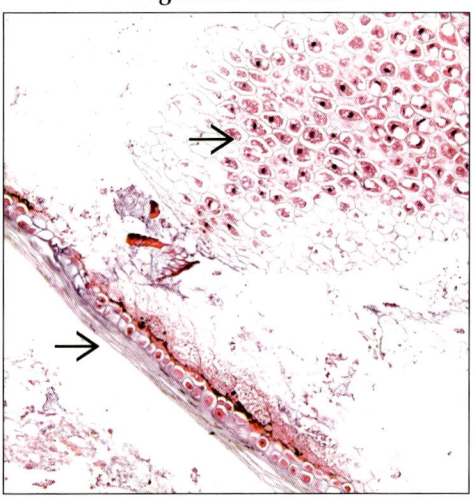

(Left) Aggressive biopsy techniques can lead to disruption of the tissue and can manifest as crypt "dropout" ⇨ &/or "peeling off" ⇨ of the epithelial surface. These specimens often show additional features of scope trauma, including telescoping, hemorrhage, or cautery. **(Right)** Fragments of vegetable matter (feces) ⇨ within the bowel lumen are a common finding in colectomy specimens in which the patient does not undergo adequate preoperative evacuative measures.

APPENDIX

Key Facts

Macroscopic Anatomy
- Tubular organ arising from cecum in right lower quadrant of abdomen
- Can range in length from < 5 cm to > 9 cm
- Mesoappendix is contiguous with mesentery of bowel

Microscopic Anatomy
- Layers are very similar to large bowel
- Mucin, fecal material, and pinworms are commonly seen in lumen
- Mucosa
  - Simple columnar epithelium, basically colonic in type
  - Crypts are more unevenly distributed and irregularly aligned than in colon
  - Paneth cells, goblet cells, and neuroendocrine cells are present
  - Large component of lymphoid tissue in children, adolescents, and young adults
  - Epithelium over lymphoid tissue may be less columnar, and crypts may be absent
  - Lamina propria contains mononuclear cells, scattered eosinophils, and neuroendocrine cells
  - Muscularis mucosa is variably developed and may appear discontinuous
  - Muscularis mucosa may be focally absent where large lymphoid aggregates are present
- Submucosa
  - Loose connective tissue containing adipose tissue, vessels, nerves, and scattered inflammatory cells
  - Lymphoid tissue may also be present within submucosa
- Muscularis propria
  - Inner circular layer, outer longitudinal layer
  - Longitudinal layer becomes continuous with taenia coli at base of appendix
  - Nerves and ganglion cells are present irregularly throughout muscular wall
- Serosa
  - Mature fibroadipose tissue with mesothelial lining (peritonealized)

Pitfalls/Artifacts
- Surface hyperplastic changes can mimic serrated polyps
- Irregular distribution and uneven alignment of crypts can raise the possibility of chronic idiopathic inflammatory bowel disease
  - Lack of architectural derangement that is much less common in normal appendix will help in making the distinction
- Appendiceal diverticula
  - Ruptured diverticula can spill mucin, mimicking a low-grade appendiceal mucinous neoplasm; however, neoplastic epithelium is absent
- Luminal mucin
  - Abundant mucin can mimic a low-grade mucinous neoplasm; however, underlying epithelium should be normal
- Müllerian elements: Endometriosis, endocervicosis, and endosalpingiosis are common
  - May mimic metastatic adenocarcinoma on frozen section

Age Variation
- Mucosal lymphoid aggregates become smaller and less confluent with increasing age
- Entire appendix becomes narrower in middle age, with increasing fibrosis

Hyperplasia
- Reactive lymphoid hyperplasia

(Left) This low-power view of the appendix demonstrates the epithelial layer ➡ and prominent lymphoid tissue ➡ of the mucosa, as well as the underlying submucosa ➡, muscularis propria ➡, and the serosa and subserosal connective tissue. Pinworms are visible in the lumen. (Right) The epithelium of the appendix resembles the colon, with columnar cells and interspersed goblet cells.

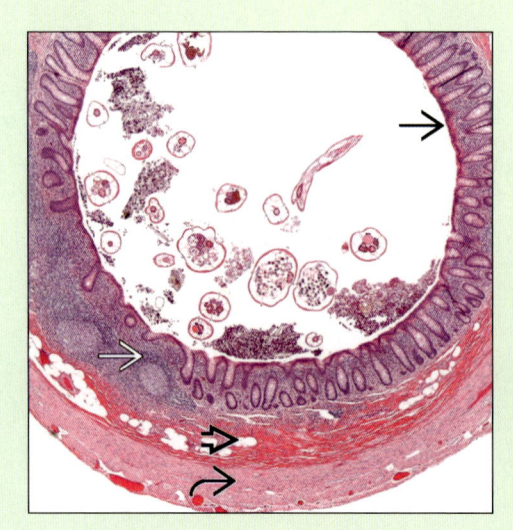

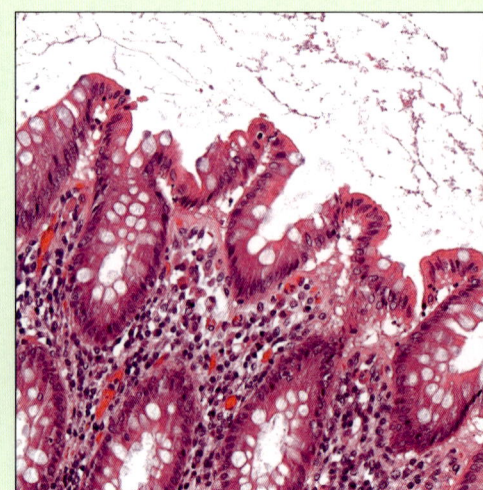

APPENDIX

Epithelium
Lamina Propria

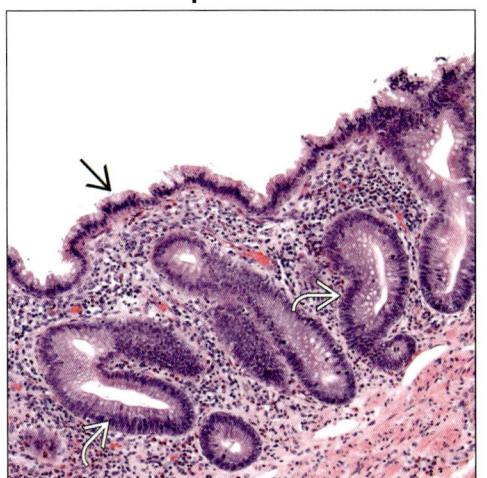

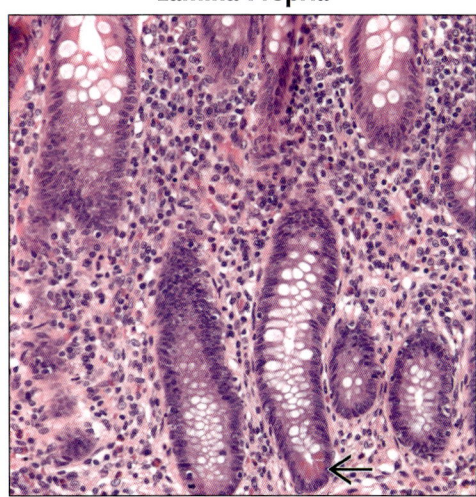

(Left) The appendiceal epithelium ➡ is a mucinous columnar lining with goblet cells, similar to the colon. The crypts ➡ in the appendix are much less orderly and more irregularly aligned than those in the colon. (Right) The lamina propria contains mononuclear cells and occasional eosinophils, similar to the colon. Note the Paneth cells in the lower right-hand corner ➡.

Lymphoid Tissue
Lymphoid Tissue

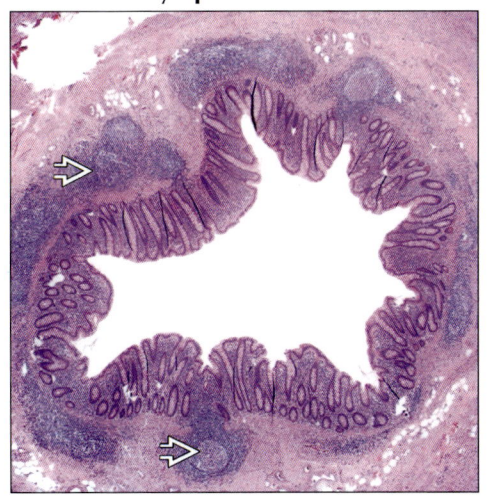

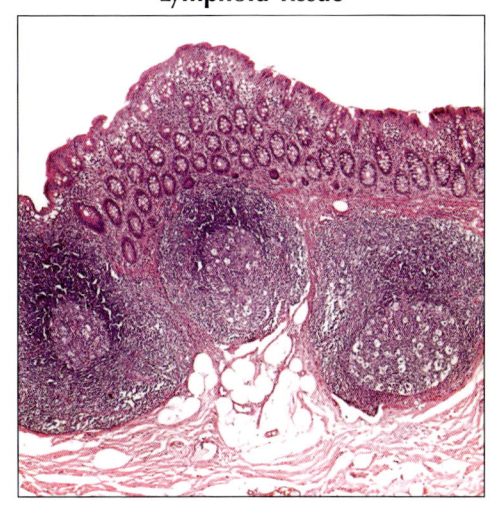

(Left) The conspicuous (and often confluent) lymphoid aggregates ➡ are a characteristic feature of the appendix. The prominent lymphoid aggregates can involve the mucosa and the submucosa. (Right) This appendix from a child shows hyperplastic lymphoid follicles with prominent germinal centers. Note that the large lymphoid follicles interrupt the muscularis mucosa.

Lymphoid Tissue
Muscularis Mucosa

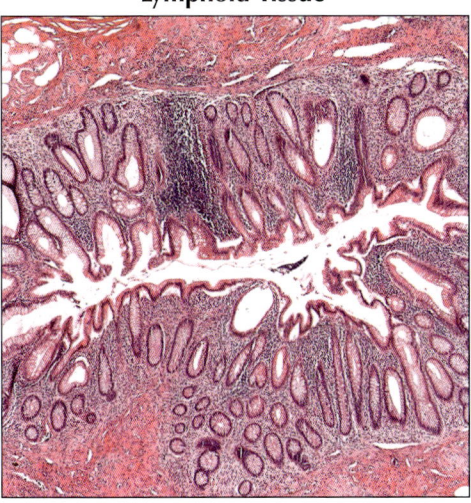

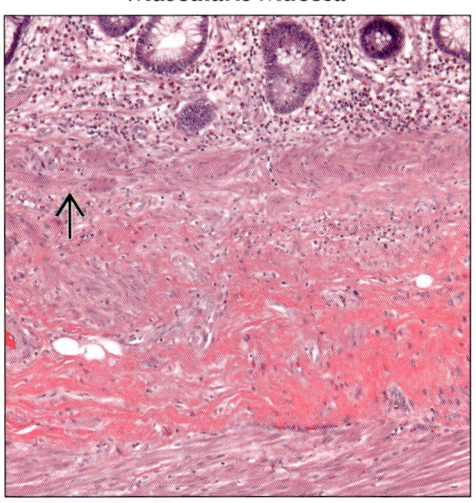

(Left) Cross section of an appendix from an adult shows marked atrophy of the lymphoid tissue, which is a common change with increasing age. (Right) This image shows a well-developed muscularis mucosa ➡. The epithelium is visible above, and the dense connective tissue of the submucosa is visible below.

APPENDIX

Musclaris Mucosa

(Left) In this image, the muscularis mucosa consists of tiny, discontinuous wisps of muscle ⇨. *(Right)* The submucosa consists of adipose tissue, vessels, lymphatics, and nerves. Lymphoid tissue may also be present.

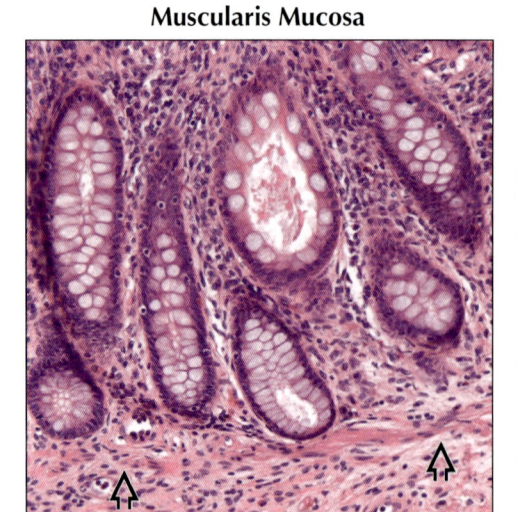

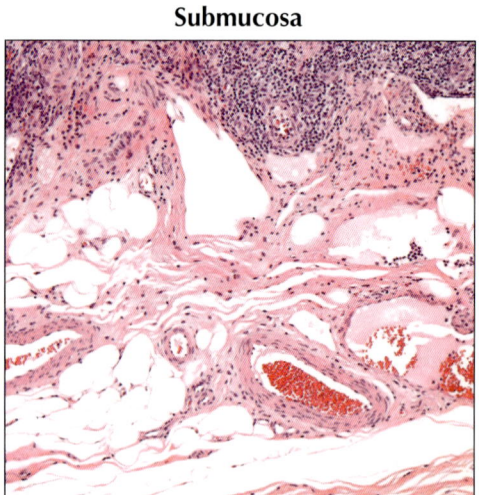

Submucosa

Muscularis Propria

(Left) The inner circular and outer longitudinal layers of the muscularis propria are illustrated here. Scattered neural elements are also visible ⇨. *(Right)* Nerves and ganglion cells ⇨ are often easily identified nestled within the inner and outer layers of the muscularis propria. Similar to those at other sites, they have prominent basophilic cytoplasm and large nucleoli.

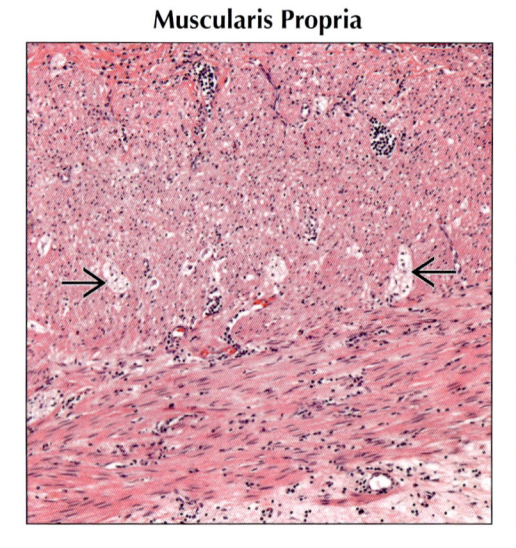

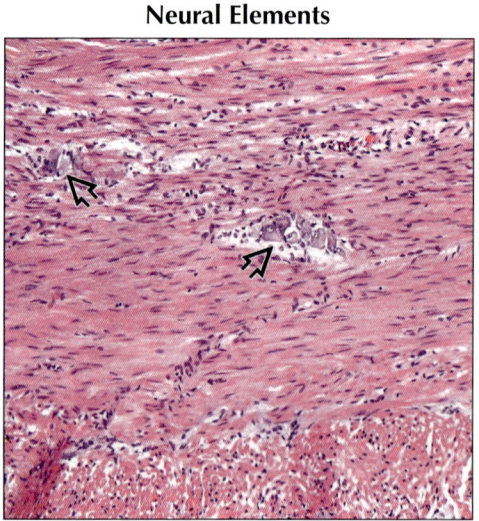

Neural Elements

Ganglion Cells

(Left) This high-power view shows the eccentrically located nucleus and prominent nucleolus of mural ganglion cells. *(Right)* The serosa consists of a thin peritoneal lining that covers the entire appendix ⇨.

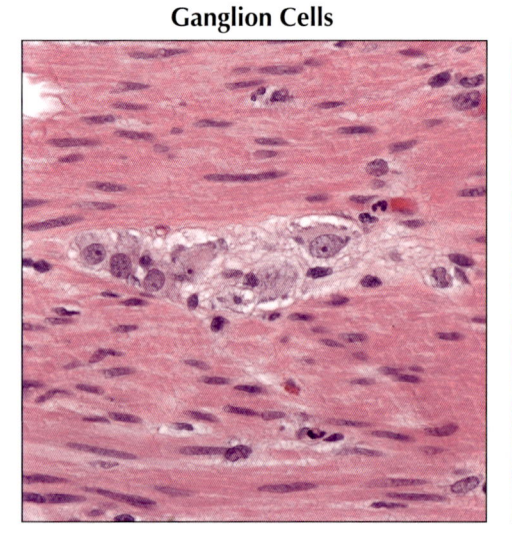

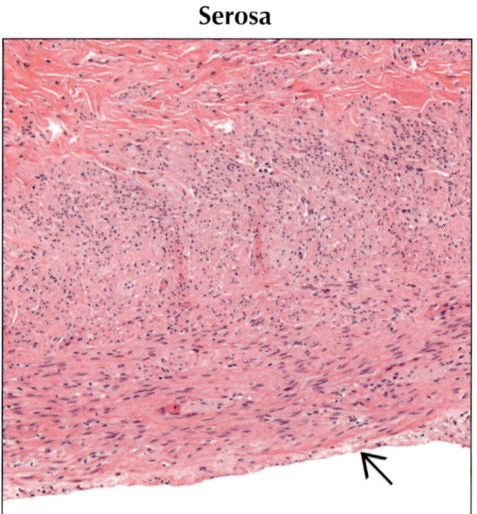

Serosa

APPENDIX

Mesoappendix

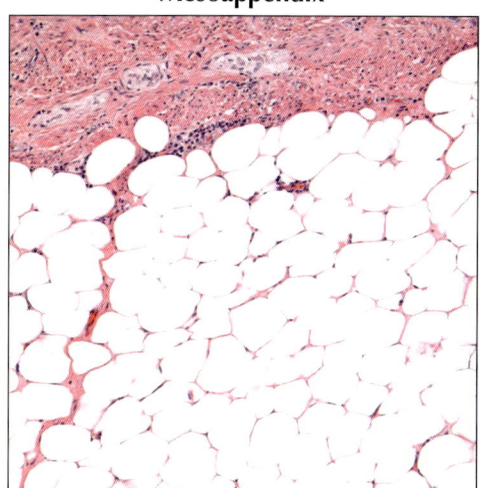

Surface Hyperplastic Changes

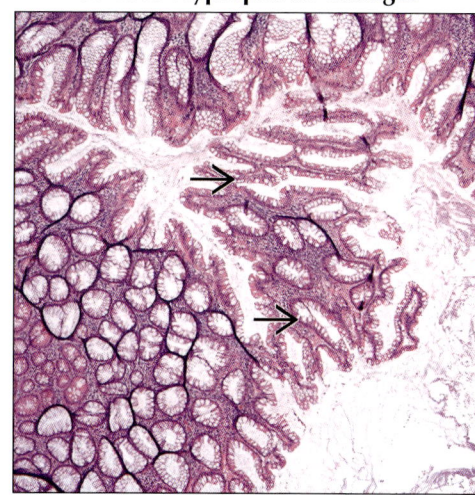

(Left) The mesoappendiceal fat is contiguous with the mesentery of the bowel. *(Right)* Mucosal irritants, such as fecaliths, can lead to hyperplastic changes ➡ in the epithelium, which may superficially resemble a serrated polyp or adenoma. Compared to these 2 entities, however, the hyperplastic change is not focal, has less architectural complexity, and does not show cytologic dysplasia.

Fibrous Obliteration of the Tip

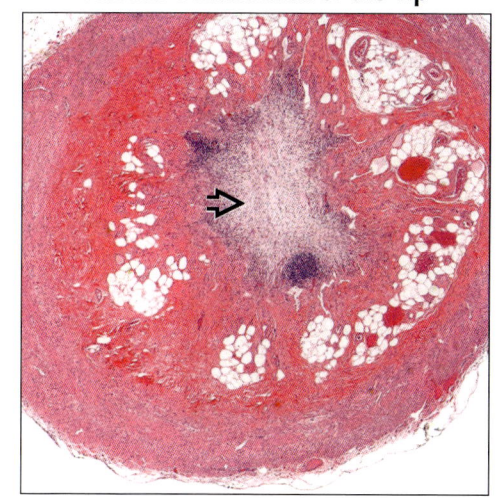

Diverticulum

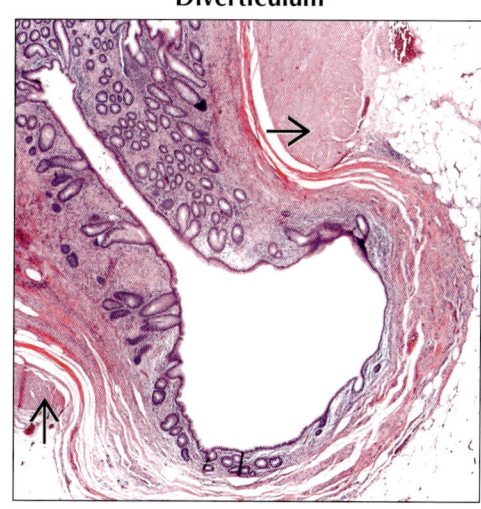

(Left) Benign neural proliferations are occasionally seen within the lamina propria or at the tip of the appendix ➡ (sometimes referred to as fibrous obliteration of the tip). They are typically of no clinical significance. *(Right)* In states of increased luminal pressure, a portion of the appendiceal mucosa may herniate through the muscularis propria ➡, creating a diverticulum. A diverticulum may become secondarily inflamed or even rupture.

Intraluminal Mucin

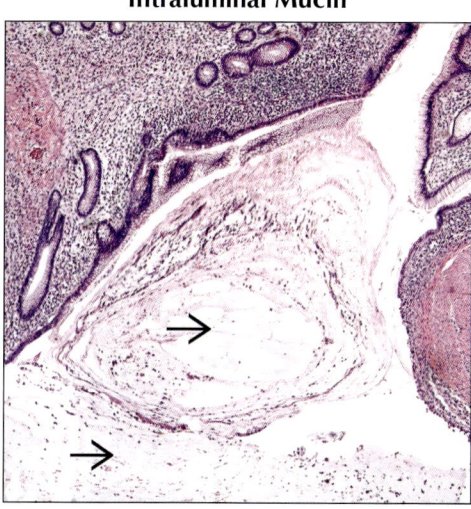

Endometriosis

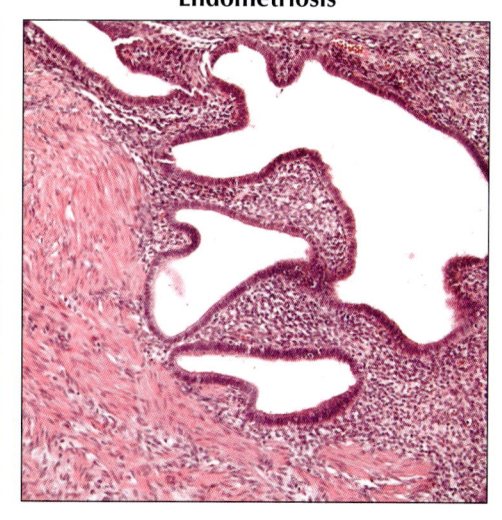

(Left) Abundant epithelial mucin may be produced secondary to trauma or inflammation ➡. Large amounts of mucin can raise the possibility of a low-grade appendiceal mucinous neoplasm, but the underlying epithelium is not neoplastic. *(Right)* In women, müllerian elements may be identified in the muscular wall or serosa. This image shows endometrial glands and stroma (endometriosis), but endocervical glands (endocervicosis) and fallopian tube epithelium (endosalpingiosis) can be seen as well.

ANUS AND ANAL CANAL

Key Facts

Macroscopic Anatomy
- Complex anatomy with controversial nomenclature
  - Extent of zones is variable, and delineations are irregular
  - Macroscopic and microscopic zones often do not correspond
- Perianal skin
- Anal canal: Squamous zone, transition zone, colorectal zone
- Dentate line lies within anal canal
  - Includes anal valves and sinuses, and bases of anal columns
  - Anal columns are vertical folds extending from mid to upper anal canal; connected at base by the small semilunar anal valves, which may appear as small papillae; anal sinuses or crypts are behind the valves
- Anal cushions: Pads of tissue outlined by the Y-shaped anal lumen; hemorrhoids represent prolapse of anal cushions
- Anal musculature: External sphincter, intersphincteric longitudinal muscle, internal sphincter, musculus submucosae ani

Microscopic Anatomy
- Colorectal zone: Continuation of rectal mucosa (CK20[+], CK7[-])
- Transition zone: Variable types of epithelium
  - CK20(-), CK7(+); CK7 staining may be very patchy
  - Anal glands open here
- Squamous zone: Nonkeratinized squamous epithelium lacking hair, appendages
- Perianal skin: Keratinizing epithelium with hair, appendages

Pitfalls/Artifacts
- Colorectal zone may have irregular crypts
- Anal transition zone epithelium may mimic high-grade anal intraepithelial neoplasia
- Ganglion cells normally absent or sparse in 1st cm above dentate line

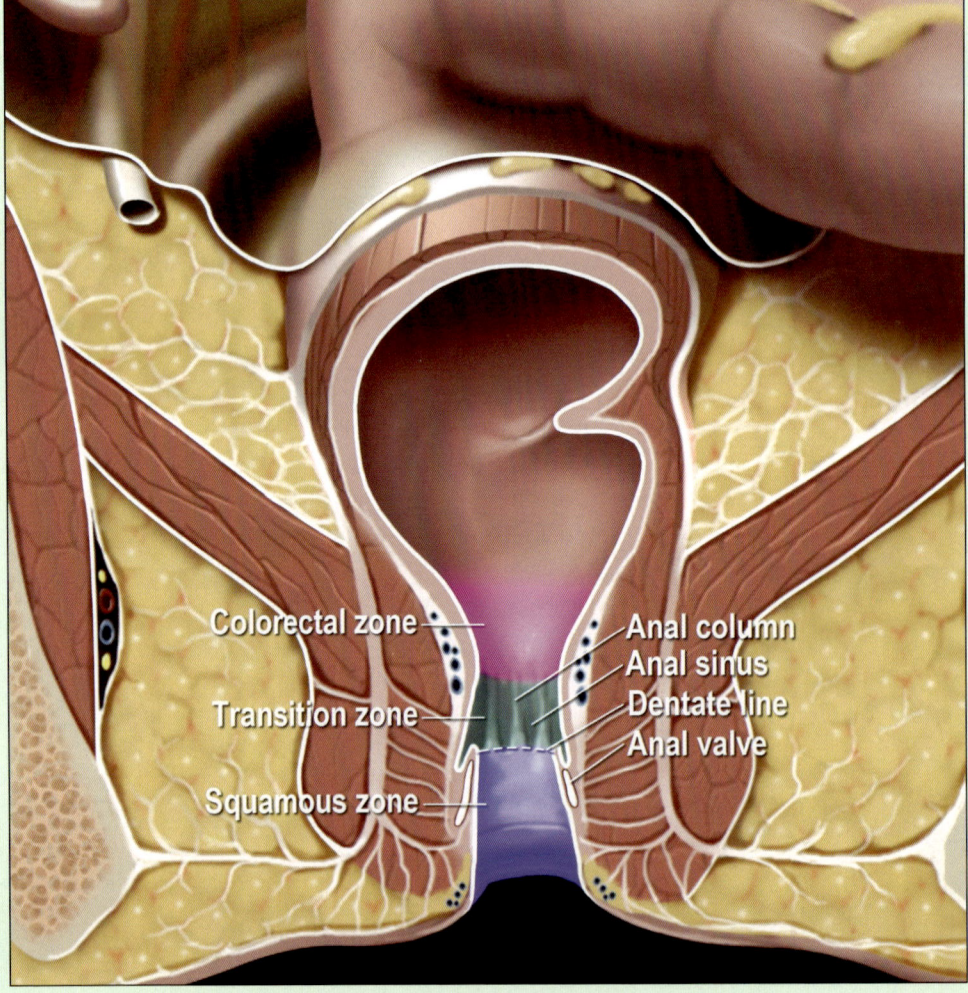

The most proximal zone of the anal canal is the colorectal zone, which is lined by uninterrupted glandular mucosa. The most distal zone is the squamous zone, lined by uninterrupted squamous mucosa. The transition zone lies in between, and contains a number of types of epithelia, including anal transition zone epithelium. The dentate line lies within the anal canal and includes the anal valves, anal sinuses, and bases of anal columns. The histologic anal canal is defined by the extent of the specialized mucosa, i.e., the transitional zone and squamous zone down to the perianal skin. The dentate line is an important anatomical landmark with respect to orientation of biopsies from this area.

ANUS AND ANAL CANAL

Perianal Skin

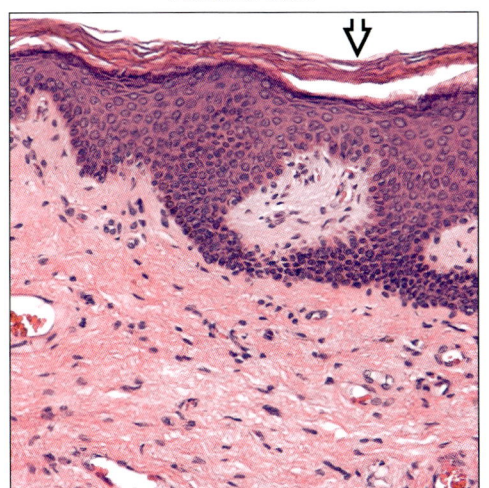

Perianal Skin and Appendages

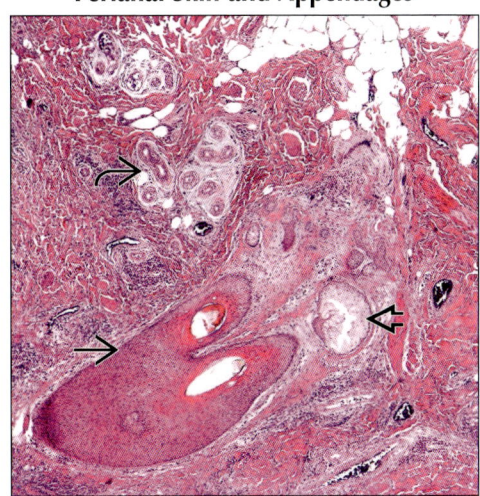

(Left) Perianal skin is keratinized ⇨, unlike the nonkeratinized squamous zone of the anal canal. *(Right)* Perianal skin contains hair follicles ➡, apocrine glands, eccrine glands ➡, and sebaceous glands ⇨. The squamous zone of the anal canal lacks hair, glands, and appendages.

Lamina Propria

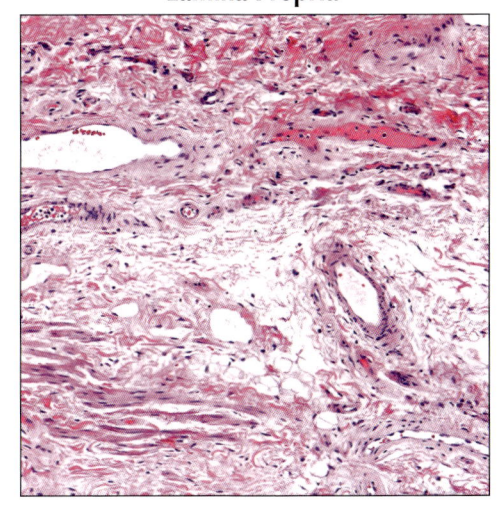

Apocrine Glands

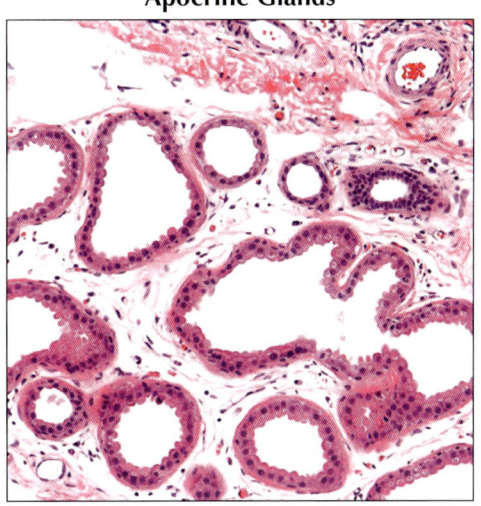

(Left) Anal canal lamina propria consists of loose connective tissue with scattered lymphocytes and mast cells. It contains vessels, lymphatics, and nerves. Ganglion cells are normally absent or sparse within 1 cm of the dentate line, which is important for evaluating patients for Hirschsprung disease. *(Right)* Apocrine glands, which can be identified by their bright pink epithelium, are commonly found in perianal skin. (Courtesy S. Shalin, MD.)

Eccrine Glands

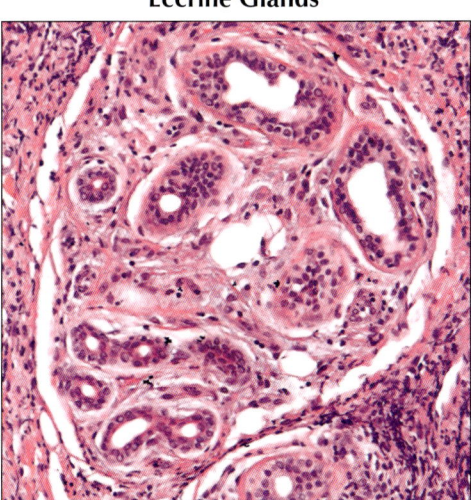

Anogenital Sweat Glands

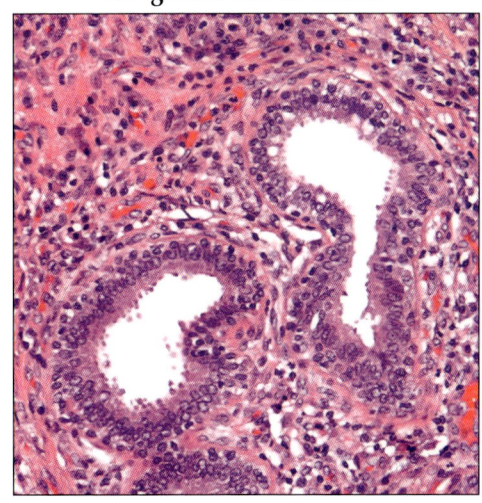

(Left) Eccrine glands are commonly found in perianal skin. They form small well-circumscribed clusters and have low cuboidal epithelium. A variably distinct myoepithelial layer is present. *(Right)* Anogenital sweat glands are another type of gland found in perianal skin. They consist of columnar epithelium with cytoplasmic "snouts" protruding into the lumen of the gland.

ANUS AND ANAL CANAL

Transition Zone

Transition Zone

(Left) Transition zone lies between squamous & colorectal zones and contains various types of epithelium, including anal transitional epithelium, which may resemble urothelium or immature squamous epithelium. Surface cells may be flat or resemble urothelial umbrella cells. *(Right)* Anal transition zone epithelium consists of basal cells with overlying columnar, cuboidal, or polygonal cells. Note cuboidal or polygonal cells on the surface. Melanocytes may be present in transition zone.

Transition Zone

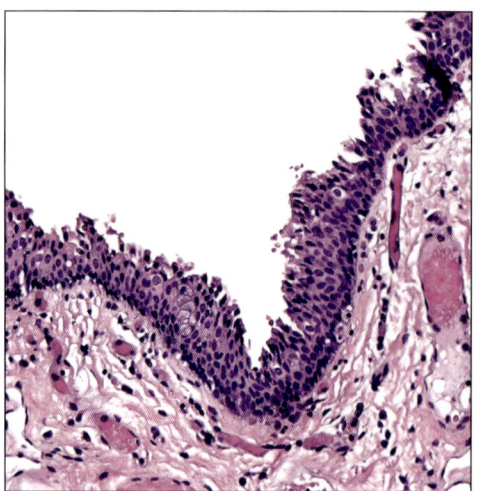

Colorectal and Transition Zones

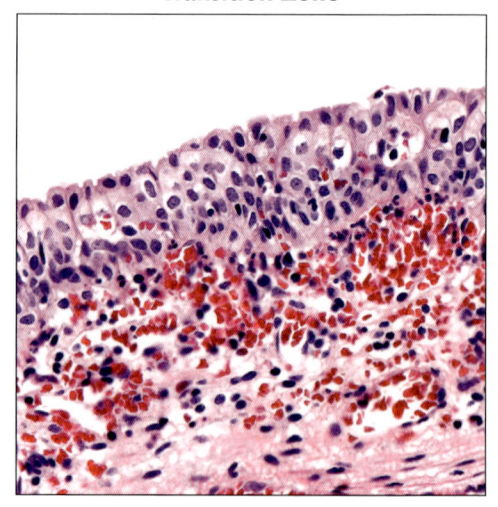

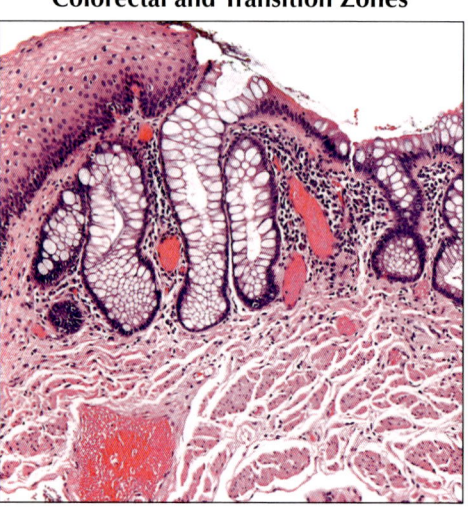

(Left) This example of transition zone epithelium more closely resembles squamous epithelium and has flattened surface epithelial cells. Scattered mononuclear cells are normally present in the lamina propria. *(Right)* The colorectal zone is a continuation of the rectal mucosa and consists of uninterrupted glandular epithelium. The muscularis mucosa extends from the rectum into the colorectal zone and upper transition zone.

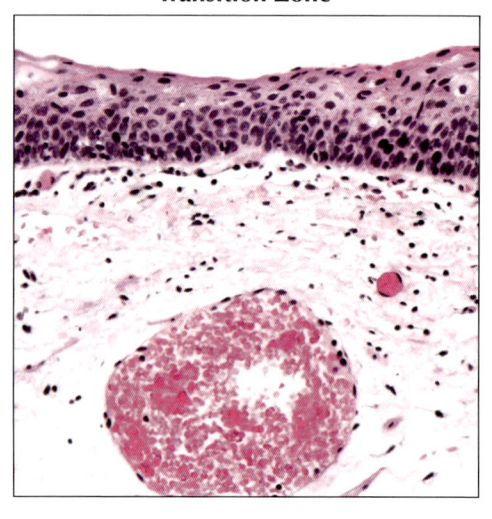

Colorectal and Transition Zones

Squamous Zone

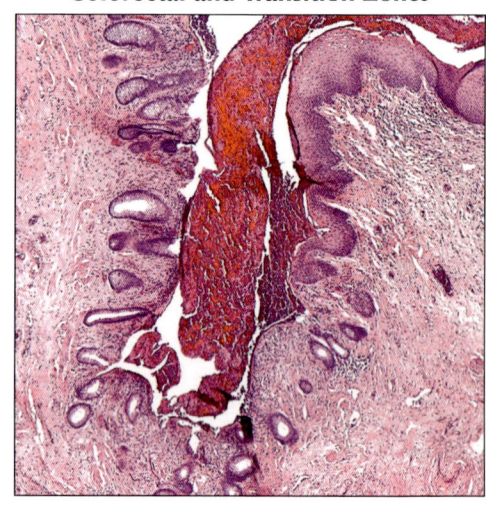

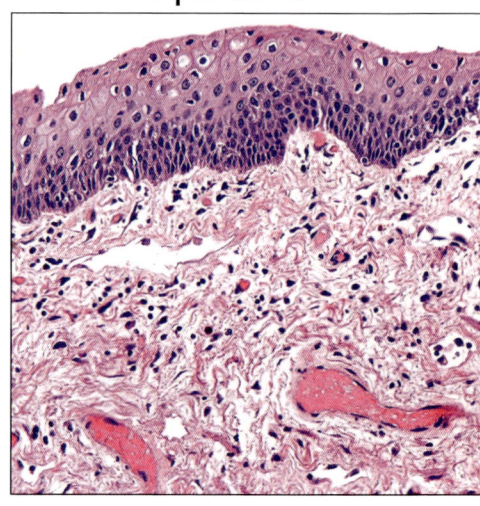

(Left) The mucosa of the colorectal zone may have shorter, more irregular crypts; this should not be mistaken for evidence of chronic inflammatory changes. *(Right)* Squamous zone consists of uninterrupted nonkeratinizing epithelium with few or no rete pegs. It lacks hair and skin appendages. Melanocytes, lymphocytes, histiocytes, and Merkel cells are present. Anal canal stroma may contain large multilobated stromal cells that should not be mistaken for a neoplastic process.

ANUS AND ANAL CANAL

Transition Zone

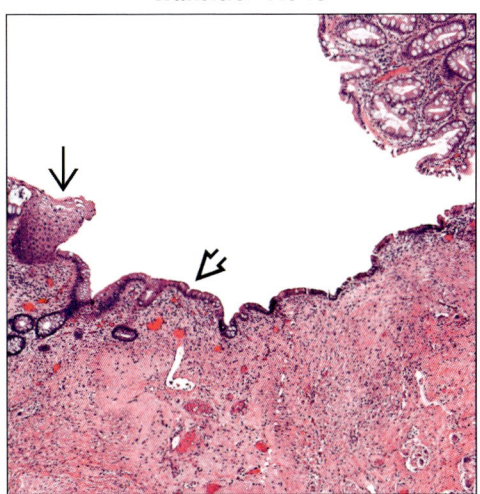

Anal Glands

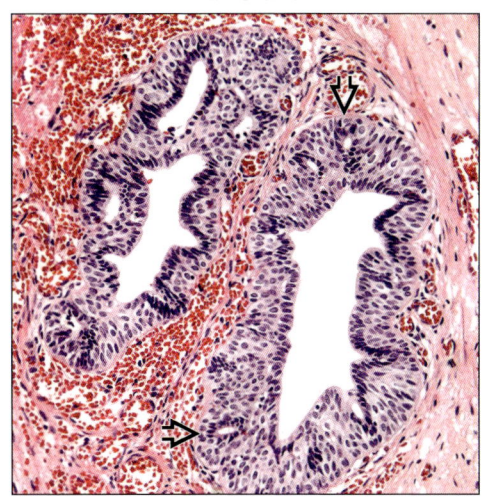

(Left) Mature squamous epithelium ➡, colorectal mucosa, and simple columnar epithelium ⇨ may also be present in the transition zone. *(Right)* Anal glands open into the transition zone. The epithelium resembles transition zone epithelium, and microcyst formation ⇨ is common. Some are present in the submucosa, but others extend into the anal musculature. The anal glands have a similar cytokeratin staining pattern to the transition zone mucosa.

Anal Glands

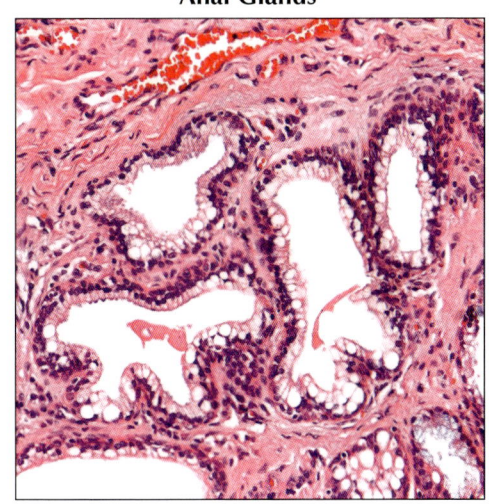

Perianal Nevus

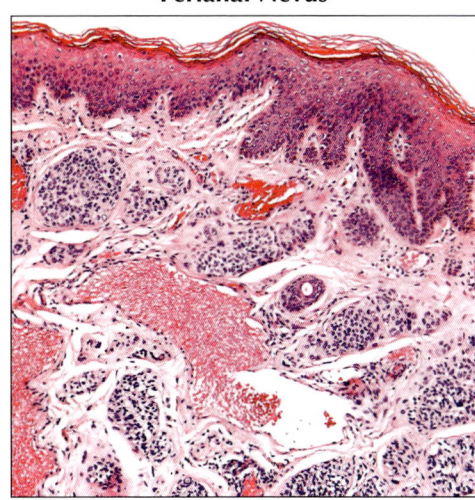

(Left) Goblet cell metaplasia is a frequent finding in anal glands. *(Right)* The melanocytes within the transition zone and perianal skin may give rise to nevi, as seen here, as well as to anal melanoma.

AIN in Transition Zone

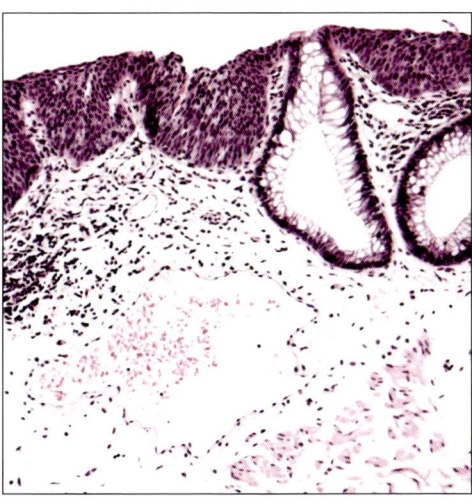

AIN in Transition Zone

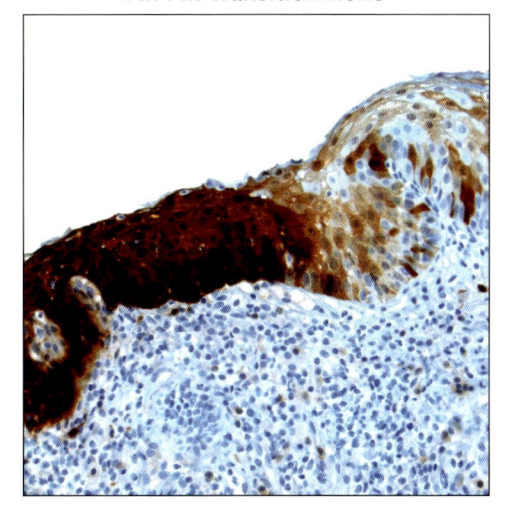

(Left) Occasionally, transition zone epithelium may be difficult to distinguish from high-grade anal intraepithelial neoplasia (AIN), which is seen here in the transition zone. *(Right)* p16 immunostaining may help distinguish high-grade AIN (full-thickness staining, on the left) from transition zone epithelium.

PERITONEAL MEMBRANES

Key Facts

Macroscopic Anatomy
- Smooth, glistening surface
- 2 layers: Parietal and visceral
  - Visceral peritoneum lines intraabdominal viscera
  - Parietal peritoneum lines surfaces of abdominal wall, diaphragm, retroperitoneum, and upper pelvis
- Visceral and parietal layers meet at mesentery
- Omentum is mature adipose tissue sandwiched between 2 double layers of visceral peritoneum

Microscopic Anatomy
- Composed of thin layer of cuboidal mesothelial cells with underlying submesothelium (connective tissue and elastic fibers)
- Normal mesothelial cells
  - Difficult to see in routine histologic sections
  - Single central nucleus with homogeneous chromatin
  - Nucleolus is typically absent

- Reactive mesothelial cells
  - Larger and more conspicuous (easily seen in histologic sections)
  - Enlarged nuclei with prominent central nucleoli
  - May show multinucleation
  - May form small papillary structures
- In reactive conditions, submesothelial layer is often thickened and more cellular

Pitfalls/Artifacts
- Reactive papillary mesothelial hyperplasia
- Endometriosis
- Endosalpingiosis
- Multilocular peritoneal inclusion cyst
- Deciduosis

(Left) When visible, the peritoneal lining appears as a relatively thin layer ⇨ of small eosinophilic cells (mesothelial cells) lining the surface of mature adipose (omental) or fibroconnective tissue. *(Right)* Mesothelial cells ⇨ are small, cuboidal eosinophilic cells that demonstrate a single central nucleus and usually lack a nucleolus. The elongated to spindled cells in the underlying connective tissue are submesothelial fibroblasts ⇨.

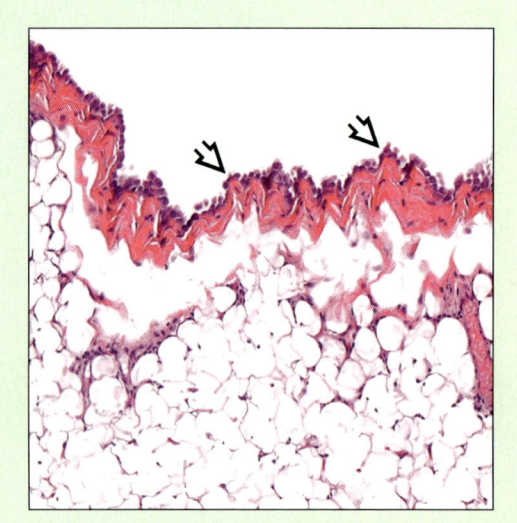

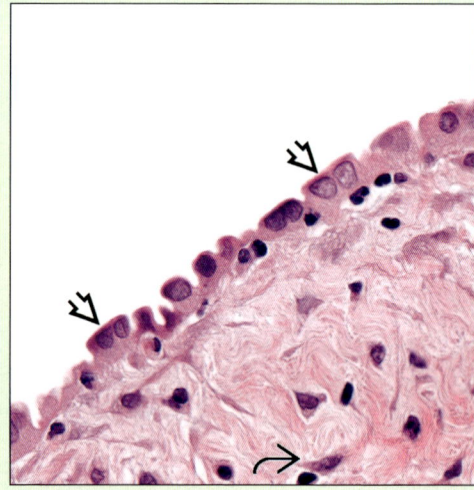

(Left) Under reactive conditions, mesothelial cells commonly adopt a plump, "hobnail" morphology ⇨ that is reminiscent of a row of tombstones or matchsticks. The lining is often also more cellular and disorganized, making it look very "busy." *(Right)* Cytologically, reactive mesothelial cells commonly show cellular and nuclear enlargement with the formation of conspicuous nucleoli ⇨. Multinucleation ⇨ and mitotic division figures ⇨ can also be seen.

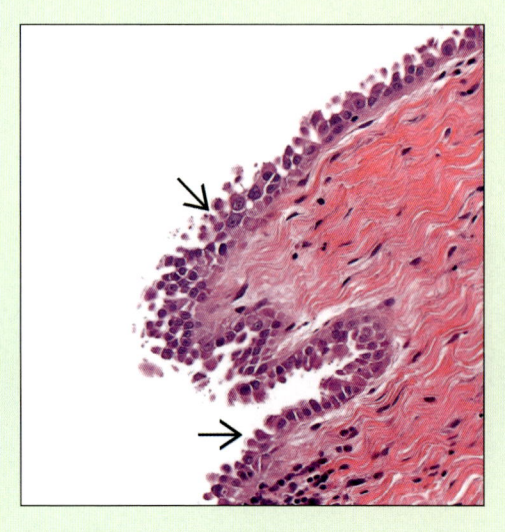

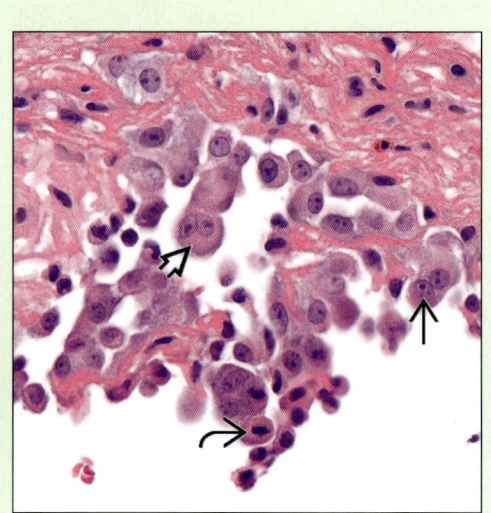

PERITONEAL MEMBRANES

Reactive Peritoneal Thickening

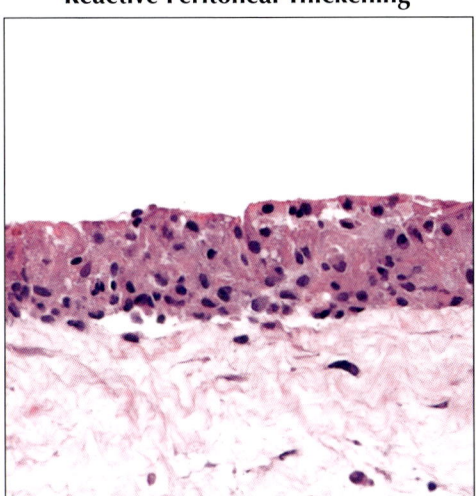

Sloughed Mesothelial Cells

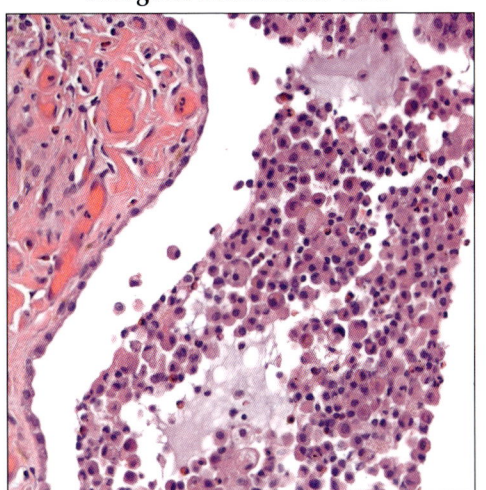

(Left) Under reactive conditions, the peritoneal lining can also become more thickened and less hobnailed. Importantly, despite their number, cells are limited to the surface and never show destructive invasion of the underlying fibroconnective tissue. *(Right)* A reactive lining can slough off of the underlying submesothelium, sometimes mimicking a neoplastic process; however, these cells are usually loosely cohesive, contain admixed inflammatory cells, and lack features of malignancy.

Sloughed Mesothelial Cells

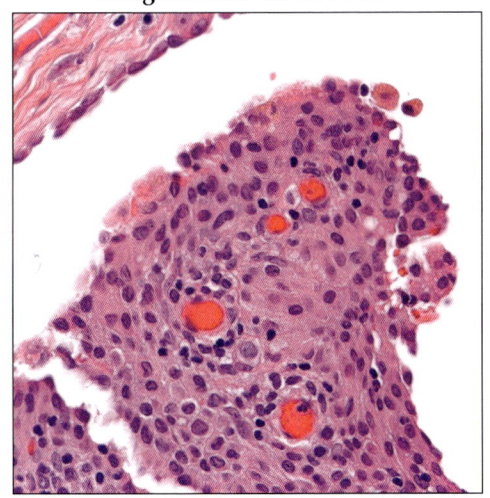

Reactive Papillary Mesothelial Hyperplasia

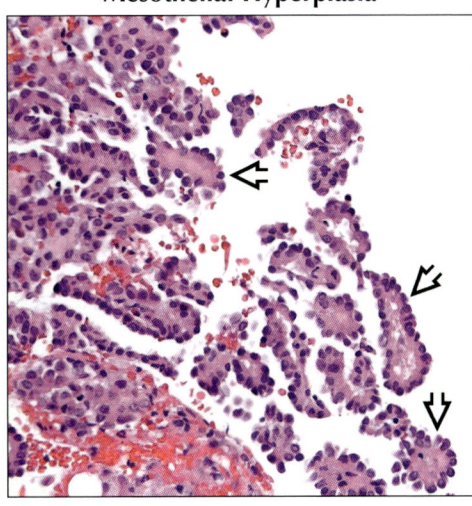

(Left) Sloughed reactive mesothelial cells are occasionally very cohesive and can mimic peritoneal involvement by carcinoma. However, reactive mesothelial cells lack malignant nuclear features, atypical mitotic figures, and coagulative necrosis. *(Right)* The peritoneal lining is capable of forming simple papillary structures (cells surrounding a central fibrovascular core) ⇨. When these structures are prominent and diffuse, a well-differentiated mesothelioma must be considered.

Multicystic Peritoneal Inclusion Cyst

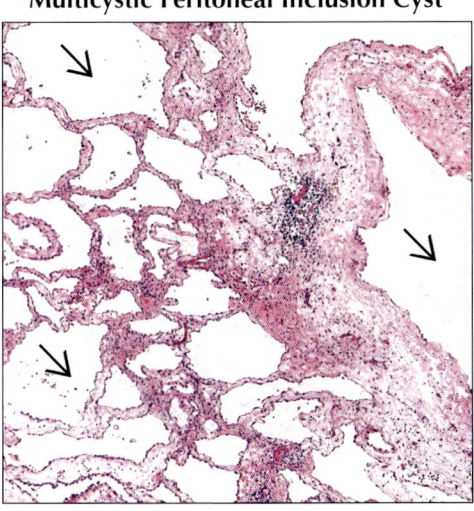

Ectopic Decidua

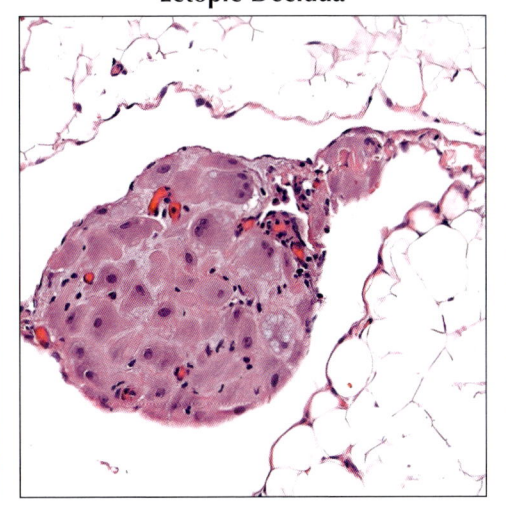

(Left) Peritoneal inclusion cysts occur almost exclusively in women and are identified by numerous dilated cystic spaces ⇨. This multicystic appearance is not typically of normal or reactive peritoneum and should suggest a pathologic diagnosis. *(Right)* Ectopic decidual tissue (deciduosis) is a rare, incidental finding in omental, mesenteric, or peritoneal tissue of postpartum women and is of no clinical significance. It can, however, morphologically mimic mesothelial cells.

SELECTED REFERENCES

ESOPHAGUS

1. Huang Q: Controversies of cardiac glands in the proximal stomach: a critical review. J Gastroenterol Hepatol. 26(3):450-5, 2011
2. Stojsic ZM et al: Histological features of gastric cardia in adults: an autopsy study. J Gastrointestin Liver Dis. 20(1):13-8, 2011
3. Ugalde PA et al: Correlative anatomy for the esophagus. Thorac Surg Clin. 21(2):307-17, x, 2011
4. Johansson J et al: Pancreatic acinar metaplasia in the distal oesophagus and the gastric cardia: prevalence, predictors and relation to GORD. J Gastroenterol. 45(3):291-9, 2010
5. Radenkovic G et al: C-kit-immunopositive interstitial cells of Cajal in human embryonal and fetal oesophagus. Cell Tissue Res. 340(3):427-36, 2010
6. Yüksel I et al: Inlet patch: associations with endoscopic findings in the upper gastrointestinal system. Scand J Gastroenterol. 43(8):910-4, 2008
7. Kilgore SP et al: The gastric cardia: fact or fiction? Am J Gastroenterol. 95(4):921-4, 2000
8. Wang HH et al: Prevalence and significance of pancreatic acinar metaplasia at the gastroesophageal junction. Am J Surg Pathol. 20(12):1507-10, 1996
9. Nakada T et al: Ectopic sebaceous glands in the esophagus. Am J Gastroenterol. 90(3):501-3, 1995
10. Dawsey SM et al: Esophageal morphology from Linxian, China. Squamous histologic findings in 754 patients. Cancer. 73(8):2027-37, 1994
11. Ohashi K et al: Melanocytes and melanosis of the oesophagus in Japanese subjects--analysis of factors effecting their increase. Virchows Arch A Pathol Anat Histopathol. 417(2):137-43, 1990
12. Goldman H et al: Mucosal biopsy of the esophagus, stomach, and proximal duodenum. Hum Pathol. 13(5):423-48, 1982
13. Al Yassin TM et al: Fine structure of squamous epitheilum and submucosal glands of human oesophagus. J Anat. 123(Pt 3):705-21, 1977
14. Weinstein WM et al: The normal human esophageal mucosa: a histological reappraisal. Gastroenterology. 68(1):40-4, 1975

STOMACH

1. Hughes C et al: Gastric pseudo-signet ring cells: a potential diagnostic pitfall. Virchows Arch. 459(3):347-9, 2011
2. Drut R et al: Omeprazole-associated changes in the gastric mucosa of children. J Clin Pathol. 61(6):754-6, 2008
3. Cats A et al: Parietal cell protrusions and fundic gland cysts during omeprazole maintenance treatment. Hum Pathol. 31(6):684-90, 2000
4. Kilgore SP et al: The gastric cardia: fact or fiction? Am J Gastroenterol. 95(4):921-4, 2000
5. Filipe MI: Mucins in the human gastrointestinal epithelium: a review. Invest Cell Pathol. 2(3):195-216, 1979

SMALL INTESTINE

1. Gramlich T et al: Small intestine. In Mills S: Histology for Pathologists. 3rd ed. Philadelphia: Lippincott Williams and Wilkins. 603-26, 2007
2. Brown I et al: Intraepithelial lymphocytosis in architecturally preserved proximal small intestinal mucosa: an increasing diagnostic problem with a wide differential diagnosis. Arch Pathol Lab Med. 130(7):1020-5, 2006
3. Kakar S et al: Significance of intraepithelial lymphocytosis in small bowel biopsy samples with normal mucosal architecture. Am J Gastroenterol. 98(9):2027-33, 2003
4. Jankowski JA et al: Maintenance of normal intestinal mucosa: function, structure, and adaptation. Gut. 35(1 Suppl):S1-4, 1994
5. Lawson HH: The duodenal mucosa in health and disease. A clinical and experimental study. Surg Annu. 21:157-80, 1989
6. Urbanski SJ et al: Pigment resembling atmospheric dust in Peyer's patches. Mod Pathol. 2(3):222-6, 1989
7. Shepherd NA et al: Exogenous pigment in Peyer's patches. Hum Pathol. 18(1):50-4, 1987
8. Sandow MJ et al: The Paneth cell. Gut. 20(5):420-31, 1979
9. Axelsson C et al: Lipohyperplasia of the ileocaecal region. Acta Chir Scand. 140(8):649-54, 1974
10. Owen RL et al: Epithelial cell specialization within human Peyer's patches: an ultrastructural study of intestinal lymphoid follicles. Gastroenterology. 66(2):189-203, 1974
11. Chacko CJ et al: The villus architecture of the small intestine in the tropics: a necropsy study. J Pathol. 98(2):146-51, 1969
12. Trier JS: The surface coat of gastrointestinal epithelial cells. Gastroenterology. 56(3):618-22, 1969
13. Cornes JS: Number, size, and distribution of Peyer's patches in the human small intestine: Part I The development of Peyer's patches. Gut. 6(3):225-9, 1965

LARGE INTESTINE

1. Lewin KJ: The endocrine cells of the gastrointestinal tract. The normal endocrine cells and their hyperplasias. Part I. Pathol Annu. 21 Pt 1:1-27, 1986
2. Hamilton SR: Structure of the colon. Scand J Gastroenterol Suppl. 93:13-23, 1984
3. Shamsuddin AM et al: Human large intestinal epithelium: light microscopy, histochemistry, and ultrastructure. Hum Pathol. 13(9):790-803, 1982

SELECTED REFERENCES

4. Kolodej P et al: Topography of the human colonic lamina propria. J Electron Microsc (Tokyo). 30(4):334-5, 1981
5. Steer HW et al: Melanosis coli: studies of the toxic effects of irritant purgatives. J Pathol. 115(4):199-205, 1975
6. Eidelman S et al: The morphology of the normal human rectal biopsy. Hum Pathol. 3(3):389-401, 1972
7. Lumb G: Normal human rectal mucosa and its mechanism of repair. Am J Dig Dis. 5:836-40, 1960

APPENDIX

1. Andreou P et al: A histopathological study of the appendix at autopsy and after surgical resection. Histopathology. 17(5):427-31, 1990
2. Spencer J et al: Gut associated lymphoid tissue: a morphological and immunocytochemical study of the human appendix. Gut. 26(7):672-9, 1985
3. Bockman DE: Functional histology of appendix. Arch Histol Jpn. 46(3):271-92, 1983
4. Vestfrid MA et al: Paneth's cells in the human appendix. A statistical study. Acta Anat (Basel). 97(3):347-50, 1977
5. Ashley DJ: Aberrant mucosa in the vermiform appendix. Br J Surg. 45(192):372-3, 1958

ANUS AND ANAL CANAL

1. Bernard JE et al: Anal intraepithelial neoplasia: correlation of grade with p16INK4a immunohistochemistry and HPV in situ hybridization. Appl Immunohistochem Mol Morphol. 16(3):215-20, 2008
2. Ramalingam P et al: Cytokeratin subset immunostaining in rectal adenocarcinoma and normal anal glands. Arch Pathol Lab Med. 125(8):1074-7, 2001
3. Williams GR et al: Keratin expression in the normal anal canal. Histopathology. 26(1):39-44, 1995
4. Seow-Choen F et al: Histoanatomy of anal glands. Dis Colon Rectum. 37(12):1215-8, 1994
5. Clemmensen OJ et al: Melanocytes in the anal canal epithelium. Histopathology. 18(3):237-41, 1991
6. van der Putte SC: Anogenital "sweat" glands. Histology and pathology of a gland that may mimic mammary glands. Am J Dermatopathol. 13(6):557-67, 1991
7. Fenger C: The anal transitional zone. Acta Pathol Microbiol Immunol Scand Suppl. 289:1-42, 1987
8. Fenger C et al: The anal transitional zone: a scanning and transmission electron microscopic investigation of the surface epithelium. Ultrastruct Pathol. 2(2):163-73, 1981
9. Aldridge RT et al: Ganglion cell distribution in the normal rectum and anal canal. A basis for the diagnosis of Hirschsprung's disease by anorectal biopsy. J Pediatr Surg. 3(4):475-90, 1968

PERITONEAL MEMBRANES

1. Sahn SA: State of the art. The pleura. Am Rev Respir Dis. 138(1):184-234, 1988
2. McFadden DE et al: Peritoneal inclusion cysts with mural mesothelial proliferation. A clinicopathological analysis of six cases. Am J Surg Pathol. 10(12):844-54, 1986
3. Rosai J et al: Nodular mesothelial hyperplasia in hernia sacs: a benign reactive condition simulating a neoplastic process. Cancer. 35(1):165-75, 1975

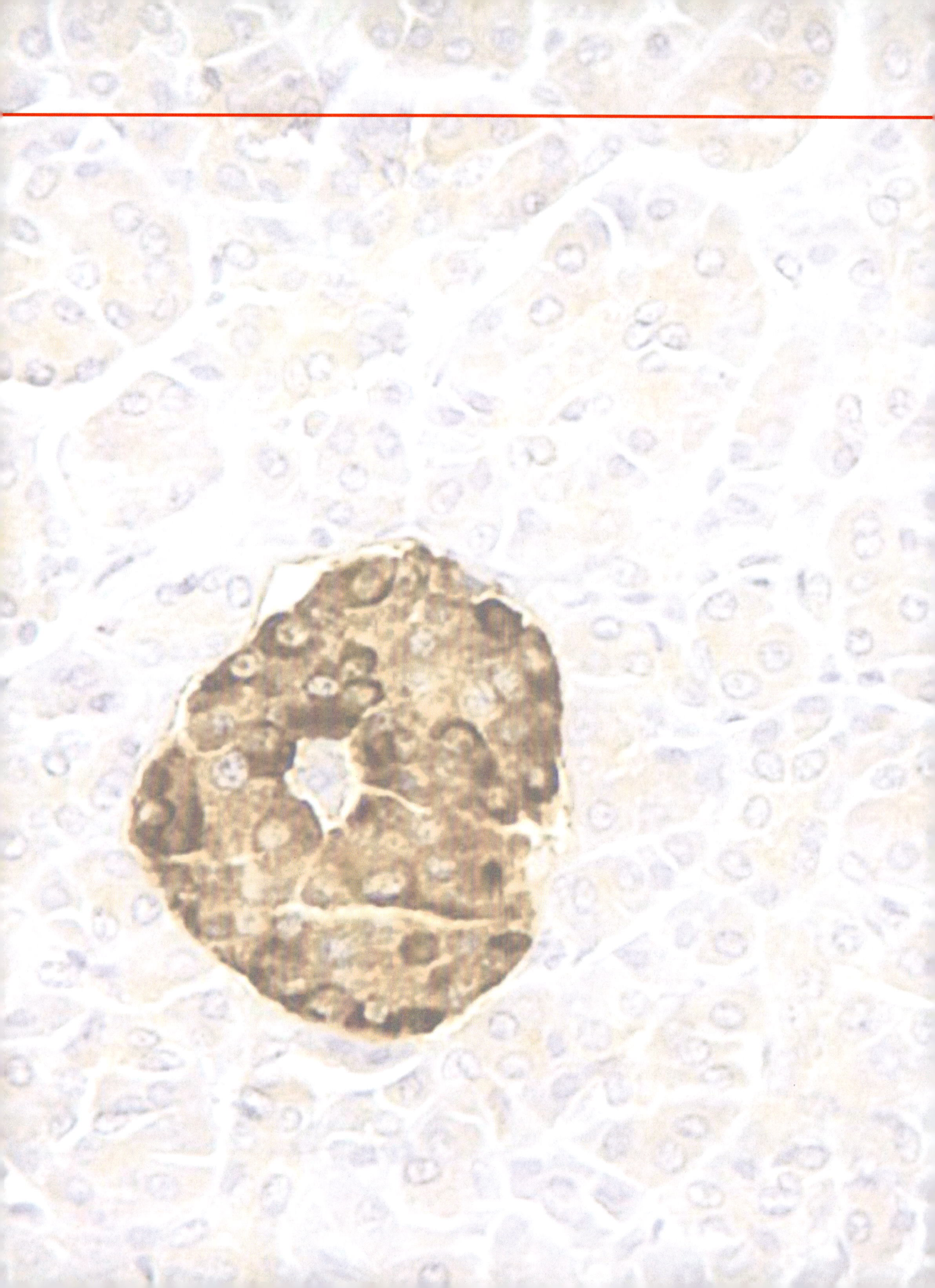

Hepatobiliary Tract and Pancreas

Liver	11-2
Gallbladder	11-10
Extrahepatic Biliary Tract	11-14
Vaterian System	11-16
Pancreas	11-18

LIVER

Key Facts

Macroscopic Anatomy
- Dual blood supply: Hepatic artery and portal vein
  - Vessels enter liver at porta hepatis (fissure at central inferior border of liver)
  - Veinous drainage: Right, middle, and left hepatic veins drain into inferior vena cava
- Bile flow: Bile canaliculi → interlobular bile ducts → right and left hepatic ducts → common hepatic duct

Microscopic Anatomy
- 2 competing conceptions of subunits: Lobule and acinus
  - Lobule: Central (hepatic) vein at center, portal tracts at periphery
  - Acinus: Portal tract is central axis, central veins at periphery; defined by liver microcirculation
- Hepatocytes
  - Polygonal cells with central nuclei and abundant cytoplasm
  - Nuclei are centrally placed, round to oval, with delicate chromatin and 1 or more nucleoli
- Portal tracts
  - Contain interlobular bile duct and bile ductules, branch of hepatic artery, branch of portal vein
  - Connective tissue framework has variably present lymphocytes and mast cells; limiting plate delineates interface with parenchyma
- Bile ducts
  - Interlobular ducts lined by cuboidal or low columnar epithelium
  - Larger septal ducts (> 100 μm in diameter) are lined by tall columnar epithelium; have denser surrounding collagen
  - 70-90% of hepatic arteries should have an attendant bile duct; unaccompanied arteries signal biliary disease
  - Nourished by hepatic arteries via peribiliary capillary plexus
- Bile ductules: Present at periphery of portal tracts, not accompanied by hepatic arteriole
  - Bile ducts drain bile from canaliculi via bile ductules and canals of Hering
  - Rarely seen in normal liver but proliferate in wide variety of pathological conditions
- Bile canaliculi
  - Formed by apposition of specialized grooves in surfaces of contributing liver cells
  - Continuous conduit that extends along hepatic plates and ultimately empties into biliary tree
- Sinusoids: Narrow vascular channels between radiating hepatic plates
  - Lined by Kupffer cells and endothelial cells
  - Supported by a delicate reticulin framework
  - Space of Disse: Not normally visible
  - Stellate cells: Store fat and vitamin A
- Central veins (terminal hepatic veins)

Pitfalls/Artifacts
- Subcapsular zone in shallow wedge biopsies
  - Elastin can cause contraction of portal areas, imitating cirrhosis
  - These changes are generally superficial, rarely extend more than 2-5 mm into liver
- Longitudinally cut large portal tracts may mimic fibrous septa
  - Comparably sized larger vessels and ducts; smooth interface between parenchyma and portal tract

Age Variation
- Infants: Extramedullary hematopoiesis common; increased stainable iron and copper
- Young children: Glycogenated nuclei common; cell plates usually 2 cells thick
- Elderly persons: Increased variation in nuclear size and hepatocyte size; prominent lipofuscin; increased portal tract hyalinization, inflammation

(Left) The classical liver lobule consists of a hexagonal structure with portal tracts at the periphery and the central venule at the center. (Right) The acinus is defined by the microcirculation of the liver. The central axis consists of the portal tract, and the hepatic plates radiate outward to the central (hepatic) venules.

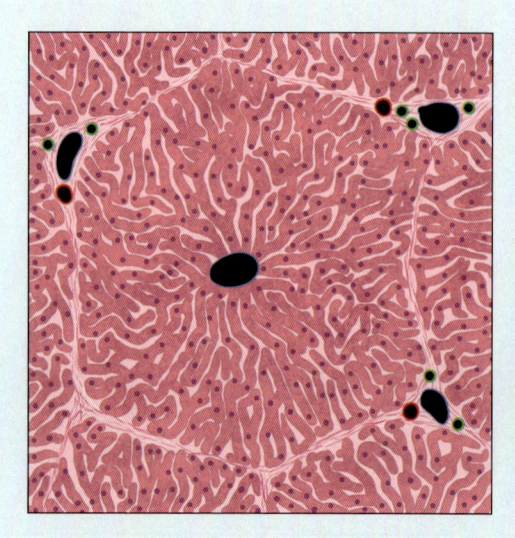

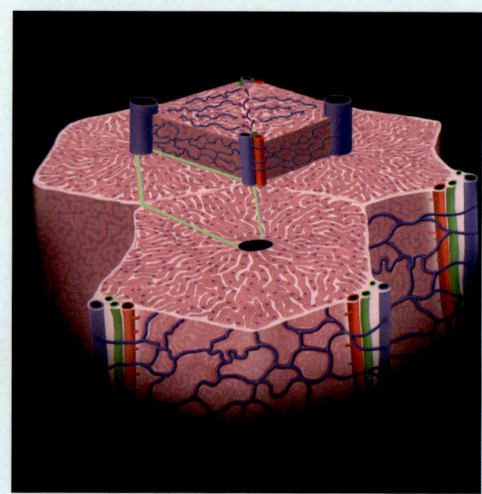

LIVER

Normal Lobule

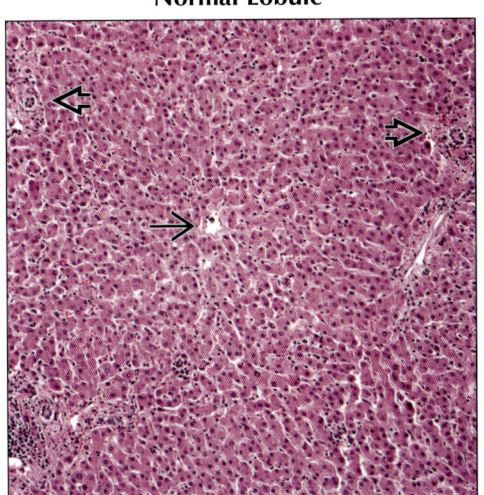

Periportal Zone/Zone 1

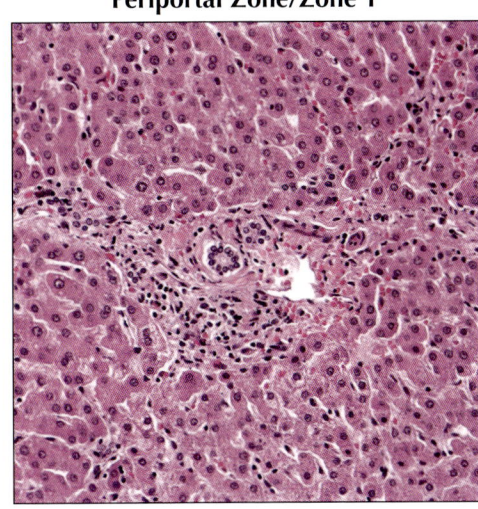

(Left) The normal lobule, which is a 2-dimensional structure, is easy to conceptualize microscopically. The central vein ➡ is the hub of the hexagon, with the portal tracts ⮕ at the periphery. *(Right)* The periportal zone in the lobule is comparable to zone 1 in the acinus. Zone 1 is best supplied with oxygen and nutrients because of the blood flow and is thus least susceptible to ischemia and toxic injury.

Midlobular Zone/Zone 2

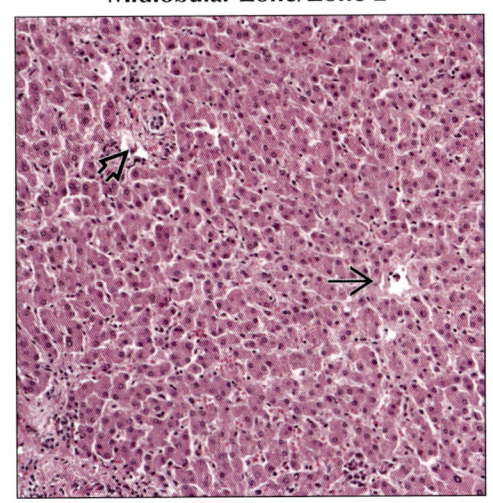

Centrilobular Zone/Zone 3

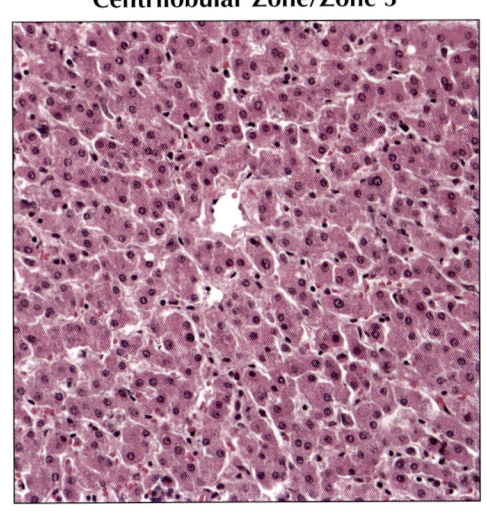

(Left) The midlobular zone, which is intermediate between the periportal (zone 1) and centrilobular (zone 3) areas, is comparable to zone 2 in the acinus. Note the portal tract ⮕ and the central venule ➡. *(Right)* The centrilobular zone around the central venule is comparable to zone 3 in the acinus. This area is the most devoid of oxygen and nutrients and is thus more susceptible to ischemia and toxic injury.

Hepatocyte Glycogen

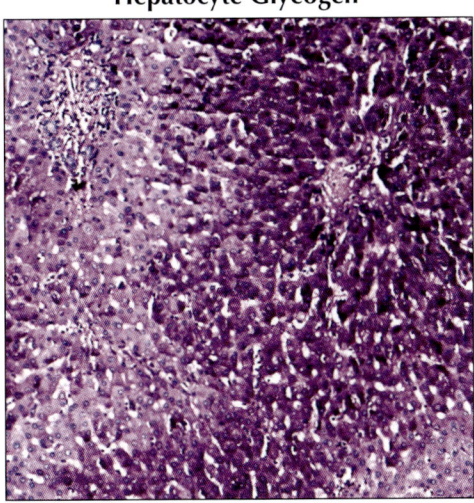

Portal Tract

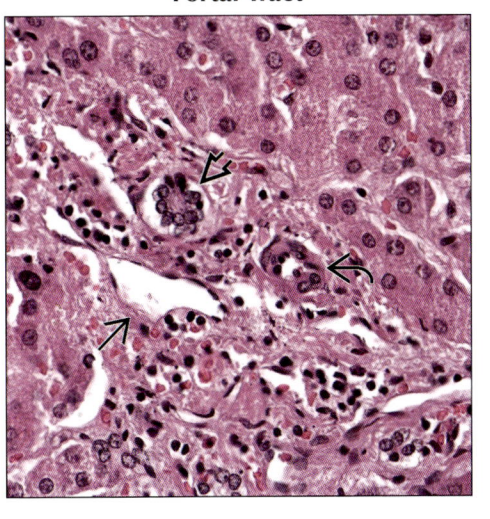

(Left) The hepatocytes contain abundant cytoplasmic glycogen (dark pink color), highlighted by a PAS stain. An irregular distribution pattern is common, as in this picture; it has no clinical significance. *(Right)* Portal tracts contain a bile duct ⮕, an accompanying small branch of the hepatic artery ➡, and a portal vein branch ➡. Occasionally, more than 1 bile duct is present per portal tract.

LIVER

Portal Tract

Portal Tract

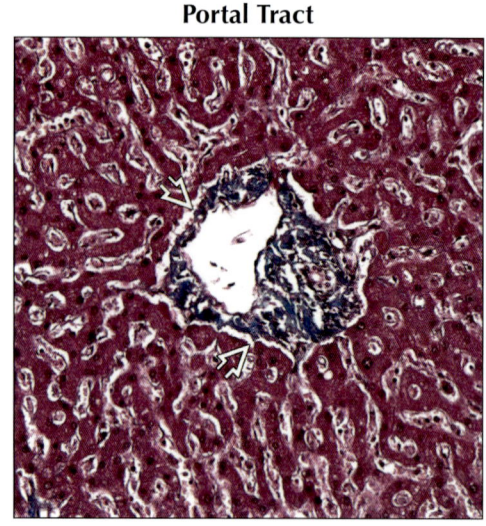

(Left) Portal tracts normally contain a variable number of lymphocytes and mast cells, and this should not be interpreted as abnormal inflammation. Neutrophils, eosinophils, and plasma cells are not usually seen in the normal liver. *(Right)* Portal tracts are supported by connective tissue stroma that becomes more coarse and dense with age. The normal interface ⇨ between the connective tissue of the portal tract and the hepatic parenchyma is smooth.

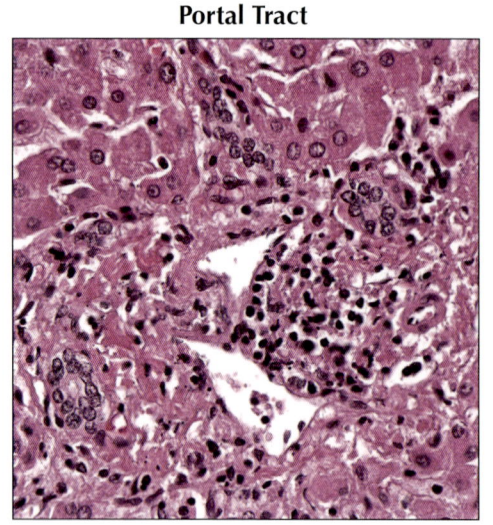

Interlobular Bile Duct

Interlobular Bile Duct Loss

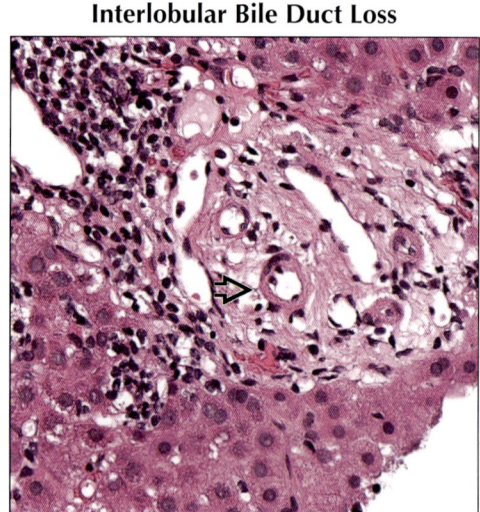

(Left) Interlobular bile ducts are lined by cuboidal or low columnar epithelium. *(Right)* 70-90% of hepatic arterioles ⇨ should be accompanied by a bile duct. When a significant percentage of arterioles lack an accompanying bile duct, loss of ducts should be suspected, as in this case of primary biliary cirrhosis.

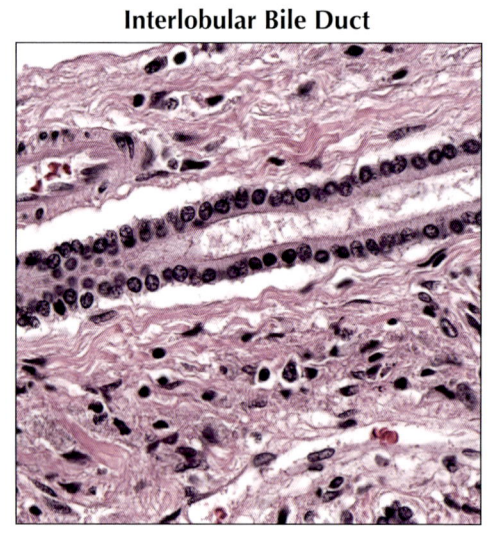

Bile Duct

Bile Ductules

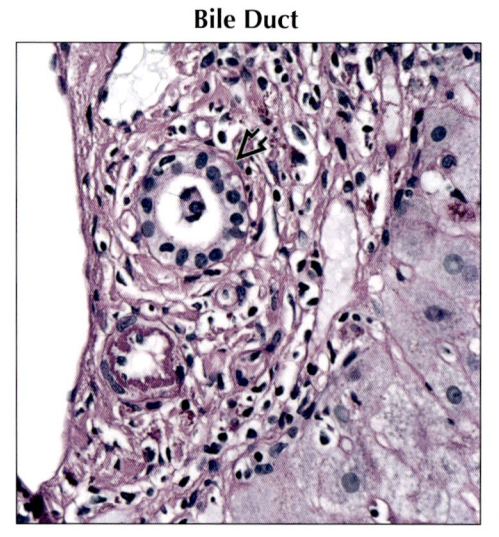

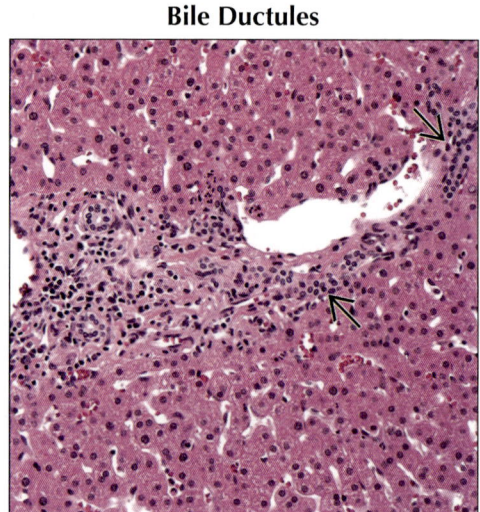

(Left) A PAS stain highlights the normal delicate basement membrane of bile ducts ⇨. Disruption of this basement membrane can be seen in bile duct damage. *(Right)* Bile ductules (cholangioles) drain bile from the canaliculi to the interlobular ducts. They are located at the periphery of the portal tracts ⇨ and lack an accompanying hepatic artery. They are seldom seen in the normal liver but proliferate in many diseases.

LIVER

Bile Duct

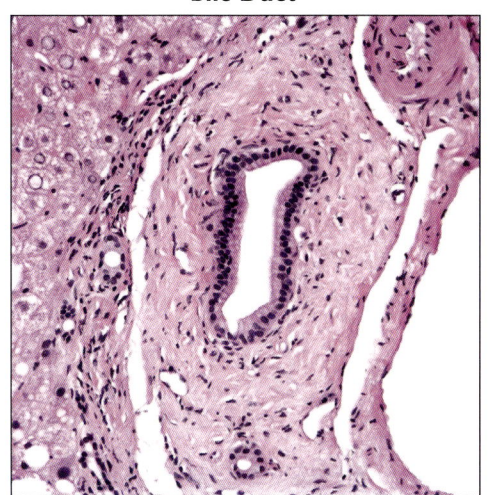

Bile Duct

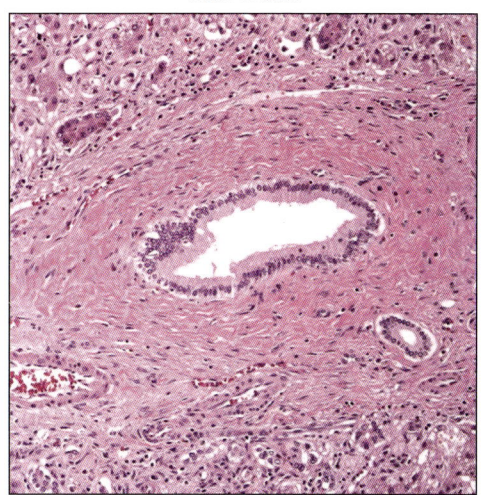

(Left) Normal larger bile ducts are lined by tall columnar epithelium. The surrounding collagen is more dense than that which surrounds the smaller interlobular bile ducts. (Right) The dense concentric collagen that surrounds larger bile ducts should not be mistaken for the "onion skin" lesion of primary sclerosing cholangitis.

Bile Duct

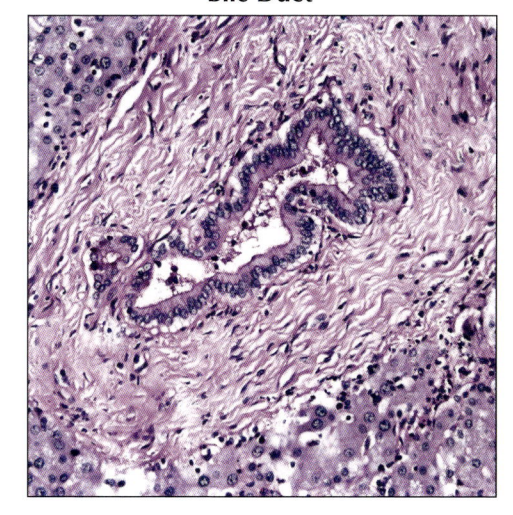

Bile Canaliculi

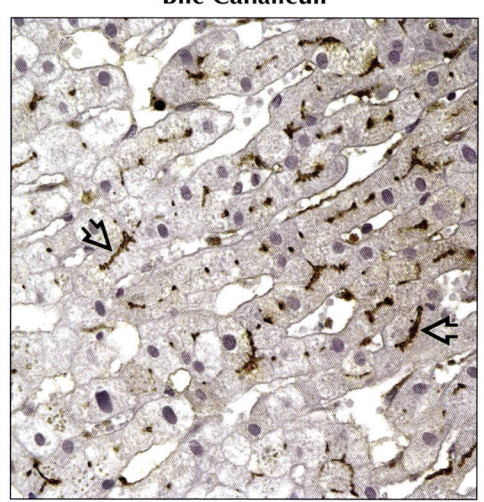

(Left) PAS stain highlights the tall columnar epithelium of larger bile ducts, as well as the dense supporting stroma. (Right) Polyclonal CEA immunostain illustrates bile canaliculi in normal liver ⇨. The canaliculi are created from grooves in hepatocytes that form a continuous conduit along the hepatic plates, which empties into the bile ductules at the edges of portal tracts. The canals of Hering link the canaliculi to the biliary tree and are not visible on routine stains.

Bile Canaliculi

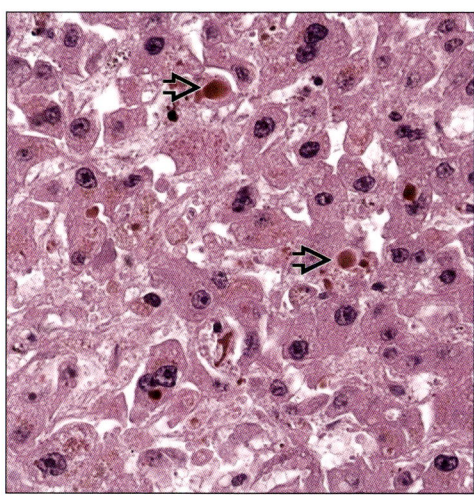

Hepatocytes

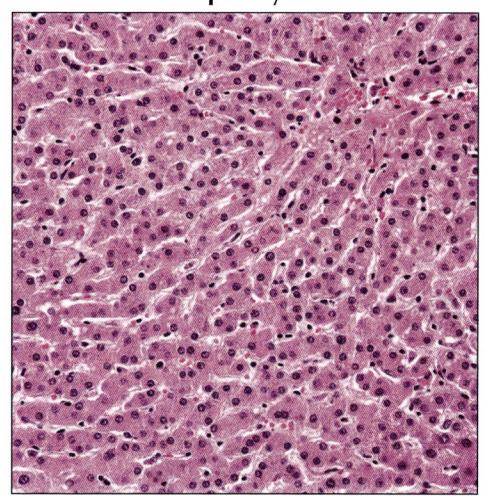

(Left) Bile canaliculi are not visible in normal liver. When bile plugs are present in cholestatic liver disease, however, they delineate the bile canaliculi ⇨. Bile may also accumulate in hepatocytes and must be distinguished from lipofuscin. Intracellular bile is less granular than iron and lipofuscin. (Right) Hepatocytes measure 25-30 μm. Normal hepatocyte cell plates are 1-2 cells thick; they may be 2 cells thick in children younger than 6 years.

LIVER

Hepatocytes

Hepatocytes

(Left) Hepatocytes are polygonal cells with abundant eosinophilic, granular cytoplasm. Improper fixation or processing can cause false hepatocyte swelling or shrinking and can produce inconsistent cytoplasmic staining. *(Right)* Hepatocyte nuclei are round, centrally placed, and frequently have a prominent nucleolus. Double nuclei are common. Variation in nuclear size increases with age. Mitotic activity is rare in the normal liver.

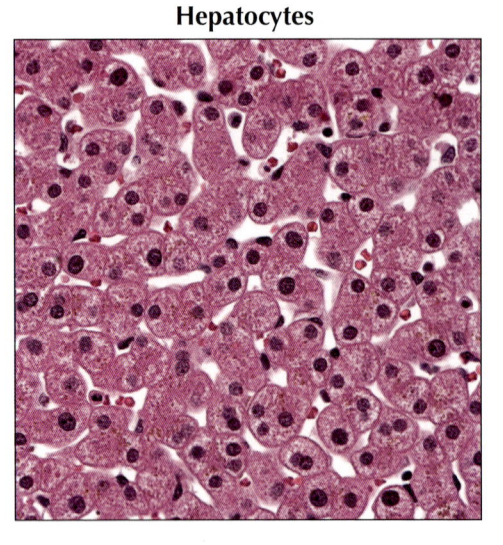

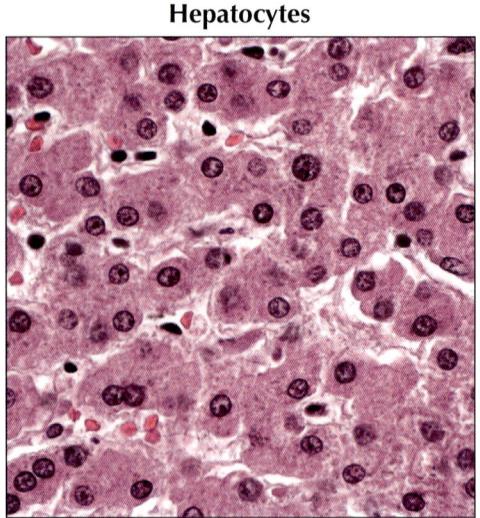

Hepatocytes

Central Vein

(Left) Glycogenated nuclei ➡ are common in children and young adults but may also be seen in pathological conditions such as fatty liver disease or Wilson disease. The enlarged nucleus has a clear, vacuolated appearance. *(Right)* Central veins (also called terminal hepatic veins) are the smallest component of venous outflow tract.

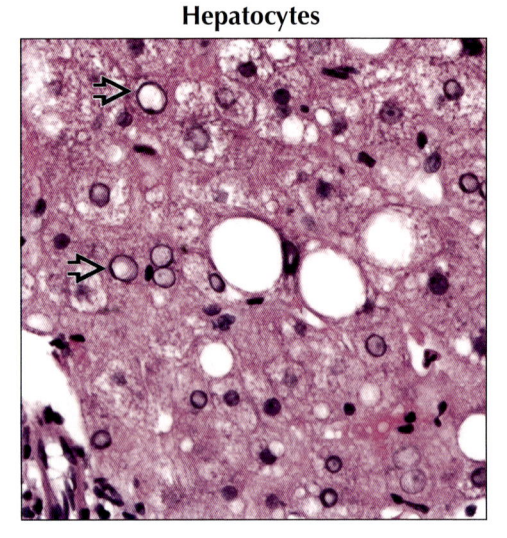

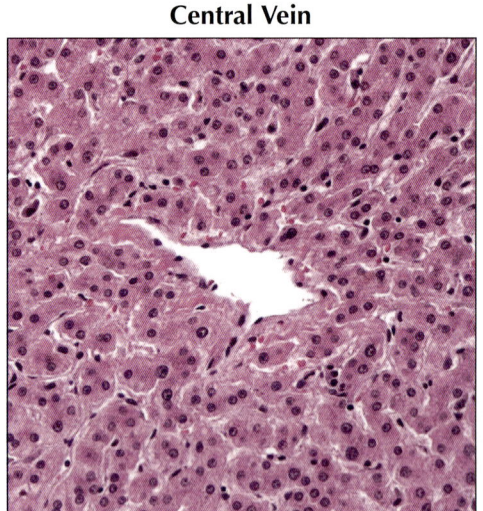

Central Vein

Sinusoids

(Left) Central veins are lined by endothelium and supported by a thin layer of collagen. They join to form the sublobular hepatic veins, and then the hepatic veins, which drain into the inferior vena cava. *(Right)* The sinusoids ➡ are the narrow vascular channels between the radiating hepatic plates. They are lined by Kupffer cells ➡ and endothelial cells. Typically, the sinusoids are empty except for a few erythrocytes.

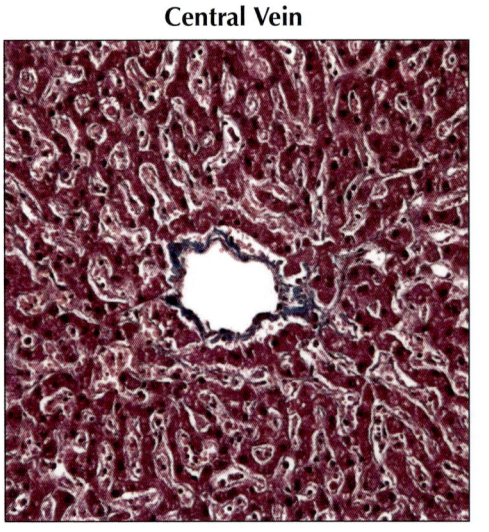

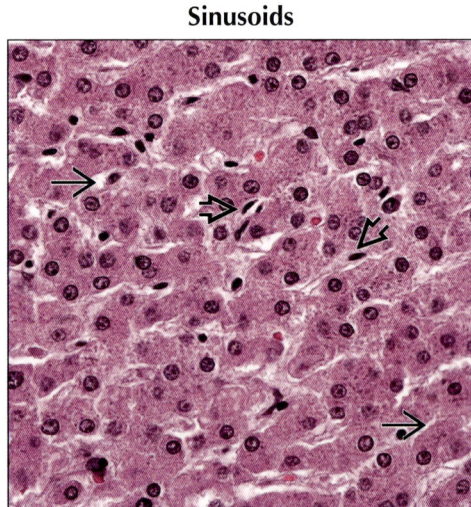

LIVER

Reticulin Framework

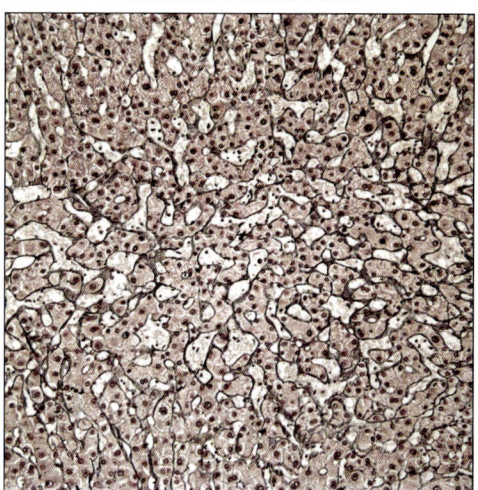

Sinusoids and Space of Disse

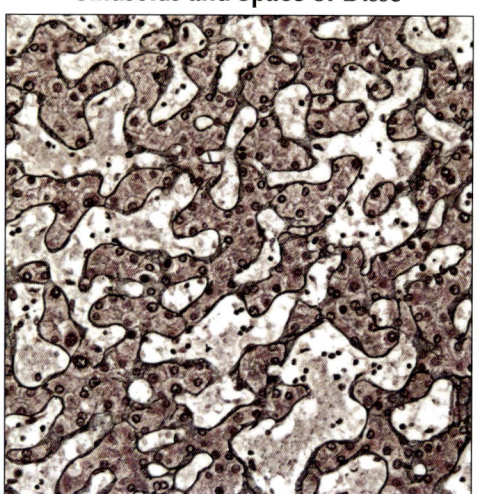

(Left) The reticulin stain highlights the normal reticulin framework of the liver. The cell plates and sinusoids form a 3-dimensional network that directs blood from portal tracts to central venules. *(Right)* The space of Disse is the zone between the endothelial cells and the hepatocytes. It is not normally visible, and it contains the reticulin framework of the liver (a continuous network of type III collagen fibers that outline the hepatic plates, as seen here).

Space of Disse

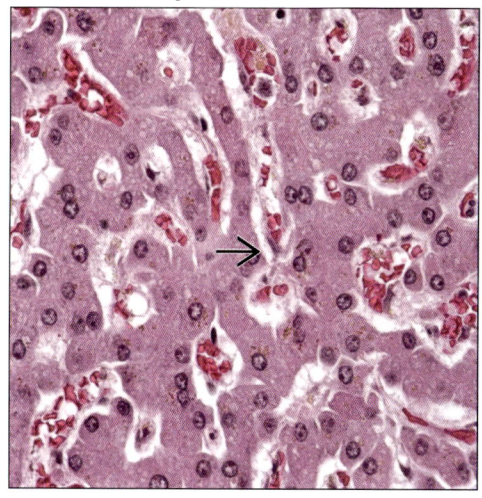

Kupffer Cells

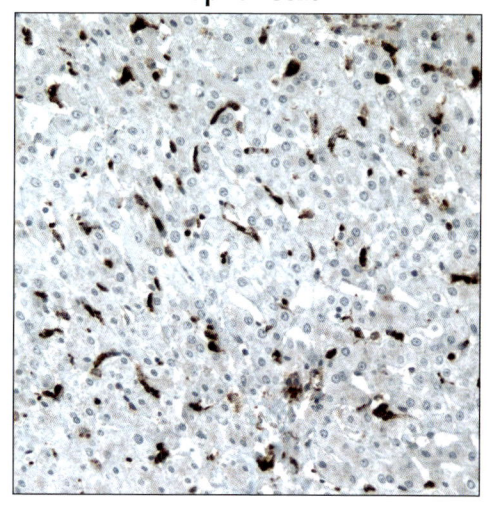

(Left) The space of Disse is the zone between the endothelial cells and the hepatocytes. It is not normally visible in routinely fixed and processed specimens, but it can be seen in suboptimally fixed autopsy material ➡. *(Right)* A CD68 immunostain highlights the numerous Kupffer cells that normally line the sinusoids. Kupffer cells are highly phagocytic macrophages which, in response to hepatocyte damage, proliferate and enlarge.

Kupffer Cells

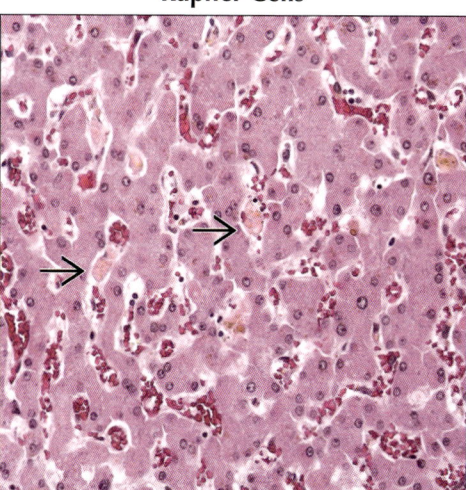

Kupffer Cells

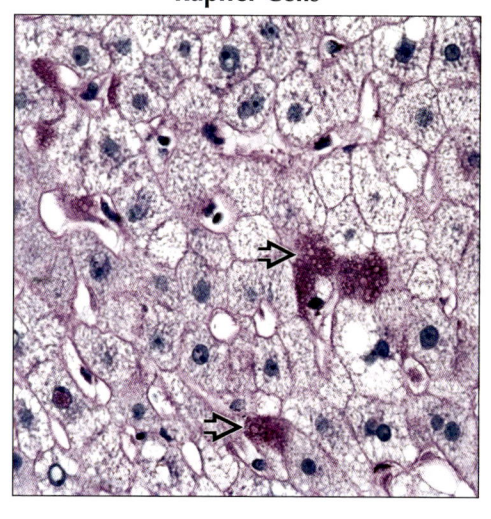

(Left) Kupffer cells may accumulate ceroid pigment ➡, a brown-yellow pigment that is composed of cellular debris. *(Right)* Ceroid pigment is strongly PAS positive, and thus this stain is useful in highlighting activated Kupffer cells ➡.

LIVER

Stellate Cells

Lipofuscin

(Left) The space of Disse contains the stellate cells (also known as Ito cells, lipocytes, or interstitial fat storing cells) ⮞, which are modified fibroblasts that store fat and vitamin A. They also have the capacity for collagen synthesis. When fat laden, they appear as multivesicular cells with cytoplasmic striations. (Right) Lipofuscin is a yellow-brown pigment that accumulates in hepatocytes, most prominently in the centrilobular area.

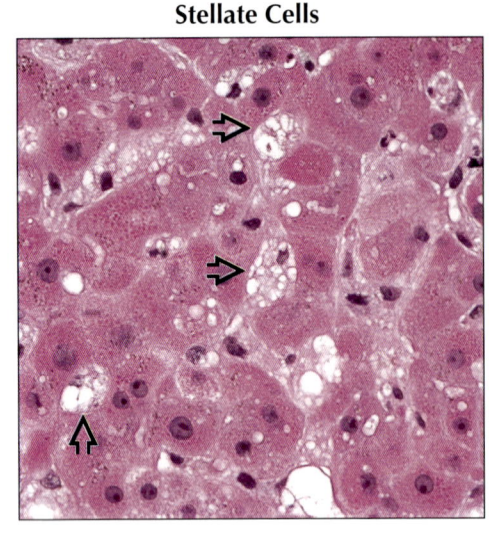

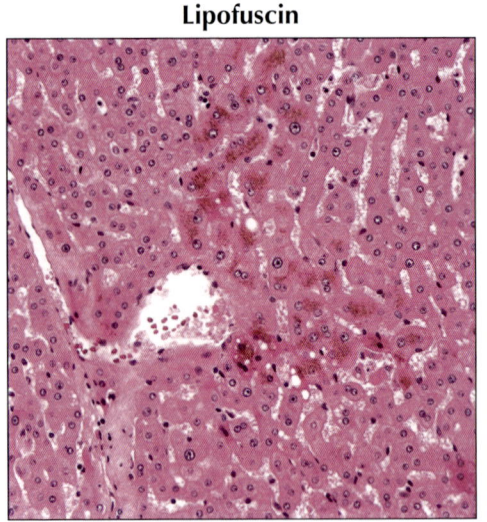

Lipofuscin

Copper

(Left) This high-power photomicrograph illustrates the yellow-brown color of lipofuscin. It is common in varying amounts in the adult liver and increases with age. It may be acid fast and PAS/diastase positive and must be distinguished from hemosiderin and hepatocellular bile. (Right) Copper is abundant in the cytoplasms of hepatocytes in infants. It gradually disappears and should be absent by 6-9 months.

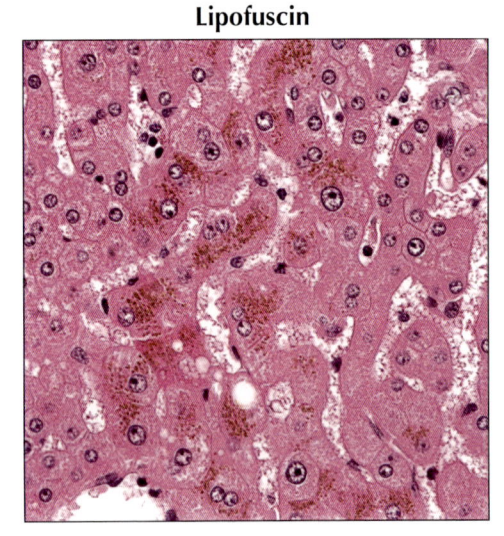

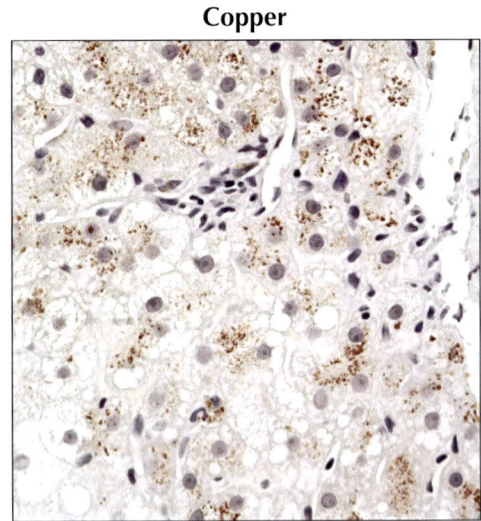

Hemosiderin

Hemosiderin

(Left) Hemosiderin is abundant in the livers of newborns and decreases over the 1st few months of life. Only minor quantities of iron are normally found in adults. Iron is most commonly found in periportal hepatocytes, where it consists of a coarse, golden-brown, refractile material. (Right) The Prussian blue stain can be used to highlight iron pigment within hepatocytes and Kupffer cells.

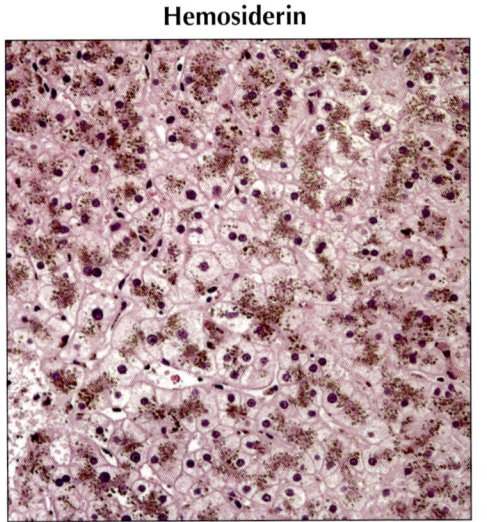

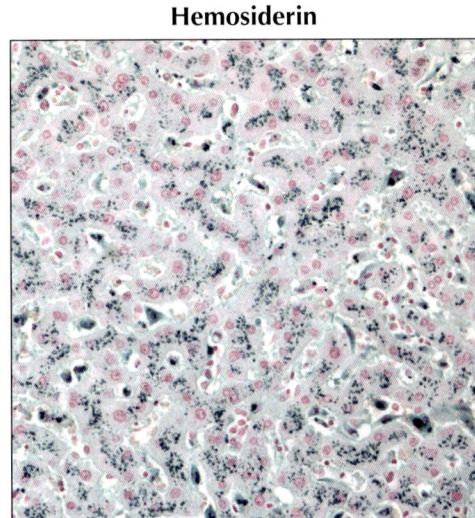

LIVER

Changes With Aging

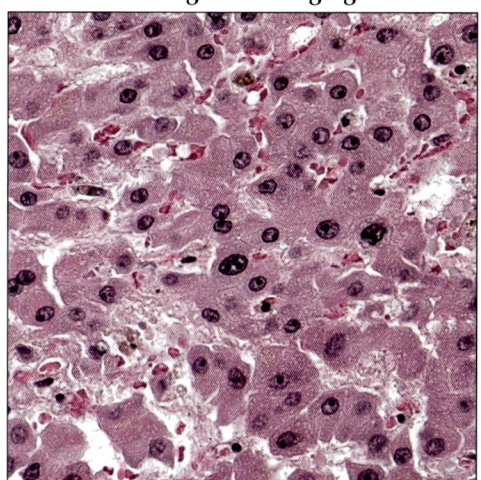

Changes With Aging

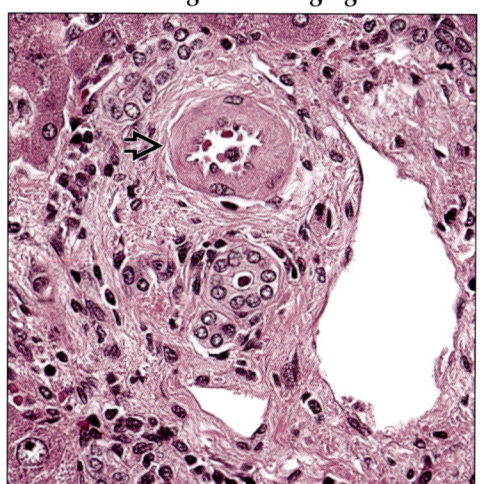

(Left) Increased variation in nuclear size and shape are commonly seen in the aging liver. *(Right)* Hepatic arterioles may become thickened with age, as shown here ⇨. These aging changes can mimic similar changes seen in the context of diabetes.

Extramedullary Hematopoiesis

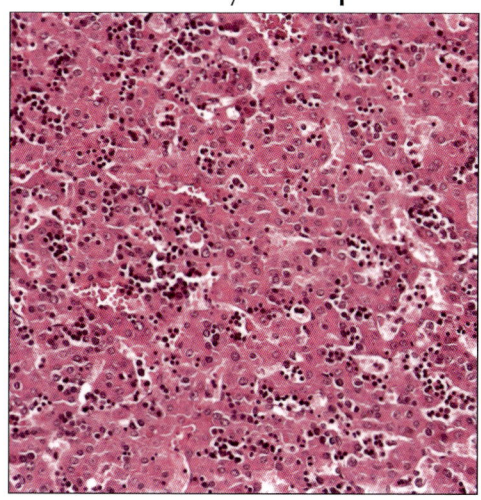

Surgical Hepatitis

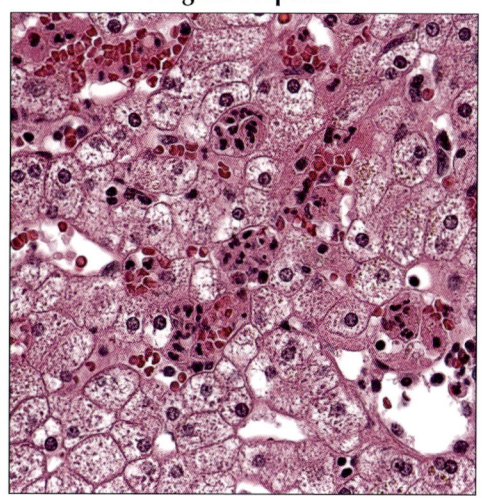

(Left) Extramedullary hematopoiesis is common in newborns, but abates within a few weeks after birth. It is largely erythropoietic, but granulocytes, megakaryocytes, and monocytes may also be seen. *(Right)* Small aggregates of neutrophils may be found within the liver in intraoperative biopsy specimens, usually those taken late during surgery. This must be distinguished from alcoholic hepatitis and other causes of pathologic neutrophilic inflammation.

Bridging Mimic

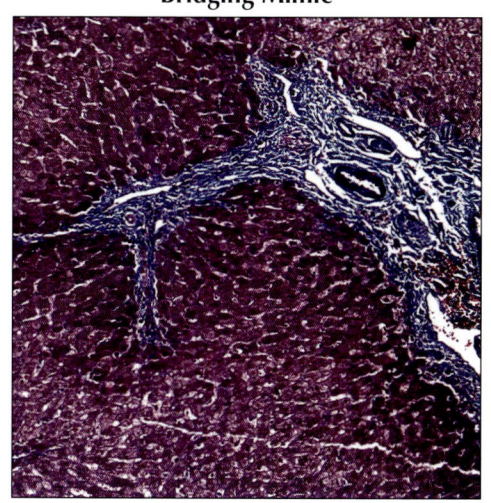

Subcapsular Artifact

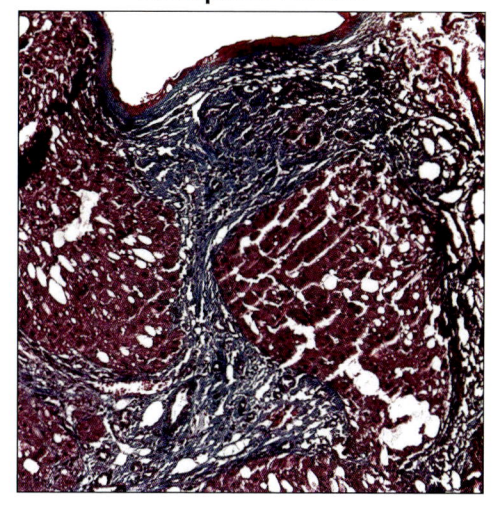

(Left) When cut at a certain angle, large portal tracts may resemble fibrous septa. The comparably sized vessels and ducts are clues that this is not a pathological change. *(Right)* Portal tracts in the subcapsular zone can appear unusually fibrotic. When wedge biopsies are taken, the capsular contraction may also form artifactual septa that isolate islands of parenchyma under the capsule and mimic cirrhosis. These changes rarely extend > 2 mm into the liver parenchyma, however.

GALLBLADDER

Key Facts

Macroscopic Anatomy
- Located in shallow depression on inferior surface of liver
  - Composed of fundus, body, and neck
  - Neck empties into cystic duct, connecting gallbladder to biliary tree
  - Cystic duct contains spiral valves of Heister, which are mucosal folds that prevent collapse
- Up to 10 cm long by 4 cm wide in adults
  - Normal wall: 1-2 mm thick
- Peritoneum reflected from liver covers free side; subserosal connective tissue of gallbladder merges with interlobular connective tissue of liver on hepatic side

Microscopic Anatomy
- Mucosa (surface epithelium plus lamina propria)
  - Cores of lamina propria lined by single layer of columnar epithelium; branching is common
  - Epithelial cells have eosinophilic cytoplasm with variably present small apical vacuoles
  - Nuclei are at base of cell or central; oval and uniform; fine chromatin and smooth nuclear membranes
  - Nucleoli are inconspicuous or absent
  - There are also scattered basal cells and narrower, darker penciloid cells admixed with biliary epithelial cells
  - A few scattered mucosal lymphocytes, plasma cells, mast cells, and histiocytes are normal
  - Lamina propria is composed of loose connective tissue and contains blood vessels, lymphatics, and elastic fibers
- Muscular wall
  - Loosely arranged bundles of circular, longitudinal, and oblique muscle fibers
  - Lacks well-formed layers seen in luminal gut
  - Fibrovascular tissue separates muscle bundles
  - Gallbladder lacks muscularis mucosa and submucosa; thus, lamina propria abuts directly onto muscularis propria
- Perimuscular connective tissue
  - Typically contains blood vessels, nerves, lymphatics, and fat
  - Occasionally contains lymph nodes, paraganglia
- Serosa
  - Peritoneum covers the part of the gallbladder not connected to liver (approximately 60%)
- Mucous glands
  - Located in neck of gallbladder
  - Cuboidal or low columnar epithelium with clear to lightly basophilic cytoplasm
  - Round, uniform, basally located nuclei
- Ducts of Luschka: Small accessory bile ducts in perimuscular connective tissue, most often on hepatic side of gallbladder
  - Supported by distinctive ring of connective tissue
  - Epithelium is similar to biliary epithelium
  - Occasionally, accessory bile ducts can be found in gallbladder bed; may leak after cholecystectomy
- Ganglion cells: Present in perimuscular connective tissue, lamina propria, muscular wall
- Ectopic liver, pancreas, adrenal, stomach, thyroid have been reported in gallbladder

Pitfalls/Artifacts
- Ducts of Luschka can be mistaken for carcinoma on frozen section
  - Look for lobular architecture
- Rokitansky-Aschoff sinuses found in almost 1/2 of normal gallbladders
  - Do not indicate chronic cholecystitis by themselves
  - Ruptured Rokitansky-Aschoff sinuses with extruded mucin can mimic cancer, as can Rokitansky-Aschoff sinuses that contain dysplastic epithelium

Metaplasia
- Pseudopyloric and intestinal metaplasia can be seen
  - Rare outside context of chronic cholecystitis

(Left) This low-power photomicrograph shows all layers of the gallbladder wall, including the mucosa (epithelium plus lamina propria), muscularis propria ⇨, and perimuscular connective tissue ➙. (Right) The nuclei of the gallbladder epithelium are uniform with fine chromatin and smooth nuclear membranes. They are located in the centers or at the bases of the cells.

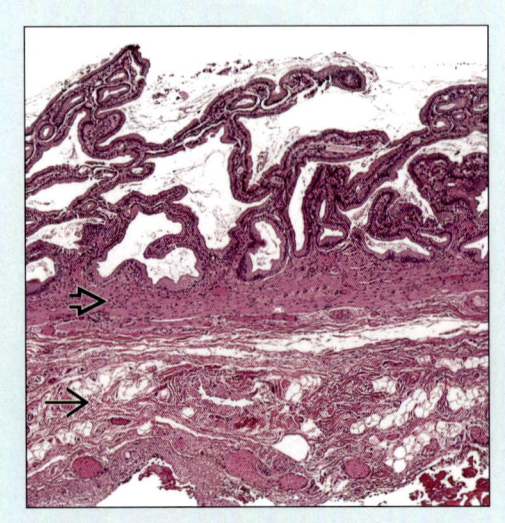

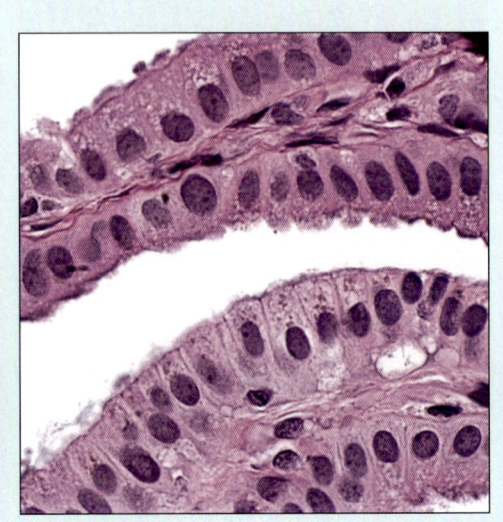

GALLBLADDER

Epithelium

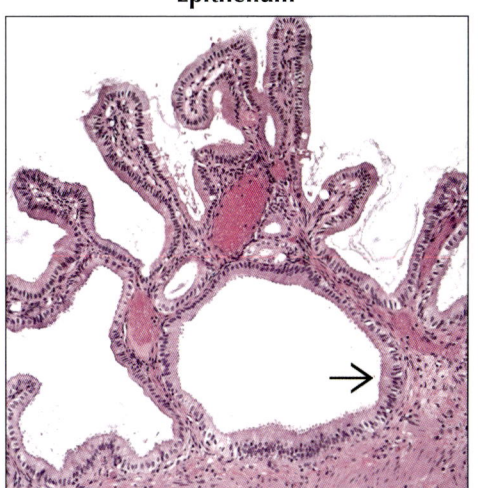

Epithelium

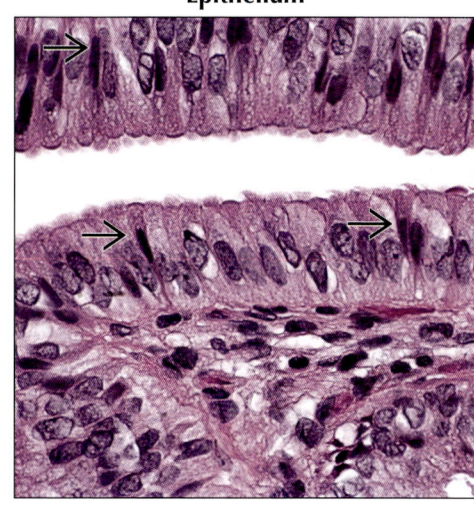

(Left) The gallbladder mucosa consists of cores of lamina propria lined by a single layer of columnar epithelium ➡. Mucosal branching is common in the normal gallbladder, as seen here. *(Right)* Dark, thin, elongated "penciloid" cells ➡, the function of which is unknown, are admixed with the biliary epithelial cells in the gallbladder mucosa.

Epithelium

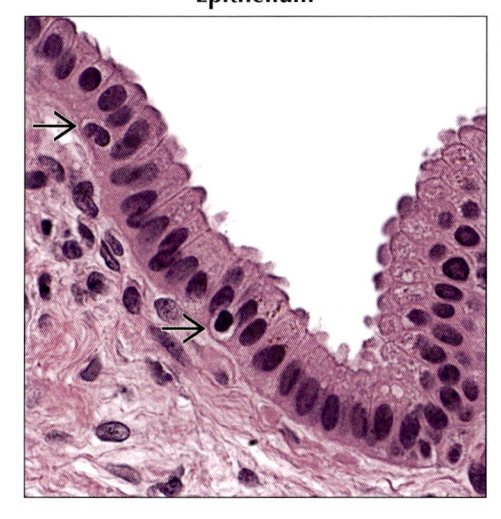

Epithelium

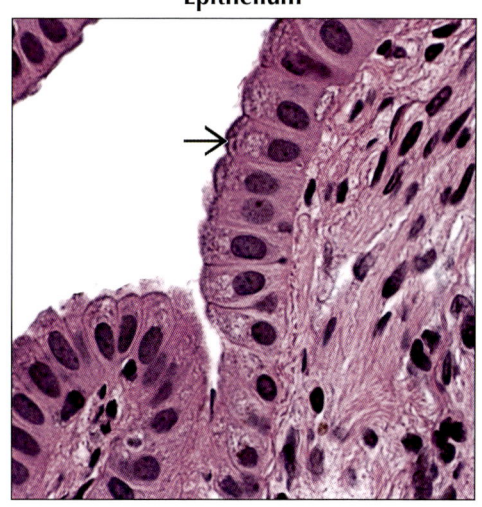

(Left) The epithelium also contains scattered basal cells ➡, which should not be mistaken for lymphocytes. *(Right)* Gallbladder epithelial cells have eosinophilic cytoplasm with variably present small apical vacuoles ➡. The nuclei are round to oval with smooth nuclear membranes. Nucleoli are inconspicuous or absent.

Lamina Propria

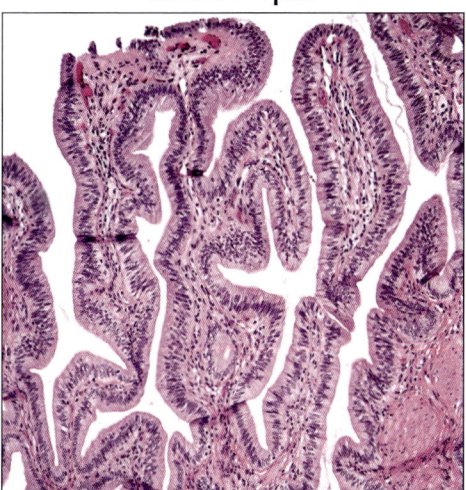

Mucosa

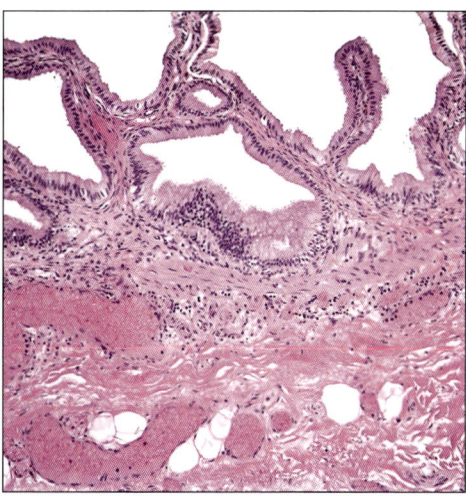

(Left) The lamina propria cores are composed of loose connective tissue and contain blood vessels, lymphatics, and elastic fibers. *(Right)* A few scattered mucosal lymphocytes, plasma cells, mast cells, and histiocytes are normally present in the gallbladder. This sparse inflammatory infiltrate alone is not diagnostic of chronic cholecystitis.

GALLBLADDER

Muscularis

Muscularis

(Left) Since the gallbladder lacks a true muscularis mucosa and submucosa, the lamina propria ⇨ abuts directly onto the muscle bundles of the muscularis propria. The muscle bundles may actually extend up into the lamina propria. *(Right)* The muscular wall consists of loosely arranged bundles of circular, longitudinal, and oblique muscle fibers. It lacks the well-developed longitudinal and circumferential layers seen in the intestine.

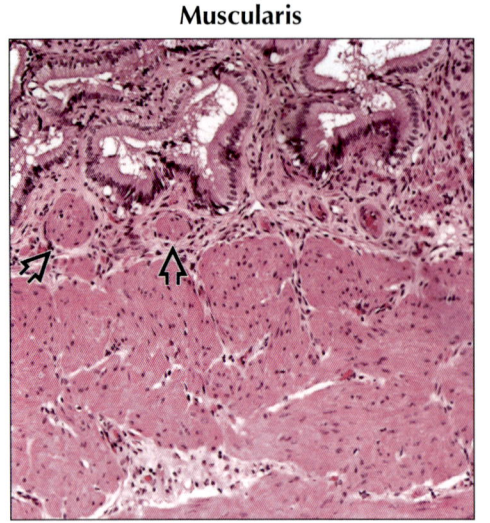

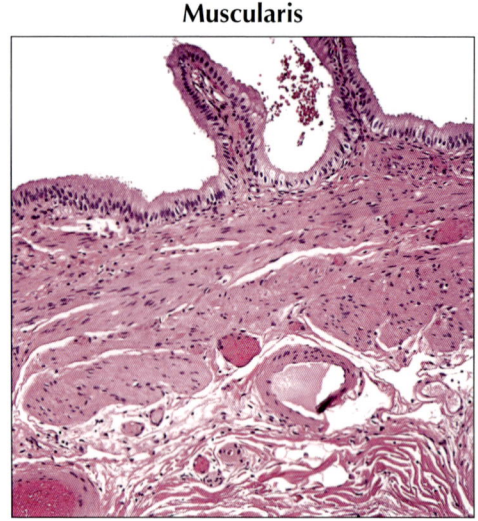

Muscularis

Ganglion Cells

(Left) Fibrovascular tissue separates the muscle bundles in the muscularis propria. *(Right)* Ganglion cells ⇨ are present in the perimuscular connective tissue, lamina propria, and muscularis propria.

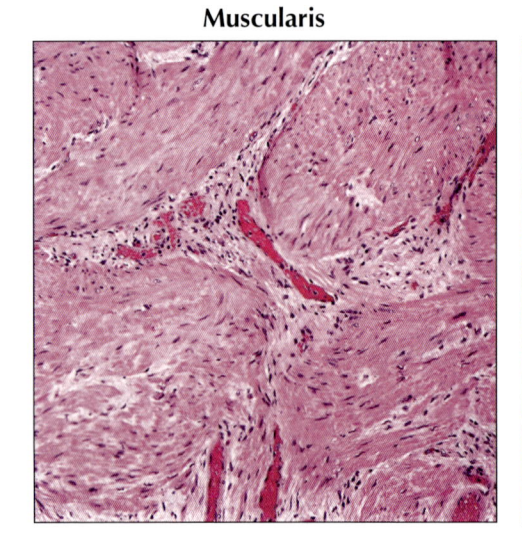

Perimuscular Connective Tissue

Mucous Neck Glands

(Left) The perimuscular connective tissue contains blood vessels, nerves, lymphatics, and fat. It occasionally contains lymph nodes and paraganglia. Peritoneum covers the portion of the gallbladder that is not connected to the liver (approximately 60%). *(Right)* Mucous neck glands are located in the neck of the gallbladder. They have cuboidal or low columnar epithelium with clear to lightly basophilic cytoplasm and round, uniform, basally located nuclei.

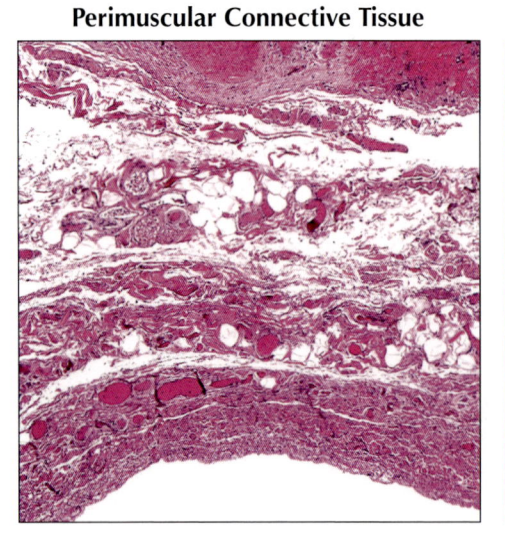

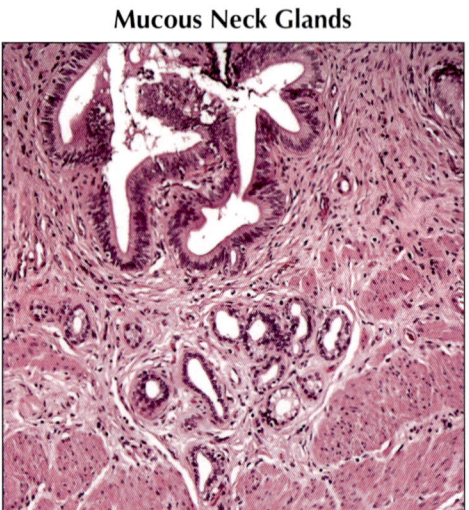

GALLBLADDER

Ducts of Luschka

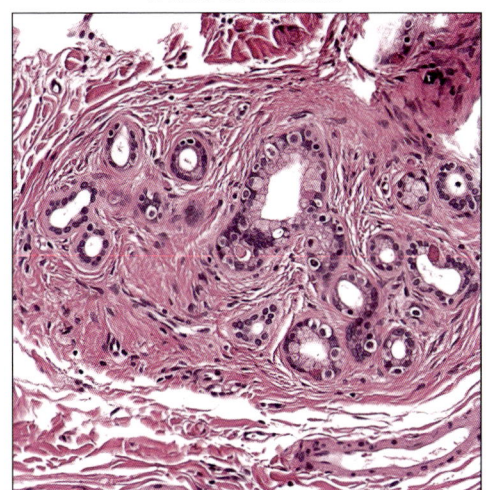

Accessory Bile Ducts

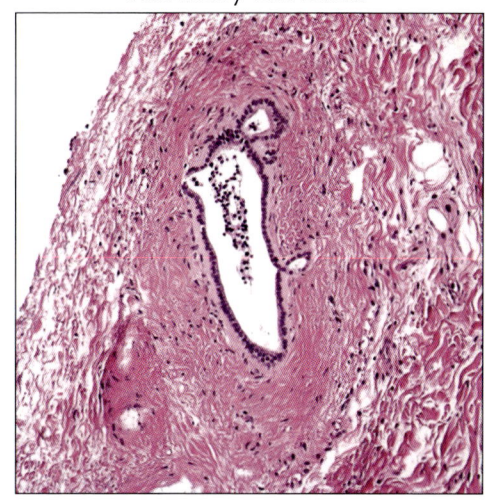

(Left) The ducts of Luschka are small accessory bile ducts in the perimuscular connective tissue, most often on the hepatic side. Note the distinctive ring of connective tissue surrounding the glands. These should not be mistaken for carcinoma on frozen sections. *(Right)* Occasionally, larger accessory bile ducts can be found in the perimuscular soft tissue in the gallbladder bed. These are significant because they may leak after cholecystectomy.

Rokitansky-Aschoff Sinuses

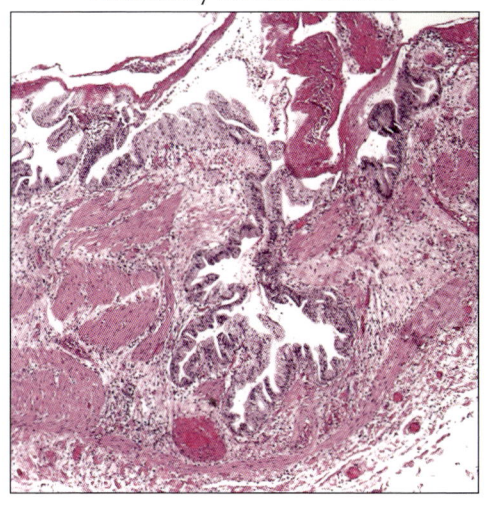

Gastric Metaplasia

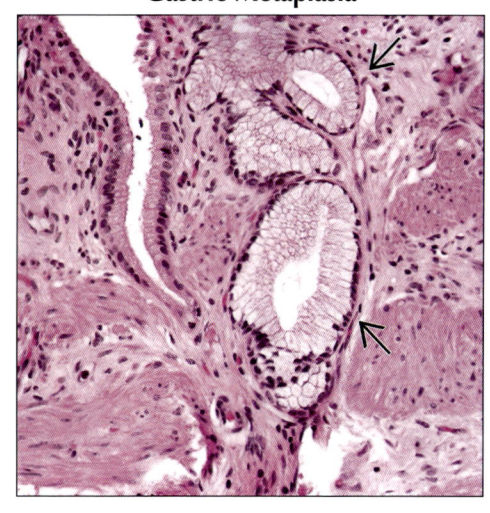

(Left) Rokitansky-Aschoff sinuses can be found in almost 1/2 of normal gallbladders and do not by themselves indicate chronic cholecystitis. *(Right)* Gastric-type or pseudopyloric metaplasia ⇨, similar to that seen in the duodenum, is a common finding in chronic cholecystitis.

Intestinal Metaplasia

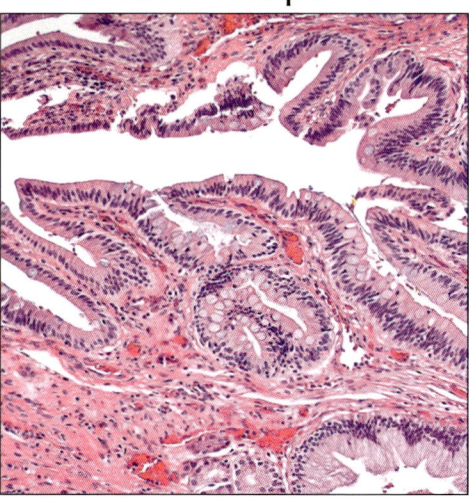

Ectopic Tissues

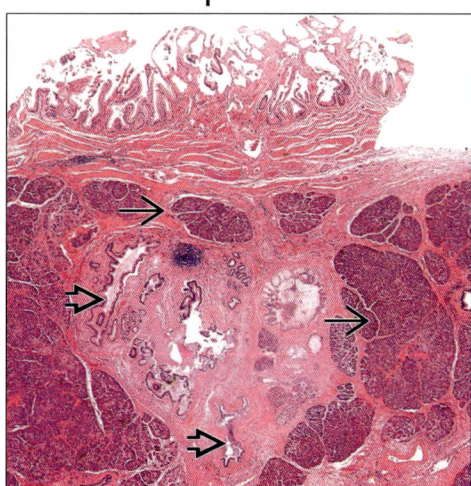

(Left) Intestinal metaplasia is also a common finding in chronic cholecystitis. (Courtesy L. Yerian, MD.) *(Right)* Ectopic liver, pancreas, adrenal, stomach, and thyroid have all been reported in the gallbladder. This photograph illustrates an example of ectopic pancreas with acinar tissue ⇨, ducts ⇨, and smooth muscle. (Courtesy L. Yerian, MD.)

EXTRAHEPATIC BILIARY TRACT

Key Facts

Macroscopic Anatomy
- Extrahepatic biliary tree is composed of **left and right hepatic ducts, common hepatic duct (CHD), cystic duct,** and **common bile duct (CBD)**; serves as conduit for bile flow
  - Left and right hepatic ducts leave liver, extend for approximately 1 cm, and fuse to become CHD
  - CHD extends for ~ 2 cm before joining cystic duct; fusion of these 2 ducts forms CBD
  - Cystic duct is ~ 3 cm in length; anatomic variability in the way cystic duct joins CHD has implications for biliary surgery
  - On average, CBD is 0.4-1.3 cm in diameter and 5 cm long
  - Lower end of CBD runs alongside and usually unites with main pancreatic duct before entering duodenum at papilla

Microscopic Anatomy
- Epithelium: Single layer of columnar epithelium
- Dense connective tissue layer (lacks muscle except for CBD and cystic duct at junction with gallbladder)
  - Upper portion of CBD contains occasional strands of muscle; thick smooth muscles invests lower 1/3
- Peribiliary connective tissue

Pitfalls/Artifacts
- Peribiliary mucous glands may be mistaken for carcinoma on frozen section
  - Perineural "invasion" by these glands has rarely been reported
  - Glands retain their lobular architecture and dense stroma; lack atypia and mitoses

Metaplasia
- Gastric and intestinal types

(Left) The left and right hepatic ducts join to become the common hepatic duct (CHD) ➡, which extends for about 2 cm before joining the cystic duct ➡. The common bile duct (CBD) ➡ is formed by the fusion of the cystic duct and CHD. The lower end of the CBD runs beside and usually unites with the main pancreatic duct before entering the duodenum at the papilla ➡. *(Right)* The subepithelial stroma is composed of dense collagen, elastic fibers, and small vessels. Inflammatory cells are sparse.

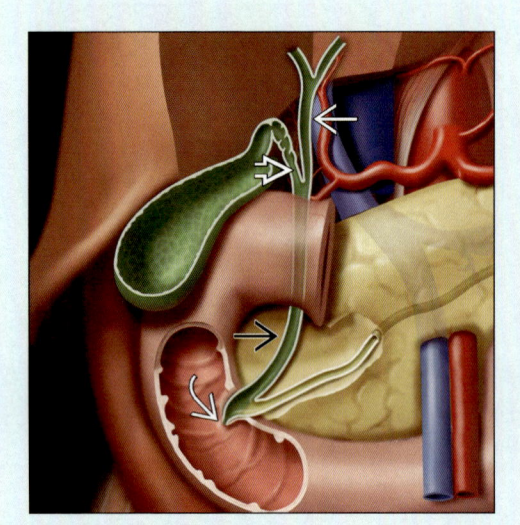

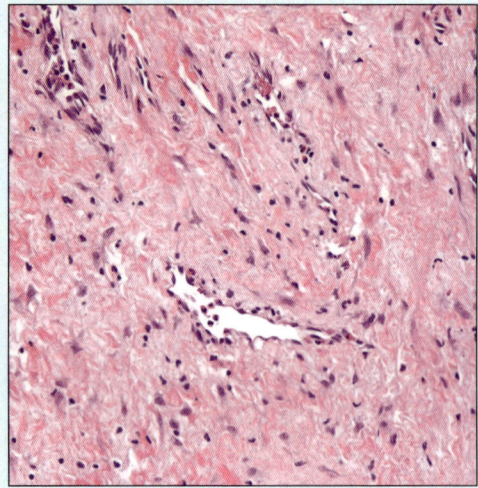

(Left) Extrahepatic bile ducts are lined by a single layer of columnar epithelium. The nuclei are round and basally located, with evenly distributed chromatin and inconspicuous nucleoli. The cytoplasm contains small amounts of mucin. Goblet cells are normally absent. Scattered neuroendocrine cells are present throughout. *(Right)* Cystic duct stroma contains muscle fibers ➡ admixed with dense connective tissue, particularly at the junction with the gallbladder (spiral valve of Heister).

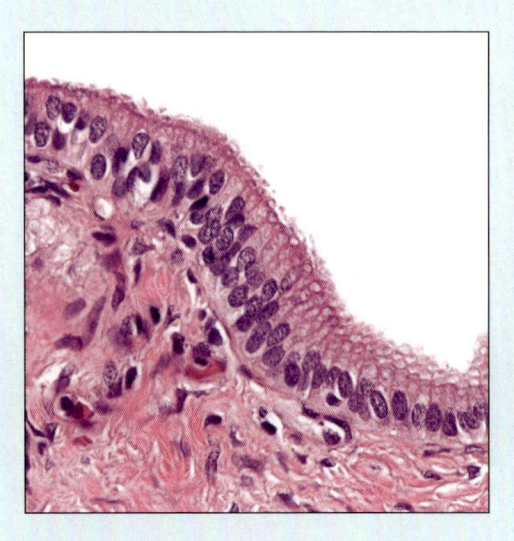

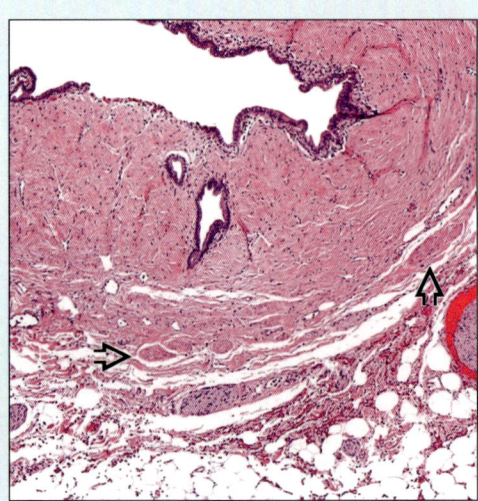

EXTRAHEPATIC BILIARY TRACT

Extrahepatic Bile Ducts: Layers

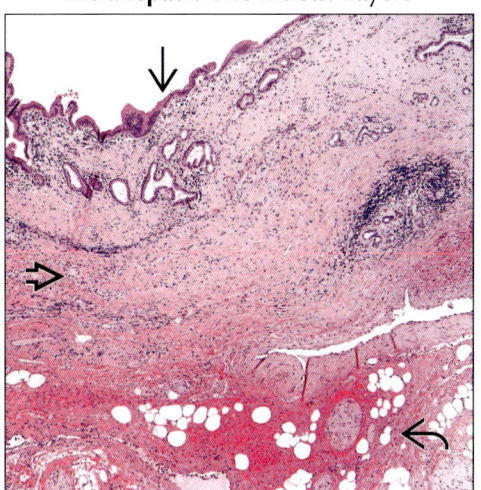

Sacculi of Beale

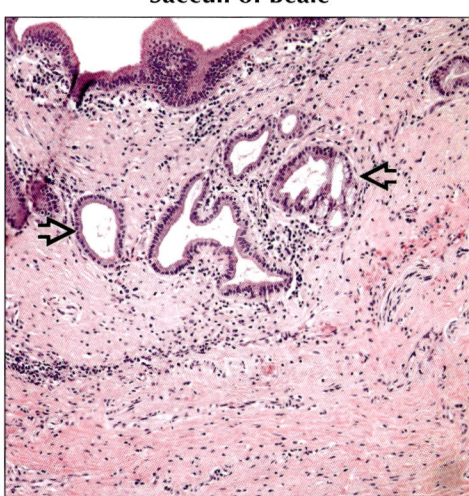

(Left) The ducts in the extrahepatic biliary tree are composed of an epithelial layer ➡️, subepithelial stroma ➡️, and the peribiliary connective tissue ➡️. The peribiliary connective tissue contains nerves, lymphatics, and vessels. *(Right)* The hepatic and common bile duct surface epithelia contain numerous regular depressions or invaginations known as the sacculi of Beale ➡️. They may appear to be isolated from the surface in tangential sections and thus may mimic carcinoma.

Lobular Mucous Glands

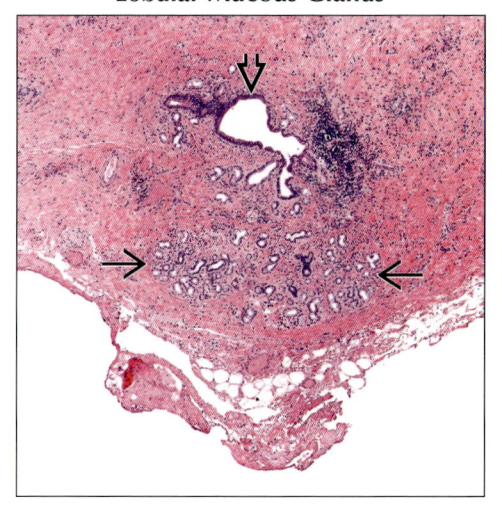

Lobular Mucous Glands

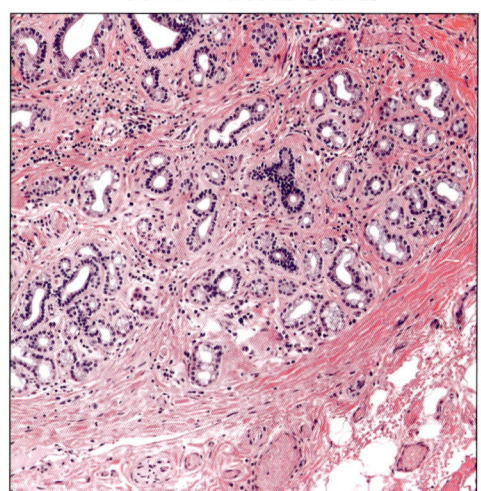

(Left) Numerous lobular mucous glands ➡️, known as peribiliary glands, biliary glands, or periductal glands, surround the sacculi ➡️ and empty into them. The more peripheral lobular mucous glands are invested by dense stroma. *(Right)* These glands are lined by low columnar or cuboidal epithelium with prominent mucin. Note the thick lobular stroma that encircles the glands; it can help differentiate normal mucous glands from an infiltrating carcinoma.

Cystic Duct

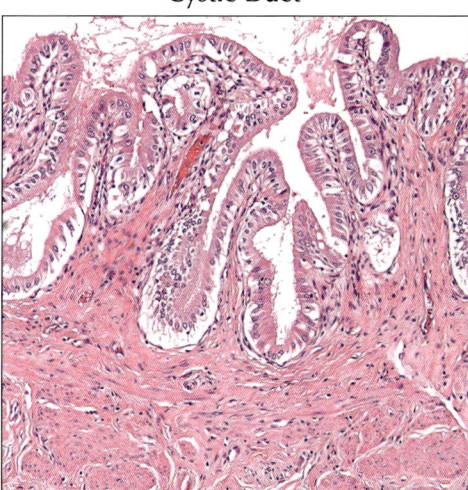

Pyloric Metaplasia

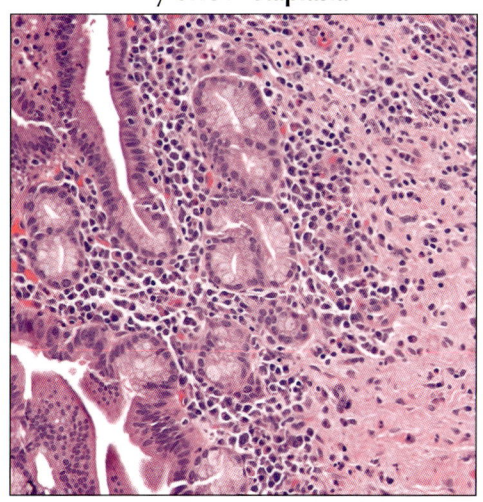

(Left) The cystic duct lining epithelium is virtually identical to that of the gallbladder and is thrown into pleats or folds. Mucous glands may be present in the lamina propria (not shown here). *(Right)* Both pyloric-type and intestinal metaplasia can be seen in the extrahepatic bile ducts, usually in association with inflammation.

VATERIAN SYSTEM

Key Facts

Macroscopic Anatomy

- Vaterian system: Distal segments of common bile duct (CBD) and main pancreatic duct, major papilla and ampulla, minor papilla, and sphincter muscle (sphincter of Oddi)
- Complex and variable anatomy
  - Common bile duct and main pancreatic duct join to form a common channel before entering duodenum in 74% of people
  - 19% of people have ducts running in parallel, with adjacent but separate openings into duodenum (bile duct opening cranial and medial to duct of Wirsung); these people usually do not have a well-developed ampulla
  - 7% of people have ducts that unite before entering duodenum, but lumina separated by connective tissue septum
- Major papilla
  - Protuberance located 8-10 cm distal to pylorus
  - Projects into 2nd portion of duodenum
- Ampulla of Vater
  - Strictly defined, ampulla of Vater is the dilated conduit present **at** the major papilla (which is the protuberance)
  - Ampulla results from union of CBD and main pancreatic duct where they open into duodenal lumen
  - Mean length: 11 mm; mean diameter: 5 mm
  - Mucosal folds or flaps are present covering ampulla in majority of people; may serve as valves
  - Only 25% of people with combined distal channel have a well-developed ampulla
- Minor papilla
  - May be difficult to appreciate macroscopically
  - Duct of Santorini usually opens into minor papilla
- Sphincter of Oddi
  - Circular and longitudinal musculature that regulates flow of bile and pancreatic enzymes into duodenum
  - Muscles held in place by muscularis propria of duodenal wall
  - Sphincter muscle fibers believed to extend up into CBD and main pancreatic duct
- Pancreatic ducts
  - Major pancreatic duct of Wirsung drains small ducts from tail of pancreas to duodenum
  - Minor pancreatic duct of Santorini joins major duct at a variety of intrapancreatic locations
- Common bile duct
  - Formed by joining of cystic duct and common hepatic duct
  - Distal CBD either runs alongside or joins with duct of Wirsung before entering duodenum at major papilla

Microscopic Anatomy

- Common bile duct and main pancreatic ducts have essentially identical epithelial linings
  - Columnar mucinous epithelium
  - No goblet cells
- Ampullary epithelium
  - Epithelium of ampulla and distal ducts consist of folds or papillae
  - Fibrovascular cores that contain sparse inflammation
  - Epithelium similar to ducts (columnar), but scattered goblet cells are common
- Associated ducts and glands
  - Numerous mucous glands present around terminal portions of ducts and ampulla
  - Morphologically similar to peribiliary mucous glands, but often larger
  - Accessory pancreatic ducts also drain into ampulla
  - Pancreatic acini may also be present
- Sphincter of Oddi
  - Muscle fibers become apparent in distal ducts (CBD and pancreatic) proximal to their entrance into the duodenum, and muscle fibers may extend up into the epithelial folds at ampulla
- Duodenal villi are few or absent at papilla
- Scattered neuroendocrine cells sometimes present around pancreatic ducts and accessory glands

(Left) The Vaterian system consists of the common bile duct ➡ and main pancreatic duct ➡ that typically join proximal to the duodenum and enter at the major papilla ➡. *(Right)* The epithelium of the ampulla and distal ducts that converge there consists of prominent folds or papillary fronds, which are supported by connective tissue stroma.

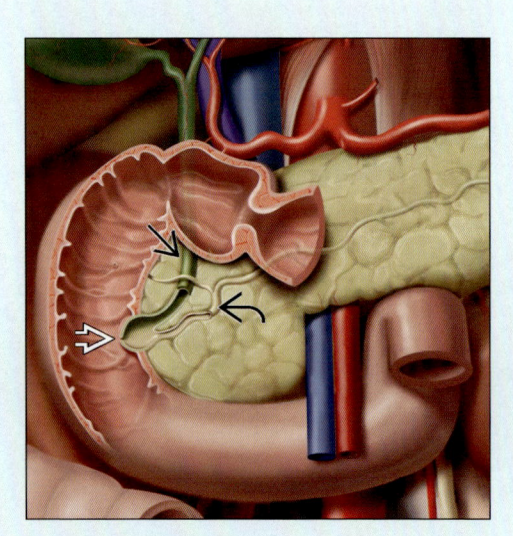

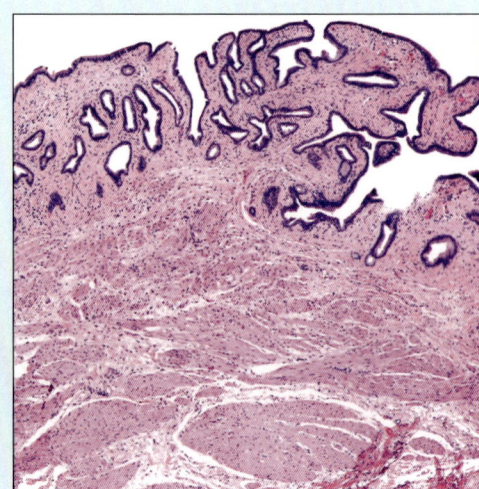

VATERIAN SYSTEM

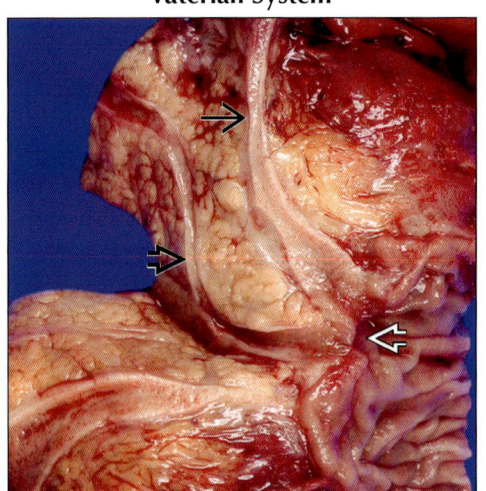

Vaterian System

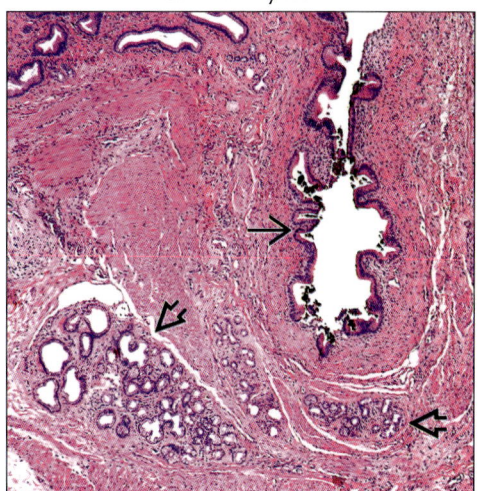

Vaterian System

(Left) This photo of a bivalved pancreas illustrates the pancreatic duct ➤ and the common bile duct ➤ entering the duodenum together at the ampulla ➤. *(Right)* This photomicrograph shows the common bile duct ➤ entering the duodenum at the ampulla. Note the numerous lobular collections of mucous glands ➤ in this area.

Ampullary Epithelium

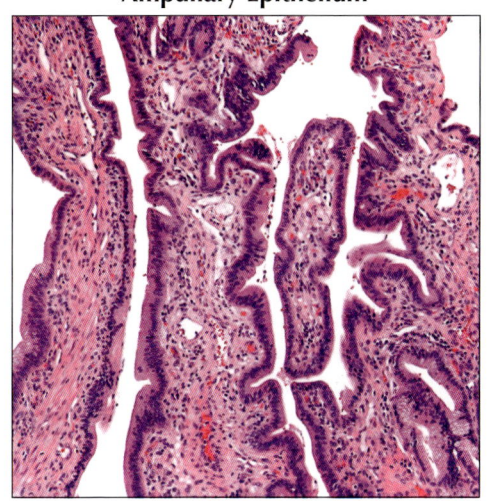

Ampullary Epithelium

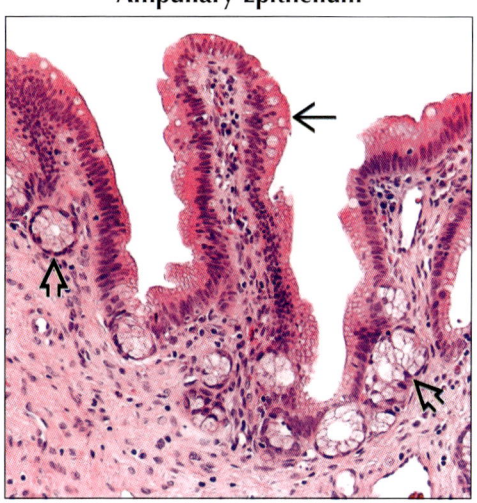

(Left) The folds or fronds of the ampullary epithelium are supported by fibrovascular cores. These cores normally contain sparse chronic inflammatory cells. *(Right)* Unlike the epithelium of the pancreatic and bile ducts, the ampullary epithelium contains scattered goblet cells ➤. Note also the mucous glands at the base of the epithelial fronds ➤.

Ductal Epithelium

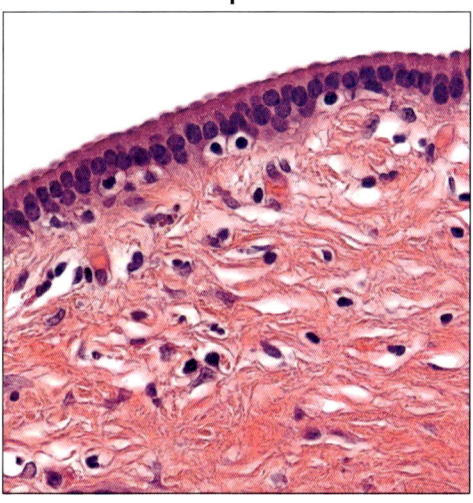

Glands and Acini

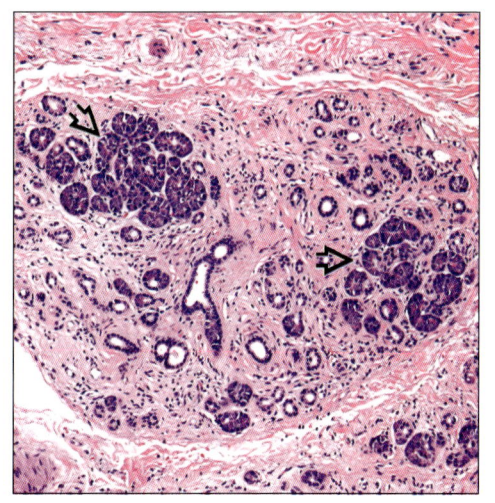

(Left) The epithelium of the terminal portions of the main pancreatic ducts and the common bile duct, which terminate in the ampulla, is a simple columnar mucinous epithelium without goblet cells. *(Right)* Numerous mucous glands are present around the ampulla and the terminal portions of the ducts. In addition, accessory pancreatic glands and pancreatic acini ➤ are often present in this area.

PANCREAS

Key Facts

Macroscopic Anatomy
- Lobular gland located in retroperitoneum behind stomach and transverse colon, and in front of aorta and vena cava
- Anterior surface is peritonealized
- 15-20 cm in length; 41-182 g on average
- No discrete capsule

Microscopic Anatomy
- Acini
  - Exocrine secretory component, comprises > 80% of pancreas
  - Spherical or tubular glands with small central lumens, surrounded by triangular secretory cells
  - Cytoplasm packed with organelles, imparting a granular appearance
  - Number of granules varies depending on secretory activity
  - Some cells have Golgi zone adjacent to nucleus
  - Variant: Acinar ectasia (focal dilatation with flattening of epithelium and inspissated secretions) is associated with obstruction, dehydration, sepsis, uremia
- Islets of Langerhans
  - Endocrine component of pancreas is present mostly within islets and comprises 1-2% of the gland in adult but 20% in neonates
  - Scattered single endocrine cells are present in ducts (mostly larger ducts) and acini, but these constitute < 10% of total number of endocrine cells in pancreas
  - 2 types of islets: Compact and diffuse
  - 4 types of endocrine cells: Beta cells, Alpha cells, Delta cells, PP cells
  - Beta cells (60-70% of islet cells) secrete insulin; at center of the islets with occasional markedly enlarged nuclei
  - Alpha cells (15-20% of islet cells) secrete glucagon
  - Delta cells (< 10% of islet cells) secrete somatostatin
  - PP cells are very rare, produce pancreatic polypeptide; mostly present in diffuse islets where they are majority of cells
- Ducts: Main ducts, interlobular ducts, intralobular ducts, intercalated ducts, centroacinar cells
  - Main ducts lined by simple columnar mucinous epithelium except in ampulla, which contains more papillary epithelium
  - Interlobular ducts are also lined by low columnar mucinous epithelium with round nuclei
  - Main and interlobular ducts are surrounded by a thick collagen layer that may contain lobular aggregates of mucous glands within wall, similar to extrahepatic bile ducts
  - Intralobular ducts have epithelium identical to intercalated ducts and have only scant surrounding collagen
  - Intercalated ducts lined by single layer of flattened cells with oval nuclei and nonsecretory cytoplasm; fuse to form intralobular ducts
  - Centroacinar cells are inconspicuous flat to cuboidal cells with pale cytoplasm in middle of acini; attach to exocrine acinar cells by tight junctions
- Connective tissue
  - Lobules separated by thin strands of loose connective tissue containing nerves and vessels
  - Adipose tissue (3-20% of gland); also present in peripancreatic soft tissue
- Pancreatic stellate cells: Similar to hepatic stellate cells, store vitamin A

Pitfalls/Artifacts
- Focal acinar transformation may mimic tumor
- Diffuse islets may be mistaken for infiltrative tumor given irregular borders

Age Variation
- Neonates have larger volume of endocrine cells and mesenchymal tissue (up to 30%)
- Ratio of hormone-producing cells in islets varies with age

(Left) The pancreas is a lobular gland located on the posterior wall of the abdomen. It lies behind the stomach and transverse colon, and in front of the aorta and vena cava. The pancreas is divided into the head, neck, body, and tail, but the demarcations are indistinct. The head lies within the curve of the duodenum, and the tail reaches to the hilum of the spleen. (Right) Delicate connective tissue septae ➡ divide the pancreatic parenchyma into lobules.

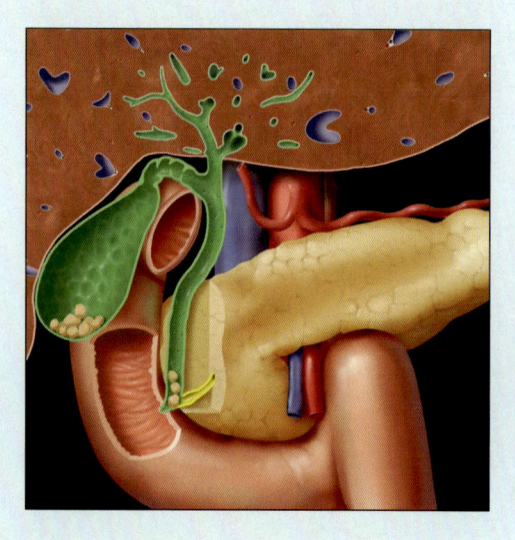

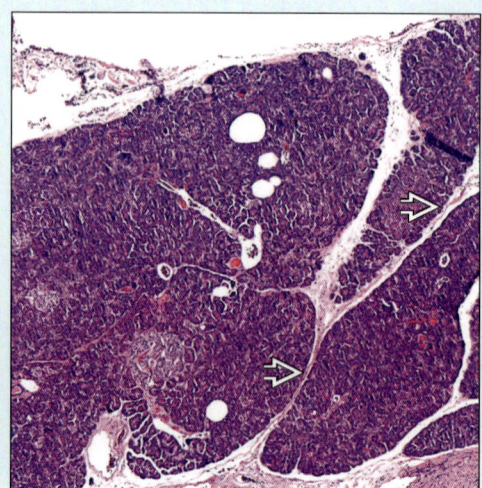

PANCREAS

Acini
Acini

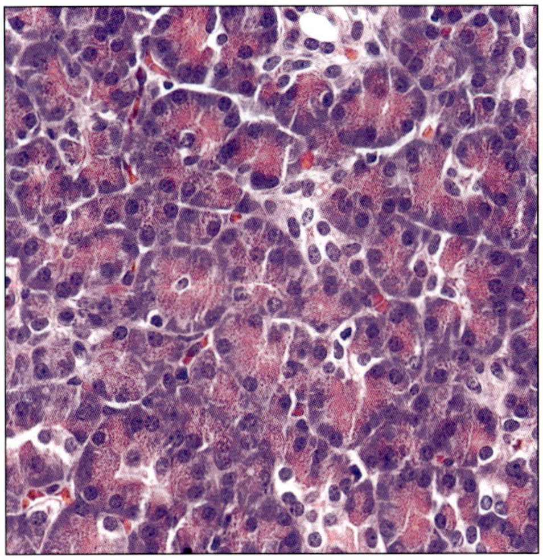

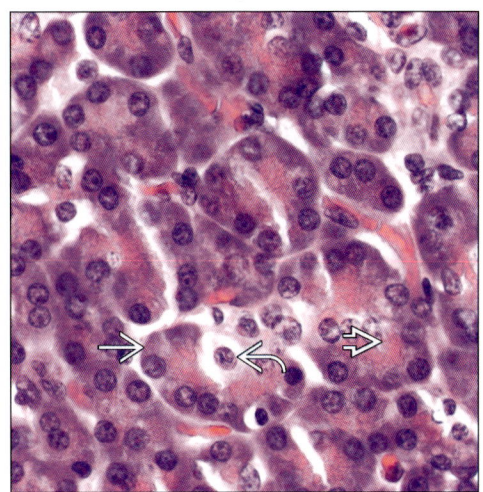

(Left) The exocrine acinar parenchyma consists of spherical or tubular glands with small central lumina, surrounded by a single layer of triangular secretory cells. There is no myoepithelial layer. Nuclei are round and basally located, with even chromatin and small nucleoli. (Right) Secretory cells have basophilic basal granules ⇒ and eosinophilic apical granules ⇒. The basal granules consist of ribosomes; the apical granules contain zymogen. A centroacinar cell, which represents the beginning of the ductal system, is visible in a lumen ⇒.

Acini
Islets of Langerhans

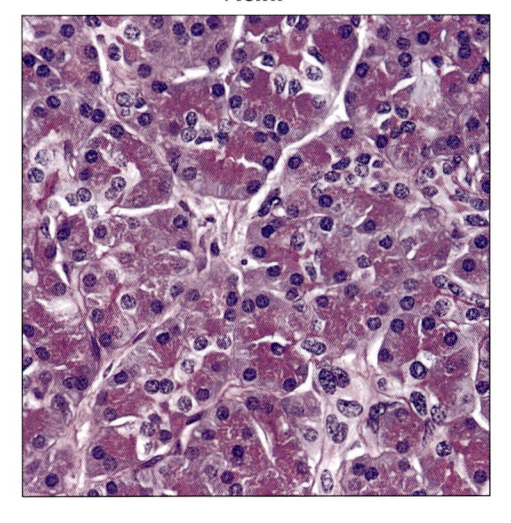

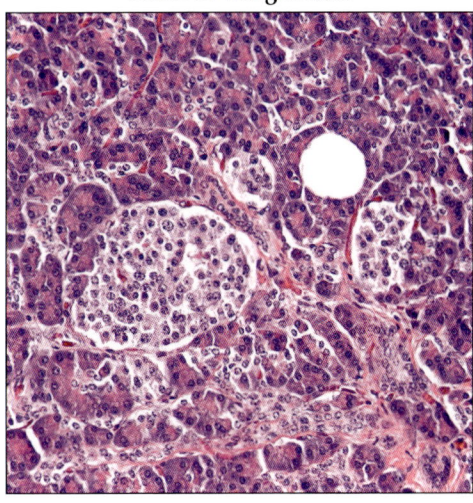

(Left) Zymogen granules are PAS positive and diastase resistant, and negative for mucin and Alcian blue because they do not contain mucin. Immunohistochemically, they are positive for pancreatic enzymes (amylase, lipase, trypsin, chymotrypsin), as well as CAM 5.2. They are negative for AE1/AE3, CK7, CK19, and CK20. (Right) Islets of Langerhans are present throughout the pancreas but are randomly distributed, with some lobules having more than others. The vast majority of the endocrine cells in the pancreas are in the islets.

Islets of Langerhans
Islets of Langerhans

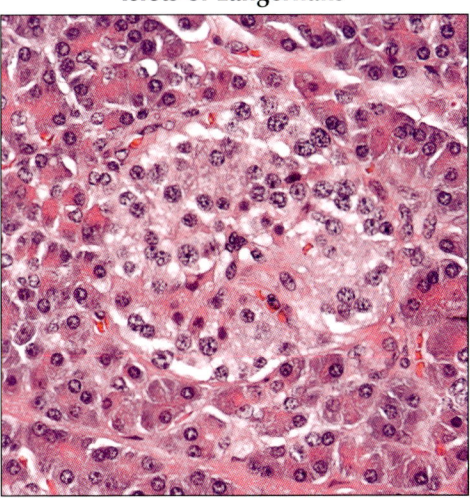

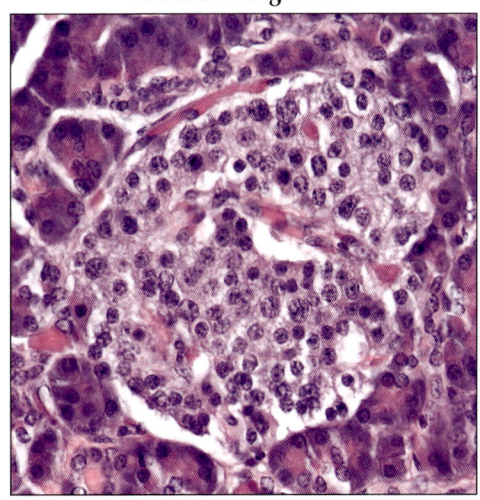

(Left) Compact islets account for 90% of the total and occur in the body and tail of the pancreas as well as the superior portion of the head. They have well-defined borders. (Right) The nuclei of compact islets have coarsely clumped or speckled chromatin.

PANCREAS

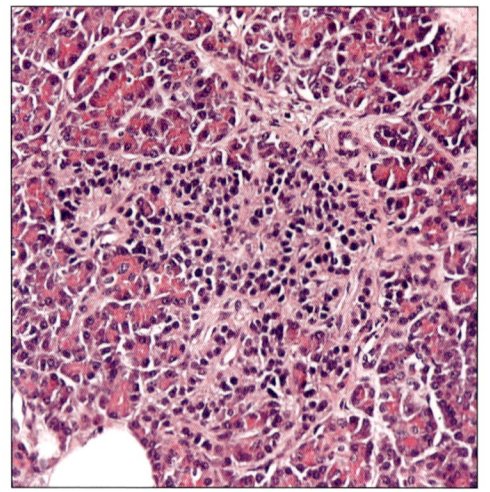

Islets of Langerhans

(Left) Diffuse islets are found in the inferior portion of the head of the pancreas, and they are much less numerous than compact islets. They have ill-defined borders, are often larger than compact islets, and have more hyperchromatic nuclei. (Right) Islets of Langerhans are not encapsulated and have a rich capillary network within them ⇨.

Islets of Langerhans / Intrapancreatic Fat

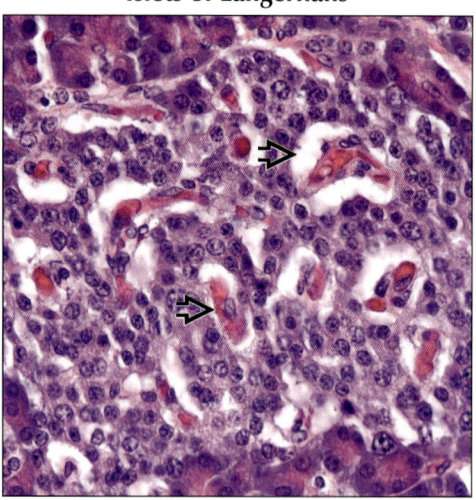

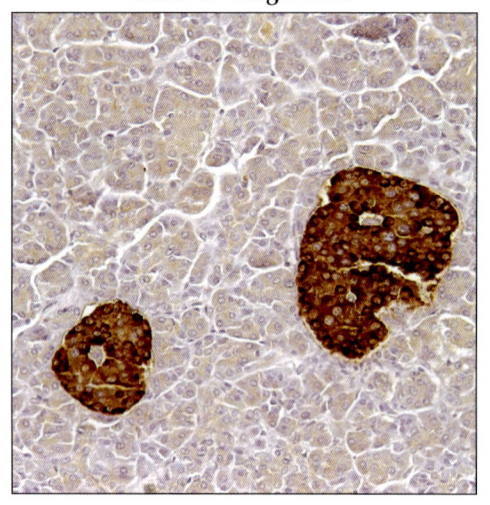

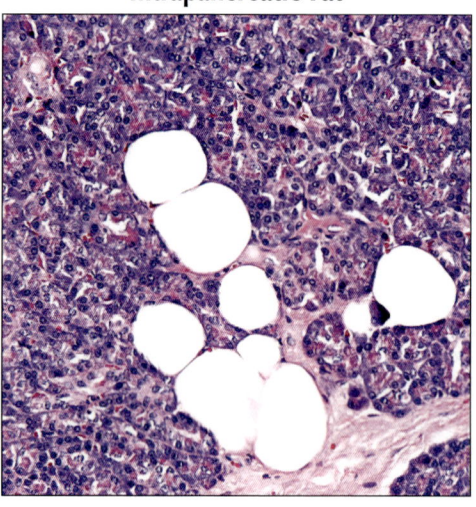

(Left) Synaptophysin immunostain highlights the islets of Langerhans. All islets produce general endocrine markers such as CD56, synaptophysin, and chromogranin. Islets are typically keratin negative. (Right) Most pancreata contain a small amount of intrapancreatic fat. The proportion of the gland composed of fat varies with age and nutritional status.

Main Pancreatic Ducts / Pancreatic Ducts

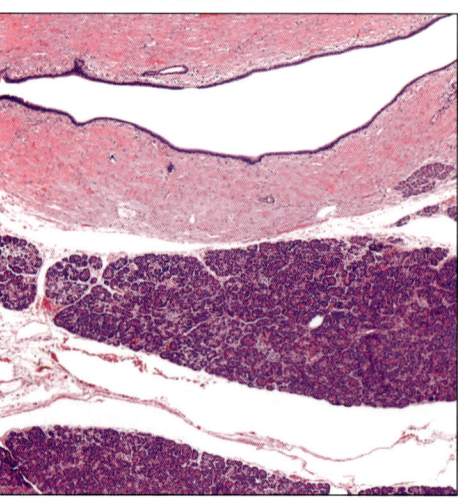

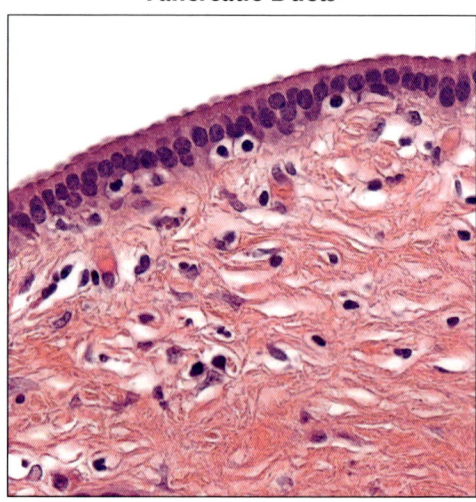

(Left) The main pancreatic ducts (also known as ducts of Wirsung and Santorini) and the interlobular ducts are surrounded by a thick collagen layer. The pancreatic ductal system transports pancreatic secretions to the duodenum. (Right) The main pancreatic ducts are lined by a simple columnar mucinous epithelium. The nuclei are round and basally located. Ductal cells are positive for keratins AE1/AE3, CAM5.2, CK7, and CK19, and are CK20 negative.

PANCREAS

Interlobular Duct

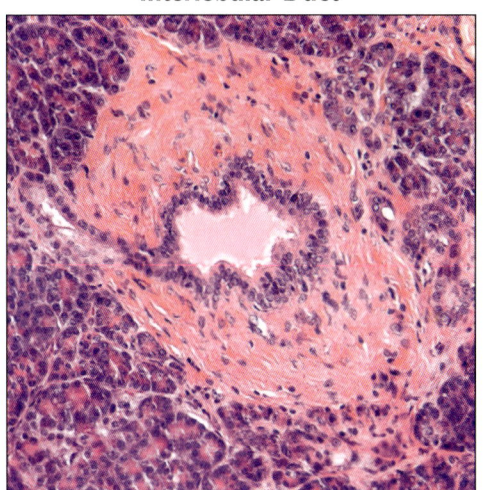

Ducts

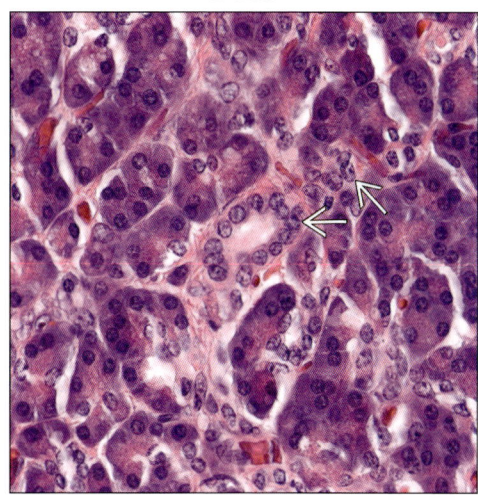

(Left) This cross section of an interlobular duct shows the surrounding thick band of supporting collagen and also contains low columnar mucinous epithelium. (Right) The intercalated ducts are the smallest ducts outside the acini. They are lined by cuboidal epithelium that does not contain mucin, and have minimal surrounding connective tissue stroma. The intercalated ducts fuse to form the intralobular ducts ➡.

Connective Tissue

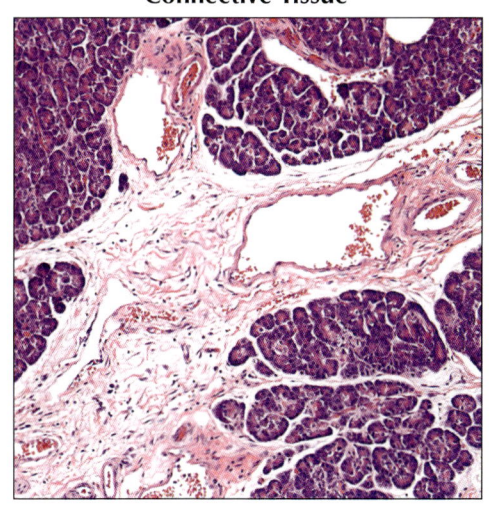

Connective Tissue

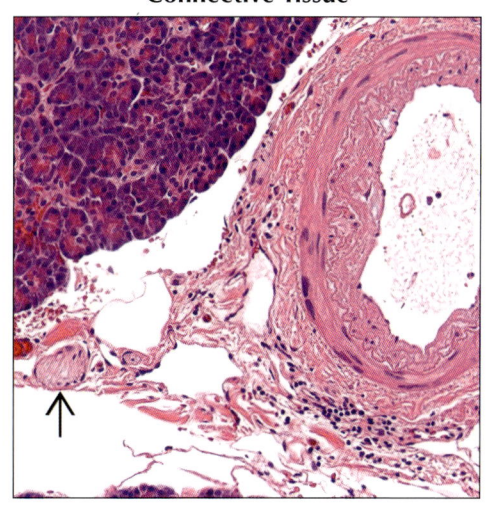

(Left) The connective tissue septae between the pancreatic lobules contain vessels and nerves. (Right) A large artery, lymphatics, veins, and a nerve ➡ are seen within this connective tissue septum.

Nerves

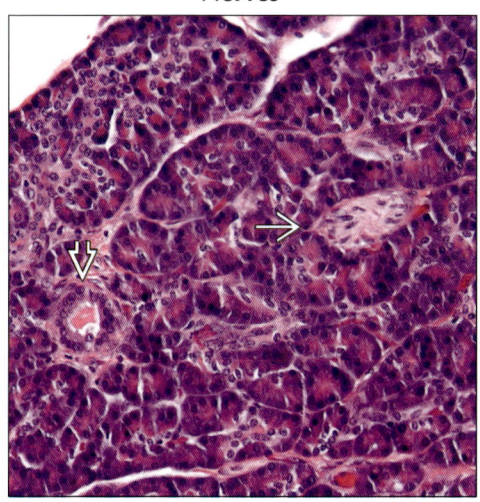

Focal Acinar Transformation

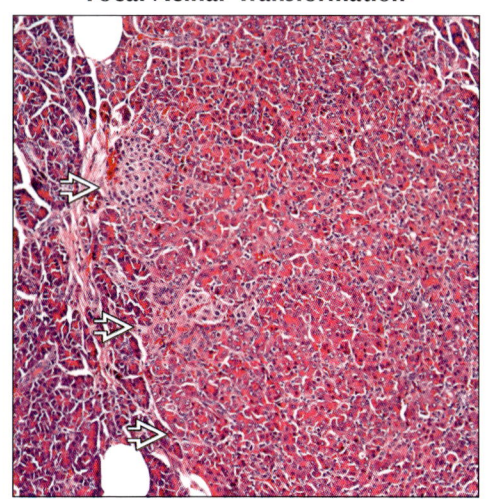

(Left) Most nerves and vessels are in the septae, but some small vessels and nerves ➡ may be present within the lobular parenchyma. Note the small duct profile at the left ➡. (Right) Focal acinar transformation consists of a pale eosinophilic nodular area ➡ that often involves an entire lobule. This change is secondary to dilatation of rough endoplasmic reticulum. The cause is unknown, but it has no pathologic significance.

SELECTED REFERENCES

LIVER

1. Roskams TA et al: Nomenclature of the finer branches of the biliary tree: canals, ductules, and ductular reactions in human livers. Hepatology. 39(6):1739-45, 2004
2. Harman D: Lipofuscin and ceroid formation: the cellular recycling system. Adv Exp Med Biol. 266:3-15, 1989
3. Gerber MA et al: Histology of the liver. Am J Surg Pathol. 11(9):709-22, 1987
4. Ogawa K et al: Sequential changes of extracellular matrix and proliferation of Ito cells with enhanced expression of desmin and actin in focal hepatic injury. Am J Pathol. 125(3):611-9, 1986
5. Watanabe T et al: Age-related alterations in the size of human hepatocytes. A study of mononuclear and binucleate cells. Virchows Arch B Cell Pathol Incl Mol Pathol. 39(1):9-20, 1982
6. Findor J et al: Structure and ultrastructure of the liver in aged persons. Acta Hepatogastroenterol (Stuttg). 20(3):200-4, 1973
7. Petrelli M et al: Variation in subcapsular liver structure and its significance in the interpretation of wedge biopsies. J Clin Pathol. 20(5):743-8, 1967
8. Rappaport AM: The structural and functional unit in the human liver (liver acinus). Anat Rec. 130(4):673-89, 1958

GALLBLADDER

1. Schnelldorfer T et al: What is the duct of luschka?: a systematic review. J Gastrointest Surg. 16(3):656-62, 2012
2. Singhi AD et al: Hyperplastic Luschka ducts: a mimic of adenocarcinoma in the gallbladder fossa. Am J Surg Pathol. 35(6):883-90, 2011
3. Albores-Saavedra J et al: Mucin-containing Rokitansky-Aschoff sinuses with extracellular mucin deposits simulating mucinous carcinoma of the gallbladder. Am J Surg Pathol. 33(11):1633-8, 2009
4. Spanos CP et al: Bile leaks from the duct of Luschka (subvesical duct): a review. Langenbecks Arch Surg. 391(5):441-7, 2006
5. Hudson I et al: Macrophages and mast cells in chronic cholecystitis and "normal" gall bladders. J Clin Pathol. 39(10):1082-7, 1986
6. Tsutsumi Y et al: Histochemical studies of metaplastic lesions in the human gallbladder. Arch Pathol Lab Med. 108(11):917-21, 1984
7. Laitio M: Morphology and histochemistry of non-tumorous gallbladder epithelium. A series of 103 cases. Pathol Res Pract. 167(2-4):335-45, 1980
8. Beilby JO: Diverticulosis of the gall bladder. The fundal adenoma. Br J Exp Pathol. 48(4):455-61, 1967
9. Burnett W et al: Some observations in the innervation of the extrahepatic biliary system in man. Ann Surg. 159:8-26, 1964
10. Evett RD et al: The fine structure of normal mucosa in human gallbladder. Gastroenterology. 47:49-60, 1964
11. Elfving G: Crypts and ducts in the gallbladder wall. Acta Pathol Microbiol Scand Suppl. 49(Suppl 135):1-45, 1960

EXTRAHEPATIC BILIARY TRACT

1. Hand BH: Anatomy and function of the extrahepatic biliary system. Clin Gastroenterol. 2(1):3-29, 1973
2. Dowdy GS Jr et al: Surgical anatomy of the pancreatobiliary ductal system. Observations. Arch Surg. 84:229-46, 1962

VATERIAN SYSTEM

1. Mirilas P et al: Benign anatomical mistakes: "ampulla of Vater" and "papilla of Vater". Am Surg. 71(3):269-74, 2005
2. Allescher HD: Papilla of Vater: structure and function. Endoscopy. 21(Suppl 1):324-9, 1989
3. DiMagno EP et al: Relationships between pancreaticobiliary ductal anatomy and pancreatic ductal and parenchymal histology. Cancer. 49(2):361-8, 1982
4. Hand BH: Anatomy and function of the extrahepatic biliary system. Clin Gastroenterol. 2(1):3-29, 1973
5. Brown JO et al: Mucosal reduplications associated with the ampullary portion of the major duodenal papilla in humans. Anat Rec. 150:293-301, 1964
6. Hand BH: An anatomical study of the choledochoduodenal area. Br J Surg. 50:486-94, 1963
7. Newman HF et al: The papilla of Vater and distal portions of the common bile duct and duct of Wirsung. Surg Gynecol Obstet. 106(6):687-94, 1958

PANCREAS

1. Innes JT et al: Normal pancreatic dimensions in the adult human. Am J Surg. 167(2):261-3, 1994
2. Akao S et al: Three-dimensional pattern of ductuloacinar associations in normal and pathological human pancreas. Gastroenterology. 90(3):661-8, 1986
3. Grube D et al: The microanatomy of human islets of Langerhans, with special reference to somatostatin (D-) cells. Arch Histol Jpn. 46(3):327-53, 1983
4. Kodama T et al: Atypical acinar cell nodules of the human pancreas. Acta Pathol Jpn. 33(4):701-14, 1983
5. Kodama T: A light and electron microscopic study on the pancreatic ductal system. Acta Pathol Jpn. 33(2):297-321, 1983

SELECTED REFERENCES

6. Stefan Y et al: The pancreatic polypeptide-rich lobe of the human pancreas: definitive identification of its derivation from the ventral pancreatic primordium. Diabetologia. 23(2):141-2, 1982

7. Rahier J et al: Cell populations in the endocrine pancreas of human neonates and infants. Diabetologia. 20(5):540-6, 1981

8. Orci L et al: Pancreatic fat. N Engl J Med. 301(23):1292, 1979

9. Pelletier G: Identification of four cell types in the human endocrine pancreas by immunoelectron microscopy. Diabetes. 26(8):749-56, 1977

10. Roberts PF et al: A histochemical study of mucins in normal and neoplastic human pancreatic tissue. J Pathol. 107(2):87-94, 1972

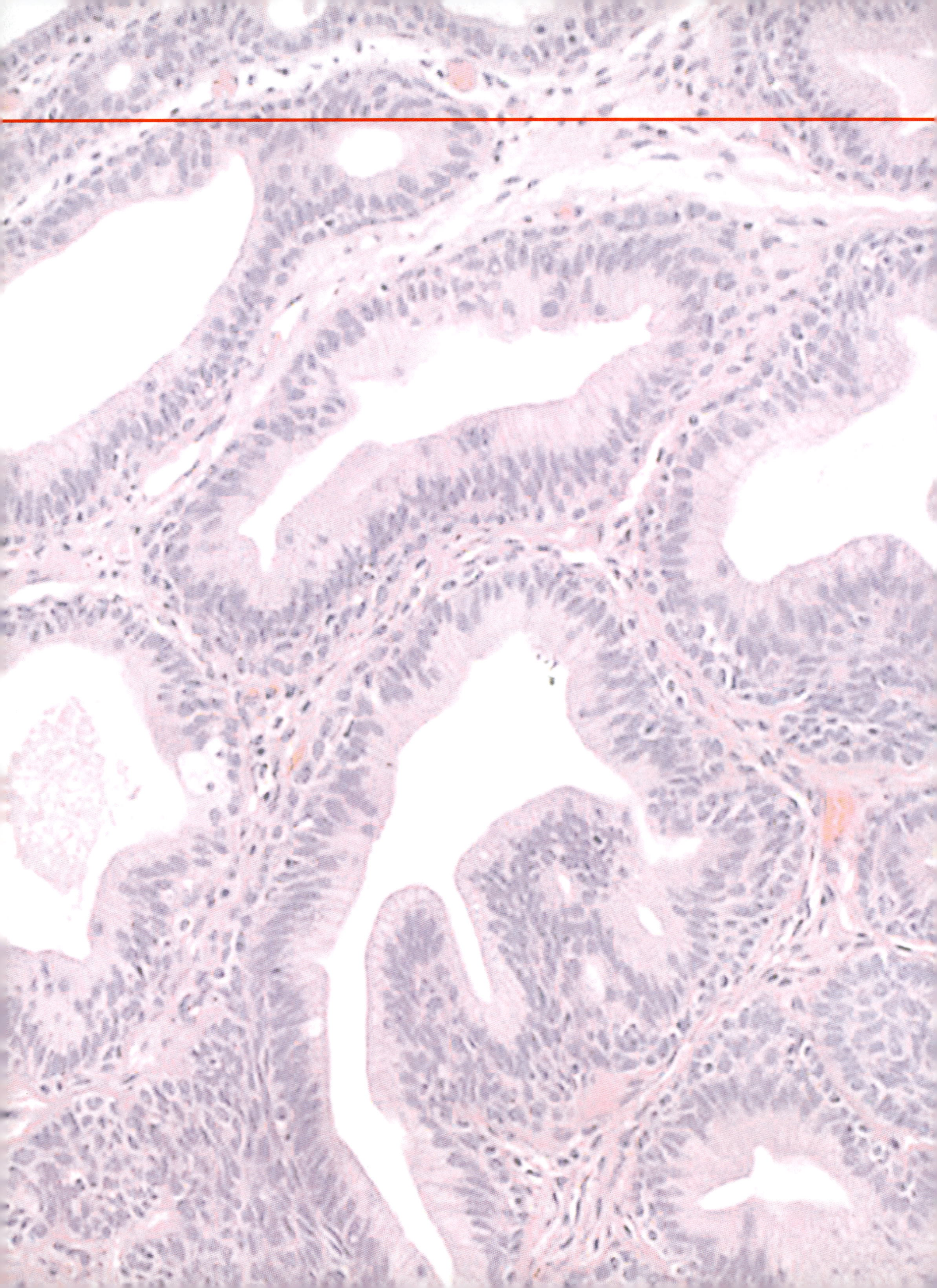

Genitourinary and Male Genital Tract

Kidney	12-2
Ureter and Renal Pelvis	12-12
Bladder	12-16
Urethra	12-22
Prostate: Regional Anatomy With Histologic Correlates	12-28
Prostate: Benign Glandular and Stromal Histology	12-38
Penis	12-48
Testis and Associated Excretory Ducts	12-52

KIDNEY

Key Facts

Macroscopic Anatomy
- Kidney
  - ~ 1 million nephrons per kidney (range: 200,000 to > 2.5 million)
  - 11-14 lobes
- Cortex
  - Cortical labyrinth
  - 10-14 generations of glomeruli
  - Medullary rays contain straight portion of proximal/distal tubules and collecting ducts
- Medulla
  - Pyramids
  - Outer medulla: Outer and inner stripe
  - Inner medulla: Papilla
- Renal pelvis
  - Calyces: Major and minor
- Renal sinus
- Renal hilum
  - Renal artery branches → interlobar → arcuate → interlobular arteries → afferent arterioles → efferent arterioles → peritubular capillaries or vasa recta
  - Renal vein

Microscopic Anatomy
- Glomeruli
  - Glomerular filtration barrier consists of visceral epithelial cells (podocytes), glomerular basement membrane, and fenestrated endothelial cells
  - Parietal epithelial cells and podocytes line Bowman capsules
  - Mesangial cells (2 nuclei per mesangial region for a 2 µm thick section) comprise stalk into which glomerular capillaries are anchored
- Juxtaglomerular apparatus
  - Consists of portions of afferent and efferent arterioles, Goormaghtigh cells, macula densa
  - Granular cells produce renin located abundantly in afferent arteriolar wall
- Proximal tubules
  - Consist of eosinophilic cytoplasm (high mitochondria content) with brush borders
- Loop of Henle
- Distal tubules
- Collecting ducts
  - Principal cells reabsorb sodium and secrete potassium
  - Intercalated cells have ↑ mitochondria content and cortical density > medulla
- Arteries: Adventitia, media, and intima lined by nonfenestrated endothelial cells
- Arterioles: Afferent and efferent
- Peritubular capillary network
- Vasa recta
- Venules
- Lymphatics
- Dendritic cell network
- Nerves

Pitfalls/Artifacts
- Renal medulla: Normal tubules not back-to-back in distribution
  - Difficult to assess interstitial fibrosis in this region
- Prominent podocytes of pediatric glomeruli not to be mistaken for collapsing glomerulopathy
- Increased extracellular matrix in perivascular regions can be mistaken for interstitial fibrosis

Age Variation
- Infants and young children
  - Weight: 13-44 g
  - Fetal lobulations
  - Smaller glomeruli and podocytes can be quite prominent
  - Low birth weight infants have lower endowment of glomeruli/nephrons
- Adults
  - Weight: 115-175 g
  - Kidneys generally larger in males than females
  - Fetal lobulations often disappear but may be retained
- Global glomerulosclerosis
  - < 40 years of age: < 10% of glomeruli (mean: 2.5%) are globally sclerotic
  - > 40 years of age: Half of the person's age minus 10 = percentage of global glomerulosclerosis that can be considered normal

(Left) Every day 1,800 L of blood (roughly 25% of the cardiac output) flow into the kidneys through the renal artery ➡, and exit the renal vein ➡. Up to 1 L of urine is produced, which exits through the ureter ➡ into the bladder. *(Right)* The cortex runs along the outer rim ➡ and extends as columns ➡ between the medullary pyramids ➡. Urine drains into the minor calices through the papillae ➡. A capsule is not present to contain tumors from gaining access to lymphatics in the sinus fat region ➡.

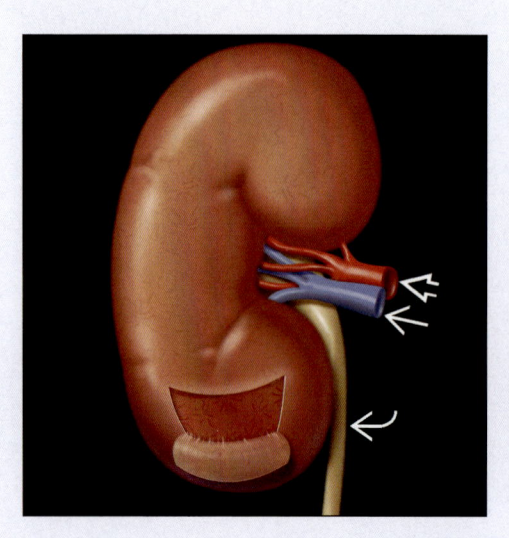

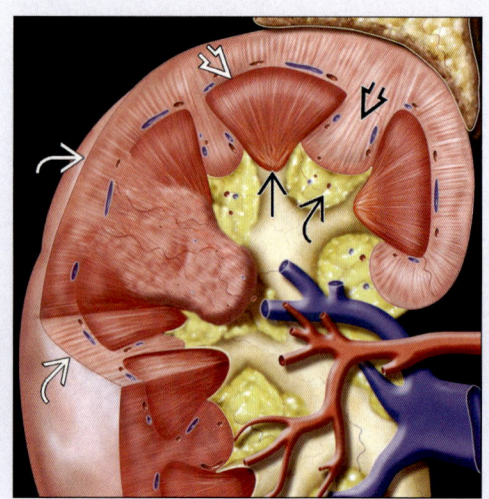

KIDNEY

Schematic of 2 Nephrons With Blood Supply

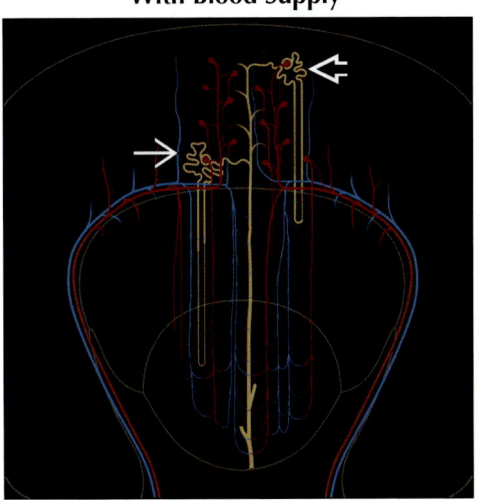

Normal Cortex

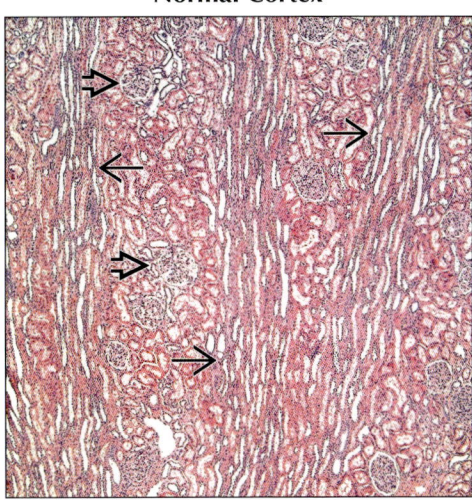

(Left) Juxtamedullary glomeruli/nephrons ➡ have a longer loop of Henle compared with cortical glomeruli/nephrons ➡. The efferent arterioles of cortical nephrons supply the peritubular capillary network while the efferent arterioles of juxtamedullary nephrons may supply the vasa recta. *(Right)* Glomeruli ➡ are present only in the cortex. Medullary rays ➡ are part of the cortex and run up toward the capsule and down toward the medulla in this photomicrograph. The tubules are closely packed in the cortex.

Schematic View of Nephron

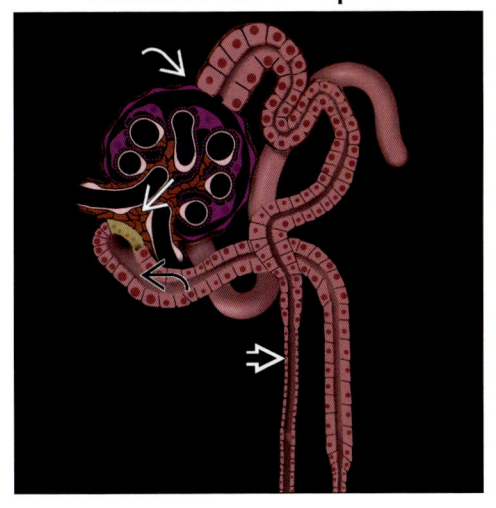

Renal Medulla

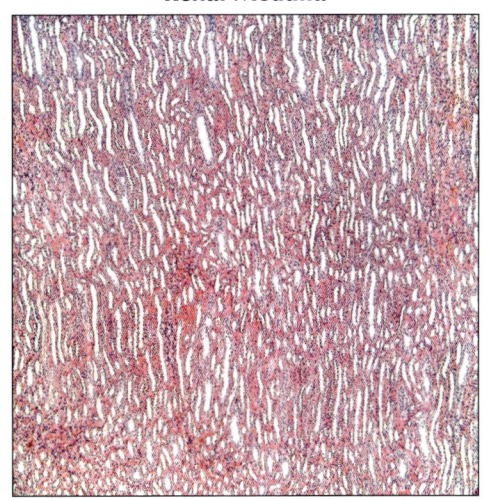

(Left) The renal corpuscle consists of a Bowman capsule and its included glomerulus. The proximal tubule joins the renal corpuscle at the urinary pole ➡. The diagram also shows the descending portion of the loop of Henle ➡, the distal tubule ➡, and the macula densa (light brown), which is in continuity with the juxtaglomerular apparatus ➡. *(Right)* The renal medulla consists of distal tubules, loops of Henle, and collecting ducts. The tubules are not as closely packed as those in the cortex. No glomeruli are present.

Schematic of 2 Nephrons

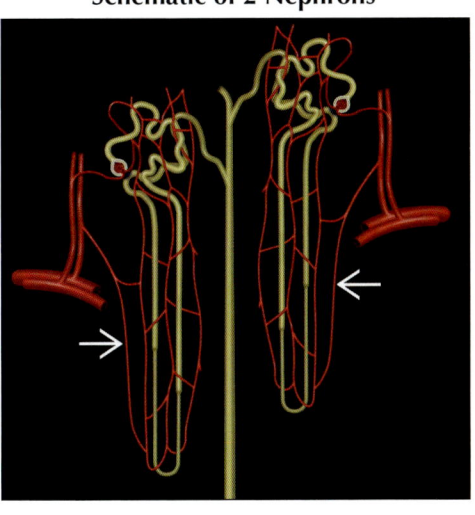

Medulla

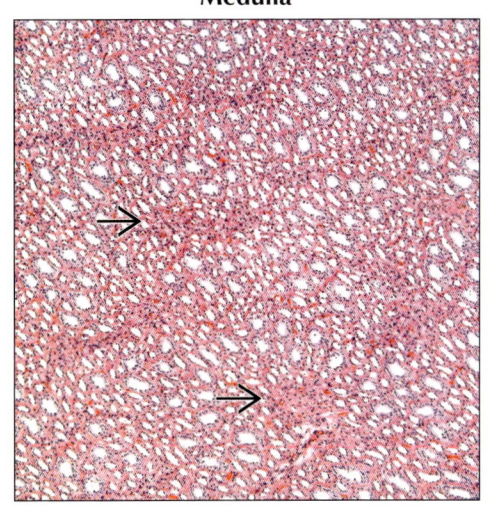

(Left) The kidney consists of approximately 1 million nephrons, and its complex vasculature is demonstrated in this schematic of 2 nephrons. The elaborate peritubular capillary network ➡ is supplied by blood from the efferent arterioles that exit the cortical glomeruli. Therefore, primary glomerular diseases will lead to secondary interstitial fibrosis and tubular atrophy when significant glomerular injury or scarring occurs. *(Right)* Efferent arterioles of juxtamedullary glomeruli become the vasa recta and form bundles ➡.

Genitourinary and Male Genital Tract

12

3

KIDNEY

Normal Glomerulus Schematic

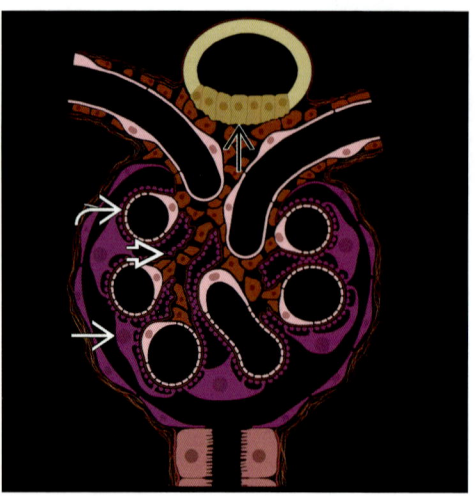

Normal Pediatric Glomerulus

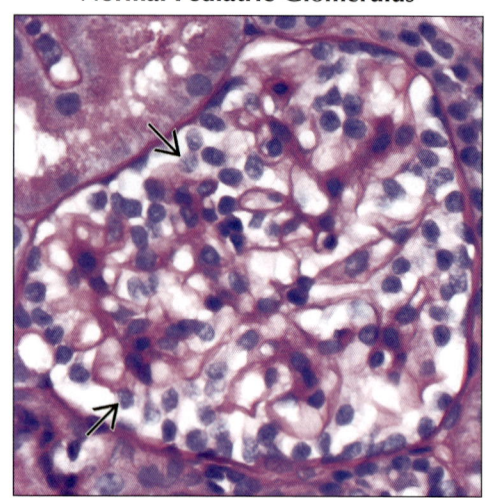

(Left) The glomerulus consists of mesangial cells ⮕, fenestrated endothelial cells ⮕, and podocytes ⮕ overlying the glomerular basement membrane. The macula densa ⮕ is adjacent to the juxtaglomerular apparatus. It is a group of densely staining cells in the distal tubule that may function as receptors that feed information to the juxtaglomerular cells. (Right) Pediatric glomeruli are smaller than adult glomeruli and have prominent podocytes ⮕ (visceral epithelial cells).

Normal Glomerulus: H&E

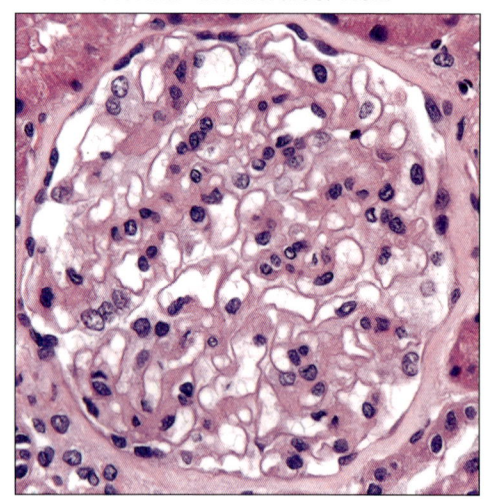

Normal Glomerulus: PAS

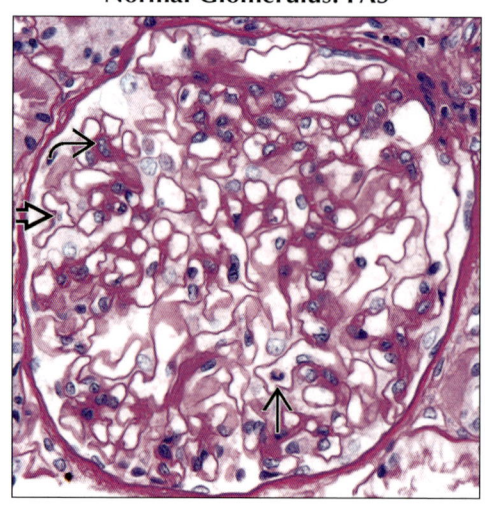

(Left) Hematoxylin and eosin is not the ideal histochemical stain for assessing structural abnormalities of the glomerulus. (Right) Periodic acid-Schiff nicely outlines the glomerular basement membrane ⮕, thereby facilitating assessment of the glomerulus. Mesangial areas ⮕ normally have < 3 nuclei per region in a 2 μm thick section. An incidental circulating neutrophil ⮕ is present in a glomerular capillary.

Normal Glomerulus: Jones Methenamine Silver

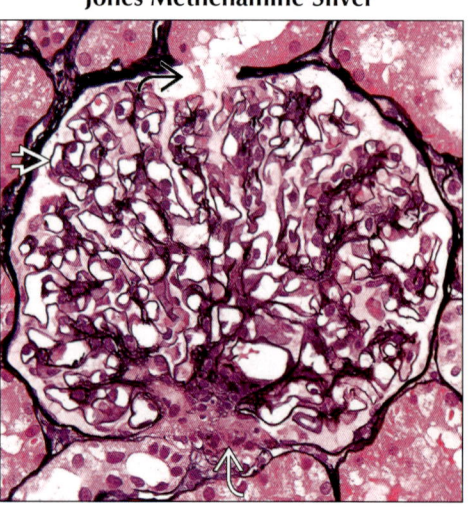

Normal Glomerulus: Masson Trichrome

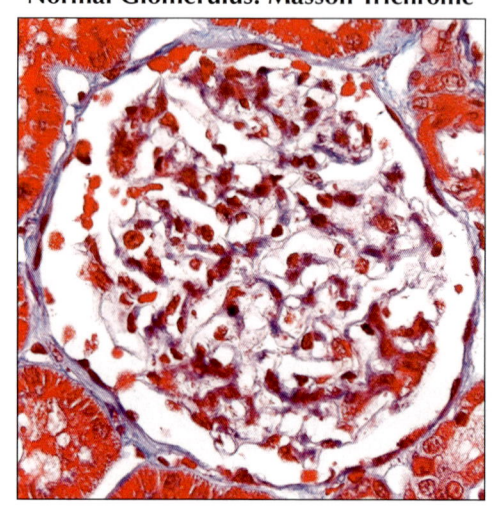

(Left) The Jones methenamine silver stain allows optimal visualization of the normal delicate glomerular basement membranes ⮕ and normal mesangial cellularity. The juxtaglomerular apparatus ⮕ is next to the hilar arteriole at the vascular pole. The tip of the glomerulus empties into the urinary pole ⮕ at the most proximal portion of the proximal tubule. (Right) Masson trichrome stains the Bowman capsule and the glomerular and tubular basement membranes blue.

KIDNEY

Schematic of Glomerular Capillaries

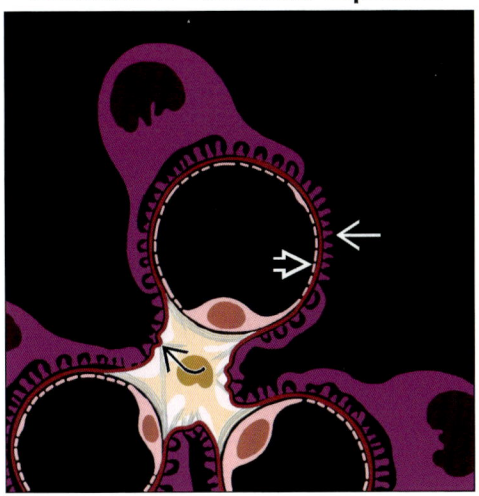

Normal Glomerular Capillaries: EM

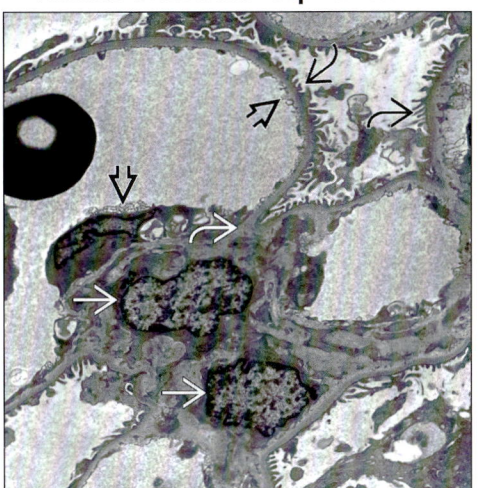

(Left) The podocytes and their foot processes ➡ cover the glomerular basement membranes. The fenestrated endothelial cells ➡ also contribute to the glomerular filtration barrier. The glomerular basement membranes are anchored to the mesangium ➡. *(Right)* The glomerular capillary basement membrane anchors in the mesangium ➡. It is lined by fenestrated endothelial cells ➡ and covered by podocytes and their foot processes ➡. Normally, 2 mesangial cells ➡ are present per mesangial region.

CD31

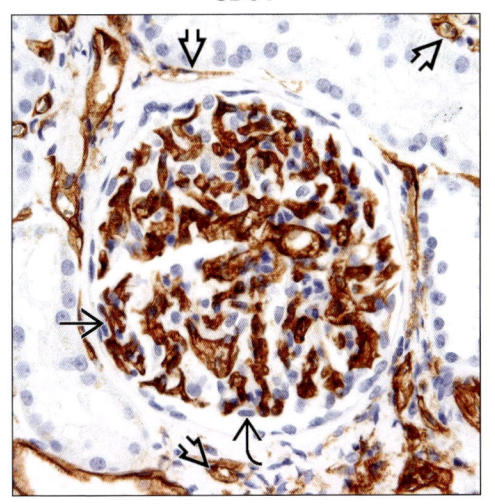

Glomerular Podocytes: CD10

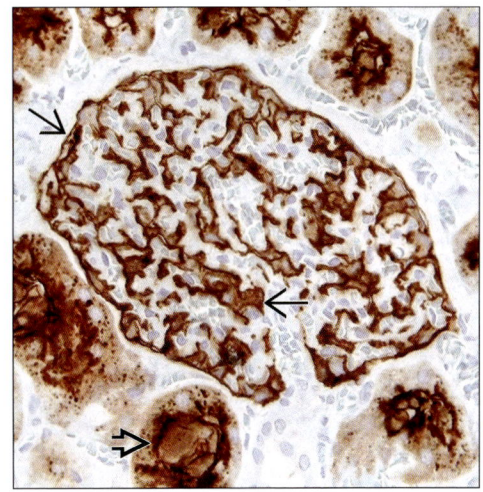

(Left) The endothelial cells within glomerular capillaries ➡ and peritubular capillaries ➡ are highlighted by CD31. Podocytes ➡ are located on the outside of the glomerular capillaries and are CD31 negative. *(Right)* CD10 (neutral endopeptidase) is expressed on podocytes (visceral glomerular epithelial cells) ➡ and the brush border ➡ of proximal tubular epithelial cells. The podocytes intricately cover the glomerular capillary surface.

Podocyte Foot Process and Slit Diaphragm Complex

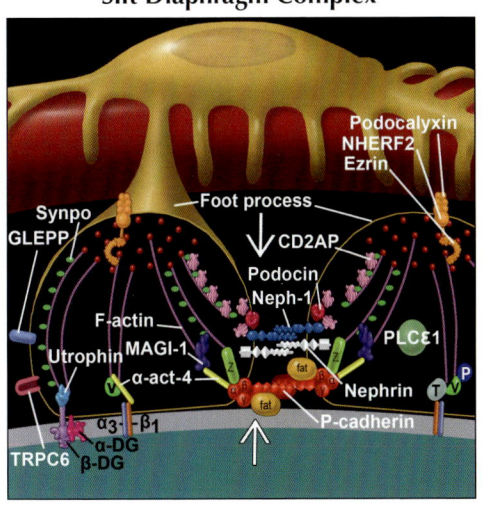

Glomerular Filtration Barrier: EM

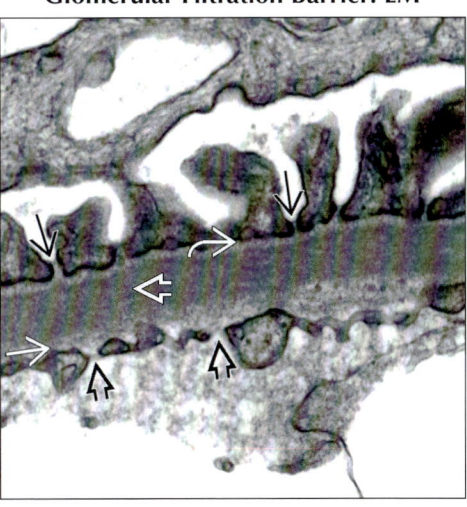

(Left) The slit diaphragm complex ➡ is a highly specialized cell junction connecting the foot processes of adjacent podocytes. It is composed of proteins (e.g., nephrin, podocin, CD2AP) expressed by the podocytes *(Right)* The glomerular basement membrane consists of the lamina densa ➡, lamina rara externa ➡, and lamina rara interna ➡. Slit diaphragms ➡ are noted. Endothelial fenestrae ➡ are 70-100 nm in diameter.

KIDNEY

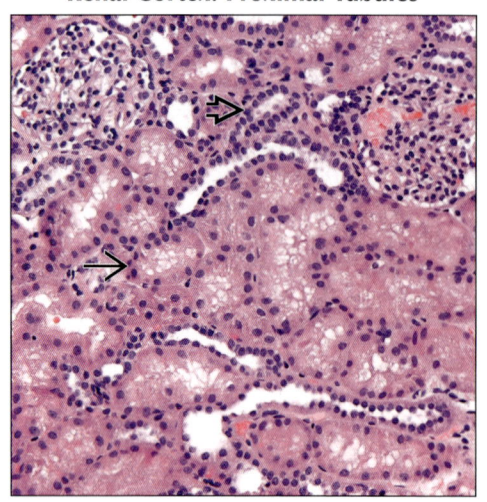

Renal Cortex: Proximal Tubules

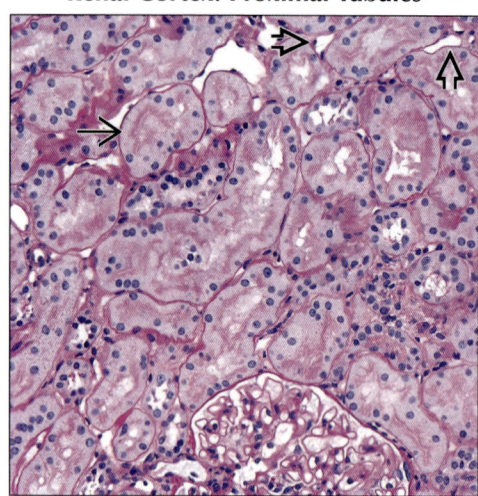

(Left) The convoluted proximal tubules ⇒ comprise the majority of tubules seen in the renal cortex. They are characterized by abundant eosinophilic cytoplasm, in contrast with the distal nephron segments ⇒ that have much smaller cells and thus more nuclei per tubule length. **(Right)** Periodic acid-Schiff stain shows the abundant cytoplasm of the proximal tubular epithelial cells ⇒. No significant space is present between tubules except for the network of peritubular capillaries ⇒.

Proximal Tubules: H&E / Proximal Tubules: PAS

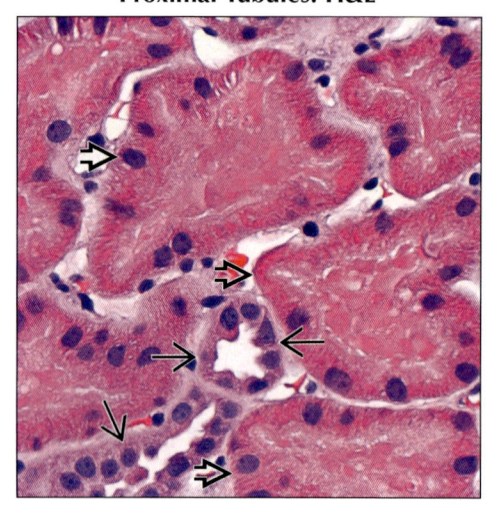

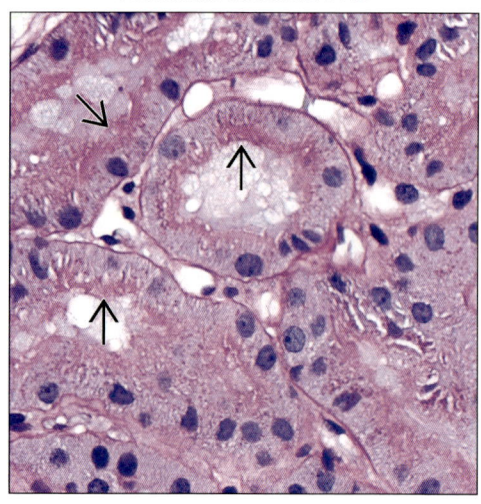

(Left) Proximal tubular cells ⇒ have abundant eosinophilic cytoplasm (due to high mitochondrial content) compared with distal tubules ⇒. 60% (~ 110 L) of the total glomerular filtrate (180 L) is reabsorbed by the proximal tubules daily. The ratio of proximal tubular profiles to distal nephron segments is roughly 3:1 in the cortex. **(Right)** The brush border ⇒ at the apical aspect of the proximal tubules is best visualized with the PAS stain and may be attenuated in acute tubular injury/necrosis.

Proximal Tubules: CD10 / Proximal Tubular Epithelial Cell: EM

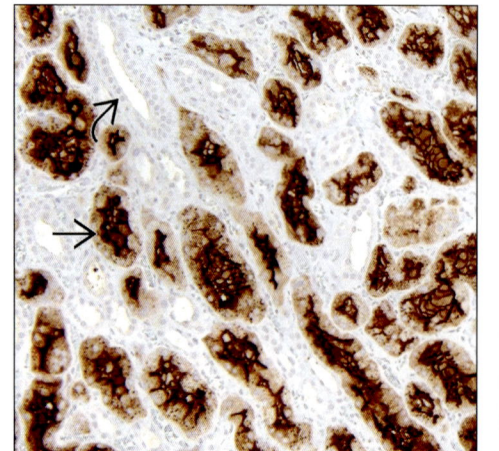

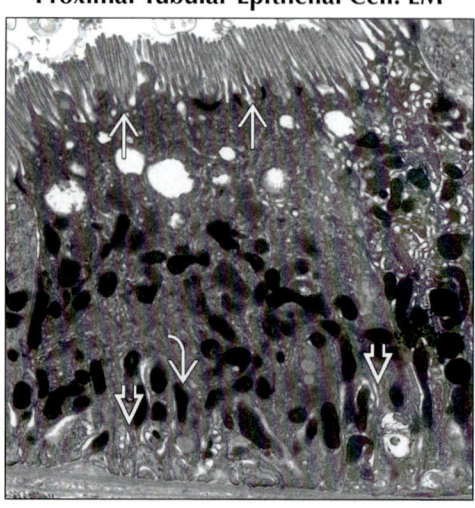

(Left) CD10 strongly stains the brush borders ⇒ on the apical aspect of the proximal tubular epithelial cells. The distal nephron segments ⇒ are negative. **(Right)** This electron micrograph shows the brush border ⇒ along the apical surface that is characteristic of proximal tubular epithelial cells. Many mitochondria ⇒ are associated with the basolateral interdigitations ⇒ along the tubular basement membrane.

KIDNEY

Distal Convoluted Tubules

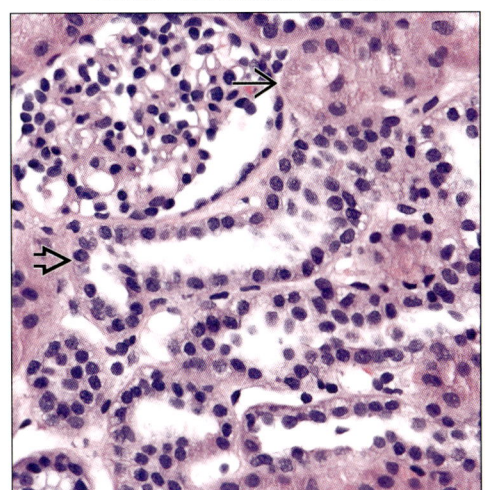

Loops of Henle

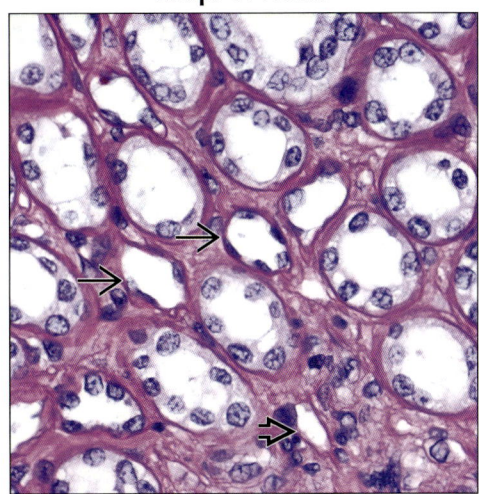

(Left) The distal tubules ⇨ are easily distinguished from the larger proximal tubular epithelial cells ⇨ as they have many more cells and nuclei per tubule length and each cell has much less cytoplasm (and thus a less eosinophilic appearance). *(Right)* Cross sections of the loops of Henle ⇨ show their nuclei protruding into the tubular lumina with attenuated cell cytoplasm. Adjacent peritubular capillaries ⇨ have a smaller caliber.

Macula Densa

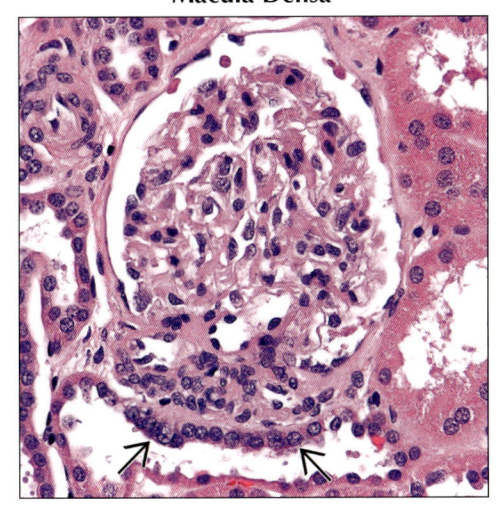

Distal Tubules and Collecting Ducts: EMA

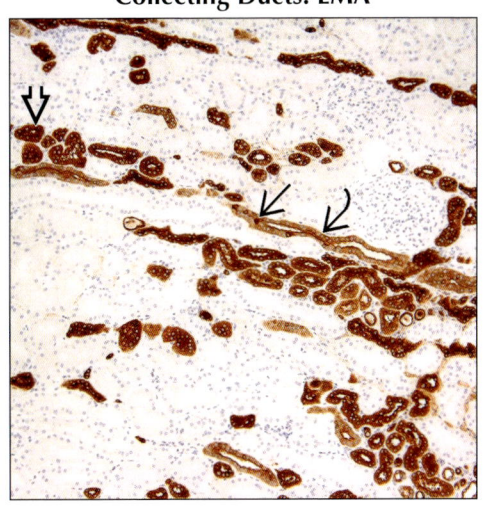

(Left) The cells of the macula densa ⇨ are columnar; they represent a specialized portion of the distal tubule that is adjacent to the juxtaglomerular apparatus and should not be mistaken for a cellular crescent. *(Right)* Epithelial membrane antigen (EMA) is expressed in the distal tubules ⇨ but not in glomeruli or proximal tubules. The principal cells of the collecting ducts ⇨ demonstrate less intense cytoplasmic staining, whereas the scattered intercalated cells ⇨ have strong staining.

Distal Tubules: EMA

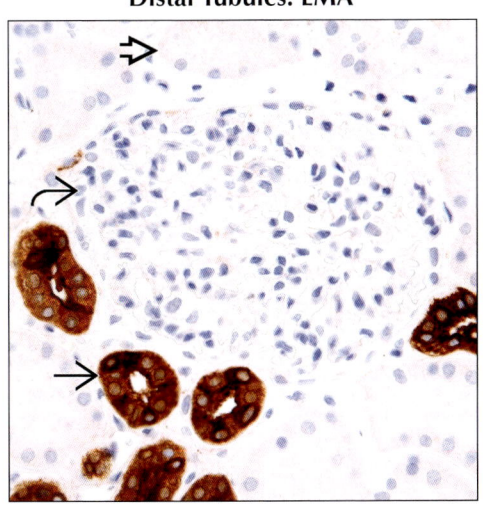

Distal Tubular Epithelial Cell: EM

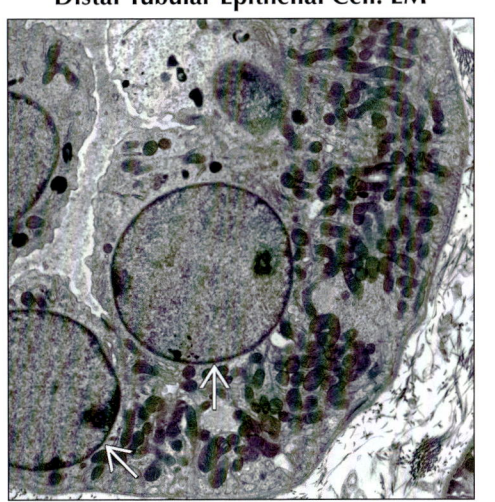

(Left) Epithelial membrane antigen highlights distal tubules ⇨, but there is no expression within the adjacent proximal tubules ⇨ or the glomerulus ⇨. *(Right)* The nuclei ⇨ of the distal tubular epithelial cells are close to the apical surface or tubular lumen. The cells are much smaller in size compared with proximal tubular epithelial cells, so many more nuclei can be seen in a cross section. No brush border is present at the apical surface, but short blunted villi may be noted.

KIDNEY

Renal Medulla: Masson Trichrome

Dolichos biflorus

(Left) Masson trichrome stains tubular basement membranes and interstitial fibrosis blue ➔. The tubules have more space between them in the medulla, where assessing the extent of interstitial fibrosis and tubular atrophy is much more difficult than in the cortex. (Right) Collecting ducts ➔ are highlighted by immunohistochemistry for the lectin Dolichos biflorus. Adjacent proximal tubules ➔ and distal tubules ➔ show no staining.

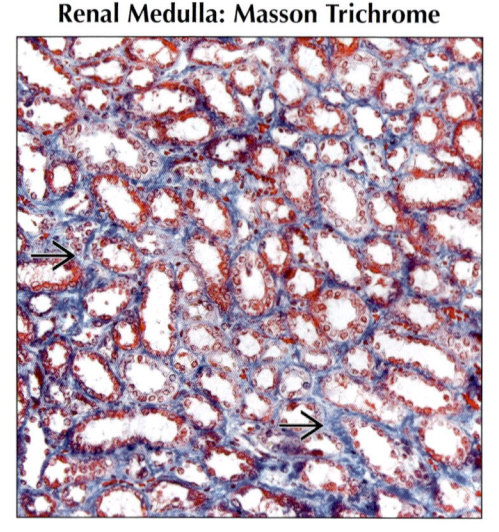

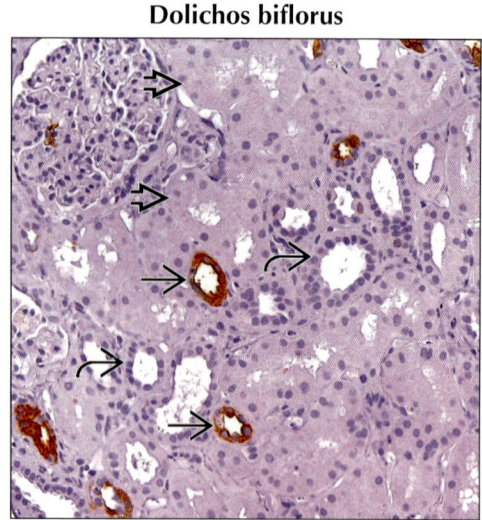

Collecting Duct: H&E

Cytokeratin 7

(Left) The lateral cell borders ➔ of the collecting ducts are often distinct, in contrast to the adjacent proximal tubular epithelial cells ➔ that lack this feature. (Right) Cytokeratin 7 highlights the distal tubules ➔ and collecting ducts ➔, but there is no expression in the proximal tubules ➔. The principal cells within the collecting ducts express cytokeratin 7 while the intercalated cells ➔ show no expression.

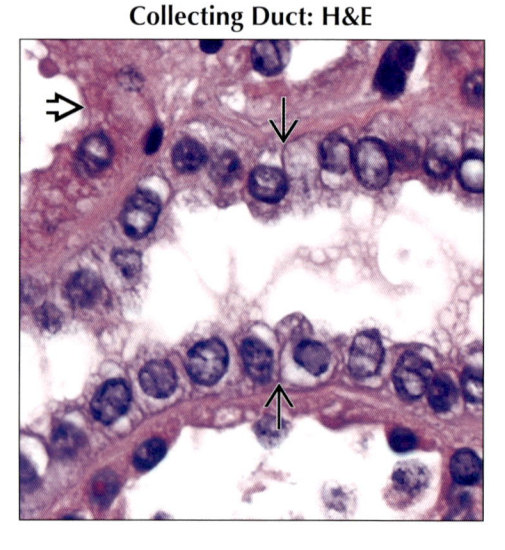

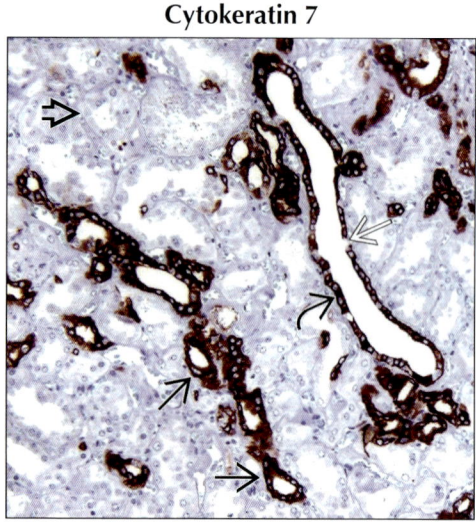

Collecting Duct: AE1/AE3

Collecting Duct: EMA

(Left) AE1/AE3 immunohistochemistry strongly stains the cytoplasm of principal cells ➔ of the collecting duct, while intercalated cells ➔ are negative. The adjacent proximal tubules ➔ demonstrate no staining. (Right) The intercalated cells ➔ show strong staining for EMA (epithelial membrane antigen), while there is a cytoplasmic blush in the principal cells ➔ of the collecting duct. Intercalated cells are specialized cells that assist in acid-base homeostasis.

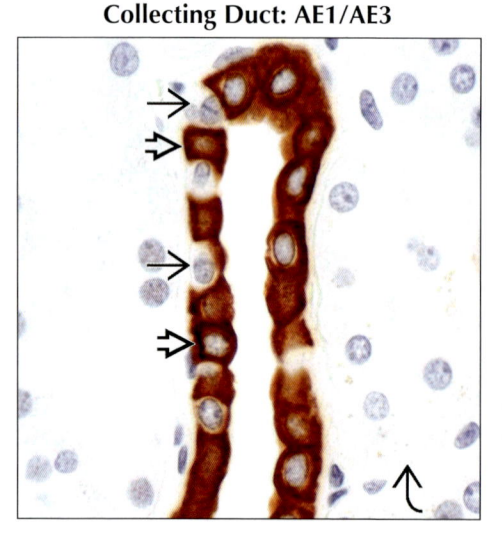

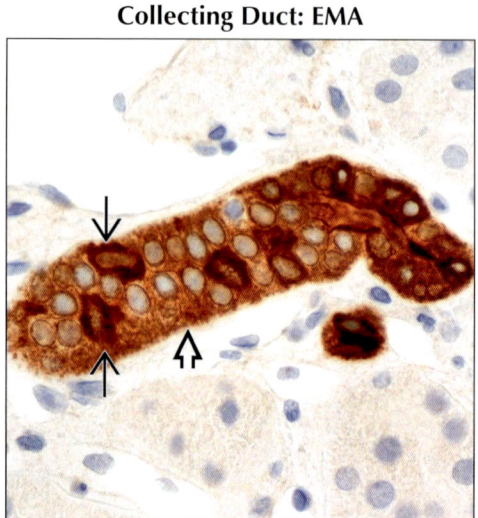

KIDNEY

Principal Cell: EM

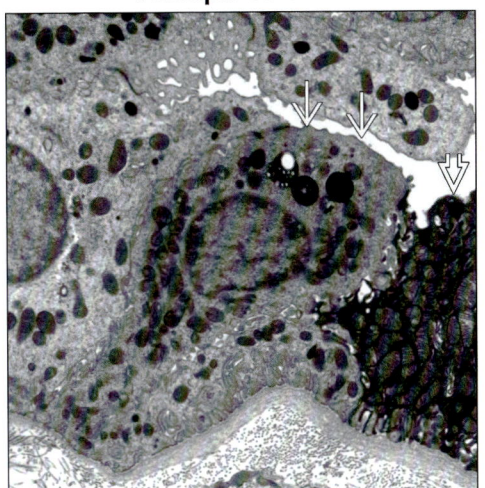

Intercalated Cell: EM

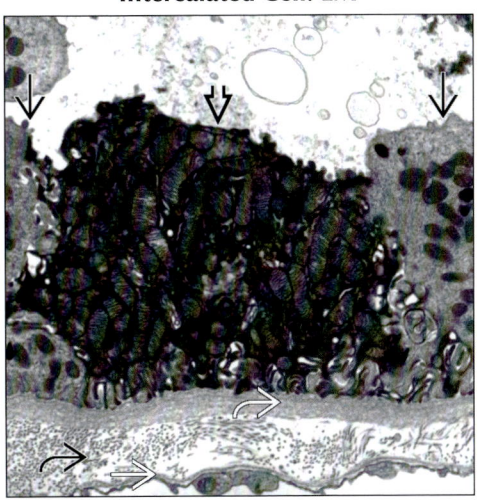

(Left) The principal cell ➡ contains fewer mitochondria and other organelles and has a distinctly lighter cytoplasmic color compared with the adjacent intercalated cell ➡. *(Right)* Abundant mitochondria are present in the cytoplasm of this intercalated cell ➡ and give the darker cytoplasmic hue seen by light microscopy. Two principal cells ➡ are adjacent in this collecting duct. Collagen fibrils ➡ are present between the tubular basement membrane ➡ and the peritubular capillary basement membrane ➡.

Nerves

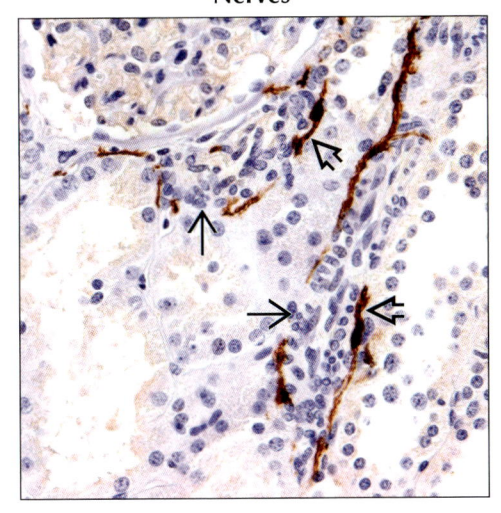

Nerves

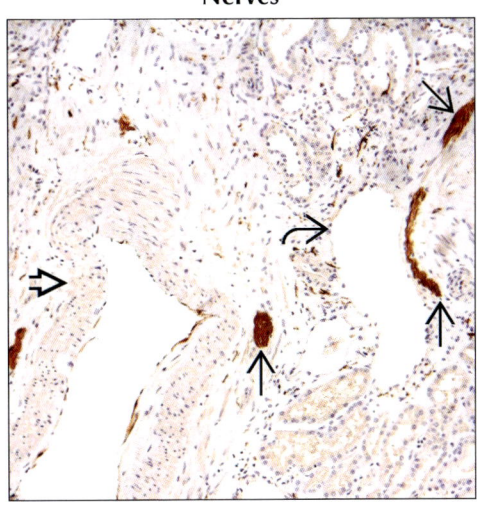

(Left) Nerves are not generally abundant in the renal cortex, but S100 highlights small nerves ➡ that course along the arterioles ➡. Renal denervation is currently gaining attention as a potential safe and effective treatment for refractory hypertension. *(Right)* S100 immunohistochemistry reveals the larger nerves ➡ that accompany large-caliber arteries ➡ and venules ➡ in the medulla and hilum of the kidney.

Renal Artery

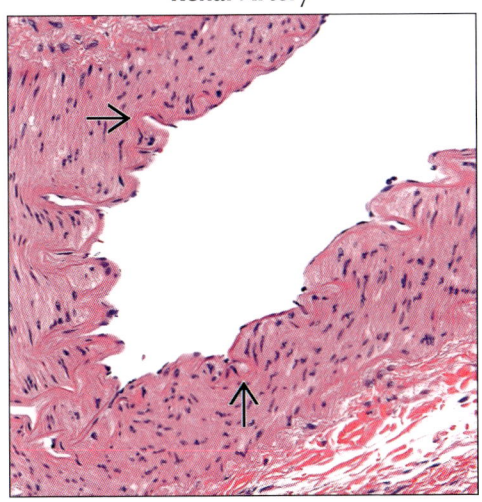

Interlobular Artery

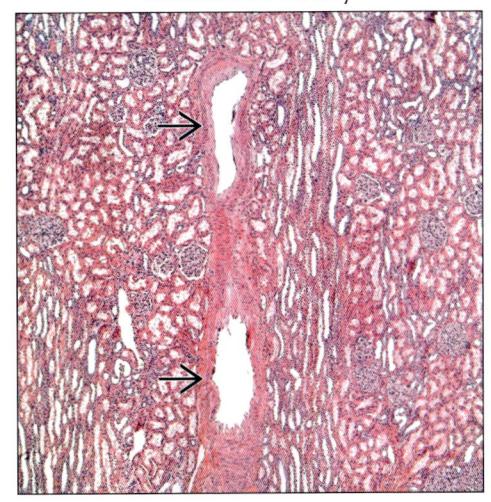

(Left) The internal elastic lamina ➡ has a refractile quality that is best appreciated when viewed under the microscope while focusing the slide up and down. This structure is not present in the veins. *(Right)* This interlobular artery ➡ extends from the arcuate artery (not shown) into the cortex adjacent to a medullary ray as afferent arterioles branch off into glomeruli.

KIDNEY

Artery and Arteriole

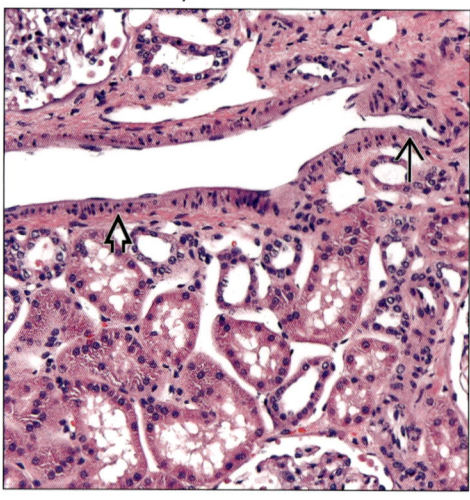

Afferent and Efferent Arterioles

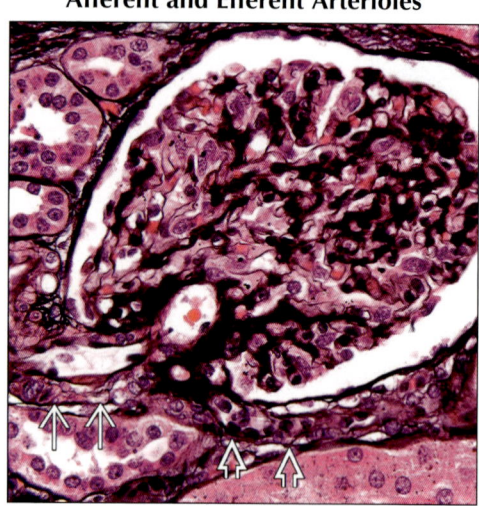

(Left) This interlobular artery ➡ branches into an afferent arteriole ➡ before entering a glomerulus (not shown). The arteriole wall thickness normally consists of ≤ 2 layers of smooth muscle cells. **(Right)** Jones methenamine silver shows an afferent arteriole ➡, which often has a thicker vessel wall and larger caliber than the efferent arteriole ➡. A fortuitous section to visualize both arterioles simultaneously may be necessary to distinguish one from the other.

Peritubular Capillary Network

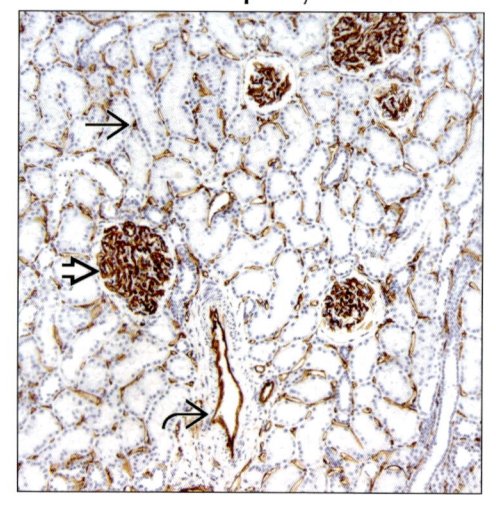

Peritubular Capillary: EM

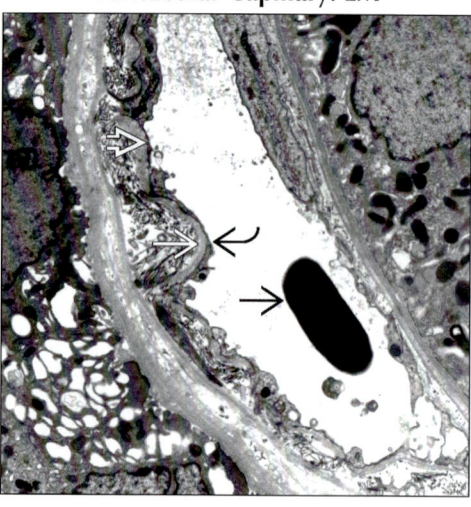

(Left) CD31 highlights the intricate peritubular capillary network ➡ as well as the glomerular capillaries ➡ and 1 artery ➡. Pathologic glomerular injury can decrease blood flow to the peritubular capillaries, which results in tubular atrophy and interstitial fibrosis. **(Right)** This peritubular capillary ➡ contains a red blood cell ➡. The endothelial cell ➡ sits atop a single basement membrane layer ➡, which may be multilayered in chronic antibody-mediated rejection in renal allografts.

CD31

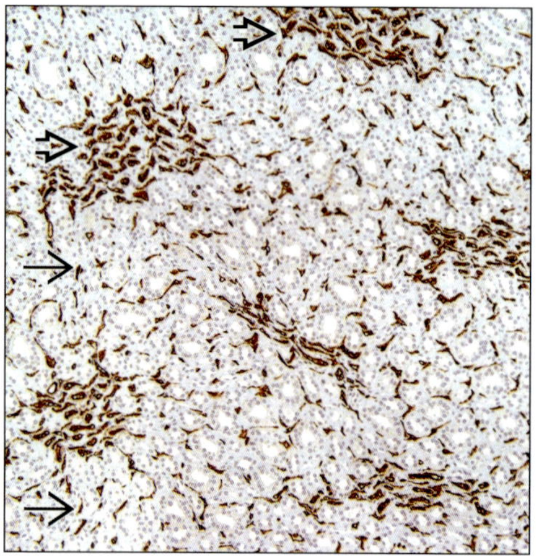

Vascular Bundle: Alpha Smooth Muscle Actin

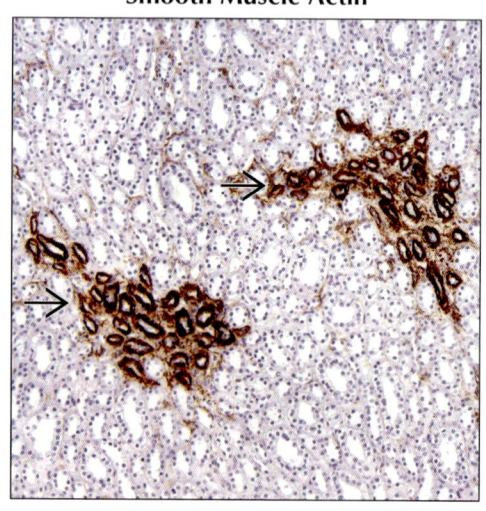

(Left) CD31 immunohistochemistry highlights the vascular bundles ➡ and individual peritubular capillaries ➡ that course through the renal medulla. **(Right)** α-smooth muscle actin highlights the vasa recta ➡, which travel in bundles through the renal medulla. Note that the peritubular capillary network that is present between the tubules is not highlighted by this immunostain.

KIDNEY

Lymphatic Vessels

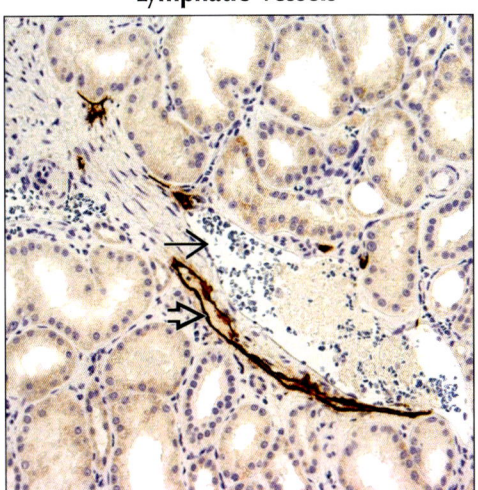

Lymphatics

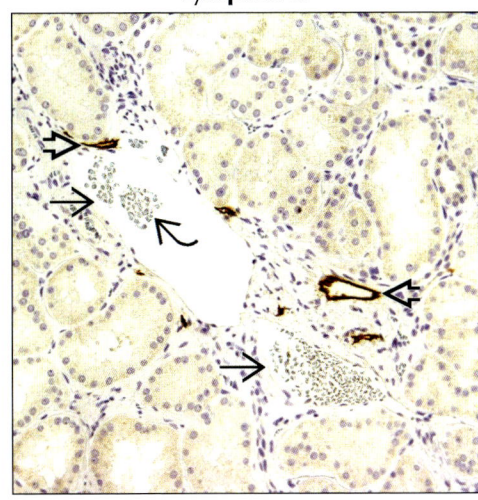

(Left) Lymphatic vessels ⇨ are sparse in the renal cortex as demonstrated by D2-40 immunohistochemistry, but they are relatively more abundant when in close proximity to renal veins and venules ⇨. Lymphatics are not present in the medulla. *(Right)* Lymphatic vessels ⇨ are sparse in the normal renal cortex as demonstrated by D2-40 immunohistochemistry but are usually present in association with renal venules ⇨ (as noted by the numerous red blood cells ⇨ in their lumina). Lymphatics are not present in the medulla.

Lymphatics

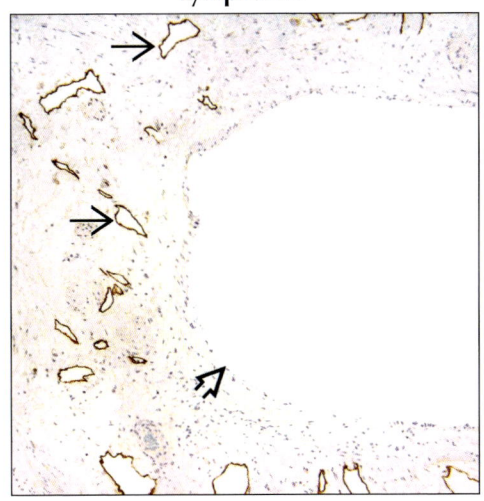

Lymphatics in Renal Sinus

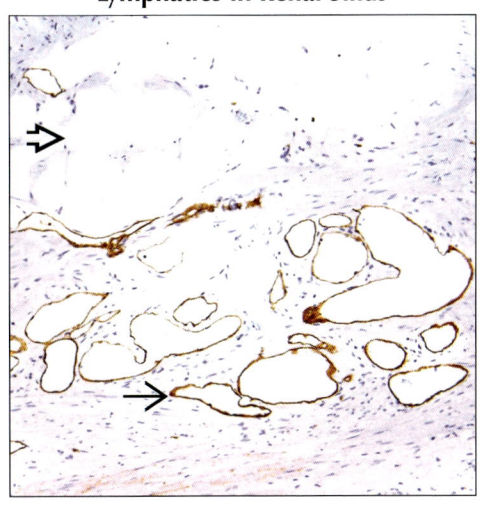

(Left) D2-40 immunohistochemistry outlines the numerous lymphatic channels ⇨ that are present in the wall of this renal vein ⇨. *(Right)* D2-40 immunohistochemistry highlights the many lymphatic vessels ⇨ that are present in close proximity to the renal sinus fat ⇨. In contrast to the outer aspect of the kidney, a capsule does not exist between the medulla and renal sinus. Therefore, large malignant renal neoplasms can extend into this region and easily gain access to these lymphatic vessels.

Resident Dendritic Cells

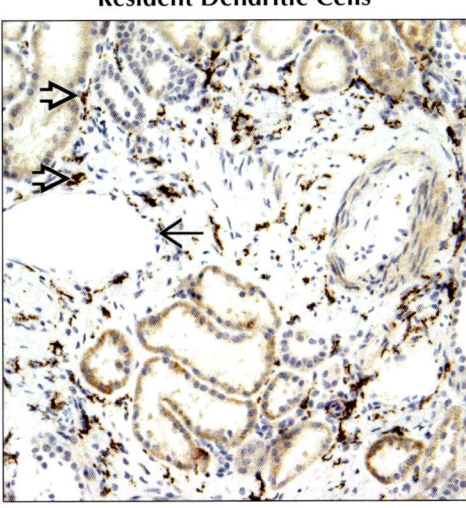

Resident Dendritic Cells

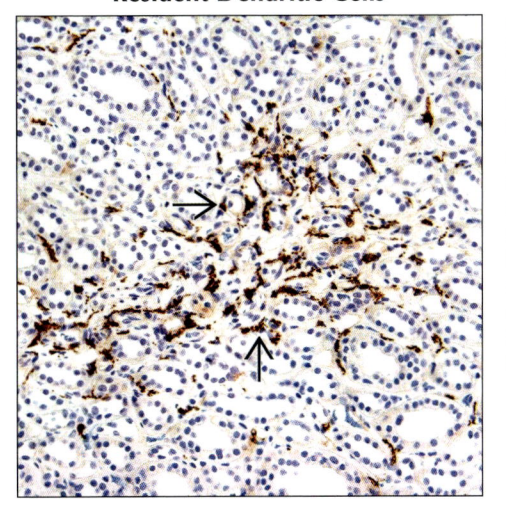

(Left) CD163 immunohistochemistry reveals numerous dendritic cells ⇨ in the normal renal cortex, which are closely approximated with venules ⇨, peritubular capillaries, and lymphatics. They may have a role in immune surveillance. *(Right)* CD163 highlights the resident dendritic cells that are present in greater density along the vascular bundles ⇨ that course through the medulla.

URETER AND RENAL PELVIS

Key Facts

Macroscopic Anatomy
- Minor calyces (calyx: Cup-shaped cavity)
  - Usually 7-14 per kidney
  - Urine from collecting ducts of renal medulla drain into minor calyces at tips of renal papilla
- Major calyces
  - Usually 2-3 per kidney
  - Collects urine from several individual minor calyces
- Renal pelvis
  - Collects urine from major calyces and drains to ureter
- Ureter
  - Conduit for urine from kidney (renal pelvis) to urinary bladder through retroperitoneum and pelvis
  - Becomes intravesical at base of bladder and empties into bladder lumen at ureteral orifices

Microscopic Anatomy
- Ureter
  - Epithelium comprised of urothelium (previously termed "transitional" epithelium)
  - Superficial umbrella cell layer is in contact with urinary space: Characterized by more eosinophilic cytoplasm and larger, sometimes multilobated nuclei
  - Intermediate cells comprise majority of urothelium (usually 3-7 cell layers); oval in shape with fine chromatin and conspicuous intranuclear grooves
  - Basal cell layer is cuboidal and lines basement membrane
  - Subepithelial connective tissue (lamina propria) is comprised of connective tissue of variable density and small blood vessels
  - Muscularis propria is comprised of smooth muscle cells, often with indistinct layers
  - Surrounding tissue is comprised of adipose tissue, blood vessels, and small peripheral nerves
- Renal pelvis and major calyces
  - Renal pelvis (and major calyceal) wall have urothelial, lamina propria, and muscularis propria layers of variable thickness
- Minor calyces
  - Renal papillae are lined by urothelium, but no underlying lamina propria or muscularis is present
  - Walls of minor calyces that abut the renal sinus fat are similar in histology to those of the pelvis and major calyces but not as thick

Pitfalls/Artifacts
- von Brunn nests in ureter may mimic invasive urothelial carcinoma
  - Urothelial nests are smaller, more confluent, and more disorganized than those of urinary bladder
  - Extend to a uniform level in lamina propria, which is distinct from invasive urothelial carcinoma (nested type)
  - Occasionally have cytoplasmic clearing that may mimic a renal cell carcinoma
- Cystitis cystica/cystitis glandularis
  - Similar to von Brunn nests, but with central luminal space
  - With cystitis glandularis, luminal cells have apically oriented cytoplasm and columnar appearance
- Cancer staging pitfall in invasive urothelial carcinoma
  - At junction with kidney in minor calyces, urothelium transitions from renal pelvis-type wall to that of renal papillae
  - Invasive urothelial carcinoma present at renal papilla will be staged higher than that of adjacent wall because "renal parenchyma" directly underlies urothelium in this anatomic location
- Cancer staging pitfall in noninvasive urothelial carcinoma
  - Urothelial carcinoma may colonize collecting ducts of renal papillae without invasion
  - This finding should not be overstaged as renal parenchymal involvement
  - Sharp, rounded architecture of urothelial neoplasia within papilla and absence of stromal response should aid in the distinction from true invasion

(Left) In this intravenous pyelogram, the course of the ureter and the organization of the collecting system of the kidney (renal pelvis and calyces) are highlighted. (Right) This schematic demonstrates the renal calyces draining into the renal pelvis. The junction of the calyces and the renal medulla has important histologic considerations.

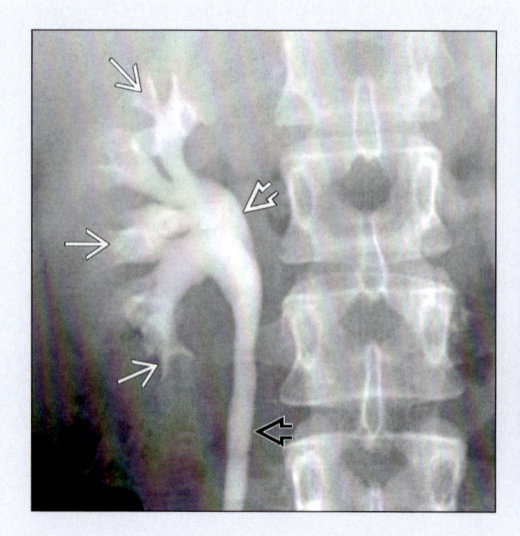

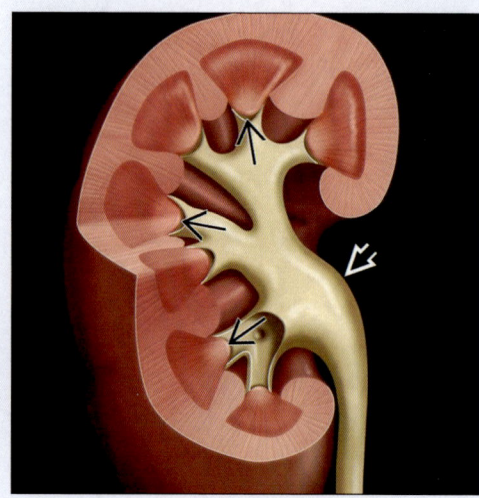

URETER AND RENAL PELVIS

Ureter

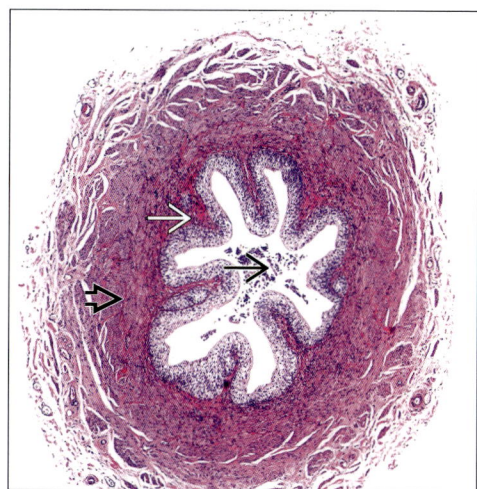

Ureter

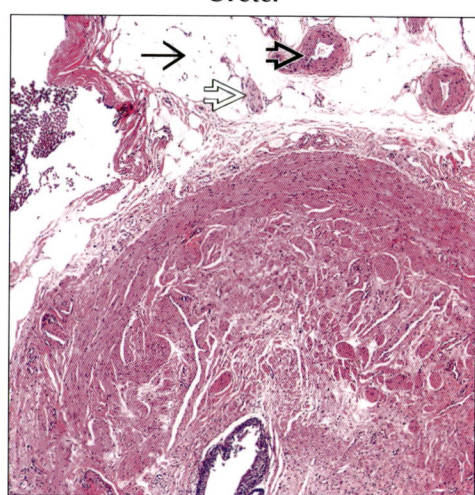

(Left) The lumen of the ureter ➔, which is lined by urothelium, typically has complex infolding near the mid portion. The lumen is surrounded by a layer of fibrous connective tissue ➔ (lamina propria/subepithelial connective tissue) and an outer layer of smooth muscle ➔ (muscularis propria). (Right) This section of ureter shows the surrounding soft tissues, which are often comprised of adipose tissue ➔, blood vessels ➔, and small peripheral nerves ➔.

Ureter

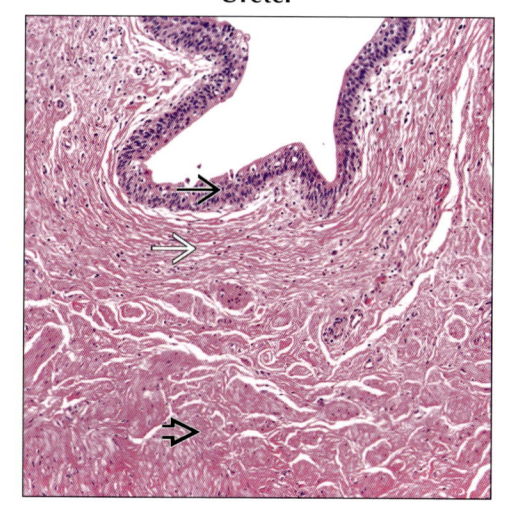

Ureter

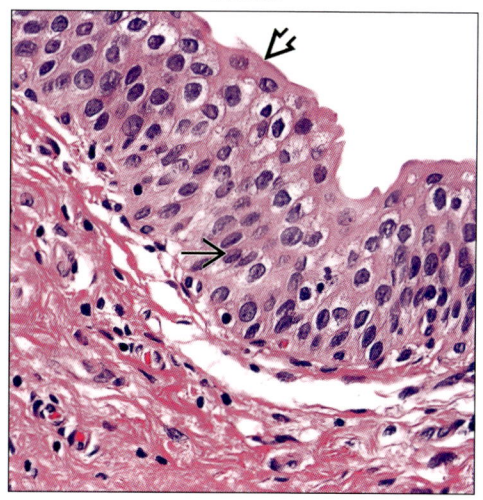

(Left) The ureter has urothelial ➔, connective tissue (lamina propria) ➔, and smooth muscle (muscularis propria) ➔ layers. (Right) The urothelium has a stratified layer of predominantly intermediate cells, organized perpendicular to the basement membrane, with fine nuclear chromatin and intranuclear grooves ➔. The superficial (umbrella) layer has more eosinophilic cytoplasm ➔. A basal cell layer, which lines the basement membrane, is often inconspicuous.

Subepithelial Connective Tissue/Lamina Propria

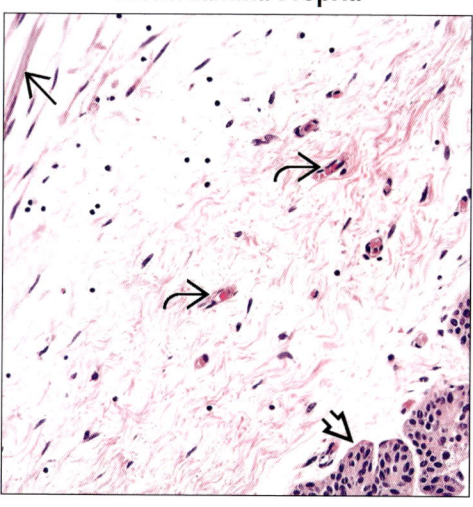

Ureter

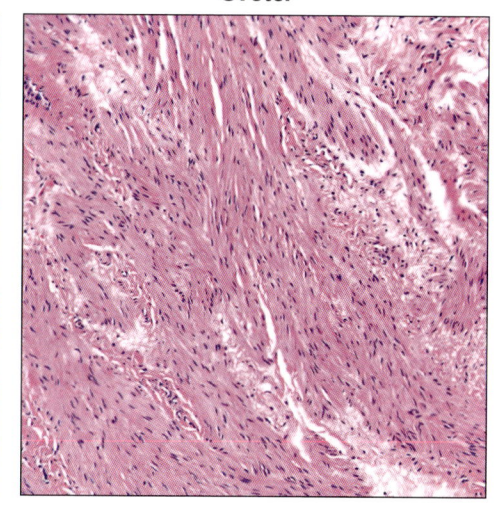

(Left) The tissue between the basement membrane of the urothelium ➔ and the smooth muscle cells of the muscularis propria ➔ is referred to as the subepithelial connective tissue (or lamina propria). In the ureter and renal pelvis, it consists of connective tissue of variable density, and small blood vessels ➔. (Right) The muscularis propria of the ureter is characterized by compact aggregates of smooth muscle.

Genitourinary and Male Genital Tract

12

13

URETER AND RENAL PELVIS

Ureter With von Brunn Nests

(Left) In the ureter, von Brunn nests are more numerous and somewhat more disorganized than typically seen in the urinary bladder. However, the nests extend to a relatively uniform level in the lamina propria ➡. (Right) These invaginated urothelial nests (von Brunn nests) are smaller and more confluent than those typically seen in the bladder; therefore, they may closely mimic invasive urothelial carcinoma (nested type) on biopsy.

Ureter With von Brunn Nests

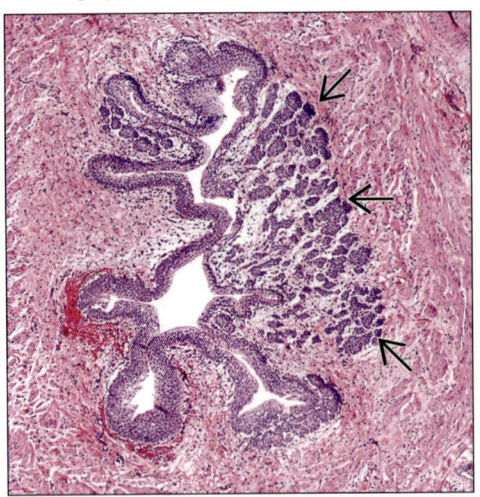

Ureter With von Brunn Nests

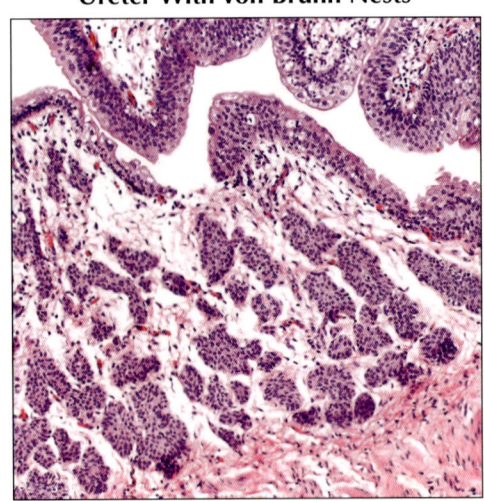

(Left) The urothelial cells within the von Brunn nests ➡ have cytologic features that are similar to those of the overlying urothelium ➡. (Right) The von Brunn nests in the ureter &/or renal pelvis occasionally have more abundant intracytoplasmic glycogen, which may histologically mimic a clear cell renal cell carcinoma in radical nephrectomy specimens. However, renal cell carcinoma does not typically extend down the wall of the ureter.

von Brunn Nests

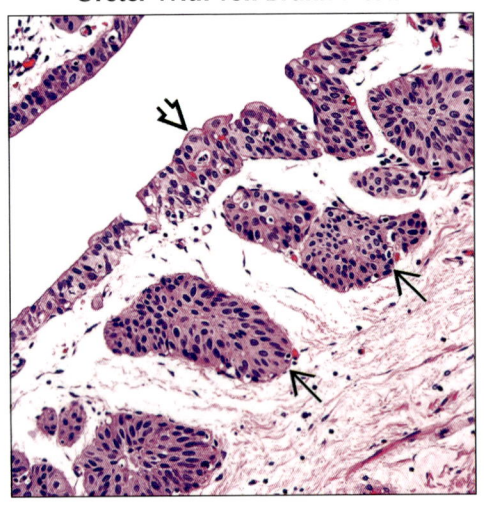

Cystitis Glandularis

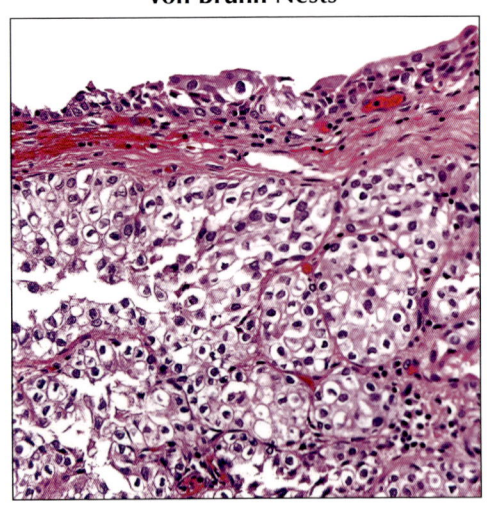

(Left) The von Brunn nests may have central cystic spaces with a more columnar luminal layer of cells and apically oriented cytoplasm (a change that is termed cystitis glandularis) ➡. This is a benign lesion that is thought to represent a reactive process secondary to prior injury or inflammation. (Right) The renal papillae ➡ bulge into the minor calyces ➡ as demonstrated in this example. The wall of the calyx ➡ is very thin in this region.

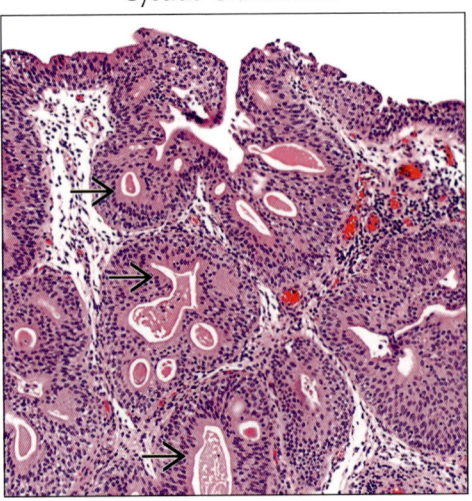

Renal Papilla

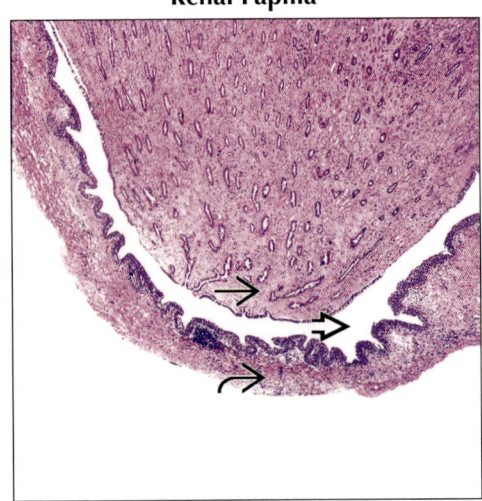

URETER AND RENAL PELVIS

Renal Calyx

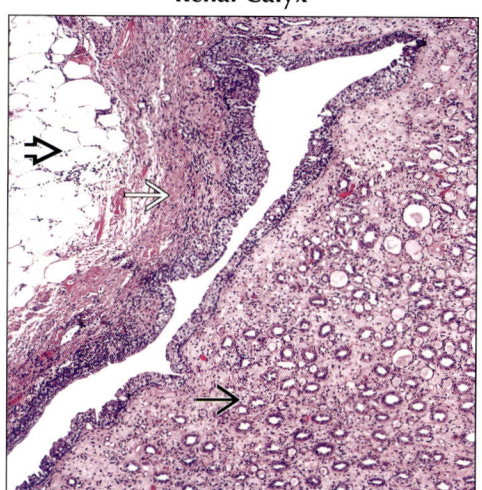

Renal Pelvis

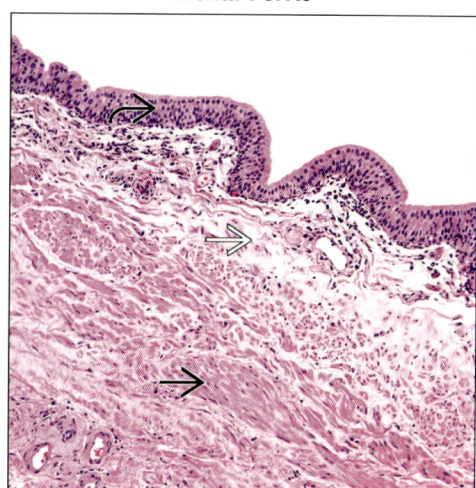

(Left) The junction of the renal papilla ⇨ with the calyx does not contain lamina propria or muscularis, which is present in the wall ⇨ of the calyx that is adjacent to the renal sinus fat ⇨. This has important implications for staging urothelial carcinoma. (Right) The renal pelvis has urothelial ⇨, lamina propria ⇨, and muscularis ⇨ layers, similar to the ureter. The wall becomes thinner in the regions of the major, and particularly the minor, calyces.

Minor Calyx Over Renal Papilla

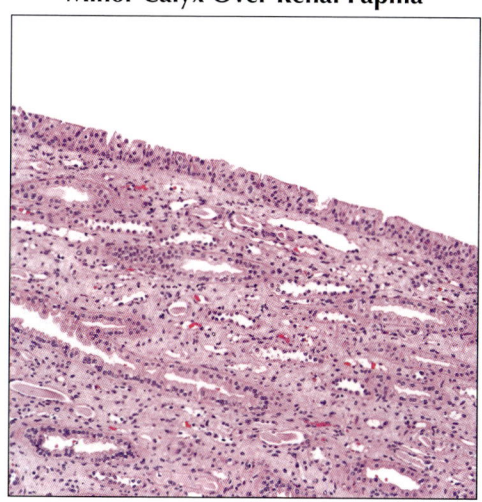

Minor Calyx Over Renal Papillae

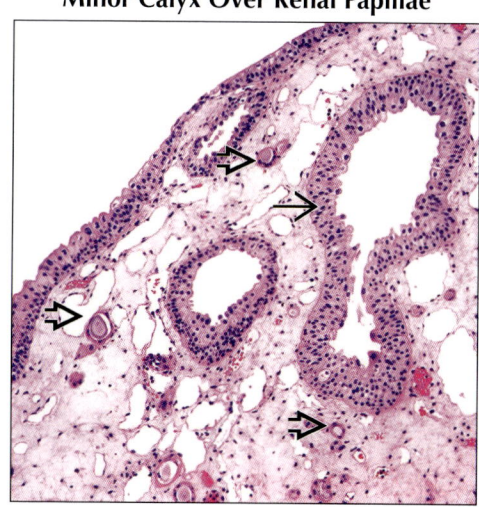

(Left) The renal papilla region of the minor calyces has distinct features, e.g., it lacks a lamina propria layer underlying the urothelium over the renal papillae. (Right) There is no subepithelial connective tissue layer (lamina propria) underlying the urothelium over the renal papillae. The underlying tissue contains urothelial-lined collecting ducts ⇨, renal tubules ⇨, and supporting stroma. This is important for staging urothelial carcinomas in this region, as even superficial invasion will be classified as renal parenchymal involvement.

Minor Calyx Over Renal Papilla

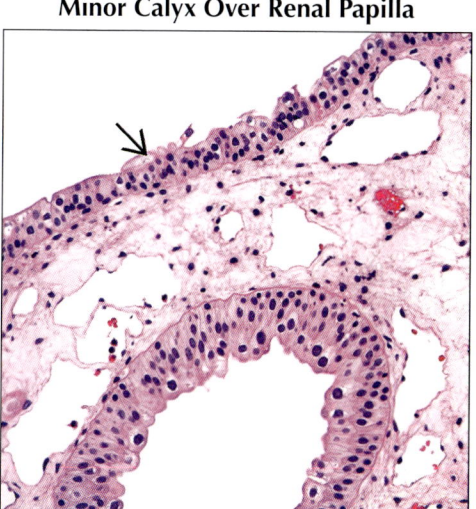

Renal Pelvis

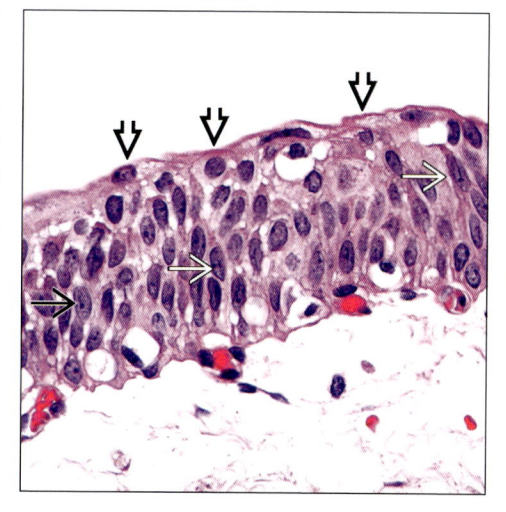

(Left) The urothelium overlying the renal papilla ⇨ may be very thin. (Right) The urothelial lining of the renal pelvis is similar to that of the urinary bladder. The intermediate cell layer is oriented with the long axis perpendicular to the basement membrane. The nuclear chromatin is fine and pinpoint nucleoli may be seen ⇨. Intranuclear grooves are also common ⇨. As in other sites, the superficial (umbrella cell) layer has variable densely eosinophilic cytoplasm ⇨.

BLADDER

Key Facts

Macroscopic Anatomy
- Inverted pyramid shape
- Adjacent structures
  - In females, cervix and superior vagina are posterior to bladder
  - In males, seminal vesicles and vas deferens are posterior to bladder
  - Levator ani muscles are lateral to bladder

Microscopic Anatomy
- Urothelium is most superficial layer, also known as transitional epithelium
- Lamina propria
  - Loose connective tissue separated from overlying urothelium by basement membrane
  - May contain a discontinuous layer of small fascicles and wisps of smooth muscle known as the muscularis mucosae
- Muscularis propria: Composed of thick bundles of smooth muscle
- Adventitia: Outermost layer, composed of fibroadipose tissue

Pitfalls/Artifacts
- Tangential sectioning of urothelium can give a false impression of urothelial hyperplasia
- Poor orientation in transurethral resection of bladder tumor (TURBT) specimens can make it difficult to distinguish between muscularis mucosae and muscularis propria
- Adipose tissue within lamina propria and muscularis propria can be mistaken for perivesicular fat

Metaplasia
- Glycogenated squamous metaplasia is a benign variation often seen in the trigone of the bladder in females

(Left) The urinary bladder lies below the peritoneum within the pelvis, and the surface of the dome is covered by pelvic parietal peritoneum. The bladder is attached at the bladder neck, with the remainder free to expand and contract as it fills with urine and empties. The seminal vesicles and vas deferens lie posterior to the bladder in the male. *(Right)* In females, the urinary bladder is separated from the rectum by the cervix and superior portion of the vagina.

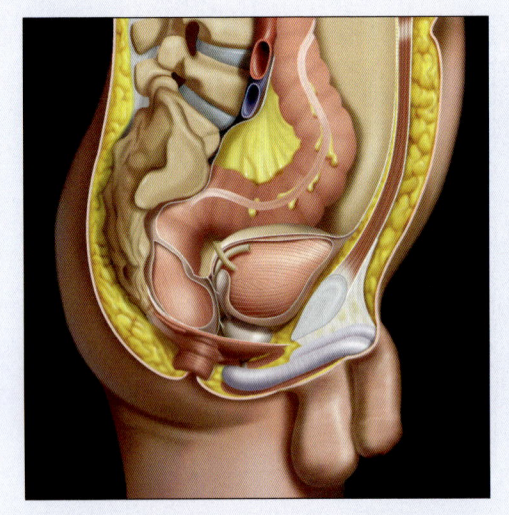

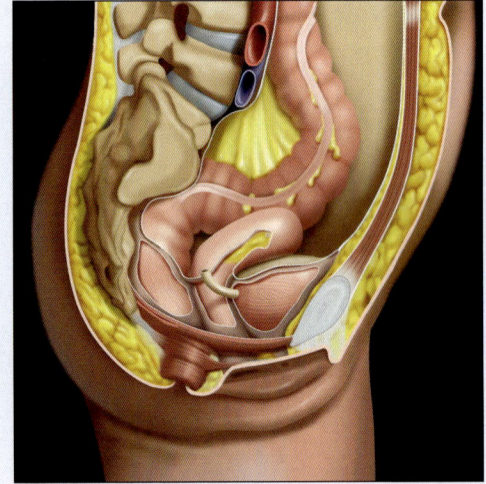

(Left) The 4 layers of the bladder can be visualized on cross section. The innermost layer is composed of the urothelium, with the underlying lamina propria ➡ separated from the urothelium by the basement membrane. Below the lamina propria lies the smooth muscle of the muscularis propria ➡. The outermost layer of the bladder consists of the perivesical fat ➡. *(Right)* Urachal remnants, which have a urothelial or glandular lining, may be present at the apex of the bladder wall ➡.

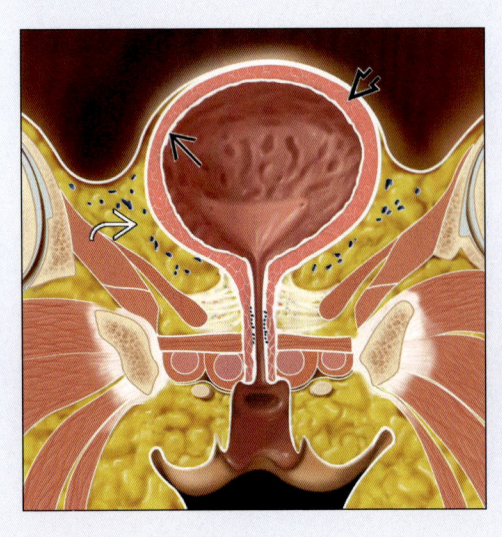

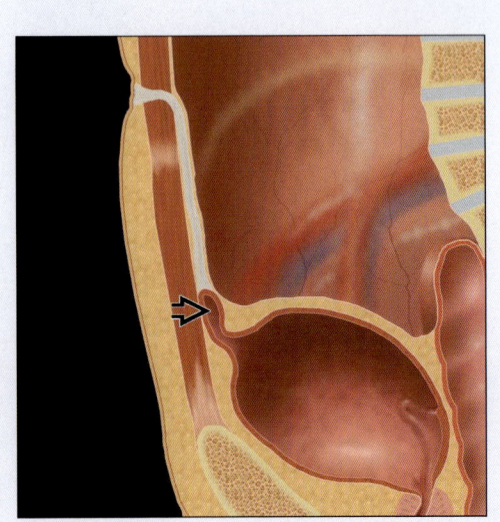

BLADDER

Normal Urothelium

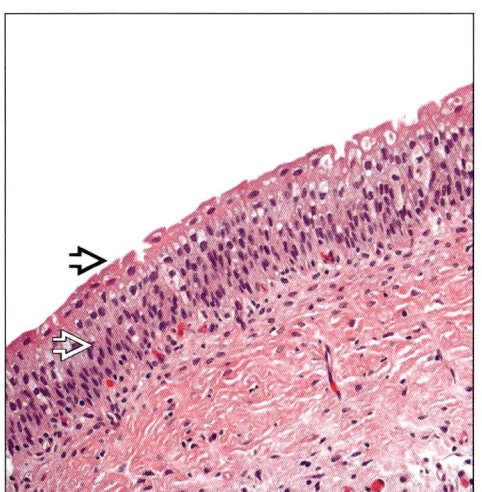

Normal Urothelium

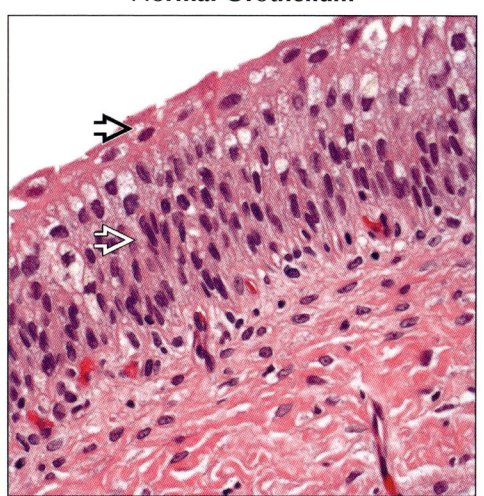

(Left) The thickness of the urothelium varies depending on the degree of distention of the bladder. The average thickness in the contracted bladder is 3-6 cell layers, while the distended bladder may only be 2-3 cell layers thick. The superficial cell layer is composed of umbrella cells ⇨. The intermediate and basal cell layers lie underneath the umbrella cells ⇨. (Right) Higher power shows the intermediate and basal cell layers ⇨ and the superficial umbrella cells ⇨.

Normal Urothelium

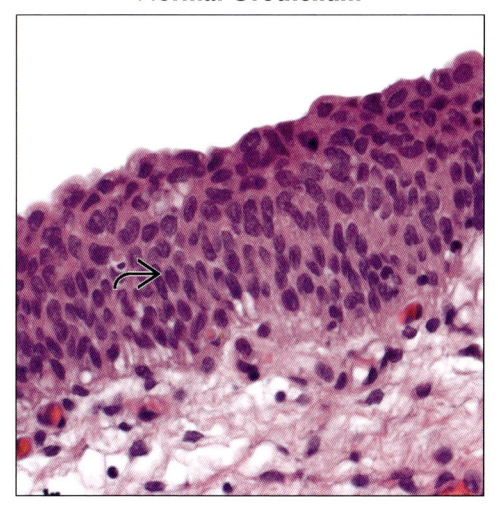

Normal Urothelium

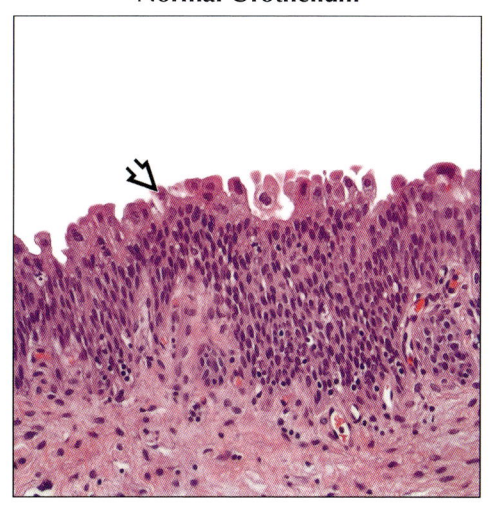

(Left) The intermediate cells may have longitudinal nuclear grooves ⇨. The nuclei are ovoid with indistinct nucleoli and display polarity, with their longitudinal axis arranged perpendicular to the basement membrane. (Right) The umbrella cells ⇨ are large with abundant eosinophilic cytoplasm and a rounded contour at the luminal surface. Invaginations of the luminal cell membrane and underlying cytoplasmic vesicles allow the cells to stretch with bladder distention.

Umbrella Cells

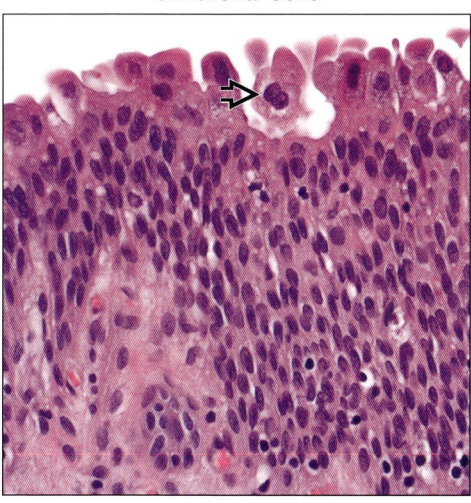

Tangential Sectioning

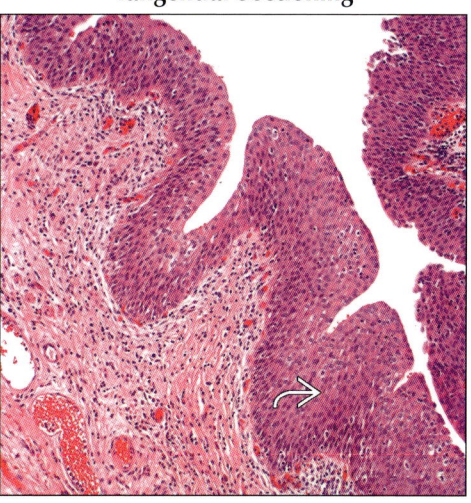

(Left) The umbrella cells may be binucleate ⇨. Although the nuclei of these cells may appear large, the cells have abundant cytoplasm, maintaining a low nuclear to cytoplasmic ratio. The presence of the umbrella cells should not be used in determining the presence of neoplasia, as in situ lesions can have an intact superficial cell layer. (Right) Tangential sectioning ⇨ may give the false impression of a thickened urothelium and should not be misdiagnosed as hyperplasia.

BLADDER

Lamina Propria

Muscularis Mucosae

(Left) The vascular plexus ⇨ is identified in the mid portion of the lamina propria and is composed of medium-sized vessels. The muscularis mucosae, when present, is often seen in association with the vascular plexus. *(Right)* The muscularis mucosae ⇨ is a thin layer of smooth muscle often associated with the vascular plexus in the lamina propria. It is composed of wisps and small fascicles of smooth muscle as opposed to the thick muscle bundles of the muscularis propria ⇨.

Muscularis Mucosae

Muscularis Mucosae

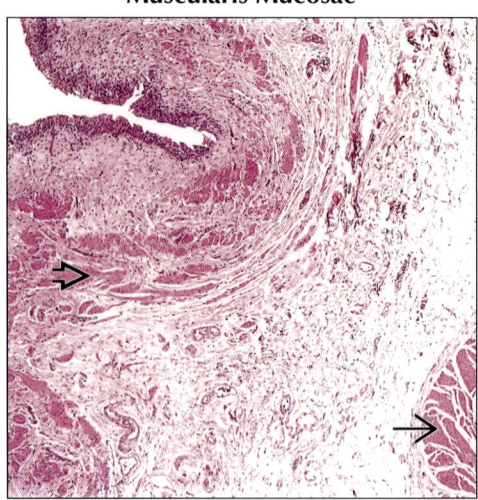

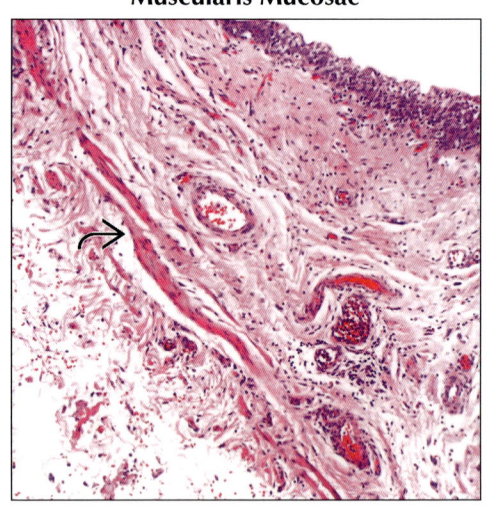

(Left) The muscularis mucosae is composed of wisps and small fascicles of smooth muscle, and when present often forms a discontinuous layer within the lamina propria ⇨. The wisps and small bundles should not be confused with the large bundles of the muscularis propria when evaluating depth of invasion of carcinoma into the bladder wall, as this will upstage the patient from a pT1 lesion to pT2. *(Right)* Wisps of smooth muscle form the muscularis mucosae ⇨ in the lamina propria.

Lamina Propria

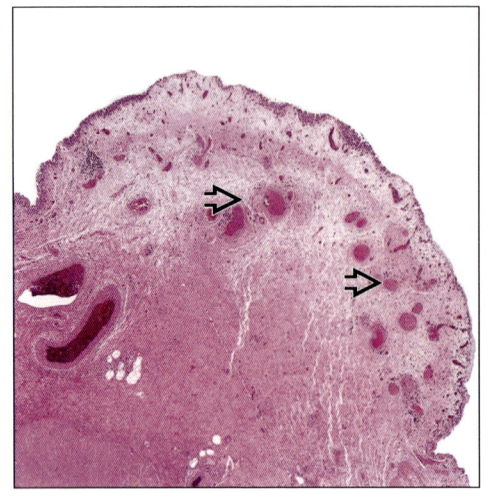

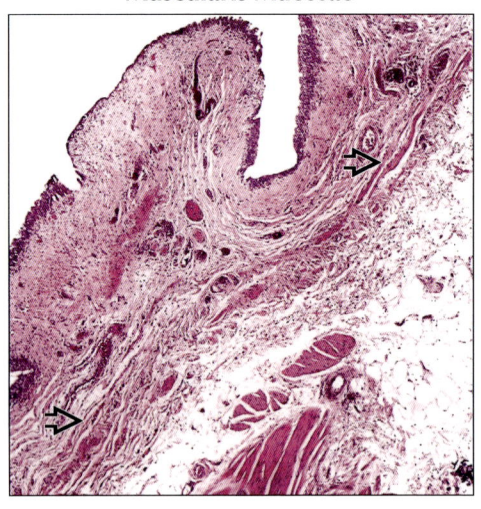

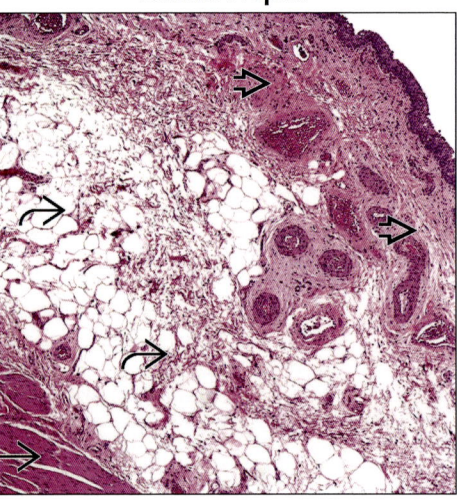

Transurethral Resection of Bladder Tumor (TURBT)

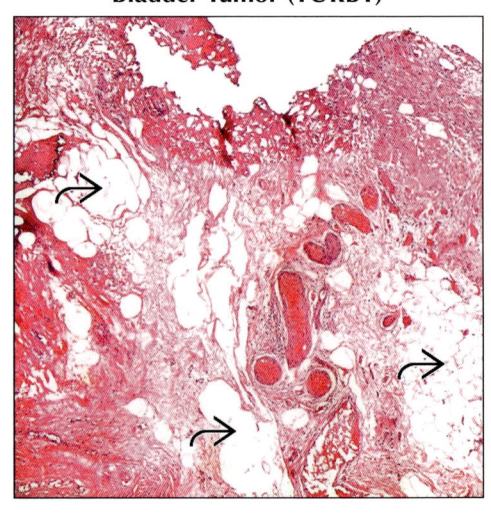

(Left) Mature adipose tissue ⇨ can be present within the lamina propria ⇨ and muscularis propria ⇨, and should not be mistaken for perivesicular fat. *(Right)* This TURBT section shows an example of mature adipose tissue ⇨ intermixed within the lamina propria and muscularis propria layers. The presence of this adipose tissue should not be confused as perivesical fat when evaluating for depth of tumor invasion.

BLADDER

Muscularis Propria
Adventitia

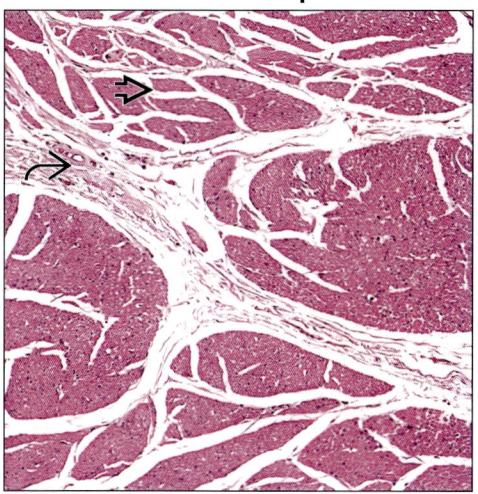

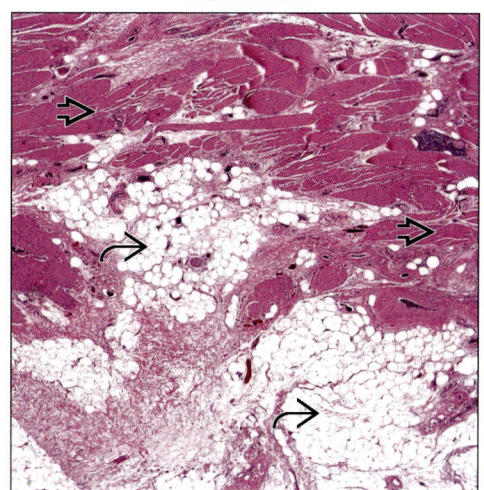

(Left) The muscularis propria is composed of large fascicles ⇨ of smooth muscle and connective tissue ⇨ containing blood vessels, lymphatic spaces, and nerves. (Right) The adventitia of the bladder is composed of fibroadipose tissue ⇨, as seen here at the interface of the adventitia with the muscularis propria ⇨. The dome of the bladder is covered by the pelvic parietal peritoneum, while other areas of the bladder lack a serosal surface.

Muscularis Propria
Muscularis Propria

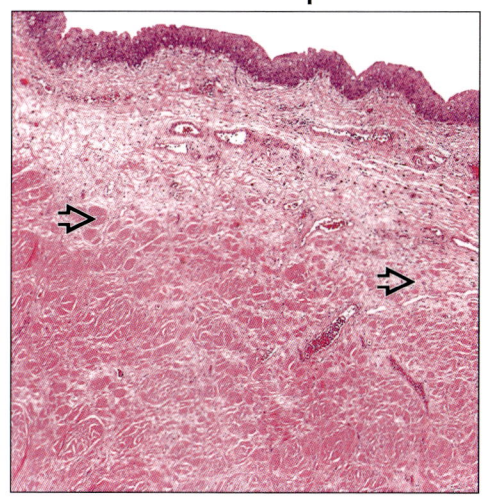

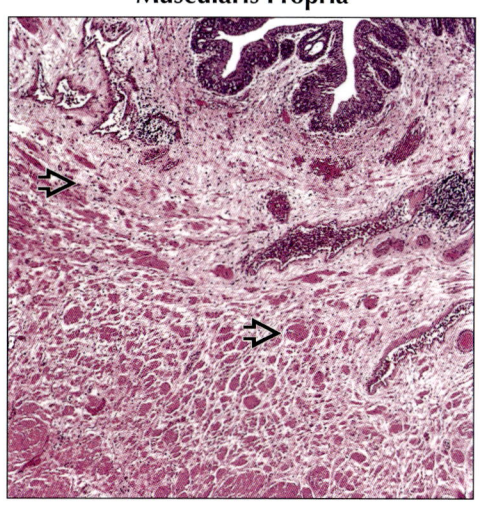

(Left) The muscularis propria in the trigone and bladder neck has unique morphological features. The muscle fascicles gradually decrease in size as they become more superficial in location ⇨ in the muscularis propria. (Right) The lamina propria is thinner in the trigone and bladder neck as the muscularis propria muscle bundles extend to a more superficial location. The muscle fascicles ⇨ become smaller and more disorganized in the superficial portions of the muscularis propria.

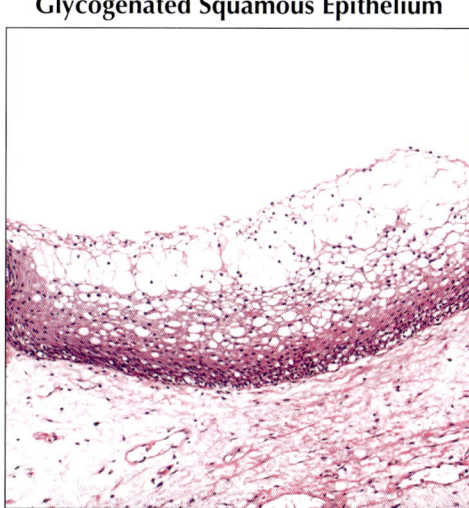

Glycogenated Squamous Epithelium
Glycogenated Squamous Epithelium

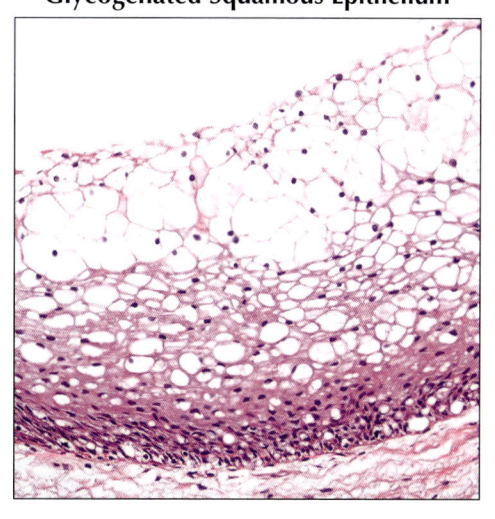

(Left) Glycogenated squamous epithelium is commonly found in the trigone area in female patients, and can be seen in male patients undergoing estrogen therapy for prostatic carcinoma. (Right) Glycogenated squamous epithelium found in the trigone area of the bladder is morphologically similar to the squamous epithelium of the cervix and vagina. The cytoplasm is abundant and clear due to the accumulation of glycogen. No nuclear atypia is present and there is no keratinization.

BLADDER

von Brunn Nests

(Left) von Brunn nests are a common normal variation present in the urothelium; they represent invaginations of the urothelium as nests into the underlying lamina propria. These lesions may occasionally be florid, causing a visible nodule on cystoscopy. The architecture shows nests with smooth contours, an orderly arrangement, and a sharp border with the lamina propria below. **(Right)** The cytologic features of von Brunn nests are bland, with no mitoses or atypia.

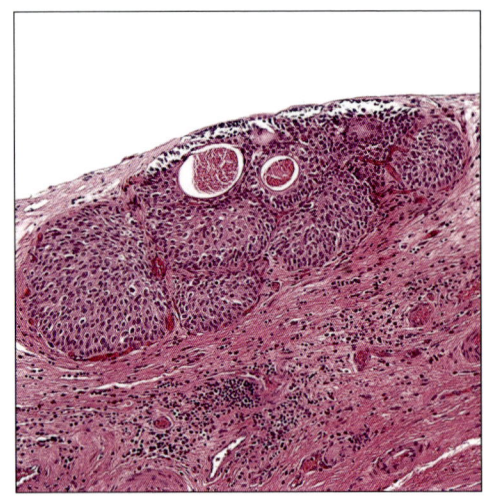

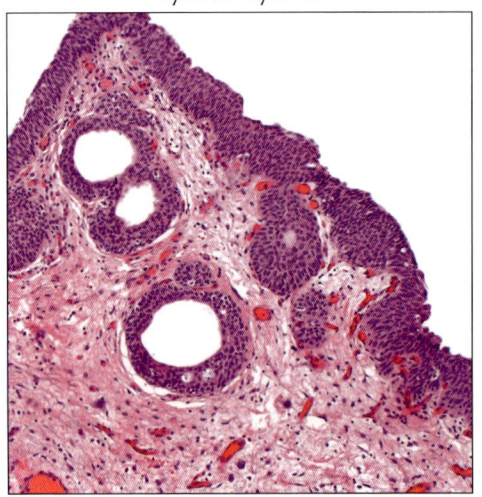

Cystitis Cystica

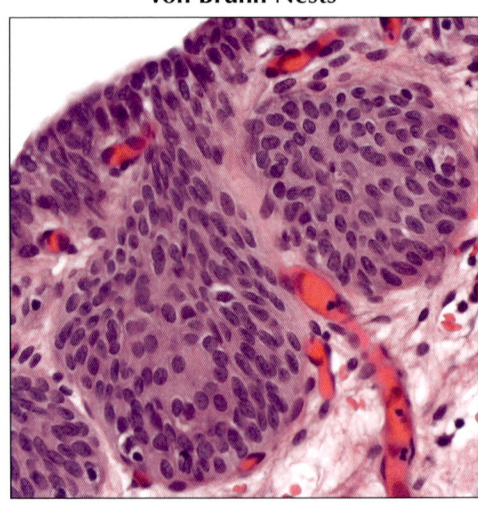

(Left) Cystitis cystica refers to von Brunn nests that have acquired a cystic lumen. The overall architecture of the nests is the same as that of von Brunn nests, with an orderly overall appearance and a sharp linear border with the underlying lamina propria. **(Right)** The epithelium lining the cysts in cystitis cystica is composed of cuboidal or flattened urothelium. The nuclei are small and lack atypia, sharing a similar morphology with the overlying urothelium.

Cystitis Glandularis

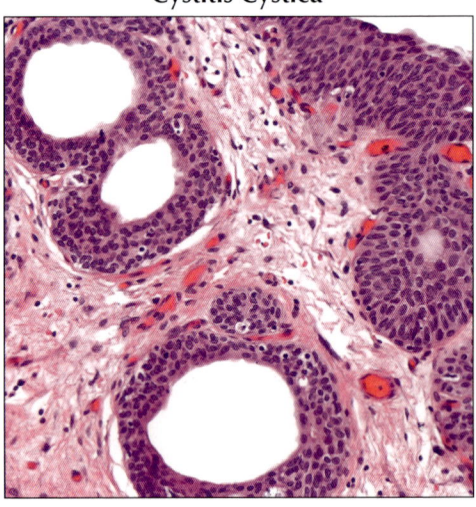

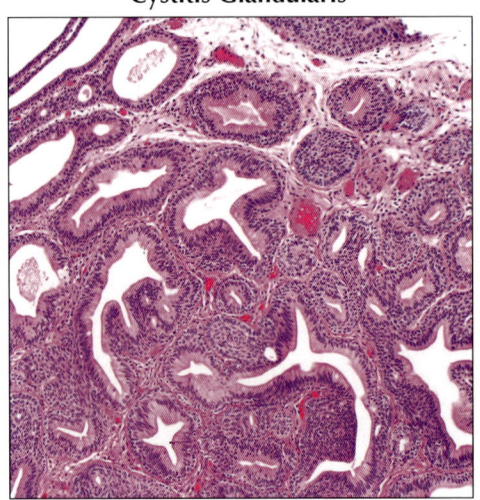

(Left) Cystitis glandularis refers to proliferations of nests of urothelial cells where the lining has undergone glandular metaplasia. The cells lining the cysts are cuboidal to columnar in shape. The overall architecture shows smooth, contoured round to branching glands with a distinct border with the lamina propria. **(Right)** The cells of cystitis glandularis lack atypia and are composed of cuboidal to columnar epithelium, which may contain mucin within the cytoplasm.

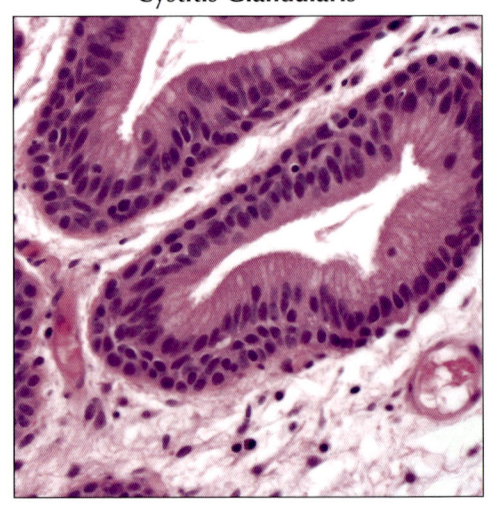

BLADDER

Cystitis Glandularis With Intestinal Metaplasia

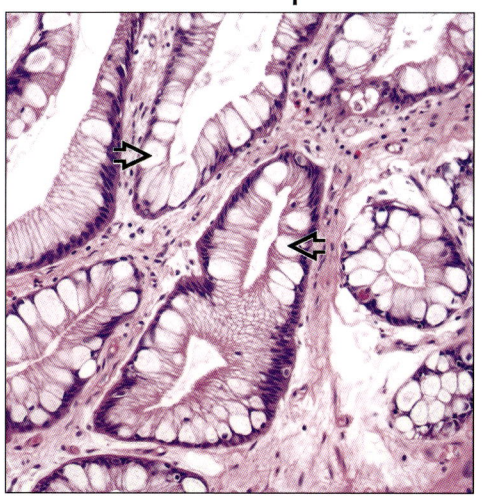

Cystitis Glandularis With Intestinal Metaplasia

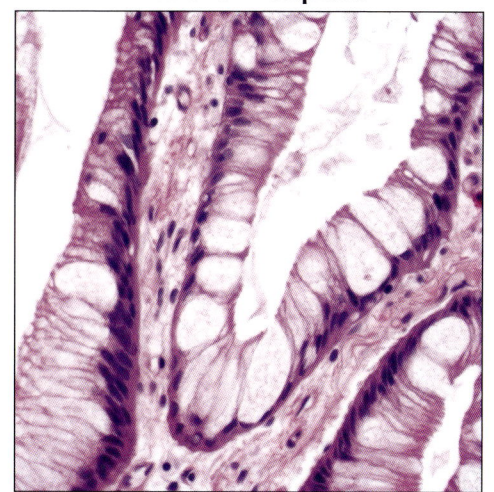

(Left) The invaginations of nests of cystitis glandularis can acquire intestinal-type goblet cells ⇨, similar to colonic epithelium. When this occurs, the proliferation is called cystitis glandularis with intestinal metaplasia. *(Right)* At higher power, the bland nuclear features of cystitis glandularis with intestinal metaplasia are apparent. No mitotic figures are present and the nuclei are small, lacking atypia.

Inverted Papilloma

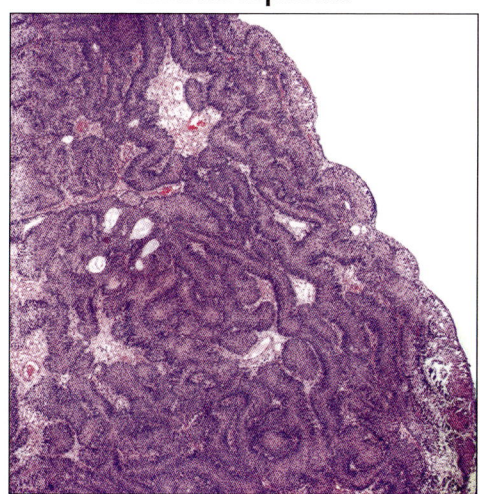

Inverted Papilloma

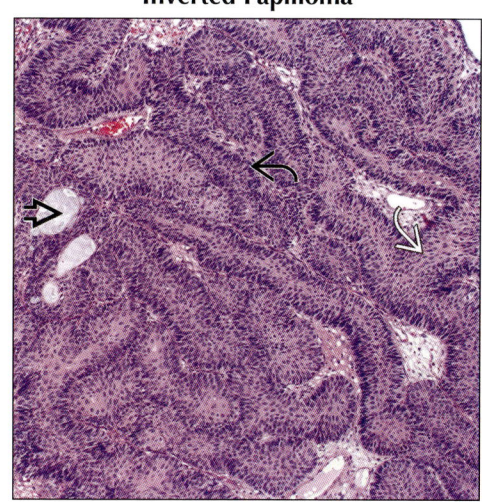

(Left) Inverted papillomas are rare, benign lesions found in the urothelial tract and may be visible on cystoscopy. The overlying surface is smooth with the lamina propria containing invaginations of cords and trabecular proliferations of cells. *(Right)* This high-power view shows peripheral palisading of darker cells ⇨ at the edges of the trabeculae, with the central cells showing a streaming pattern ⇨ with occasional cystic dilation ⇨.

Paraganglia

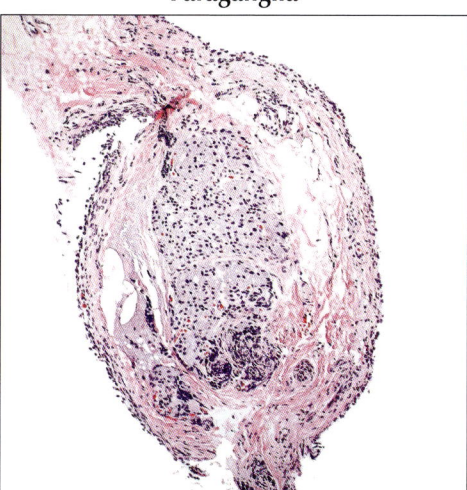

Paraganglia

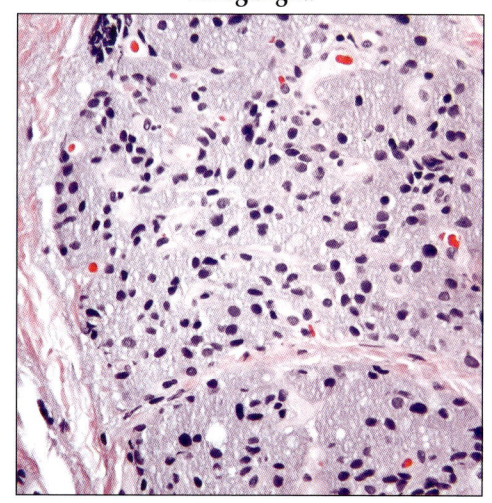

(Left) Paraganglia may be seen within the lamina propria, where they may be confused for invasive carcinoma or paraganglioma. The paraganglia are often seen in association with nerves and small-caliber vessels. *(Right)* A higher power view of the paraganglia shows an aggregate of cells with basophilic cytoplasm and bland-appearing small to medium-sized nuclei. Immunohistochemical staining will show positive staining for chromogranin or synaptophysin and negative cytokeratin staining.

URETHRA

Key Facts

Macroscopic Anatomy
- Male urethra (15-20 cm)
  - Preprostatic: Intramural segment (within wall of urinary bladder)
  - Prostatic: Receives secretions from prostatic and ejaculatory ducts at verumontanum
  - Membranous (Intermediate): Passes through pelvic and urogenital diaphragm
  - Penile or spongy (subdivided: Bulbar, pendulous, fossa navicularis)
- Female urethra (4 cm)
  - Proximal: Extends from bladder to mid urethra
  - Distal: Exits body between clitoris and vagina
- Paraurethral/periurethral glands also present
  - Female: Skene
  - Male: Cowper (membranous) and Littré (penile)

Microscopic Anatomy
- In males, preprostatic, prostatic, and membranous urethra lined by stratified urothelium with superficial umbrella cell layer
- In males, bulbar and pendulous regions of penile urethra lined by distinctive stratified columnar layer
- In males, most distal aspect (fossa navicularis) lined by nonkeratinizing squamous epithelium
- In females, proximal 1/3 is lined by stratified urothelium that transitions to nonkeratinizing squamous epithelium distally
- Paraurethral and periurethral glands
  - Ducts lined by stratified columnar/cuboidal epithelial layer
  - Acini comprised of cells with intracytoplasmic mucin
  - Prostatic-type glands may also be seen
- Intraepithelial glandular structures
  - Small collections of intraepithelial cells with intracytoplasmic mucin

Pitfalls/Artifacts
- Florid von Brunn nests
  - Numerous rounded invaginations of benign urothelium into underlying connective tissue
  - Invaginations extend to a uniform depth (unlike nested urothelial carcinoma)
- Polypoid/papillary urethritis
  - Papillae and polypoid excrescences with broad base
  - No complex hierarchical branching (unlike papillary urothelial neoplasia)
- Nephrogenic adenoma
  - Generally considered a regenerative/reparative lesion
  - May have papillary, tubular, cystic, solid/diffuse, or flat pattern
- Urethral caruncle
  - Inflammatory lesion at urethral meatus, usually in postmenopausal women
  - Consists of inflammatory cells, blood vessels, and varying edematous to fibrotic stroma
  - Rare cases may contain atypical stromal cells
  - Lining epithelium may be urothelial or squamous
- Fibroepithelial polyp
  - Rare, but may occur in children
  - Most common in posterior urethra
  - Loose fibrous stroma lined by urothelium, sometimes with reactive epithelial atypia
- Prostatic-type polyp
  - Polypoid lesion lined by an admixture of benign urothelial and prostatic secretory-type cells

Metaplasia
- Nonkeratinizing glycogenated squamous metaplasia
  - Common in proximal urethra and bladder trigone of women
- Glandular metaplasia
  - May be seen with chronic irritative conditions

Hyperplasia
- "Transitional" cell hyperplasia
  - Prominent thickened urothelial layer within periurethral ducts and glands
- Lobular hyperplasia of Cowper gland
  - Only rare case reports

(Left) In this dissection of the male pelvis (midsagittal view), the lumen of the urethra is not present at every level, but the anatomic distribution of its course is highlighted: Bladder ⇨, intramural ⇨, prostatic ⇨, membranous ⇨, and penile ⇨. (Right) In this dissection of the female pelvis (midsagittal view), the lumen of the urethra ⇨ is seen in continuity with the bladder ⇨. Compared to the male urethra (15-20 cm), the female urethra is relatively short in length (4 cm).

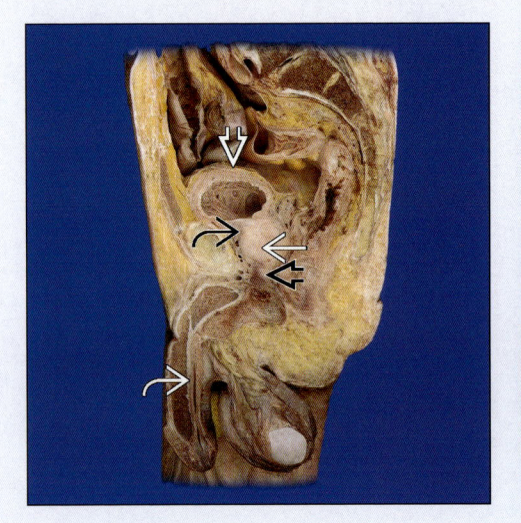

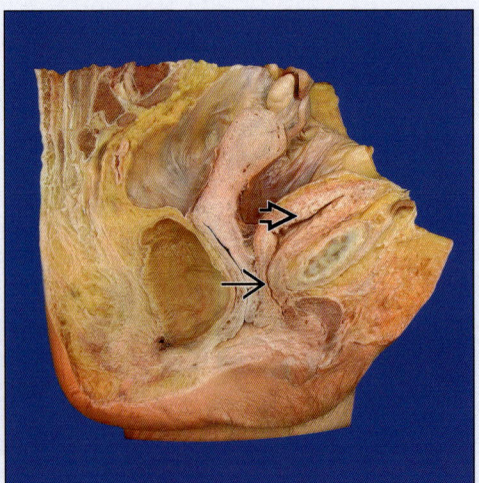

URETHRA

Male Urethra Anatomy

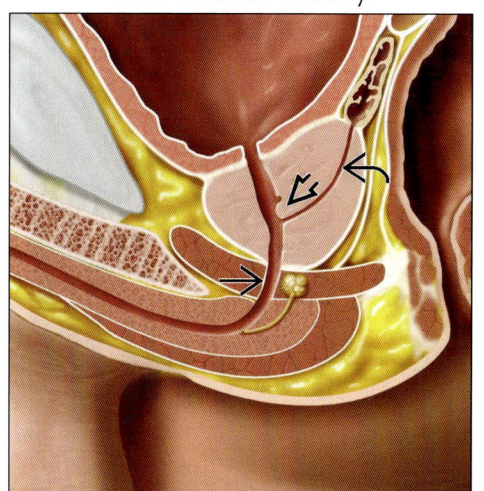

Male: Membranous Urethra

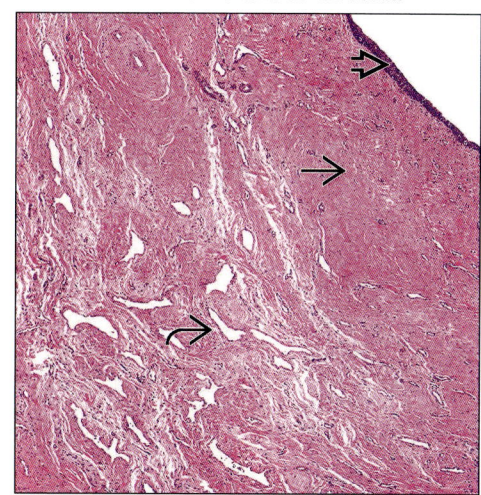

(Left) This diagram of the male pelvis highlights the location of the verumontanum ⇨, where the ejaculatory ducts ⇨ empty into the prostatic urethra. The membranous urethra ⇨ (1-2 cm) courses from the apex of the prostate to the perineal membrane at the bulb of the penis within the deep perineal space. (Right) The membranous urethra has an epithelial lining ⇨, an underlying lamina propria ⇨, and a region rich in vascular channels ⇨.

Male: Membranous Urethra

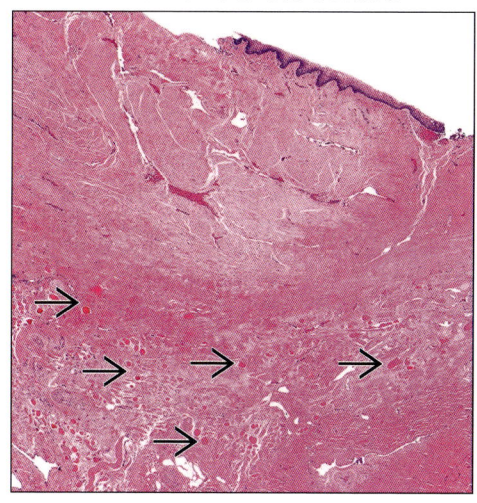

Urethra: Urothelium

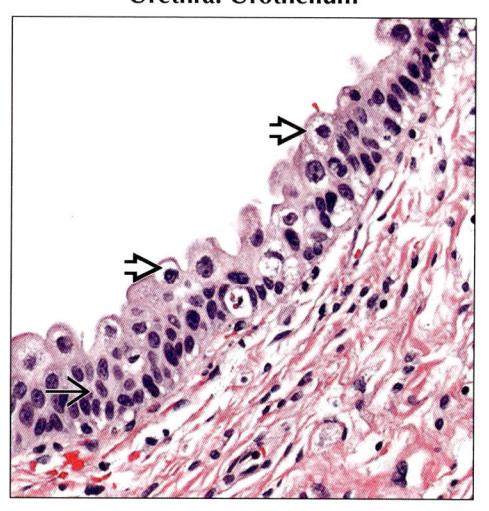

(Left) Skeletal muscle ⇨ may be seen deep in the wall of the membranous urethra because it traverses the pelvic floor musculature, which is composed of muscle fibers of the levator ani and the coccygeus (just distal to the apex of the prostate gland). (Right) The proximal portions of the urethra may have urothelium (transitional epithelium) identical to that of the bladder. The elongated intermediate cells with intranuclear grooves ⇨ are the predominant type, but an umbrella cell layer is also seen ⇨.

Male: Prostatic Urethra (Verumontanum)

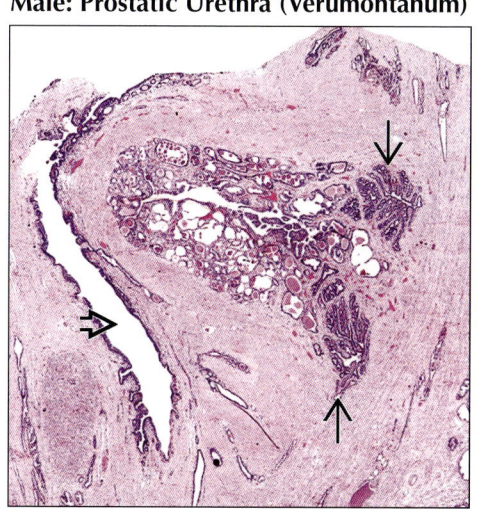

Male: Prostatic Urethra

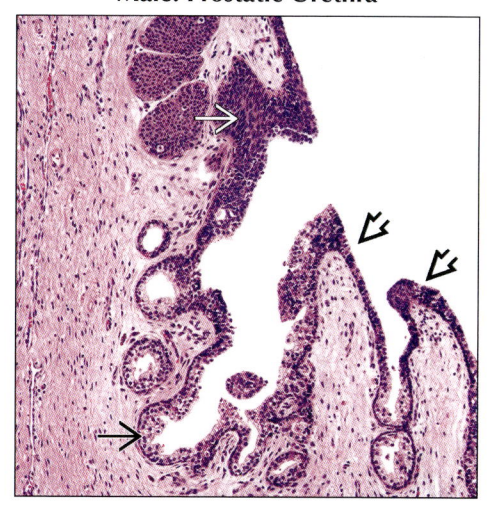

(Left) The verumontanum (or colliculus seminalis) is a posterior protuberance into the prostatic urethral lumen ⇨ that represents the site where the prostatic and ejaculatory ducts ⇨ enter the urethra. (Right) The normal prostatic urethra has an irregular surface with small polypoid projections ⇨ that may mimic a neoplastic process. The lining epithelial cells of the prostatic urethra are an admixture of urothelial ⇨ and prostatic secretory ⇨ cells.

URETHRA

Male Urethra

Penile Urethra

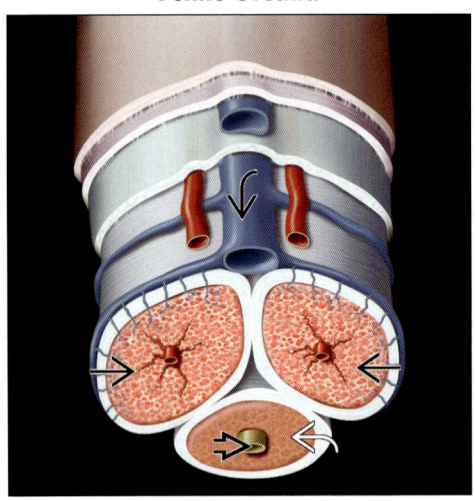

(Left) This schematic diagram highlights the anatomic regions of the male urethra: Intramural ➡, prostatic ➡, membranous ➡, and penile (including bulbar ➡ and pendulous ➡).
(Right) This diagram represents a cross section of the penis and highlights the urethra ➡, which travels through the corpus spongiosum ➡. The location of the corpora cavernosa ➡ and deep dorsal vein ➡ are also highlighted for comparison.

Male: Penile Urethra

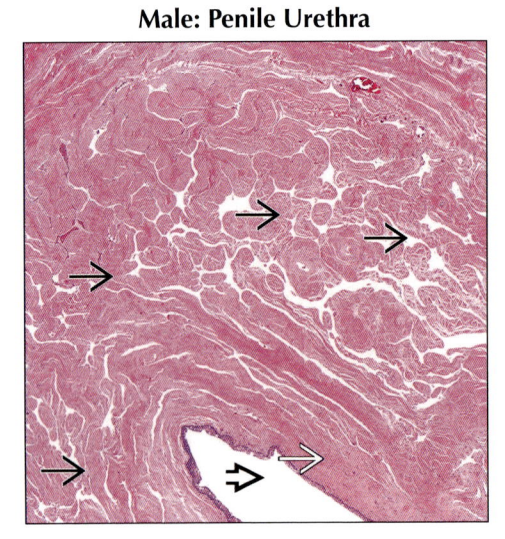

Male: Penile Urethra

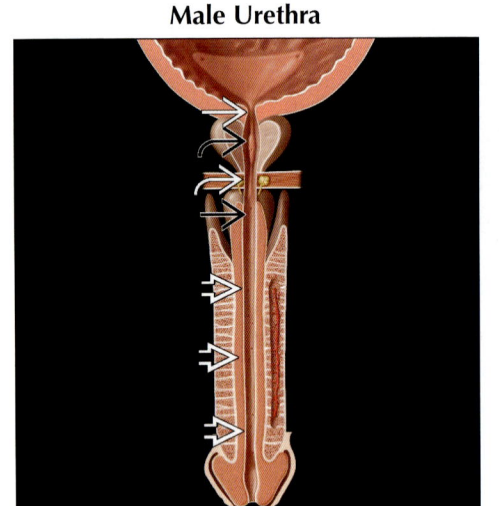

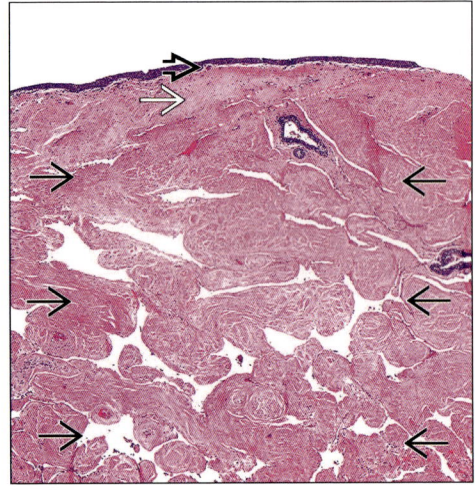

(Left) The lumen of the penile urethra ➡ is surrounded by a thin layer of fibrous connective tissue (the lamina propria) ➡ and then by the periurethral corpus spongiosum ➡. (Right) The corpus spongiosum ➡, which underlies the lamina propria ➡ and the epithelial layer ➡ of the penile urethra, consists of interconnected, branching vascular spaces that are surrounded by smooth muscle and connective tissue.

Male: Penile Urethra (Distal/Pendulous)

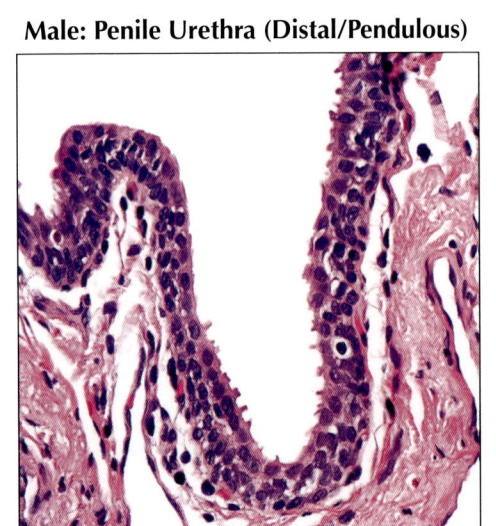

Male: Penile Urethra (Fossa Navicularis)

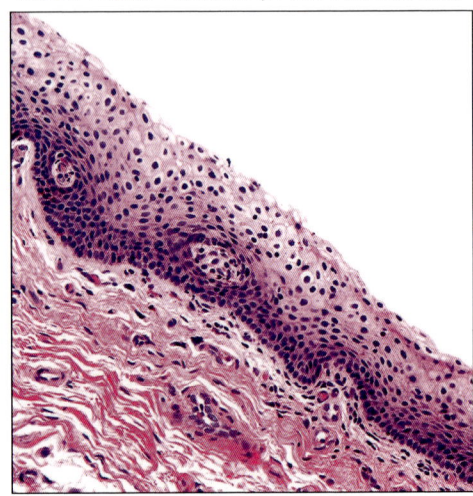

(Left) The epithelium of the penile urethra has been referred to as a stratified or pseudostratified columnar layer, and ranges from approximately 4-15 layers of cells. (Right) The most distal portion of the male urethra, a saccular dilatation called the fossa navicularis, is lined by nonkeratinizing squamous epithelium that becomes continuous with the epithelium of the glans penis.

URETHRA

Female Urethral Anatomy

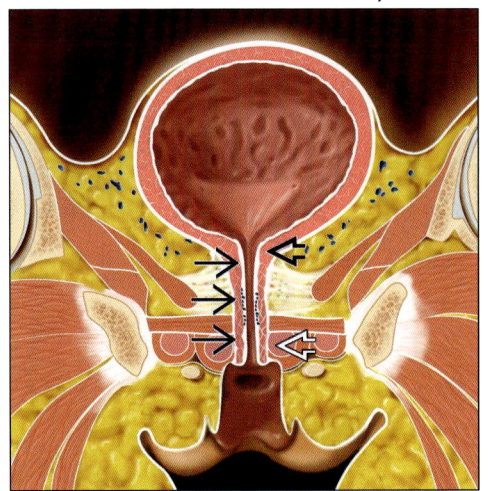

Female Urethra

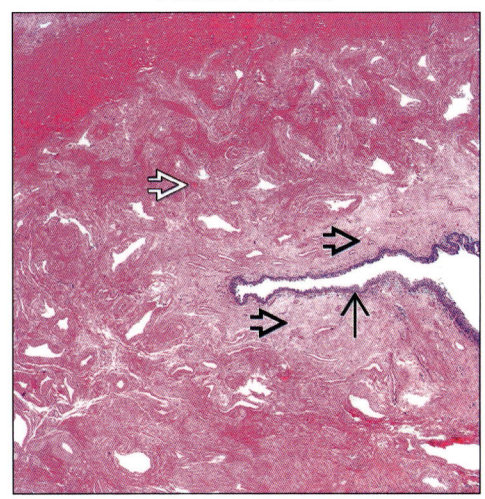

(Left) The female urethra ➡ has a much shorter course compared to that of the male. It is divided simply into the proximal and distal regions. The internal ➡ and external ➡ sphincters are also labeled. *(Right)* The female urethra is composed of an epithelial layer ➡, underlying fibrous connective tissue with small capillary-sized vessels (lamina propria) ➡, and surrounding larger "erectile type" vascular spaces ➡.

Female Urethra

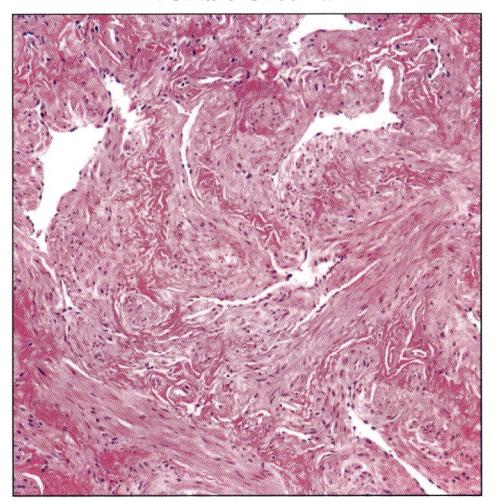

Female Urethra: Squamous Metaplasia

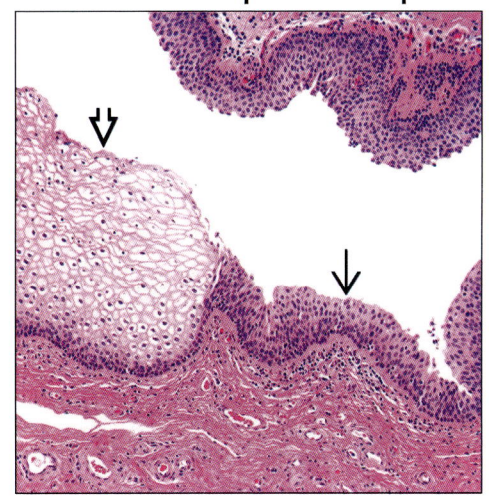

(Left) These large venous-like spaces with surrounding smooth muscle stroma are typically seen beneath the lamina propria in the female urethra. *(Right)* Nonkeratinizing squamous epithelium ➡ is commonly seen in the proximal urethra and trigone of females, and is typically considered normal. It typically contains abundant glycogen, lending the squamous cells a pale appearance. Note the adjacent urothelium ➡.

Female Urethra: Distal

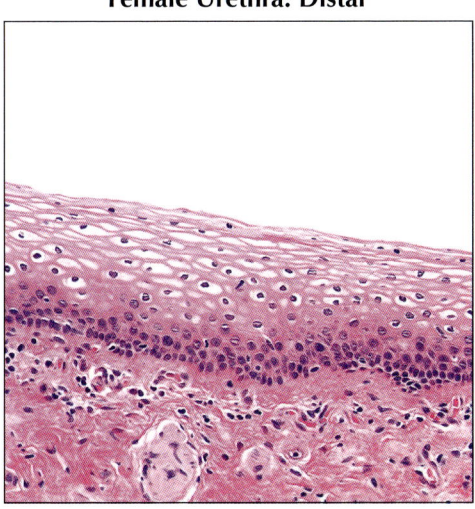

Female Urethra: Squamous Metaplasia

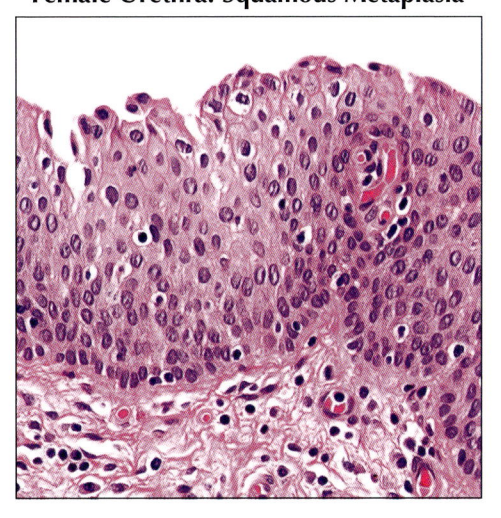

(Left) The distal region of the female urethra is typically lined by nonkeratinizing squamous epithelium, as shown here. *(Right)* A urothelial lining is typically present in the proximal portions of the female urethra, but this may be replaced by metaplastic epithelium, especially nonkeratinizing glycogenated squamous epithelium in regions near the urinary bladder.

URETHRA

Keratinizing Squamous Metaplasia

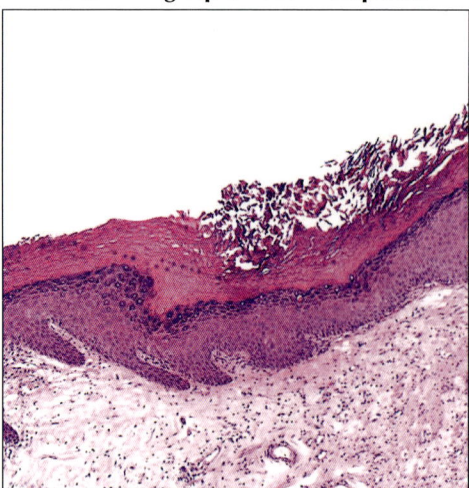

Mucinous Intraepithelial Cells

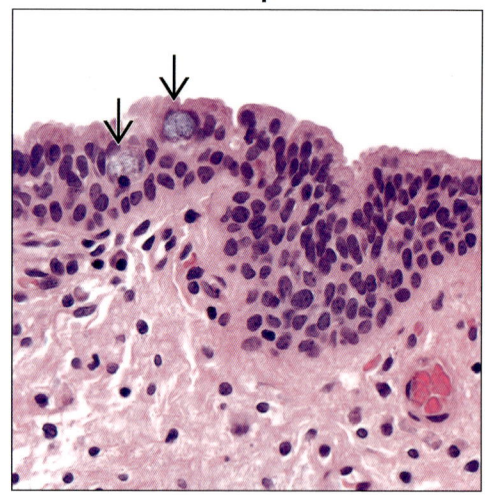

(Left) Keratinizing squamous metaplasia is an abnormal process that is most commonly associated with states of chronic irritation secondary to a variety of etiologies. (Right) The urothelium may occasionally show individual cells with mucinous features ⇒, especially in states of chronic irritation or inflammation. These metaplastic cells are characterized by intracytoplasmic intestinal-type mucin ⇒. This is not generally regarded as a preneoplastic condition.

Intestinal Metaplasia

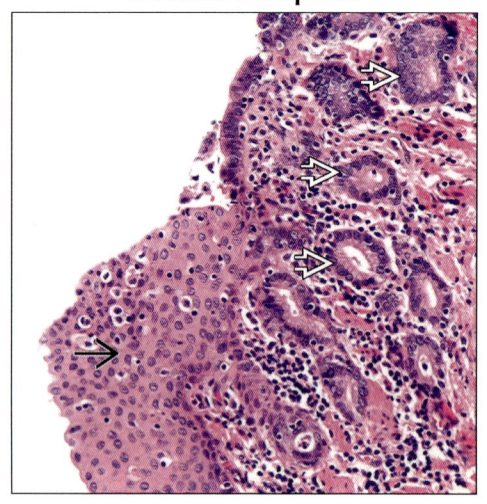

Intestinal Metaplasia

(Left) In this section of urethral epithelium in a patient with a long history of urethral diverticula and infections, there is well-developed intestinal metaplasia ⇒, which may be contrasted with the adjacent urothelium ⇒. (Right) Intestinal metaplasia of the urethra has a histologic appearance (and immunophenotype) that is identical to that of enteric type mucosa from any anatomic site.

von Brunn Nests

von Brunn Nests

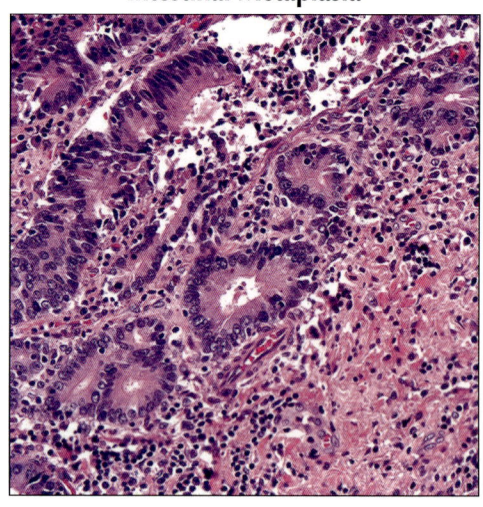

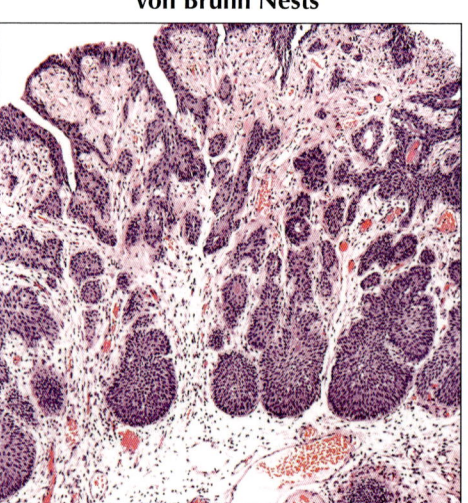

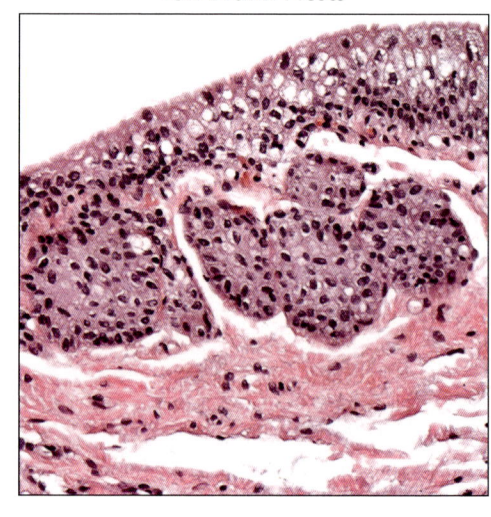

(Left) von Brunn nests are invaginations of benign urothelium into the lamina propria. Unlike cytologically bland forms of invasive urothelial carcinoma, such as nested type, these benign urothelial nests extend to a relatively uniform level within the lamina propria. (Right) The urothelial cells within von Brunn nests are cytologically bland with histologic features similar to those in the overlying flat urothelium.

URETHRA

Urethral Ducts

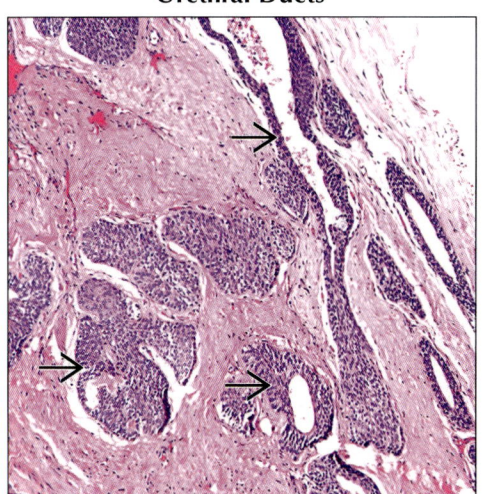

Periurethral/Paraurethral Glands

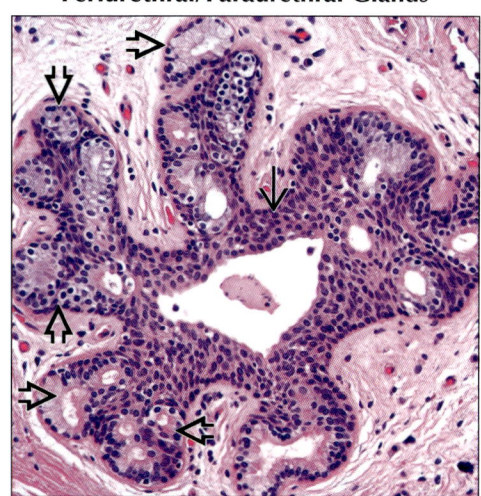

(Left) Numerous ducts ➡ of varying caliber are frequently identified within the wall of the urethra; they connect the surrounding glands to the urethral lumen and are typically lined by cuboidal or urothelial-type epithelium. *(Right)* This section from the penile urethra shows periurethral glands with a tubuloacinar arrangement, consisting of columnar epithelium ➡ and peripherally placed mucinous-type epithelium ▷.

Periurethral/Paraurethral Glands

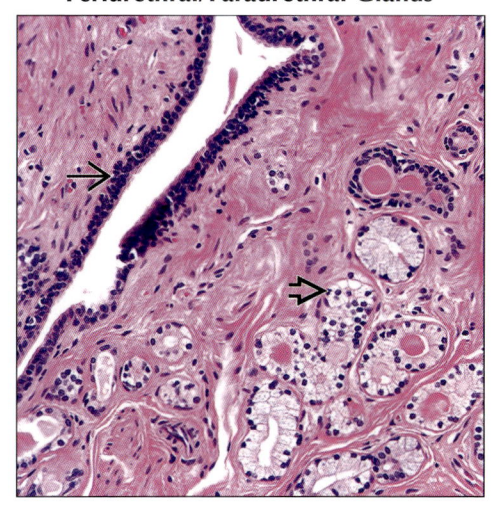

Periurethral/Paraurethral Glands

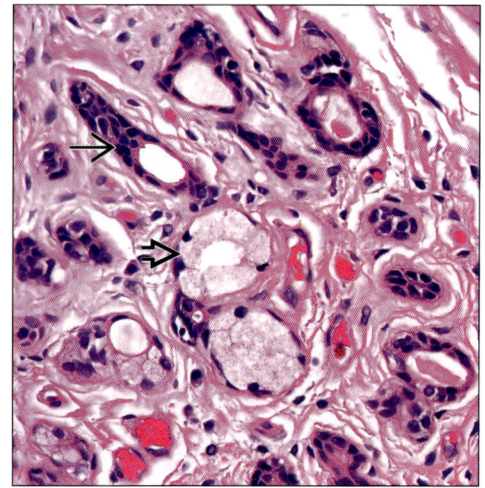

(Left) This deeper, large-caliber duct ➡ is present adjacent to a collection of mucinous acini ▷. This architectural arrangement is typical of the benign glandular structures that are frequently identified adjacent to the urethra. *(Right)* The accessory glands that are present within the wall of the urethra or in surrounding tissues may consist of an admixture of small acini lined by both mucinous ▷ and cuboidal ➡ epithelium.

Periurethral/Paraurethral Glands

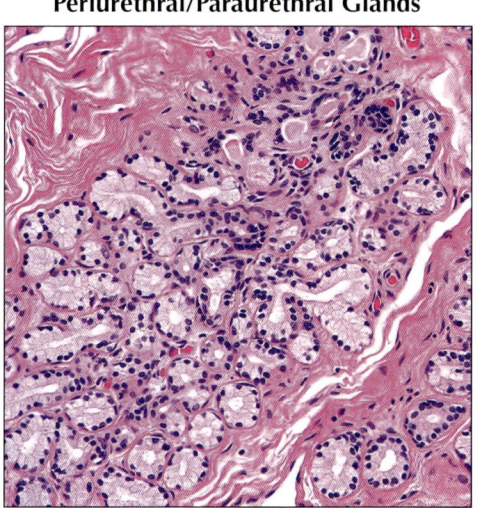

Intraepithelial Glandular Cells

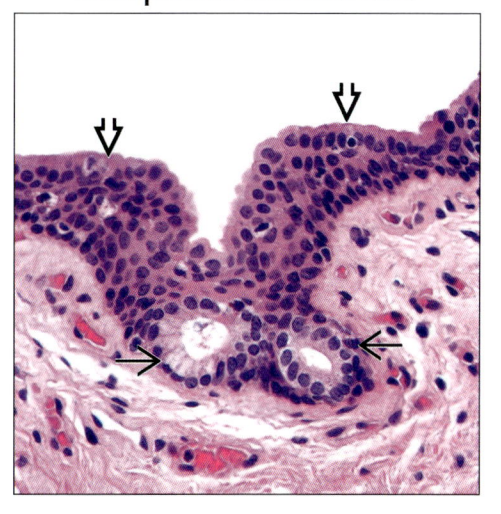

(Left) This collection of acini with mucinous epithelium is typical of the glands identified within the wall of the urethra. The lobular/circumscribed architectural arrangement aids in their recognition as a normal benign structure. *(Right)* Intraepithelial glandular cells ➡ may also be seen within the otherwise normal epithelium ▷ that lines the urethra, as in this example. These are usually seen within the vicinity of underlying ducts and accessory glands.

PROSTATE: REGIONAL ANATOMY WITH HISTOLOGIC CORRELATES

Key Facts

Macroscopic Anatomy
- Prostate divided into regional zones of McNeal
  - Transition zone surrounds prostatic urethra
  - Central zone extends from bladder base to mid prostate (inverted pyramidal shape)
  - Peripheral zone extends from superior prostate to apex & surrounds both central & transition zones

Microscopic Anatomy
- Peripheral zone
  - Glands show variable caliber and often follow contour of prostate gland surface
- Transition zone
  - More nodular aggregates of prostate glands
- Central zone
  - Distinct histology with intraluminal epithelial bridging and papillae
  - Often have more eosinophilic cytoplasm

Pitfalls/Artifacts
- Normal anatomic variation may mimic adenocarcinoma histologically
  - Central zone glands
  - Urothelium within prostate glands

Age Variation
- Benign prostatic hyperplasia may distort normal anatomy in older adults
  - Transition zone may extend into apex, and stromal hyperplasia may extend to bladder base

Metaplasia
- Urothelial (transitional) metaplasia
  - Common in periurethral region, rarely extends into peripheral zone

Hyperplasia
- Benign prostatic hyperplasia (BPH)

(Left) The prostate gland ⇒ is inferior to the bladder ⇒, superior to the pelvic floor musculature ⇒, and anterior to the rectum ⇒. Urine flows to the prostatic urethra, starting at the bladder neck ⇒. (Right) This gross radical prostatectomy specimen shows anterior ⇒, posterior ⇒, and posterolateral ⇒ views. The paired seminal vesicles ⇒ and vas deferentia ⇒ are seen posteriorly and superiorly (probe through prostatic urethra). (Courtesy G. Paner, MD.)

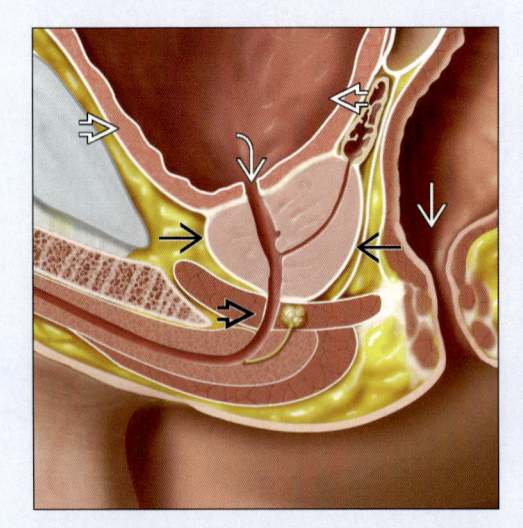

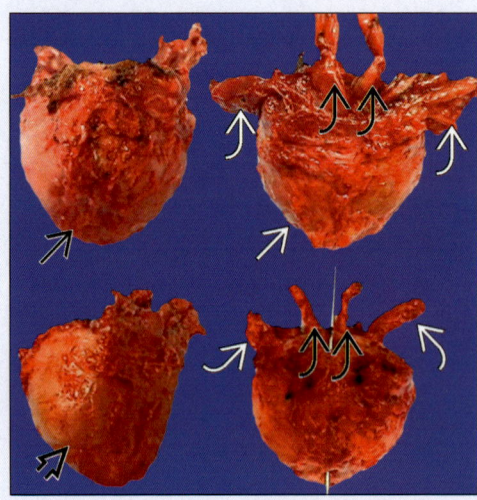

(Left) This graphic demonstrates the anatomic zones of the prostate. The central zone is an inverted pyramid shape at the superior aspect (orange), the transition zone is in the periurethral region (blue), and the surrounding tissue is the peripheral zone (green). Yellow represents the anterior fibromuscular stroma. (Right) The microscopic anatomy of the prostate varies from superior to inferior, depending on the anatomic zones that are present in a given cross section level.

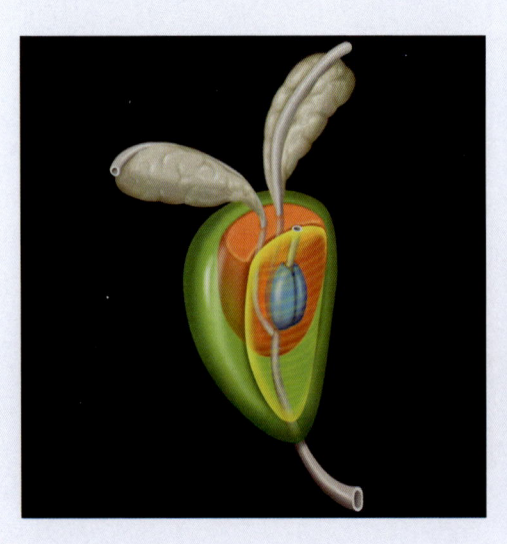

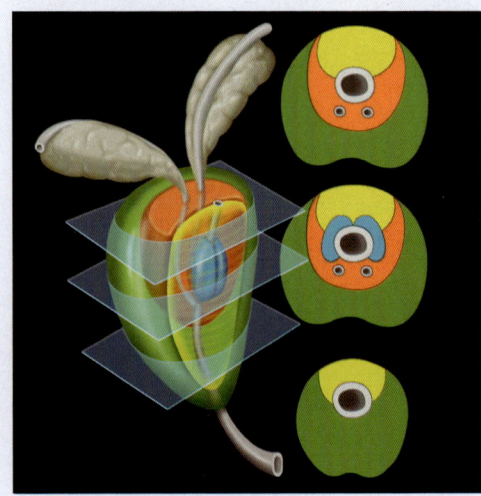

PROSTATE: REGIONAL ANATOMY WITH HISTOLOGIC CORRELATES

Apical Cross Section of Prostate

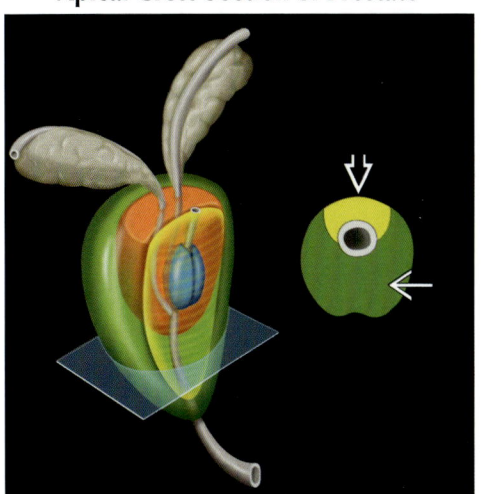

Apical Prostate

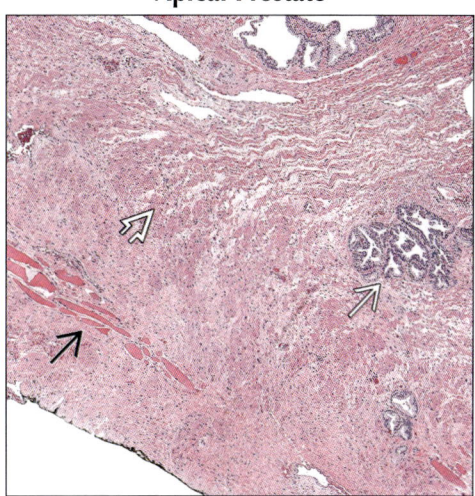

(Left) Apical cross sections of the prostate gland typically show peripheral zone prostatic tissue ⇨ and anterior fibromuscular stroma ⇨. In severe benign prostatic hyperplasia, the transition zone glands and stroma may extend inferiorly into the apical tissues. *(Right)* The apical prostate typically consists of peripheral zone prostatic glands ⇨, fibromuscular stroma ⇨, and admixed skeletal muscle ⇨ from the pelvic floor &/or anterior soft tissues.

Apical Prostate

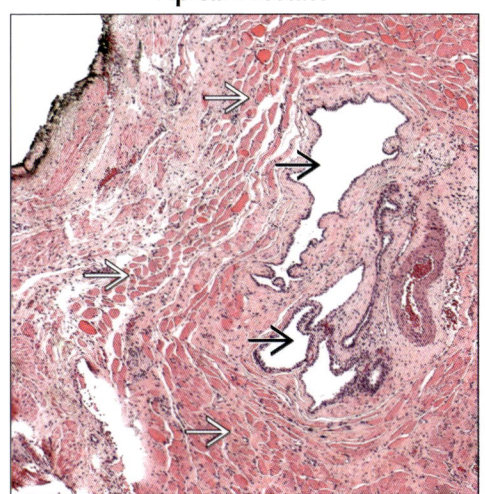

Apical Prostate

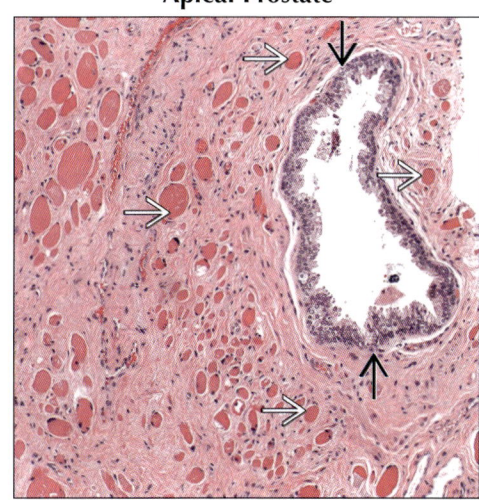

(Left) The benign prostate glands of the apex ⇨ are often intermixed with scattered skeletal muscle fibers ⇨; therefore, skeletal muscle fibers should not be considered to be extraprostatic tissue in the apex. *(Right)* On higher-power magnification, this benign prostate gland ⇨ is completely surrounded by skeletal muscle ⇨. This underscores the fact that skeletal muscle is often intraprostatic in histologic sections taken from the prostatic apex.

Anteriormost Aspect of Apex

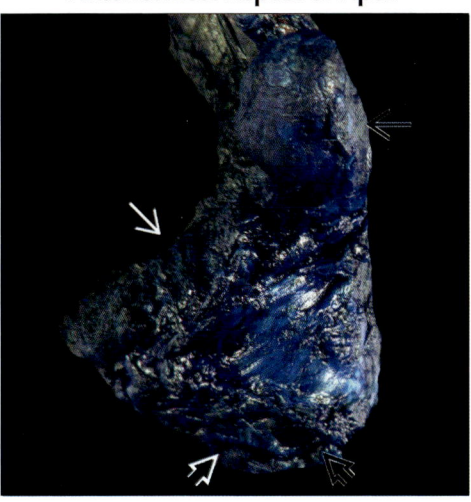

Apical Prostate

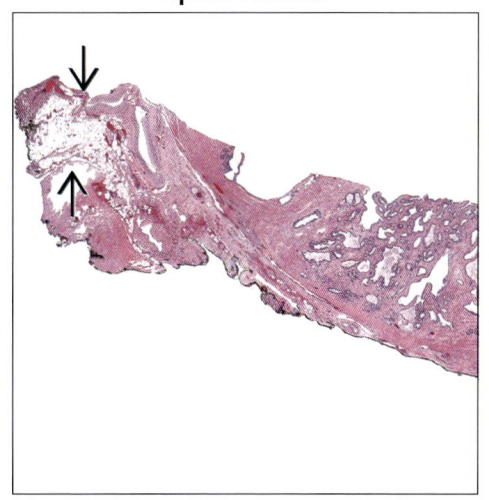

(Left) This lateral view of an inked gross prostate specimen can be oriented by the following landmarks: Posterior seminal vesicles ⇨, base ⇨, and apex ⇨. When a thick section of the apex is amputated, the most anterior aspect ⇨ may contain adipose tissue from the anterior stroma. *(Right)* In this single section from the prostatic apex, which was serially sectioned in an anterior/posterior plane after amputation, adipose tissue is identified anteriorly ⇨.

PROSTATE: REGIONAL ANATOMY WITH HISTOLOGIC CORRELATES

Mid-Level Section of Prostate

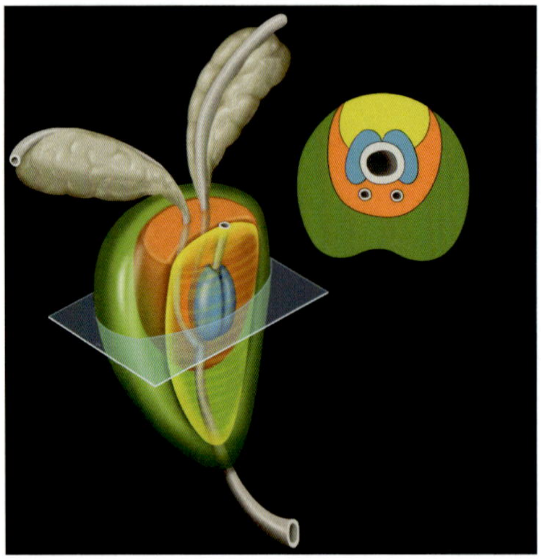

Mid Prostate Peripheral Zone

(Left) A mid-level macroscopic cross section of the prostate gland typically contains peripheral zone (green) and transition zone (blue) tissue, but the central zone (orange) may also be seen depending on the exact level of the section and anatomic variation between patients. *(Right)* This normal posterolateral quarter section from the mid prostate shows a typical low-power distribution of the prostate glands. The outer contour of the prostate is highlighted by the arrows ⇨.

Mid Prostate Peripheral Zone

Mid Prostate Peripheral Zone

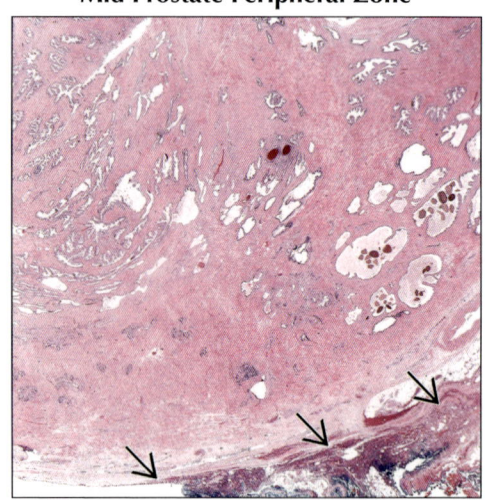

(Left) The benign prostate glands of the peripheral zone at the mid level have a variable orientation. A linear arrangement of the glands ⇨ that runs parallel to the outer contour of the prostate gland is common. *(Right)* This mid-level section shows the boundary of the extraprostatic tissue at the posterolateral aspect, which is defined as the level of the adipose tissue ⇨. The benign prostate glands show a typical caliber and distribution.

Mid Prostate Peripheral Zone

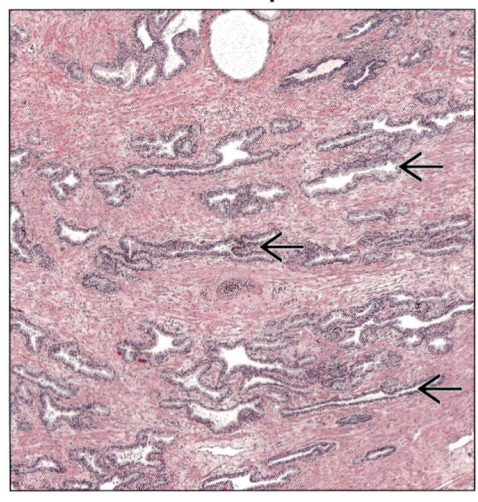

Mid Prostate Peripheral Zone

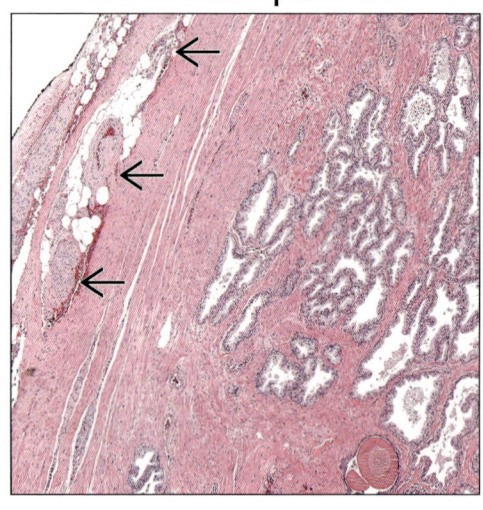

(Left) Normal prostate glands may show marked dilatation and a nearly complete loss of cytoplasm; this pattern is referred to as cystic atrophy. The large size of the glands is more appreciable by comparison to adjacent normal-sized glands ⇨. In some patients, this type of cystic change may fill the peripheral zone. *(Right)* In this example of the mid peripheral zone, there is more heterogeneous gland morphology with an admixture of both dilated cystic ⇨ and smaller round glands ⇨.

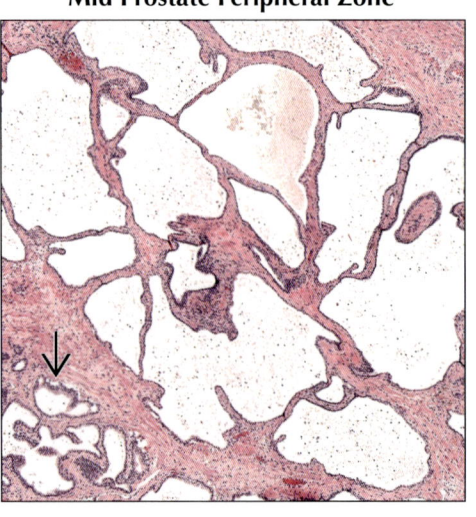

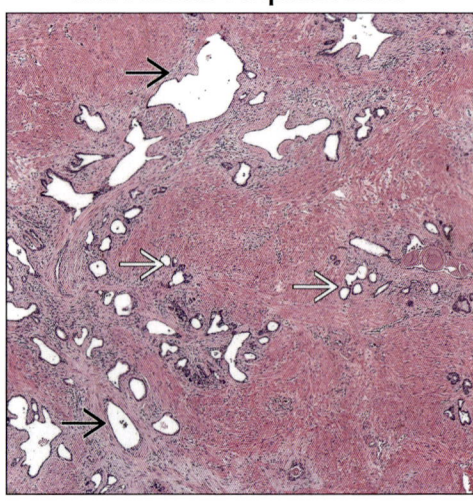

PROSTATE: REGIONAL ANATOMY WITH HISTOLOGIC CORRELATES

Mid Prostate Transition Zone

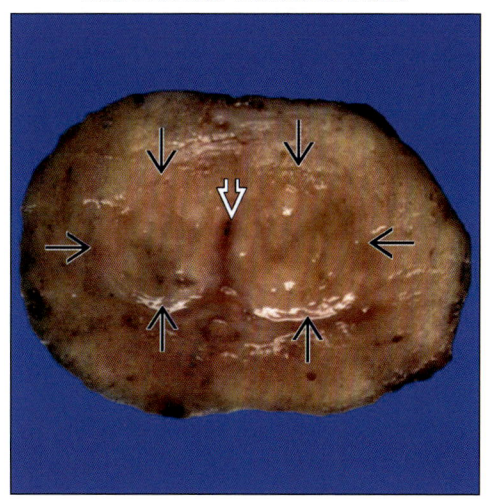

Transition Zone Boundary With Peripheral Zone

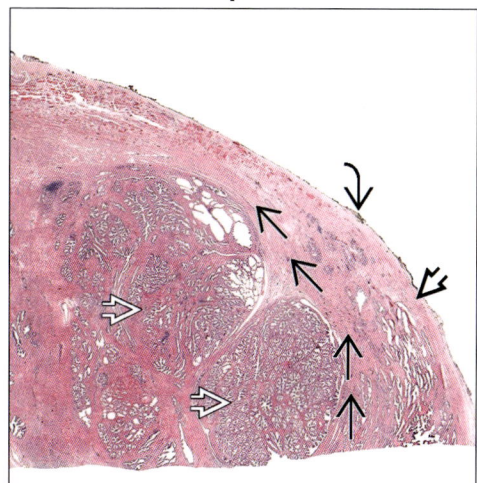

(Left) This gross macrosection of the mid prostate is from a patient with benign prostatic hyperplasia. The transition zone, which surrounds the urethra ⇨, is prominent ⇨. *(Right)* A lobular arrangement of the prostate glands ⇨ is typical of the transition zone. The boundary with the peripheral zone is fairly distinct in this section ⇨. The peripheral zone glands ⇨ have a more linear arrangement that follows the outer contour of the prostate gland ⇨.

Transition Zone

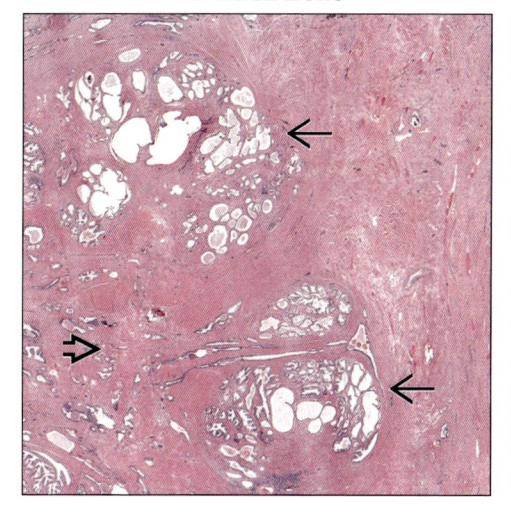

Transition Zone

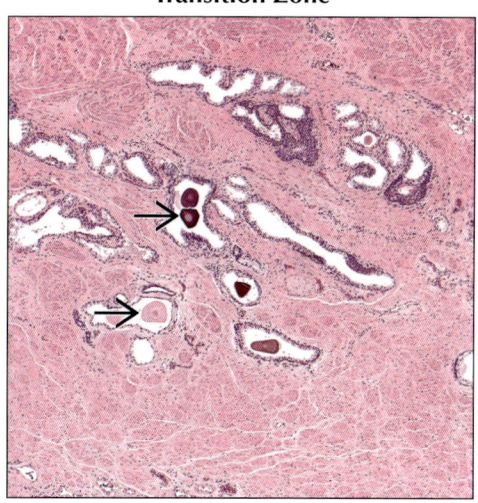

(Left) The transition zone is commonly composed of circumscribed nodules of glands with an increased epithelial to stromal ratio ⇨, as seen in this example. There is architectural variation with other foci showing fewer glands of less pronounced organization ⇨. *(Right)* In the transition zone, the density of the glands and the nodular architecture vary considerably depending on the presence of BPH. Intraluminal corpora amylacea ⇨ are common.

Periurethral Prostate

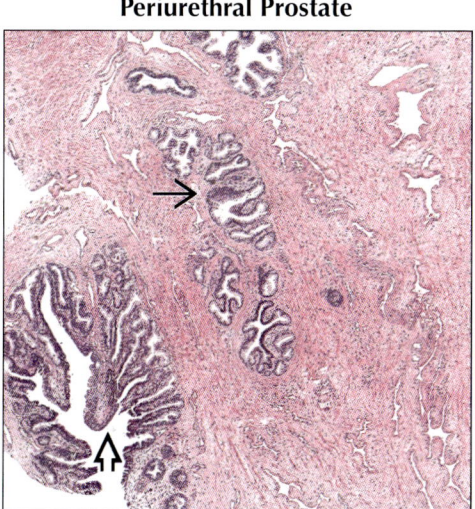

Periurethral Area

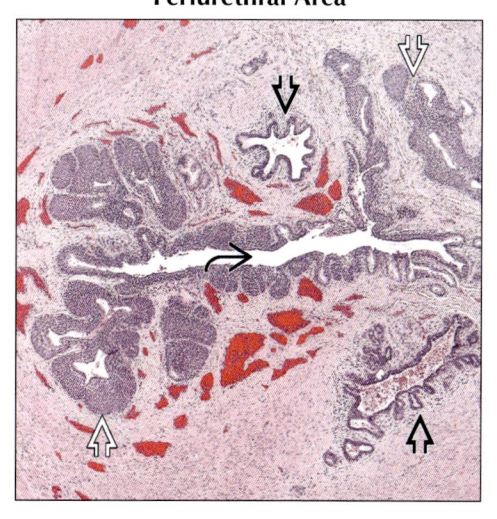

(Left) The prostatic glands ⇨ directly underlying the prostatic urethra ⇨ are less lobular in architecture and are more commonly lined by an admixture of prostatic epithelium and urothelium. *(Right)* The lumen of the prostatic urethra ⇨ is lined predominantly by urothelium. The surrounding prostatic glands ⇨ are variably lined by a stratified urothelium ⇨, a feature that has been referred to as transitional (urothelial) metaplasia.

PROSTATE: REGIONAL ANATOMY WITH HISTOLOGIC CORRELATES

Extraprostatic Tissue: Posterolateral

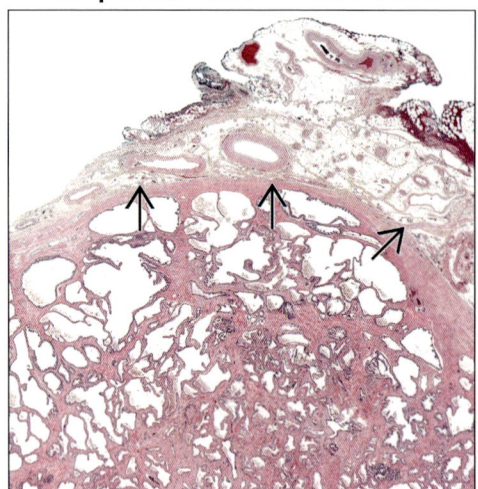

Extraprostatic Tissue: Posterolateral

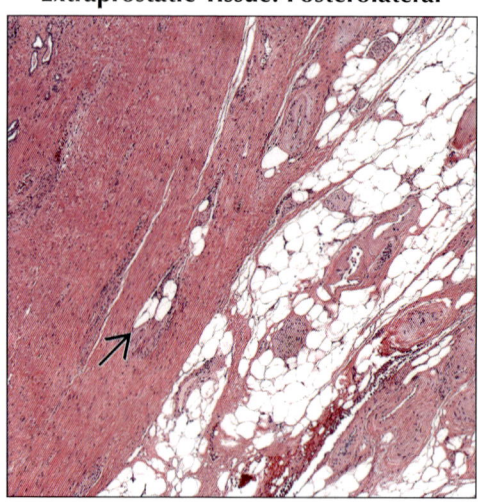

(Left) Often, there is a distinct junction between the prostate and the extraprostatic tissue at the posterolateral aspect of the prostate, which is the location of the neurovascular bundles. Even at low-power magnification, the sharp line at the start of the extraprostatic adipose tissue is evident ➡. *(Right)* The extraprostatic tissue begins at the plane with the 1st identifiable adipose tissue ➡. This is the most reproducible landmark for the prostatic/extraprostatic junction.

Extraprostatic Tissue: Posterolateral

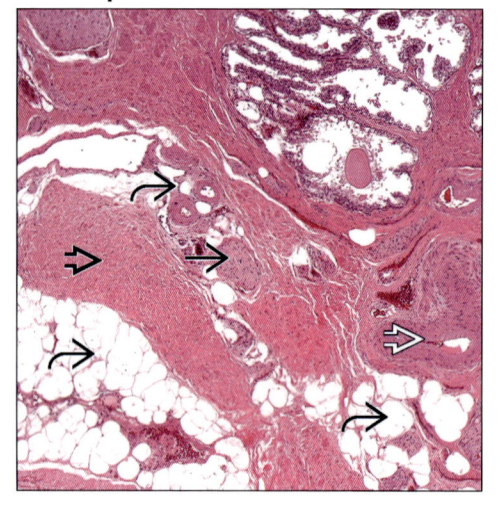

Extraprostatic Tissue: Posterolateral

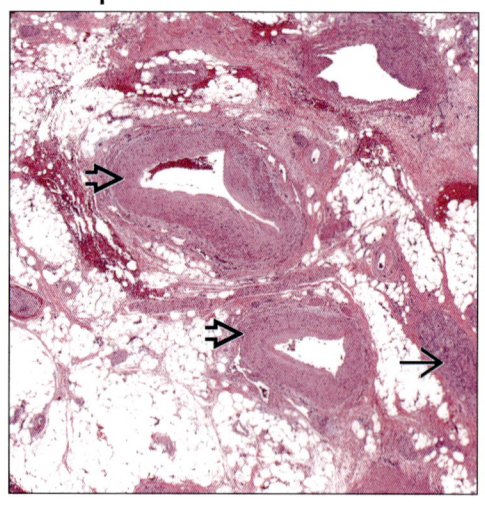

(Left) An admixture of fibrous tissue ➡, adipocytes ➡, large-caliber blood vessels ➡, and peripheral nerves ➡ are commonly seen in the extraprostatic tissues, particularly in the posterolateral region. *(Right)* Large-caliber blood vessels ➡ and peripheral nerves ➡ are often prominent in the posterolateral extraprostatic soft tissue when the neurovascular bundle is not surgically spared.

Extraprostatic Tissue: Posterolateral

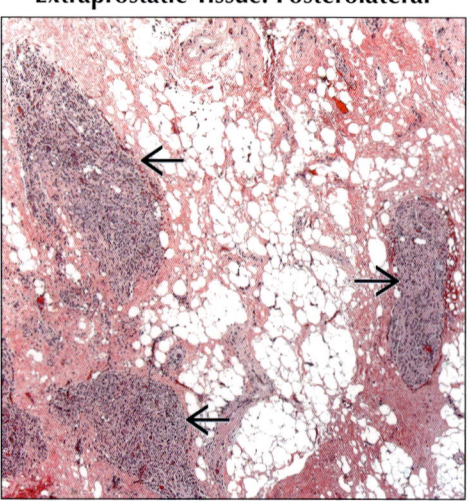

Ganglion

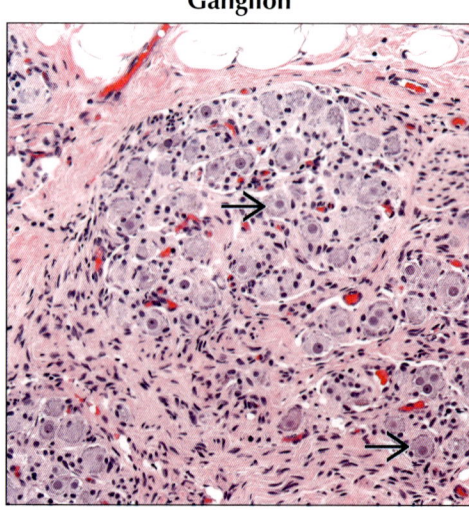

(Left) Collections of ganglion cells are commonly found admixed with adipose tissue in the extraprostatic tissues ➡. They may mimic high-grade prostatic carcinoma because of the sheet-like arrangement and the presence of nucleoli at higher-power magnification. *(Right)* Ganglia are common in the periprostatic tissues. They are composed of collections of ganglion cells ➡, which are characterized by large nuclei, prominent nucleoli, and cytoplasmic granules.

PROSTATE: REGIONAL ANATOMY WITH HISTOLOGIC CORRELATES

Anterior Soft Tissue

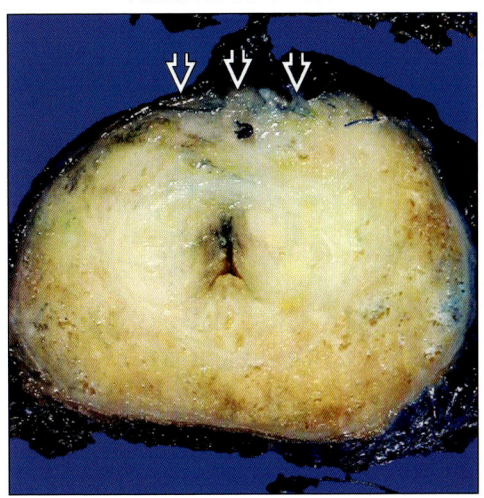

Anterior Prostate

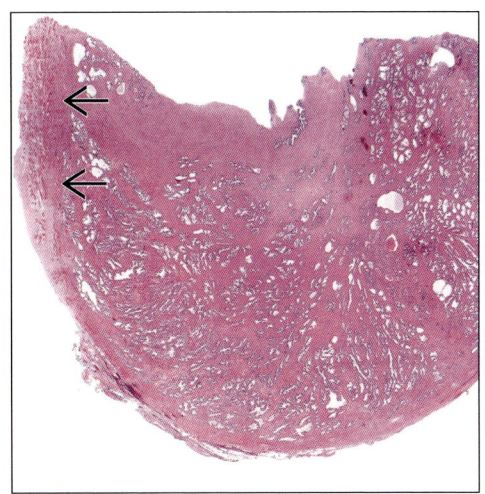

(Left) This macroscopic cross section from a radical prostatectomy specimen is oriented with the anterior soft tissue facing upward ➡. Knowledge of the composition of these anterior tissues and their boundary with the prostatic tissues can greatly facilitate cancer staging. (Courtesy G. Paner, MD.) *(Right)* This image of a half macrosection from a radical prostatectomy specimen shows the anterior stromal tissues, which are identified by skeletal muscle fibers ➡.

Anterior Prostate

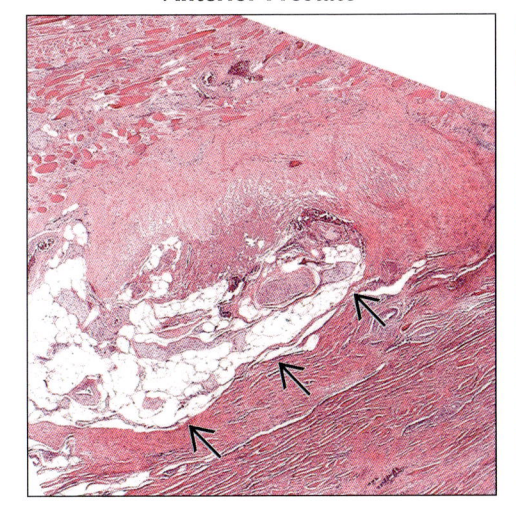

Anterior Prostate

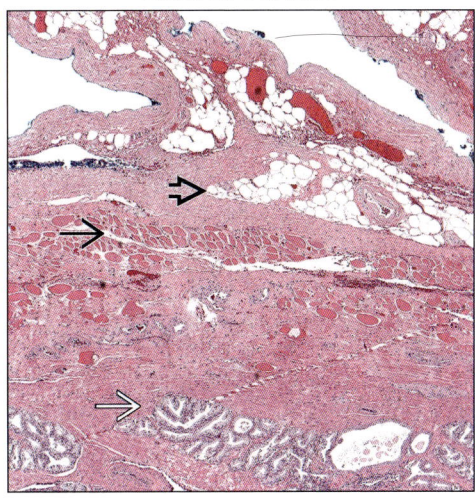

(Left) In the anterior zone of the prostate, the extraprostatic tissue is defined by the plane in which the adipose tissue is first seen ➡. Skeletal muscle may be seen on both the intra- and the extraprostatic sides of this line. *(Right)* This example of the anterior region highlights the presence of intraprostatic skeletal muscle ➡ admixed with benign glands ➡. The extraprostatic tissue would begin at the adipose tissue ➡ in this section.

Anterior Prostate

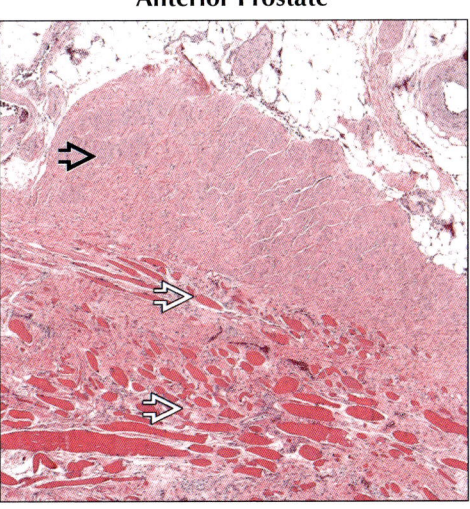

Anterior Prostate

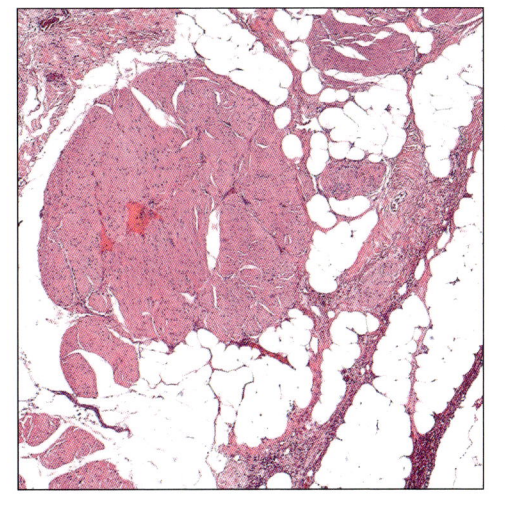

(Left) In the more superior regions of the prostate, the anterior soft tissue contains large compact bundles of smooth muscle ➡ that may be intermixed with skeletal muscle ➡. *(Right)* Large compact smooth muscle bundles within the anterior extraprostatic soft tissue may become continuous with the bladder neck musculature as one moves superiorly. Large amputations of the bladder base that extend too anteriorly may contain these bundles and, occasionally, some skeletal muscle fibers.

PROSTATE: REGIONAL ANATOMY WITH HISTOLOGIC CORRELATES

Superior Prostate Cross Section

Central Zone

(Left) The central zone glands are typically seen in sections from the bladder base. The central zone comprises a larger proportion of each macrosection as one moves superiorly. In this schematic, the paired ejaculatory ducts ➔, which course towards the urethra ➔, are also seen within the central zone. *(Right)* This section shows the unique morphology of the central zone glands, which are characterized by epithelial bridging ➔ and intraluminal papillary tufts ➔.

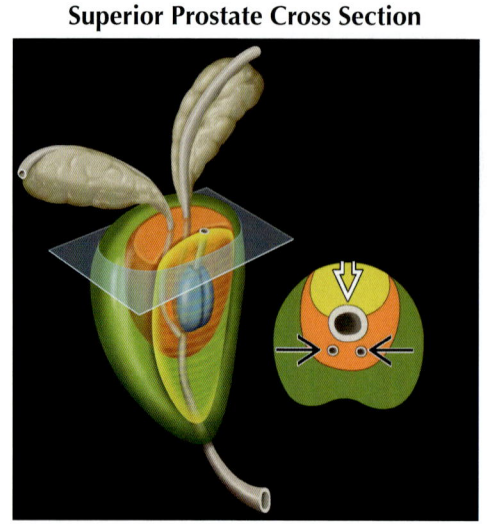

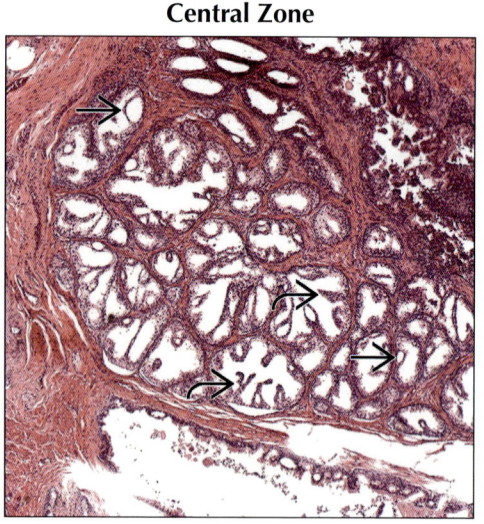

Central Zone

Central Zone

(Left) This example of central zone glands shows the characteristic epithelial bridging that forms so-called lacunar spaces ➔ and the increased number of elongated intraluminal papillary excrescences ➔. These features may be mistaken for prostatic neoplasia due to the degree of epithelial complexity. *(Right)* Immunohistochemical evaluation has demonstrated that these lacunar spaces ➔ of the benign central zone glands contain lactoferrin.

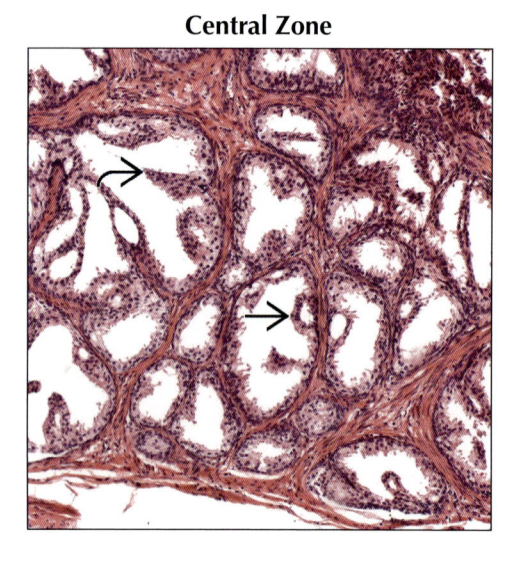

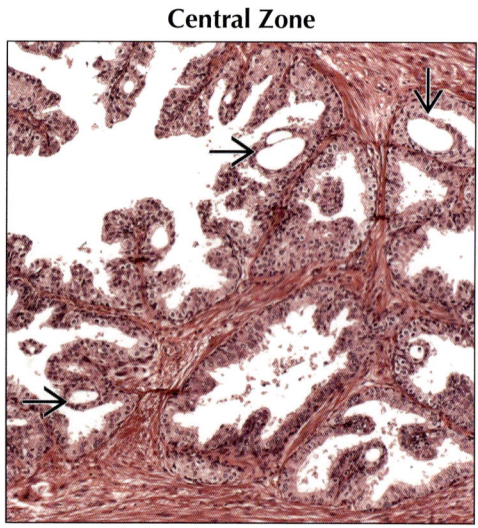

Central Zone

Central Zone

(Left) The central zone of the prostate gland may occasionally have a focal cribriform appearance ➔ that may mimic high-grade prostatic intraepithelial neoplasia or other intraductal proliferations. Typical epithelial bridging with lacunae is also seen ➔. *(Right)* This benign prostate gland was seen in a transrectal needle core biopsy labeled "bladder base." The papillary excrescences and lacunae are typical histologic features of the central zone.

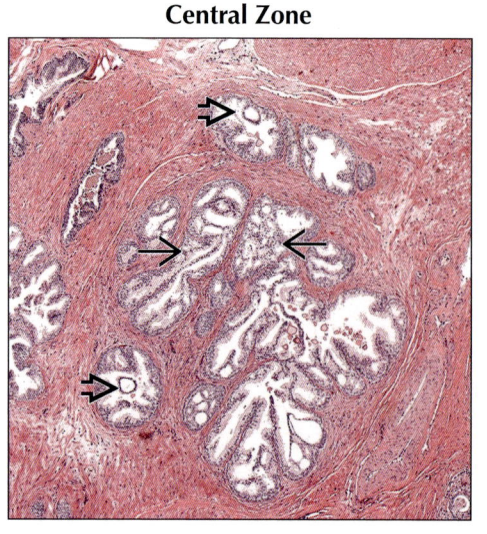

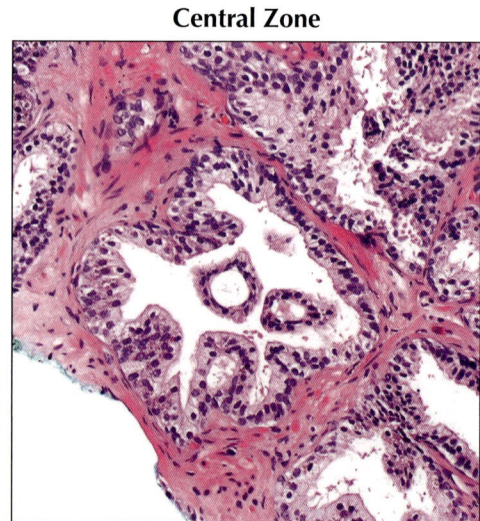

PROSTATE: REGIONAL ANATOMY WITH HISTOLOGIC CORRELATES

Course of Ejaculatory Ducts

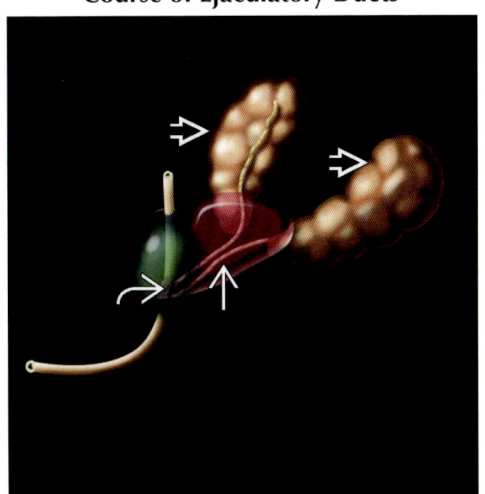

Paired Ejaculatory Ducts

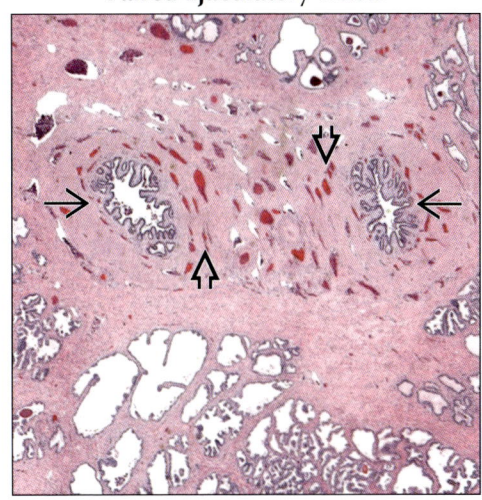

(Left) This schematic shows the relationship of the seminal vesicles ⇨ to the ejaculatory ducts ➡ and urethra ➡. The paired ejaculatory ducts course through the central zone to the urethra, where the ejaculatory contents are emptied. *(Right)* The paired ejaculatory ducts ➡ are seen in this section from a radical prostatectomy specimen. These ducts are typically surrounded by loose fibrous stroma containing numerous thin-walled blood vessels ⇨.

Ejaculatory Duct

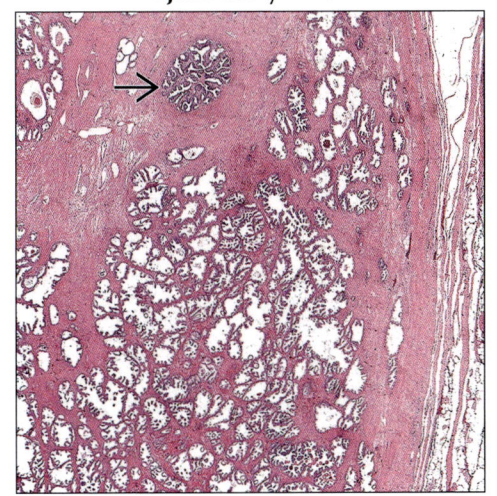

Ejaculatory Duct

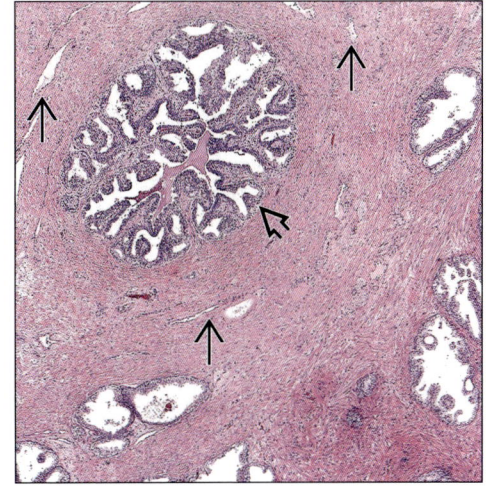

(Left) The ejaculatory duct ➡ is readily appreciable on low-power evaluation due to the central lumen with complex intraluminal epithelial infolding, which is very similar to that of the seminal vesicle. Note the surrounding rim of loose fibrous stroma. *(Right)* As shown here, each ejaculatory duct ➡ typically has a complex intraluminal papillary architecture. The rim of fibrous tissue with associated thin-walled blood vessels ⇨ is also a characteristic feature.

Paired Ejaculatory Ducts Near Urethra

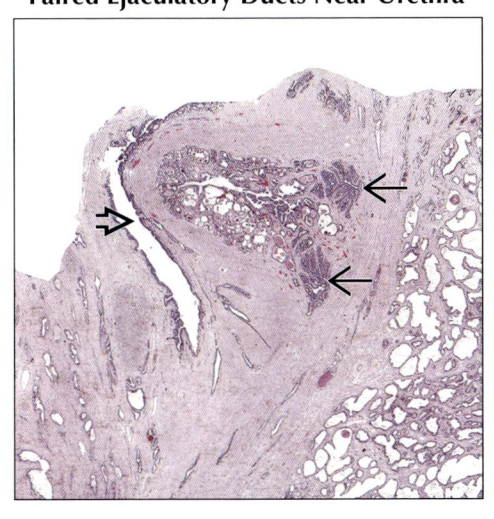

Paired Ejaculatory Ducts Near Urethra

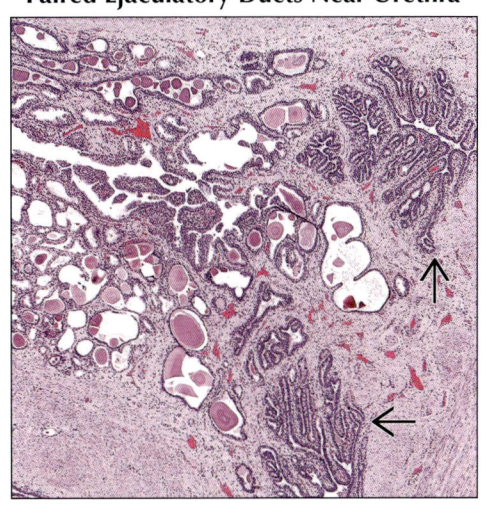

(Left) In this low-power photomicrograph of the prostatic urethra ⇨ near the verumontanum, the paired ejaculatory ducts ➡ end their course through the central zone and begin to connect with the prostatic urethral lumen, where their ejaculatory products are emptied. *(Right)* At higher power, the typical complex papillary infolding of the ejaculatory ducts ➡ is appreciated. The ejaculatory duct epithelium gradually admixes with prostatic secretory and urothelial epithelium.

PROSTATE: REGIONAL ANATOMY WITH HISTOLOGIC CORRELATES

Seminal Vesicles Attached to Prostate

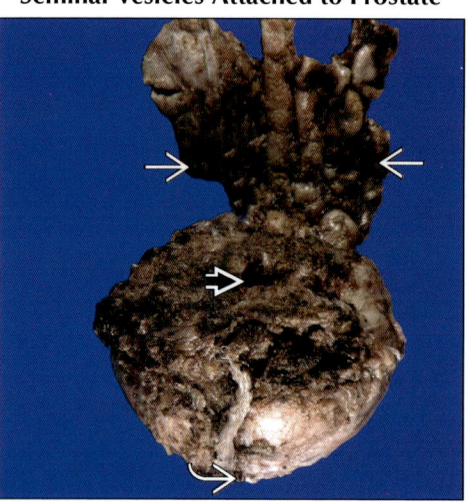

Seminal Vesicle

(Left) This prostate gland gross specimen may be oriented by the seminal vesicles ➡, the urethral opening at the bladder base ➡, and the apex ➡. The paired seminal vesicles are attached to the prostate at the superior and posterior-most aspect of the gland. *(Right)* On low-power magnification, the tortuosity of the seminal vesicle lumen may be appreciated. The surrounding thick layer of smooth muscle ➡ is a characteristic feature of the seminal vesicle as well.

Seminal Vesicle

Seminal Vesicle

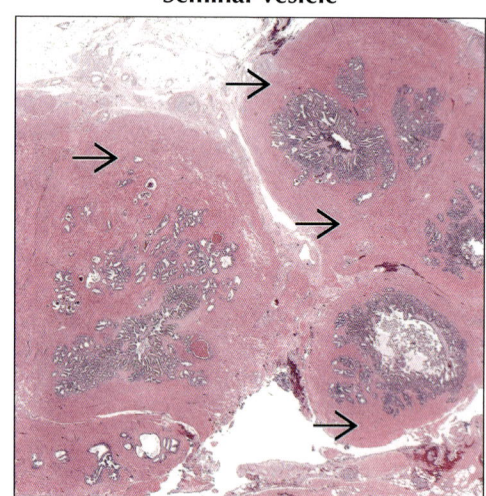

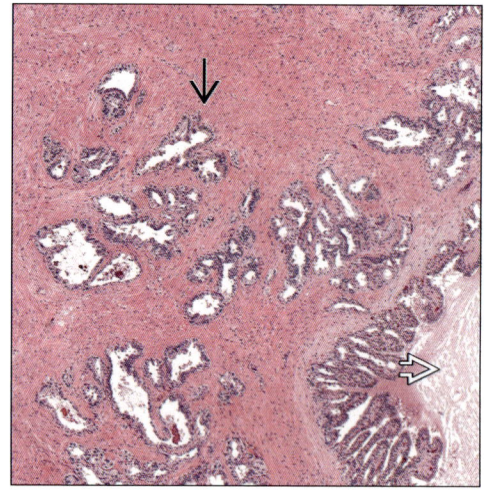

(Left) The thick muscular wall that surrounds the epithelial lined lumen is characteristic of the seminal vesicle. If carcinoma involves this muscular wall, it should be regarded as seminal vesicle involvement. *(Right)* Invaginations of seminal vesicle epithelium may form small glandular structures ➡ surrounding the central lumen ➡. This finding may occasionally mimic prostatic carcinoma glands. High-power examination will confirm seminal vesicle-type epithelium.

Seminal Vesicle Adjacent to Prostate

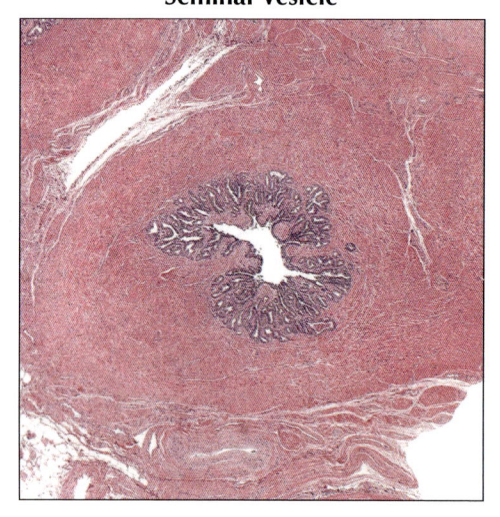

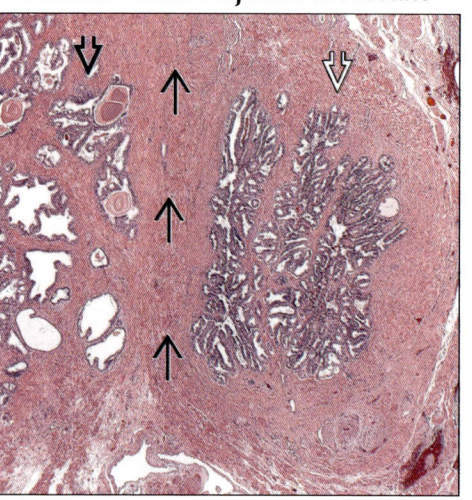

Seminal Vesicle With Prostatic Tissue in Wall

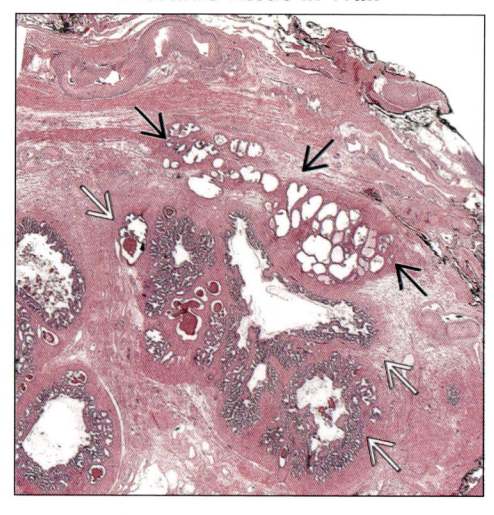

(Left) This is the normal junction ➡ between the seminal vesicle ➡ and the prostate gland ➡. Because of the very complex infolding of the seminal vesicle epithelium, the central lumen may be difficult to appreciate in some sections. *(Right)* In some prostates, collections of benign prostate glands ➡ may be found in the wall of the seminal vesicle ➡. This may be due to the proposed shared embryogenesis of the seminal vesicle and central zone of the prostate.

PROSTATE: REGIONAL ANATOMY WITH HISTOLOGIC CORRELATES

Bladder Neck

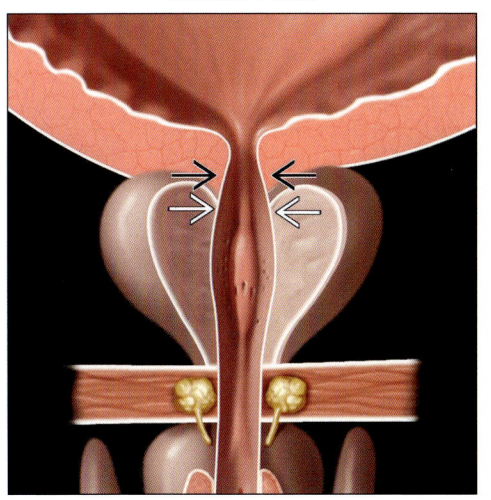

True Bladder Neck

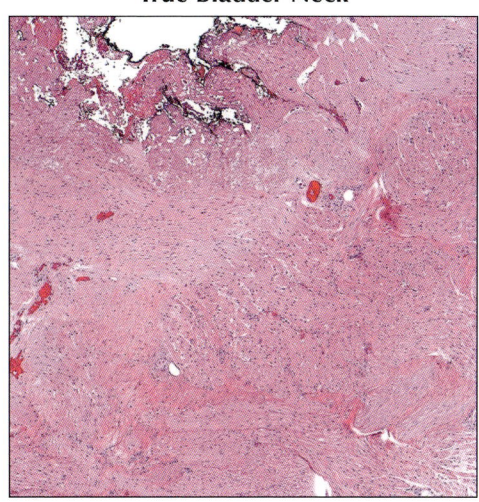

(Left) The resection plane of a prostatectomy procedure determines the type of tissue seen in the bladder base margin. A plane through the true bladder neck ➡ will produce smooth muscle, while a more inferior plane ➡ yields prostate glands. This plane may be distorted by BPH. *(Right)* This tissue taken as a margin from the bladder base of a prostatectomy specimen shows thick smooth muscle without prostate glands. This histology is diagnostic of microscopic bladder neck tissue.

True Bladder Neck

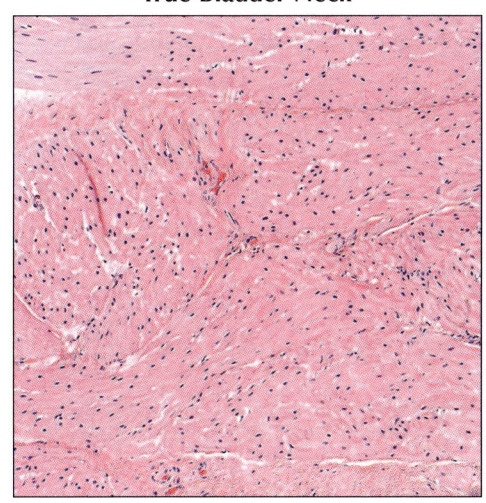

Prostate Tissue Near Bladder Base

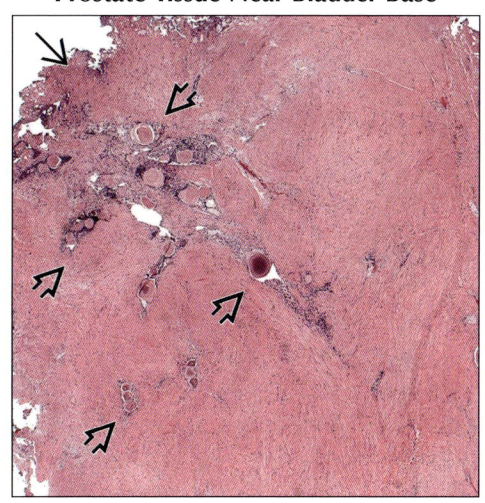

(Left) The compact smooth muscle bundles (without admixed normal prostate glands) are characteristic of the bladder neck. If carcinoma involves this tissue, it should be regarded as microscopic bladder neck invasion for staging (AJCC, 7th edition: T3a). *(Right)* Taken at the bladder base region (superior aspect) of a radical prostatectomy, this tissue should not be regarded as bladder neck for staging purposes, because of the admixed benign prostate glands ➡ (the true margin is inked ➡).

Prostate Tissue Near Bladder Base

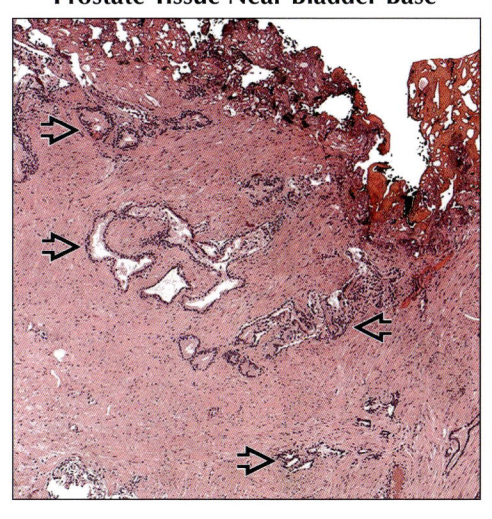

Prostate Tissue Near Bladder Base

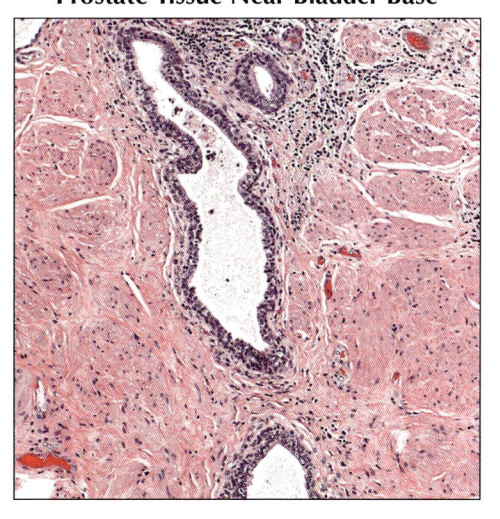

(Left) This tissue from the bladder base of a radical prostatectomy specimen also contains admixed benign prostate glands ➡ and should therefore not be regarded as bladder neck musculature. *(Right)* On high-power magnification, these glands in the bladder base margin tissue are prostatic in appearance. This represents prostatic tissue in the bladder base due to a resection plane inferior to the true bladder neck. Carcinoma involving such tissue should be staged as intraprostatic.

PROSTATE: BENIGN GLANDULAR AND STROMAL HISTOLOGY

Key Facts

Macroscopic Anatomy
- Prostate gland
  - Located inferior to urinary bladder, superior to pelvic floor, and anterior to rectum
- Seminal vesicles
  - Paired glandular structures located in superior/posterior region of prostate
  - Extend superiorly along posterior aspect of bladder
- Cowper (bulbourethral) glands
  - Paired glandular structures located just distal to prostate gland in periurethral region

Microscopic Anatomy
- Prostate glands are composed of 2 cell layers
  - Secretory cells are luminal facing and have clear to eosinophilic, sometimes vacuolated cytoplasm
  - Secretory cells show immunoreactivity for PSA and PSAP but not for p63 or high molecular weight cytokeratin
  - Basal cells located adjacent to underlying stroma, beneath secretory cells, with high nuclear to cytoplasmic ratios and frequent small nucleoli
  - Basal cells show immunoreactivity for p63 &/or high molecular weight cytokeratin but not for PSA and PSAP
- Prostatic stroma
  - Histologic appearance depends on presence or absence of hyperplasia
  - Normal stroma has fibromuscular appearance
  - Cytologically bland spindled cells with varying collagenous to myxoid stroma and associated small blood vessels in transition zone with hyperplasia
- Periurethral tissue
  - Complex glandular tissue with admixture of prostatic secretory epithelium and urothelium

Pitfalls/Artifacts
- Normal variation in prostate histology may mimic malignancy (benign lesions typically show at least focally retained basal cell layer)
  - Simple atrophy
  - Cystic atrophy
  - Partial atrophy
  - Sclerotic atrophy
  - Adenosis
  - Inflammatory changes
  - Mesonephric remnants
  - Nephrogenic adenoma
  - Clear cell cribriform hyperplasia
  - Sclerosing adenosis
- Radiation atypia in benign glands
  - Glands with scattered pleomorphic cells
  - Atrophic eosinophilic cytoplasm

Age Variation
- Benign prostatic hyperplasia is common with increasing age with resultant enlargement of transition zone
  - Leads to urinary obstructive symptoms
- Atrophy appears to be more common in older individuals

Metaplasia
- Transitional (urothelial)
  - Extension of urothelium into prostatic glands, typically of transition zone
  - Stratified epithelium with frequent longitudinal nuclear grooves
- Mucinous metaplasia
  - Rare cells with intracytoplasmic mucin may be present in benign glands

Hyperplasia
- Benign prostatic glandular and stromal hyperplasia in periurethral transition zone
  - Stromal hyperplasia with cellular nodules of benign spindled cells
  - Lobular glandular hyperplasia with increased gland density
- Basal cell hyperplasia
  - Cellular aggregates of basophilic cells at periphery of prostate glands
  - Basal cells may entirely fill glands
  - Fairly common in transition zone

(Left) Normal glands typically show an undulating epithelial/luminal interface. The secretory cells ➡ have pale, sometimes vacuolated cytoplasm. The basal cell layer ➡ is prominent in this example. (Right) Normal prostate glands are typically of medium to large caliber and are aggregated into loose groups surrounded by fibromuscular stroma. Corpora amylacea ➡ are common in the lumina of benign glands.

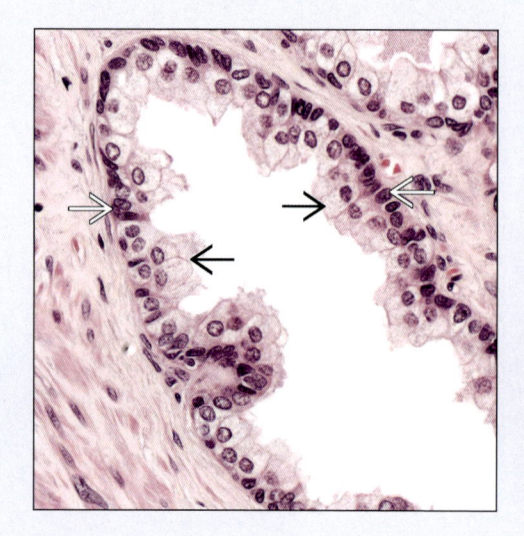

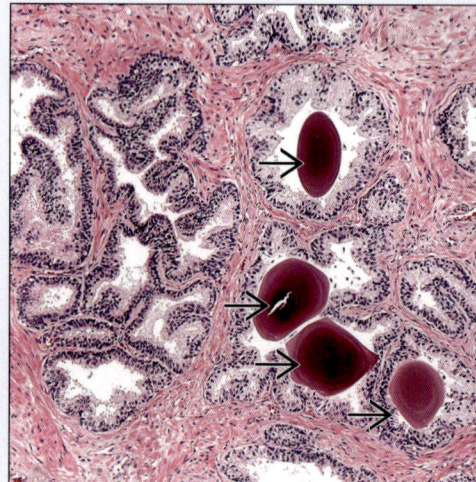

PROSTATE: BENIGN GLANDULAR AND STROMAL HISTOLOGY

Architecture

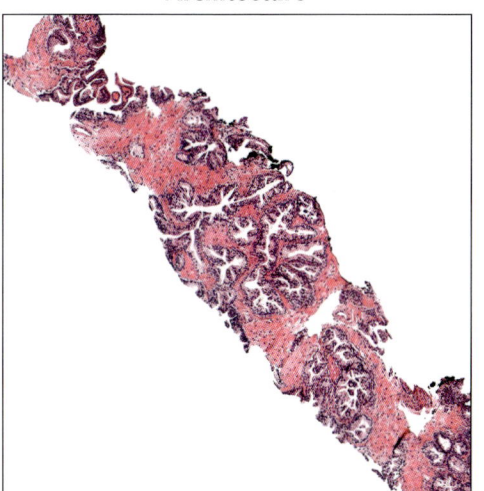

Architecture

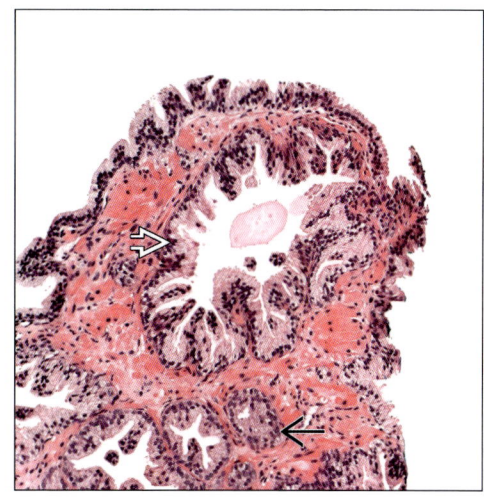

(Left) At low power, benign nonatrophic prostate glands are typically of similar caliber and are evenly distributed or arranged into vague aggregates. Glands may be rounded or elongated, arranged in a branching configuration. Elongated branching glands are sometimes referred to as "ducts." (Right) This benign gland demonstrates the typical undulating or tufted secretory cell layer ➡. Glands of smaller caliber may be seen at the edge of larger glands ➡ due to tangential sectioning.

Glands

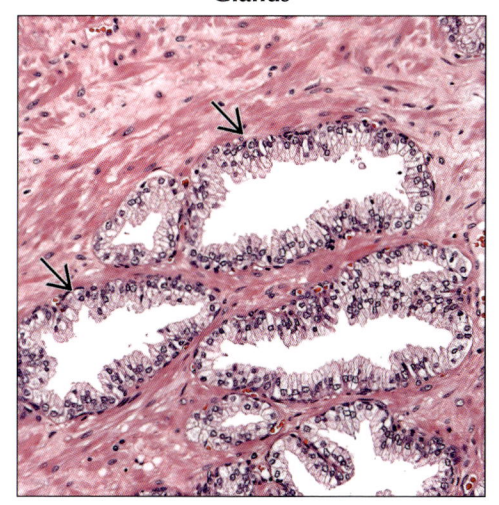

Glands

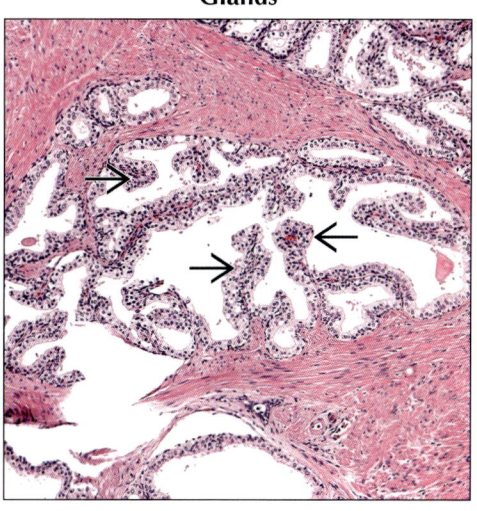

(Left) Some benign glands are of a smaller caliber and have less intraluminal complexity; however, the luminal surface still has some subtle undulation ➡. In contrast, prostatic adenocarcinoma glands often have a very sharply defined luminal surface. (Right) Benign prostate glands may have larger intraluminal papillary excrescences ➡, particularly in certain regions, such as the prostatic central zone. These large luminal infoldings are less common in carcinoma glands.

Nuclei

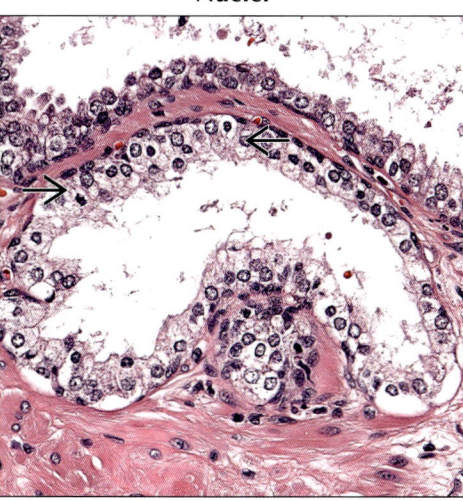

Nuclei/Cytoplasm

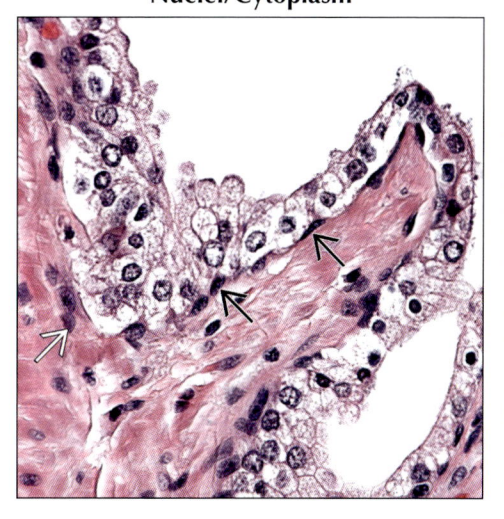

(Left) In normal glands, the distance between a nucleus and the basement membrane is variable ➡. Many carcinomas are characterized by nuclei that are more uniformly basal in location. (Right) The pale to clear cytoplasm of the secretory cells in this gland is typical, as are the round nuclei that vary in distance from the basement membrane. A flattened basal cell layer ➡ is variably seen in benign glands, which may resemble adjacent stromal cells ➡ by routine H&E morphology.

PROSTATE: BENIGN GLANDULAR AND STROMAL HISTOLOGY

Benign Prostatic Hyperplasia

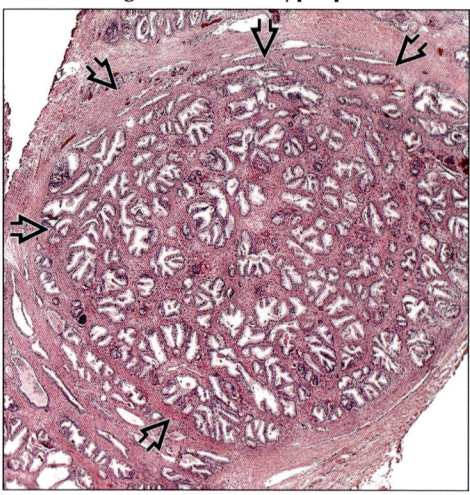

Benign Prostatic Hyperplasia

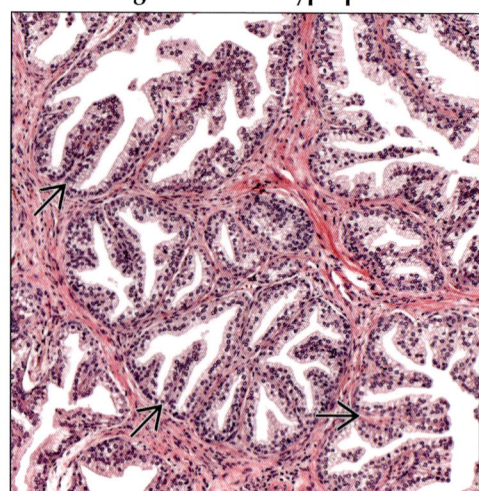

(Left) In this transurethral prostate resection specimen, the nodular, circumscribed arrangement of these glands is characteristic of benign prostatic hyperplasia ⇨. Even on low-power examination, some intraluminal infolding within the glands is appreciable. *(Right)* This degree of intraluminal infolding with resultant papillary excrescences → is typical of the benign prostatic glands often seen in glandular hyperplasia.

Benign Prostatic Hyperplasia

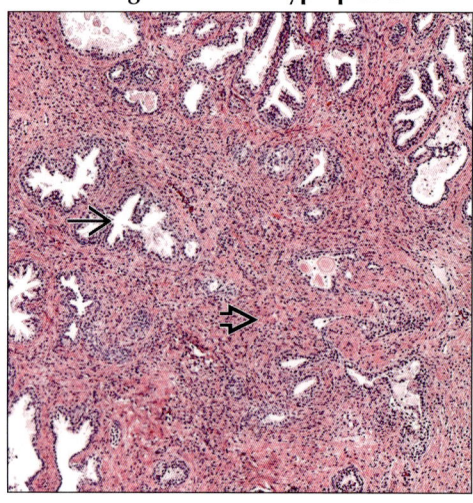

Benign Prostatic Hyperplasia

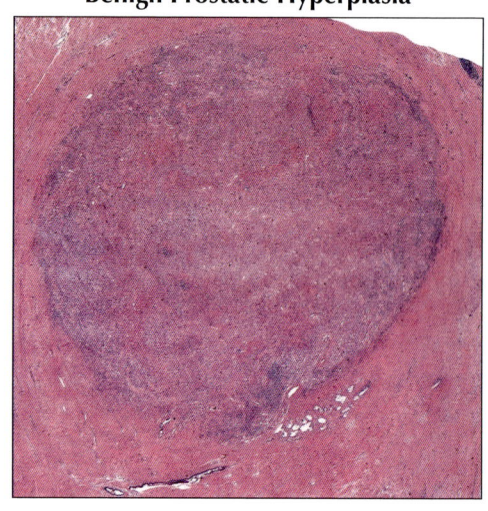

(Left) In this example of benign prostatic hyperplasia, there is an equal admixture of benign prostatic glands → and prostatic stroma ⇨. One may see a varying admixture of glands and stroma within an individual specimen. *(Right)* This well-circumscribed nodule is characteristic of a pure hyperplastic stromal nodule, which is part of the spectrum of benign prostatic hyperplasias. These nodules are frequent incidental findings in radical prostatectomy specimens.

Stromal Hyperplasia

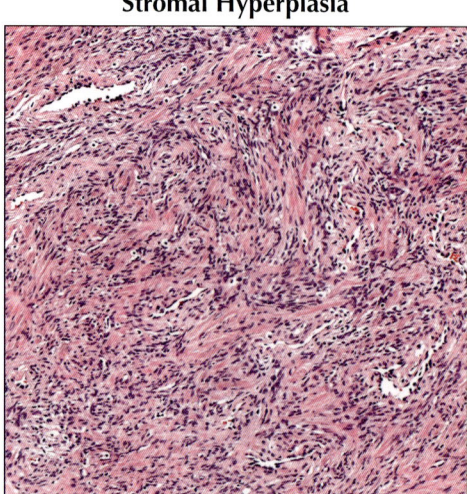

Stromal Hyperplasia

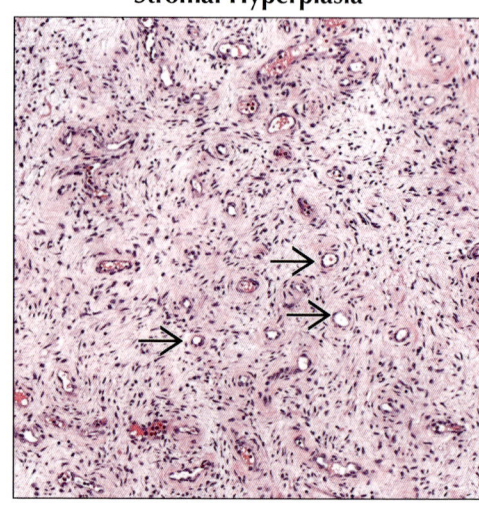

(Left) Cellular foci of pure prostatic stromal cells without glands are seen in areas of nodular stromal hyperplasia. The spindle cells are monomorphic without the degree of nuclear size variation or hyperchromasia often seen in a stromal neoplasm. *(Right)* Small caliber blood vessels → admixed with loose myxoid stroma are characteristic features of a benign hyperplastic stromal nodule.

PROSTATE: BENIGN GLANDULAR AND STROMAL HISTOLOGY

Basal Cell Hyperplasia

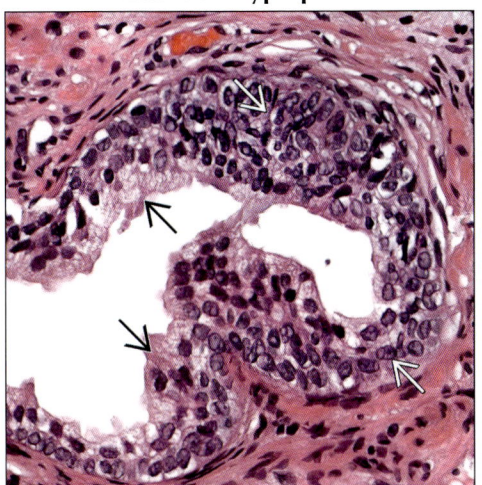

Prominent Basal Cells

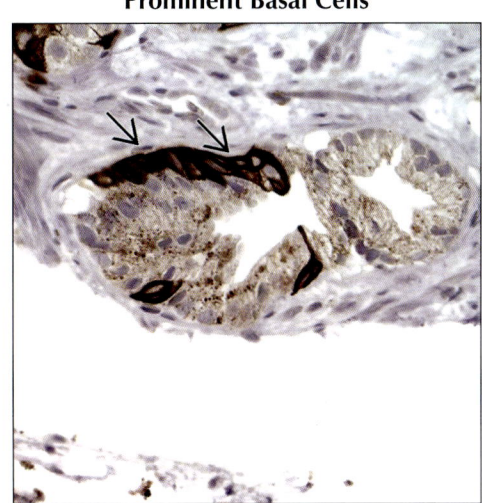

(Left) This benign prostate gland with basal cell hyperplasia highlights the distinction between the basal cells and secretory cells. The secretory cells have more abundant cytoplasm ⇒ and are luminally oriented. The basal cells form nodular aggregates along the basement membrane side of the gland ⇒. *(Right)* The basal cells are highlighted by strong cytoplasmic immunoreactivity for high molecular weight cytokeratin ⇒. The secretory cell layer is nonreactive with this antibody.

Basal Cell Hyperplasia in BPH

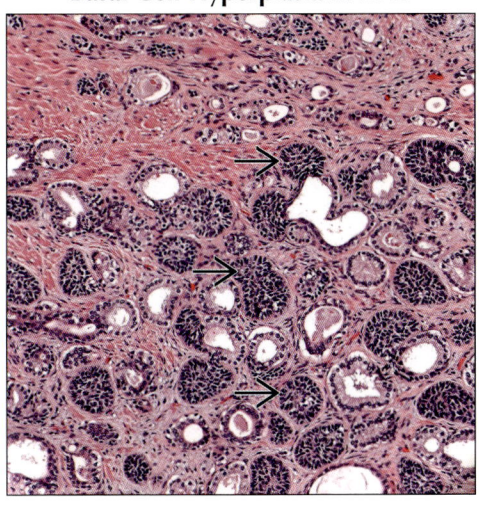

Simple Atrophy

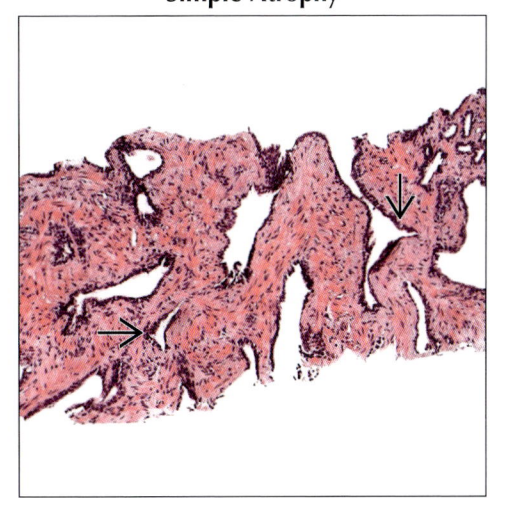

(Left) In this photograph, multiple glands contain peripheral nodules of basal cells or appear completely filled by dark basophilic cells with a high N:C ratio ⇒, typical of basal cell hyperplasia. The presence of nests of basal cells within a population of otherwise normal glands can mimic an infiltrative process. *(Right)* In simple prostate gland atrophy, there is a marked loss of cytoplasm in the individual prostatic secretory cells. Frequently, the atrophic glands also have a more angulated shape ⇒.

Simple Atrophy

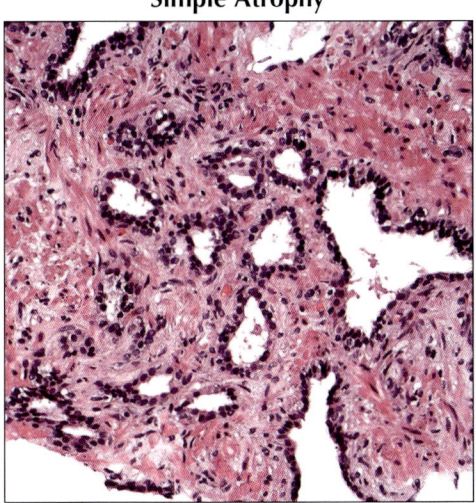

Cystic Atrophy

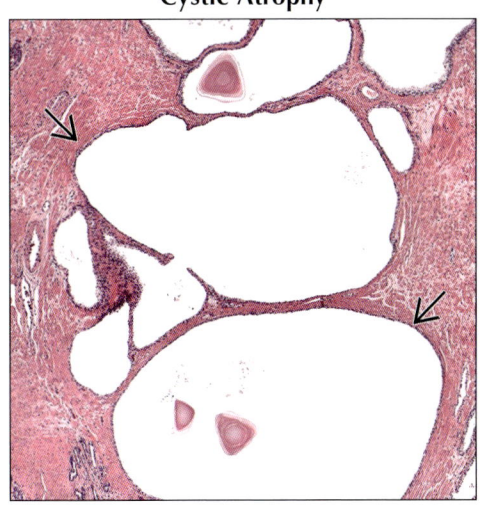

(Left) On higher power magnification, these atrophic glands have a uniform loss of cytoplasm that imparts a very basophilic appearance to the glands. When the benign atrophic glands are crowded, as in this example, they may mimic a low-grade adenocarcinoma. *(Right)* In cystic atrophy, the benign prostatic glands become markedly dilated and often have a rounded shape ⇒. Similar to the cells of simple atrophy, the individual prostatic secretory cells have a loss of luminal cytoplasm.

PROSTATE: BENIGN GLANDULAR AND STROMAL HISTOLOGY

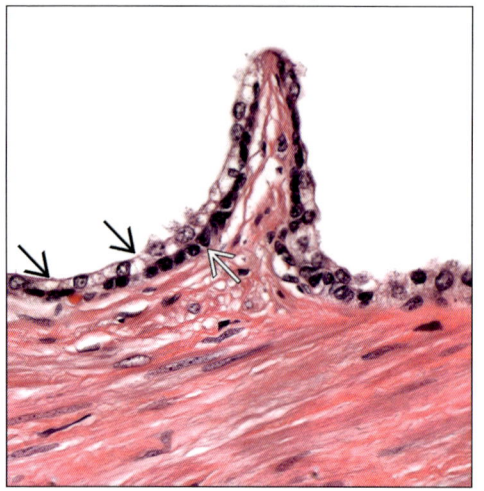

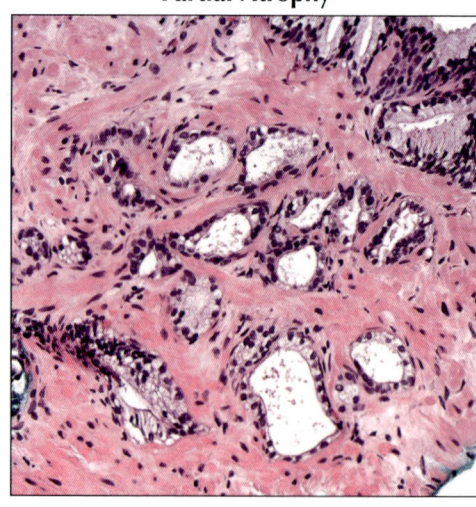

(Left) On evaluation of the lining epithelium in a large gland with cystic atrophy, the secretory cells contain no luminal cytoplasm, but there is some residual cytoplasm lateral to the nucleus ➡. A distinct basal cell layer is evident in this example ➡. **(Right)** The small glands of partial atrophy are typically crowded. There is loss of luminal cytoplasm and some gland angulation.

Cystic Atrophy

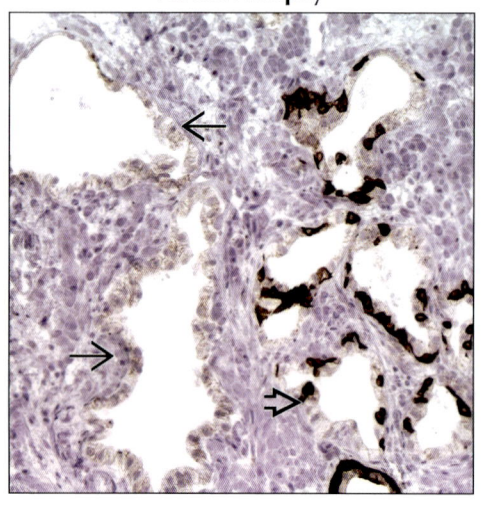

Partial Atrophy

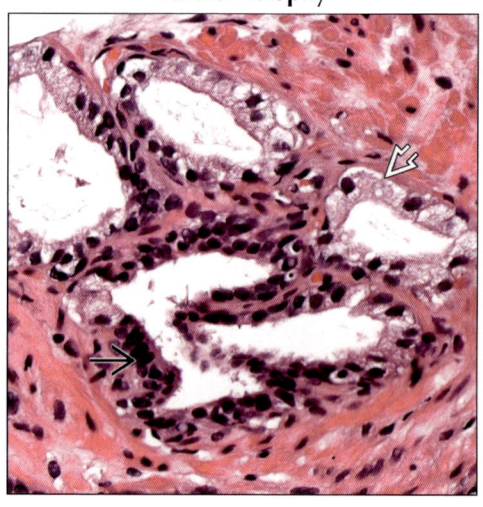

(Left) In this high molecular weight cytokeratin antibody immunostain, a patchy discontinuous basal cell layer is highlighted ➡ in a subset of the glands, while some of the glands do not show a basal cell layer ➡. This finding is typical of benign partial atrophy. **(Right)** On higher power magnification, the secretory cells in partial atrophy typically have variable areas of complete atrophy ➡ and areas with residual cytoplasm located lateral to the nucleus ➡.

Partial Atrophy

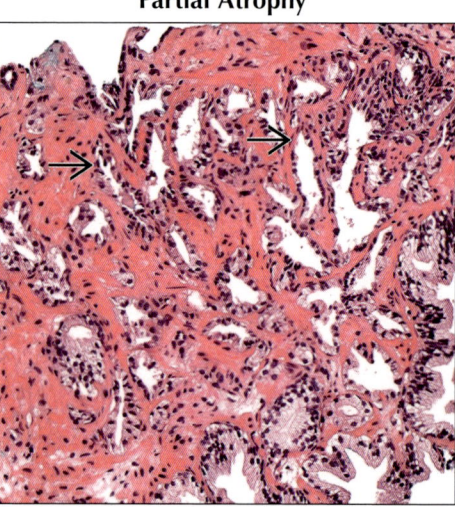

Partial Atrophy

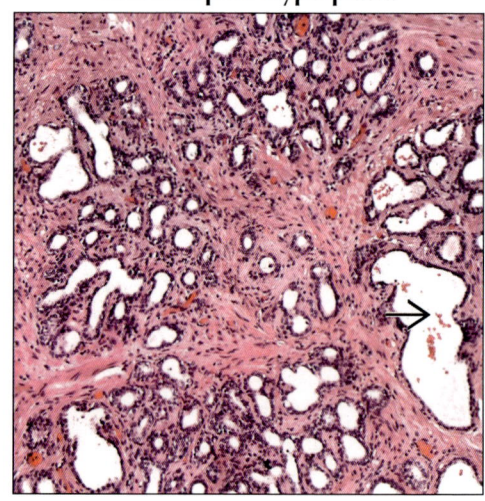

(Left) In this example of partial atrophy, the glands have a more disorganized pseudoinfiltrative appearance. Atrophic glands often have a more angulated contour ➡. In partial atrophy, the glands have variable amounts of luminal cytoplasm. **(Right)** Post-atrophic hyperplasia is characterized by vaguely circumscribed collections of small rounded atrophic glands, often with associated larger-caliber ducts/glands ➡.

Partial Atrophy

Post-Atrophic Hyperplasia

PROSTATE: BENIGN GLANDULAR AND STROMAL HISTOLOGY

Post-Atrophic Hyperplasia

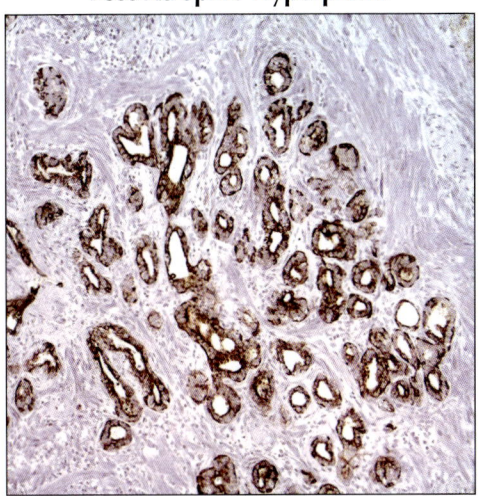

Sclerotic Atrophy

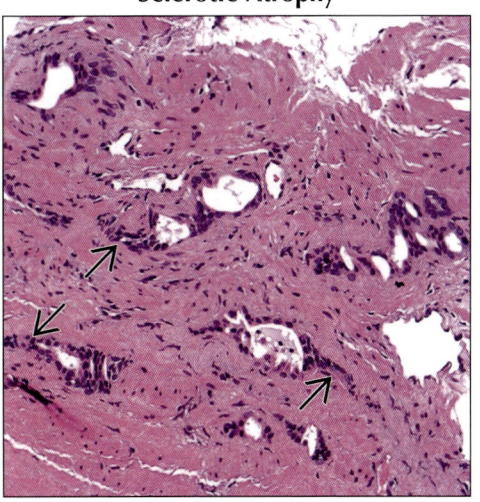

(Left) In contrast to partial atrophy, post-atrophic hyperplasia has a very prominent basal cell population that can be easily demonstrated by immunohistochemical markers, such as high molecular weight cytokeratin (as shown here), cytokeratin 5/6, or p63. *(Right)* Sclerotic atrophy is a benign change that can closely mimic invasive carcinoma in other organ systems. The glands are often angulated with pointed ends ⇒, and the surrounding stroma appears more densely collagenized.

Sclerotic Atrophy

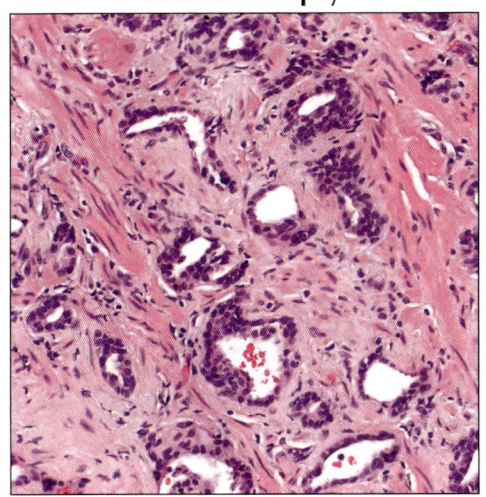

Clear Cell Cribriform Hyperplasia

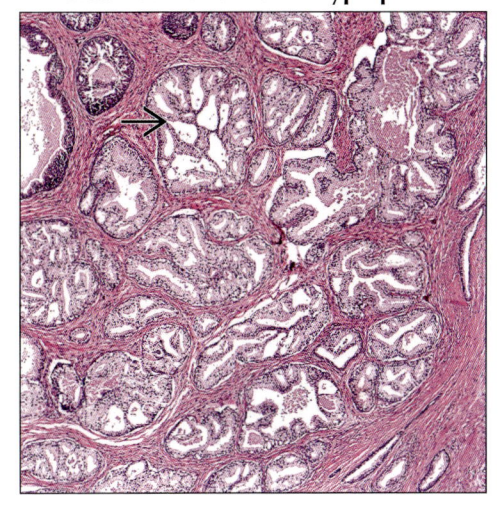

(Left) The surrounding changes seen in sclerotic atrophy resemble the stromal responses that may be seen in invasive carcinomas in other organs; however, this type of stromal response is rare in prostate cancer. *(Right)* In the transition zone, a benign cribriforming process may be encountered that is termed clear cell cribriform hyperplasia. The epithelial cells may bridge the entire gland ⇒, a feature that mimics neoplastic intraductal lesions. (Courtesy G. Paner, MD.)

Clear Cell Cribriform Hyperplasia

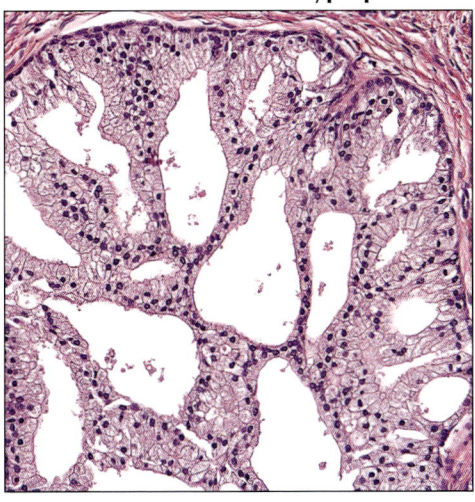

Mesonephric Remnants

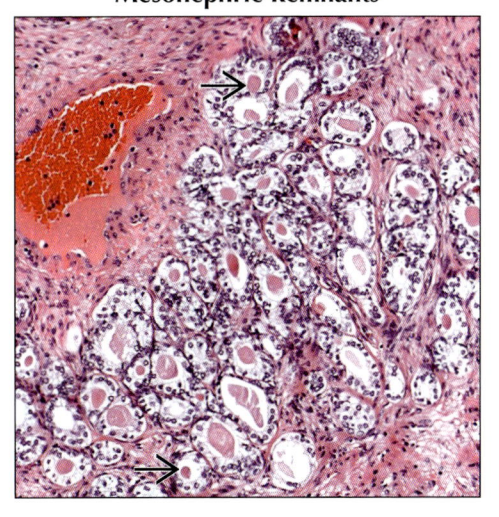

(Left) Clear cell cribriform hyperplasia, unlike intraductal carcinoma or cribriform high grade prostatic intraepithelial neoplasia, has bland cytologic features without nucleomegaly &/or prominent nucleoli. (Courtesy G. Paner, MD.) *(Right)* Mesonephric remnants are identical to those commonly found in the uterine cervix. They are characterized by small glandular structures, which typically contain a densely eosinophilic rounded intraluminal concretions ⇒.

PROSTATE: BENIGN GLANDULAR AND STROMAL HISTOLOGY

(Left) With associated inflammatory infiltrates (both acute ⇒ and chronic ⇒), the benign prostatic glands may appear more crowded with a pseudoinfiltrative appearance, and darker due to the loss of cytoplasm. **(Right)** In the presence of intraluminal neutrophils ⇒, benign prostatic glands may show some degree of nucleomegaly and may contain small nucleoli. These features should not be attributed to neoplasia in this inflammatory setting.

Inflammatory Changes

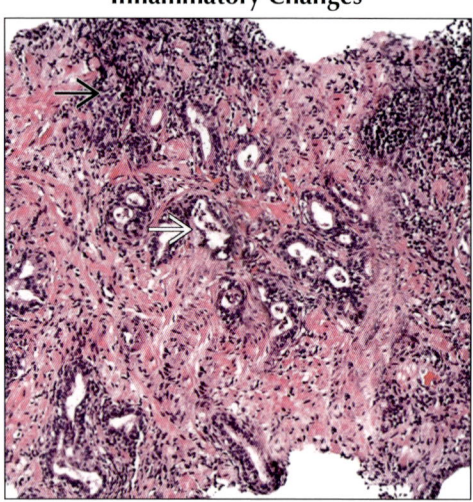

Inflammatory Changes

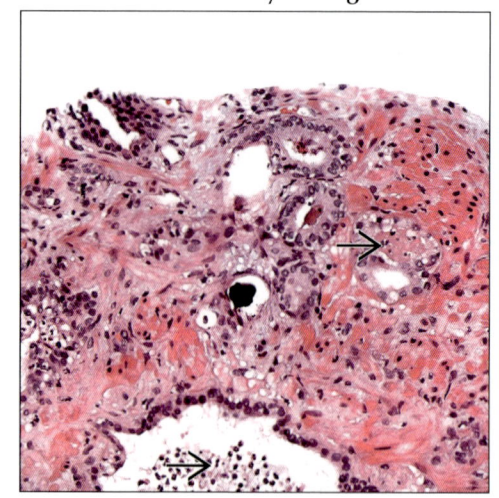

(Left) In prostates that contain a dense chronic inflammatory infiltrate, a pseudocribriform epithelial pattern ⇒ may be seen that can mimic a neoplastic process, such as cribriform adenocarcinoma. **(Right)** In this example of benign glands with associated chronic inflammation, the dense intraepithelial lymphocytic infiltrate imparts a pseudocribriform pattern with an increased basophilic appearance.

Inflammatory Changes

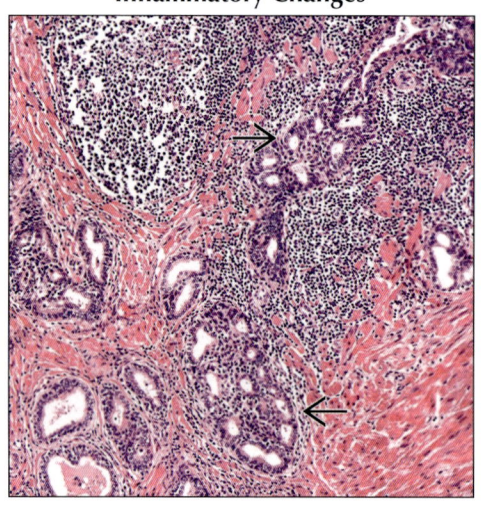

Inflammatory Changes

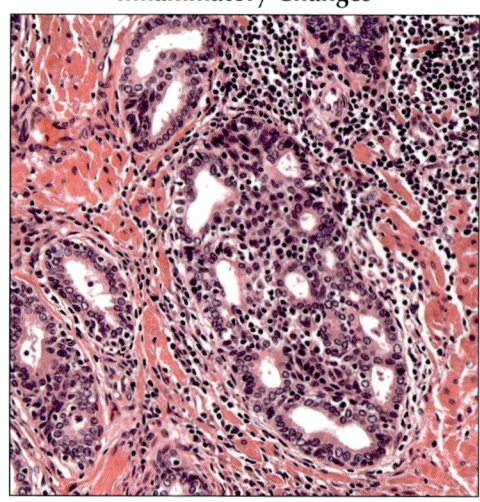

(Left) Benign prostatic glands may contain thin epithelial bridges in the setting of marked inflammatory infiltrates ⇒. This is 1 of the few benign cribriforming lesions. **(Right)** Inflamed benign prostate glands have a more basophilic appearance due to the loss of cytoplasm (higher nuclear to cytoplasmic ratio) and the increased number of cells per unit area. Cytologic features should be interpreted cautiously in the presence of intraluminal acute inflammation ⇒.

Inflammatory Changes

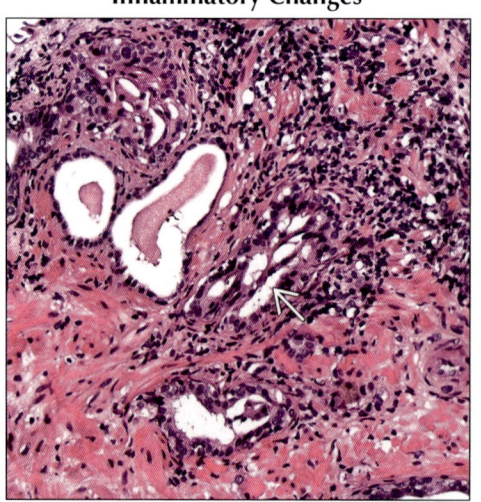

Inflammatory Changes

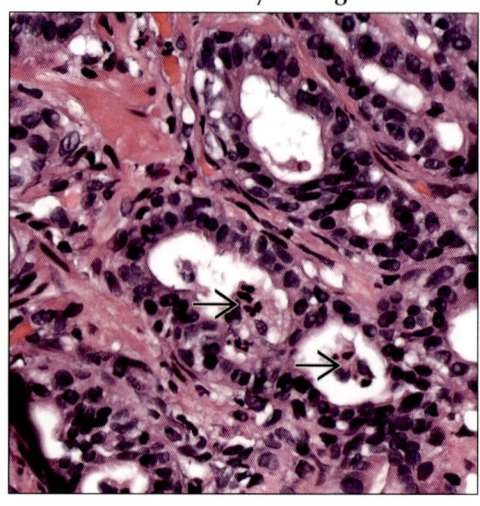

PROSTATE: BENIGN GLANDULAR AND STROMAL HISTOLOGY

Ejaculatory Duct

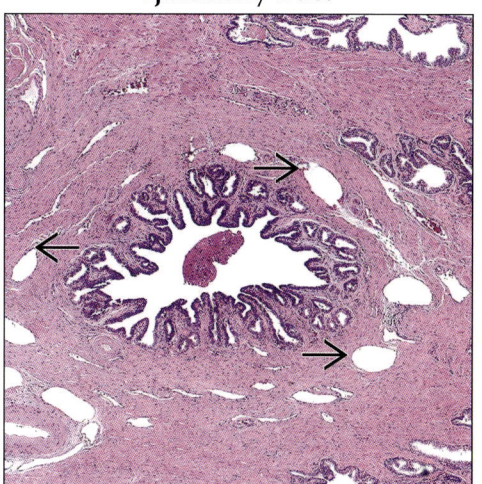

Ejaculatory Duct

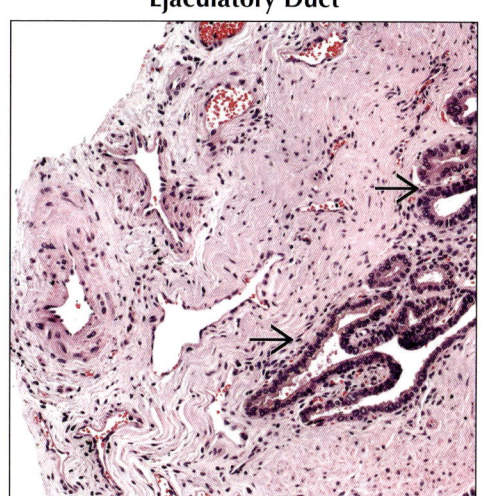

(Left) In contrast to the dense smooth muscle of the seminal vesicle, the ejaculatory duct is surrounded by a loose collagenous stroma, which often contains delicate thin-walled blood vessels ➡. This structure is seen within the prostate gland, coursing toward the prostatic urethra. *(Right)* The loose fibrous stroma and dilated thin-walled vessels in this biopsy tissue are characteristic of the soft tissue surrounding the ejaculatory duct ➡.

Ejaculatory Duct

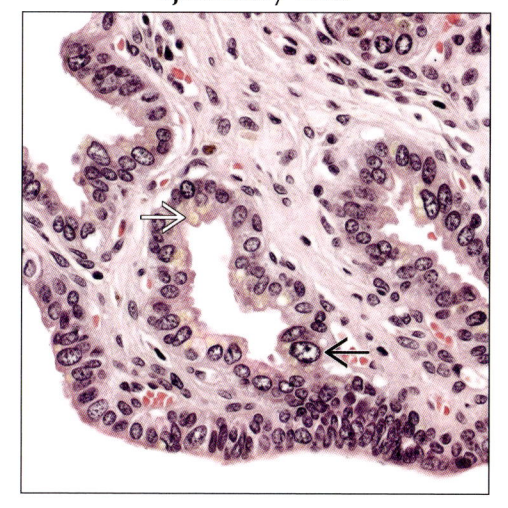

Cowper Gland

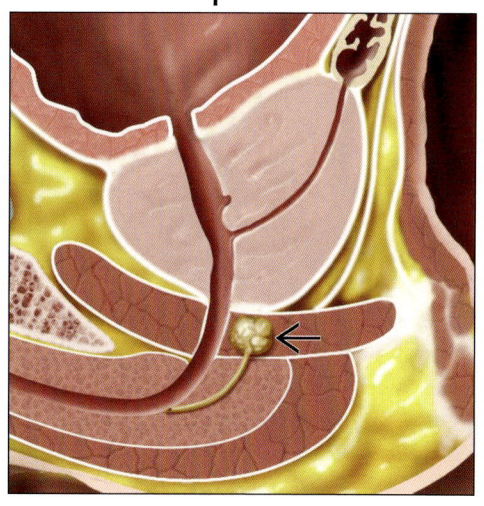

(Left) The epithelium that lines the ejaculatory duct is histologically indistinguishable from that of the seminal vesicle. It contains both the characteristic intracytoplasmic lipochrome pigment ➡ and scattered pleomorphic nuclei ➡. *(Right)* The Cowper (or bulbourethral) glands are paired glandular structures located just distal to the prostate gland ➡. They are typically intermixed with the surrounding skeletal muscle.

Cowper Gland

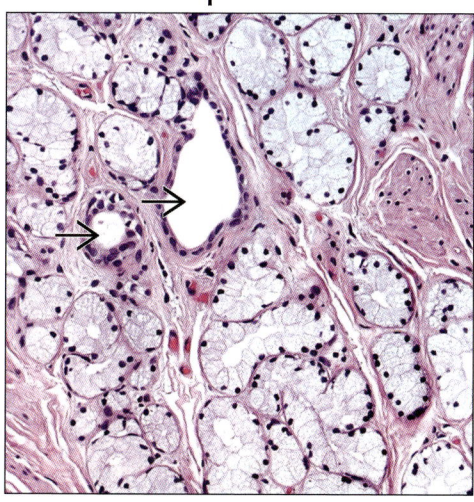

Cowper Gland

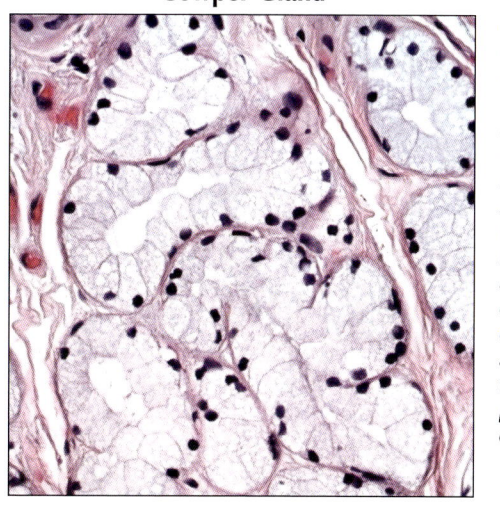

(Left) The Cowper gland is characterized by a lobular arrangement with a central duct ➡ that is surrounded by acini that are filled with cells containing intracytoplasmic mucin. This appearance is similar to minor salivary glands. *(Right)* The small cytologically bland nuclei and the lobular architectural arrangement of Cowper gland aid in its distinction from prostatic adenocarcinoma. In addition, the mucin associated with prostate cancer is commonly extracellular/intraluminal.

PROSTATE: BENIGN GLANDULAR AND STROMAL HISTOLOGY

Seminal Vesicle

Seminal Vesicle

(Left) The seminal vesicles, which are paired structures, are located at the superiormost aspect of the prostate gland and are attached posteriorly. Both have a compact layer of dense smooth muscle ⇒ that surrounds the luminal epithelium. Adjacent prostatic tissue ⇒ is often present in histologic sections. *(Right)* On high-power magnification, the dense smooth muscle wall ⇒ of the seminal vesicle is seen underlying the invaginations of epithelium ⇒.

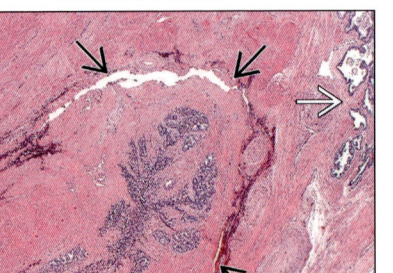

Seminal Vesicle

Seminal Vesicle

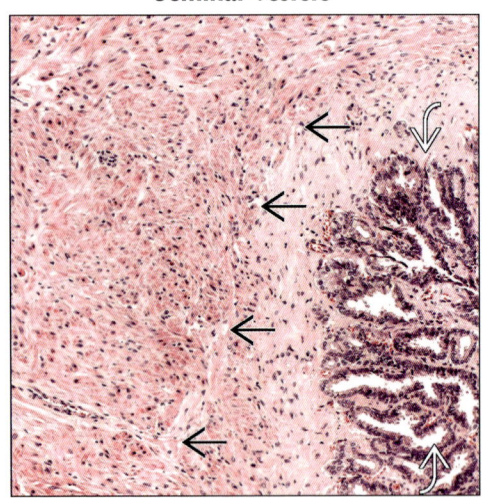

(Left) The seminal vesicle typically has a central lumen (right lower edge of the field) ⇒ surrounded by a layer of epithelium with complex invaginations into the surrounding stroma. *(Right)* At the periphery of the large central lumen of the seminal vesicle, the epithelium is frequently tangentially sectioned, imparting the appearance of infiltrative small glands. This appearance may closely mimic prostatic adenocarcinoma.

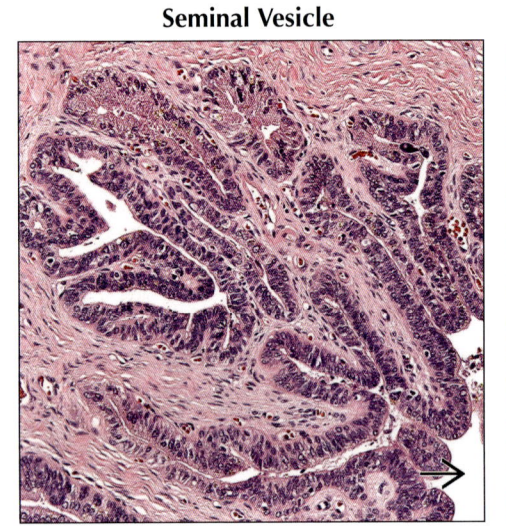

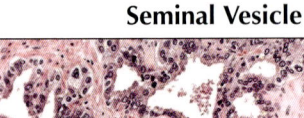

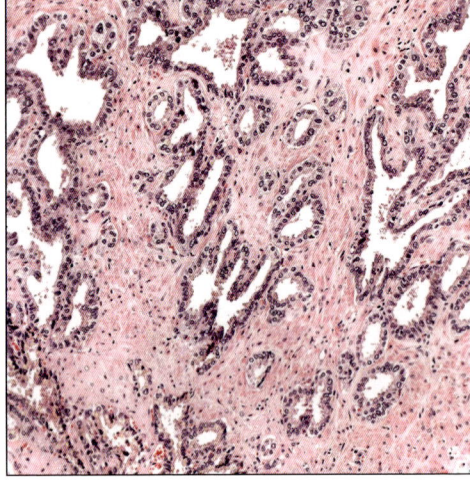

Seminal Vesicle

Seminal Vesicle

(Left) Seminal vesicle epithelium is characterized by cells with scattered pleomorphic nuclei ⇒. In contrast, prostatic adenocarcinoma is composed of cells with more monomorphic round nuclei. *(Right)* The combination of pleomorphic nuclei ⇒ and intracytoplasmic lipochrome pigment ⇒ helps to confirm seminal vesicle epithelium. In difficult cases, the nuclear expression of pax-8 is also characteristic of seminal vesicle epithelium.

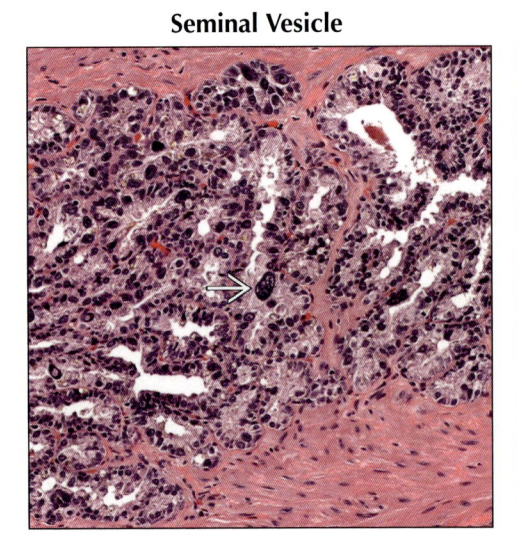

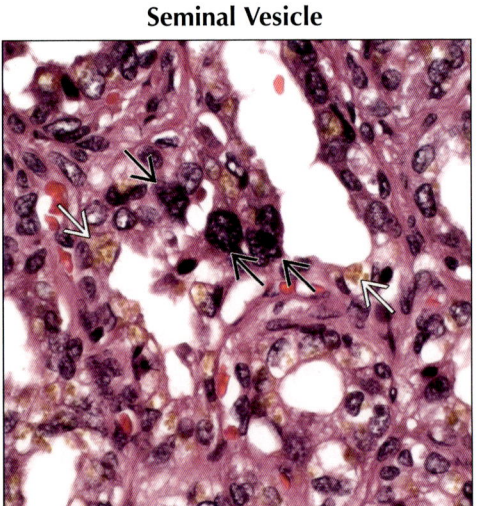

PROSTATE: BENIGN GLANDULAR AND STROMAL HISTOLOGY

Extraprostatic Tissues

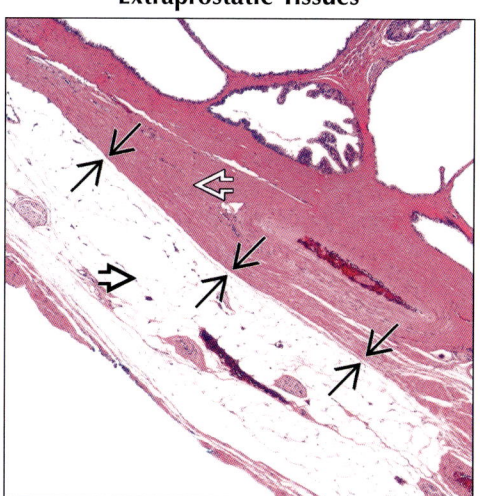

Extraprostatic Tissues: Peripheral Nerves

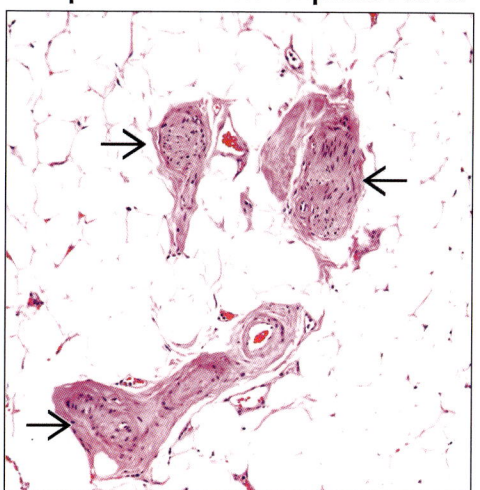

(Left) This section from a radical prostatectomy specimen highlights the extraprostatic tissue, defined as the soft tissue peripheral/external to the plane ⇒ between the prostatic stroma ⇒ and the adipose tissue ⇒. The plane is very distinct in this section, but it may be less well developed in other areas. *(Right)* Varying sized peripheral nerves ⇒ are frequently encountered in the extraprostatic connective tissues.

Extraprostatic Tissues: Blood Vessels

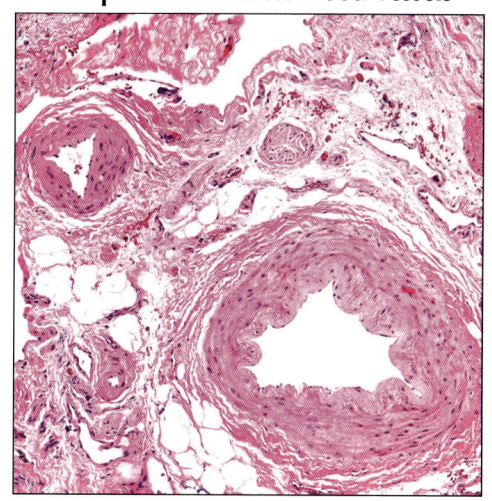

Extraprostatic Tissues: Paraganglia

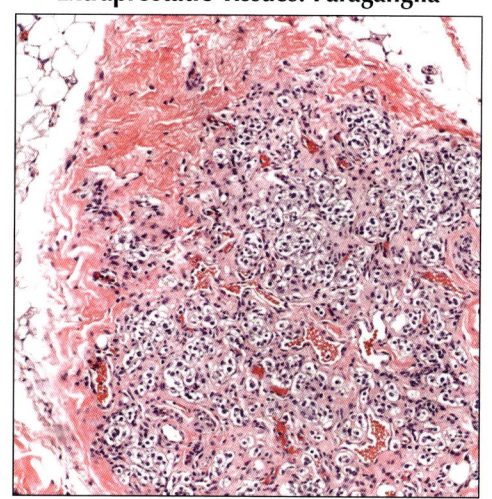

(Left) Blood vessels of varying caliber are common in the extraprostatic tissues. *(Right)* Normal paraganglia are occasionally found in extraprostatic tissues. The cells are often round and have clear to amphophilic cytoplasm. The cells may grow as small nests or have a more sheet-like arrangement. These paraganglia may easily be mistaken for high-grade prostatic adenocarcinoma. By immunohistochemistry, they are cytokeratin negative and synaptophysin/chromogranin positive.

Extraprostatic Tissues: Ganglion

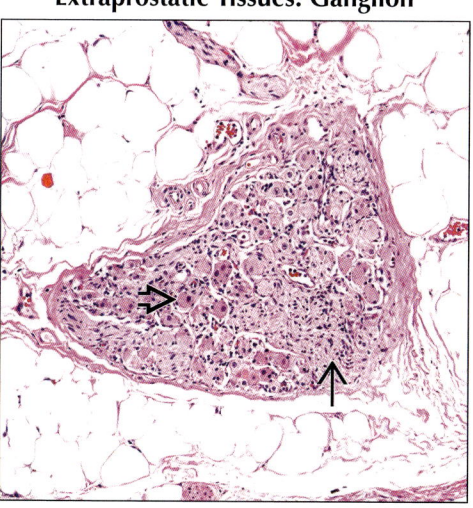

Extraprostatic Tissues: Ganglion

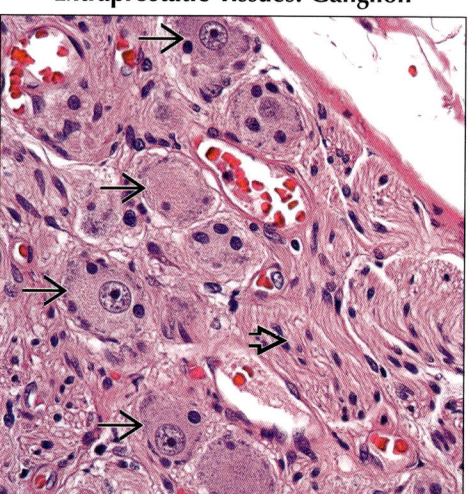

(Left) Ganglia are also frequently found in the extraprostatic tissues around the prostate gland. They are composed of admixtures of peripheral nerve ⇒ and collections of plump ganglion cells ⇒. *(Right)* At high-power evaluation, the ganglion cells ⇒ are characterized by round cells with abundant eosinophilic cytoplasm, large round nuclei, and large prominent nucleoli. These cells are admixed with peripheral nerve ⇒.

PENIS

Key Facts

Macroscopic Anatomy
- Shaft (proximal portion) is predominantly composed of paired corpora cavernosa and ventrally situated corpus spongiosum
- Distal portion is composed of glans, foreskin, and distal-most portions of corpus spongiosum and corpora cavernosa
  - Corpus spongiosum expands into cone-like shape at distal portion of penis to form majority of glans
  - Urethral meatus is located centrally on tip of glans
  - Corona: Elevated ridge of tissue present circumferentially at base of glans
  - Coronal sulcus: Indentation that lies adjacent and proximal to corona
  - Corona and coronal sulcus are replaced by frenulum (fold of tissue fixing foreskin to glans) on ventral-most aspect
  - Foreskin, or prepuce, covers glans in uncircumcised persons

Microscopic Anatomy
- Shaft or body
  - Paired corpora cavernosa and single corpus spongiosum are composed of interconnecting networks of vascular spaces that fill with blood upon erection
  - Urethra is located centrally within corpus spongiosum
  - Tunica albuginea: Dense layer of fibrous tissue that surrounds each structure; prominent around each corpus cavernosum, thinner around corpus spongiosum
  - Median raphe: Where tunica albuginea surrounding each corpus cavernosum meets and fuses at midline
  - Buck fascia: Layer of loose connective tissue rich in elastic fibers, which completely surrounds corpora cavernosa and corpus spongiosum and their associated tunics
  - Dartos muscle: Thin, irregular layer of smooth muscle bundles interspersed within loose connective tissue and located around Buck fascia
  - Layer of skin forms outermost layer of penile shaft
- Glans
  - Outermost layer: Thin layer of stratified squamous epithelium that lacks adnexal structures and melanocytes
  - Lamina propria: Lies beneath squamous epithelium; consists of a layer of loose connective tissue of varying thickness (1-2 mm) that separates epithelial layer from corpus spongiosum
  - Corpus spongiosum is expanded at glans, forming cone-shaped structure composed of rich network of vascular spaces
  - In a portion of the population, distal-most parts of corpora cavernosa and tunica albuginea can extend into proximal portion of glans
- Foreskin or prepuce
  - Flap of tissue circumferentially covering glans
  - Composed of outer skin layer and inner mucosal layer
  - Outer epidermal layer consists of keratinizing stratified squamous epithelium and underlying dermis
  - Underlying dermis contains occasional associated adnexal structures
  - Inner mucosal layer is histologically similar to that of glans and has underlying lamina propria
  - Dartos smooth muscle is located centrally within foreskin and is an extension of smooth muscle layer found in shaft of penis

(Left) The shaft, or body of the penis is composed predominantly of 3 elongated tubular structures of erectile tissue: The paired corpora cavernosa ⊃ and the corpus spongiosum →, which surrounds the urethra. (Right) The corpus spongiosum expands and acquires a cone-like shape at the distal-most portion of the penis, forming the majority of the glans. The foreskin can be seen surrounding the glans.

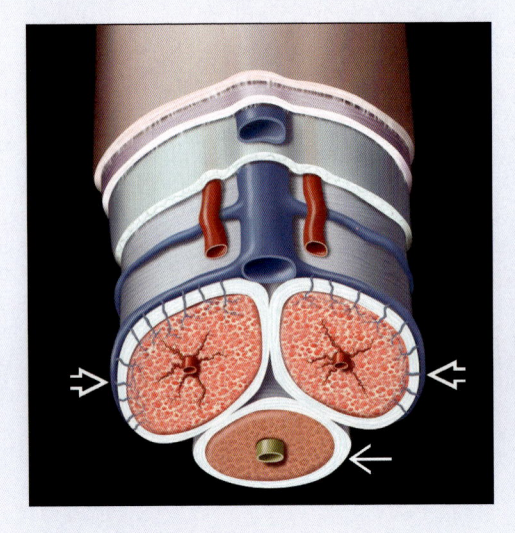

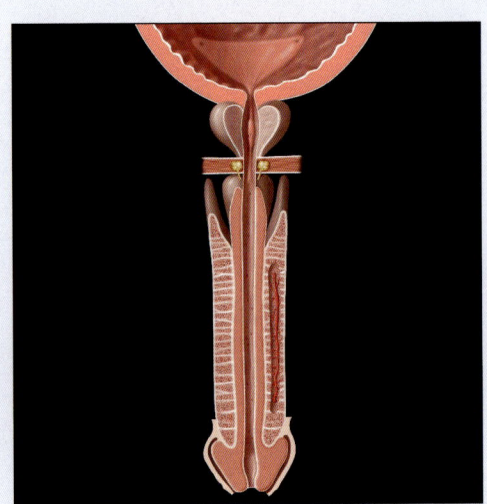

PENIS

Corpora Cavernosa
Corpora Cavernosa

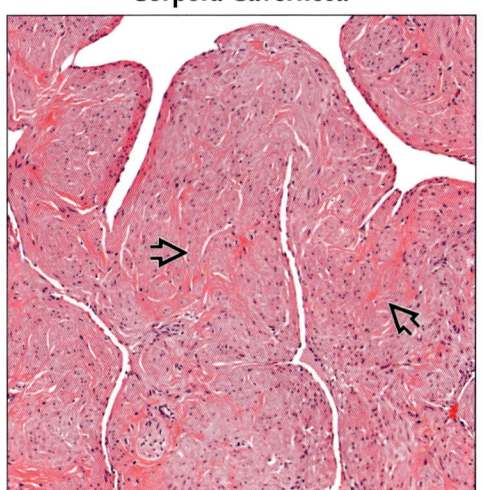

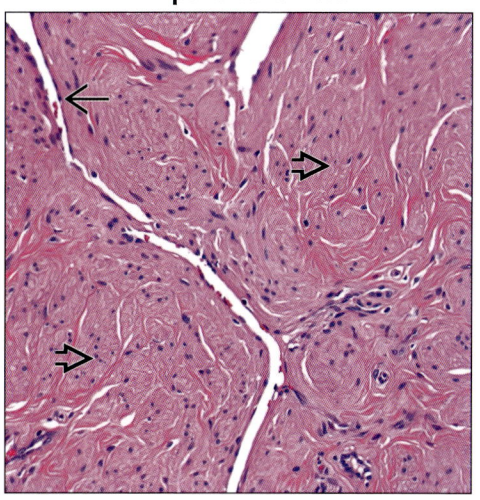

(Left) The corpora cavernosa are the paired main erectile tissues of the penis. They consist of an interanastomosing vascular network with intervening trabeculae ⇨ composed of smooth muscle and fibrous tissue. The trabeculae of the corpora cavernosa tend to have a more predominant smooth muscle component than that seen in the corpus spongiosum. *(Right)* The trabeculae ⇨ of the corpora cavernosa are lined by a single layer of endothelial cells ⇨.

Corpora Cavernosa
Tunica Albuginea

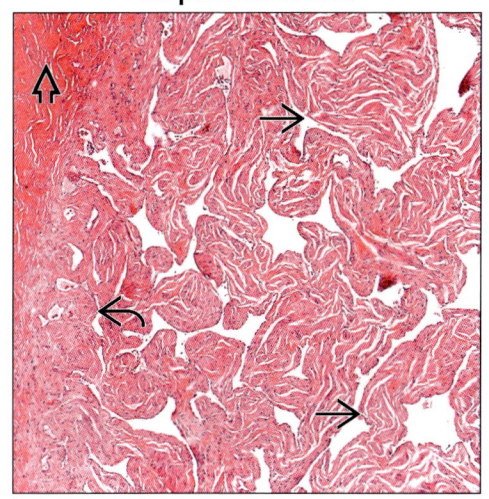

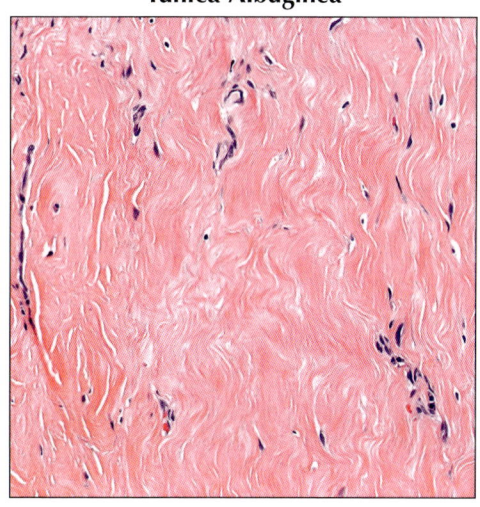

(Left) The corpora cavernosa are surrounded by a layer of thick connective tissue called the tunica albuginea ⇨. Note that the vascular trabeculae at the periphery ⇨ are of a smaller caliber and appear less prominent than those seen within the central portions of the corpora cavernosa ⇨. *(Right)* The tunica albuginea consists of a poorly vascularized layer of fibrous connective tissue composed predominantly of thick collagen fibers.

Tunica Albuginea
Corpus Spongiosum

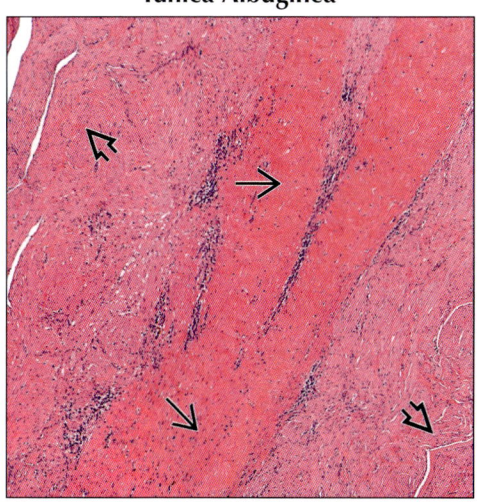

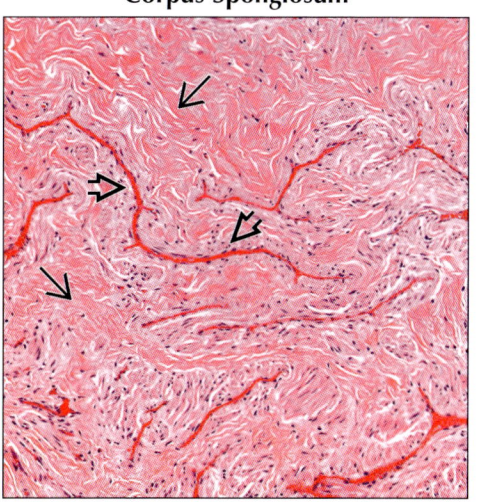

(Left) The tunica albuginea encasing the 2 corpora cavernosa ⇨ fuse at the midline, forming a fibrous septum ⇨. A complete septum is present in the more proximal portion of the shaft but becomes discontinuous within the distal portion. *(Right)* The endothelial-lined channels ⇨ of the corpus spongiosum are surrounded by trabeculae ⇨ composed of smooth muscle and fibrous tissue. The trabeculae of the corpus spongiosum tend to have less smooth muscle than those of the cavernosa.

PENIS

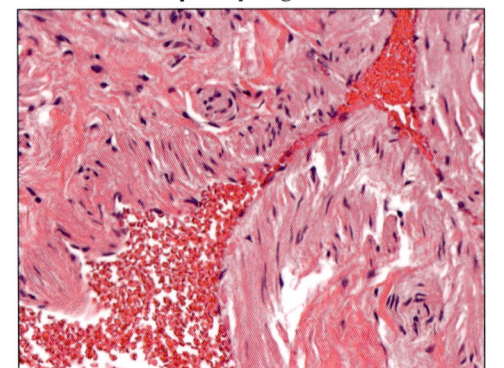

Corpus Spongiosum

(Left) The vascular spaces of the corpora spongiosum are lined by a layer of endothelial cells surrounded by the fibrous trabeculae. *(Right)* The urethra ➡ and its associated periurethral glands ➡ are located centrally within the corpus spongiosum. The vascular network and fibrous trabecula of the corpus spongiosum ➡ can be seen surrounding the urethra.

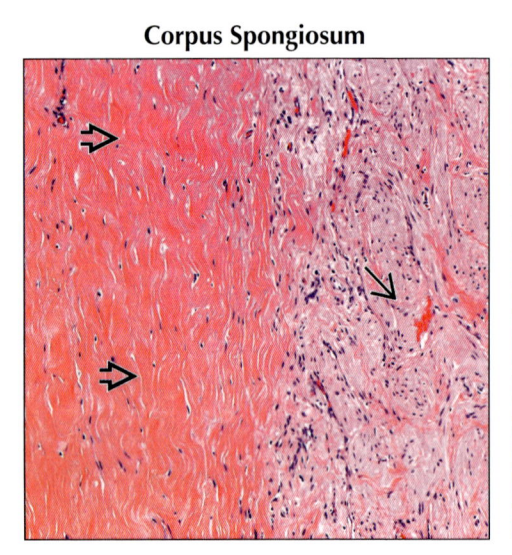

Corpus Spongiosum / Buck Fascia

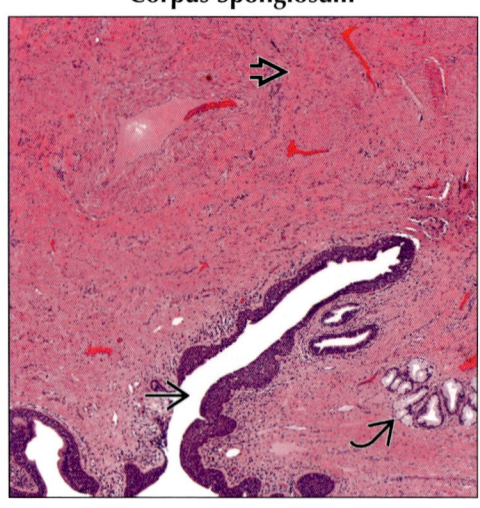

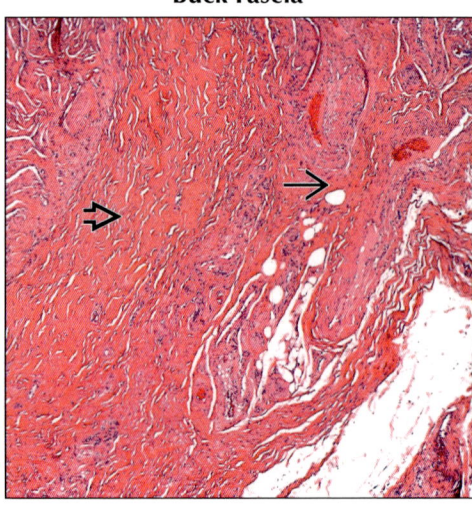

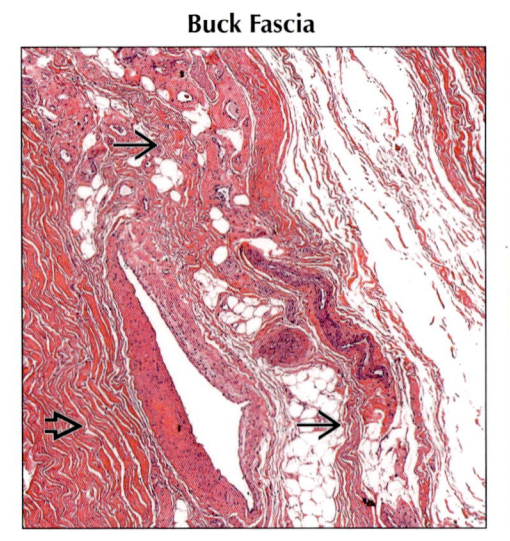

(Left) The tunica albuginea ➡ of the corpus spongiosum is thinner than that of the corpora cavernosa. Unlike the corpora cavernosa, the vascular spaces of the corpus spongiosum ➡ do not tend to decrease in caliber toward the periphery of the structure and are of fairly uniform size throughout. *(Right)* The loose connective tissue of Buck fascia ➡ surrounds the dense layer of collagen fibers that make up the tunica albuginea ➡.

Buck Fascia / Glans

(Left) Buck fascia ➡, seen here at higher power, is a layer of loose connective tissue with interspersed blood vessels and nerves that surrounds the thick layer of collagen that makes up the tunica albuginea ➡. *(Right)* The squamous epithelium ➡ of the glans lacks adnexal structures, such as hair follicles or sebaceous glands. The lamina propria ➡ separates the glans from the network of vascular channels that make up the corpus spongiosum ➡.

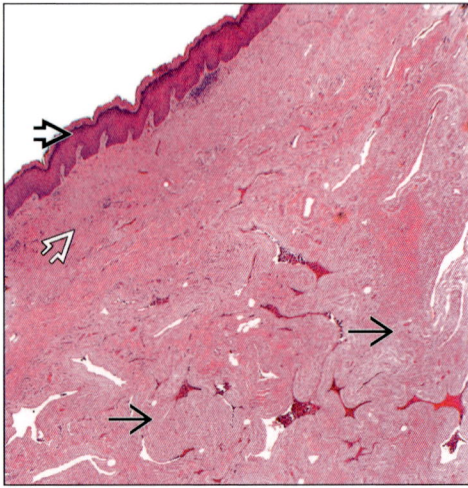

PENIS

Glans

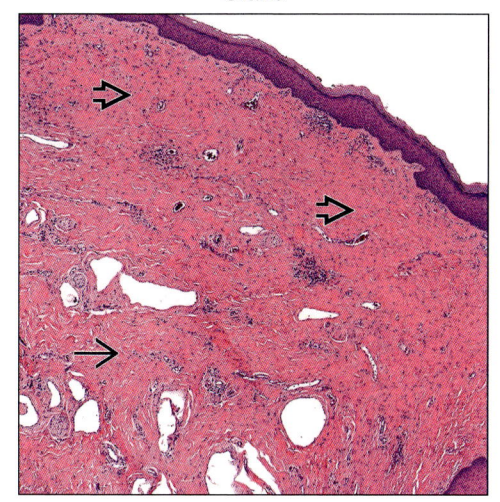

Glans

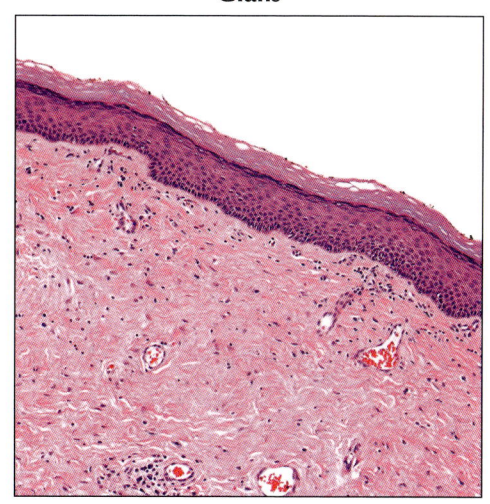

(**Left**) The connective tissue layer comprising the lamina propria ➤ varies in thickness, and its border with the underlying corpus spongiosum ➤ is often ill-defined in histologic sections. (**Right**) The squamous epithelial layer of the glans may have a thin layer of keratinization in circumcised males. Note the lack of adnexal structures associated with the epithelium, as well as the lack of melanocytes within the basal layer of the squamous epithelium.

Foreskin

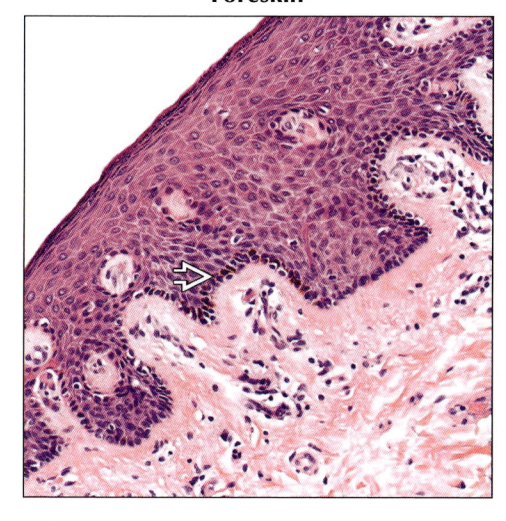

Foreskin

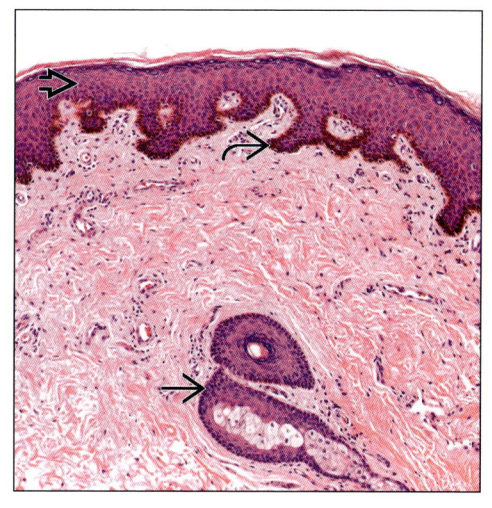

(**Left**) The outer epidermal layer of the foreskin is composed of keratinizing stratified squamous epithelium. Melanocytes and pigmentation ➤ can often be seen in the basal layer. (**Right**) The keratinizing squamous epithelium ➤ of the foreskin epidermis may have occasional adnexal structures ➤ identified within the underlying dermis. Note the pigmentation of the basal layer ➤, which is in contrast with the squamous epithelium of the glans.

Foreskin

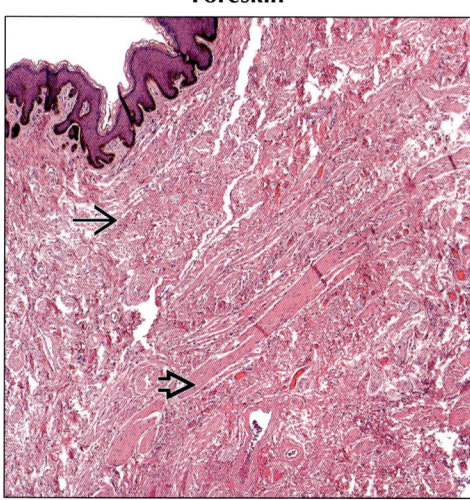

Dartos

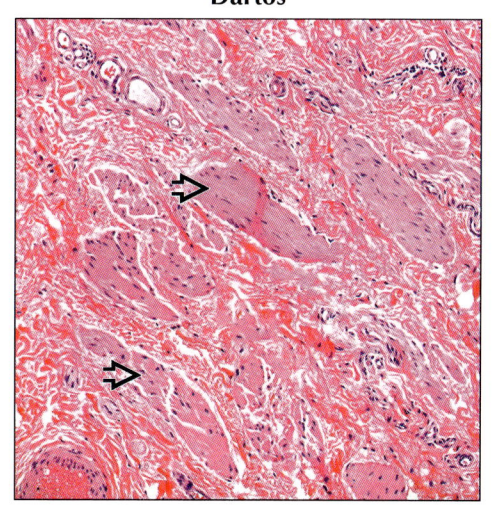

(**Left**) Underlying the dermis ➤ of the foreskin is the layer of dartos smooth muscle ➤, which is located centrally within the foreskin, separating the cutaneous epidermis and dermis from the inner mucosal squamous epithelium and lamina propria. (**Right**) The dartos smooth muscle layer in the foreskin is continuous with that of the penile shaft and consists of bundles of smooth muscle ➤ interspersed within a fibrous connective tissue with associated nerves and blood vessels.

TESTIS AND ASSOCIATED EXCRETORY DUCTS

Key Facts

Macroscopic Anatomy
- Paired male gonads
  - Weigh approximately 15-20 g each
- Suspended within scrotal sac by spermatic cord
  - Spermatic cord contains vas deferens and blood vessels that supply testis
- Scrotum consists of 4 layers
  - Outer skin
  - Dartos muscle
  - Colles fascia
  - Parietal layer of tunica vaginalis

Microscopic Anatomy
- Outermost testicular capsule has 3 layers
  - Tunica albuginea is thick fibrous layer
  - Tunica vasculosa is the loose connective tissue layer that projects fibrous septa into the testicular parenchyma, dividing it into lobules
  - Tunica vaginalis (visceral) is mesothelial lining layer
- Interstitium
  - Composed of loose connective tissue containing Leydig cells that surrounds the seminiferous tubules
  - Also contains nerves, lymphatics, vessels
  - Leydig cells are seen in greatest quantity in interstitium of testes and produce androgens
- Seminiferous tubules
  - Highly convoluted tubular structures that contain germ cells and Sertoli cells
  - Sertoli cells lie near basal aspect of seminiferous tubules and form blood-testis barrier
  - Germ cells comprise about 90% of cells within the seminiferous tubules
  - The most immature cells (spermatogonia) form the basal-most layer
  - The most mature cells aggregate along luminal surface
  - Germ cell maturation occurs in approximately 70 days and proceeds through an orderly maturation process: Spermatogonia, primary spermatocytes, secondary spermatocytes, spermatids, and mature spermatozoa
- Rete testis
  - Receives contents from the seminiferous tubules
  - Characterized by its cavernous-appearing channels lined by flat to low columnar epithelium
- Efferent ductules
  - Receive contents of rete testis
  - Luminal surface has undulating configuration and is lined by columnar epithelium
- Epididymis
  - Composed predominantly of columnar cells with apical stereocilia, known as principal cells
- Vas deferens
  - Transports spermatozoa from epididymis to ejaculatory duct

Age Variation
- At birth, testicle is composed of loose, immature mesenchymal tissue with small seminiferous tubules often lacking lumina
  - Majority of cells within seminiferous tubules of fetal and prepubertal testis are immature Sertoli cells, which have oval nuclei and inconspicuous nucleoli
  - Immature germ cells are only occasionally seen
- Decrease in spermatogenesis and fibrosis of seminiferous tubules are seen in elderly population

(Left) The testes are suspended within the scrotal sac by the spermatic cord. The cord contains the blood supply of the testis and the vas deferens, which transports the spermatozoa from the testis to the ejaculatory duct. (Right) Septa ➢ from the testicular capsule ➢ divide the testis into separate lobules. The epididymis, efferent ductules, and the rete testis are the tubular structures ➢ present at the mediastinum with adjacent blood vessels.

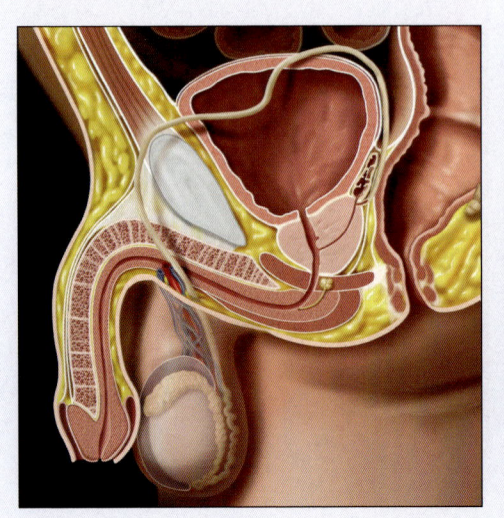

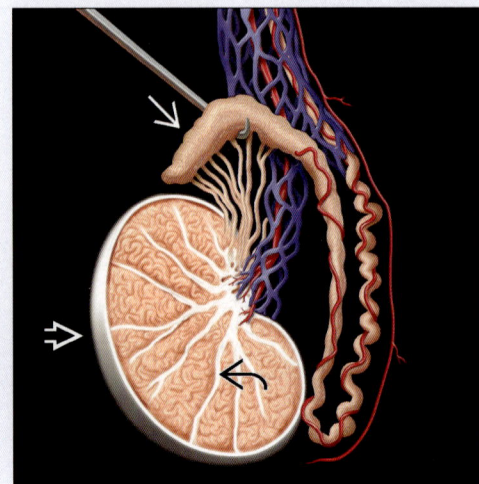

TESTIS AND ASSOCIATED EXCRETORY DUCTS

Outer Surface

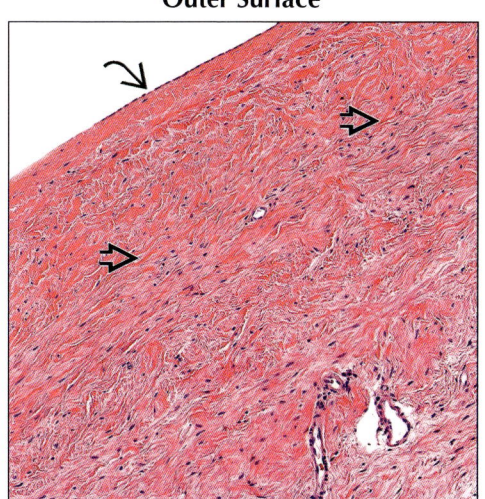

Tunica Vaginalis and Tunica Albuginea

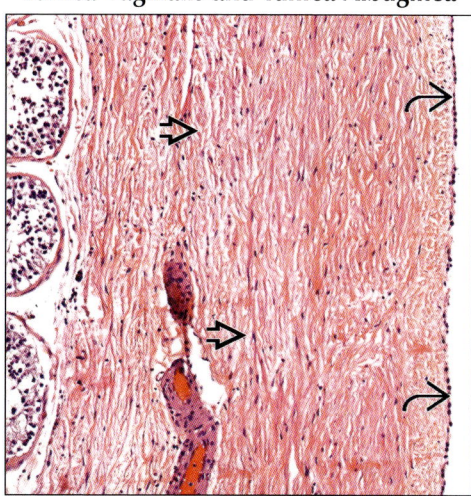

(Left) Beneath the flattened mesothelial layer of the tunica vaginalis ➔ lies the thick layer of dense collagen called the tunica albuginea ➔, which forms a capsule surrounding the testis. *(Right)* The visceral portion of the tunica vaginalis ➔ consists of a single layer of flattened mesothelial cells that make up the outermost layer of the testicle, external to the tunica albuginea ➔. The parietal counterpart of the tunica vaginalis lines the innermost layer of the scrotum.

Tunica Vasculosa

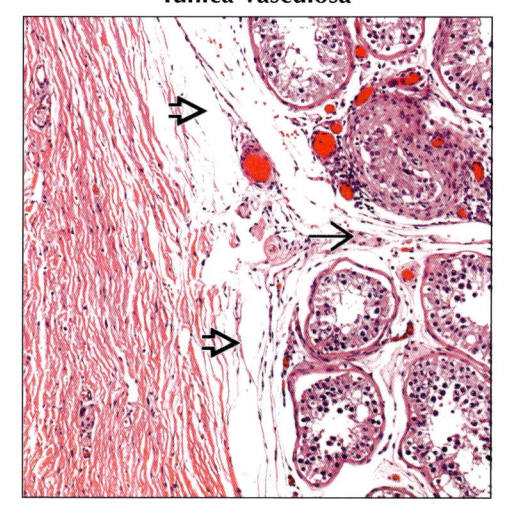

Interstitium

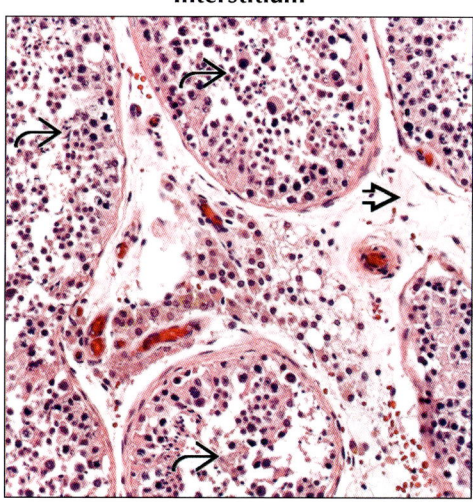

(Left) The tunica vasculosa ➔ is a layer of loose connective tissue containing numerous lymphatic spaces and blood vessels that lies beneath the tunica albuginea. The septa ➔, which separate the testis into approximately 250 lobules, arise from the tunica vasculosa. *(Right)* The loose connective tissue between the seminiferous tubules ➔ is known as the interstitium ➔. Interspersed within the interstitial tissue are blood vessels, mast cells, nerves, and Leydig cells.

Interstitium

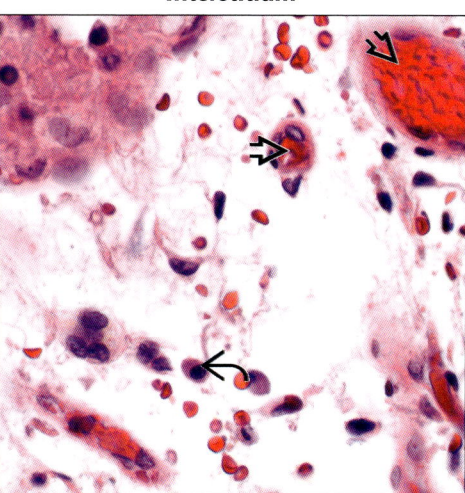

Interstitium

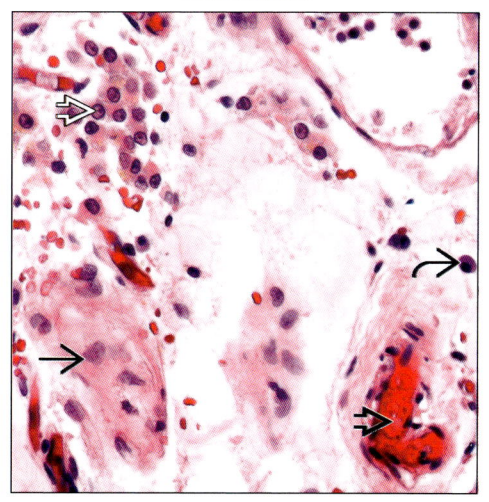

(Left) The loose connective tissue of the interstitium contains blood vessels ➔ and scattered mast cells ➔. *(Right)* Along with blood vessels ➔, nerves ➔, and scattered mast cells ➔ are Leydig cells ➔, which produce testosterone. Leydig cells are present as single cells, or more commonly, small clusters of cells with abundant eosinophilic cytoplasm and a round vesicular nucleus.

TESTIS AND ASSOCIATED EXCRETORY DUCTS

Leydig Cells

Leydig Cells

(Left) Leydig cells ⇨ have eosinophilic cytoplasm, single vesicular nuclei, and often lie in close proximity to blood vessels ⇨ and adjacent to the seminiferous tubules in the interstitium. Intracytoplasmic lipid droplets and lipofuscin pigment ⇨ are commonly present in Leydig cells. (Right) Lipid droplets ⇨ and brown pigment known as lipofuscin ⇨ begin to accumulate within the brightly eosinophilic cytoplasm of the Leydig cells ⇨ at puberty and increase with age.

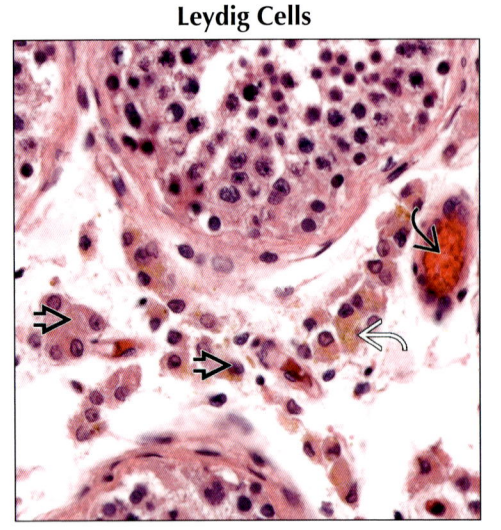

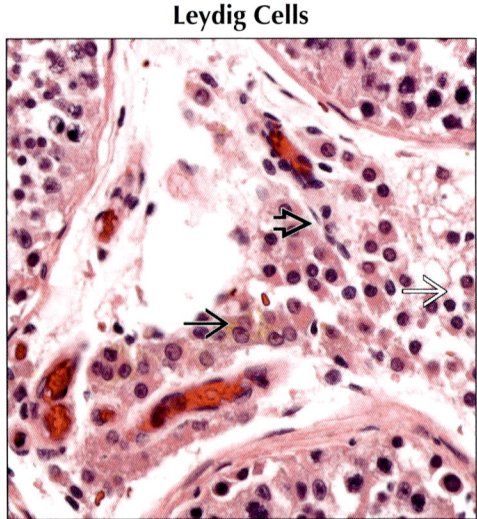

Reinke Crystals

Leydig Cells

(Left) Intracytoplasmic crystalloids known as Reinke crystalloids ⇨ can occasionally be found within Leydig cells. The crystalloids are only identified in postpubertal testes. (Right) Leydig cells can be identified outside of the testicular interstitium, often within nerve fibers. The epididymis, spermatic cord, and hilar soft tissue are common sites where Leydig cells may be present. A cluster of Leydig cells ⇨ is identified surrounding a nerve fiber ⇨ adjacent to the epididymis.

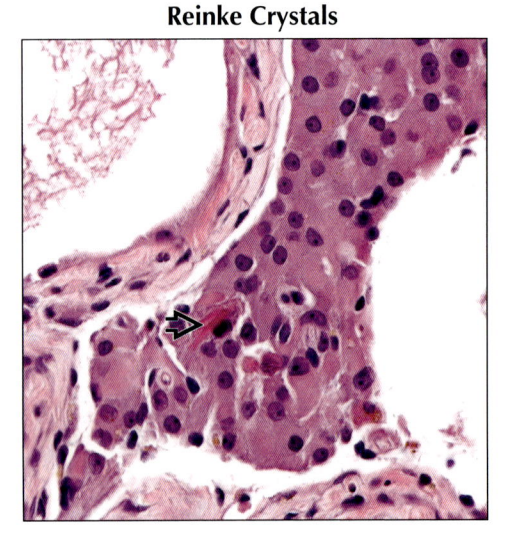

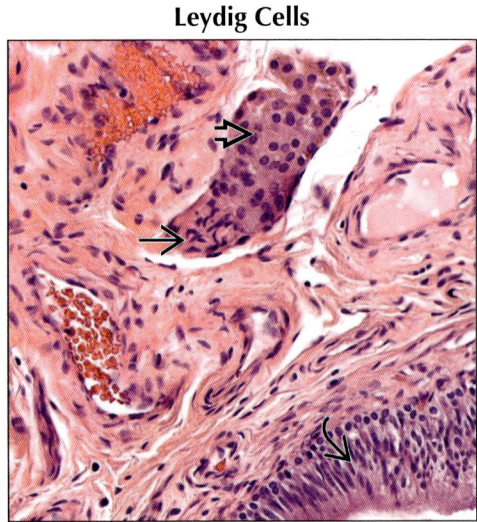

Seminiferous Tubules

Seminiferous Tubules

(Left) The seminiferous tubules ⇨ are convoluted tubular structures containing the germ cells and Sertoli cells. A basement membrane and lamina propria surround each tubule, separating it from the adjacent interstitium ⇨ of the testis. (Right) Each lobule of the testis houses between 1 and 4 long, convoluted seminiferous tubules, which contain the maturing germ cells ⇨ within the testis before emptying their contents into the rete testis.

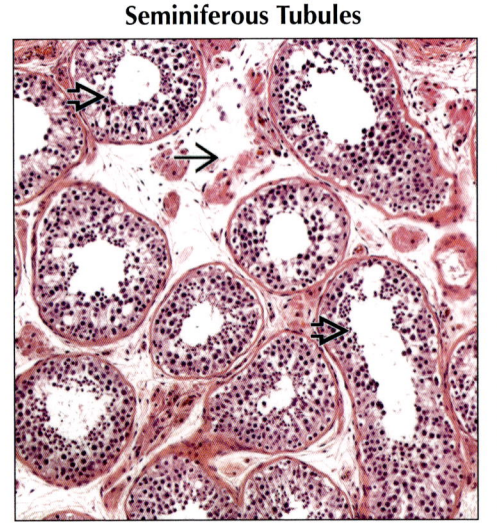

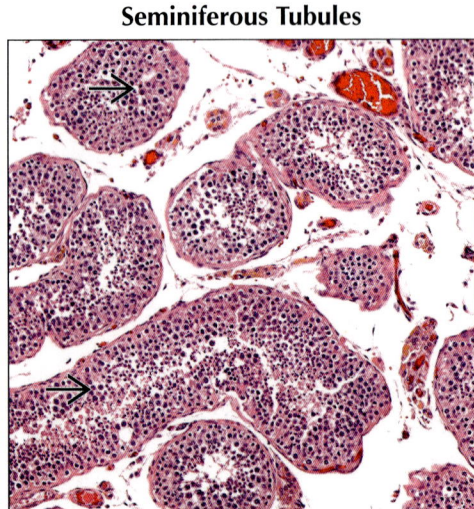

TESTIS AND ASSOCIATED EXCRETORY DUCTS

Sertoli Cells

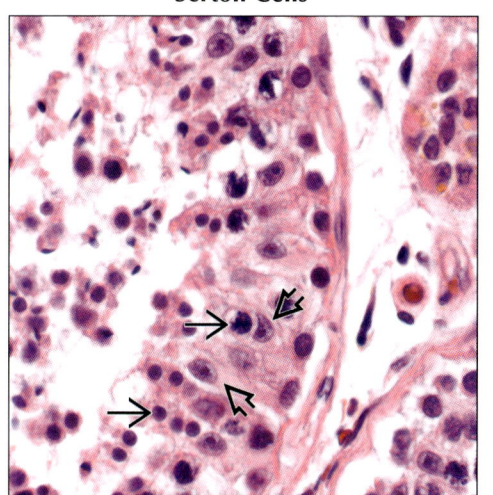

Sertoli Cells

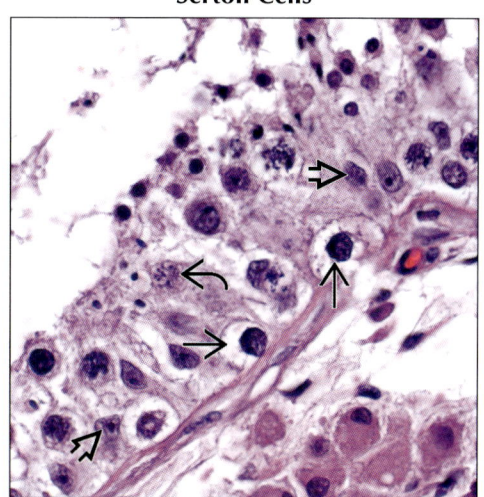

(Left) Sertoli cells are irregular columnar cells with inconspicuous cytoplasmic borders, round or slightly irregular nuclei, folded nuclear membranes, and prominent nucleoli. The cytoplasm forms extensions to support the adjacent germ cells. *(Right)* Sertoli cells lie between the spermatogonia and primary spermatocytes, with the base of the cell attached to the underlying basement membrane. Tight junctions between Sertoli cells form the blood-testis barrier.

Sertoli Cells

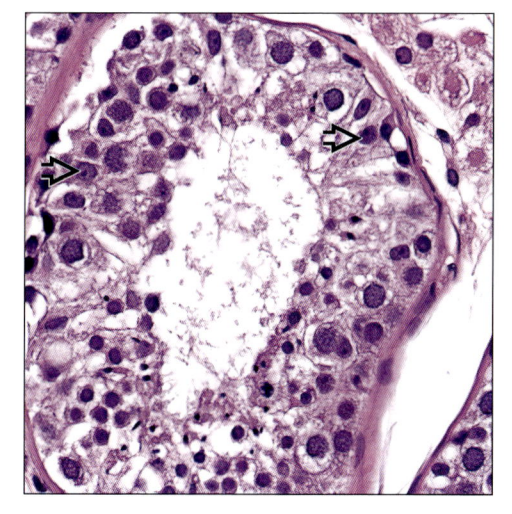

Spermatogonia

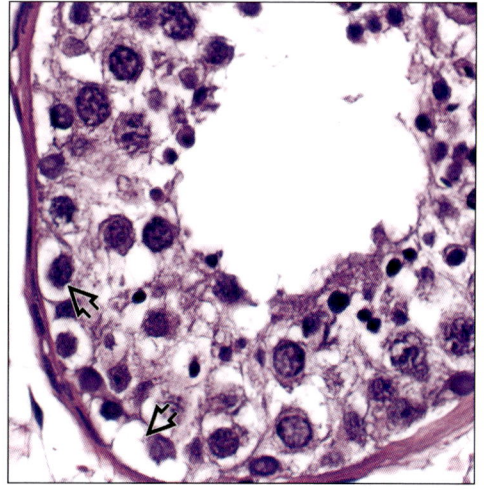

(Left) Sertoli cells support the surrounding germ cells and form the blood-testis barrier. It separates the tubular contents into a luminal compartment, which contains primary spermatocytes, secondary spermatocytes, and spermatids, and an underlying compartment, which contains spermatogonia and primary spermatocytes. *(Right)* Spermatogonia are the most undifferentiated of the germ cells in the seminiferous tubules.

Spermatogonia

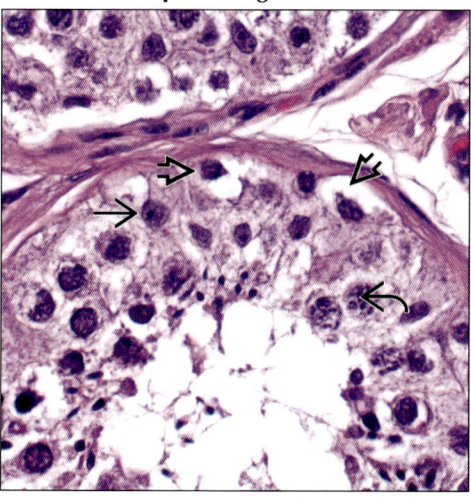

Primary Spermatocytes

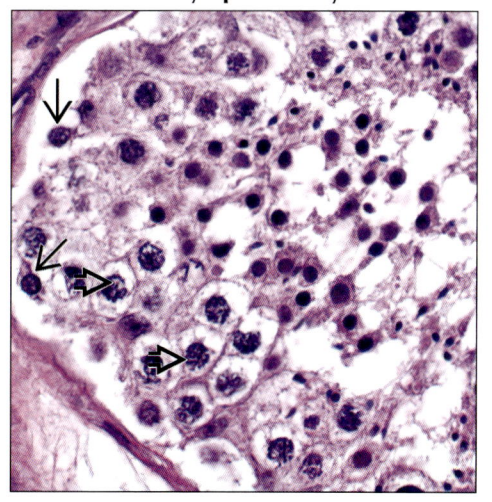

(Left) The small spermatogonia have round to ovoid nuclei and lie against the basement membrane of the tubule within the basal compartment. The spermatogonia proliferate both to replenish their population and to give rise to primary spermatocytes. Sertoli cells can be found adjacent to the spermatogonia. *(Right)* Primary spermatocytes have larger nuclei than the spermatogonia and occupy a more central location within the tubule.

TESTIS AND ASSOCIATED EXCRETORY DUCTS

Primary Spermatocytes

(Left) Spermatogonia ➡ give rise to primary spermatocytes ➡, which are larger and have characteristically coarse chromatin. The primary spermatocytes move from the basal compartment of the tubule to the luminal compartment soon after their maturation from spermatogonia. **(Right)** Nuclei of primary spermatocytes ➡ are large, with coarse, clumped chromatin. Sertoli cells ➡ and spermatogonia ➡ occupy a more basal location in the tubule.

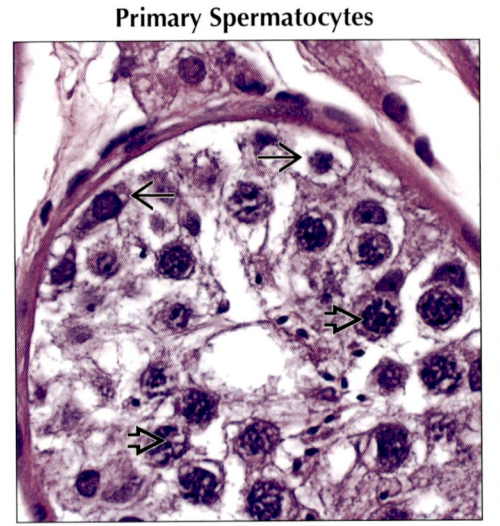

Spermatids

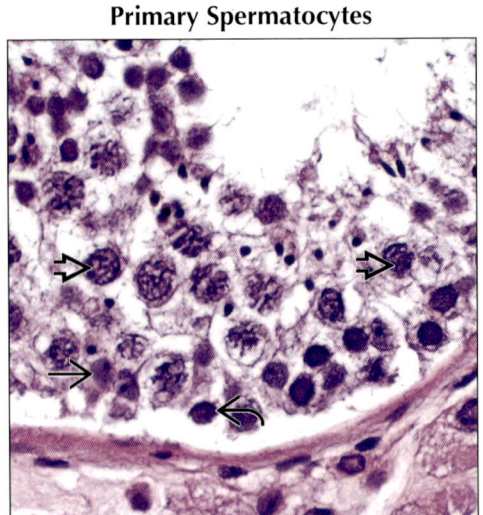

(Left) Primary spermatocytes ➡ mature into secondary spermatocytes, which quickly mature into spermatids. Secondary spermatocytes and early spermatids ➡ are morphologically similar, with round nuclei much smaller than those of the primary spermatocytes. **(Right)** Spermatids vary morphologically as they mature into spermatozoa. Early forms have round nuclei with more abundant cytoplasm ➡, whereas late spermatids have ovoid to elongated nuclei ➡ and much less cytoplasm.

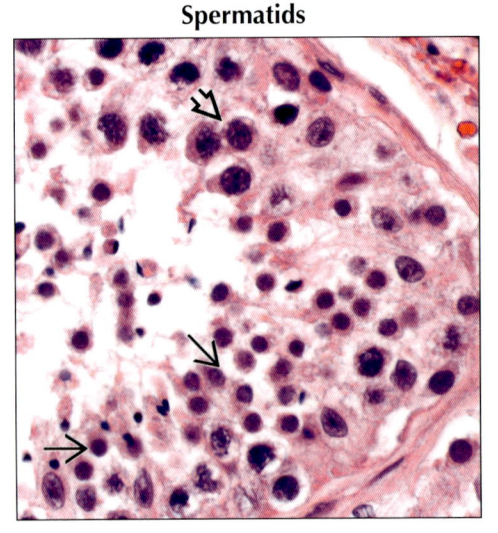

Rete Testis

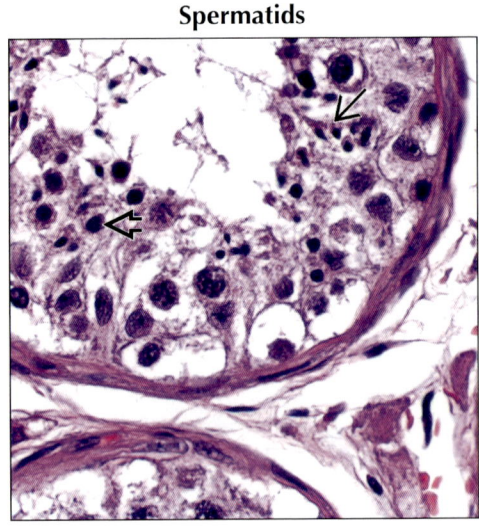

(Left) The seminiferous tubules empty their contents into the rete testis, a network of channels in the mediastinum of the testis. The tubules of the rete testis are surrounded by stroma containing collagen and elastic fibers with occasional myoid and fibroblastic cells. **(Right)** The flattened, low columnar epithelium of the rete testis has microvilli and a single flagellum on the luminal aspect although these structures are not apparent on routine histologic sectioning.

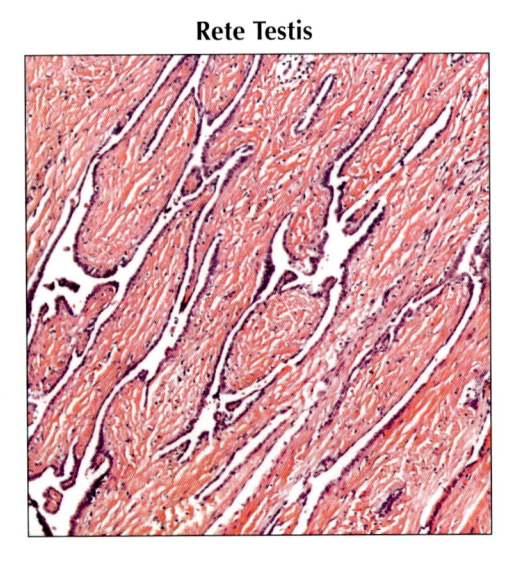

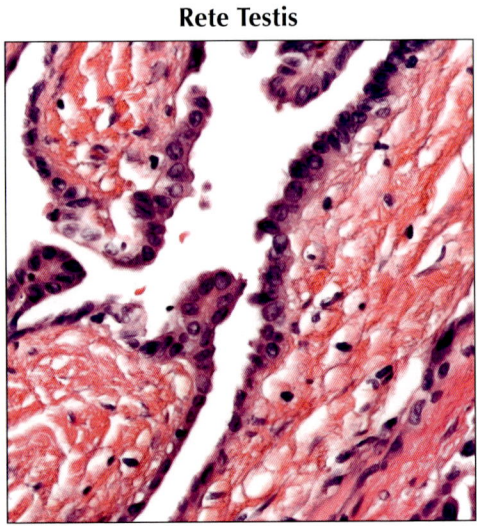

TESTIS AND ASSOCIATED EXCRETORY DUCTS

Rete Testis

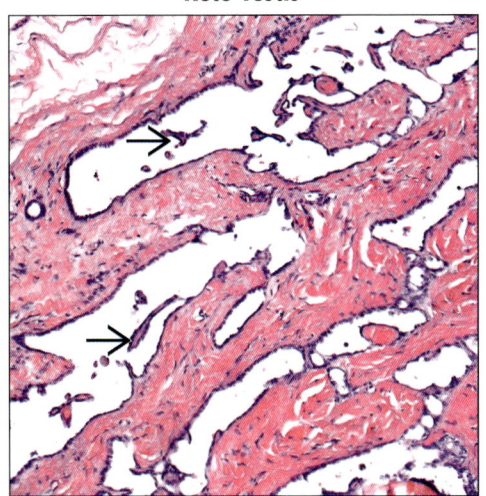

Rete Testis

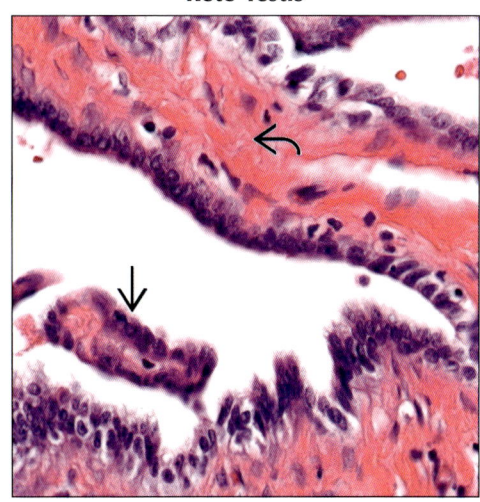

(Left) The chordae retis ➔ are columns of tissue that serve to connect the opposing walls of the rete testis. When viewed on cross sectioning, these structures appear as intraluminal islands of epithelial-lined fibrous tissue. (Right) The chordae retis ➔ are lined by the same flattened, low columnar epithelium as the walls of the rete testis. Thick collagen fibers with occasional myoid and fibroblastic cells can be seen in the surrounding stroma ➔.

Efferent Ductules

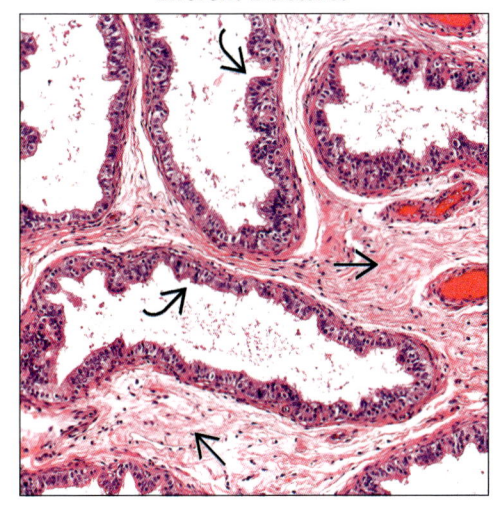

Efferent Ductules

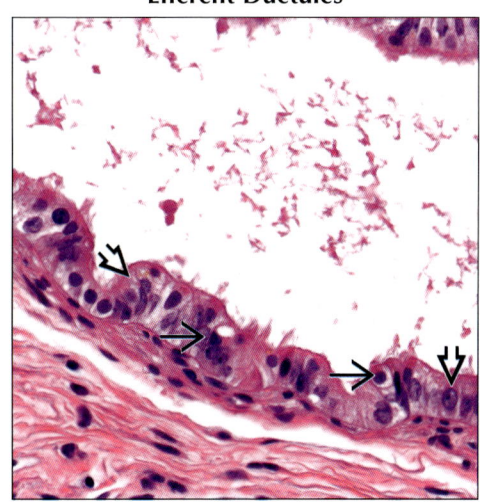

(Left) The efferent ductule luminal surface has an undulating architecture ➔. The surrounding stroma contains smooth muscle and fibroblasts ➔. (Right) The epithelium of the efferent ductules is composed of columnar cells ➔, which may be ciliated, and basal cells. Lymphocytes ➔ may be identified within the epithelium, and the admixture of columnar and basal cells with lymphocytes results in an overall pseudostratified appearance to the epithelium.

Efferent Ductules

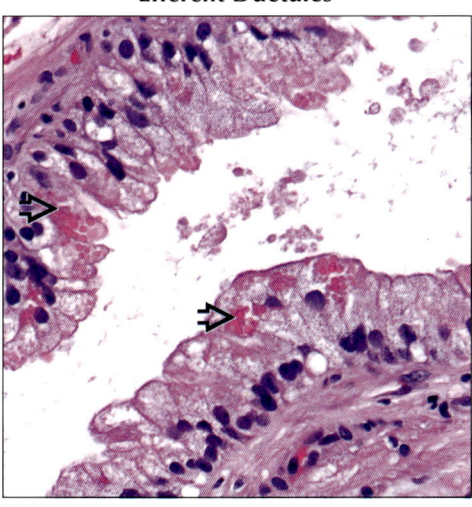

Epididymis

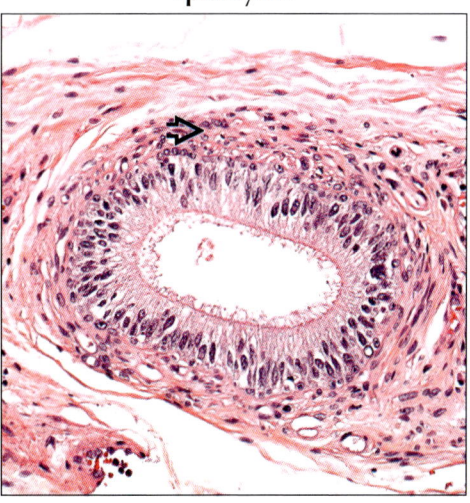

(Left) Cells with intracytoplasmic collections of brightly eosinophilic, PAS-positive globules ➔ are occasionally seen in the efferent ductules and, less commonly, in the epididymis. (Right) The tubules of the epididymis are more regular in shape and have a smoother, less undulating luminal surface when compared to the tubules of the efferent ductules. Surrounding the tubule is a well-defined layer of smooth muscle ➔.

TESTIS AND ASSOCIATED EXCRETORY DUCTS

Epididymis

Epididymis

(Left) A cribriform pattern ➡ can be seen in the epididymis in about 1/2 of the population and should not be mistaken for a pathologic process. A well-defined layer of smooth muscle surrounds each tubule ➡. *(Right)* The epithelium of the epididymis is composed of principal cells ➡, basal cells ➡, apical cells, and clear cells. The majority of the cells are the tall columnar principal cells, which have apical stereocilia ➡. Lymphocytes are scattered throughout the epithelium.

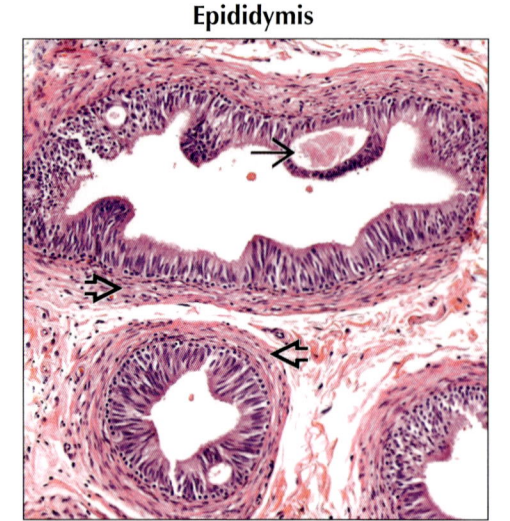

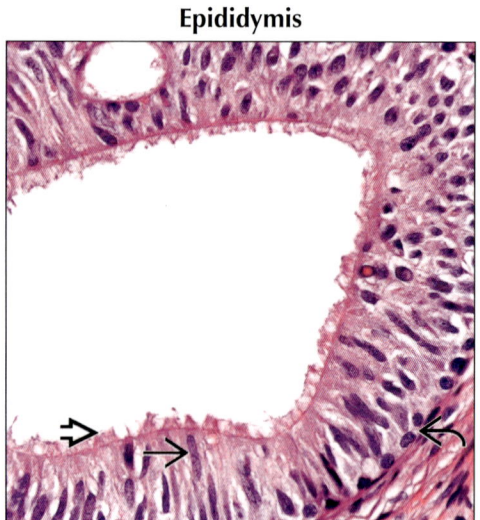

Epididymis

Vas Deferens

(Left) Eosinophilic inclusions ➡ can be identified within the nuclei of the tall columnar cells in the epididymis and in the cells of the vas deferens. Intracytoplasmic golden brown lipofuscin pigment can also be seen in the epididymis. *(Right)* The vas deferens is a long (approximately 35 cm) muscular-coated structure that receives contents from the epididymis. The distal portion (ampulla) of the vas deferens joins with the seminal vesicle excretory duct to form the ejaculatory duct.

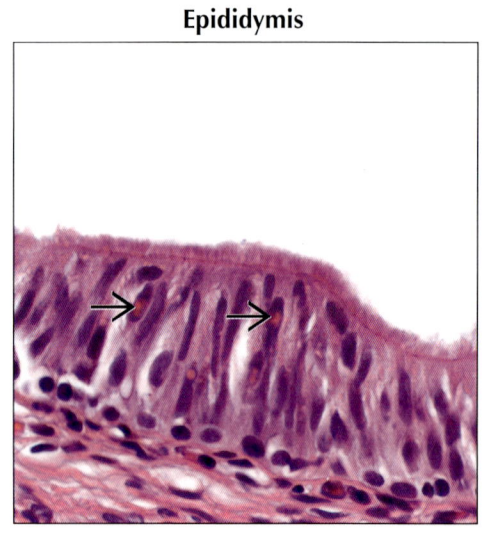

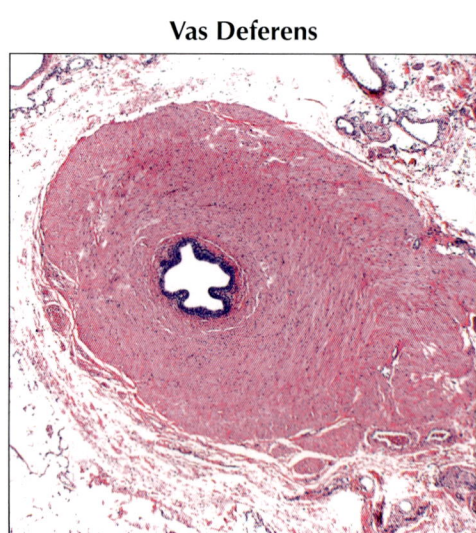

Vas Deferens

Vas Deferens

(Left) The thick muscular wall of the vas deferens in composed of 3 layers: An inner longitudinal layer ➡, a middle circular layer ➡, and an outer longitudinal layer ➡. The epithelial surface may have a folded architecture ➡, particularly in the more distal portion. *(Right)* The epithelium of the vas deferens is composed of columnar cells ➡ and basal cells ➡. The columnar cells have stereocilia ➡ on the apical aspect, which can be seen on the luminal surface.

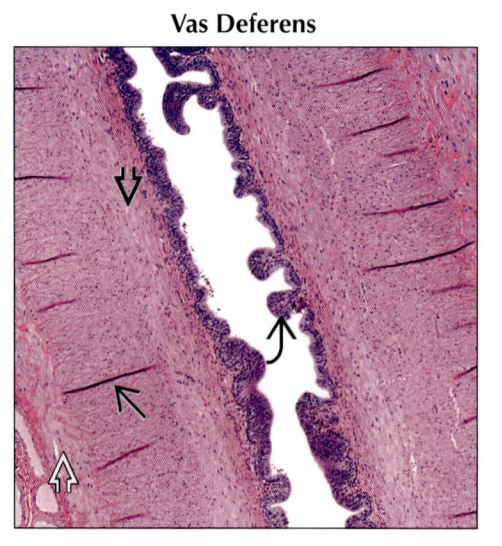

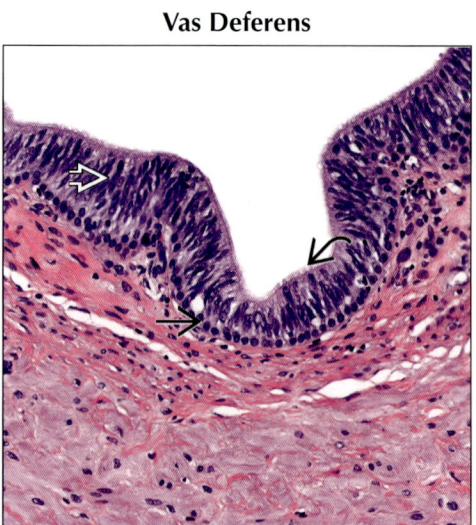

TESTIS AND ASSOCIATED EXCRETORY DUCTS

Prepubertal Testis

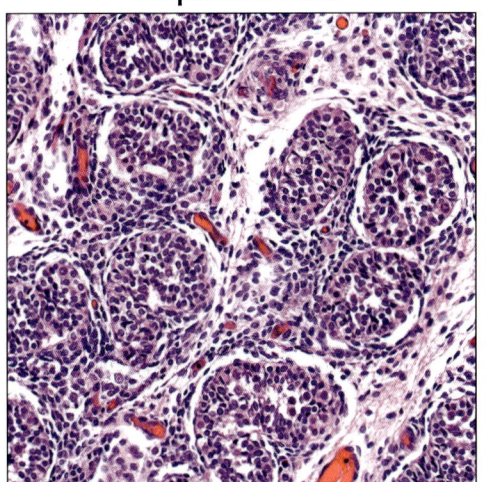

Prepubertal Testis

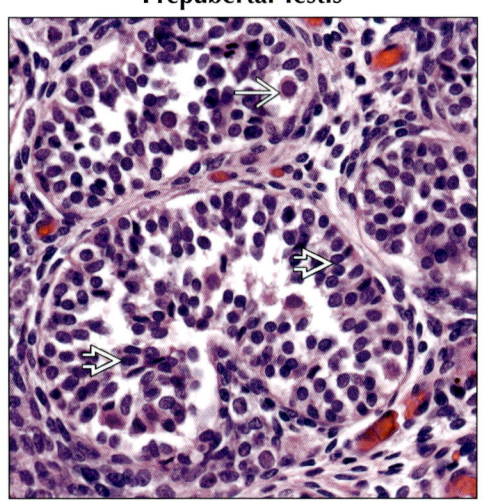

(Left) At birth, the testis is composed of loose, immature mesenchymal tissue with small seminiferous tubules, the majority of which lack lumina. (Right) At birth, the majority of the seminiferous tubules appear solid, lacking a central lumen. Immature Sertoli cells ➡, with oval to elongated nuclei and inconspicuous nucleoli, comprise the majority of the cells within the tubules. Rare immature germ cells can be identified ➡.

Peritubular Fibrosis

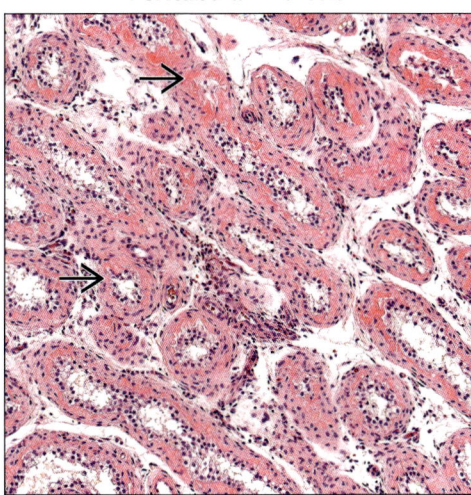

Testicular Appendages

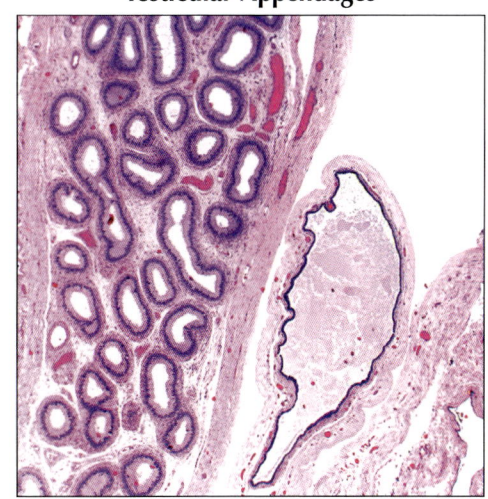

(Left) Thickening of the wall of the seminiferous tubules ➡ may be identified in focal areas as men age. More widespread thickening and hyalinization of the seminiferous tubules can be seen in cryptorchid testicles, in which the testicles fail to completely descend from the abdomen. (Right) The testicular appendages are mesonephric or paramesonephric duct remnants. The pictured appendix epididymis is a remnant of the mesonephric duct and is lined by columnar epithelium, which may be ciliated.

Adrenal Cortical Rest

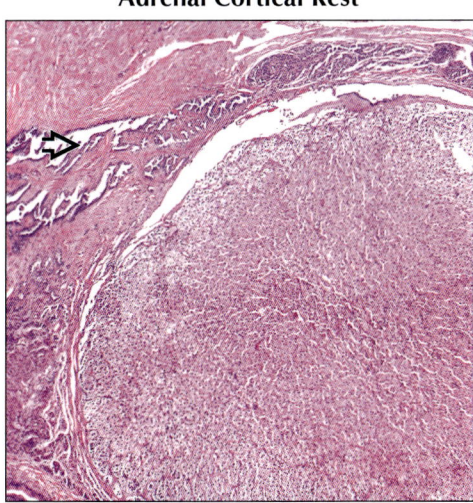

Adrenal Cortical Rest

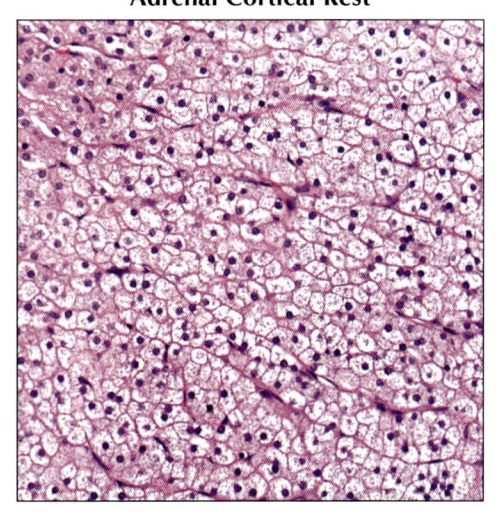

(Left) Adrenal cortical rests may be found in the spermatic cord or in the hilar soft tissue adjacent to the epididymis or rete testis. The adrenal tissue in this case is present within the hilar soft tissue, with normal rete testis ➡ identified in the upper left corner. (Right) Histologically unremarkable adrenal cortical tissue, with vacuolated, lipid-filled, lightly eosinophilic cytoplasm, is identified within adrenal cortical rests.

SELECTED REFERENCES

KIDNEY

1. Kambham N: Normal kidney structure. In Colvin RB et al: Diagnostic Pathology: Kidney Diseases. Salt Lake City: Amirsys Publishing. 1-30, 2011
2. Clapp WL: Renal anatomy. In Zhou XJ et al: Silva's Diagnostic Renal Pathology. New York: Cambridge University Press. 1-46, 2009
3. Smith SM et al: Low incidence of glomerulosclerosis in normal kidneys. Arch Pathol Lab Med. 113(11):1253-5, 1989
4. Kasiske BL et al: The influence of age, sex, race, and body habitus on kidney weight in humans. Arch Pathol Lab Med. 110(1):55-60, 1986

URETER AND RENAL PELVIS

1. Olgac S et al: Urothelial carcinoma of the renal pelvis: a clinicopathologic study of 130 cases. Am J Surg Pathol. 28(12):1545-52, 2004
2. Volmar KE et al: Florid von Brunn nests mimicking urothelial carcinoma: a morphologic and immunohistochemical comparison to the nested variant of urothelial carcinoma. Am J Surg Pathol. 27(9):1243-52, 2003
3. Kaye KW et al: Applied anatomy of the kidney and ureter. Urol Clin North Am. 9(1):3-13, 1982
4. Notley RG: Ureteral morphology: anatomic and clinical considerations. Urology. 12(1):8-14, 1978
5. Notley RG: The musculature of the human ureter. Br J Urol. 42(6):724-7, 1970
6. Morse HD: The etiology and pathology of pyelitis cystica, ureteritis cystica and cystitis cystica. Am J Pathol. 4(1):33-50, 1928

BLADDER

1. Paner GP et al: Further characterization of the muscle layers and lamina propria of the urinary bladder by systematic histologic mapping: implications for pathologic staging of invasive urothelial carcinoma. Am J Surg Pathol. 31(9):1420-9, 2007
2. Guo CC et al: Noninvasive squamous lesions in the urinary bladder: a clinicopathologic analysis of 29 cases. Am J Surg Pathol. 30(7):883-91, 2006
3. Philip AT et al: Intravesical adipose tissue: a quantitative study of its presence and location with implications for therapy and prognosis. Am J Surg Pathol. 24(9):1286-90, 2000
4. Grignon DJ et al: Paraganglioma of the urinary bladder: immunohistochemical, ultrastructural, and DNA flow cytometric studies. Hum Pathol. 22(11):1162-9, 1991
5. Ro JY et al: Muscularis mucosa of urinary bladder. Importance for staging and treatment. Am J Surg Pathol. 11(9):668-73, 1987
6. Goldstein AM et al: New concepts on formation of Brunn's nests and cysts in urinary tract mucosa. Urology. 11(5):513-7, 1978
7. Tanagho EA et al: The trigone: anatomical and physiological considerations. 2. In relation to the bladder neck. J Urol. 100(5):633-9, 1968 53, 1984

URETHRA

1. Lane Z et al: Polypoid/papillary cystitis: a series of 41 cases misdiagnosed as papillary urothelial neoplasia. Am J Surg Pathol. 32(5):758-64, 2008
2. Moore KL et al. Clinically Oriented Anatomy. 5th ed. Philadelphia: Lippincott Williams & Wilkins. 2005
3. Pavlica P et al: Imaging of male urethra. Eur Radiol. 13(7):1583-96, 2003
4. Young RH et al: Urethral caruncle with atypical stromal cells simulating lymphoma or sarcoma--a distinctive pseudoneoplastic lesion of females. A report of six cases. Am J Surg Pathol. 20(10):1190-5, 1996
5. Oliva E et al: Nephrogenic adenoma of the urinary tract: a review of the microscopic appearance of 80 cases with emphasis on unusual features. Mod Pathol. 8(7):722-30, 1995
6. Young RH: Nephrogenic adenomas of the urethra involving the prostate gland: a report of two cases of a lesion that may be confused with prostatic adenocarcinoma. Mod Pathol. 5(6):617-20, 1992
7. Carlile A et al: Age changes in the human female urethra: a morphometric study. J Urol. 139(3):532-5, 1988
8. Maung R et al: Intestinal metaplasia and dysplasia of prostatic urethra secondary to stricture. Urology. 32(4):361-3, 1988
9. Young RH: Papillary and polypoid cystitis. A report of eight cases. Am J Surg Pathol. 12(7):542-6, 1988
10. Tokunaga S et al: Benign prostatic epithelial polyp of urethra. Urology. 29(1):73-5, 1987
11. Remick DG Jr et al: Benign polyps with prostatic-type epithelium of the urethra and the urinary bladder. A suggestion of histogenesis based on histologic and immunohistochemical studies. Am J Surg Pathol. 8(11):833-9, 1984
12. McCallum RW: The adult male urethra: normal anatomy, pathology, and method of urethrography. Radiol Clin North Am. 17(2):227-44, 1979
13. Packham DA: The epithelial lining of the female trigone and urethra. Br J Urol. 43(2):201-5, 1971
14. Powell NB et al: The female urethra; a clinico-pathological study. J Urol. 61(3):557-70, 1949
15. Deter RL et al: A clinical and pathological study of the posterior female urethra. J Urol. 55:651-62, 1946
16. Lintgen C et al: A clinico-pathological study of 100 female urethras. J Urol. 55:298-305, 1946

SELECTED REFERENCES

PROSTATE: REGIONAL ANATOMY WITH HISTOLOGIC CORRELATES

1. Fine SW et al: Anatomy of the prostate revisited: implications for prostate biopsy and zonal origins of prostate cancer. Histopathology. 60(1):142-52, 2012
2. Selman SH: The McNeal prostate: a review. Urology. 78(6):1224-8, 2011
3. Fine SW et al: Anatomy of the anterior prostate and extraprostatic space: a contemporary surgical pathology analysis. Adv Anat Pathol. 14(6):401-7, 2007
4. McNeal J: Central zone histology of the prostate. Hum Pathol. 34(3):298; author reply 298-9, 2003
5. Srodon M et al: Central zone histology of the prostate: a mimicker of high-grade prostatic intraepithelial neoplasia. Hum Pathol. 33(5):518-23, 2002
6. McNeal J: Pathology of benign prostatic hyperplasia. Insight into etiology. Urol Clin North Am. 17(3):477-86, 1990
7. Villers A et al: Ultrasound anatomy of the prostate: the normal gland and anatomical variations. J Urol. 143(4):732-8, 1990
8. McNeal JE: Normal anatomy of the prostate and changes in benign prostatic hypertrophy and carcinoma. Semin Ultrasound CT MR. 9(5):329-34, 1988
9. McNeal JE: Normal histology of the prostate. Am J Surg Pathol. 12(8):619-33, 1988
10. McNeal JE: Anatomy of the prostate and morphogenesis of BPH. Prog Clin Biol Res. 145:27-53, 1984
11. McNeal JE et al: Anatomy of the prostatic urethra. JAMA. 251(7):890-1, 1984
12. McNeal JE: Normal and pathologic anatomy of prostate. Urology. 17(Suppl 3):11-6, 1981
13. McNeal JE: The zonal anatomy of the prostate. Prostate. 2(1):35-49, 1981
14. McNeal JE: Anatomy of the prostate: an historical survey of divergent views. Prostate. 1(1):3-13, 1980
15. McNeal JE: Regional morphology and pathology of the prostate. Am J Clin Pathol. 49(3):347-57, 1968

PROSTATE: BENIGN GLANDULAR AND STROMAL HISTOLOGY

1. Chen YB et al: Mesonephric remnant hyperplasia involving prostate and periprostatic tissue: findings at radical prostatectomy. Am J Surg Pathol. 35(7):1054-61, 2011
2. Wang W et al: Partial atrophy on prostate needle biopsy cores: a morphologic and immunohistochemical study. Am J Surg Pathol. 32(6):851-7, 2008
3. Hosler GA et al: Basal cell hyperplasia: an unusual diagnostic dilemma on prostate needle biopsies. Hum Pathol. 36(5):480-5, 2005
4. McNeal J: Central zone histology of the prostate. Hum Pathol. 34(3):298; author reply 298-9, 2003
5. Rioux-Leclercq NC et al: Unusual morphologic patterns of basal cell hyperplasia of the prostate. Am J Surg Pathol. 26(2):237-43, 2002
6. Srodon M et al: Central zone histology of the prostate: a mimicker of high-grade prostatic intraepithelial neoplasia. Hum Pathol. 33(5):518-23, 2002
7. Oppenheimer JR et al: Partial atrophy in prostate needle cores: another diagnostic pitfall for the surgical pathologist. Am J Surg Pathol. 22(4):440-5, 1998
8. Epstein JI: Adenosis (atypical adenomatous hyperplasia): histopathology and relationship to carcinoma. Pathol Res Pract. 191(9):888-98, 1995
9. Gagucas RJ et al: Verumontanum mucosal gland hyperplasia. Am J Surg Pathol. 19(1):30-6, 1995
10. Gaudin PB et al: Verumontanum mucosal gland hyperplasia in prostatic needle biopsy specimens. A mimic of low grade prostatic adenocarcinoma. Am J Clin Pathol. 104(6):620-6, 1995
11. Gaudin PB et al: Adenosis of the prostate. Histologic features in transurethral resection specimens. Am J Surg Pathol. 18(9):863-70, 1994
12. Grignon DJ et al: Sclerosing adenosis of the prostate gland. A lesion showing myoepithelial differentiation. Am J Surg Pathol. 16(4):383-91, 1992
13. Jones EC et al: Sclerosing adenosis of the prostate gland. A clinicopathological and immunohistochemical study of 11 cases. Am J Surg Pathol. 15(12):1171-80, 1991
14. Villers A et al: Anatomy of the prostate: review of the different models. Eur Urol. 20(4):261-8, 1991
15. McNeal J: Pathology of benign prostatic hyperplasia. Insight into etiology. Urol Clin North Am. 17(3):477-86, 1990
16. Young RH et al: Sclerosing adenosis of the prostate. Arch Pathol Lab Med. 111(4):363-6, 1987
17. McNeal JE: The prostate and prostatic urethra: a morphologic synthesis. J Urol. 107(6):1008-16, 1972
18. McNeal JE: Regional morphology and pathology of the prostate. Am J Clin Pathol. 49(3):347-57, 1968

PENIS

1. Velazquez EF et al: Preputial variability and preferential association of long phimotic foreskins with penile cancer: an anatomic comparative study of types of foreskin in a general population and cancer patients. Am J Surg Pathol. 27(7):994-8, 2003

SELECTED REFERENCES

2. Cubilla AL et al: Anatomic levels: important landmarks in penectomy specimens: a detailed anatomic and histologic study based on examination of 44 cases. Am J Surg Pathol. 25(8):1091-4, 2001
3. Cold CJ et al: The prepuce. BJU Int. 83(Suppl)1:34-44, 1999
4. Fitzpatrick T: The corpus cavernosum intercommunicating venous drainage system. J Urol. 113(4):494-6, 1975

TESTIS AND ASSOCIATED EXCRETORY DUCTS

1. Bouman A et al: Prevalence of testicular adrenal rest tissue in neonates. Horm Res Paediatr. 75(2):90-3, 2011
2. Srigley JR: The paratesticular region: histoanatomic and general considerations. Semin Diagn Pathol. 17(4):258-69, 2000
3. Rey R: The prepubertal testis: a quiescent or a silently active organ? Histol Histopathol. 14(3):991-1000, 1999
4. Shah VI et al: Histologic variations in the epididymis: findings in 167 orchiectomy specimens. Am J Surg Pathol. 22(8):990-6, 1998
5. Sahni D et al: Incidence and structure of the appendices of the testis and epididymis. J Anat. 189 (Pt 2):341-8, 1996
6. Waters BL et al: Development of the human fetal testis. Pediatr Pathol Lab Med. 16(1):9-23, 1996
7. Trainer TD: Histology of the normal testis. Am J Surg Pathol. 11(10):797-809, 1987

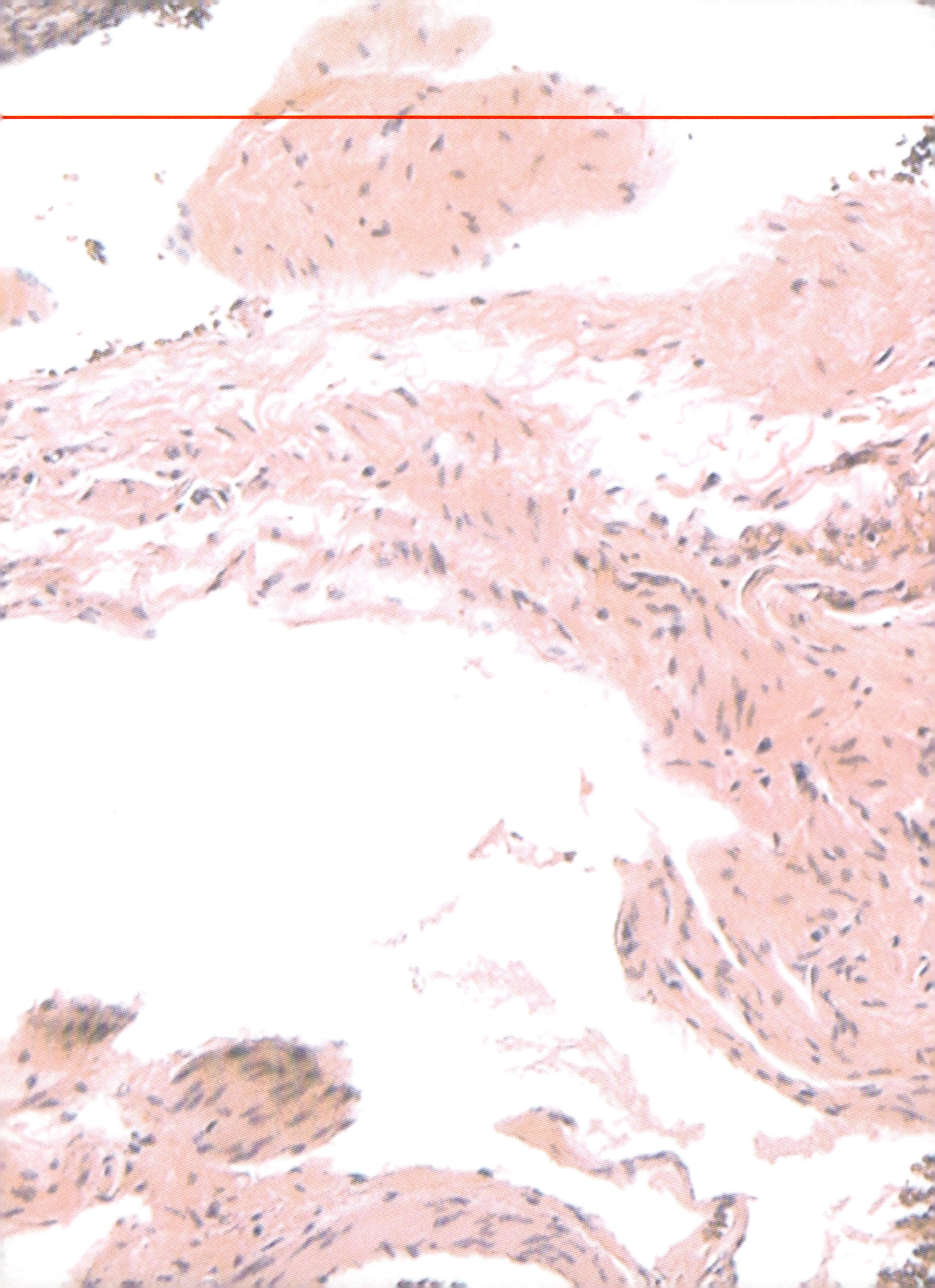

Female Genital Tract

Vulva — 13-2

Vagina — 13-6

Uterus — 13-10

Fallopian Tube — 13-24

Ovary — 13-30

Placenta — 13-40

VULVA

Key Facts

Macroscopic Anatomy
- General anatomic landmarks of vulva
  - Female genitalia external to hymen
  - Anteriorly limited by (and including) mons pubis
  - Posteriorly delimited by anus
  - Laterally, extends to inguinal-gluteal folds
- Mons pubis
  - Prominence over pubic symphysis that is composed of adipose tissue
  - Anteriormost region of vulva
- Hymen
  - Border of distal-most extent of vagina and posterior aspect of vulvar vestibule
- Labia majora
  - Located lateral (and parallel) to labia minora
- Labia minora
  - Present lateral to vulvar vestibule and medial to labia majora
- Clitoris
  - Located anterior to frenulum at junction of labia minora
- Vulvar vestibule
  - Extends from exterior surface of hymen to clitoris anteriorly, fourchette posteriorly, labia minora anterolaterally, and Hart line posterolaterally
  - Includes vaginal opening and urethral orifice
  - Also includes openings for paired Skene ducts, vestibular glands, and Bartholin glands
- Bartholin glands
  - Paired mucin-secreting glands located posterolaterally in vulva
- Hart line
  - Inferior junction between vulvar vestibule and perineal skin

Microscopic Anatomy
- Epithelium
  - Covered by stratified squamous epithelium
  - Keratinized in labia majora and minora
  - Nonkeratinized in vestibule where it may be glycogenated
  - Keratinization generally increases laterally toward surrounding skin
- Stroma
  - Stromal cell can be spindled, fusiform, or stellate, and may have nuclear multilobation
- Adnexal structures
  - Labia majora contains eccrine glands, sebaceous glands, and hair follicles, similar to those found in skin at other locations
  - Labia minora is devoid of adnexal structures in most women
- Clitoris
  - Contains vascular erectile tissue
- Mammary-like anogenital glands
  - Located within sulcus between labia majora and minora
  - Lined by luminal cuboidal/columnar epithelial cells that have underlying myoepithelium
  - Luminal cells may have apocrine appearance
- Minor vestibular glands
  - Superficial glands that enter mucosal surface of vestibule
  - Mucinous-type epithelium that may be admixed with squamous epithelium
- Bartholin glands
  - Acini consist of mucinous cells
  - Main duct lined by transitional-type epithelium

Pitfalls/Artifacts
- Multinucleated atypia
  - Multinucleated epithelial cells without viral cytopathic effect
  - May mimic squamous dysplasia
- Vulvar stromal cells with atypia
  - Normal stromal cells may have large multilobated nuclei

Metaplasia
- Squamous metaplasia of underlying vestibular glands
  - May mimic invasive squamous cell carcinoma

(Left) The major anatomic landmarks of the vulva include the mons pubis ⇨, clitoris ⇨, labia minora ⇨, labia majora ⇨, and vestibule ⇨. The urethral meatus ⇨ is present within the vulvar vestibule. (Right) The vulva is covered by stratified squamous epithelium. The basal cell layer ⇨ has a higher nuclear to cytoplasmic ratio, and the cells gradually mature toward the surface.

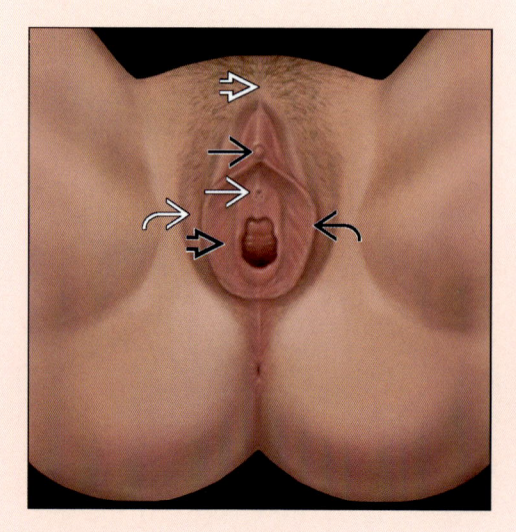

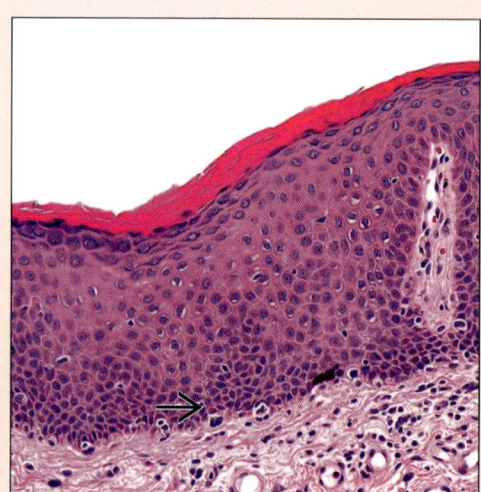

VULVA

Labia Majora
Labia Majora

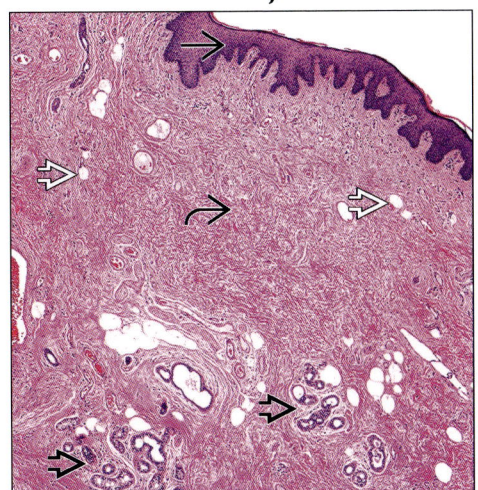

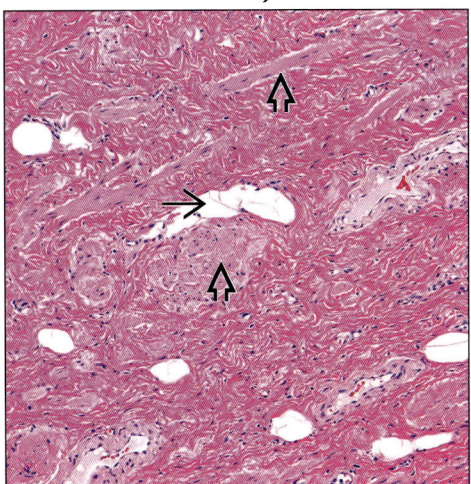

(Left) In the labia majora, the tissue underlying the epithelium ➡ contains collagen ➡, adipose tissue ➡, and adnexal structures ➡. Adnexal structures and adipose tissue are typically absent in the labia minora. (Right) The dermis of the labia majora typically contains superficial adipose tissue ➡ and smooth muscle bundles ➡, as well as an admixture of cutaneous adnexal structures that extend to deeper layers.

Labia Majora (Eccrine Glands)
Labia Majora (Sebaceous Glands)

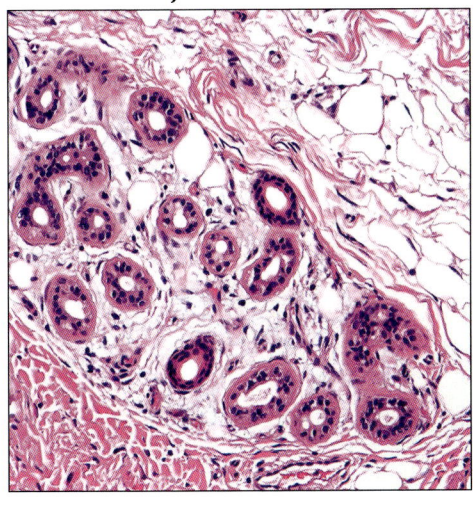

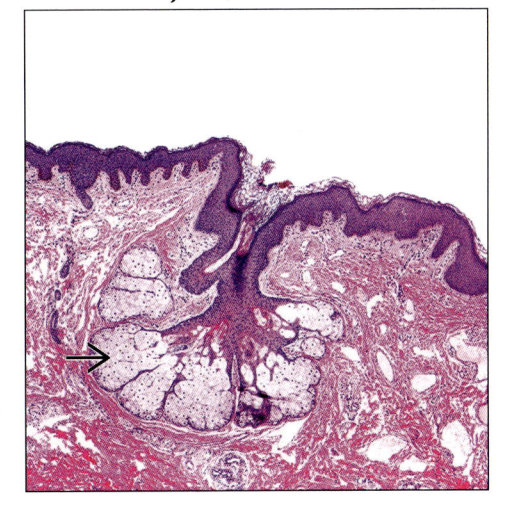

(Left) Eccrine-type glands are typically found in small circumscribed clusters. The secretory cells are a low cuboidal epithelium with scant eosinophilic cytoplasm. An indistinct surrounding myoepithelial layer is also present. (Right) Sebaceous glands ➡, ± associated hair follicles, are commonly identified at various levels within the labia majora. As in other areas of the body, the sebaceous glands contain clear vacuolated cytoplasm.

Labia Majora (Hair Follicle)
Labia Majora (Apocrine Glands)

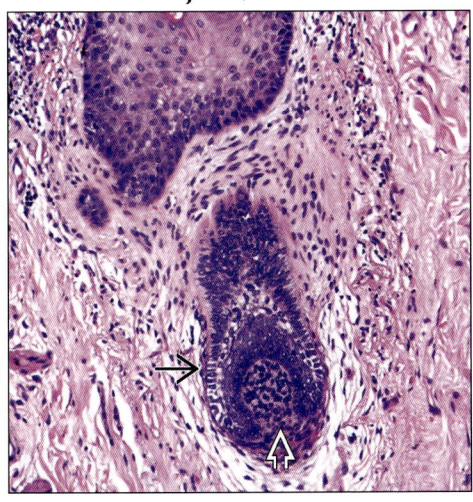

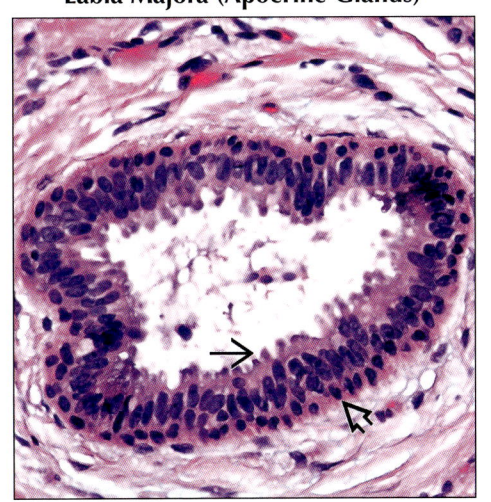

(Left) Hair follicles ➡ are also seen in the labia majora. This photomicrograph shows the base of the follicle (the bulb) with the invaginated papilla ➡. (Right) Apocrine-type glands are also commonly identified within the labia majora. The secretory cells have more abundant eosinophilic cytoplasm with characteristic apical blebbing ➡. A distinct myoepithelial layer ➡ is seen in this example.

VULVA

Labia Majora

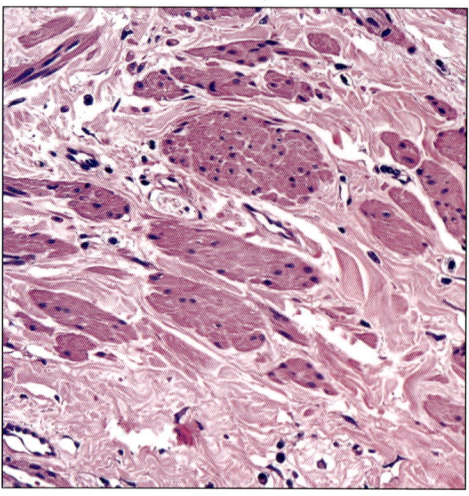

Vulvar Stromal Cells

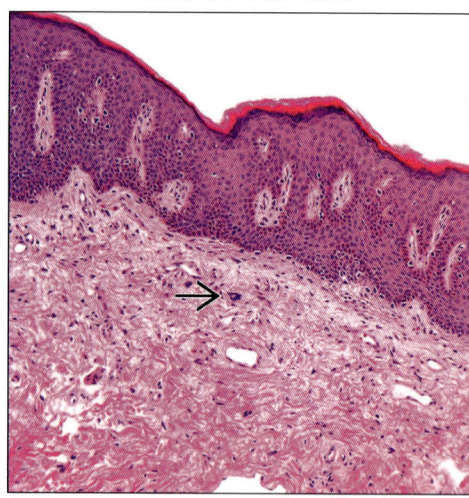

(Left) Dense bundles of smooth muscle are also commonly identified in the labia majora, but they are not typically seen in the labia minora. *(Right)* The superficial stroma underlying the epithelium of the vulva may contain a focal zone with somewhat increased stromal cellularity. This stroma may contain a subset of larger atypical cells ➡ that are visible even on low-power magnification.

Vulvar Stromal Cells

Labia Minora

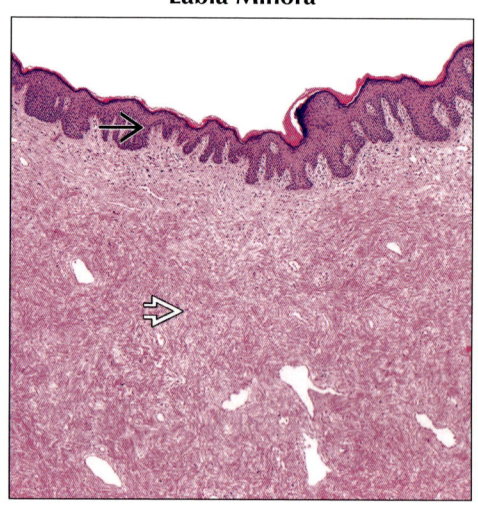

(Left) As in the vagina, the stromal cells of the vulva may have multilobated nuclei ➡ that can resemble a variety of neoplastic processes. These normal stromal cells are identical to those seen in fibroepithelial polyps. *(Right)* The squamous epithelium ➡ and the underlying stroma ➡ of the labia minora are demonstrated in this photomicrograph. The majority of the labia minora is devoid of adnexal structures and adipose tissue.

Labia Minora

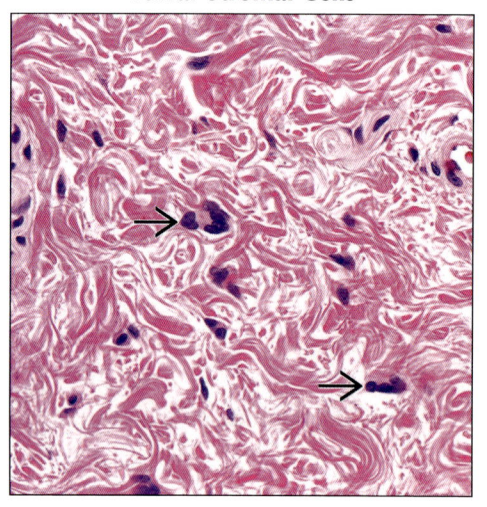

Labia Minora

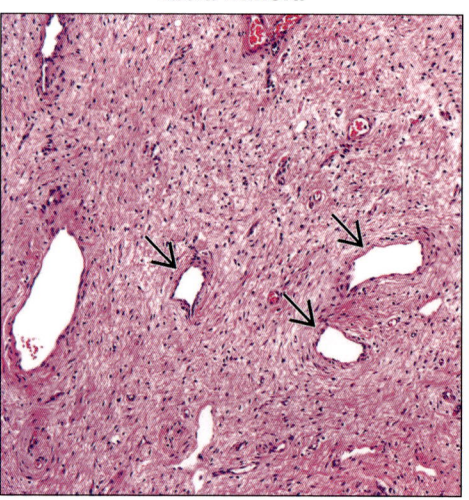

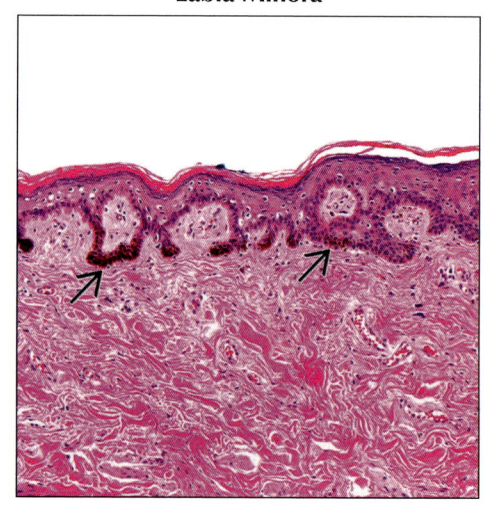

(Left) The stroma of the labia minora is rich in blood vessels ➡ and elastic fibers. Unlike the labia majora, the stroma of the labia minora does not usually contain admixed adipose tissue, smooth muscle, or adnexal structures. *(Right)* In the lateral and posterior regions of the labia minora, the epithelium may be pigmented ➡. The epithelium of the labia majora in the region peripheral to the Hart line may also be pigmented.

VULVA

Mammary-Like Anogenital Glands

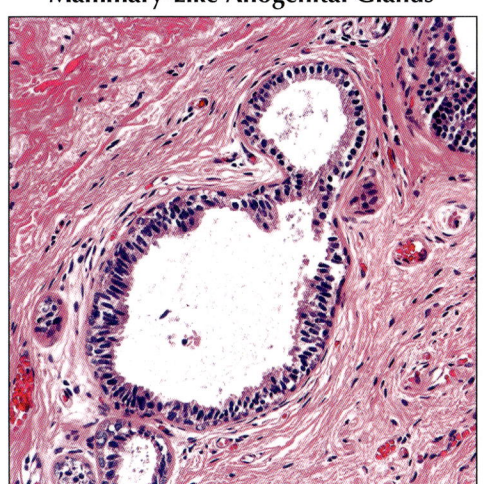

Mammary-Like Anogenital Glands

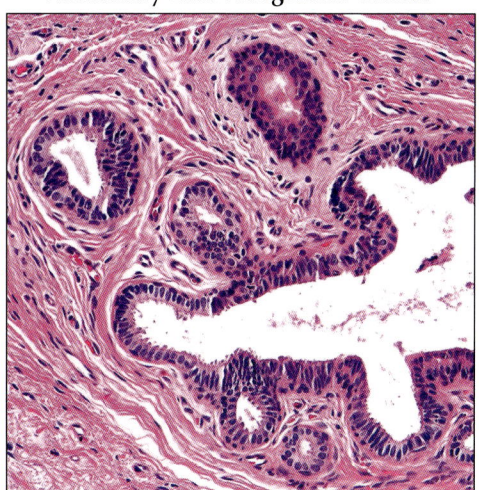

(Left) The sulcus between the labia majora and minora contains "mammary-like anogenital" glands. These glands may be the origin of breast-like lesions in the vulva, such as fibroadenoma and hidradenoma papilliferum. (Right) The mammary-like anogenital glands are morphologically similar to apocrine glands with eosinophilic cytoplasm and apical snouts. These glands are distinguished from vestibular, müllerian, or Bartholin glands by the absence of mucinous or ciliated epithelium.

Bartholin Duct

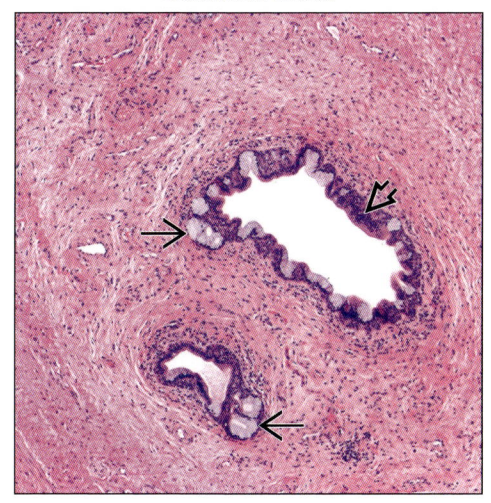

Bartholin Duct Epithelium

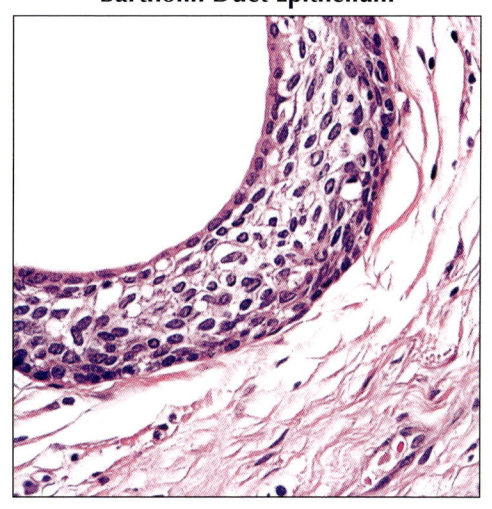

(Left) The Bartholin (bulbourethral) duct enters the vulvar vestibule posterolaterally, adjacent to the hymen. The duct often has a urothelial-type (transitional) epithelium ➡ with peripheral foci of mucinous-type glandular epithelium ➡. (Right) The Bartholin (bulbourethral) duct epithelium has a histologic appearance similar to urothelium (transitional epithelium). Cystic change may occur in these ducts and may produce a clinically apparent mass lesion.

Bartholin Gland

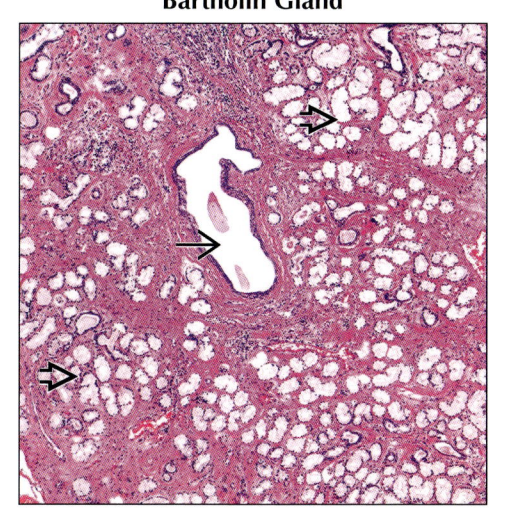

Bartholin Gland

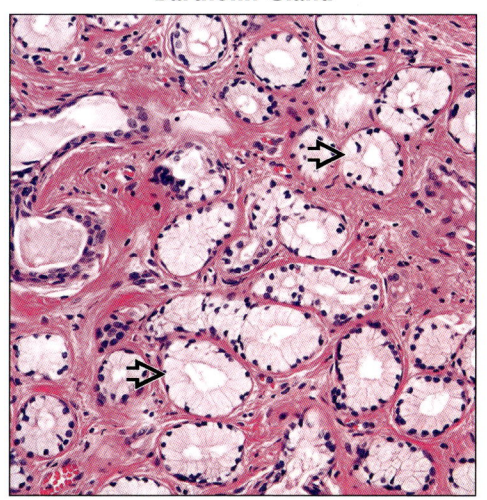

(Left) The ductal epithelium in the Bartholin (bulbourethral) gland ducts ➡ that are located near the main acini has a flattened appearance with scant cytoplasm, while the mucinous glands have abundant blue-gray cytoplasm ➡. (Right) The mucinous epithelium ➡ of the Bartholin (bulbourethral) glands is characterized by small, cytologically bland, pyknotic nuclei with abundant pale cytoplasm. The intervening stroma is typically densely collagenized.

VAGINA

Key Facts

Macroscopic Anatomy
- Fibromuscular tube extending from vestibule of vulva, between the labia minora, to uterine cervix
  - Located posterior (dorsal) to urinary bladder and anterior (ventral) to rectum
  - Anteriorly, vagina is separated from the bladder by fibroadipose tissue, but urethra enters vaginal wall distally
  - Posteriorly, upper 1/4 is adjacent to the rectouterine space
  - Middle portion is separated from rectum by rectovaginal septum, a layer of fibroadipose tissue
  - Distal portion is separated from anal canal predominantly by sphincter musculature

Microscopic Anatomy
- Stratified nonkeratinizing squamous epithelium
  - Basal cell layer comprised of single columnar epithelial layer with high nuclear to cytoplasmic ratio
  - Parabasal layer comprised of approximately 2 cell layers, above basal layer, with higher nuclear to cytoplasmic ratio than more superficial layers
  - Intermediate cell layer is most prominent with more abundant cytoplasm that is sometimes glycogenated
  - Superficial cell layer appears flattened with cells showing pyknotic nuclei and dense eosinophilic cytoplasm with occasional keratohyalin granules
- Subepithelial stroma (lamina propria)
  - Elastic fibers
  - Venous and lymphatic network
  - Loose connective tissue
  - Scattered spindled to stellate stromal cells (nuclei may be multilobated)
- Muscle
  - Outer longitudinal layer of smooth muscle is continuous with uterus
  - Thin inner circular smooth muscle layer
  - Fewer smooth muscle fibers anteriorly due to urethra
- Adventitia
  - Inner dense connective tissue layer adjacent to muscularis
  - Outer loose connective tissue layer contains peripheral nerves, blood vessels, and lymphatics

Pitfalls/Artifacts
- Epithelial proliferation and maturation varies with menstrual cycle
  - Predominance of thick glycogenated squamous epithelium just prior to ovulation
  - Gradual decrease in cell layers (and cytoplasm) after ovulation until start of next cycle
- Atrophic epithelial changes
  - Fewer cell layers and loss of cytoplasm imparts a basophilic appearance
  - Closely mimics a high-grade squamous intraepithelial lesion
- Wolffian (mesonephric) duct remnants (most commonly in lateral walls)
  - Collection of round to elongated glands with central eosinophilic secretion (± central duct)
  - Lined by short cuboidal layer of cytologically bland epithelial cells with little cytoplasm
  - May mimic adenocarcinoma, but remnants typically retain some lobular architecture
- Adenosis
  - Glandular epithelium located at stromal-epithelial interface, due to persistence of embryonic müllerian glandular tissue
  - Epithelium may be mucinous, tuboendometrioid, or embryonal type
  - Majority of adenosis in adults due to intrauterine exposure to diethylstilbestrol (DES)

Age Variation
- After menopause, vaginal epithelium atrophies due to low estrogenic state
- In newborns, vaginal epithelium is often fully mature due to maternal estrogen

Metaplasia
- Parakeratosis of epithelium may be seen with uterine prolapse

(Left) This sagittal dissection of the female pelvis (anterior on the right) shows the urinary bladder ⊳ anterior to the uterus ➔. The vagina ⇨ is located posterior to the urethra ➔. (Right) This schematic diagram shows the anatomic relationships between the urinary bladder ⊳, uterus ➔, vagina ⇨, and rectum ➔. The uterine cervix ➔ is present at the junction between the uterus and the vagina.

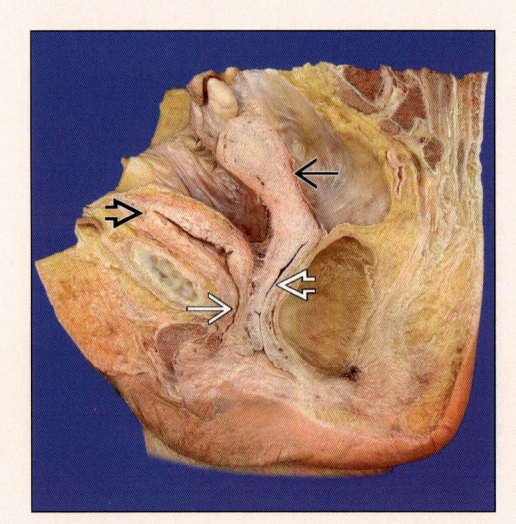

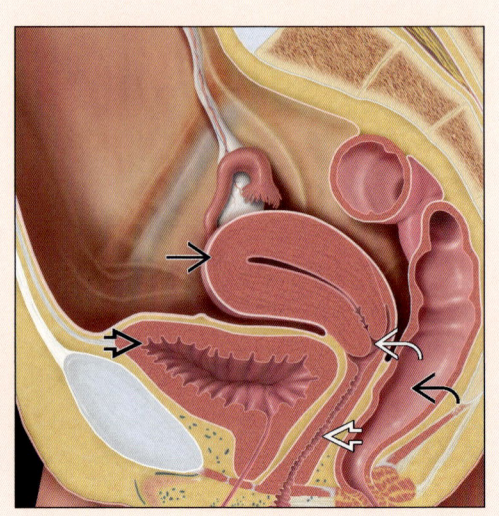

VAGINA

Mucosa

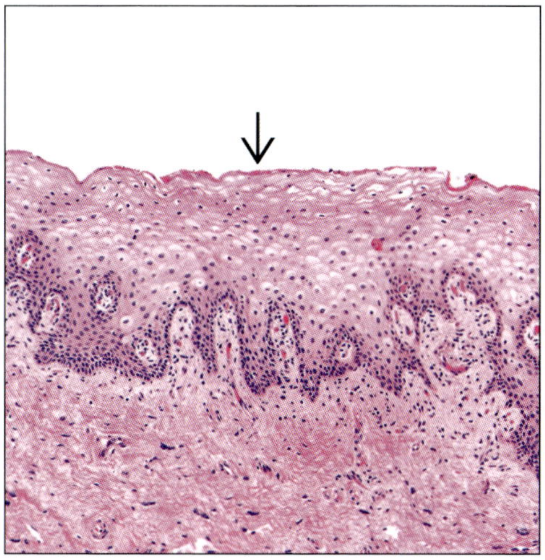

Epithelium

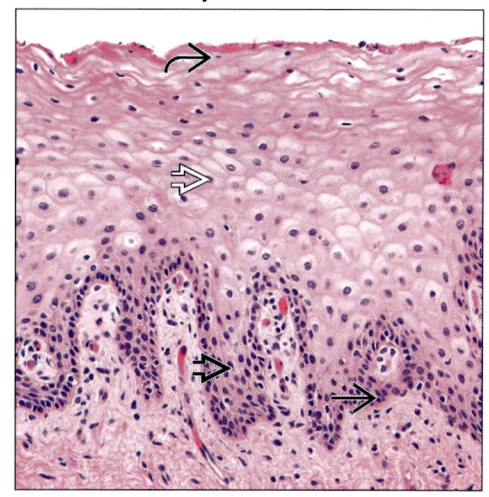

(Left) The vaginal mucosa consists of an epithelial layer ⇒ and underlying lamina propria. (Right) The epithelium consists of 4 layers. The basal layer ⇒ is a single layer of columnar cells with scant cytoplasm. The parabasal layer ⇒ is approximately 2 cell layers thick with slightly more cytoplasm. Intermediate cells ⇒ are the predominant cell type, and they have abundant eosinophilic cytoplasm. The superficial cells ⇒ appear flattened, with pyknotic nuclei.

Epithelium

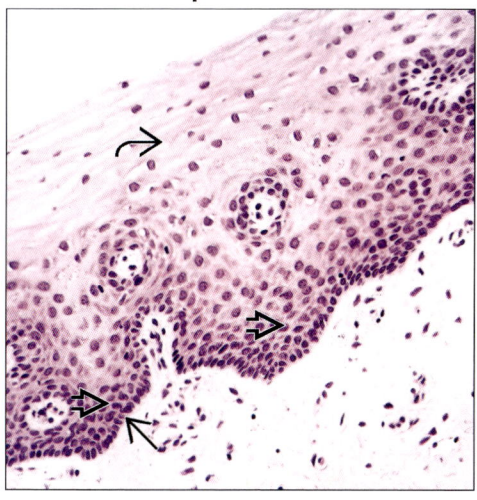

Epithelium

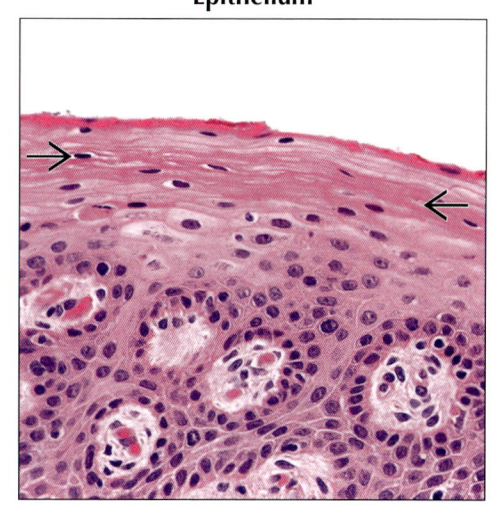

(Left) This section of epithelium shows a distinct basal cell layer ⇒ at the epithelial-stromal junction. The parabasal cells ⇒ have slightly more cytoplasm, and the intermediate cells ⇒ typically have the most cytoplasm. (Right) This section of vaginal epithelium has a more prominent superficial cell layer ⇒, which is characterized by flattened cells with pyknotic nuclei arranged in a plane parallel to the basement membrane.

Epithelium (Glycogenated)

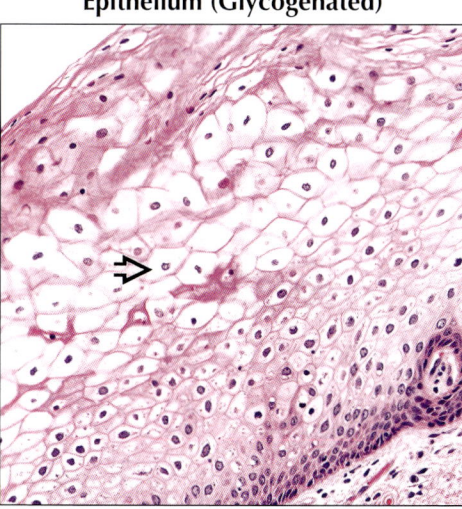

Epithelium (Atrophic)

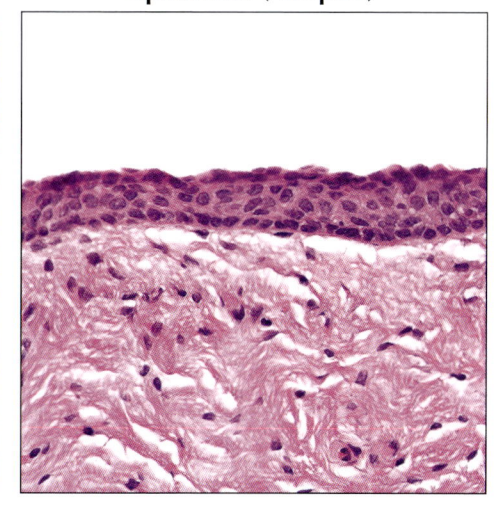

(Left) The intermediate cells may contain abundant intracytoplasmic glycogen ⇒ that can potentially mimic the koilocytic changes of HPV infection. (Right) After menopause, reduced estrogen often leads to marked vaginal atrophy. Atrophic squamous epithelium has fewer cell layers, and the individual cells have less cytoplasm; these features impart a more basophilic appearance. These histologic changes may mimic a high-grade squamous intraepithelial lesion.

VAGINA

(Left) The lamina propria ➡ lies directly beneath the squamous epithelium ➡, and consists of collagen fibers of variable density, elastic fibers, sparse stromal cells, and varying numbers of venous and lymphatic channels. The lamina propria is typically more dense in deeper areas adjacent to the muscularis. **(Right)** The lamina propria of the vagina may have a very loose, hypocellular stroma with an edematous appearance.

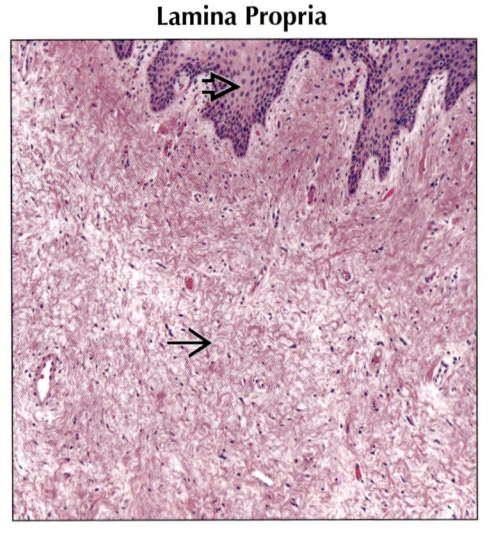

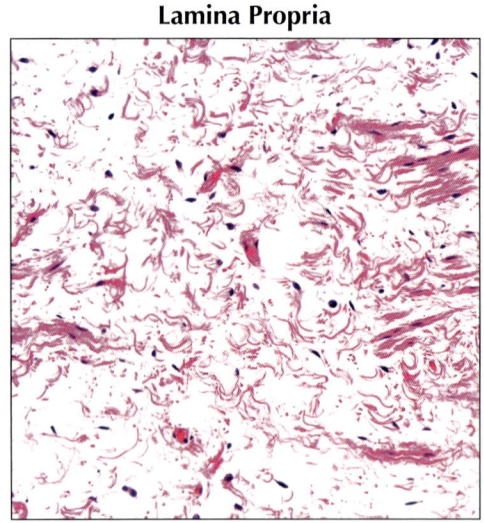

(Left) The lamina propria may also contain venous channels ➡ that are similar to the erectile tissue seen in other anatomic sites. **(Right)** The vaginal lamina propria is typically very hypocellular. The individual stromal cells may be spindled, fusiform, or stellate. A subset of these stromal cells may have multilobated nuclei ➡.

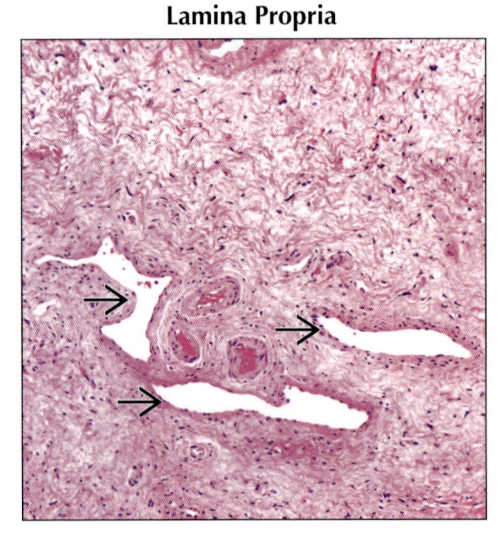

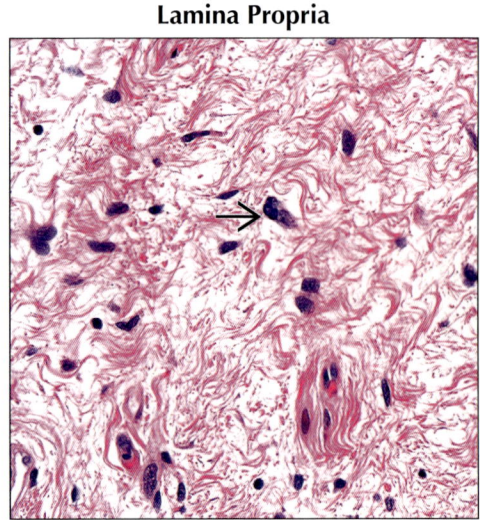

(Left) The multilobated stromal cells ➡ of the vaginal lamina propria may be striking, even on low-power scanning magnification. Similar cells may also be seen in the cervix and vulva. **(Right)** The presence of these multilobated nuclei ➡ in the vaginal lamina propria stromal cells may suggest the possibility of a neoplastic process, but this degree of atypia is within the spectrum of normal. These cells are identical to those seen in a fibroepithelial polyp.

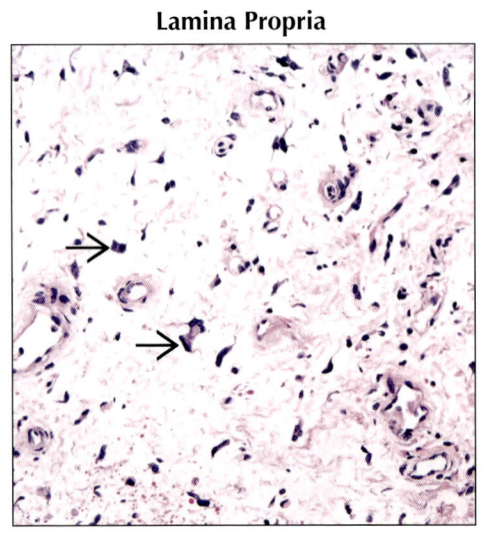

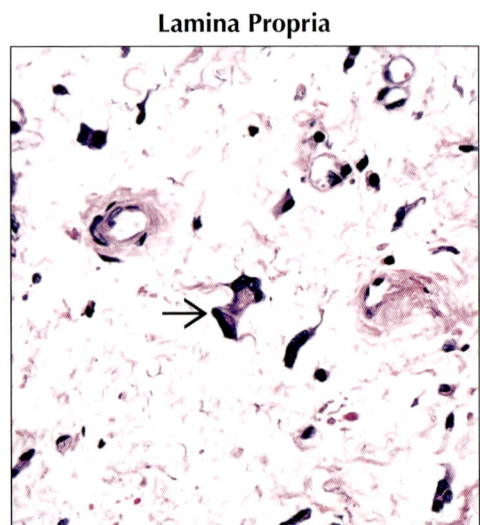

VAGINA

Muscularis
Muscularis

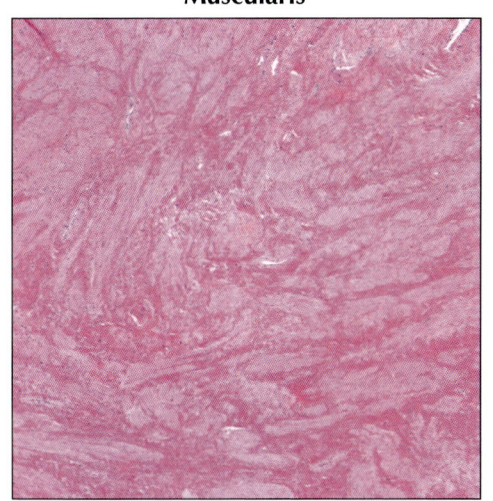

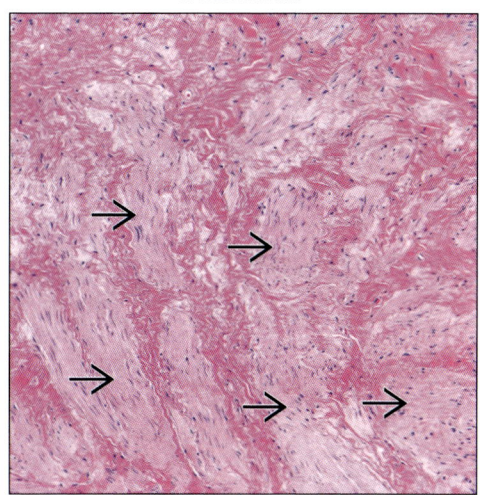

(Left) The muscularis of the vagina is composed of inner circular and outer longitudinal smooth muscle layers, but these 2 layers may be relatively indistinct. The outer longitudinal layer of the vaginal muscularis, which is thicker and more conspicuous, is continuous with the muscularis of the uterus. (Right) The muscularis is comprised of variably arranged fascicles of normal smooth muscle ⇨.

Rectovaginal Septum
Distal Vaginal Wall

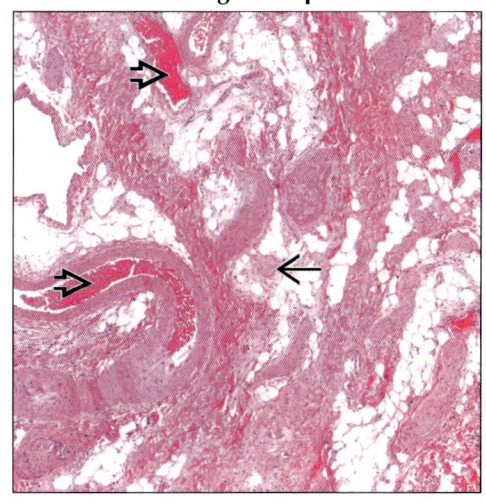

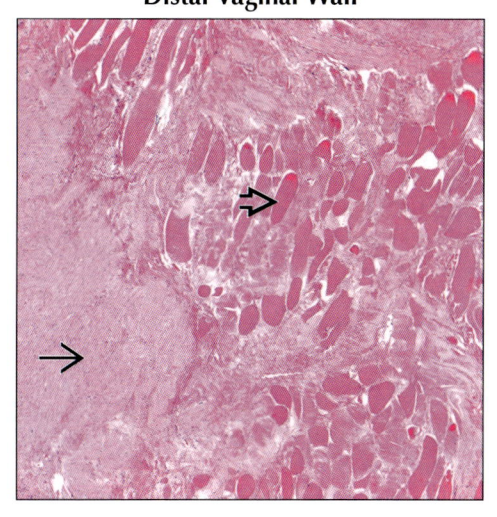

(Left) In the the middle segment of the vagina, the rectum is separated from the posterior aspect of the the vagina by a rim of fibroadipose tissue (the rectovaginal septum) that also contains blood vessels ⇨ and small nerves ⇨. (Right) In the distal vagina near the introitus, the muscularis ⇨ of the vaginal wall may merge and become admixed with the skeletal muscle fibers ⇨ of the sphincter musculature (bulbospongiosus muscle).

Wolffian Duct Remnants
Müllerian Remnants

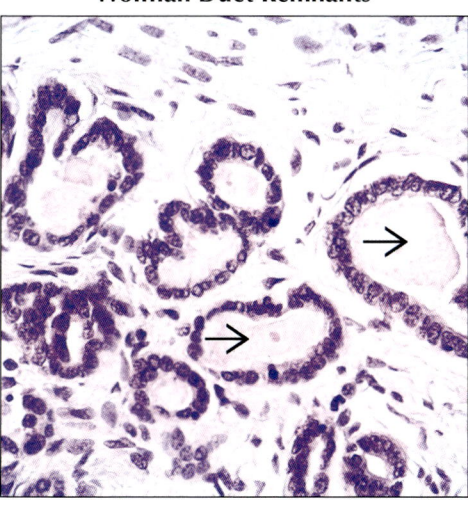

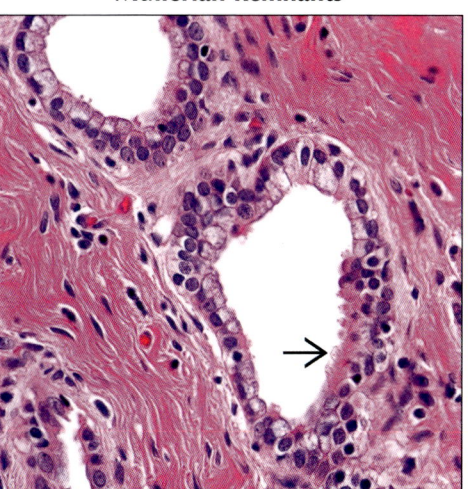

(Left) Wolffian duct (also called mesonephric or Gartner duct) remnants are not infrequently identified in the vagina. These glandular structures are typically lined by a cuboidal epithelial layer with little cytoplasm, and the lumen is often filled with eosinophilic secretions ⇨. (Right) Although rarely seen outside the setting of DES exposure, remnants of müllerian ducts may occasionally be seen in the vagina. This example has a ciliated ⇨ tubal-type epithelium.

UTERUS

Key Facts

Macroscopic Anatomy
- Complex organ with multiple regions: Ectocervix, endocervix, lower uterine segment, endometrium, myometrium, and serosa
  - Ectocervix: Distal end of uterus, typically covered by stratified squamous epithelium
  - Endocervix: Tunnel-like lumen of uterine cervix, lined by mucin-secreting pits
  - Lower uterine segment: Triangle-shaped transition from endocervix to uterine corpus
  - Endometrium: Uterine mucosa composed of glands and stroma
  - Myometrium: Muscular wall of uterus composed of layers of smooth muscle
  - Serosa: Thin lining of body and fundus of uterus; covers portions of uterus that are not retroperitoneal

Microscopic Anatomy
- Ectocervix: Stratified squamous epithelium overlying fibrous stroma
- Transformation zone: Squamocolumnar junction that lies between ectocervix and endocervix
  - Transformation zone identified by squamous metaplasia of endocervix; migrates during reproductive years
- Endocervix: Simple, columnar mucinous epithelial cells line endocervical pits that extend into fibrous stroma
- Lower uterine segment: Transition between endocervix and endometrium; admixtures of endometrial and endocervical glands and stroma may be seen in this region
- Endometrial glands
  - Columnar epithelial cells that vary from simple to pseudostratified
  - Epithelium may contain vacuoles (secretory) or be ciliated
  - Functionalis: Superficial endometrial layer, lost during menstruation
  - Basalis: Deep layer of more monomorphic glands that regenerates functionalis after shedding
- Endometrial stroma
  - Densely cellular supporting stroma composed of spindle cells with elongated nuclei admixed with blood vessels (spiral arterioles)
  - Stromal cells range from small and spindled (proliferative phase) to large, eosinophilic, and polygonal (secretory phase, pregnancy, hormone effect)
- Myometrium: Smooth muscle wall of uterus, composed of 3 layers (inner longitudinal, middle circular, and outer longitudinal)
  - Middle circular layer heavily vascularized and contains arcuate arteries
- Serosa: Thin mesothelial lining of uterine corpus and fundus

Pitfalls/Artifacts
- Glandular compression, simulating hyperplasia, may be seen following biopsy
- Suction created by biopsy instruments may lead to "gland in gland" artifact
- Exfoliation artifact leads to epithelial shedding, which can mimic serous carcinoma
- Arias-Stella effect may closely resemble carcinoma due to marked atypia and glandular crowding

Age Variation
- During puberty, endocervical epithelium migrates toward ectocervix (ectropion) and then is slowly replaced by squamous epithelium during reproductive years
- Endometrial atrophy: Inactive, cystically dilated glands may be present after menopause

Metaplasia
- Squamous metaplasia: Occurs along transformation zone
- Ciliated (tubal) metaplasia: Common; occurs in endocervix and endometrial glands
- Mucinous metaplasia: Uncommon metaplasia of endometrium; typically consists of simple to stratified, columnar mucinous epithelial cells

(Left) The uterus lies in the pelvis and comprises the ectocervix ➔, endocervix ➔, endometrium ➔, and myometrium ➔. (Right) The ectocervical mucosa consists of stratified, nonkeratinizing squamous epithelium composed of 3 layers: Basal/parabasal ➔, stratum spongiosum ➔, and superficial ➔.

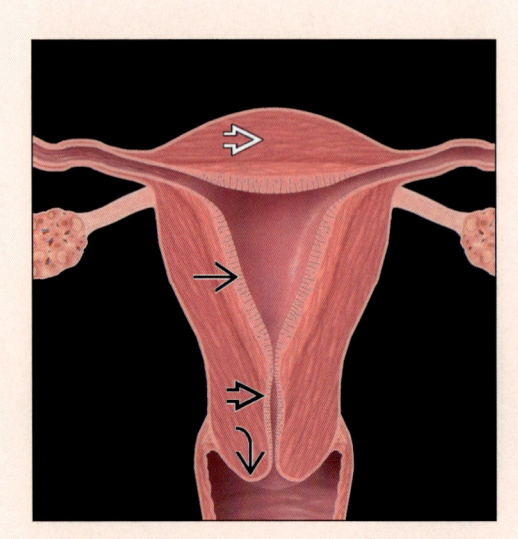

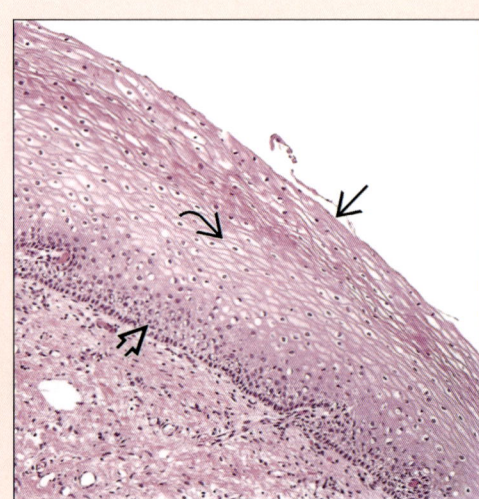

UTERUS

Ectocervix: Basal Layer

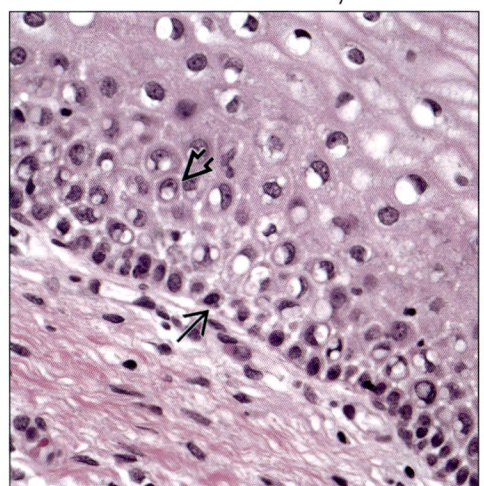

Ectocervix: Superficial

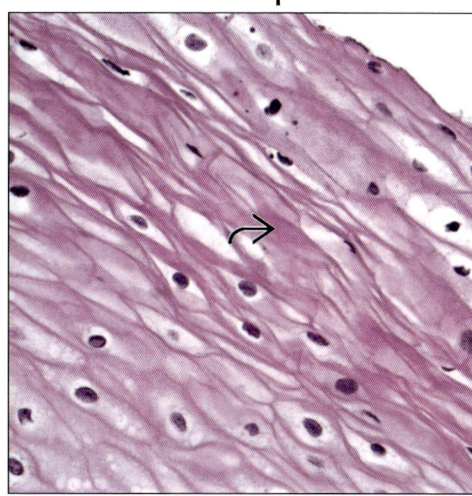

(Left) The basal/parabasal layers are composed of round to cuboidal cells. Basal cells ⇨ have scant cytoplasm and dark nuclei, whereas parabasal cells ⇨ are slightly larger and with more cytoplasm. Scattered mitotic figures may be seen. *(Right)* The stratum spongiosum and superficial layers compose the majority of the squamous epithelium. As cells mature, the nuclei become smaller and darker while the cells become flat. Superficial cells may not have visible nuclei ⇨.

Ectocervix: Atrophy

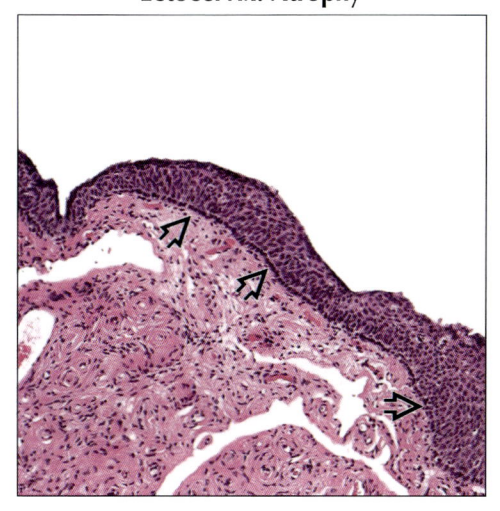

Ectocervix: Atrophy

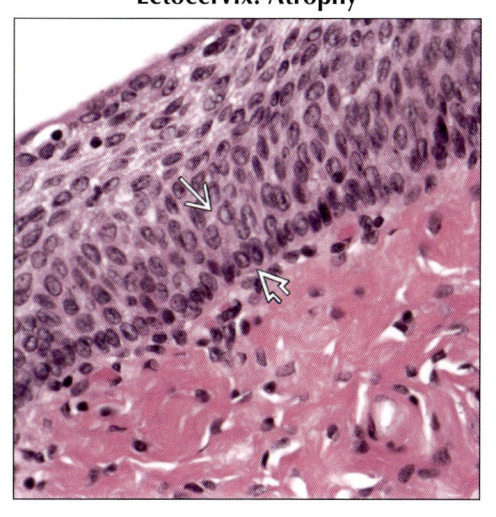

(Left) As patients age, the cervical epithelium may undergo atrophic changes. In atrophy, the epithelium is composed predominately of basal and parabasal cells. An easily apparent and orderly basal layer ⇨ is usually present. *(Right)* This photograph of atrophy shows the basal ⇨ and parabasal ⇨ layers along with a thinned stratum spongiosum and superficial layer. Loss of glycogen leads to decreased cytoplasm relative to the nucleus, which may mimic dysplasia. Mitotic figures should be absent.

Cervix: Transformation Zone

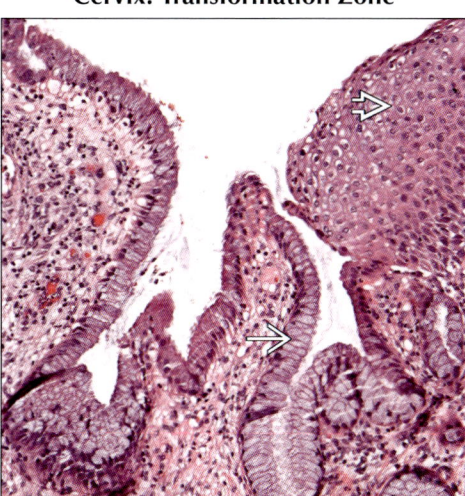

Endocervix: Endocervical Glands

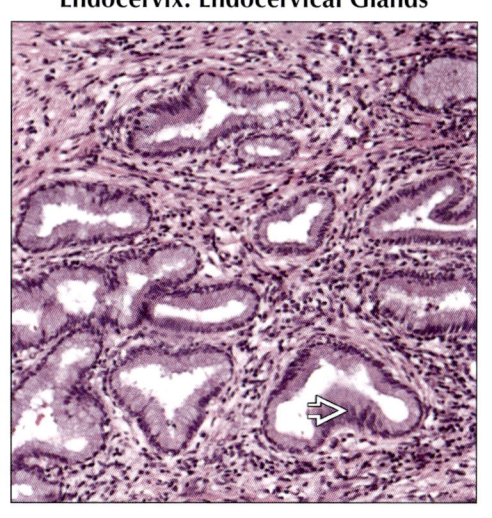

(Left) The transformation zone is an irregularly defined junction of squamous ⇨ and mucinous ⇨ epithelium. This squamocolumnar junction migrates to the ectocervix during puberty. As females age, squamous metaplasia causes the junction to migrate back into the endocervical canal. *(Right)* Endocervical "glands" (technically crypts, as they connect to the surface) are composed of a simple columnar mucinous epithelium ⇨ with basally oriented nuclei and amphophilic cytoplasm.

UTERUS

Endocervix: Stroma

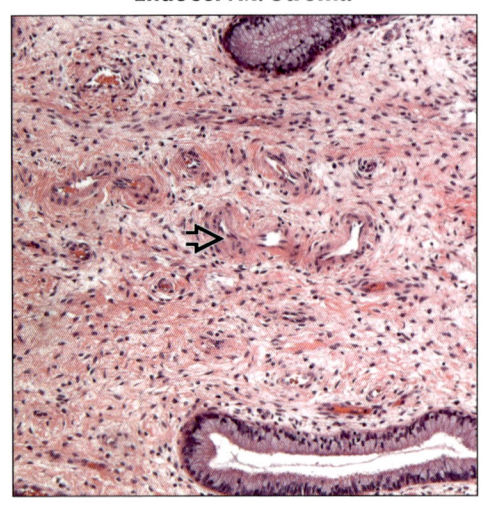

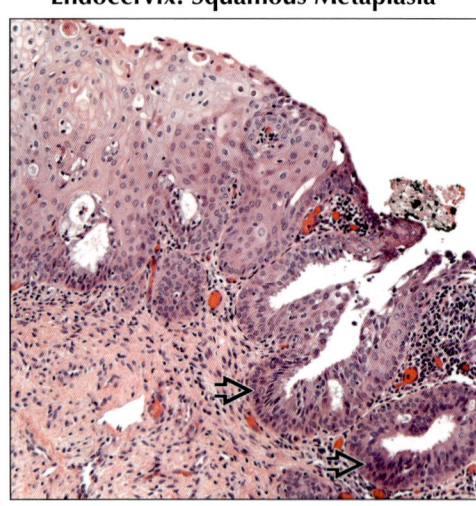

(Left) Cervical stroma is predominantly composed of fibrous tissue and blood vessels ⇨. Small wisps of smooth muscle may be present but are rarer than in the rest of the uterus. Scattered lymphocytes and plasma cells are normal. **(Right)** Squamous metaplasia occurs at the transformation zone and can extend along the surface of the endocervix. The metaplasia may involve glands, causing thickening of the epithelium and loss of normal mucinous cells ⇨.

Endocervix: Squamous Metaplasia

Endocervix: Squamous Metaplasia

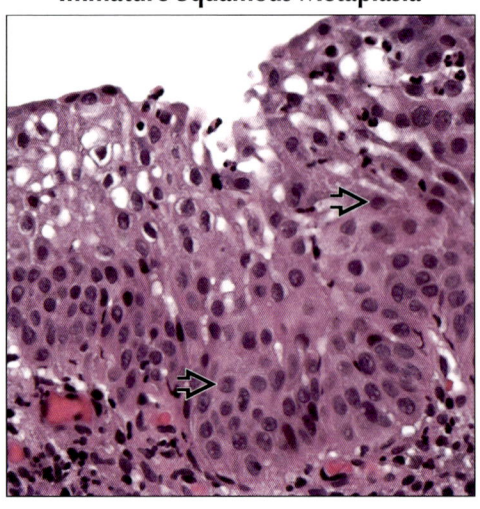

(Left) Squamous metaplasia can fill the endocervical glands ⇨, causing obliteration of the gland lumen. These glands typically appear as round nests of normal squamous epithelium. **(Right)** Immature squamous epithelium may occupy the transformation zone. This epithelium contains less glycogen than typical cervical epithelium and is composed of immature keratinocytes ⇨ throughout all levels. These immature cells may mimic dysplasia; however, true atypia and atypical mitotic activity are absent.

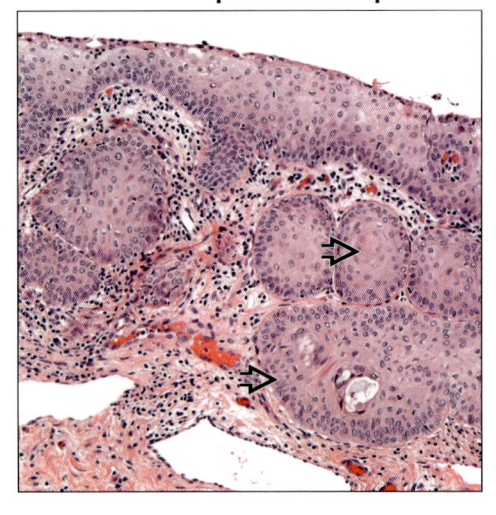

Immature Squamous Metaplasia

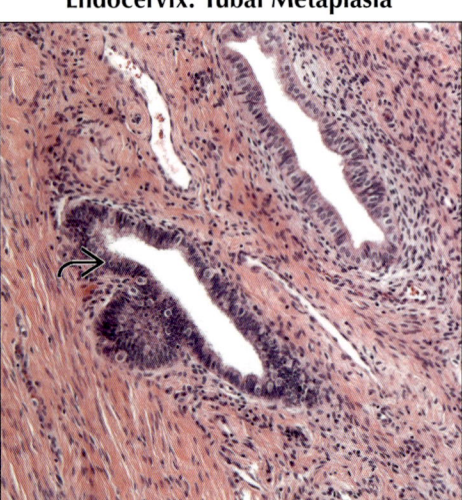

Endocervix: Tubal Metaplasia

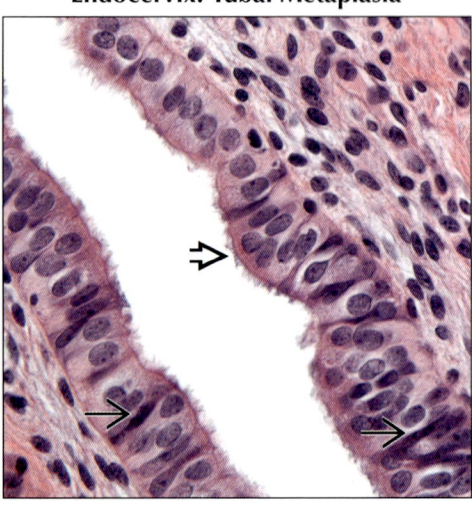

(Left) The columnar ⇨ mucinous cells of the endocervix may also undergo metaplasia to tubal epithelium. Involved glands may appear more hyperchromatic at low power, at times resembling endometrial glands or glands involved by adenocarcinoma in situ. **(Right)** High-power examination of areas of tubal metaplasia will reveal tubal-type epithelium composed of both ciliated ⇨ and secretory cells ⇨. Note the lack of atypia, mitotic activity, and apoptotic debris seen in adenocarcinoma in situ.

Endocervix: Tubal Metaplasia

UTERUS

Endocervix: Tunnel Clusters

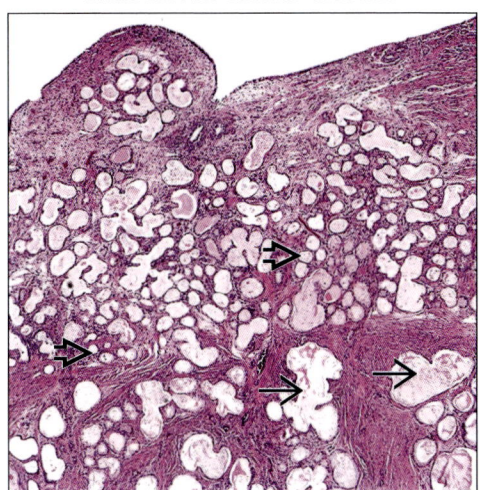

Endocervix: Tunnel Clusters

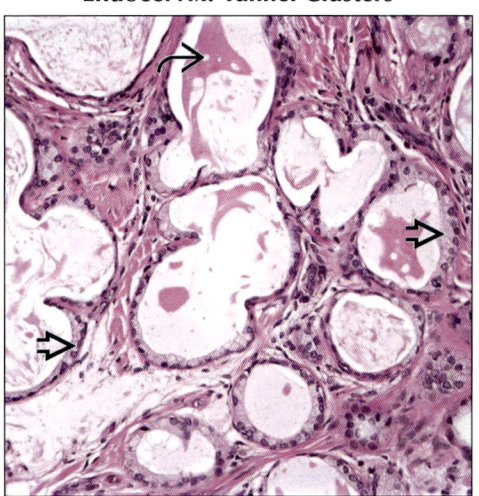

(Left) As squamous epithelium covers the openings to the endocervical glands, the glands become dilated and filled with mucinous material. Type A tunnel clusters ⇨ are small, whereas type B tunnel clusters ⇨ are dilated. Frequently, the 2 patterns are intermixed. *(Right)* Type A tunnel clusters have an attenuated simple cuboidal lining of mucinous cells ⇨ and inspissated, eosinophilic, mucinous material ⇨ in the lumina.

Endocervix: Nabothian Cyst

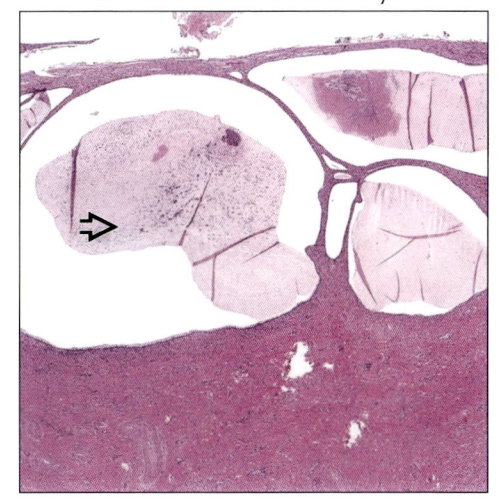

Endocervix: Nabothian Cyst

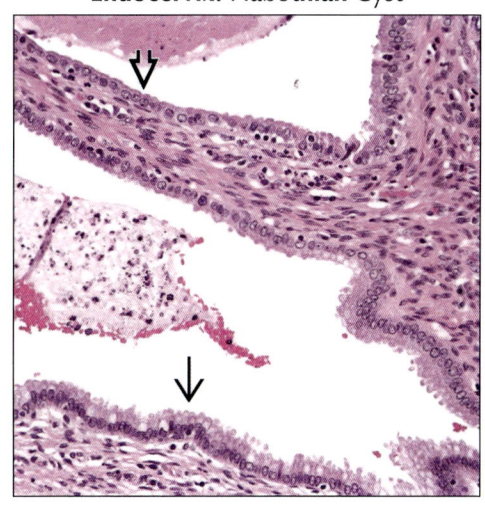

(Left) Occasionally, endocervical glands occluded by the process of squamous epithelialization will expand, forming cystic spaces filled with mucin ⇨. These cysts are known as nabothian cysts and may become large enough to form a cervical mass. *(Right)* The lining of a nabothian cyst is typically composed of endocervical columnar mucinous epithelium ⇨. The lining may become attenuated and assume a low cuboidal morphology ⇨.

Endocervix: Microglandular Hyperplasia

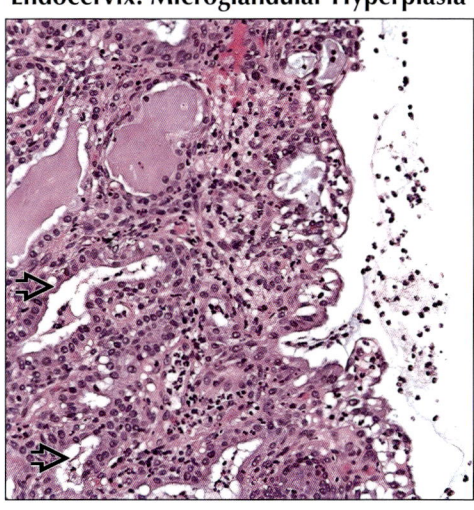

Endocervix: Microglandular Hyperplasia

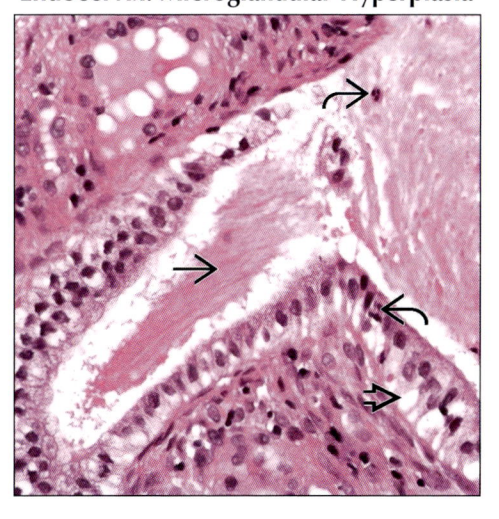

(Left) Microglandular hyperplasia of the cervix is composed of an increased number of small glands ⇨ that proliferate in the endocervix. This phenomenon has been associated with oral contraceptive use. *(Right)* The glands that make up microglandular hyperplasia often have irregular contours, columnar mucinous epithelium with subnuclear vacuoles ⇨, and inspissated mucin ⇨. Scattered neutrophils ⇨ can be seen in both the mucin and the epithelium.

UTERUS

Cervix: Mesonephric Remnant

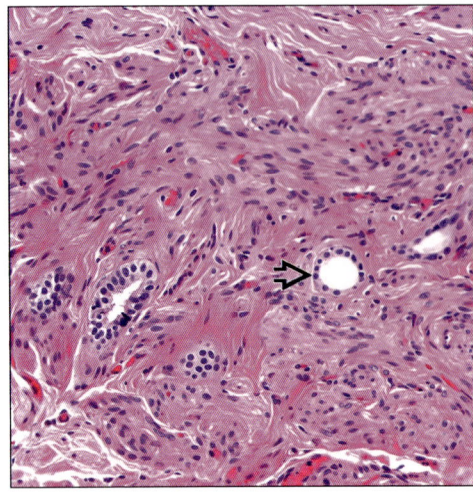

Cervix: Mesonephric Remnant

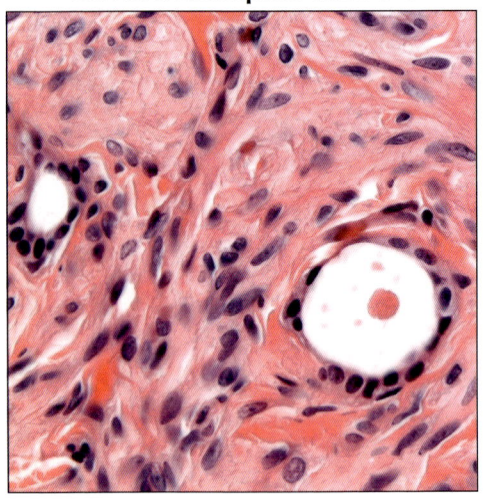

(Left) Scattered small tubular glands may be seen deep within the cervical stroma. These glands are composed of low cuboidal epithelium ⇨ and generally lack atypia and mitotic activity. Occasionally, they may be associated with a long cleft-like space. (Courtesy A. Cole, MD.)
(Right) Mesonephric remnants are composed of bland, low cuboidal epithelium. Eosinophilic, PAS-positive secretions can commonly be identified within the lumen. (Courtesy A. Cole, MD.)

Cervix: Decidua

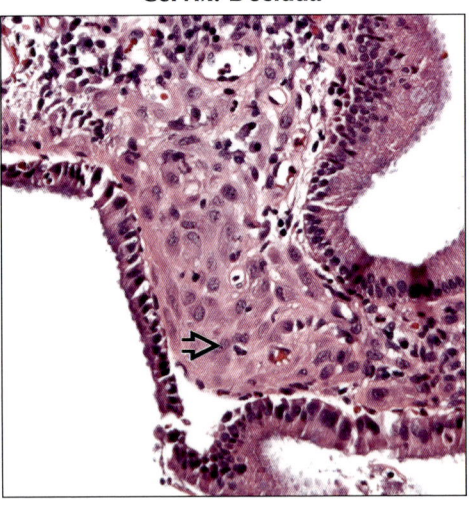

Cervix and Lower Uterine Segment

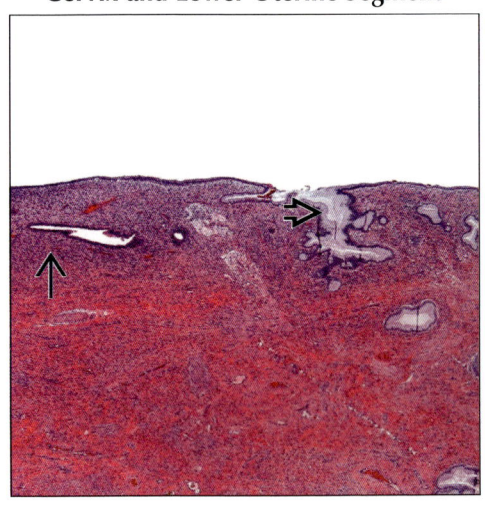

(Left) In pregnant patients, a stromal decidual reaction may occur. Ectopic decidua is composed of large, polygonal, eosinophilic cells ⇨ with bland nuclei. Nests of these cells may mimic squamous metaplasia or invasive squamous cell carcinoma but can be distinguished from the latter by the lack of atypia.
(Right) As the endocervix transitions to the lower uterine segment, the glands lose their basophilic mucin ⇨ and the stroma becomes more spindled and basophilic ⇨.

Lower Uterine Segment

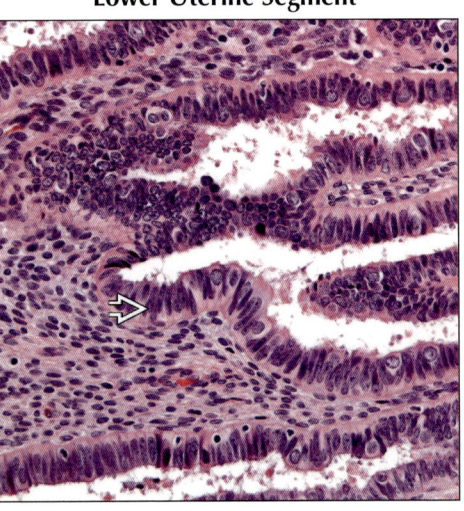

Lower Uterine Segment

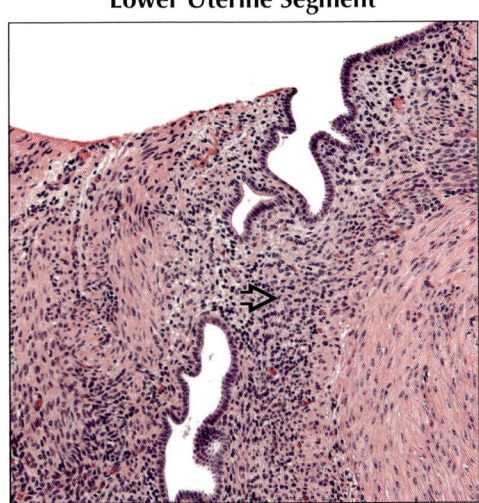

(Left) The lower uterine segment displays glandular and stromal changes that are intermediate between the endocervix and the endometrium. These endocervical glands are composed of columnar epithelium ⇨ that lost the basophilic mucin seen in endocervical epithelium.
(Right) The endometrial lining of the lower uterine segment is thinner than the uterine corpus endometrial lining. The stroma becomes more cellular and basophilic ⇨ as it approaches the endometrium.

UTERUS

Endometrium

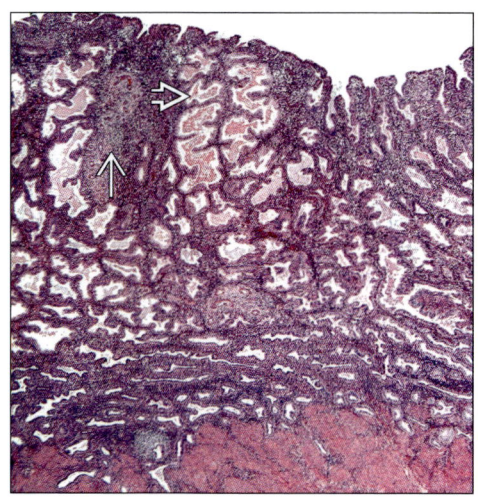

Endometrial Layers

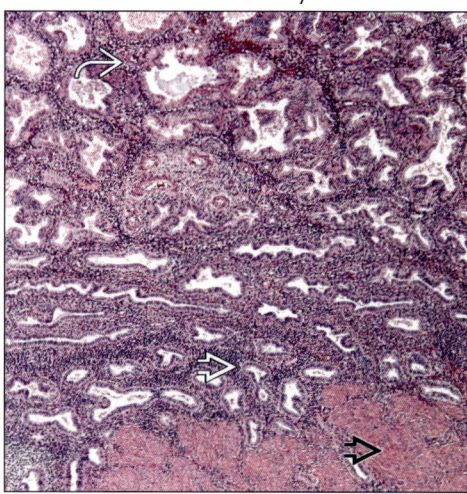

(Left) The endometrial lining of the uterine corpus is much thicker than that of the lower uterine segment. It is composed of glands ➡ with intervening stroma ➡. **(Right)** Two distinct layers of endometrium can be identified. The layer adjacent to the myometrium ➡ is known as the basalis ➡. The basalis is the reserve cell layer of the endometrium that regenerates the functionalis ➡ after menses. The basalis, as opposed to the functionalis, is only slightly hormonally responsive.

Endomyometrium: Irregular Junction

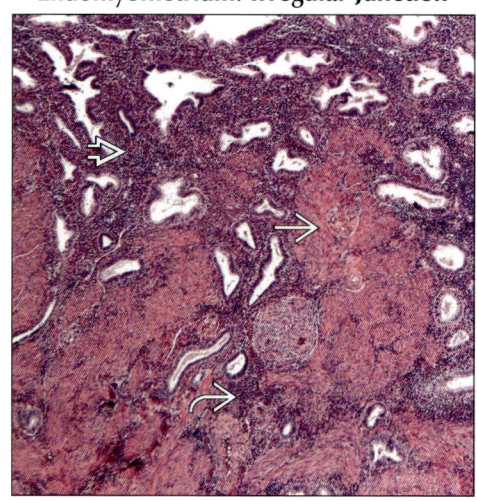

Endometrium: Lymphoid Aggregate

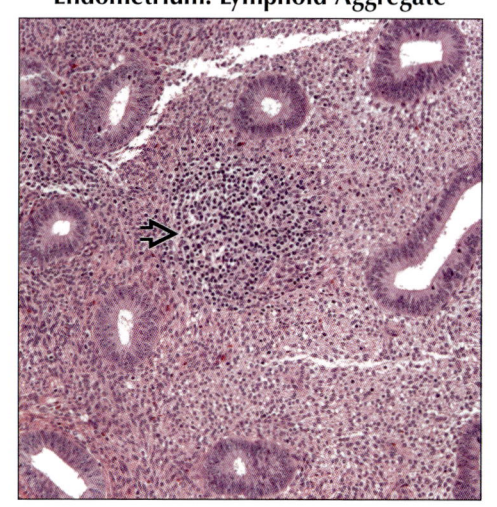

(Left) The interface between the endometrium ➡ and the myometrium ➡ may be irregular, which may cause difficulty in determining the depth of invasion in endometrial adenocarcinoma. The presence of endometrial stroma ➡ may help identify an irregular endometrial/myometrial interface involved by tumor as opposed to true invasion. **(Right)** Scattered lymphoid aggregates ➡ are normally seen within the endometrial stroma. These are a normal finding and not diagnostic of chronic endometritis.

Endometrium: Chronic Endometritis

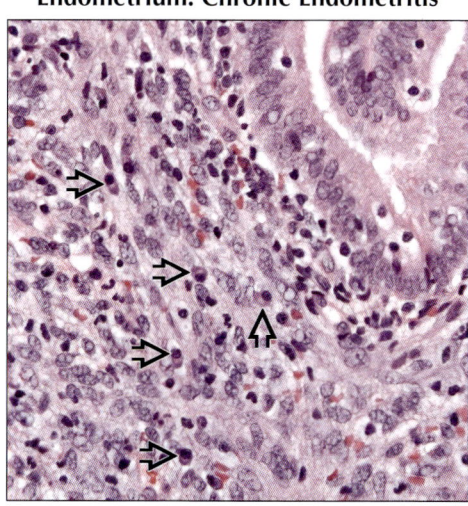

Proliferative Endometrium

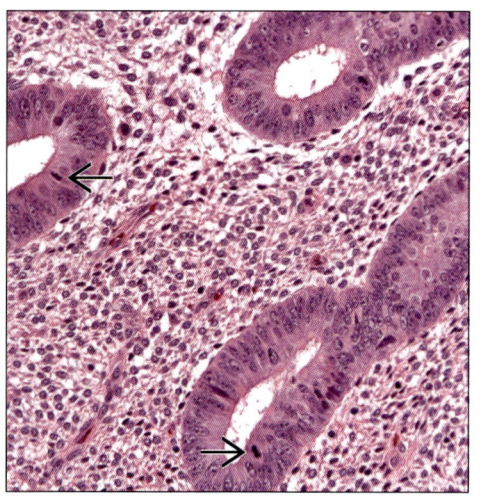

(Left) Plasma cell infiltrates ➡ are not a normal finding within the endometrium and are generally diagnostic of chronic endometritis. Endometrial polyps may contain rare plasma cells; however, this alone does not warrant a diagnosis of chronic endometritis. **(Right)** Proliferative endometrial glands have a rounded contour and are composed of pseudostratified columnar cells. Scattered mitotic figures ➡ should be readily apparent. Stromal mitoses may be identified.

UTERUS

Proliferative Gland

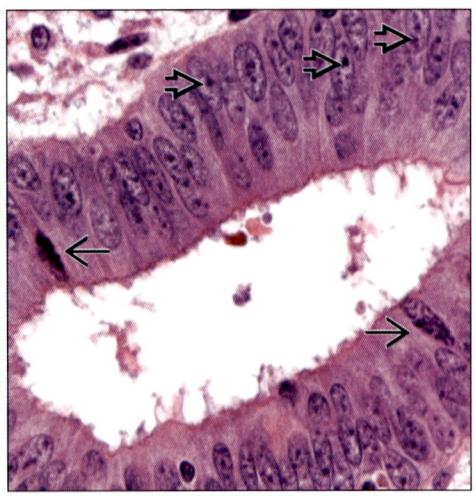

Proliferative Stroma

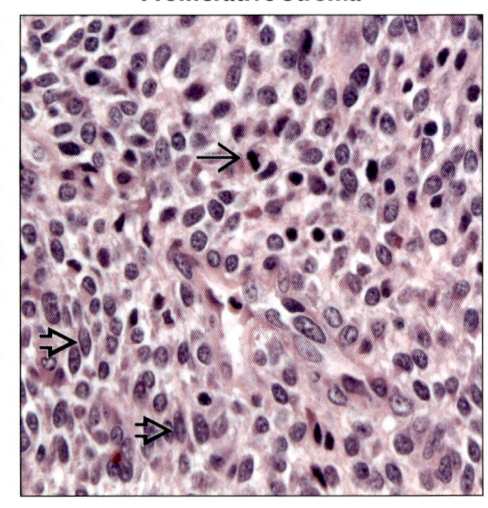

(Left) Proliferative glands are composed of pseudostratified columnar cells with mitotic figures ➡. The nuclei are elongated (cigar-shaped) and contain vesicular chromatin and multiple small nucleoli ▷. In the early proliferative phase, the glands are uncoiled, and as they grow, they become more convoluted. (Right) During the proliferative phase, the stromal cells have round to spindled nuclei ▷ and scant cytoplasm. Mitotic figures are typically easy to identify ➡.

Interval Phase Endometrium

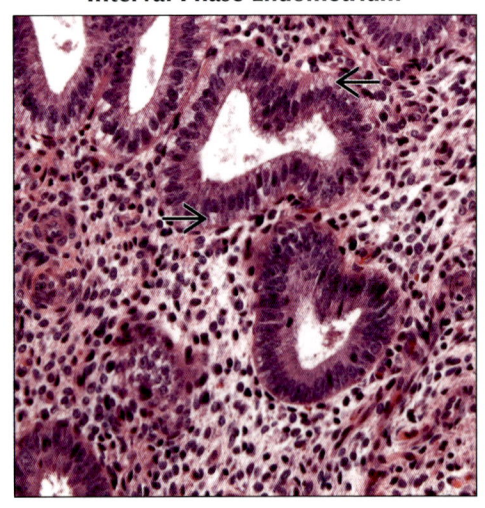

Early Secretory Endometrium

(Left) Around day 10 or 11 of the menstrual cycle, small subnuclear vacuoles ➡ begin to form. These vacuoles will become more pronounced, peaking at day 17. The glandular contours become more irregular as the gland grows. Scattered proliferative type glands and rare mitotic figures may be identified. (Right) At least 1/2 of the glands should contain subnuclear vacuoles ▷ in early secretory endometrium (around day 16). (Courtesy A. Cole, MD.)

Secretory Endometrium

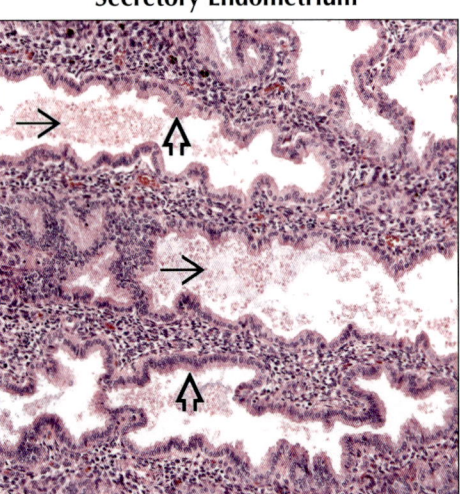

Secretory Endometrium: Crowding

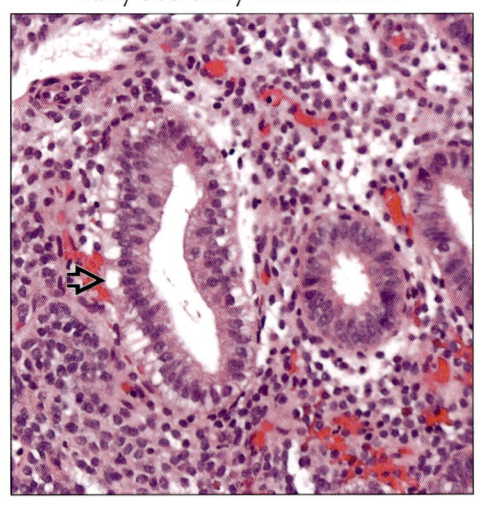

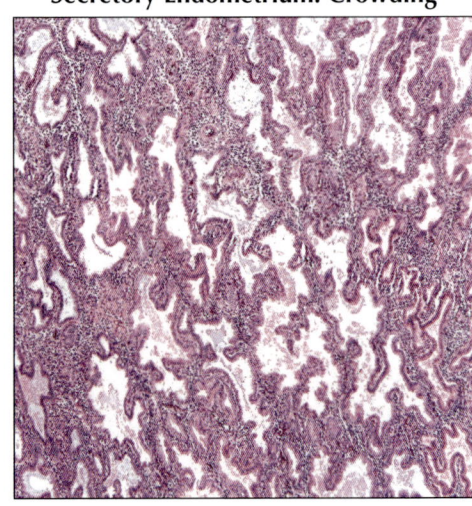

(Left) The middle of the secretory phase is marked by glands that lack cytoplasmic vacuoles but have abundant luminal secretions ➡. The glandular epithelium is composed of a simple columnar epithelium with abundant eosinophilic cytoplasm ▷. (Right) During the secretory phase, extensive glandular crowding may be present. This crowding must be distinguished from the glandular crowding seen in hyperplasia, which usually carries a proliferative morphologic profile.

UTERUS

Late Secretory Endometrium

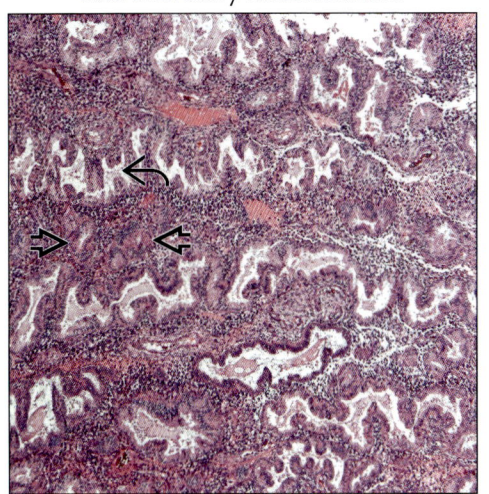

Late Secretory Endometrium

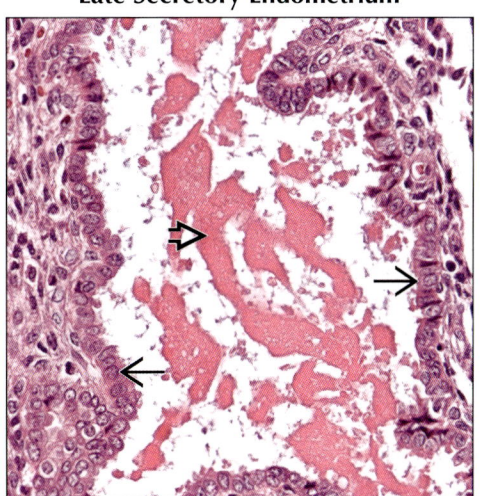

(Left) As the glands progress through the secretory phase, the glandular lumina become more convoluted (or "saw-toothed") ➡. The spiral arterioles ➡ become more pronounced due to the presence of an early predecidual cuff surrounding the vessels. *(Right)* A late secretory gland with a dilated lumen contains inspissated eosinophilic secretions ➡. Note the absence of vacuoles. The lining epithelium is columnar to cuboidal with rounded vesicular nuclei ➡.

Secretory Endometrium: Surface

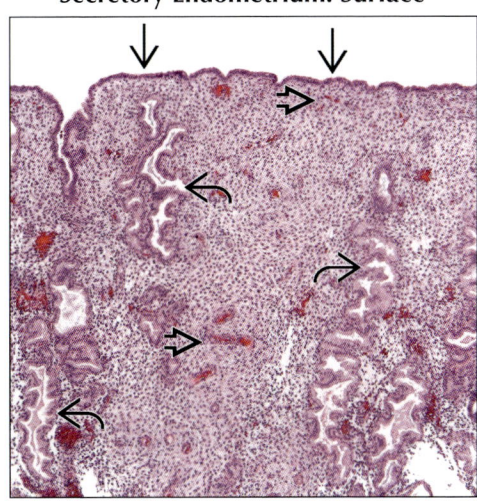

Spiral Arterioles

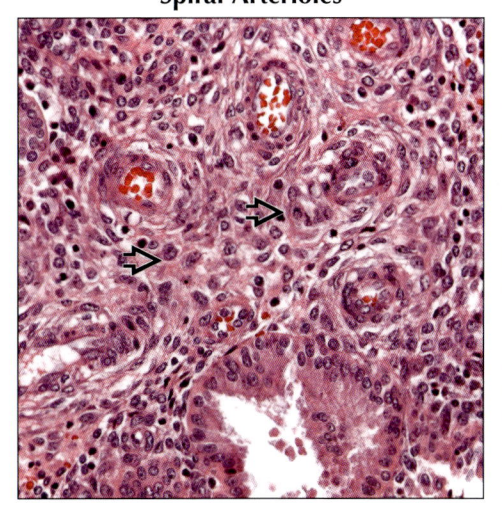

(Left) Stromal changes mark progression into the late secretory phase. These changes consist of the development of predecidua surrounding the superficial spiral arterioles ➡. This predecidual change then expands and begins to coalesce beneath the endometrial surface ➡. Exhausted, serrated secretory glands are present ➡. *(Right)* These superficial spiral arterioles are surrounded by a cuff of relatively large, polygonal, eosinophilic predecidual cells ➡.

Predecidua

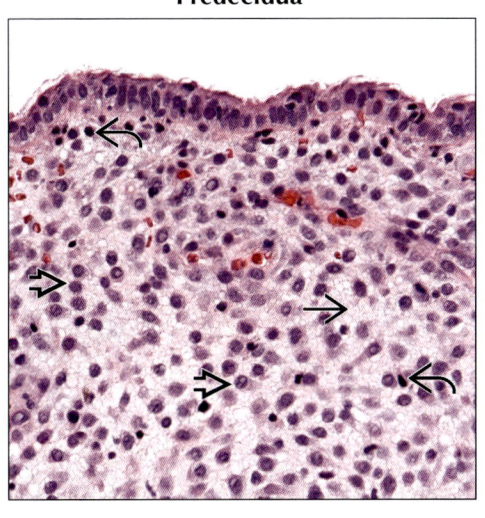

Menstrual Endometrium

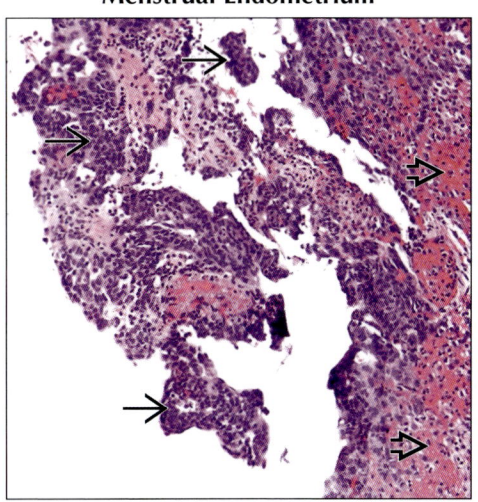

(Left) The predecidual cells coalesce beneath the endometrial surface. The "pseudodecidualized" cells contain abundant eosinophilic cytoplasm ➡ and are separated by increasing amounts of stromal edema ➡. Scattered stromal inflammatory cells (granulocytes) ➡ are present and will increase in number as menstruation is approached. *(Right)* The superficial endometrium begins to fragment. Stromal hemorrhage ➡ and condensation (clumping) ➡ are present as well. (Courtesy A. Laury, MD.)

UTERUS

Menstrual Endometrium

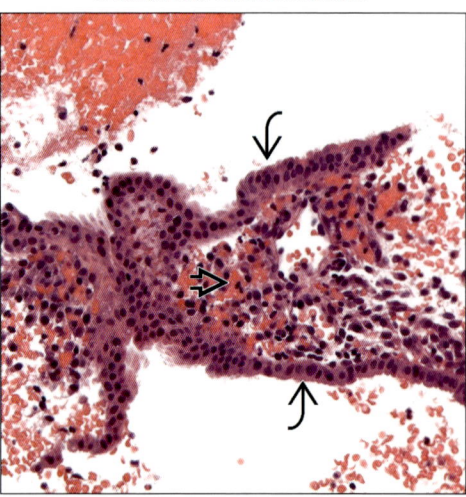

(Left) A fragment of superficial endometrium during menstruation shows marked eosinophilia ➡. Stromal fragmentation and hemorrhage ➡ are apparent. **(Right)** As the endometrium breaks down, the stromal cells condense, forming rounded aggregates ➡. Typically, a rim of eosinophilic epithelium ➡ can be seen adherent to the stromal fragments. This epithelium may contain nuclear atypia and should not be confused with malignancy.

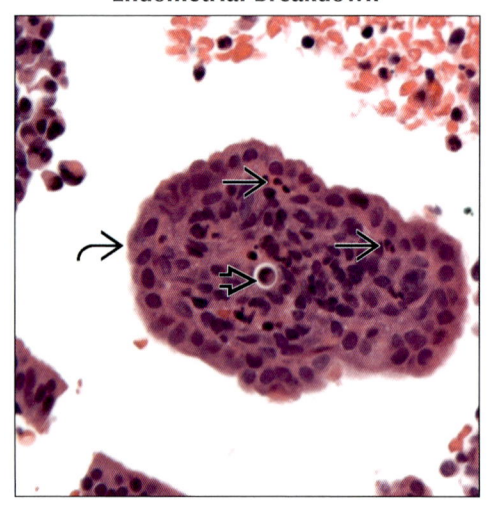

Endometrial Breakdown

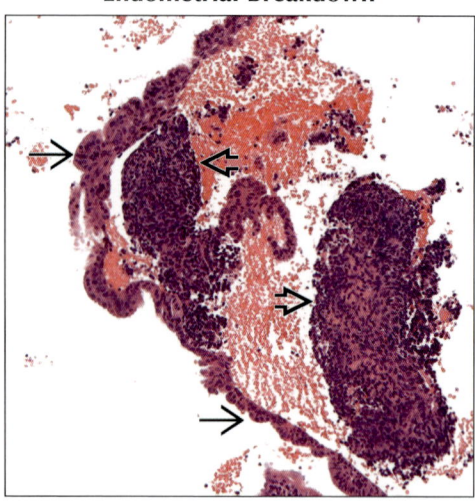

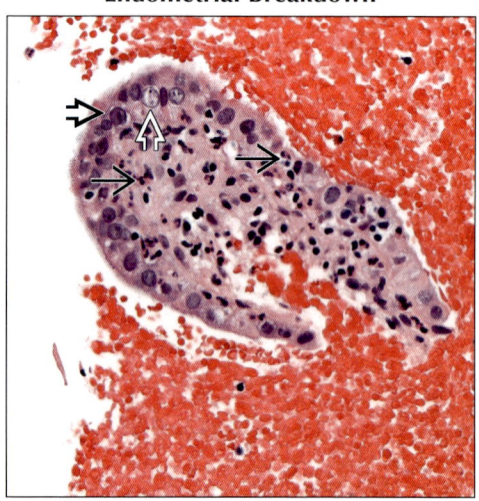

(Left) Stromal fragments, also known as "blue balls," are common in stromal breakdown. An apoptotic cell ➡ and scattered inflammatory cells ➡ can be seen within the stroma. Note the rim of eosinophilic glandular epithelium ➡. **(Right)** This endometrial stromal fragment is extensively permeated by stromal granulocytes ➡. The lining of epithelium has mild atypia consisting of variation of nuclear size and shape ➡ as well as variable nuclear chromasia ➡.

Endometrial Polyp

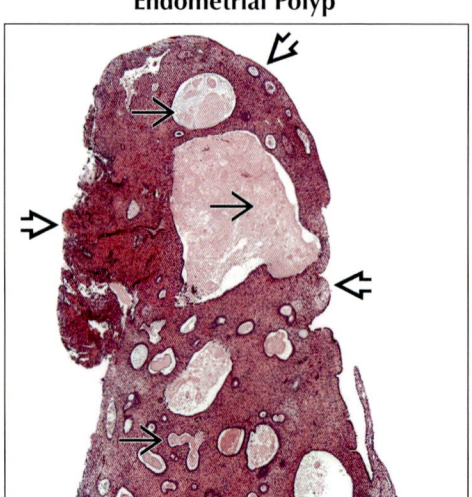

(Left) Endometrial polyps are common findings when examining uterine samples. In an intact specimen, one can appreciate the lining of the polyp along 3 sides by surface epithelium ➡. Altered endometrial glands ➡ are another common finding. **(Right)** In addition to a polypoid shape and irregular endometrial glands ➡, the stroma ➡ of the polyp differs from the stroma of the nonpolypoid endometrium. Typically, the stroma is less cellular and has a fibrotic, eosinophilic appearance.

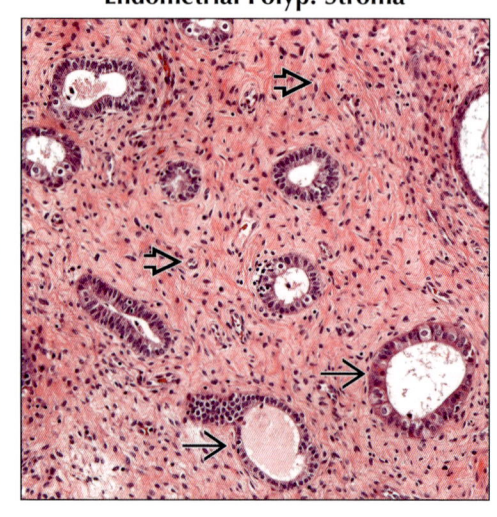

UTERUS

Endometrial Polyp: Glands

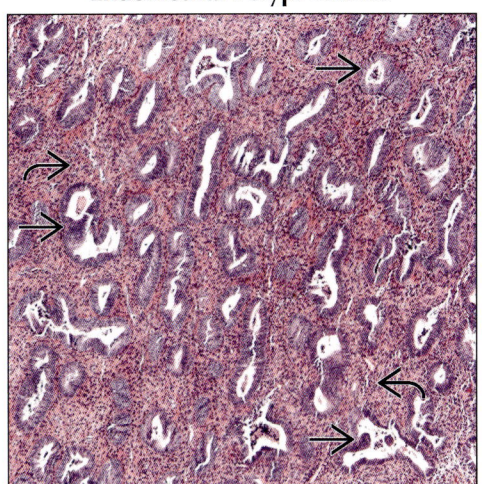

Endometrial Polyp: Blood Vessels

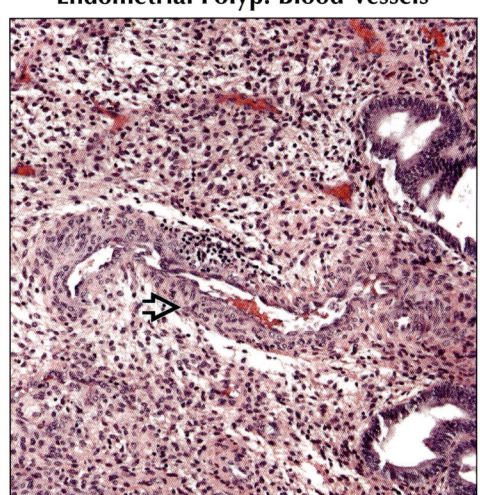

(Left) The morphology of endometrial glands ➡ in polyps is highly variable. The glands may be irregular or cystically dilated. The amount of stroma ➡ between the glands is variable as well, leading to glands that are widely spaced or slightly crowded, as seen in this example. (Right) Frequently, thick-walled blood vessels ➡ may be seen in the polyp stroma. Note the presence of relatively acellular stroma that is more eosinophilic than typical endometrial stroma.

Ciliated Cells

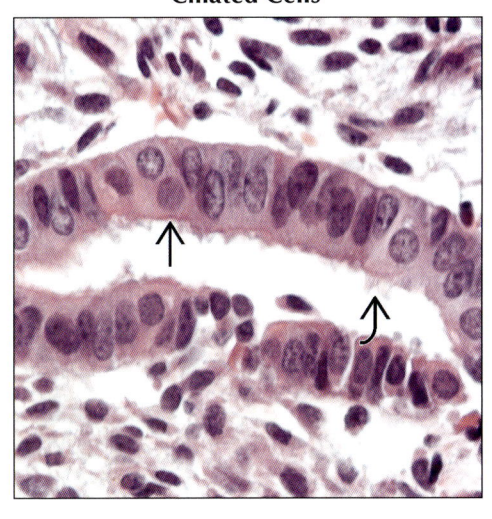

Decidualized Endometrium

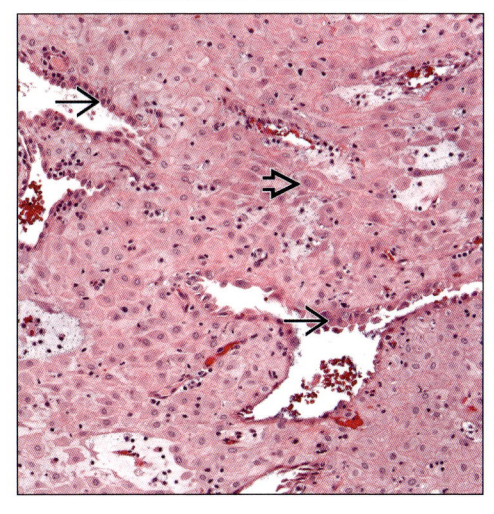

(Left) Ciliated cells ➡ can occasionally be found within endometrial glands. These cells are pear-shaped, with round nuclei and abundant eosinophilic cytoplasm and apical cilia ➡. (Right) During pregnancy, the endometrial glands and stroma become altered, or decidualized. The glandular epithelium ➡ becomes thinned and either simple cuboidal or hobnailed. Endometrial stromal cells ➡ become enlarged and hypereosinophilic.

Decidualized Endometrium

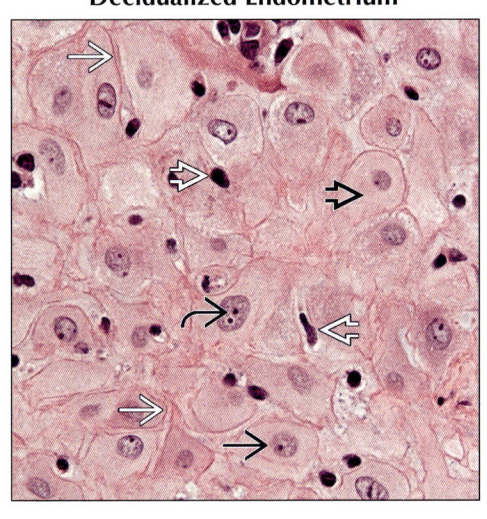

Decidualized & Secretory Endometrium

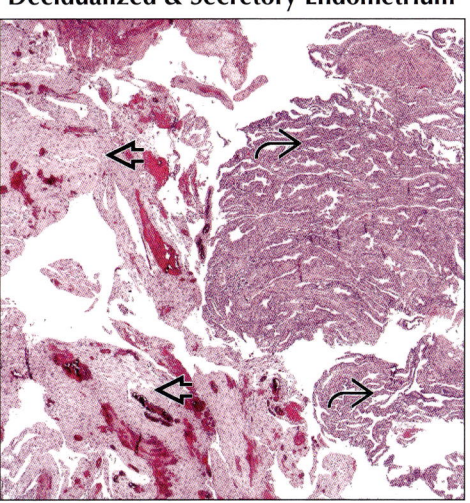

(Left) Decidualized stromal cells contain abundant eosinophilic cytoplasm ➡ and centrally placed, round nuclei ➡ with pinpoint nucleoli ➡. The cells have a well-demarcated eosinophilic border ➡. Scattered inflammatory cells (granulocytes) ➡ can be seen interspersed among the stromal cells. (Right) Decidualized endometrium ➡ with its abundant stroma can be seen on the left. Secretory endometrium with numerous, crowded glands ➡ occupies the right half of this image.

UTERUS

Arias-Stella Effect

(Left) During pregnancy, hypersecretory changes may occur in the glandular epithelium ⇨. These changes have been termed "Arias-Stella effect." The changes are highly variable and may be markedly atypical and confused with carcinoma. **(Right)** In Arias-Stella effect, the cells project into the endometrial glandular lumen (hobnailing ⇨) and have vesicular, optically clear nuclei ⇨. Only scant amounts of endometrial stroma ⇨ may be present.

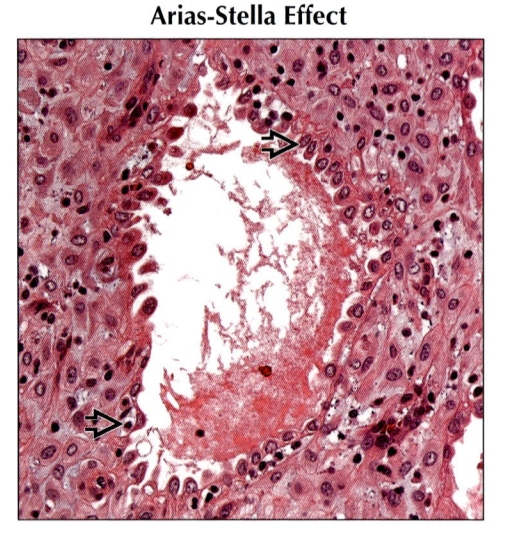

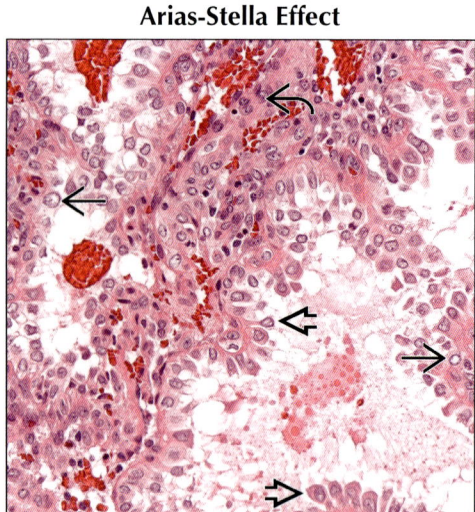

Arias-Stella Effect

(Left) Glands involved by Arias-Stella effect may have markedly pleomorphic features. Enlarged cells can project and shed into the lumen ⇨. Additionally, the nuclei may become enlarged and hyperchromatic, having a "glassy" appearance ⇨. Mitotic figures should be essentially absent. (Courtesy A. Laury, MD.) **(Right)** A hypersecretory, enlarged gland ⇨ involved by Arias-Stella effect is seen adjacent to a normal endometrial gland ⇨. (Courtesy A. Laury, MD.)

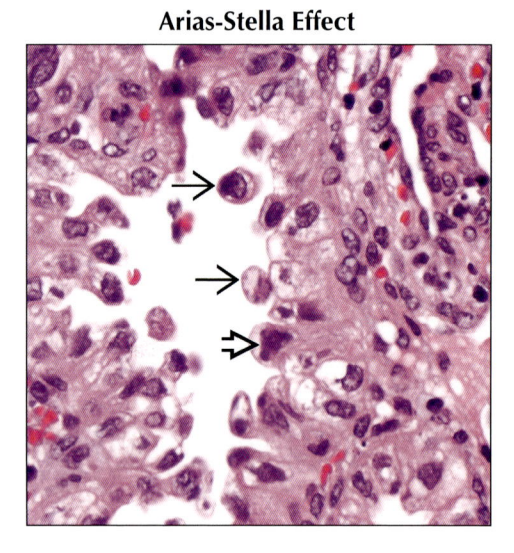

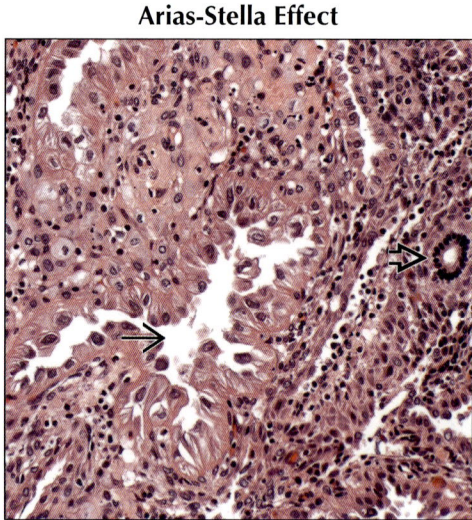

Implantation Site / Implantation Site: Vessel

(Left) Examination of a uterine specimen from a pregnant patient may reveal the placental implantation site. This site is marked by the presence of extravillous, intermediate trophoblasts ⇨ within a hypereosinophilic substance termed "fibrinoid" or "Nitabuch fibrin" ⇨. **(Right)** Intermediate trophoblasts ⇨ remodel the decidual spiral arterioles ⇨, replacing the smooth muscle wall. This helps to facilitate oxygen transfer from the maternal to the fetal blood.

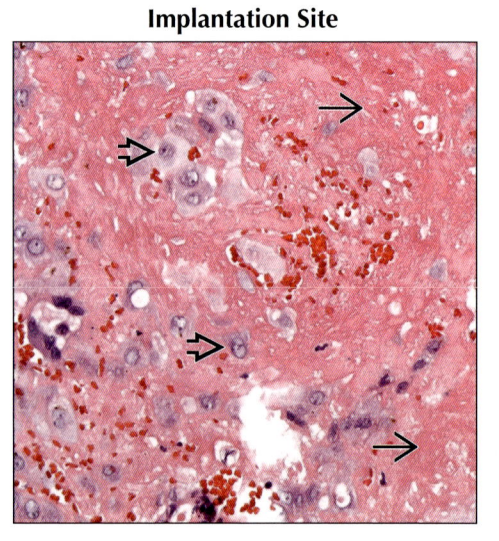

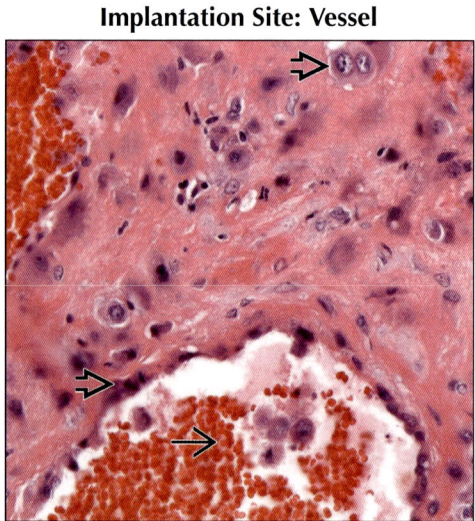

UTERUS

Disordered Proliferative Endometrium

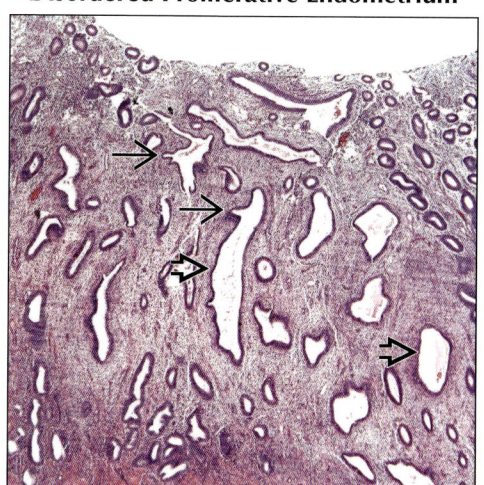

Disordered Proliferative Endometrium

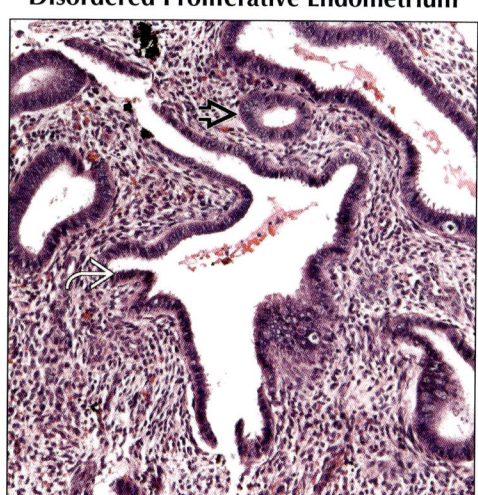

(Left) Disordered proliferative endometrium is common around perimenarche and perimenopausal years. It can be identified by the presence of scattered cystically dilated glands ⇨ with irregular contours and outpouchings ⇨. This change is commonly attributed to unopposed estrogen. (Right) The glands in disordered proliferative endometrium may be normal ⇨ or dilated ⇨. The stroma is similar to that seen in the proliferative phase. Mitotic figures and ciliated cells are usually present.

Anovulatory Endometrium

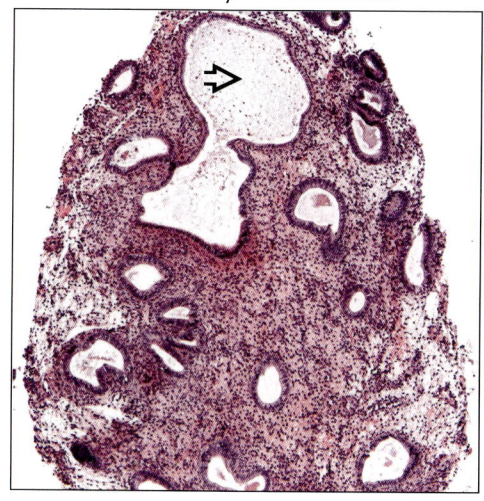

Atrophic Endometrium

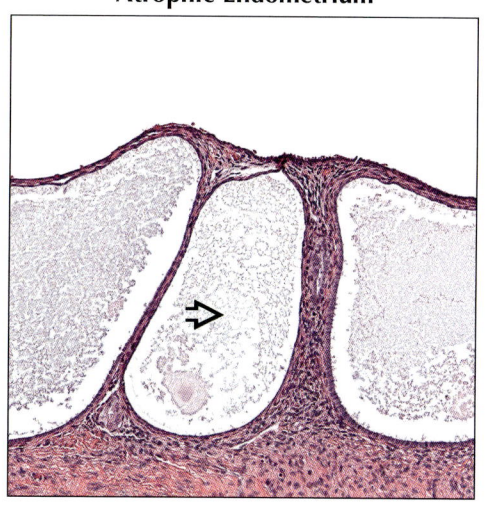

(Left) Anovulatory endometrium and disordered proliferative endometrium are terms that are often used interchangeably. In the presence of estrogen, the glands become cystically dilated ⇨. When estrogen is absent, dilation may be minimal; however, gland and stromal breakdown and tubal metaplasia may be present. (Right) Atrophic endometrium is composed of mitotically inactive, often cystically dilated glands ⇨ lined by a simple cuboidal lining. Crowding should not be evaluated in the setting of atrophy.

Atrophic Polyp

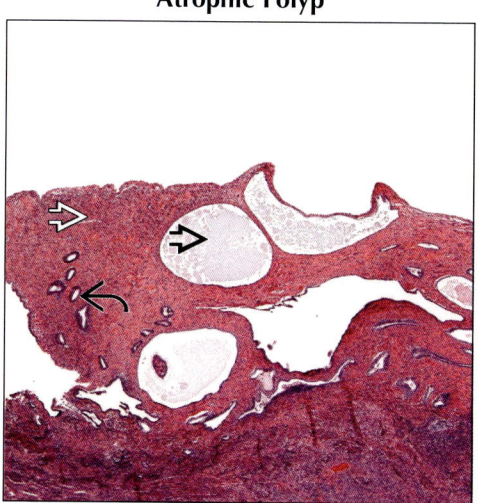

Atrophic Polyp

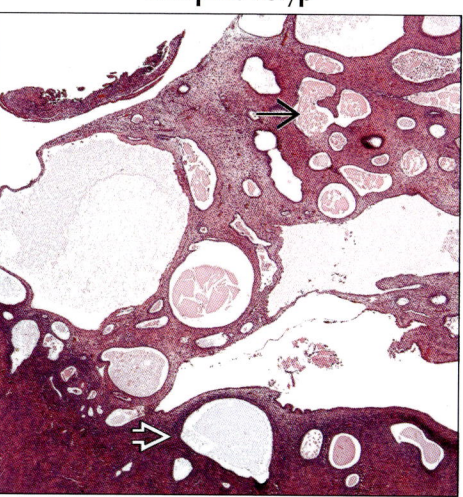

(Left) A mixture of atrophic small glands ⇨ and cystic glands ⇨ may be seen in cases of atrophy. Here, the glands are set in the fibrotic stroma ⇨ of an atrophic endometrial polyp. (Right) Atrophic, cystically dilated glands can be seen both in an endometrial polyp ⇨ and in the background endometrium ⇨. Although the area of glands relative to stroma is increased, this is not considered evidence of hyperplasia.

UTERUS

Atrophic Polyp

Adenomyosis

(Left) The lining of an atrophic endometrial gland is typically composed of a single lining of cuboidal ⇨ to columnar epithelium with a high nuclear to cytoplasmic ratio. No mitotic activity should be present. (Right) Adenomyosis is defined as the presence of endometrial glands ⇨ and stroma ⇨ beyond the border of the endomyometrial junction. A minimum distance of 1-2 mm has been suggested to avoid overdiagnosis. Normal physiologic changes may occur in adenomyosis.

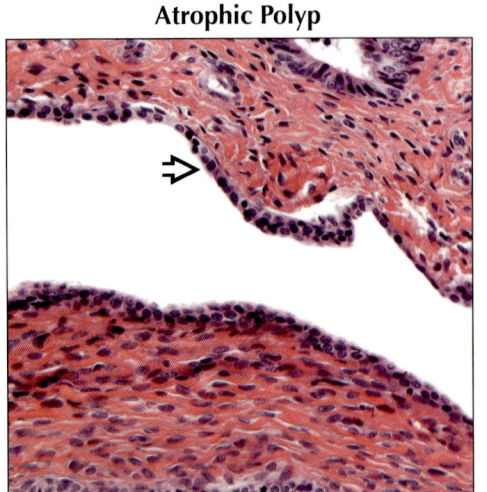

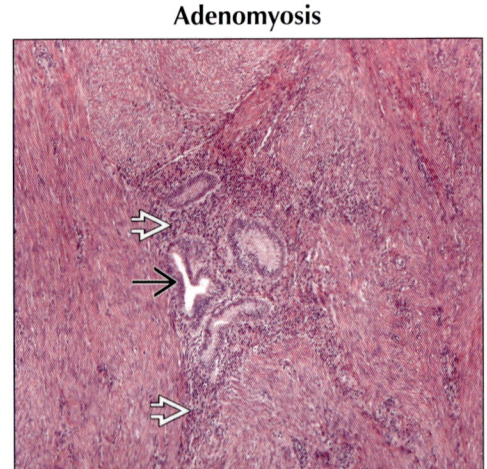

Superficial Myometrium

Arcuate Arteries

(Left) The myometrium is composed predominately of smooth muscle cells with elongated, cigar-shaped nuclei ⇨. Collagen and elastin fibers are present as well. The cells may greatly enlarge during pregnancy, and variable mitotic activity may be found, especially during the secretory phase. (Right) Deeper within the myometrium are the arcuate arteries ⇨. These arteries may be a helpful landmark when evaluating for possible myometrial invasion in cases of endometrial adenocarcinoma.

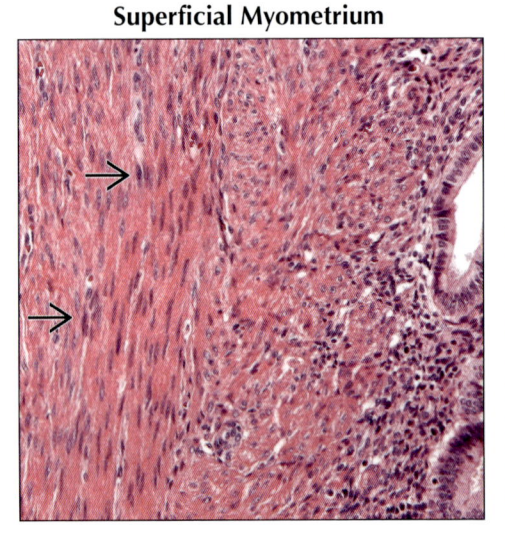

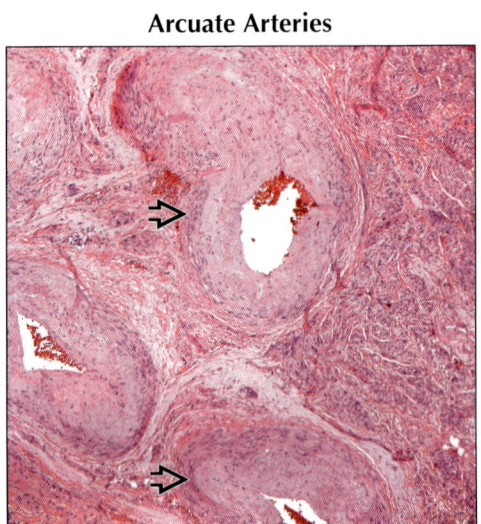

Arcuate Arteries

Uterine Serosa

(Left) The arcuate arteries may contain changes, such as atherosclerosis, medial calcification ⇨, or thrombosis. In multiparous patients, the uterine vasculature is more pronounced (as seen here) than that seen in a nulliparous patient. (Right) The deep myometrium ⇨ is covered by a thin serosal lining ⇨. The serosa is composed of a thin layer of mesothelial cells with flattened nuclei ⇨.

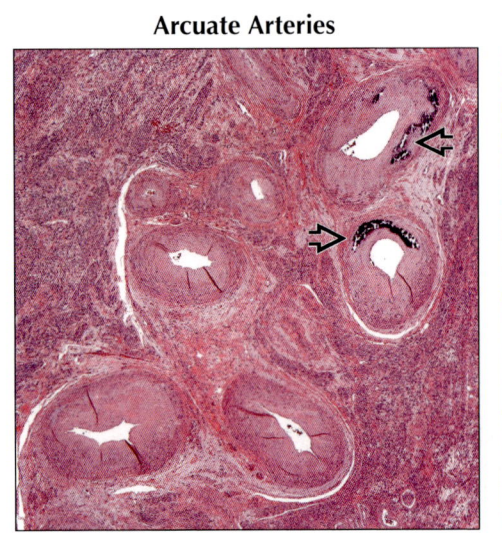

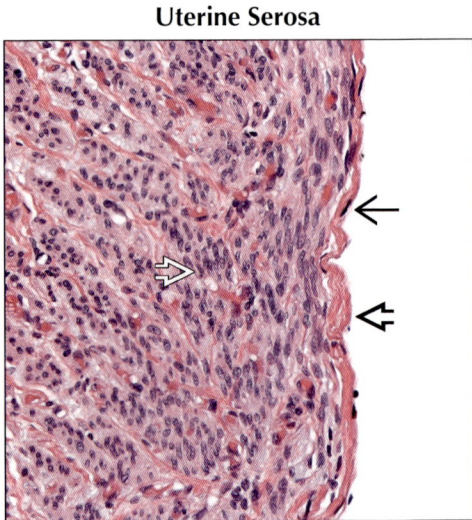

UTERUS

Serosal Adhesion

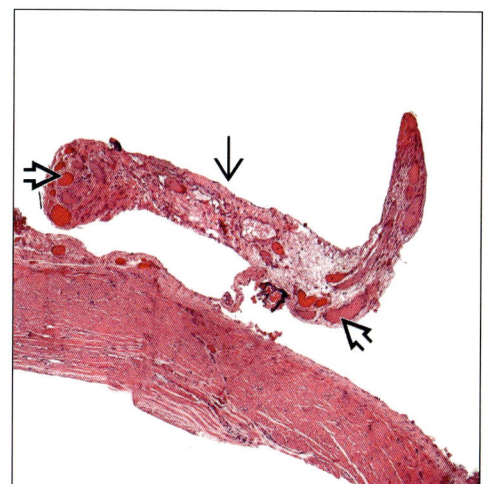

Exfoliation Artifact

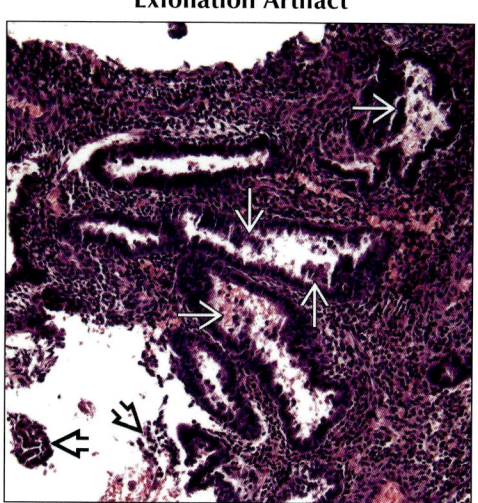

(**Left**) Fibrous adhesions ➡ may be present in patients who have had abdominal surgery or other causes of pelvic irritation. The presence of vascular growth ➡ in the adhesion is a helpful identifying feature. (**Right**) The instillation of fluids during hysteroscopy has a caustic effect on the endometrium. This is manifested by stromal fragmentation ➡ and hemorrhage and exfoliation of epithelial cells into the glandular lumen ➡, particularly near the surface. (Courtesy C. Crum, MD.)

Fragmentation and Pseudocrowding

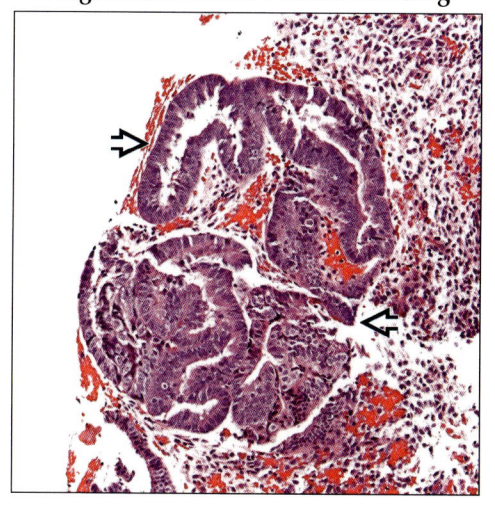

Telescoping Artifact

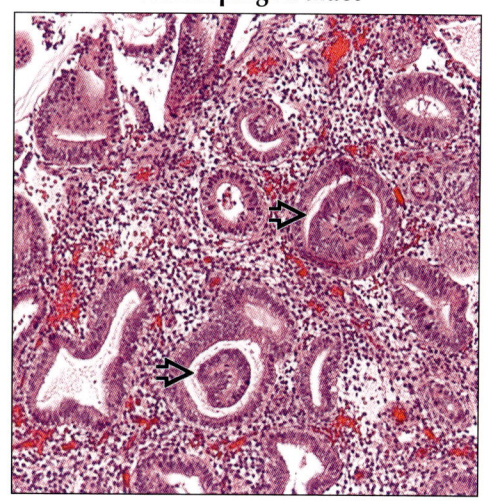

(**Left**) Fragmentation of endometrial tissue is often due to biopsy instruments. Strips of endometrial glandular epithelium without intervening stroma ➡ may appear markedly convoluted and should not be used to evaluate the presence of glandular crowding. (**Right**) Suction created by biopsy tools may lead to intussusception of glandular epithelium ➡, leading to a "gland in gland" phenomenon that should be recognized as a benign artifact. (Courtesy A. Cole, MD.)

Telescoping Artifact

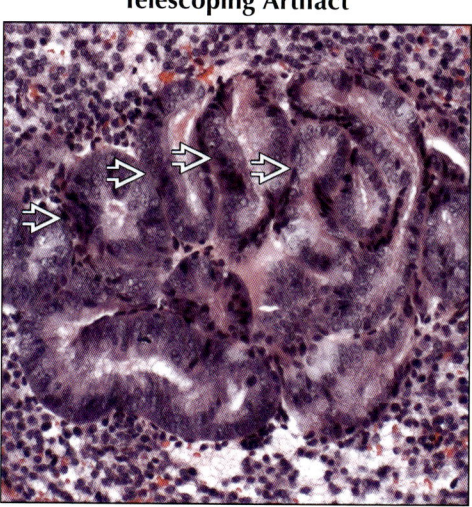

Hormone Effects

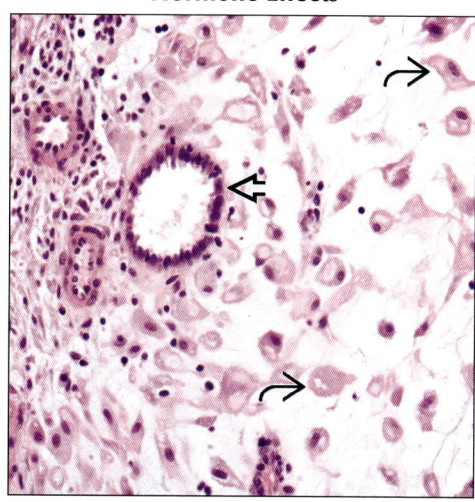

(**Left**) Severe telescoping artifact may lead to the compression of a single gland tract, noted by a ribbon-like reduplication of the gland ➡. This is another benign artifact that must not be interpreted as evidence of malignancy. (Courtesy A. Laury, MD.) (**Right**) Many cases of abnormal/dysfunctional bleeding are treated with progestin therapy. Progestins lead to small, tubular endometrial glands with an inactive lining ➡ as well as decidual change of the stroma cells ➡.

FALLOPIAN TUBE

Key Facts

Macroscopic Anatomy
- 3 regions: Isthmus, ampulla, and fimbriated end
  - Isthmus: Extends from wall of uterus
  - Ampulla: Mid portion of fallopian tube that is more tortuous and dilated than isthmus
  - Fimbriated end: Composed of delicate, finger-like projections extending into pelvic cavity adjacent to ovary
- Broad ligament
  - Contains fallopian tube as well as blood vessels and supporting connective tissue
  - Predominately composed of fibroadipose tissue
  - Walthard rests, paratubal cysts, and endosalpingiosis frequently seen here

Microscopic Anatomy
- Epithelium: Varying admixture of secretory and ciliated cells
  - Number of ciliated cells believed to increase with increasing levels of estrogen
  - Regional variation in number of secretory and ciliated cells exists
- Stroma: Composed of smooth muscle and fibroconnective tissue
  - Thickest in the isthmus; thins as fimbriated end is approached
  - 3 layers of smooth muscle are present in isthmus adjacent to uterine wall
  - Remainder of tube wall contains 2 layers of smooth muscle
- Outermost mesothelial cell layer
  - Reactive mesothelial cells may be present in inflammatory or malignant conditions
  - Reactive mesothelial cells identified by "hobnail" morphology, polygonal shape, and presence of nucleoli
- Regional microscopic variation
- Isthmus
  - Thick smooth muscle wall (3 layers) with muscle fibers in parallel and perpendicular orientation
  - Projections inside tube (plica) have minimal complexity
  - Secretory cells predominate
- Ampulla
  - Muscular wall thins and loses organization (2 layers)
  - Increase in number of plica and their complexity
- Fimbriated end
  - No muscular wall is present
  - Finger-like plica project into abdominal cavity
  - Ciliated cells predominate

Pitfalls/Artifacts
- Tangential sections through epithelium may mimic hyperplasia and malignancy
- Hydrosalpinx may mimic an ovarian cyst, paratubal cyst or endometriosis

Age Variation
- Atrophic changes can be seen after menopause

Metaplasia
- Squamous: Stratified, nonkeratinizing
- Mucinous: Columnar, mucin-containing cells
  - Rare phenomenon that may be associated with Peutz-Jeghers syndrome
- Transitional: Urothelial (bladder-like) epithelium
- Decidual change: Pregnant or postpartum patients

Hyperplasia
- Tubal epithelial hyperplasia is relatively unstudied and is an evolving concept
- Hyperplasia most commonly involves secretory cells and likely leads to pelvic serous carcinogenesis

(Left) The isthmus ➡ is closest to the body of the uterus. The ampulla ➡ comprises the midportion of the tube, and the fimbriated end ➡ is located at the opening of the tube into the pelvis. *(Right)* The ampulla is seen with its numerous plica, or finger-like projections, into the lumen of the tube. This area of the tube provides the environment that supports fertilization of the egg.

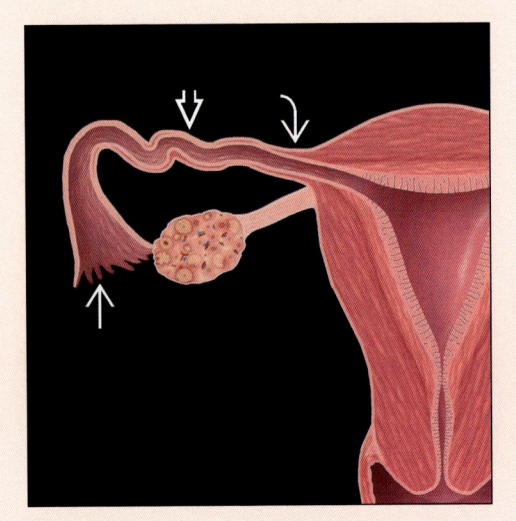

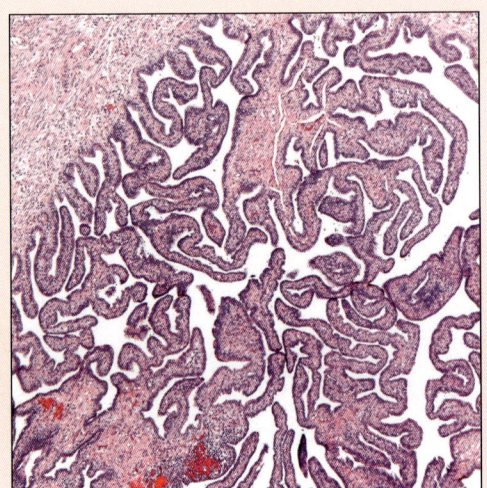

FALLOPIAN TUBE

Isthmus

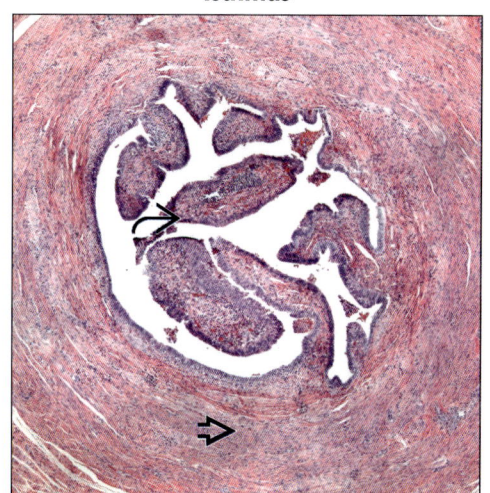

Isthmus

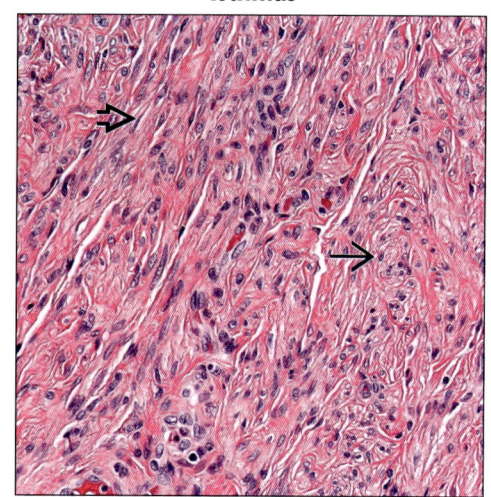

(Left) The isthmus has few plica ⇨ and is predominately composed of a thick muscular wall composed of smooth muscle ⇨. *(Right)* The wall of the isthmus of the tube is composed of fascicles of smooth muscle that can be seen running perpendicularly ⇨ and parallel ⇨ to the long axis of the fallopian tube lumen.

Mid Portion

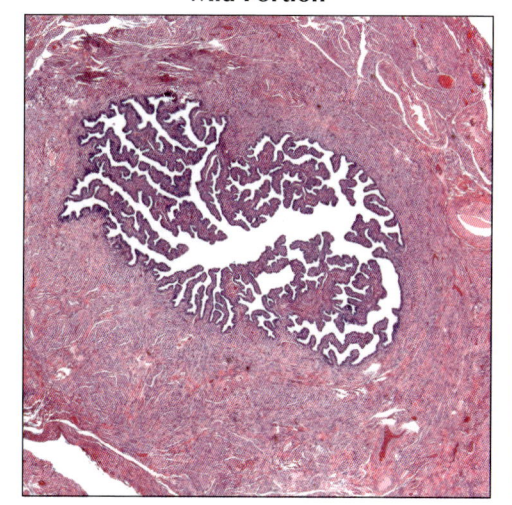

Mid Portion

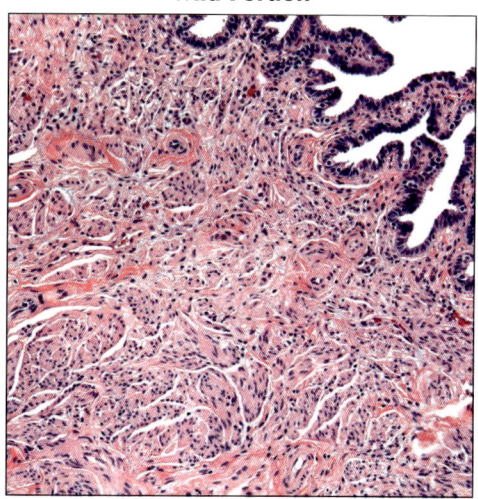

(Left) Toward the fimbriated end of the tube, the muscular wall of the tube becomes more attenuated, and the number and complexity of the plica increases. This photo was taken in the mid portion between the isthmus and the ampulla. *(Right)* The muscular wall of the ampulla becomes thinner, and the organization of the smooth muscle cells decreases as one approaches the fimbriated end of the tube.

Ampulla

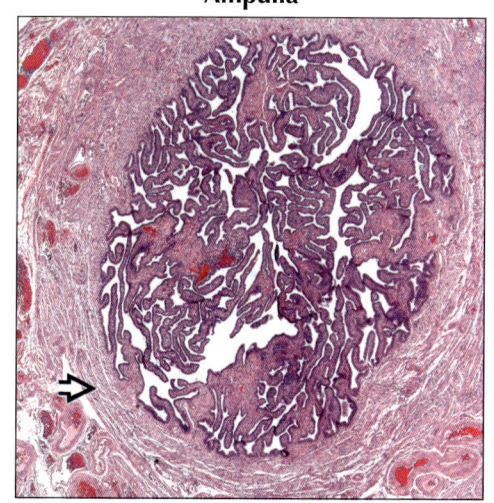

Ampulla

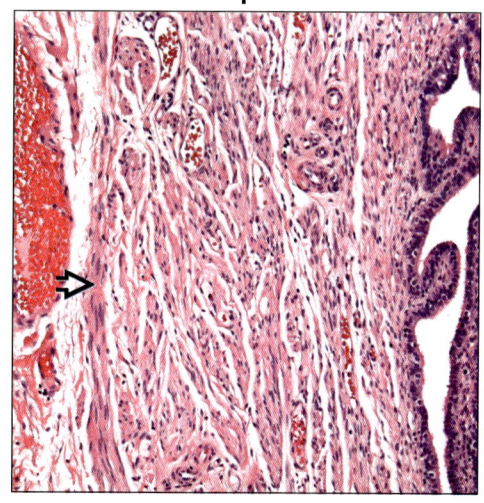

(Left) The ampulla of the fallopian tube has a much thinner muscular wall ⇨ with numerous plica projecting into the tubal lumen. *(Right)* The wall of the ampulla is composed of wispy smooth muscle fibers that are no longer organized in large fascicles ⇨.

FALLOPIAN TUBE

Fimbriated End

Fimbriated End

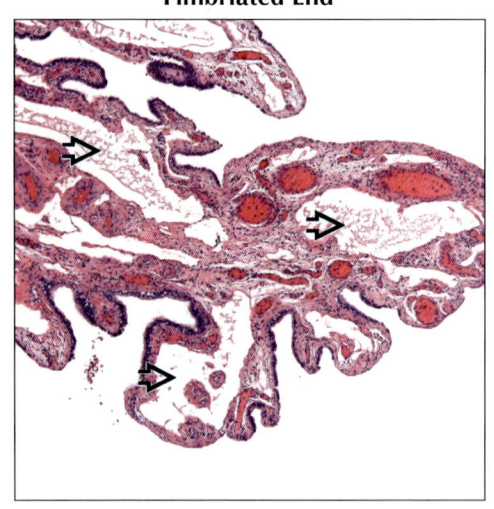

(Left) The fimbriated end of the fallopian tube consists of plica that project into the pelvic cavity. These plica often appear as "islands" of stroma that are lined by tubal epithelial cells. *(Right)* In this section of fallopian tube, numerous dilated lymphatic channels ⇨ can be seen in the plical stroma.

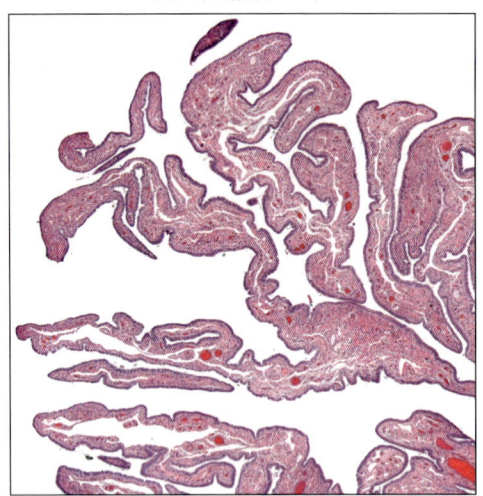

Epithelium

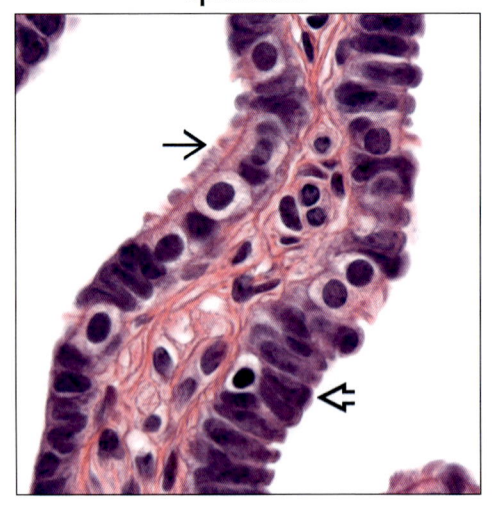

Epithelium: Secretory Cells

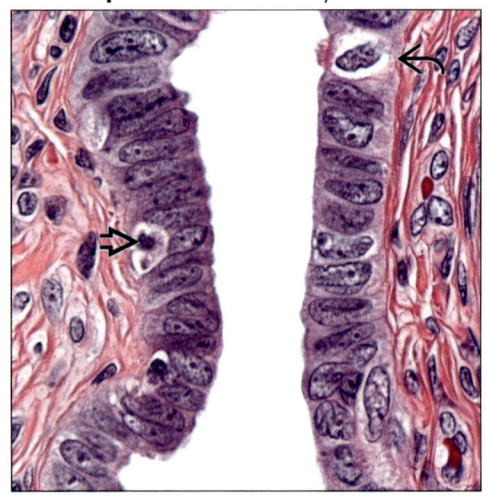

(Left) Tubal epithelium is composed of varying numbers of secretory cells ⇨ and ciliated cells ➔. The proportions of these cells vary in response to hormonal status. It is believed that the secretory cells can differentiate into ciliated cells. *(Right)* Occasionally, secretory cells are the predominant cell type, as seen here. Lymphocytes ⇨ can be identified within the lining epithelial cells. Note the single ciliated cell ➔. The intercalated cell (not pictured) is thought to represent a type of secretory cell.

Epithelium: Ciliated Cells

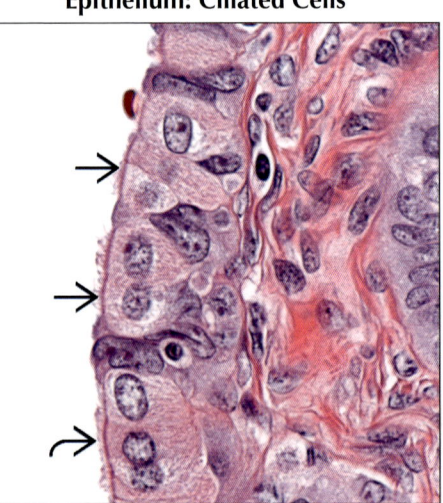

Paratubal Cyst

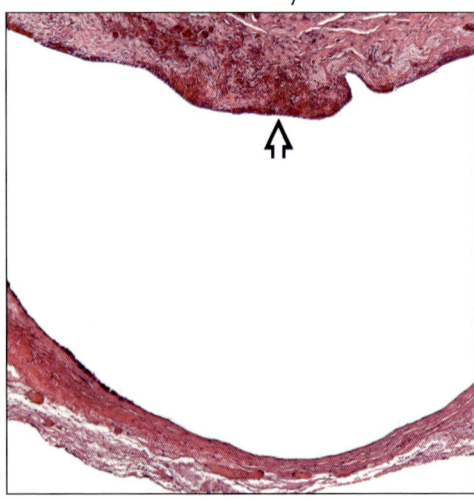

(Left) Note the bright pink terminal bar ➔ that can be identified under the cilia ➔. Ciliated cells are typically rounder and contain much more cytoplasm than secretory cells; they have been likened to fried eggs. *(Right)* Cysts may form at the periphery of the tube. These cysts may vary in size from microscopic to many centimeters in diameter. They are usually full of clear, thin fluid. This cyst has focal hemorrhage into the wall ⇨.

FALLOPIAN TUBE

Paratubal Cyst

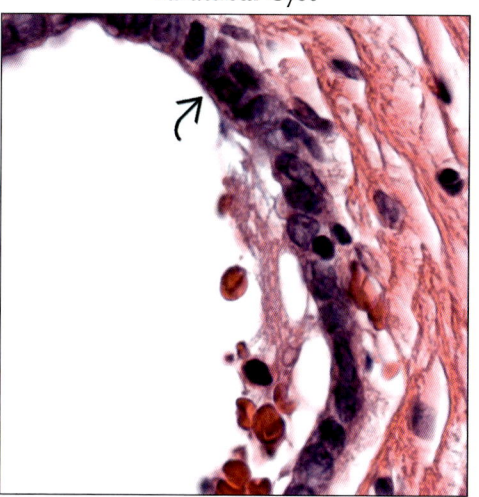

Paratubal Cyst

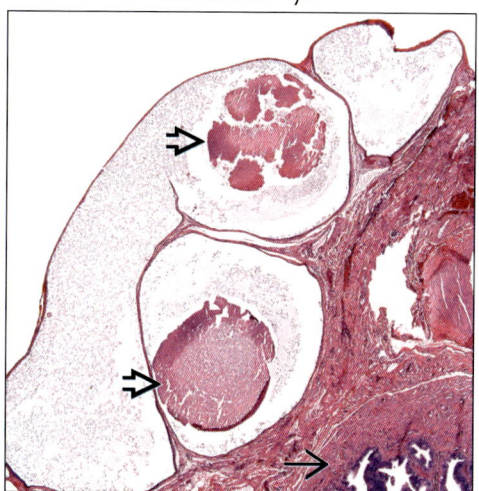

(Left) Paratubal cysts are typically lined by a simple, low cuboidal epithelium ⇨. The wall surrounding the cyst should be thin and devoid of muscle. *(Right)* This photomicrograph shows multiple thin-walled, paratubal cysts. Note the eosinophilic secretions that may accumulate within the cysts ⇨. The fallopian tube lumen and muscular wall can be identified in the bottom right corner ⇨. The lining epithelium may be so attenuated that it may be difficult to see.

Squamous Metaplasia

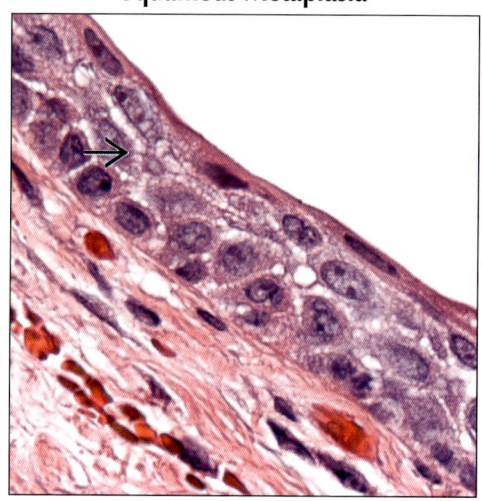

Walthard Rest

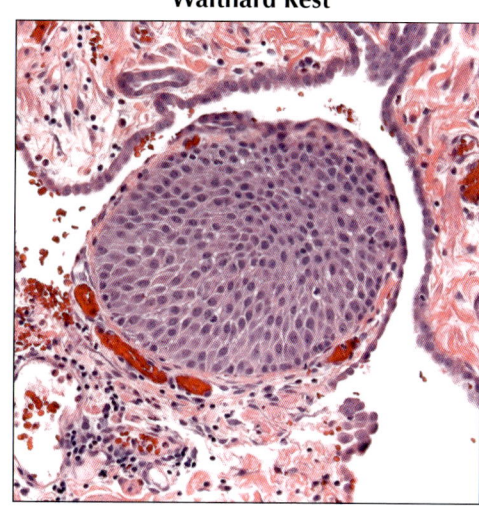

(Left) Squamous metaplasia of the tubal epithelium frequently occurs in the setting of inflammation or trauma. The normal lining is replaced by stratified squamous lining. Intercellular bridges (present as thin, pink lines ⇨) between the keratinocytes can be observed at high power. *(Right)* Walthard rests are a common finding in the fallopian tube. They are composed of transitional epithelium, similar to the epithelium found in the bladder.

Walthard Rest

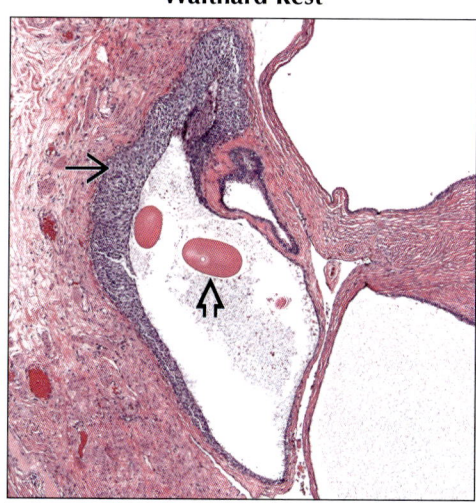

Multiple Walthard Rests

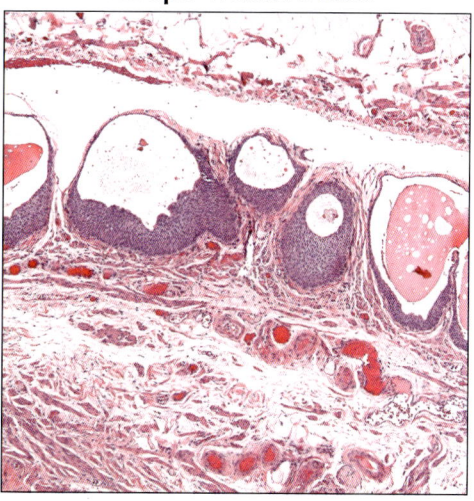

(Left) Walthard rests may become cystically dilated. The lining epithelium ⇨ bears a resemblance to that seen in the bladder. Frequently, eosinophilic secretions may be seen in the lumen ⇨. *(Right)* This photomicrograph shows multiple cystic Walthard rests within the supporting connective tissue of the fallopian tube.

FALLOPIAN TUBE

Mesonephric Remnant

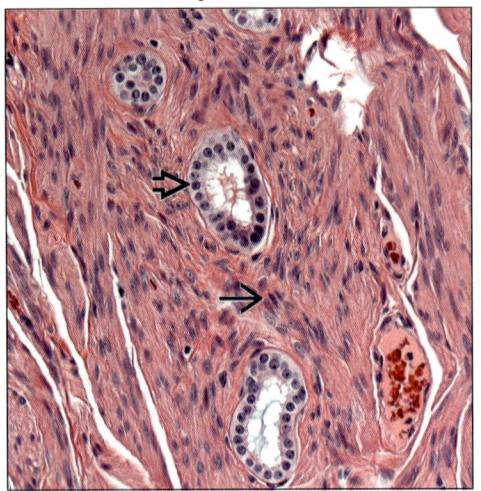

Walthard Rest: Epithelium

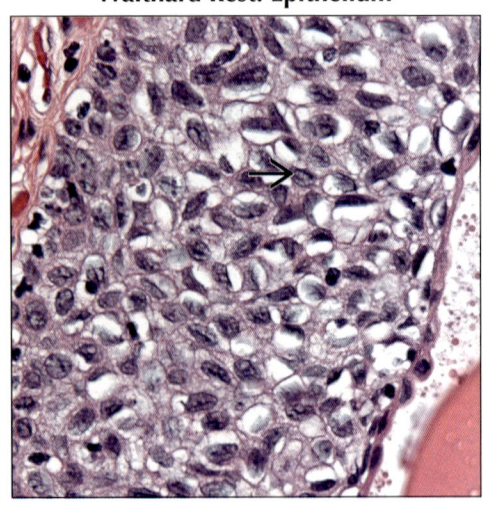

(Left) Mesonephric remnants are commonly found in the tubal wall. They are composed of small, gland-like structures with a simple cuboidal lining ⇨. They are surrounded by a dense fibromuscular stroma ➔. *(Right)* Close examination of the lining of a Walthard rest shows elongated epithelial cells with scattered grooved nuclei ➔. The nuclei are often found streaming perpendicularly to the lumen of the cyst.

Artifact: Tangential Sectioning

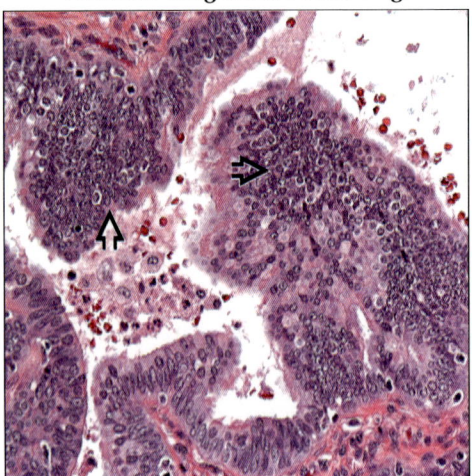

Reactive Mesothelium

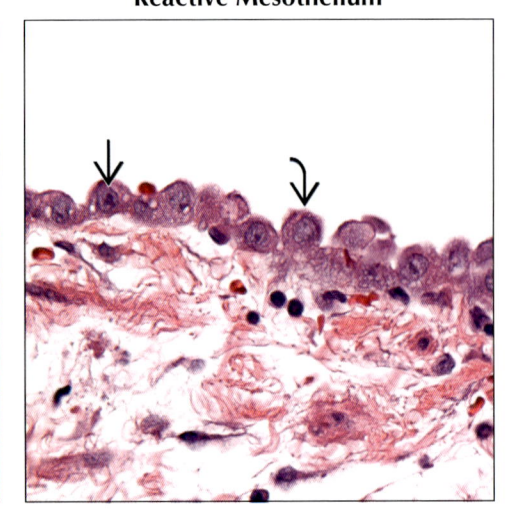

(Left) Tangential sectioning of the epithelium of the fallopian tube ⇨ may create areas that appear to be hyperplastic (so-called papillary hyperplasia of the fallopian tube). No significant nuclear atypia is seen. *(Right)* The outermost lining of the tube is composed of mesothelial cells that may become reactive. Reactive mesothelial cells are polygonal and often possess a "hobnail" morphology ➔. Single, prominent nucleoli can be identified ➔.

Decidual Change

Tubal Pregnancy

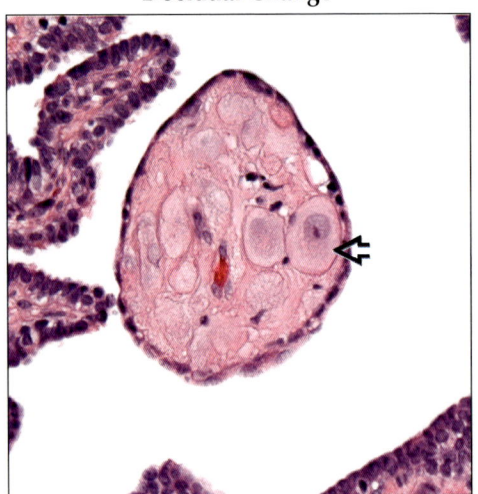

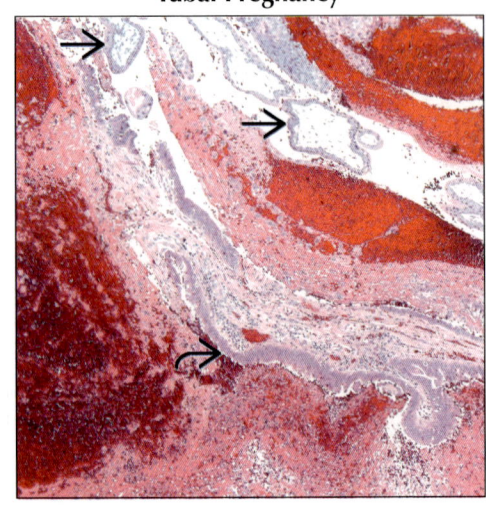

(Left) Decidual change, marked by enlarged cells with abundant eosinophilic cytoplasm ⇨, may occur in patients who are pregnant or have recently been pregnant. *(Right)* Tubal pregnancies may contain placental villi ➔ adjacent to fallopian tube plica ➔. There is often abundant hemorrhage within the tube (hematosalpinx). In advanced cases, rupture of the wall of the tube may occur.

FALLOPIAN TUBE

Hydrosalpinx

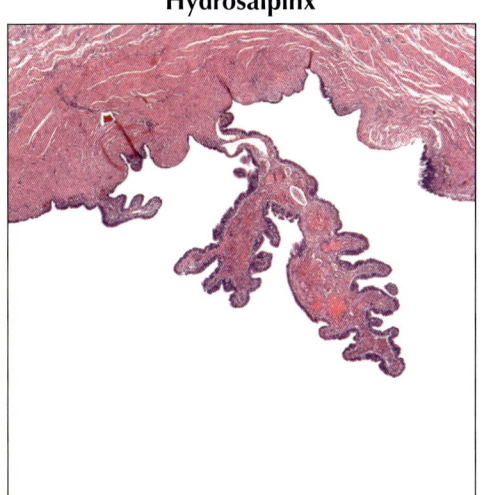

Hydrosalpinx

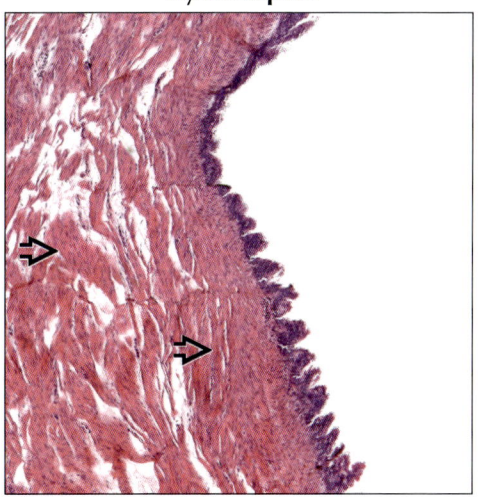

(Left) The tube may become cystically dilated, usually due to previous infection or inflammation; this is termed hydrosalpinx. In hydrosalpinx, the plica are often decreased in number or not present at all. *(Right)* In this example of hydrosalpinx, no plica are present. Note the muscular wall ⇨, which can help to differentiate a hydrosalpinx from a paratubal cyst or serous cyst microscopically.

Endosalpingiosis

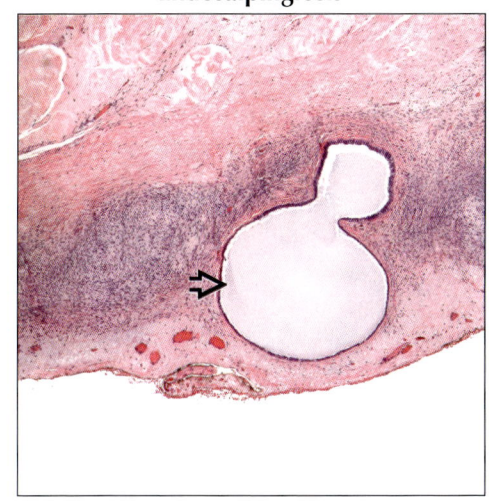

Endosalpingiosis

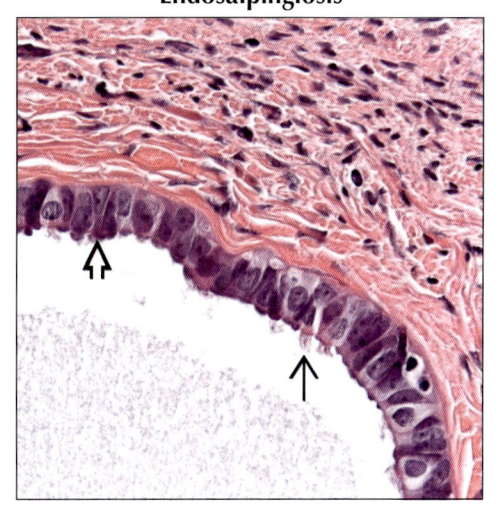

(Left) Endosalpingiosis is the presence of cystic, normal tubal epithelium outside of the fallopian tube lumen. It may be seen in the wall of the fallopian tube and resemble a paratubal cyst, or, in extreme cases, hydrosalpinx. In this figure, endosalpingiosis is seen involving the ovary ⇨. *(Right)* The lining of an endosalpingiotic cyst is composed of normal tubal epithelium consisting of secretory ⇨ and ciliated cells ⇨.

Atrophy

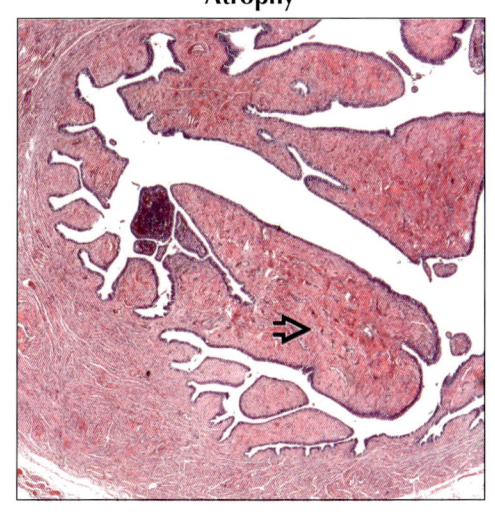

Atrophy

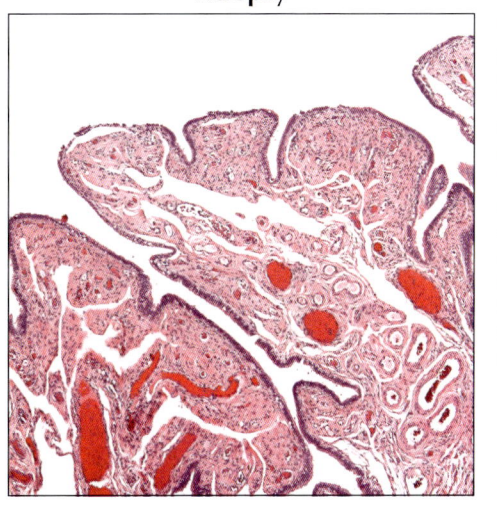

(Left) In postmenopausal patients, the fallopian tube undergoes atrophic changes. These changes consist of large, fibrous plica ⇨ with a simple lining of normal tubal epithelium. The number of plica and fimbria are often decreased. *(Right)* Atrophy of the fimbriated end leads to a decrease in number and complexity of the individual fimbria. There is a predominance of stroma compared to the epithelium.

OVARY

Key Facts

Macroscopic Anatomy
- Cortex
  - Outer layer of ovary
  - Composed of stroma; contains developing follicles
- Medulla
  - Mid portion of ovary
  - Composed predominantly of stroma, with blood vessels and nerves
- Hilum (also known as hilus)
  - Where blood vessels and nerves enter the parenchyma

Microscopic Anatomy
- Surface epithelium
  - Delicate single layer of cuboidal to columnar cells that cover outermost surface of ovary
- Cortex
  - Stroma composed of stromal cells (fibroblast-like cells) and developing follicles
  - Primordial follicle: Single layer of flat follicle cells surrounding the oocyte
  - Primary follicle: 1-2 layers of follicular cells surrounding the oocyte
  - Secondary (preantral) follicle: Multiple layers of granulosa cells as well as the development of zona pellucida and beginning of a fluid-filled cyst (antrum)
  - Mature (Graafian) follicle: Eccentrically located oocyte and granulosa cells as well as a well-developed antrum; established presence of a theca interna and externa
- Medulla
  - Stroma composed of fibroblasts, collagen, and elastic fibers
  - Clusters of blood vessels transgressing from hilum
  - Occasionally, smooth muscle, fat, decidual or luteinized cells may be identified
- Hilum
  - Connective tissue with large-caliber blood vessels and nerves
  - Scattered nests of hilus cells, resembling Leydig cells of the testis, may be present; Reinke crystals or cytoplasmic pigment may aid in their identification
  - Rete ovarii: Tubules and slit-like spaces analogous to rete testis

Pitfalls/Artifacts
- Endosalpingiosis: Small cystic structures lined by tubal-type epithelium
- Benign ovarian cysts (corpus luteum of pregnancy or follicle cysts) may clinically resemble a neoplasm
- Surface papillation may be confused with surface serous tumors (adenofibromas)
- Endometriosis, especially with reactive atypia, may simulate malignancy both clinically and histologically

Age Variation
- At birth, ovaries are much smaller than they are around beginning of puberty
- Ovaries increase 20-30x in size before onset of puberty
- At onset of puberty, ovaries have reached their full size
- Ovarian surface becomes more convoluted throughout reproductive life
- After menopause, ovaries lose about 50% of their size and weight

Metaplasia
- Cortical inclusion glands or cysts may undergo metaplasia
  - Serous, mucinous, or transitional types
  - Nests of transitional epithelium are known as Walthard rests

Hyperplasia
- Varying amounts of stromal hyperplasia may be seen in peri- and postmenopausal patients
- Cortical stromal hyperplasia may be diffuse, or form discreet nodules

(Left) In this photograph of an ovary and the adjacent fallopian tube ➜, the outer cortex ➜ of the ovary is visible. The convolution of the cortex increases with age. The fallopian tube has a fimbriated end ➜. (Right) Small follicle cysts ➜ can be seen in the cortex on the cut surface of the ovary. The medulla ➜ lies under the cortex and is composed of stroma. The hilum comprises the most central portion ➜.

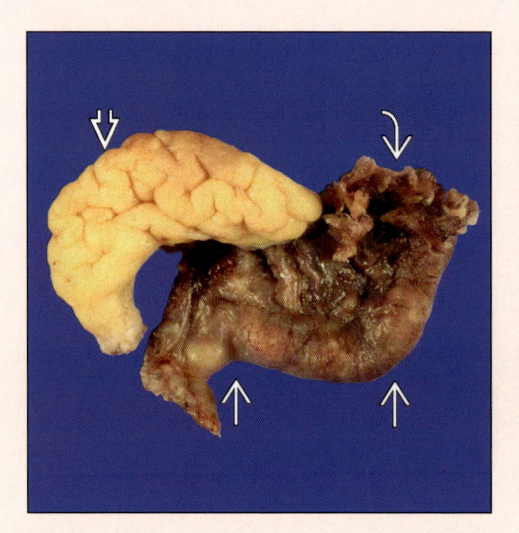

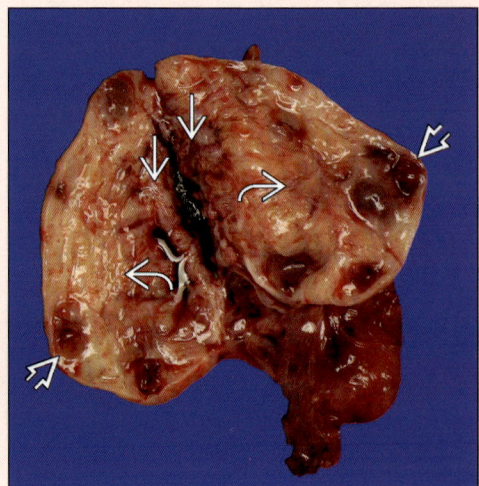

OVARY

Hilar Vessels

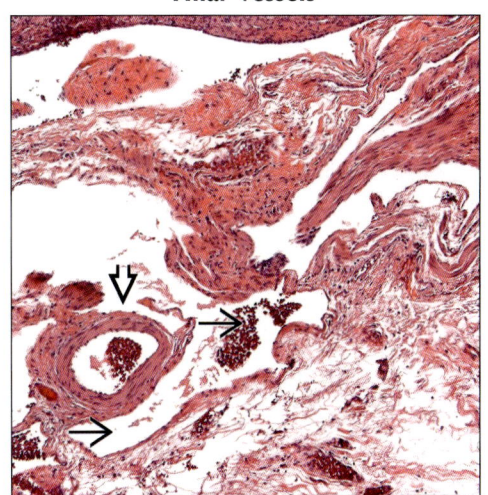

Medullary Vessels

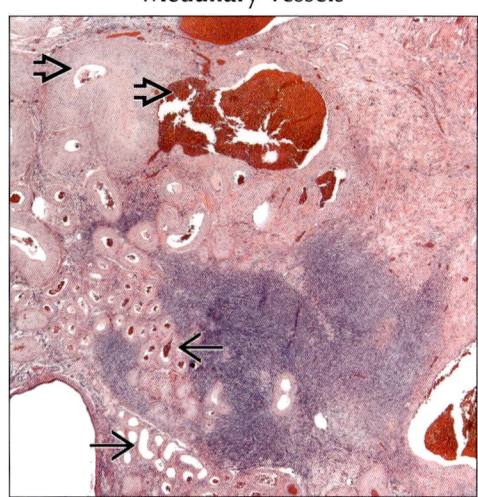

(*Left*) Numerous large blood vessels and abundant connective tissue are present at the hilum. The arteries ⇨ and veins ➔ that supply the ovary enter here. (*Right*) Large medullary vessels ⇨ become smaller and more coiled ➔ as they progress deeper into the medulla. In postmenopausal patients, the relative lack of stroma may give the false impression of an increase in the number of vessels, which may mimic a benign vascular tumor or malformation.

Medullary Vessels

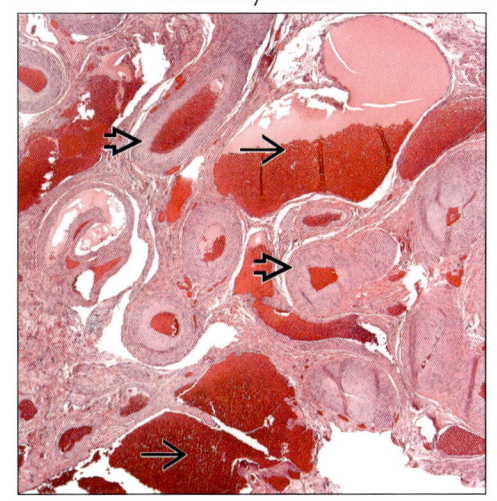

Hilum: Nerve

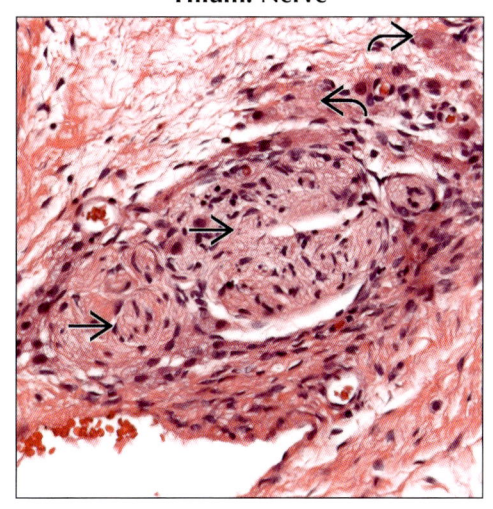

(*Left*) As the arteries ⇨ and veins ➔ progress into the ovary, they become more convoluted. With age, changes such as atherosclerosis, calcification, or amyloid deposition may be seen in these vessels. (*Right*) Nerves of the sympathetic nervous system ➔ also enter the ovary at the hilum. Hilus cells ➔, analogous to Leydig cells of the testis, may be seen in and around these nerves and around blood vessels.

Hilus Cells

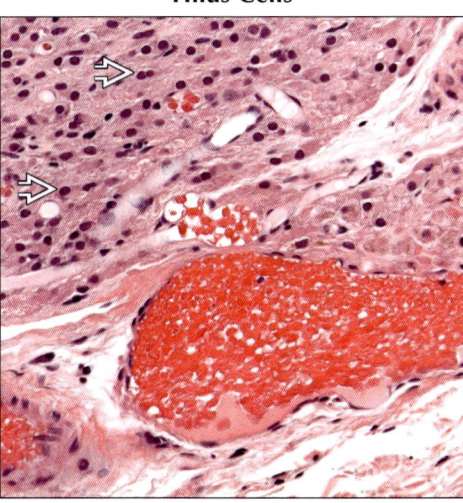

Hilus Cells: Reinke Crystal

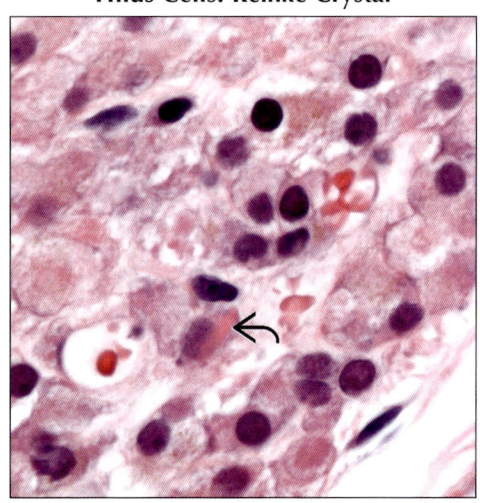

(*Left*) Hilus cells are polygonal, eosinophilic cells ⇨ present within the ovarian hilum and abutting the medulla. These cells are absent during childhood; they begin to appear around puberty and increase in number throughout life. (*Right*) Eosinophilic crystals of Reinke ➔ may be identified within the cytoplasm of the ovarian hilus cells although they are often absent. A Masson trichrome stain may aid in their detection.

OVARY

Hilus Cells: Pigment

Rete Ovarii

(Left) The presence of a fine, brown, granular pigment ➡ in the cytoplasm of hilus cells may aid in their identification. These hilus cells are adjacent to a blood vessel ➡. (Right) The rete ovarii ➡ can be found in the hilum of the ovary. The rete ovarii are analogous to the rete testis and are composed of round to slit-like tubules with occasional luminal papillae ➡. They are lined by epithelium that may appear flat to columnar.

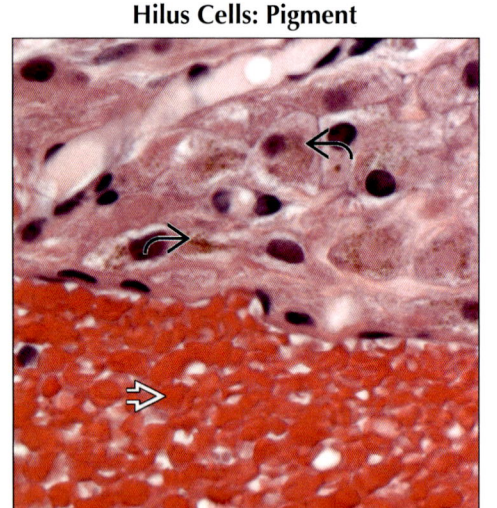

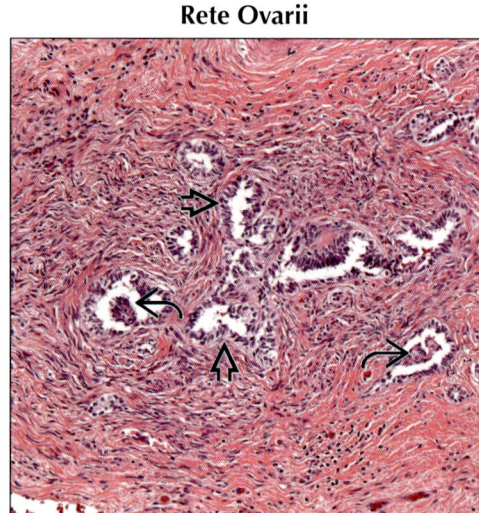

Rete Ovarii and Hilus Cells

Wolffian Ducts

(Left) The rete ovarii is often surrounded by a well-demarcated cuff of spindled stroma ➡. This stroma is similar to, but not contiguous with, the ovarian stroma. Clusters of hilus cells ➡ may be seen in association with the rete ovarii. (Right) Wolffian duct remnants ➡ may be identified throughout the gynecologic tract. They are most common in the vagina but can be identified in the hilum of the ovary. They should not be mistaken for metastatic carcinoma.

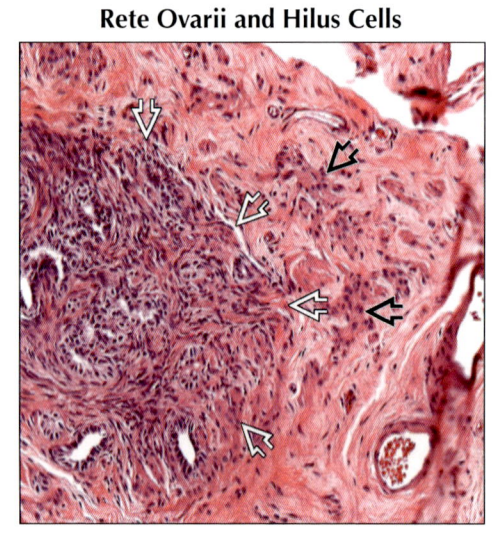

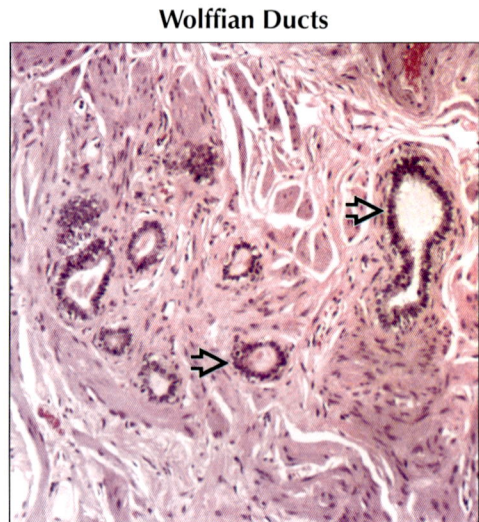

Wolffian Duct

Ovarian Stroma

(Left) Wolffian ducts may be confused with the rete ovarii, but the presence of eosinophilic luminal secretions ➡ and the absence ➡ of a well-developed surrounding spindle cell stroma can aid in this distinction. The cells lining a Wolffian duct are typically cuboidal with round nuclei. (Right) Spindled stromal cells are present within the medulla and the ovarian cortex. These cells have scant cytoplasm and elongated, tapered nuclei, often forming fascicles ➡ or whorls.

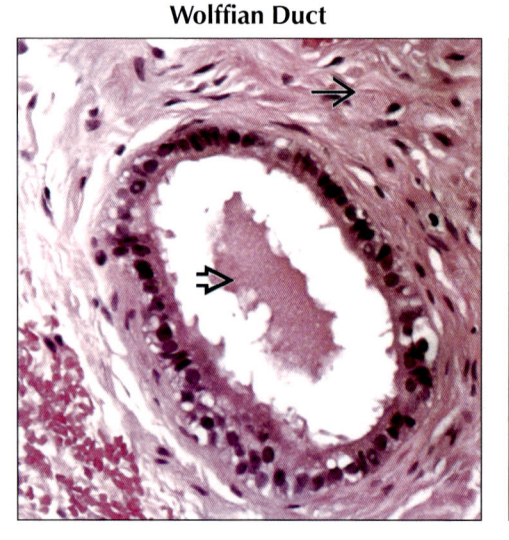

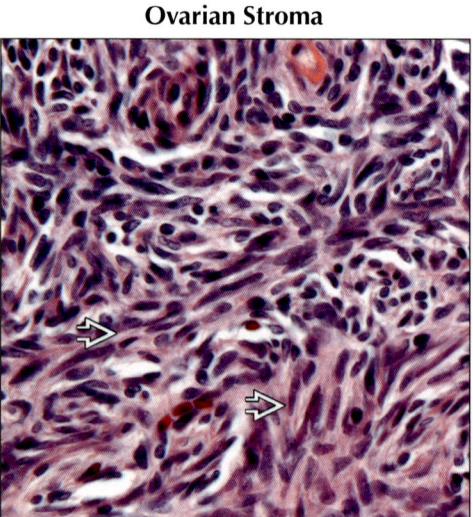

OVARY

Stroma: Luteinized Cells

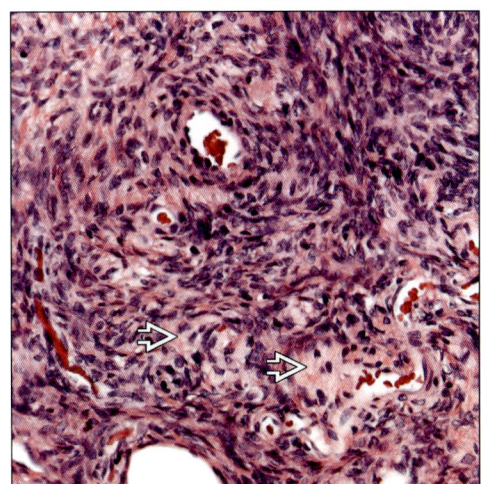

Stroma: Fat

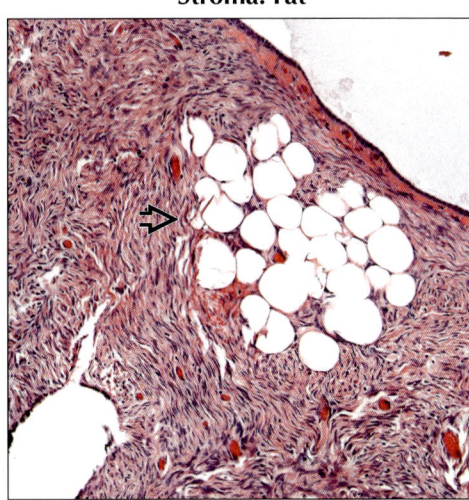

(Left) Luteinized cells ⇨ may be seen interspersed within the medullary stroma. These cells can be recognized by their ample, eosinophilic cytoplasm and the presence of round, centrally placed nuclei. These cells increase in number throughout reproductive life. (Right) Heterotopic tissues may be identified within the stroma. Here, a collection of fat cells ⇨ is present within the cortical stroma. Bundles of smooth muscle may be present as well.

Stroma: Endosalpingiosis

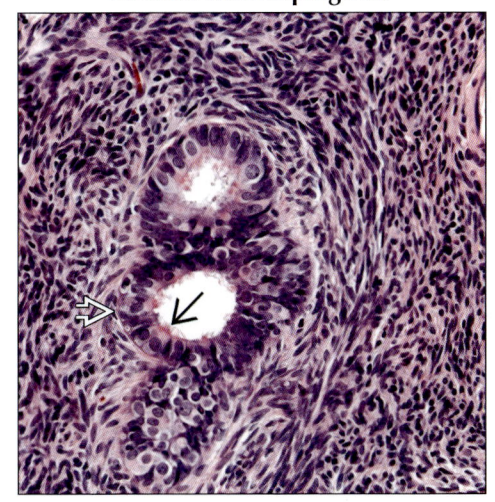

Ovarian Stroma

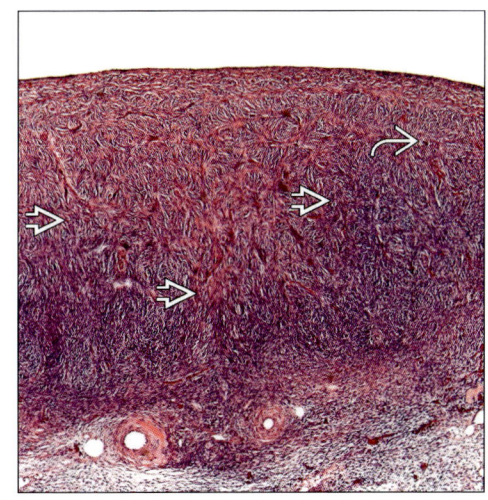

(Left) Within the stroma, scattered cortical inclusion cysts may be present. These cysts increase in number with age and are thought to be a result of ovulation. They may be lined by simple cuboidal epithelium or by tubal epithelium (endosalpingiosis) ⇨. The presence of cilia ⇨ can be helpful in identifying the latter. (Right) The junction ⇨ between the medulla and the cortex is ill defined, and the 2 may blend ⇨ and become indistinguishable.

Primordial Follicle

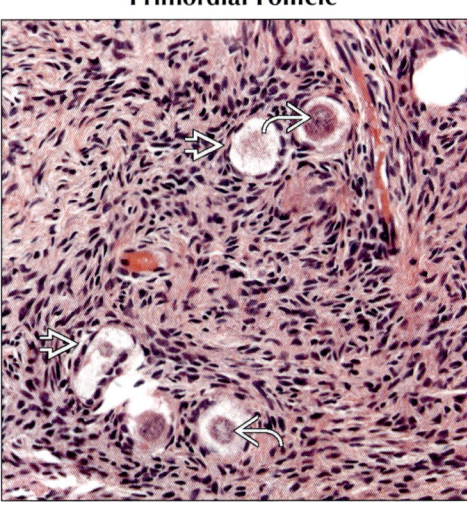

Primary Follicle

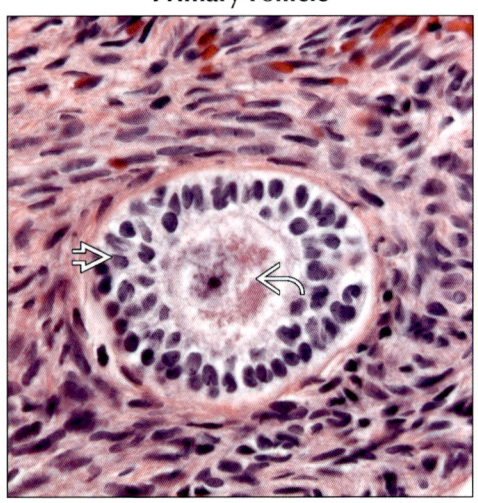

(Left) Primordial follicles ⇨ are found in a linear distribution in the superficial cortex. They are lined by a single flattened layer of granulosa cells. In younger patients, oocytes ⇨ may be identified within the center of the primordial follicle. (Right) As the follicle matures, the granulosa cells ⇨ assume a cuboidal or columnar shape. In the primary follicle, 1-2 distinct layers of granulosa cells are present. The oocyte ⇨ begins to enlarge as well.

OVARY

Preantral Follicle

Mature Follicle

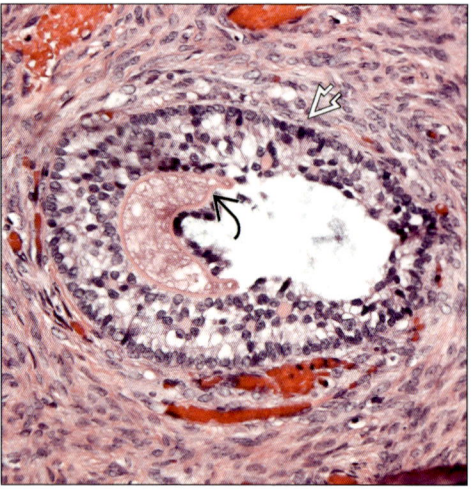

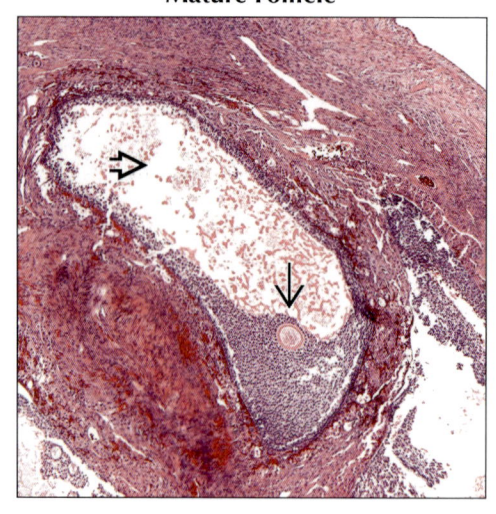

(Left) As follicles mature, they migrate deeper into the cortex. The preantral follicle is characterized by 3-5 layers of granulosa cells ⇨ and the development of a thin, eosinophilic layer surrounding the oocyte: The zona pellucida ⇨. **(Right)** Granulosa cells secrete fluid, eventually forming the antrum ⇨, or the portion filled with follicular "liquor." At this point, the oocyte is mature and surrounded by an increased number of granulosa cells, forming the cumulus oophorous ⇨.

Mature Follicle: Oocyte

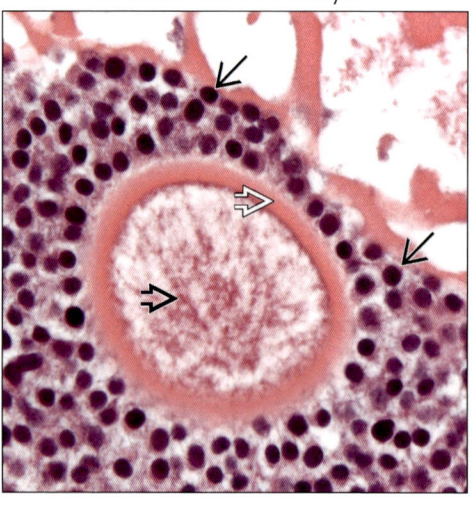

Mature Follicle: Granulosa and Theca Interna Layers

(Left) The mature oocyte ⇨, with its thickened zona pellucida ⇨, is surrounded by granulosa cells ⇨. **(Right)** As the maturing follicle progresses deeper into the cortex, the stromal cells differentiate into 2 specialized layers of theca cells. The granulosa cell layer ⇨ abuts the inner of these 2 layers, the theca interna ⇨. Cystic Call-Exner bodies ⇨ may be identified within the granulosa cell layer and recapitulate those found in granulosa cell tumors.

Theca Interna and Externa

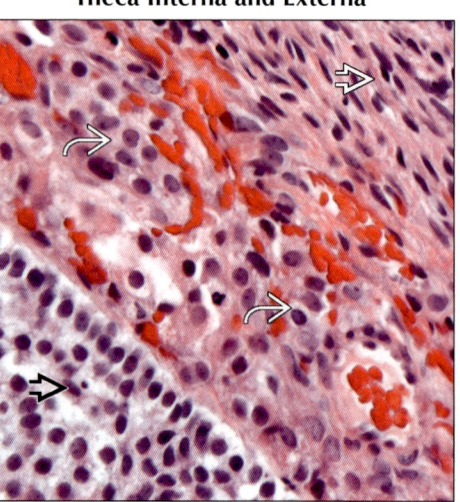

Corpus Luteum

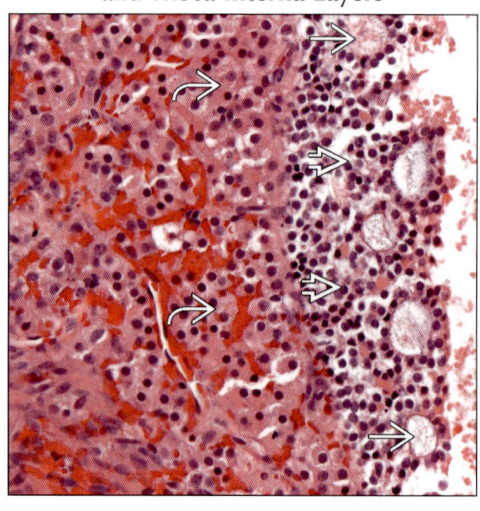

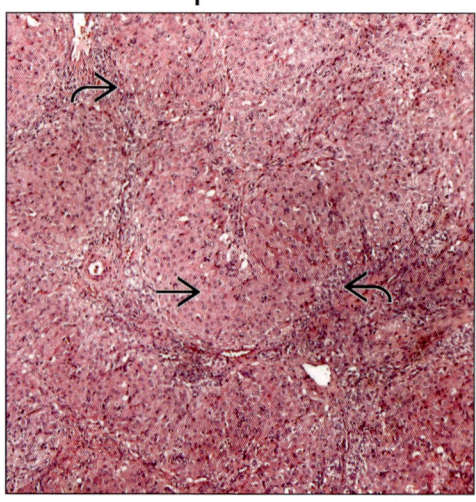

(Left) The theca externa layer comprises the outermost layer of the fully mature follicle. The theca interna ⇨ is composed of round, eosinophilic cells with round nuclei, whereas the theca externa ⇨ is composed of spindled, eosinophilic cells with elongated nuclei. Compare granulosa cells ⇨. **(Right)** After ovulation, the corpus luteum forms. The corpus luteum is composed of granulosa lutein cells ⇨ and theca lutein cells ⇨, remnants of the granulosa and theca interna layers, respectively.

OVARY

Corpus Luteum: Menstruation

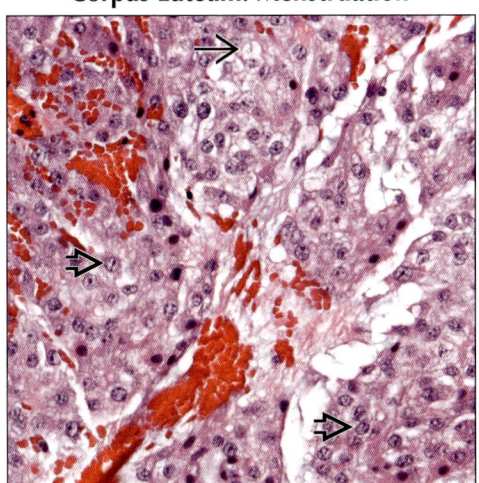

Corpus Luteum: Menstruation

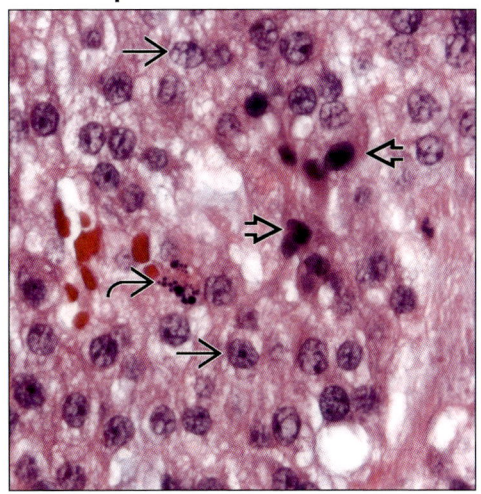

(Left) Within the corpus luteum, the granulosa cells become luteinized are are termed granulosa lutein cells. Granulosa lutein cells ⊃ are enlarged, polygonal cells with ample eosinophilic cytoplasm and scattered lipid droplets →. **(Right)** The nucleus of the granulosa lutein cell is round and vesicular with easily discernible nucleoli →. Apoptotic debris → and K cells ⊃, noted by their darkly staining cytoplasm and nuclei, may be identified as well.

Hemorrhagic Corpus Luteum

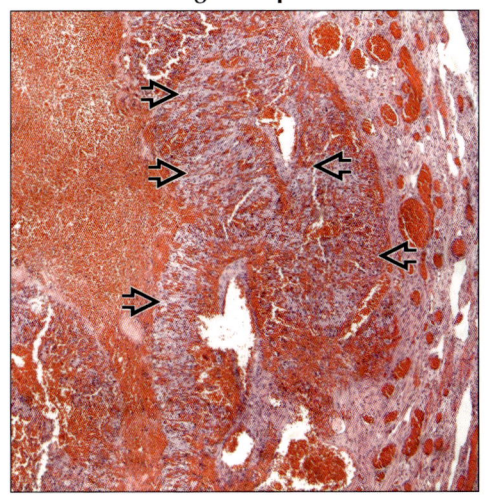

Hemorrhagic Corpus Luteum

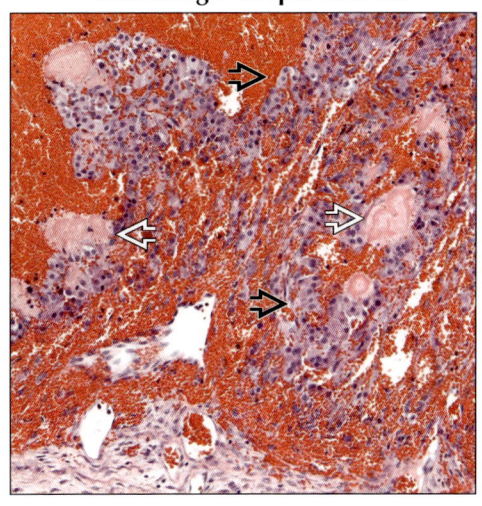

(Left) One of the most common complications associated with an otherwise normal corpus luteum is associated hemorrhage. Additionally, exceptionally large luteal cysts may mimic ovarian neoplasms and be excised. The undulating lining ⊃ of this luteal cyst can be seen admixed with abundant hemorrhage. **(Right)** Fragments of granulosa lutein cells ⊃ and fibrin thrombi → can be helpful features when considering the differential diagnosis of a hemorrhagic ovarian cyst.

Involuting Corpus Luteum

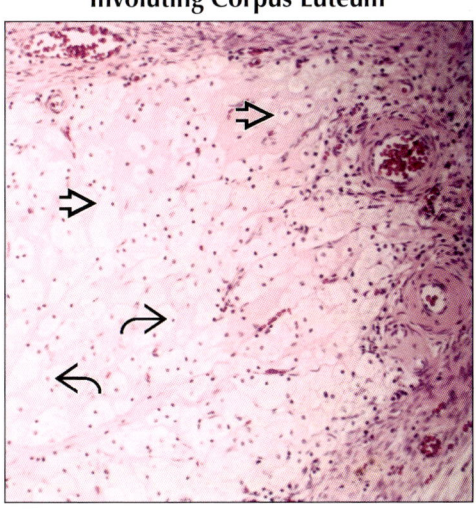

Corpora Albicans

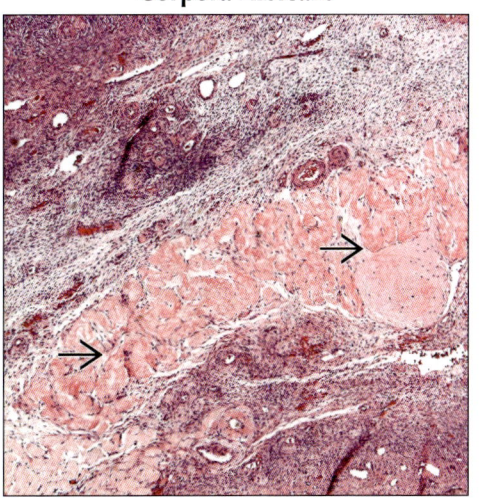

(Left) When a corpus luteum undergoes routine involution, the granulosa lutein cells accumulate abundant cytoplasmic lipid ⊃, which leads to pale staining. The cells become smaller and have pyknotic nuclei →. **(Right)** The involuting corpus luteum is replaced by collagen and fibroblasts and eventually forms a scar known as a corpus albicans →. Occasional macrophages may be identified in and around these structures. Corpora albicans may become resorbed and may disappear completely.

OVARY

Corpus Luteum: Pregnancy

Corpus Luteum: Pregnancy

(Left) During pregnancy, the corpus luteum may enlarge to form a variably sized cystic structure with a yellow lining. In striking cases, such as the one pictured, multiple, large cysts filled with fibrin & blood may form. *(Right)* During pregnancy, involution of the corpus luteum does not occur. The cells continue to enlarge, reaching a maximum size of around 55 μm. One histologic feature of pregnancy is the development of cytoplasmic vacuoles in the corpus luteum ⇨, which enlarge throughout pregnancy.

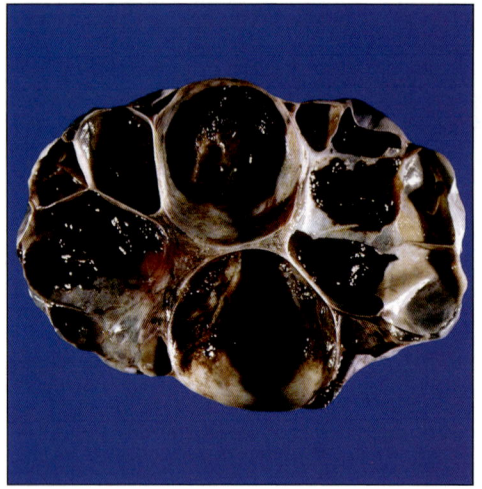

Corpus Luteum: Pregnancy

Involuting Follicle

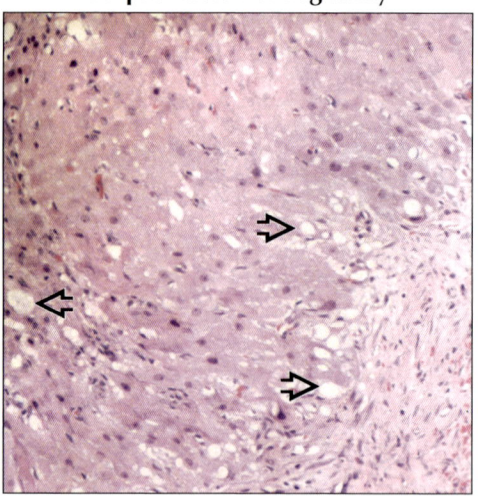

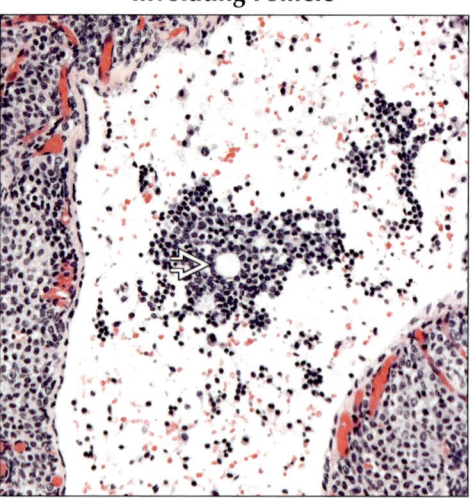

(Left) Another histologic feature seen during pregnancy (and rarely in the corpus luteum of menstruation) are hyaline bodies ⇨. Hyaline bodies increase in number throughout gestation. *(Right)* The vast majority of follicles undergo atresia. Primordial and primary follicles involute completely and leave no evidence of their existence. Mature follicles (follicles that reach the antral stage) that involute are recognizable. The earliest sign is the degeneration of the oocyte ⇨.

Involuting Follicle: Lining

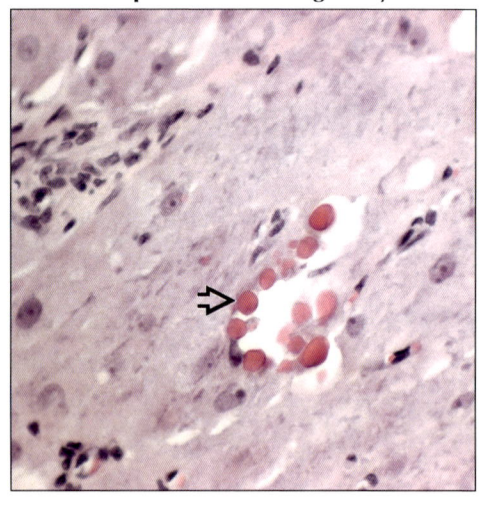

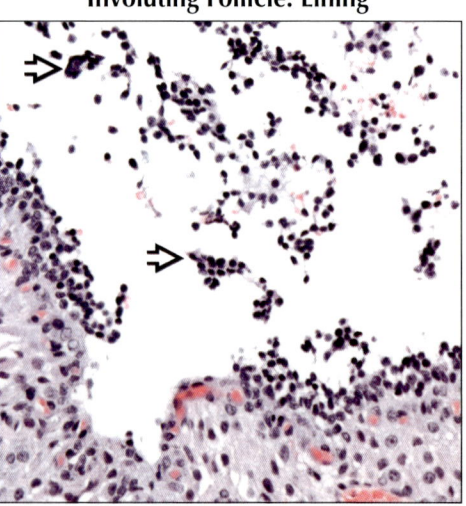

Involuting Follicle

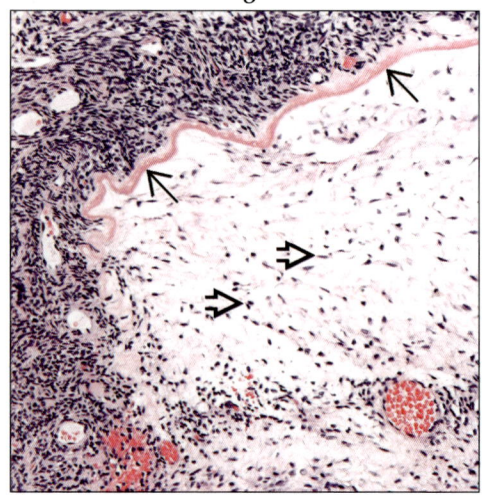

(Left) Following the degeneration of the oocyte, the granulosa cells become mitotically inert and decrease in size. This is followed by shedding of the granulosa cells ⇨ into the antral cavity. *(Right)* In the involuting follicle, the cystic cavity is eventually filled with loose, vascular stroma composed of connective tissue and fibroblasts ⇨. The undulating follicular basement membrane becomes thickened ⇨, and at this stage is known as the "glassy membrane."

OVARY

Involuting Follicle: Late

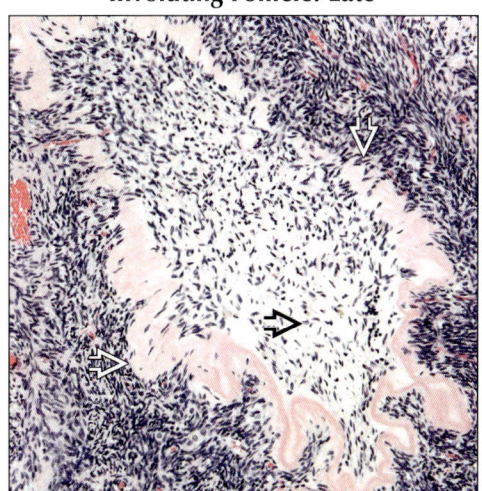

Follicle Cyst

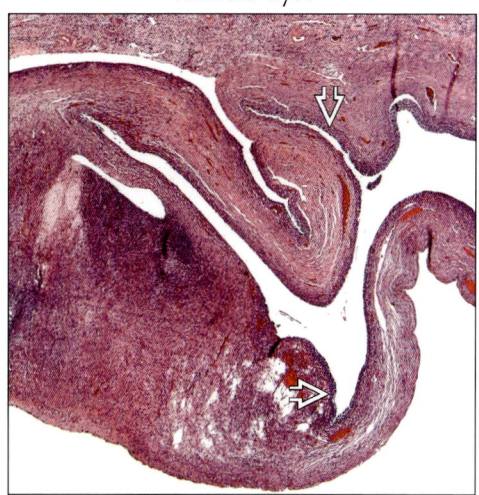

(Left) The "glassy membrane" ⇨ represents the heretofore histologically inapparent basement membrane that lies between the granulosa cell layer and theca interna. Most mature follicles completely fill with fibrous connective tissue ⇨ and form scars. (Right) Occasionally, the cystic portion of a follicle will persist. A thin lining of granulosa cells ⇨ can usually be identified. When the cyst is > 3 cm in diameter, it is termed a follicle cyst.

Hyaline Scar

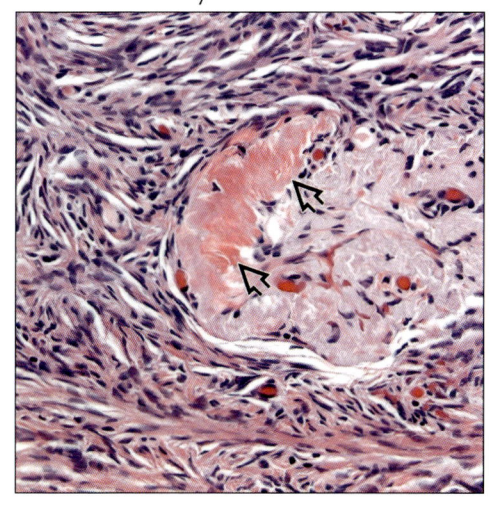

Corpora Fibrosa

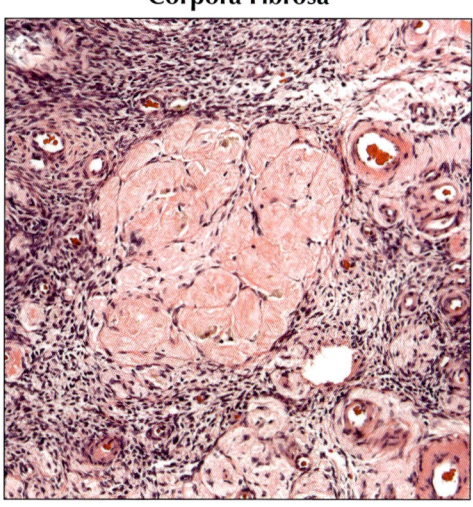

(Left) The majority of follicles do not form cysts and become known as corpora fibrosa. As the involuting follicle shrinks, it becomes hyalinized, which can be seen occurring in the left portion ⇨ of the pictured follicle. (Right) Once complete hyalinization has occurred, the resulting corpora fibrosa is formed. The corpora fibrosa is composed of an undulating band of hyaline tissue. Most of the resulting corpora fibrosa are eventually resorbed into the ovarian stroma.

Ovarian Surface

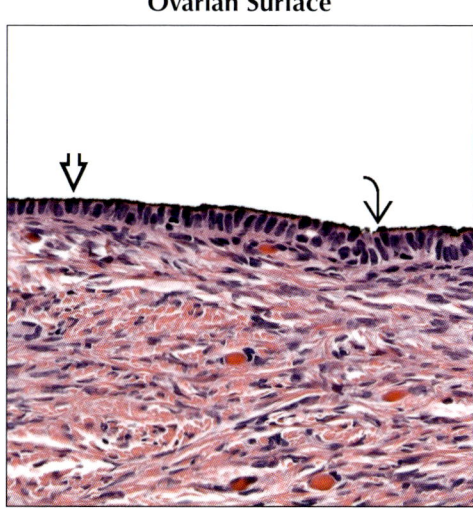

Cortical Inclusion Cyst

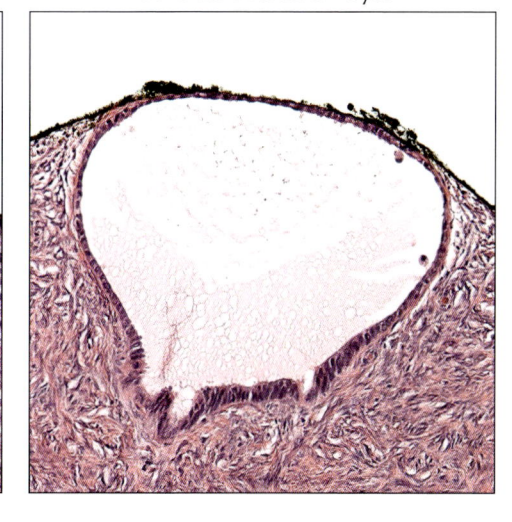

(Left) The surface epithelium of the ovary is a simple cuboidal to columnar lining ⇨ with occasional areas of pseudostratification ⇨. This epithelium is very delicate and is typically avulsed during handling of the ovary during surgery or pathologic examination. (Right) Cortical inclusion cysts or glands are commonly found beneath the cortical surface. These glands (or cysts, if > 1 cm) represent invaginations of the surface epithelium that no longer communicate with the surface.

OVARY

Cortical Inclusion Gland

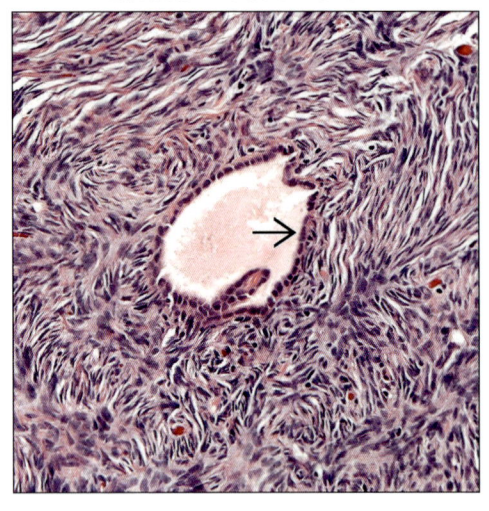

(Left) Cortical inclusion cysts and glands may be found deeper within the cortical stroma. The lining is typically simple cuboidal to columnar epithelium ➡, similar to that found on the ovarian surface. **(Right)** Surface papillation, or micropapillomatosis, is composed of finger-like projections of cortical stroma ➡ covered by otherwise unremarkable ovarian surface epithelium. The simple papillae and lack of epithelial atypia and stratification differentiate these from surface tumors.

Surface Papillation

Surface Adhesion

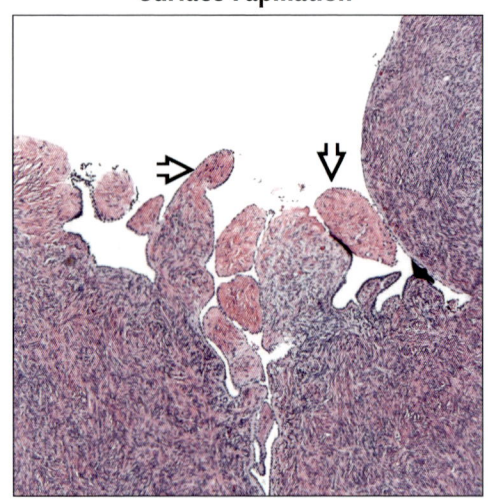

(Left) Delicate bands of fibrous tissue ➡, termed adhesions, may be seen originating from the ovarian surface. Adhesions may be more numerous in patients with a history of abdominal surgery or pelvic trauma. They are associated with an increased risk of pelvic pain. **(Right)** Small collections of urothelial (transitional)-type epithelium ➡ may be seen within the ovary or broad ligament. These Walthard rests may contain small centrally located cysts ➡.

Walthard Rest

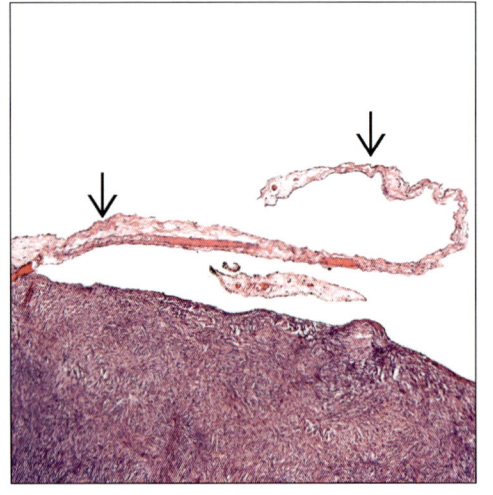

Walthard Rest

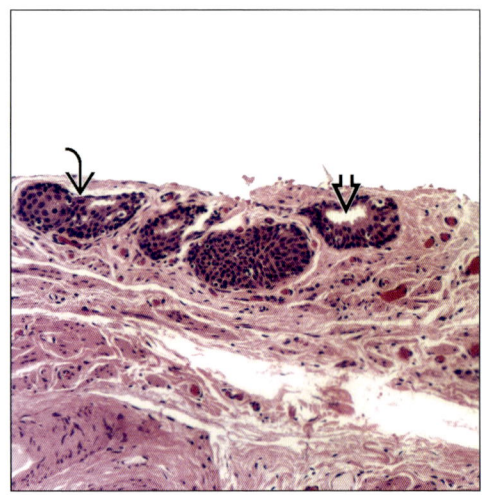

(Left) Walthard rests are composed of transitional epithelium that bears a striking similarity to bladder epithelium. A well-defined basal layer ➡ underlies a stratified epithelium that appears to "stream" toward the surface ➡. **(Right)** A not-uncommon finding is the presence of otherwise unremarkable endometrial glands ➡ and stroma ➡ within the ovary, termed endometriosis. The glands or stroma may range in amount from abundant, as pictured, to completely absent.

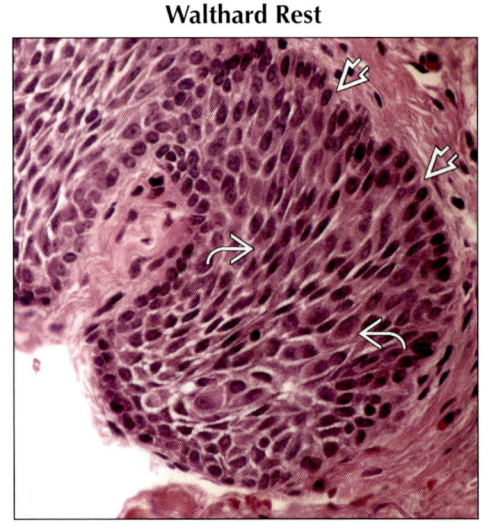

Endometriosis

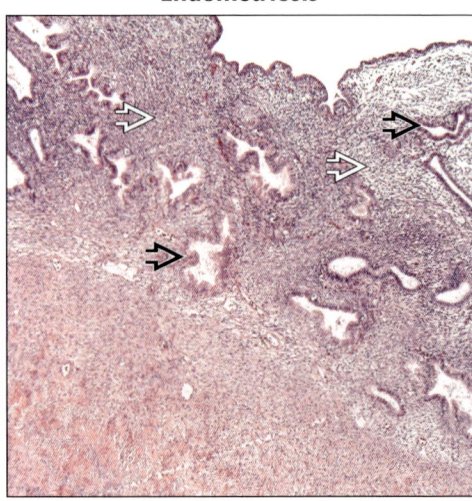

OVARY

Endometriosis: Gland Poor
Endometriosis: Stromal Hemorrhage

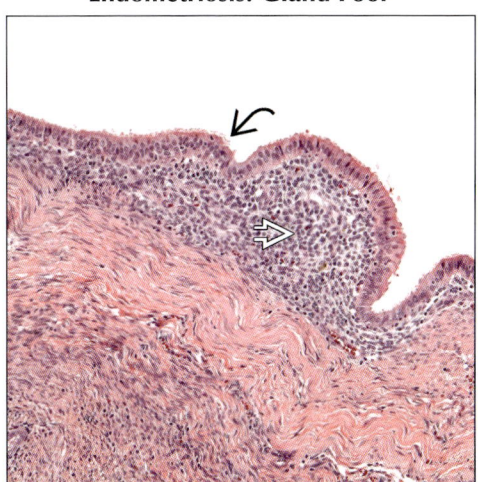

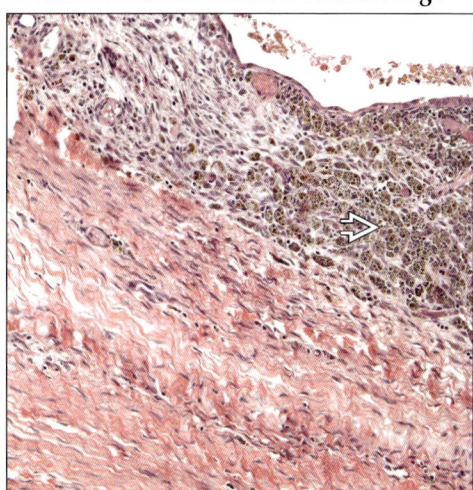

(Left) Some examples of endometriosis may lack endometrial glands and be composed of endometrial stroma ⇨. An epithelial lining ⇨ may or may not be visible. (Right) Another helpful histologic feature of endometriosis is the presence of pigmented macrophages ⇨. These pigmented macrophages ingest the blood associated with endometriosis and may occupy the stromal compartment. In cases that lack glands or stroma, stromal hemorrhage may suggest the presence of endometriosis.

Atrophic Ovary
Atrophic Ovary

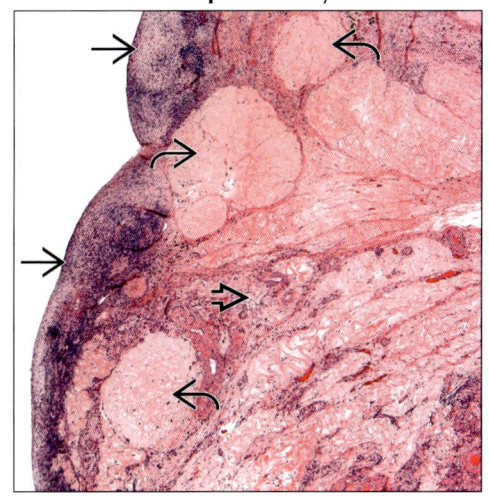

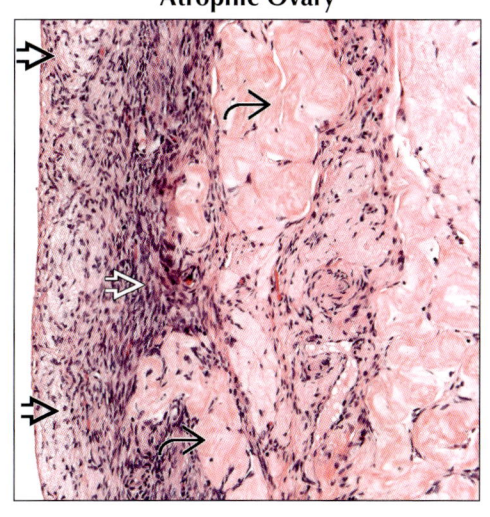

(Left) Peri- and postmenopausal patients' ovaries can display a range of atrophic changes. Examination typically reveals thinning of the cortex ⇨ and scant medullary and hilar stroma ⇨. In some patients, numerous corpora albicantia may be present ⇨. (Right) This atrophic ovary displays a markedly thinned cortex ⇨ with very scant stroma ⇨. Two corpora albicantia ⇨ are present.

Stromal Hyperplasia
Stromal Hyperplasia

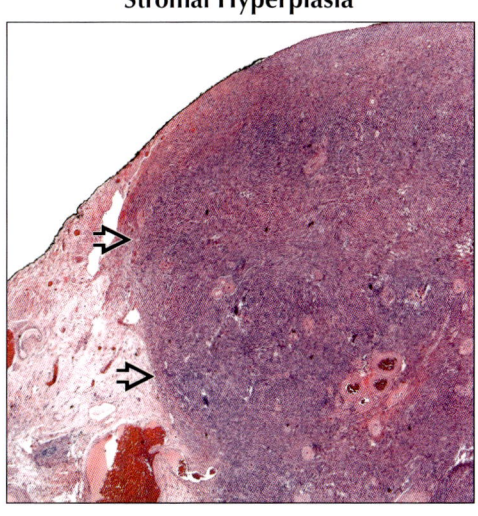

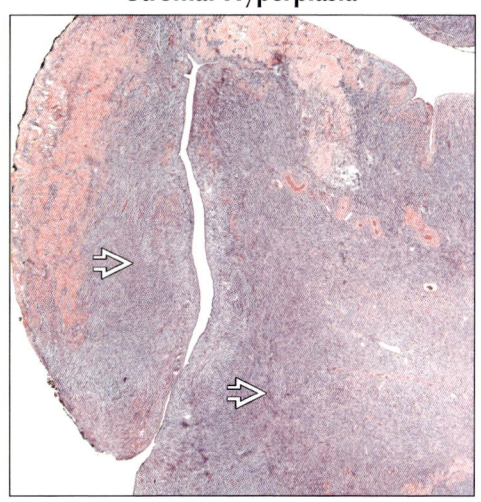

(Left) In some peri- and postmenopausal patients, there are varying degrees of stromal hyperplasia. In some patients, the stromal hyperplasia may have well-circumscribed borders ⇨ and mimic sex cord-stromal neoplasms (fibroma). Occasionally, multiple nodules may be present and efface the normal ovarian architecture. (Right) This atrophic ovary displays a moderate amount of stromal hyperplasia ⇨. In this example, however, a discreet nodule is not formed.

PLACENTA

Key Facts

Macroscopic Anatomy
- Umbilical cord: Rope-like structure housing 2 arteries and 1 vein, surrounded by Wharton Jelly
- Amniotic membranes: Sac-like structure containing fetus and amniotic fluid
  - 2 layers: Amnion and chorion
- Placental disk: Flat, disc-shaped organ composed of villi; has fetal surface (chorionic plate) and maternal surface (cotyledons)

Microscopic Anatomy
- Amnion: Single-cell lining with underlying basement membrane
- Chorion: Lies outside amnion and is composed predominately of trophoblastic cells (X cells) and stroma
- Stem villi: Large villi extending from chorionic plate that give rise to secondary villi
- Secondary villi: Intermediate-sized villi arising from stem villi, which give rise to terminal villi
- Tertiary villi: Small villi that are rich with capillaries: Where maternal-fetal oxygen exchange takes place

Age Variation
- Immature villi: Large villi with abundant villous mesenchyme, centrally located vessels, and prominent trophoblastic linings
- Mature villi: Comparatively smaller and increased in number when compared to less mature villi
  - Vessels are more peripheral and trophoblasts are less pronounced

Metaplasia
- Squamous metaplasia may occur normally or in presence of chorionic irritation

---

(Left) A normal umbilical cord contains 3 vessels: An umbilical vein, shown here, and 2 umbilical arteries. *(Right)* The umbilical artery is composed of 2 muscular layers (inner ➡ and outer ➡) and endothelium ➡. All 3 vessels in the umbilical cord lack an adventitial layer, differentiating them from other blood vessels in the body. As the adventitia is absent, so too are the lymphatics and vasa vasorum that are typically present in this layer.

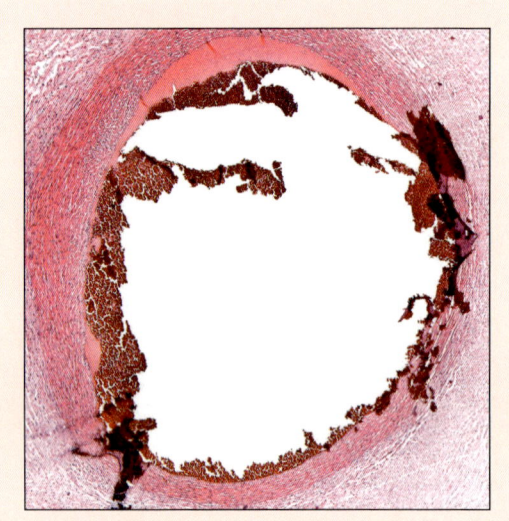

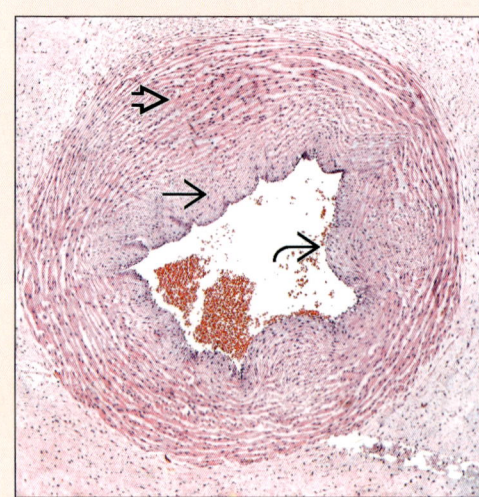

(Left) The majority of the umbilical cord is composed of stroma, designated Wharton jelly. This stroma is composed of mucopolysaccharides and sparse, spindled cells ➡, and scant collagen. The purpose of the Wharton jelly is to cushion and protect the vascular structures within the cord. *(Right)* A not uncommon finding is that of a single umbilical artery ➡. Although these neonates may have no complications, there is an association with congenital anomalies, namely of the urinary tract.

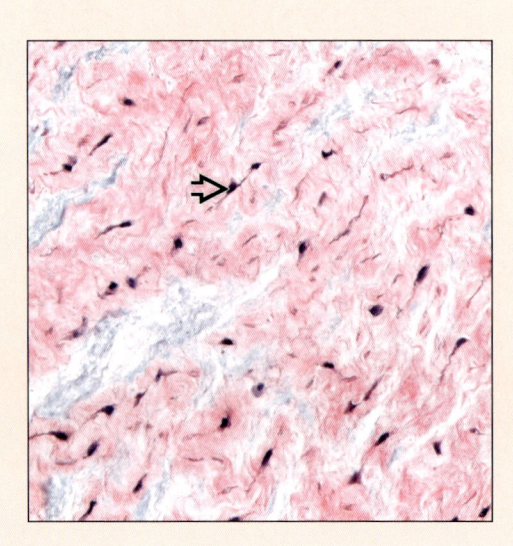

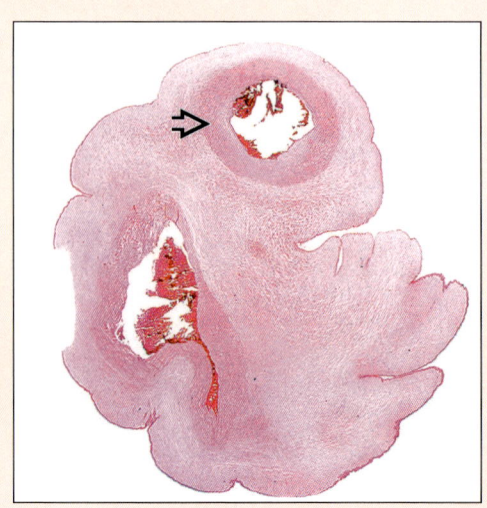

PLACENTA

Cord: Omphalomesenteric Duct Remnant

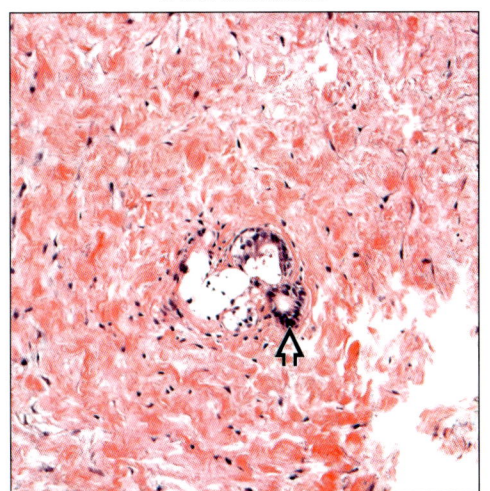

Cord: Omphalomesenteric Duct Remnant

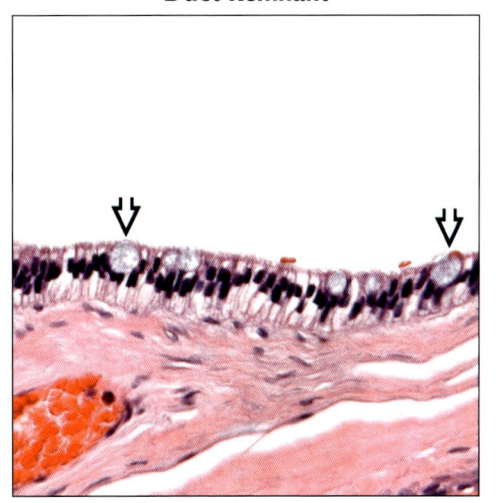

(Left) The omphalomesenteric duct represents the remnant connection of the yolk sac to the developing midgut. This structure is tubular and lined by columnar to cuboidal epithelium ⇨ that may secrete mucin. Heterotopic tissue may be present, including gastric, pancreatic, or bowel. *(Right)* The lining epithelium of an omphalomesenteric may contain heterotopic tissue, such as mucinous epithelium with scattered goblet cells ⇨.

Cord: Allantoic Remnant

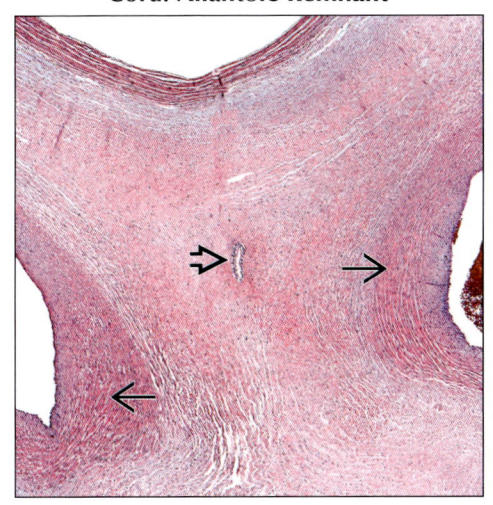

Cord: Allantoic Remnant

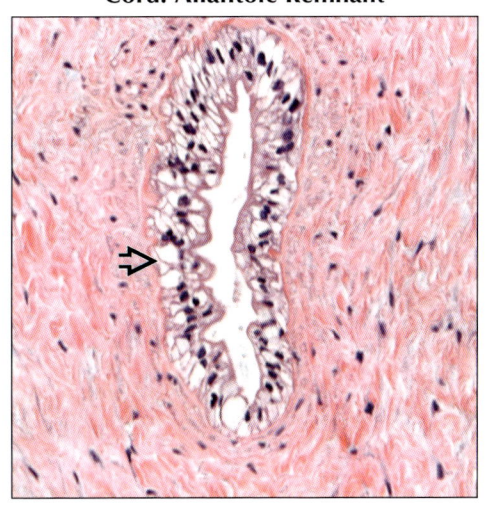

(Left) The allantoic remnant ⇨ (duct) represents the involuted allantois. This remnant can be encountered in the proximal portion of the umbilical cord, typically between the umbilical arteries ⇨. *(Right)* Various types of lining epithelium may be seen within allantoic remnants, including transitional epithelium, simple cuboidal epithelium (seen here ⇨ with vacuolar change), and yolk sac-like cells. The allantoic remnant and its epithelial lining are rarely clinically significant.

Cord: Allantoic Remnant

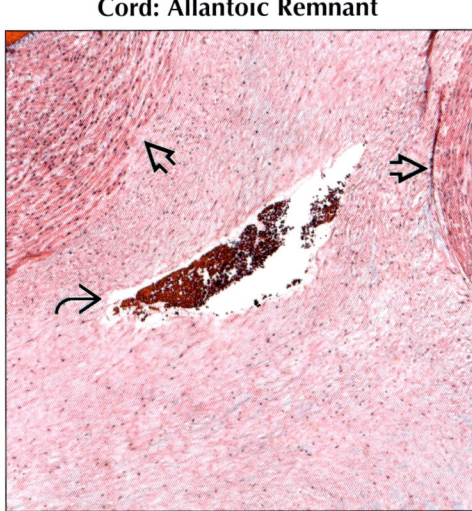

Cord: Hemorrhage

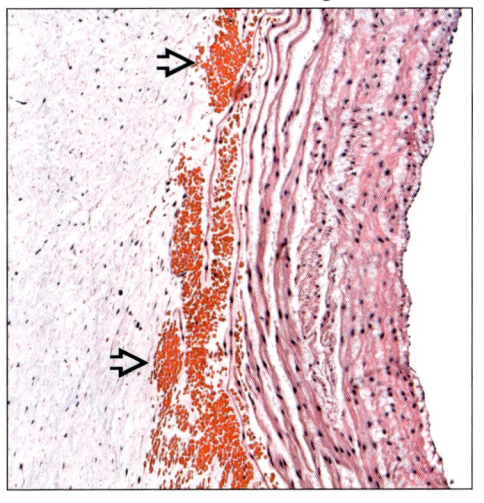

(Left) The lining epithelium of an allantoic remnant ⇨ may not be present; however, they may be identified due to their location between the umbilical arteries ⇨. *(Right)* Occasionally, perivascular hemorrhage ⇨ may be identified in the umbilical cord. If a grossly identified hematoma is not present, these areas likely represent artifactual extravasation of blood into the perivascular tissue (usually due to traction or cord clamps) and is of no clinical significance.

PLACENTA

Amnion

Amnion and Chorion

(Left) The amniotic epithelium is usually composed of a single layer of cuboidal cells ⇨ that may display squamoid features. The epithelium lies on a homogeneous, eosinophilic basement membrane ⇨. A layer of fibroblasts ⇨ lies directly beneath the basement membrane. (Right) Chorionic "X cells" ⇨ compose the 1st cellular layer of the chorion. These cells are typically seen admixed with the underlying maternal decidual cells ⇨.

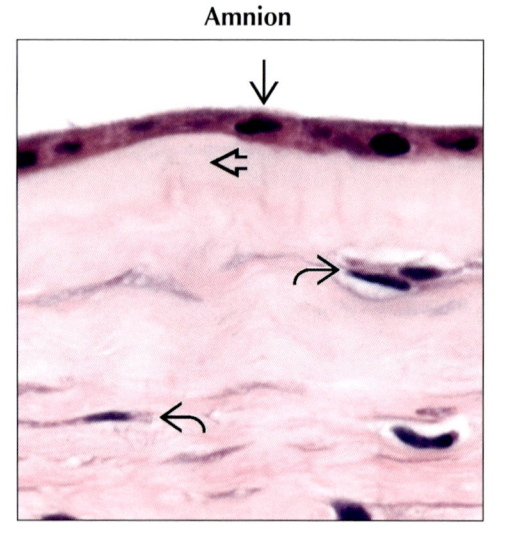

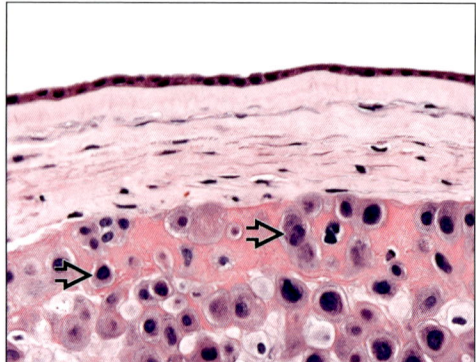

Chorion: Superficial Layers

Subamniotic Clefts

(Left) The chorion consists of multiple layers. The spongy layer ⇨ is relatively acellular and separates the amnion and chorion. Scattered macrophages and fibroblasts may be seen beneath the spongy layer. The next layer is the reticular zone ⇨, followed by a false basement membrane ⇨. Beneath this are the X cells ⇨ and decidua ⇨. (Right) Artifactual subamniotic clefts ⇨ and subchorionic fibrin ⇨ may be present and have no clinical significance.

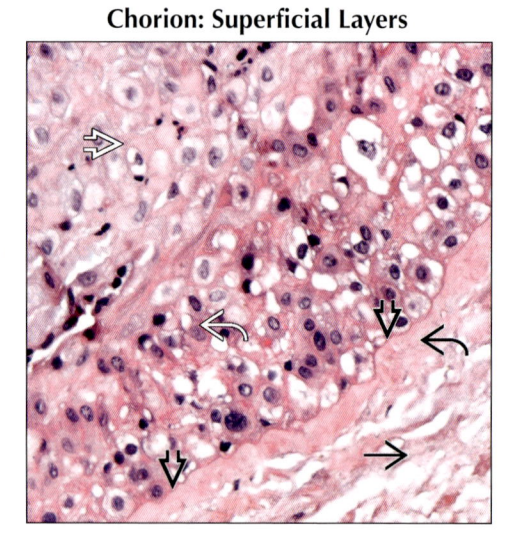

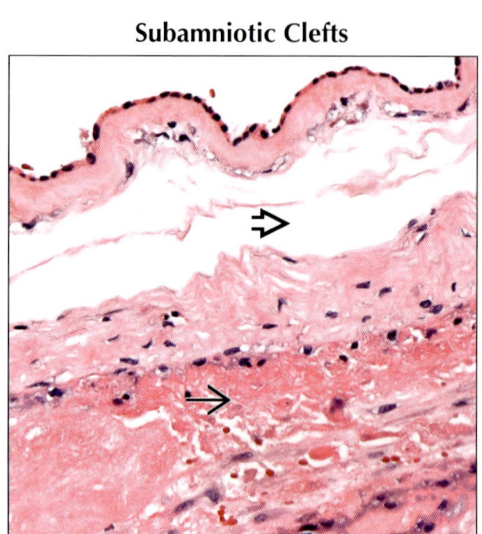

Membrane: Sclerotic Villi

Subamniotic Macrophages

(Left) Scattered sclerotic villous remnants ⇨ may be seen within the chorionic portion of the placental membranes. (Right) Scattered macrophages may be identified beneath the amnion, within the chorion or the artifactual cleft that may form. Here, a macrophage contains abundant globular brown pigment seen in meconium staining.

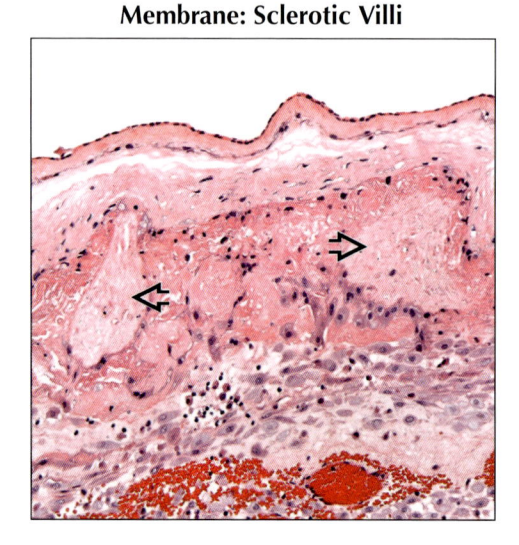

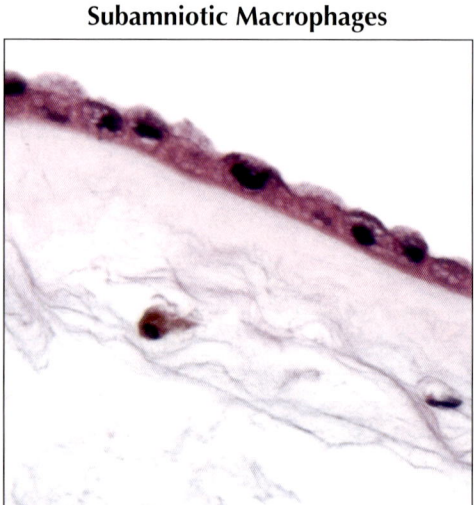

PLACENTA

Amnion: Squamous Metaplasia

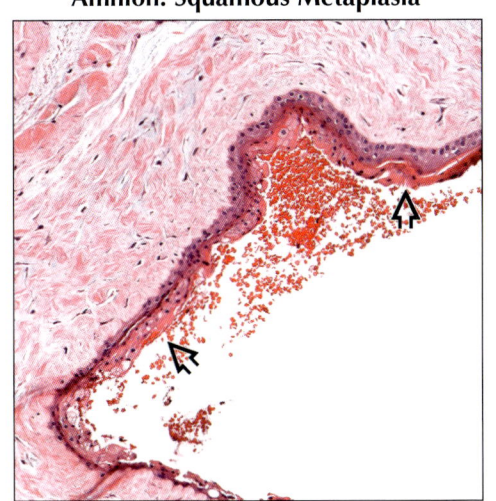

Diamniotic Monochorionic Membranes

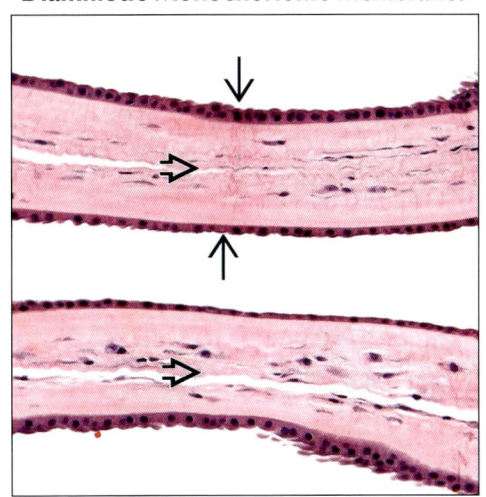

(Left) As can be seen in the umbilical cord, the amniocytes of the membranes and chorionic (fetal) surface may undergo squamous metaplasia ⇨. This finding has no clinical implications for the developing fetus. (Right) Several variations of membranes may be seen in multiple-gestation pregnancies. The presence of 1 chorion ⇨, which is relatively attenuated and acellular, and 2 amniotic sacs ⇨ leads to the diamniotic monochorionic membranes pictured here.

Diamniotic Dichorionic Membranes

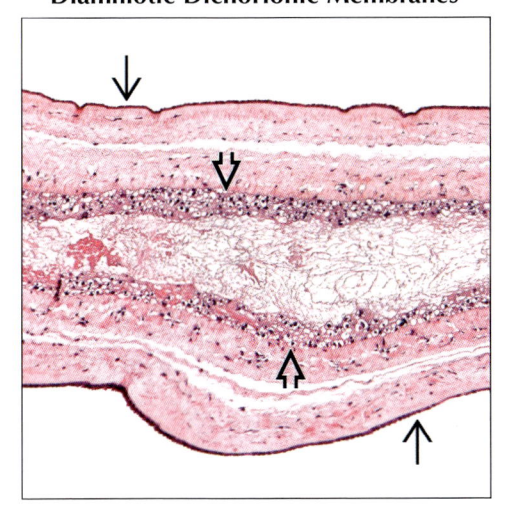

Immature Villi

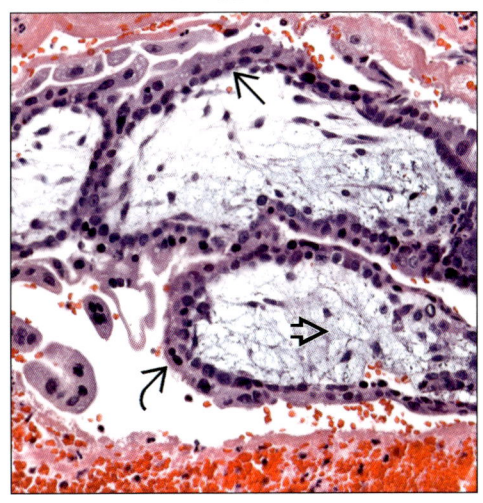

(Left) Twin pregnancies with 2 complete sets of amniotic membranes lead to the appearance of fused membranes (the membrane T zone). These "di-di" membranes are composed of 2 distinct chorionic ⇨ and amniotic ⇨ layers. (Right) Villi around 6 weeks of age are round to oval, with basophilic stroma ⇨ and a relative lack of stromal vessels. The cytotrophoblastic ⇨ and syncytiotrophoblastic ⇨ layers are distinct and highly cellular compared to later in gestation.

Immature Villi and Trophoblasts

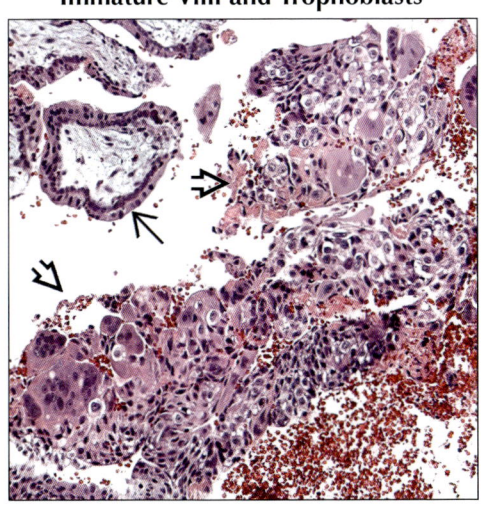

Fetal Blood Elements

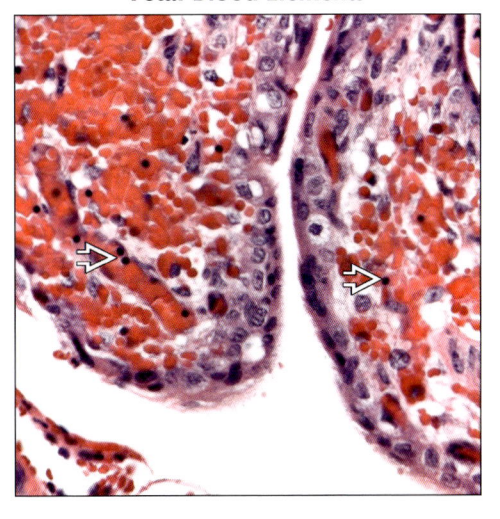

(Left) Extravillous trophoblasts ⇨ (intermediate and syncytiotrophoblasts) may be relatively increased in number and clustered in close approximation. The presence of extremely immature villi ⇨ should argue against a misdiagnosis of choriocarcinoma. (Right) Capillaries will begin to proliferate within the immature villi starting after the 6th week. Between this time and the 10th to 12th weeks, nucleated fetal red blood ⇨ cells may be identified in otherwise normal placentas.

PLACENTA

Immature Villi

Placental Villi

(Left) Immature villi are larger with a more cellular stroma ⇨ than their mature counterparts. The vessels ➔ within the villi tend to be more centrally located. The villi become progressively smaller throughout pregnancy. **(Right)** Within the mature placenta, 3 types of villi may be identified. As the villi extend from the chorionic plate, the stem villi ⇨, which give rise to the secondary villi, ➔ will branch to form the tertiary villi ⇨.

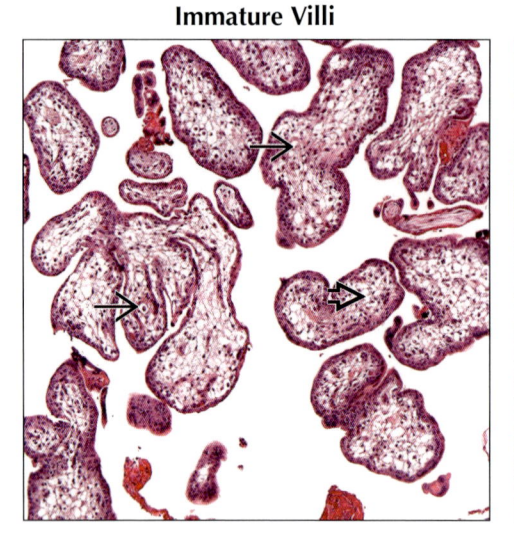

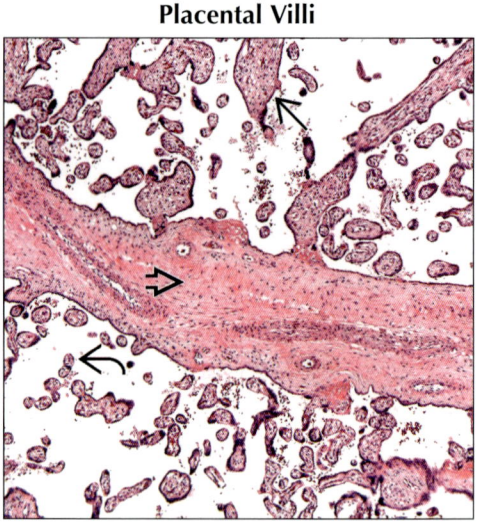

Placental Villi

Placental Villi

(Left) A large stem villus can be seen in the upper right corner. The stem villi contain the large caliber stem vessels ⇨, which coalesce in the chorionic plate and eventually, the umbilical cord. **(Right)** Numerous secondary villi ⇨ can be seen giving rise to scattered tertiary, or terminal villi ➔. These secondary villi can be differentiated from stem villi based on the lack of large, thick-walled, arteries and veins.

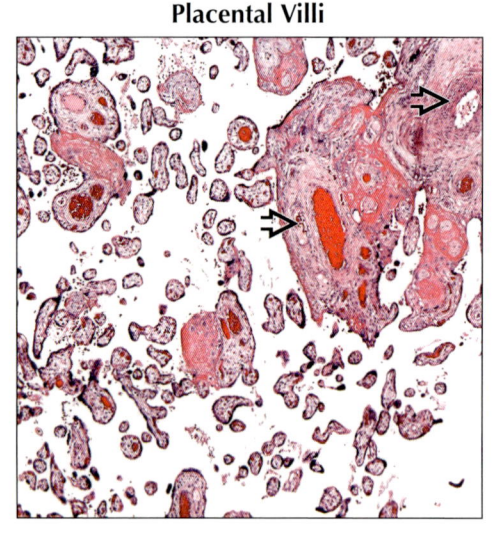

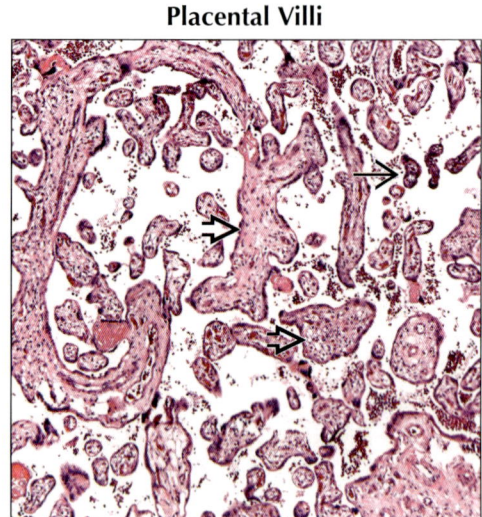

Secondary Villus

Tertiary Villi

(Left) Secondary villi typically contain multiple capillaries that tend to be centrally located ⇨. In addition to having more vascular structures, the secondary villi are larger and contain more stroma ➔ when compared to their terminal counterparts. **(Right)** Tertiary villi vary in size, but are generally smaller than secondary villi. The peripheral location of the villous capillaries ⇨ helps to facilitate the transfer of oxygen from mother to fetus.

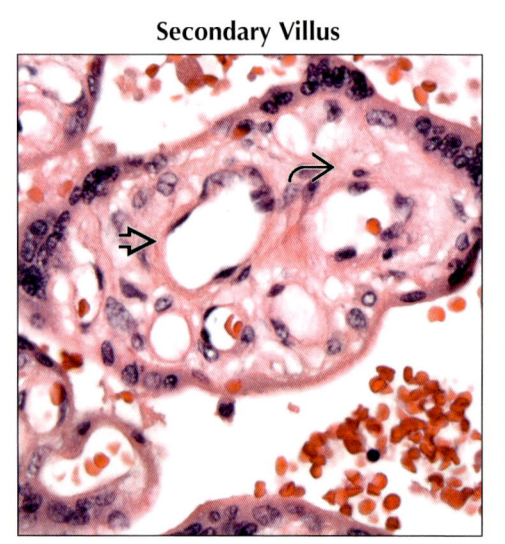

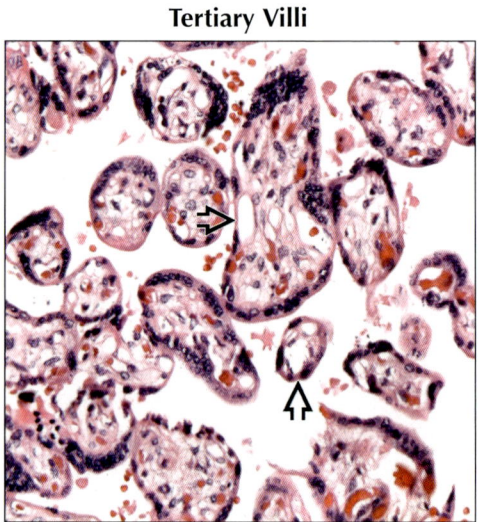

PLACENTA

Tertiary Villi

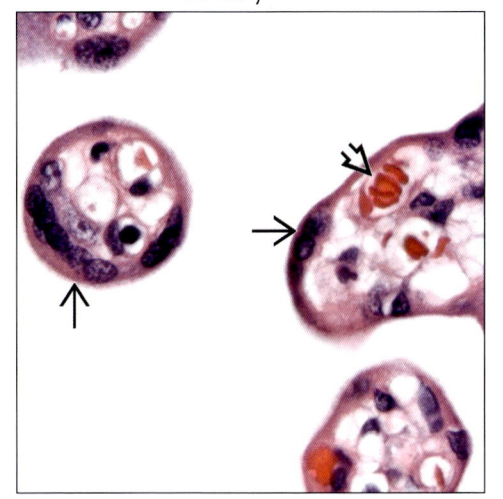

Perivillous Fibrin

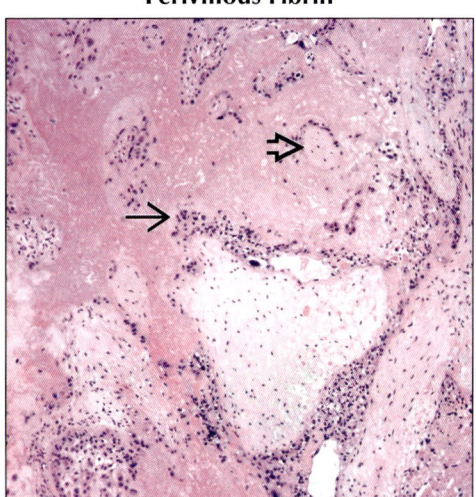

(Left) In mature tertiary villi, the cytotrophoblastic layer is typically not visible. The syncytiotrophoblastic layer is thin and irregular, and clusters of darkly staining syncytiotrophoblastic nuclei ⇉ may be the only evidence of its presence. Fetal blood ⇉ may be seen in the terminal villi capillaries. (Right) Scattered pockets of perivillous fibrin may be seen in otherwise normal placentas. The fibrin encases the villi ⇉, leading to their involution; however, trophoblasts ⇉ may persist.

Decidua

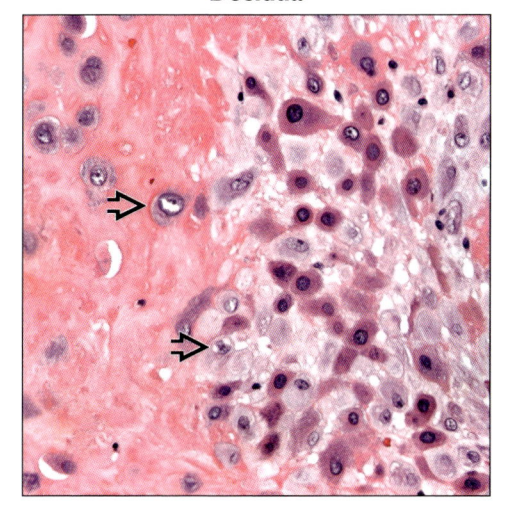

Decidualized Endometrium

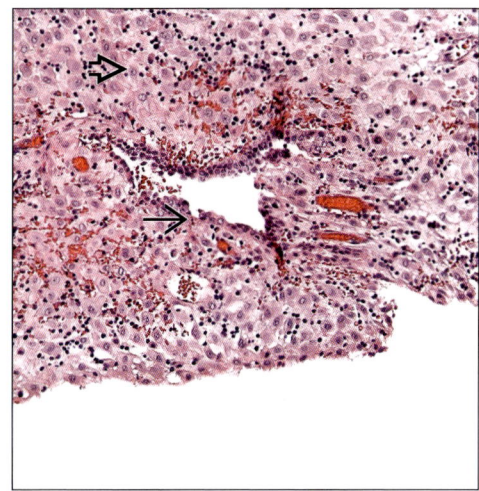

(Left) Endometrial stromal cells undergo a process of "decidualization," leading to the so-called decidua ⇉. These cells can be identified by their abundant eosinophilic cytoplasm, centrally located vesicular nuclei, and well-defined cell borders. (Right) Occasionally, large fragments of accompanying decidualized endometrial glands ⇉ and stroma ⇉ may be present with the placenta. This may be the predominant component of so-called "products of conception" seen in cases of missed abortions or previable pregnancies.

Calcification

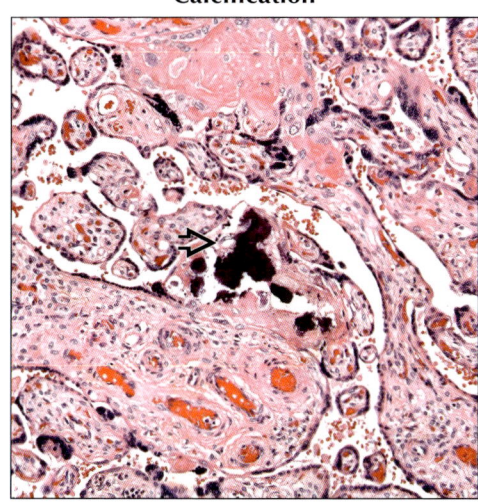

Implantation Site

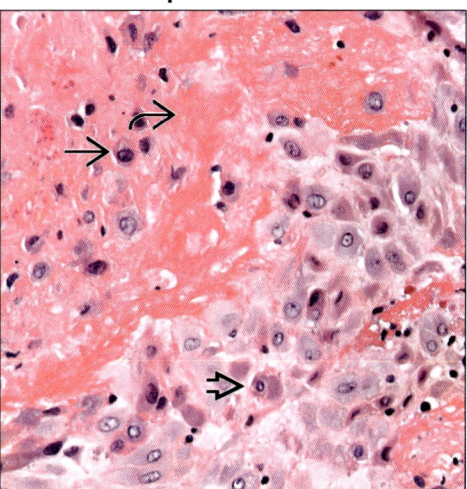

(Left) Scattered calcifications ⇉ are commonly identified in or around placental villi in mature placentas. Calcification is often normal. It may be abnormal, however, if excessive for gestational age, and may be a sign of ischemia. (Right) The implantation site is composed of maternal decidua ⇉, extravillous trophoblastic cells ⇉, and Nitabuch fibrinoid ⇉. Identification of the implantation site may serve as proof of intrauterine pregnancy when villi are absent.

SELECTED REFERENCES

VULVA

1. Scurry J et al: Mammary-like gland adenoma of the vulva: review of 46 cases. Pathology. 41(4):372-8, 2009
2. van der Putte SC et al: Cysts of mammarylike glands in the vulva. Int J Gynecol Pathol. 14(2):184-8, 1995
3. McLachlin CM et al: Multinucleated atypia of the vulva. Report of a distinct entity not associated with human papillomavirus. Am J Surg Pathol. 18(12):1233-9, 1994
4. van der Putte SC: Mammary-like glands of the vulva and their disorders. Int J Gynecol Pathol. 13(2):150-60, 1994
5. van der Putte SC: Ultrastructure of the human anogenital "sweat" gland. Anat Rec. 235(4):583-90, 1993
6. van der Putte SC: Anogenital "sweat" glands. Histology and pathology of a gland that may mimic mammary glands. Am J Dermatopathol. 13(6):557-67, 1991
7. McLean M. Anatomy and physiology of of the vulva. In Ridley CM et al: The Vulva. New York: Churchill Livingstone. 39-65, 1988
8. Rorat E et al: Human bartholin gland, duct, and duct cyst. Histochemical and ultrastructural study. Arch Pathol. 99(7):367-74, 1975

VAGINA

1. Eschenbach DA et al: Influence of the normal menstrual cycle on vaginal tissue, discharge, and microflora. Clin Infect Dis. 30(6):901-7, 2000
2. Patton DL et al: Epithelial cell layer thickness and immune cell populations in the normal human vagina at different stages of the menstrual cycle. Am J Obstet Gynecol. 183(4):967-73, 2000
3. Abdul-Karim FW et al: Atypical stromal cells of lower female genital tract. Histopathology. 17(3):249-53, 1990
4. Ferry JA et al: Mesonephric remnants, hyperplasia, and neoplasia in the uterine cervix. A study of 49 cases. Am J Surg Pathol. 14(12):1100-11, 1990
5. O'Brien PC et al: Vaginal epithelial changes in young women enrolled in the National Cooperative Diethylstilbestrol Adenosis (DESAD) project. Obstet Gynecol. 53(3):300-8, 1979
7. Robboy SJ et al: Intrauterine diethylstilbestrol exposure and its consequences: pathologic characteristics of vaginal adenosis, clear cell adenocarcinoma, and related lesions. Arch Pathol Lab Med. 101(1):1-5, 1977
8. Ulfelder H et al: The embryologic development of the human vagina. Am J Obstet Gynecol. 126(7):769-76, 1976

UTERUS

1. Lindhard A et al: Ultrasound characteristics and histological dating of the endometrium in a natural cycle in infertile women compared with fertile controls. Fertil Steril. 86(5):1344-55, 2006
2. de Ziegler D et al: Understanding endometrial physiology and menstrual disorders in the 1990s. Curr Opin Obstet Gynecol. 5(3):378-88, 1993
3. Novotny DB et al: Tubal metaplasia. A frequent potential pitfall in the cytologic diagnosis of endocervical glandular dysplasia on cervical smears. Acta Cytol. 36(1):1-10, 1992
4. Lauchlan SC: Metaplasias and neoplasias of Müllerian epithelium. Histopathology. 8(4):543-57, 1984
5. Kearns M et al: Life history of decidual cells: a review. Am J Reprod Immunol. 3(2):78-82, 1983
6. Masterton R et al: The cyclical variation in the percentage of ciliated cells in the normal human endometrium. J Reprod Fertil. 42(3):537-40, 1975
7. Singer A: The uterine cervix from adolescence to the menopause. Br J Obstet Gynaecol. 82(2):81-99, 1975
8. Forsberg JG: Cervicovaginal epithelium: its origin and development. Am J Obstet Gynecol. 115(7):1025-43, 1973
9. McLennan CE et al: Extent of endometrial shedding during normal menstruation. Obstet Gynecol. 26(5):605-21, 1965

FALLOPIAN TUBE

1. Rabban JT et al: Transitional cell metaplasia of fallopian tube fimbriae: a potential mimic of early tubal carcinoma in risk reduction salpingo-oophorectomies from women with BRCA mutations. Am J Surg Pathol. 33(1):111-9, 2009
2. Hunt JL et al: Histologic features of surgically removed fallopian tubes. Arch Pathol Lab Med. 126(8):951-5, 2002
3. Peters WM: Nature of "basal" and "reserve" cells in oviductal and cervical epithelium in man. J Clin Pathol. 39(3):306-12, 1986

OVARY

1. Hirschowitz L et al: Ovarian hilus cell heterotopia. Int J Gynecol Pathol. 30(1):46-52, 2011
2. Sidawy MK et al: Endosalpingiosis in female peritoneal washings: a diagnostic pitfall. Int J Gynecol Pathol. 6(4):340-6, 1987
3. McNatty KP et al: Follicular development during the luteal phase of the human menstrual cycle. J Clin Endocrinol Metab. 56(5):1022-31, 1983
4. Blaustein A: Surface cells and inclusion cysts in fetal ovaries. Gynecol Oncol. 12(2 Pt 1):222-33, 1981

SELECTED REFERENCES

5. Mulligan RM: A survey of epithelial inclusions in the ovarian cortex of 470 patients. J Surg Oncol. 8(1):61-6, 1976

6. Reeves G: Specific stroma in the cortex and medulla of the ovary. Cell types and vascular supply in relation to follicular apparatus and ovulation. Obstet Gynecol. 37(6):832-44, 1971

7. Boss JH et al: Structural Variations in the adult ovary. Clinical signficance. Obstet Gynecol. 25:747-64, 1965

8. Pinkerton JH et al: Development of the human ovary--a study using histochemical technics. Obstet Gynecol. 18:152-81, 1961

9. Joel RV et al: Fate of the corpus albicans: a morphologic approach. Am J Obstet Gynecol. 80:314-6, 1960

10. Bigelow B: Comparison of ovarian and endometrial morphology spanning the menopause. Obstet Gynecol. 11(5):487-513, 1958

11. Teoh TB: The structure and development of Walthard nests. J Pathol Bacteriol. 66(2):433-9, 1953

PLACENTA

1. van Diik CC et al: The umbilical coiling index in normal pregnancy. J Matern Fetal Neonatal Med. 11(4):280-3, 2002

2. Yeh IT et al: Vacuolated cytotrophoblast: a subpopulation of trophoblast in the chorion laeve. Placenta. 10(5):429-38, 1989

3. Naeye RL: Umbilical cord length: clinical significance. J Pediatr. 107(2):278-81, 1985

4. Kurman RJ et al: Intermediate trophoblast: a distinctive form of trophoblast with specific morphological, biochemical and functional features. Placenta. 5(4):349-69, 1984

5. Freese UE: The uteroplacental vascular relationship in the human. Am J Obstet Gynecol. 101(1):8-16, 1968

6. Pierce GB Jr et al: The Origin and function of human syncytiotrophoblastic giant cells. Am J Pathol. 43:153-73, 1963

7. Arts NF: Investigations on the vascular system of the placenta. I. General introduction and the fetal vascular system. Am J Obstet Gynecol. 82:147-58, 1961

8. Bourne GL: The microscopic anatomy of the human amnion and chorion. Am J Obstet Gynecol. 79:1070-3, 1960

9. Danforth D et al: The microscopic anatomy of the fetal membranes with particular reference to the detailed structure of the amnion. Am J Obstet Gynecol. 75(3):536-47; discussion 548-50, 1958

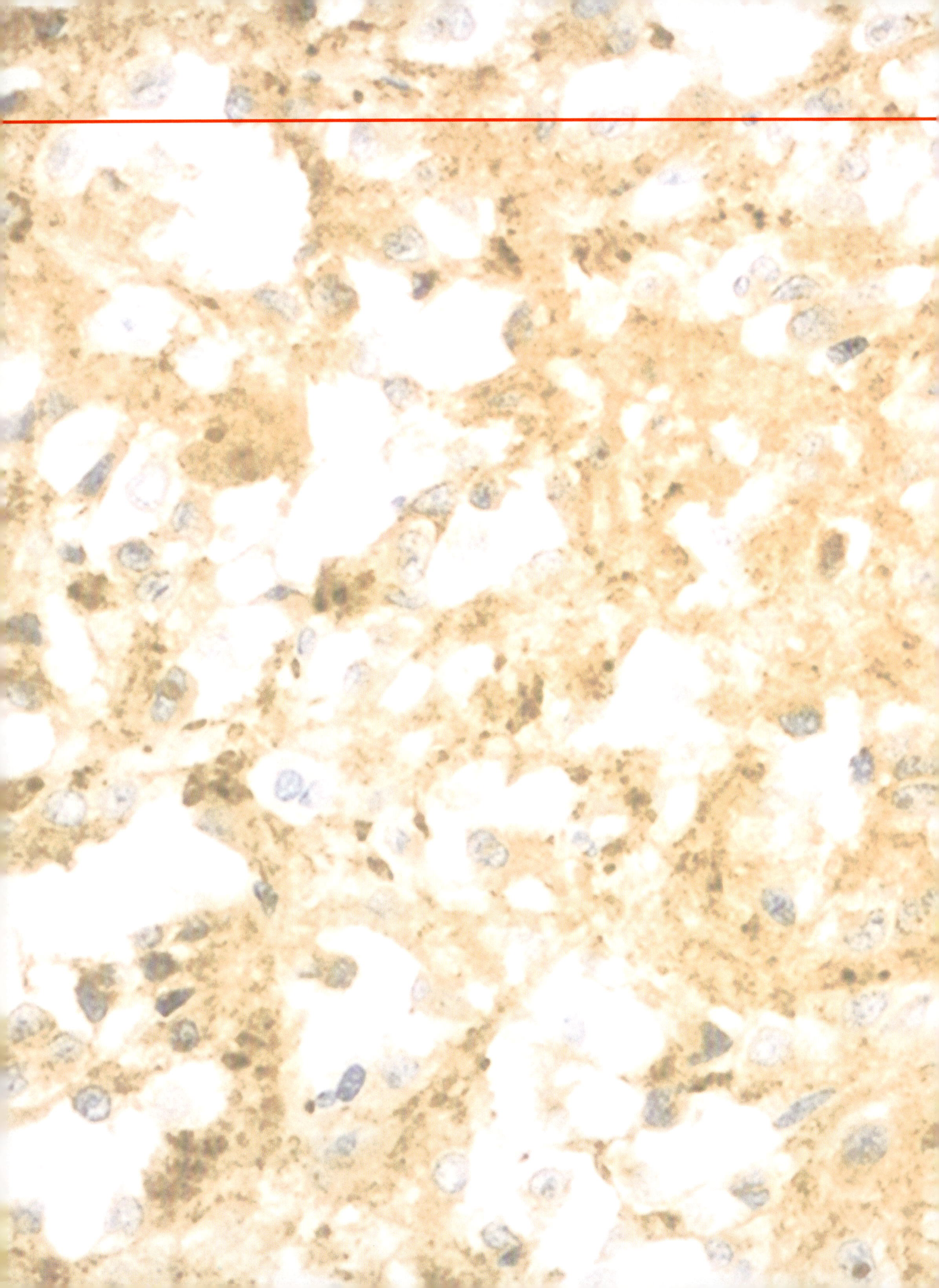

Endocrine

Adrenal Gland	14-2
Paraganglia	14-6
Thyroid	14-8
Parathyroid	14-12
Pineal Gland	14-16
Pituitary	14-18

ADRENAL GLAND

Key Facts

Macroscopic Anatomy
- Located in retroperitoneum, superior and medial to kidneys
- Right adrenal gland is pyramidal; left adrenal gland is crescent-shaped
- On cut section, 3 zones are visible grossly
  - Outermost layer: Thick and bright yellow; mostly composed of zona fasciculata
  - Middle layer: Thin and brown, composed of zona reticularis
  - Innermost layer: Gray, composed of adrenal medulla

Microscopic Anatomy
- Adrenal cortex is histologically divided into 3 layers (from outermost to innermost)
  - Zona glomerulosa
  - Zona fasciculata
  - Zona reticularis

- Adrenal medulla
  - Central portion of adrenal gland
  - Present in head and body of gland but absent in tail

Age Variation
- In neonates, majority of adrenal cortex is composed of provisional (or fetal) cortex with an outer thin rim of definitive cortex
  - After birth, provisional cortex involutes and the definitive cortex becomes the adult adrenal cortex

Hyperplasia
- Nodular adrenocortical hyperplasia consists of areas of hyperplastic adrenocortical cells that occur with increasing frequency with age

---

(Left) The adrenal glands are in the retroperitoneum superior to the kidneys. The right adrenal gland is pyramidal in shape; the left adrenal has a crescent-shaped appearance. Each adrenal is supplied by the superior (arising from the inferior phrenic artery), middle (arising from the aorta), and inferior (arising from the renal artery) arteries. (Right) The innermost layer of the adrenal gland, the medulla ➡, is composed of gray glistening tissue and is surrounded by the outer bright yellow cortical tissue.

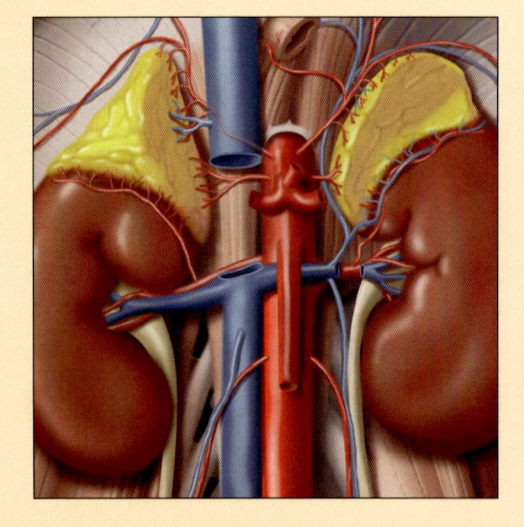

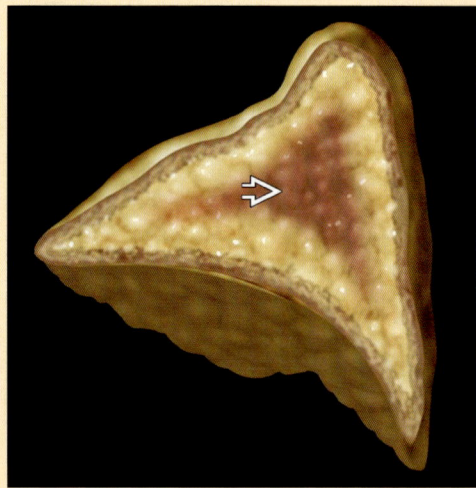

(Left) The adrenal cortex is composed of 3 layers. The zona glomerulosa ➡ lies directly beneath the capsule. The zona fasciculata ➡ forms the middle layer of the cortex. The zona reticularis ➡ forms the innermost layer. (Right) The thin, discontinuous layer of zona glomerulosa cells ➡ lie directly beneath the capsule. The vacuolated cells of the zona fasciculata ➡ are underneath the zona glomerulosa and form the majority of the cortex. The deeply eosinophilic zona reticularis ➡ lies deepest.

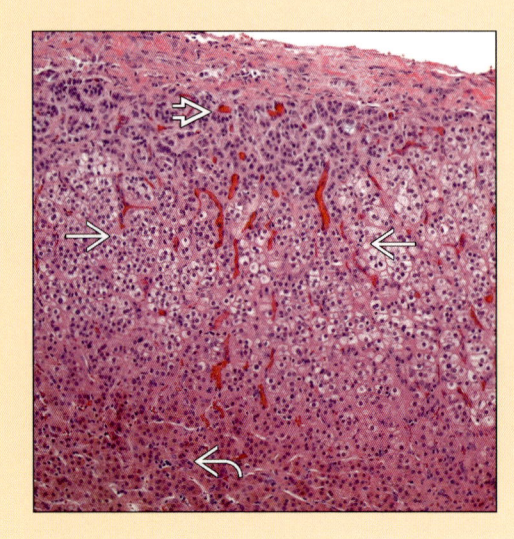

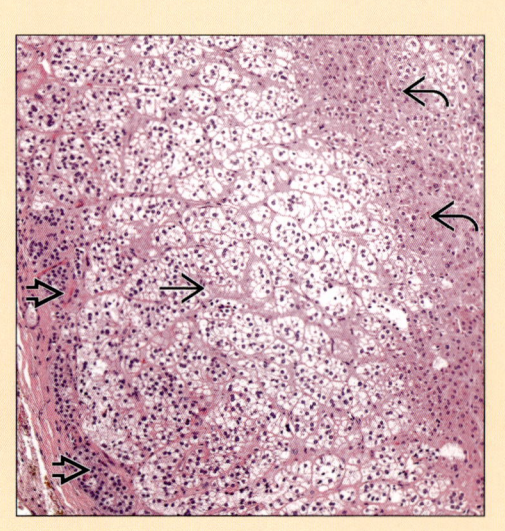

ADRENAL GLAND

Zona Glomerulosa

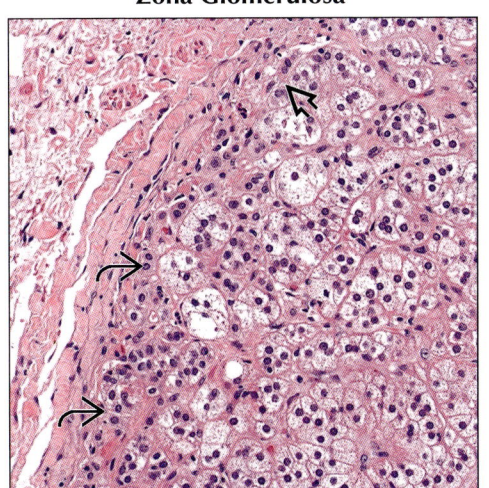

Zona Glomerulosa

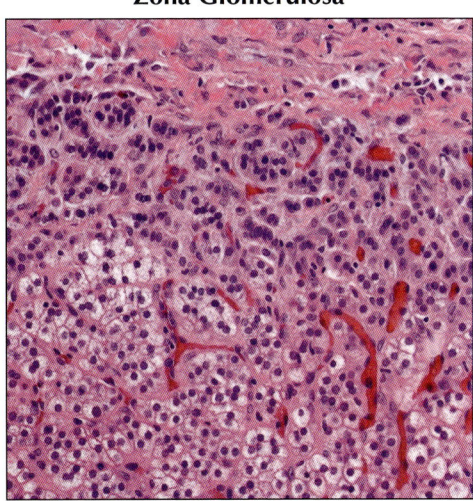

(Left) Zona glomerulosa cells ⇨ are located directly beneath the adrenal capsule. This thin layer of the cortex is discontinuous, and in some areas gaps allow for the cells of the zona fasciculata ⇨ to lie directly against the adrenal capsule. *(Right)* The cells of the zona glomerulosa are arranged in small clusters and balls. They have slightly eosinophilic to amphophilic cytoplasm that is sparse compared to that of the zona fasciculata cells.

Zona Fasciculata

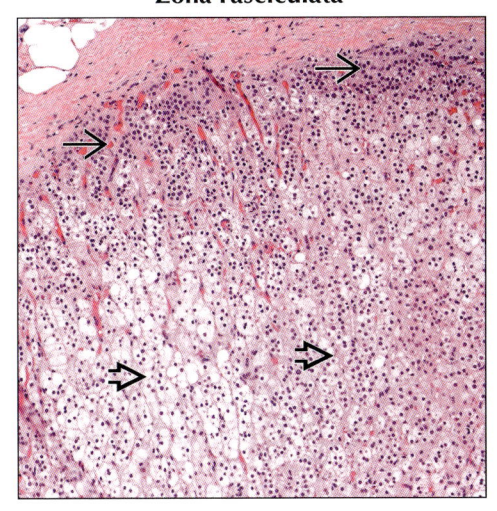

Zona Fasciculata

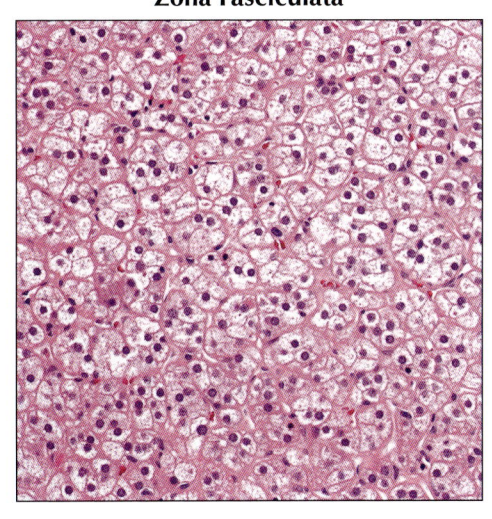

(Left) The zona fasciculata ⇨ lies beneath the zona glomerulosa ⇨ and accounts for the majority of the adrenal cortex. The cells have abundant lipid-laden cytoplasm, which produces the finely vacuolated appearance of the cells microscopically and the bright yellow color of the adrenal cortex macroscopically. *(Right)* This high-power photomicrograph illustrates the abundant, finely vacuolated cytoplasm of the cells of the zona fasciculata.

Zona Reticularis

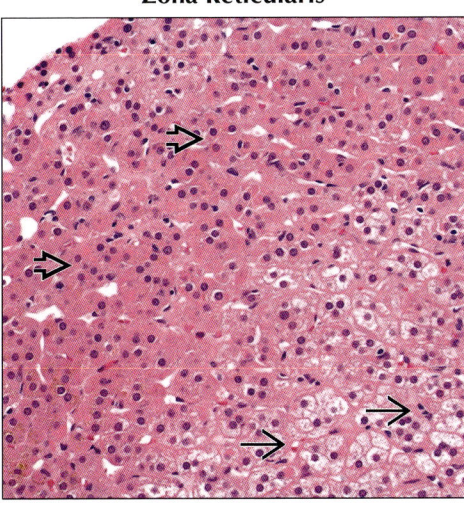

Zona Reticularis

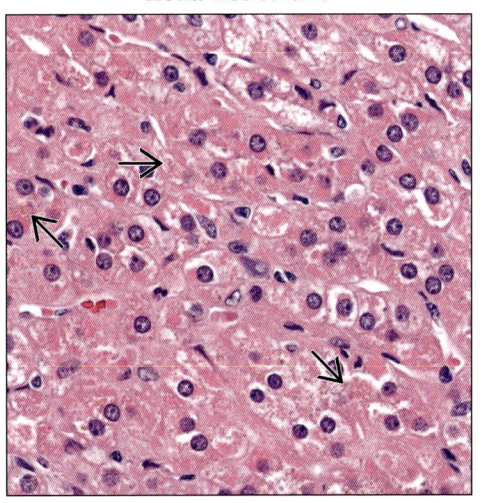

(Left) The zona reticularis ⇨ forms the innermost layer of the adrenal cortex. The cytoplasm is more eosinophilic when compared to the cells of the adjacent zona fasciculata ⇨. *(Right)* The cells of the zona reticularis may occasionally contain intracytoplasmic accumulations of golden brown lipochrome pigment ⇨. This pigment is often most abundant within the deeper cells of the zona reticularis along the corticomedullary junction.

ADRENAL GLAND

Cortical-Medullary Junction

Adrenal Capsule

(Left) The junction of the zona reticularis layer ▷ of the adrenal cortex and the underlying adrenal medulla ➔ is irregular. The cytoplasm of the zona reticularis cells along the junction contain lipochrome pigment ➔. (Right) Collections of adrenal cortical cells ➔ can be identified outside of the adrenal capsule ▷ within the periadrenal fat. These collections of benign cortical cells are normal and should not be confused with a neoplastic process.

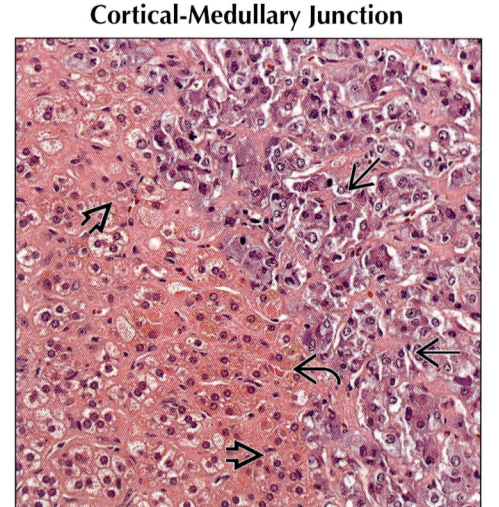

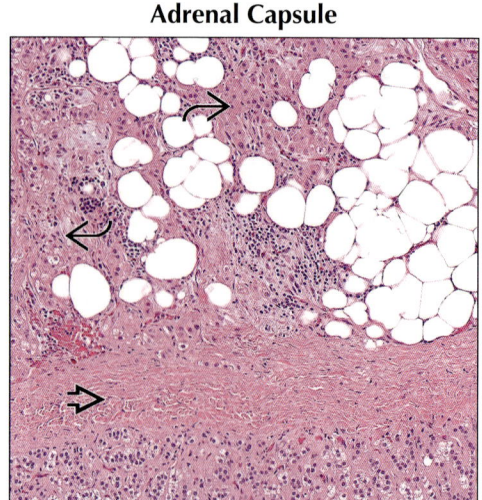

Adrenal Medulla

Adrenal Medulla

(Left) The cells of the adrenal medulla are arranged in nests and are surrounded by fibrovascular septa. The cytoplasm is basophilic to amphophilic, with focal vacuolization. (Right) The cytoplasm of the adrenal medulla cells is basophilic and granular in appearance ▷, in contrast to the lightly eosinophilic and heavily vacuolated cytoplasm of the adrenal cortical cells ➔. The cells of the adrenal medulla are larger than the cells of the adjacent adrenal cortex.

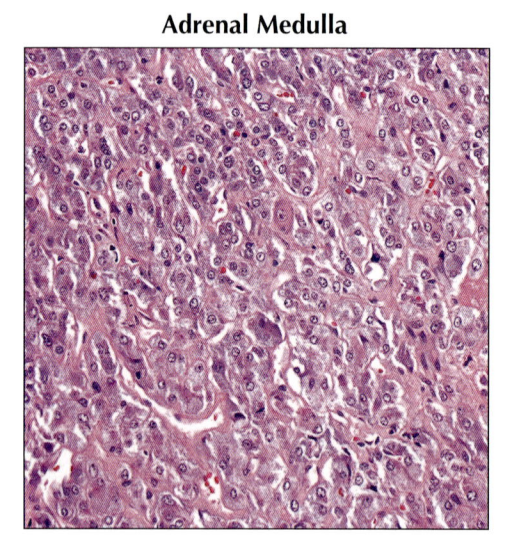

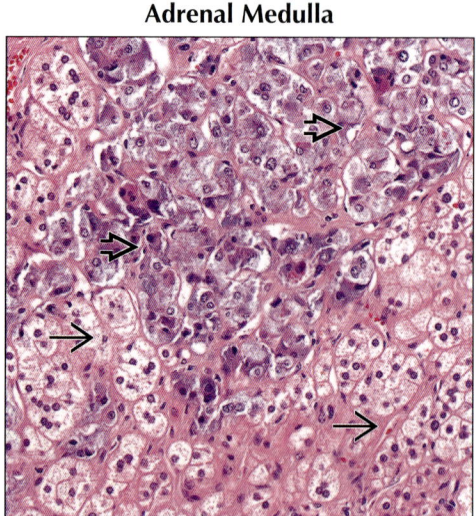

Adrenal Medulla

Adrenal Medulla

(Left) The nuclei of the adrenal medulla cells appear vesicular, with clumped chromatin and peripheral condensation along the nuclear membrane. A central nucleolus may be present, and the nuclei are often eccentrically located. Intracytoplasmic globules ▷ are sometimes identified within the cells and stain with PAS histochemical staining (PAS stain not shown). (Right) Rare ganglion cells ➔ can be seen interspersed among the adrenal medulla cells and can occur either singly or in small clusters.

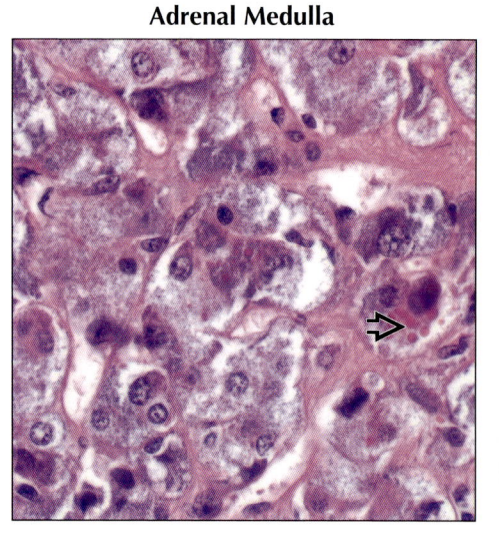

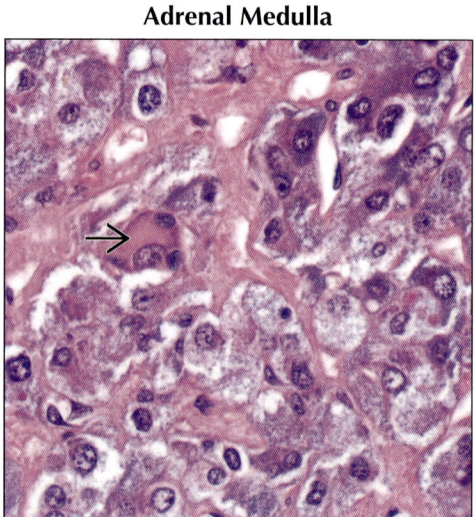

ADRENAL GLAND

Adrenal Medulla

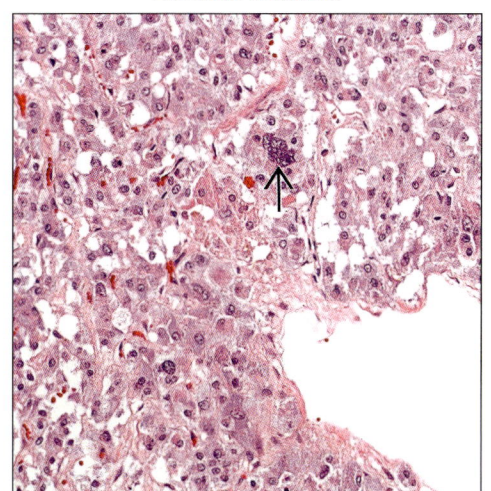

Central Adrenal Vein

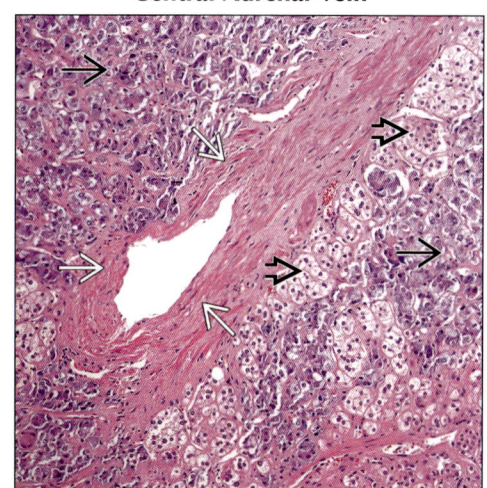

(Left) The cells of the adrenal medulla can appear atypical, with nuclear enlargement and hyperchromasia ⇒. This atypia is normal and does not represent a neoplastic process. *(Right)* The central adrenal vein is centrally located within the medulla ⇒. It has an uneven muscular layer ⇒ surrounding it, which may be completely absent in areas, allowing cells to be separated from the lumen by the intima only. Invaginated cortical cells ⇒ can be seen surrounding the vein.

Adrenal Cortex, 1 Week After Birth

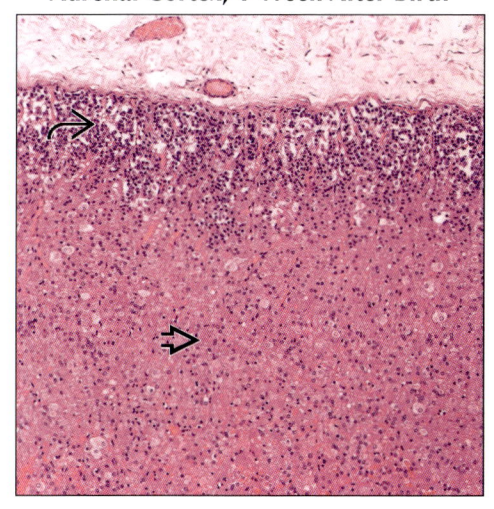

Adrenal Cortex, 1 Week After Birth

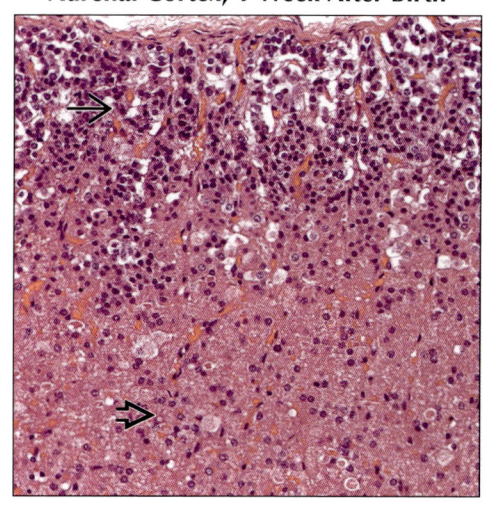

(Left) Directly beneath the adrenal capsule there is a thin band of small, hyperchromatic cells arranged in cords ⇒ that overlies the provisional (or fetal) cortex ⇒. As the provisional cortex involutes, this outer layer will proliferate to become the definitive (or adult) adrenal cortex. *(Right)* The provisional cortex ⇒ is composed of large cells with abundant eosinophilic cytoplasm and vesicular nuclei, as opposed to the smaller, hyperchromatic cells of the definitive cortex ⇒.

Adrenal Cortex, 3 Weeks After Birth

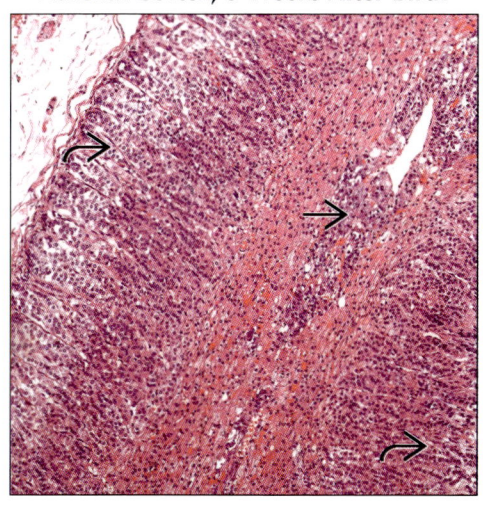

Adrenal Cortex, 3 Weeks After Birth

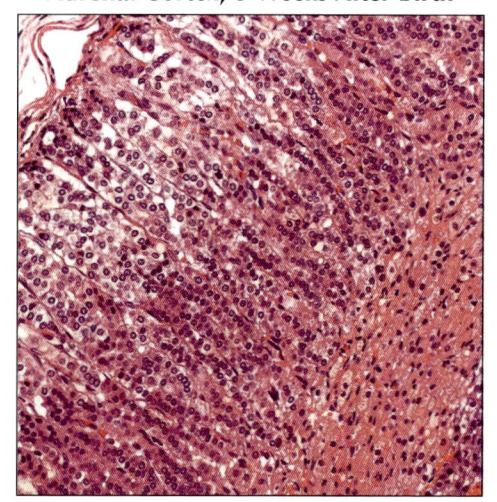

(Left) By 3 weeks after birth, the provisional cortex has largely involuted. The cells in the definitive cortex, which began as a thin subcapsular rim of cells, have now proliferated to form the adult adrenal cortex ⇒. Within the central portion of the gland, the adrenal medulla ⇒ is visible. *(Right)* At 3 weeks after birth, the cells of the definitive adrenal cortex have expanded as the provisional cortex involuted, and now form the cords and nests of the adult cortex.

PARAGANGLIA

Key Facts

Macroscopic Anatomy
- Small, generally microscopic neuroendocrine organs associated with autonomic nervous system
  - Sympathetic paraganglia are located along prevertebral and paravertebral sympathetic chains and in connective tissue surrounding pelvic organs
  - Parasympathetic paraganglia are located along cervical and thoracic branches of glossopharyngeal and vagus nerves

Microscopic Anatomy
- Paraganglia contain 2 cell types
  - Neuroendocrine cells: Small round cells with clear to amphophilic cytoplasm organized into nests (*zellballen*) and cords
  - Supporting (sustentacular) cells: Partially or completely surround neuroendocrine cells and are usually flattened and inconspicuous

Pitfalls/Artifacts
- Paraganglia, particularly when identified in organ resection specimens, may closely mimic nests of carcinoma

Age Variation
- Adrenal medulla and carotid bodies enlarge with age; other paraganglia decrease in size

Hyperplasia
- Hyperplasia of carotid body may occur in some conditions, particularly hypoxic states (e.g., high altitude, pulmonary disorders, or hypertension)

(Left) The sympathetic paraganglia are along the prevertebral and paravertebral sympathetic chains, and include the adrenal medulla ➡ and the organ of Zuckerkandl ➡. They are numerous around pelvic organs such as the bladder ➡. The parasympathetic paraganglia are along the cranial and thoracic branches of the glossopharyngeal and vagus nerves, and include the carotid bodies ➡. *(Right)* The adrenal medulla has a solid architecture with a vaguely nested pattern.

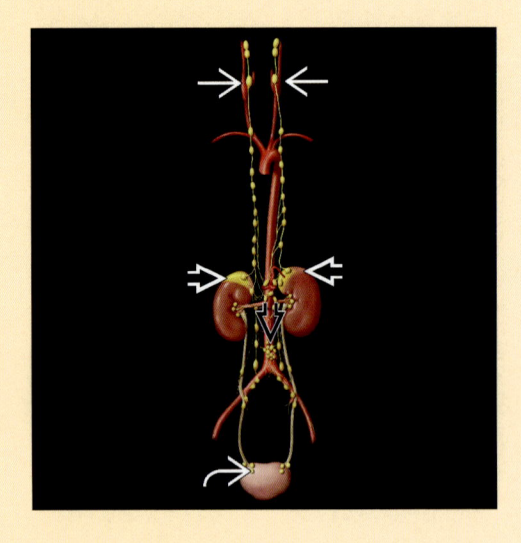

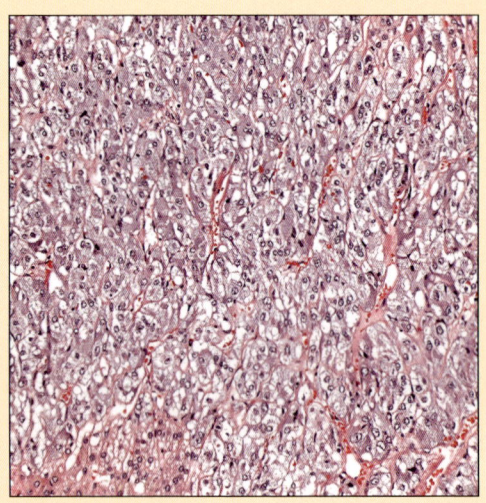

(Left) In adults, extraadrenal paraganglia are less conspicuous, with scattered nests of neuroendocrine cells with clear cytoplasm ➡ separated by fibrous stroma. They are often found adjacent to peripheral nerves and ganglia ➡. *(Right)* On high-power magnification, the paraganglia are characterized by nests of neuroendocrine cells with clear to amphophilic cytoplasm and round, uniform nuclei. The sustentacular cells are generally not identifiable.

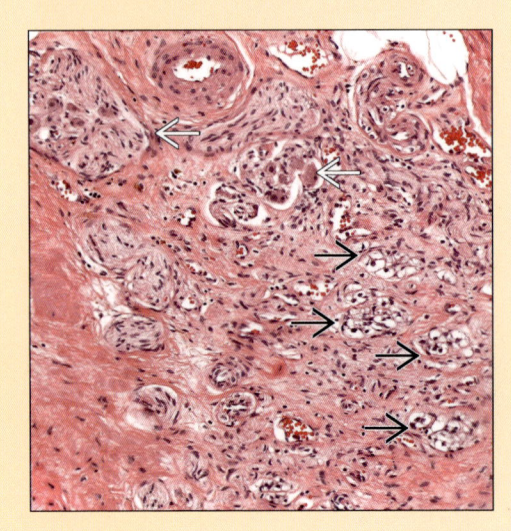

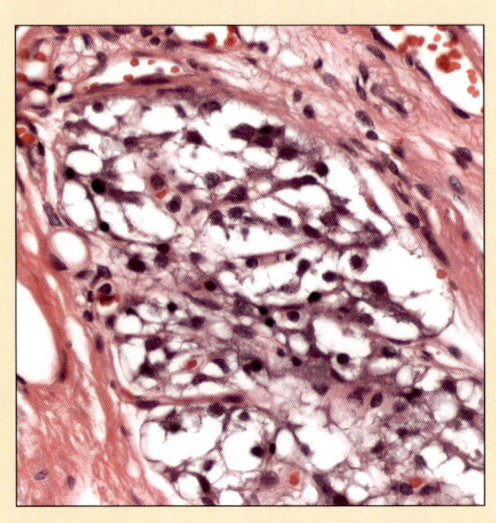

PARAGANGLIA

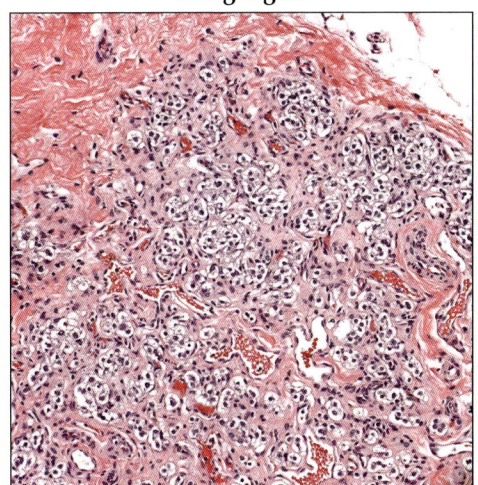

Paraganglia

Paraganglia

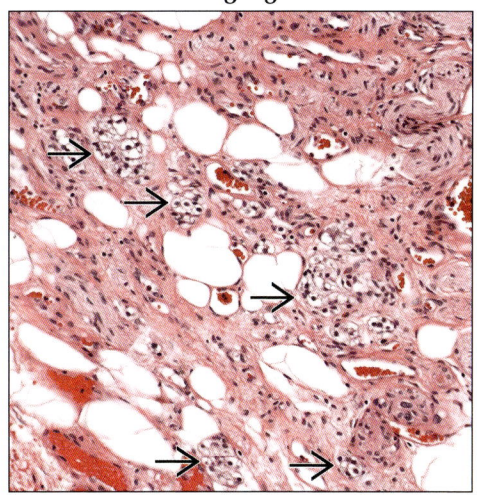

(Left) This example of a paraganglion (carotid body) is more cellular, but is still comprised of tight nests of neuroendocrine cells surrounded by fibrous stroma. *(Right)* Some paraganglia, especially those in connective tissue adjacent to parenchymal organs, are comprised of very few nests ⇒ scattered amongst fibrous tissue, nerves, and fat; therefore, they may be easily overlooked. In resection specimens, these paraganglia may be confused with nests of carcinoma cells.

Paraganglia

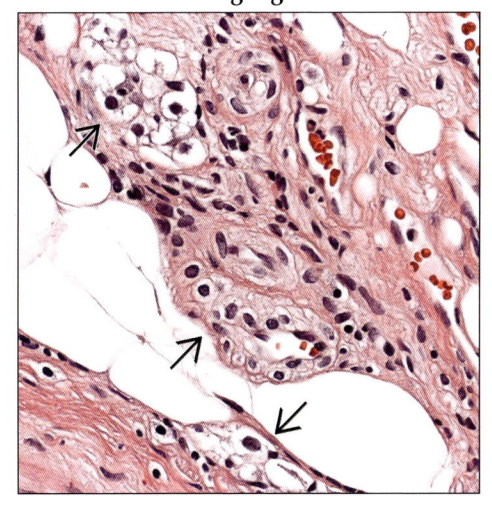

Paraganglia (Chromogranin)

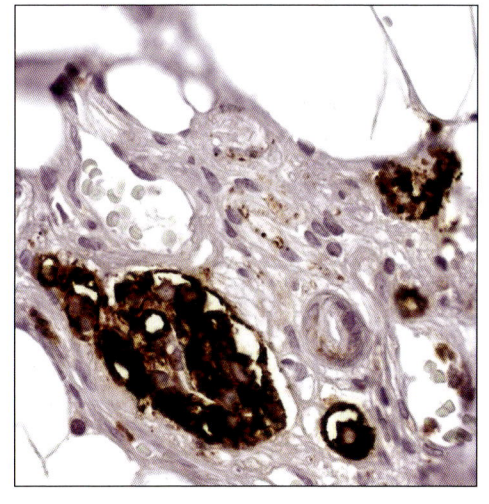

(Left) These typical nests of paraganglionic cells ⇒ show predominantly clear cytoplasm in the neuroendocrine cells with the typical small uniform nuclei. The sustentacular cells are not conspicuous. *(Right)* The nests of paraganglionic cells are highlighted by immunostains for chromogranin, which typically show strong cytoplasmic staining in the neuroendocrine cell component. In contrast to nests of carcinoma cells, the paraganglia are cytokeratin negative.

Paraganglia (Synaptophysin)

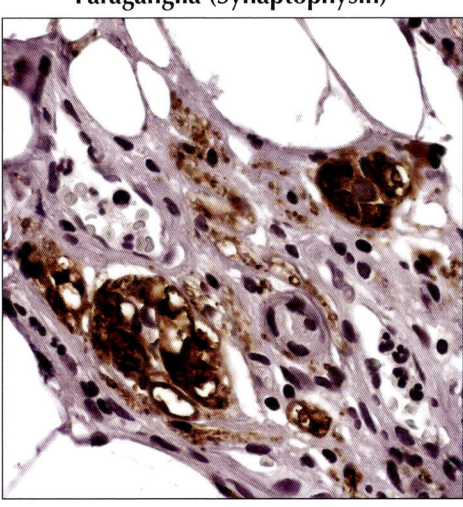

Paraganglia (S100 Protein)

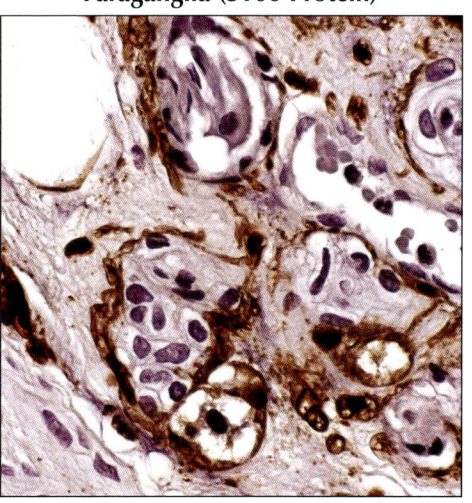

(Left) Synaptophysin immunostains characteristically show diffuse cytoplasmic immunoreactivity in the neuroendocrine cell component. *(Right)* Immunostains for S100 protein typically demonstrate strong cytoplasmic immunoreactivity in the flattened supporting (sustentacular) cells that surround the neuroendocrine cells. These cells are generally inconspicuous on H&E stain, and have also been referred to as "type 2" or "satellite" cells.

THYROID

Key Facts

Macroscopic Anatomy
- H-shaped endocrine organ (15-25 g) composed of 2 lateral lobes (each approximately 5 cm long, 2.5 cm wide, 2 cm deep) connected by a central isthmus
  - Located anterior to upper trachea, just below laryngeal cricoid cartilage
  - Lobes have pointed superior and blunt inferior poles
  - 40% have a pyramidal lobe, which extends cephalad from the isthmus
  - Size varies with stature, age, sex, iodine intake, hormonal status, and gland functional status
- Invested by a delicate fibrous capsule that extends into the gland dividing it into lobules (thyromeres)
- Cut surface is red-brown and firm; nodules seen in 10% of nongoitrous euthyroid individuals
- Paired superior and inferior parathyroid glands are attached to posterior thyroid capsule
- Small lymph nodes can be seen around isthmus, including the pretracheal (Delphian) lymph node
- Embryologically derived from a median anlage and 2 lateral anlagen
- Median anlage derived from 1st and 2nd branchial pouch endoderm at base of primitive pharynx during 4th week
  - Descends into neck, passing anterior to hyoid bone and larynx
  - Remains connected to foramen cecum by thyroglossal duct, which subsequently involutes
  - Failure of duct to involute can result in thyroglossal duct cysts
- Lateral anlagen (ultimobranchial bodies) derive from 4th and 5th branchial pouches during 7th week and provide the parafollicular C cells
  - Ultimobranchial bodies provide C cells, which disperse throughout mid to upper 1/3 of the lateral thyroid lobes
  - Ultimobranchial body remnants, so-called solid cell nests, can be seen in lateral lobes of most thyroids

Microscopic Anatomy
- Functional unit of thyroid gland is the follicle
- Follicles are spherical cyst-like structures of variable size (0.2-1 mm on average) and shape
  - Follicles surrounded by an extensive capillary network
- Lined by a monolayer of flat to columnar follicular epithelial cells (thyrocytes)
  - Cell size varies by functional status of follicle; flat cells are inactive, cuboidal cells secrete colloid, and columnar cells resorb colloid
- Colloid is an eosinophilic to basophilic secretion composed mostly of thyroglobulin
  - Thyroglobulin is an iodinated glycoprotein and serves as an inactive storage form of active thyroid hormones T3 and T4
  - Resorption vacuoles are present in follicles resorbing colloid
  - Calcium oxalate crystals are often present in colloid
- Sanderson polsters are small aggregates of follicles at 1 end of a follicle that may have a papillary or undulating appearance
  - Seen in normal thyroids but increased in hyperplastic conditions
- So-called palpation thyroiditis is common; represents disrupted follicles replaced by macrophages, chronic inflammatory cells
- Focal areas of stromal adipose tissue can be seen in normal thyroids
- Intrathyroidal skeletal muscle, cartilage, parathyroid glands, thymic tissue are occasionally present
- Parafollicular C cells account for a small proportion of thyroid mass; difficult to see in normal thyroids
  - Restricted to mid and superior lateral lobes
  - Located between follicular cells and basement membrane
  - Cuboidal cells with pale cytoplasm with coarse nuclear chromatin; secrete calcitonin
- Solid cell nests are small (0.1-2 mm) multilobed clusters of oval basaloid cells interspersed among follicles; small numbers of C cells present
  - Restricted to mid and superior lateral lobes
  - Squamous metaplasia and cystic change not uncommon

(Left) As the median thyroid anlage descends into the neck, it is attached to its origin at the foramen cecum ➡ by the thyroglossal duct ➡. Failure to involute can result in thyroglossal duct cyst. (Right) Normal thyroid gland is composed of 2 lateral lobes connected by a central isthmus ➡ and invested by a thin fibrous capsule with numerous small surface vessels. 40% of thyroid glands will have a pyramidal lobe ➡.

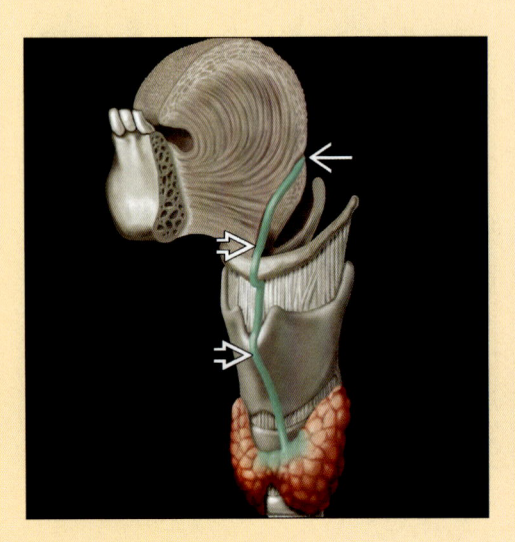

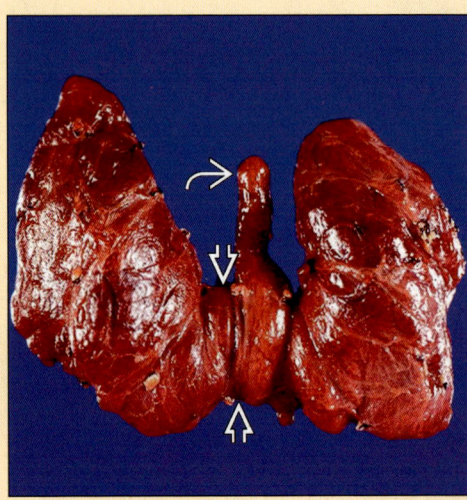

THYROID

Capsule and Extracapsular Thyroid Tissue

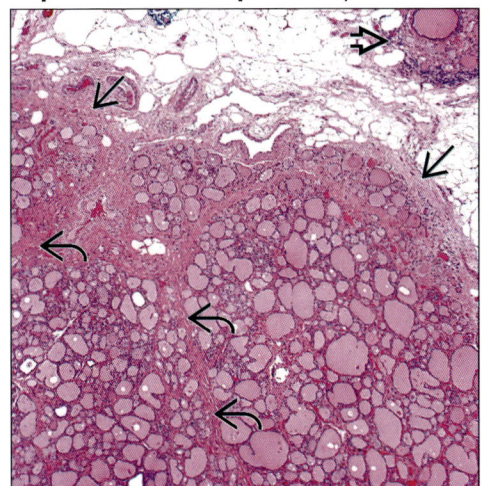

Incidental Nodules

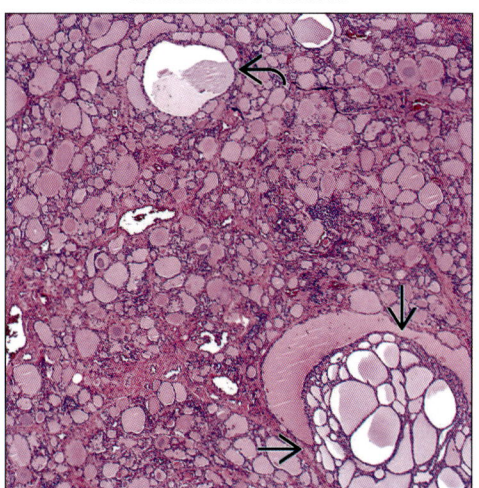

(Left) The thyroid gland is covered by a delicate fibrous capsule ➡ that extends into the parenchyma ➡, dividing the gland into vague lobules (thyromeres). Small nodules of otherwise unremarkable thyroid tissue are often present outside of the capsule proper ➡. *(Right)* Incidental nodules can be seen macroscopically in about 10% of nongoitrous thyroid glands. Microscopic nodules ➡ and colloid cysts ➡ are also frequently seen in nongoitrous and euthyroid individuals.

Follicular Epithelial Cells

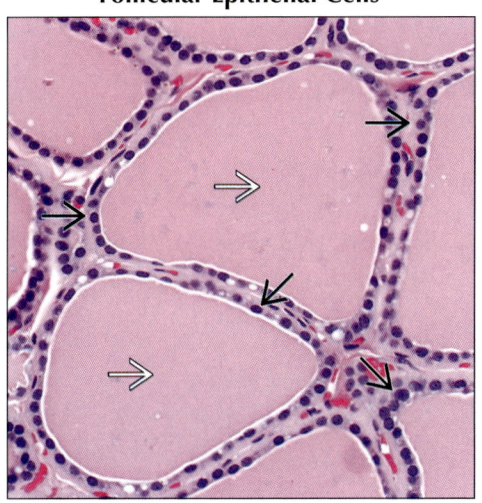

Thyroid Hormone Synthesis

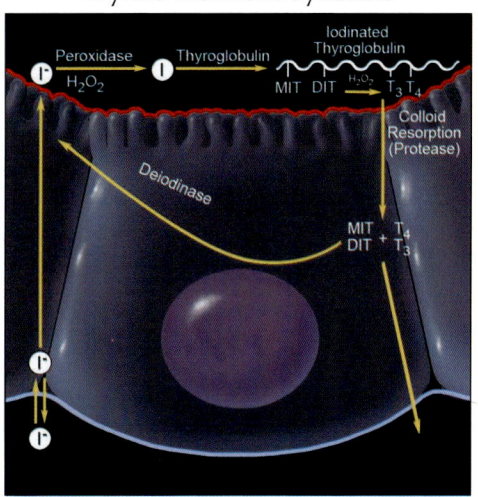

(Left) Follicles are lined by a monolayer of follicular cells surrounding a mass of colloid ➡. Cuboidal follicular cells ➡ synthesize colloid. Flat follicular cells are inactive. *(Right)* Colloid consists mostly of thyroglobulin, an iodinated glycoprotein that serves as the storage form of the active thyroid hormones T3 and T4. In response to pituitary TSH, follicular cells resorb thyroglobulin and convert it to T3 and T4, which are released into the perifollicular capillaries.

Resorption Vacuoles

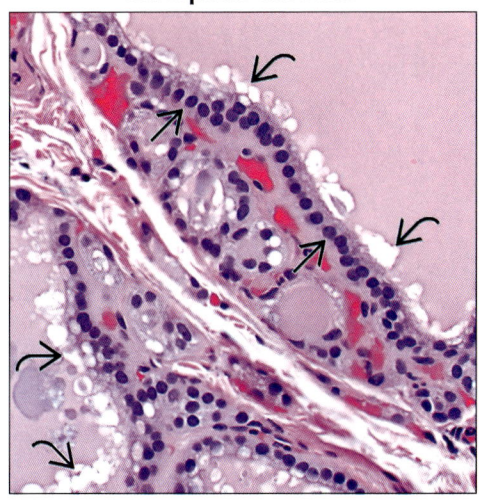

Sanderson Polster

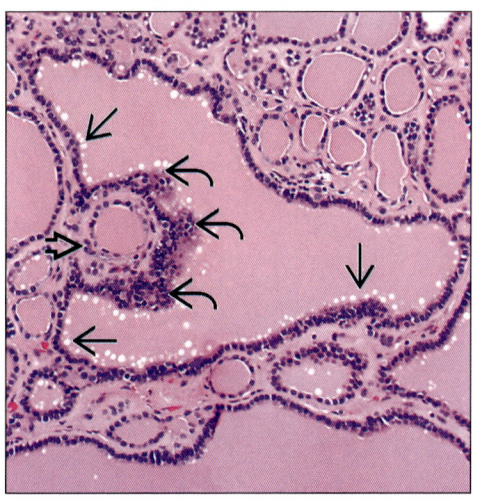

(Left) Follicles actively resorbing colloid are usually lined by more columnar follicular epithelial cells ➡ and demonstrate resorption vacuoles. These appear as a row of small vacuoles at the colloid and epithelial cell interface ➡. *(Right)* Sanderson polsters ➡ are intraluminal collections of follicles at 1 end of a larger follicle and often have an undulating or papillary ➡ appearance. They are more common in active follicles, as evidenced by the resorption vacuoles ➡.

THYROID

Colloid Calcium Oxalate Crystals

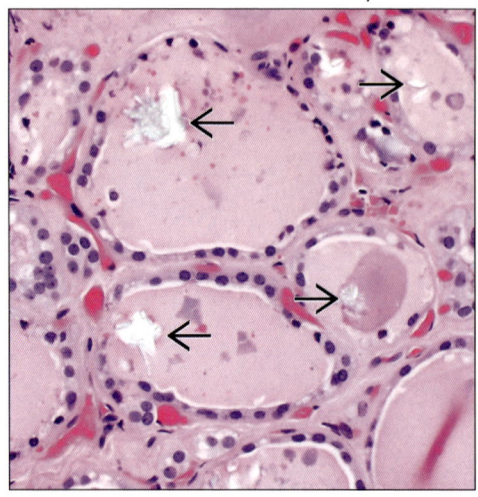

Calcium Oxalate Crystals, Polarized Light

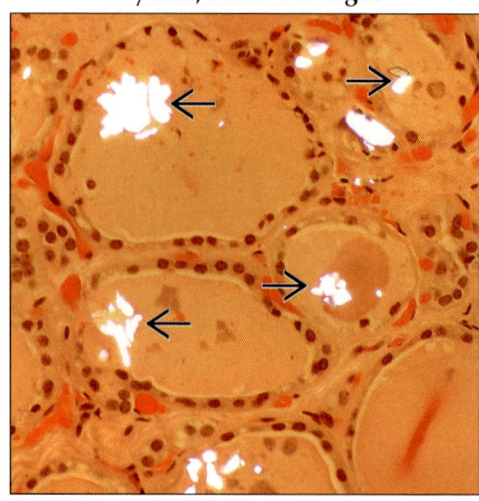

(Left) Irregular, rhomboidal, anisotropic calcium oxalate crystals ➡ can be seen within the colloid of most (~ 85% in autopsy studies) thyroid glands. They can be present in normal follicles but are more frequent with age, in renal failure patients on dialysis, and in inactive follicles. They are uncommon in cases of chronic thyroiditis. *(Right)* Although calcium oxalate crystals can be easily identified using routine light microscopy, they are more readily identified using polarized light ➡.

Palpation Thyroiditis

Intrathyroidal Parathyroid Tissue

(Left) Ruptured follicles incite a granulomatous reaction referred to as palpation thyroiditis. These are seen in most resected thyroids and are characterized by macrophages and lymphocytes ➡ replacing the damaged follicle to varying degrees. Although most cells are mononuclear macrophages, multinucleated cells can be seen as well. *(Right)* Intracapsular &/or intrathyroidal parathyroid tissue ➡ or glands are not uncommonly seen in otherwise normal thyroid glands.

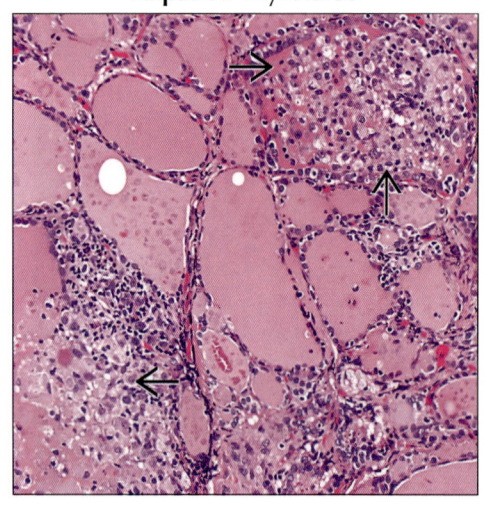

Stromal Adipose Tissue

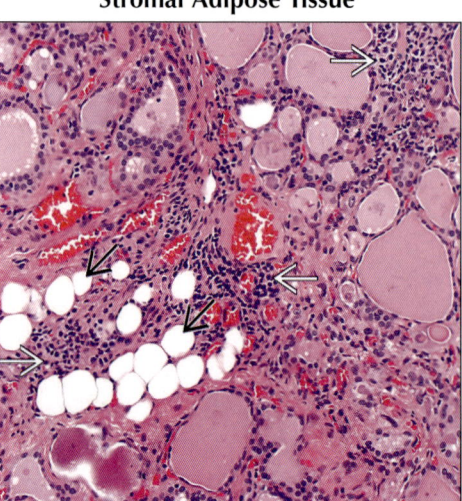

Intrathyroidal Skeletal Muscle

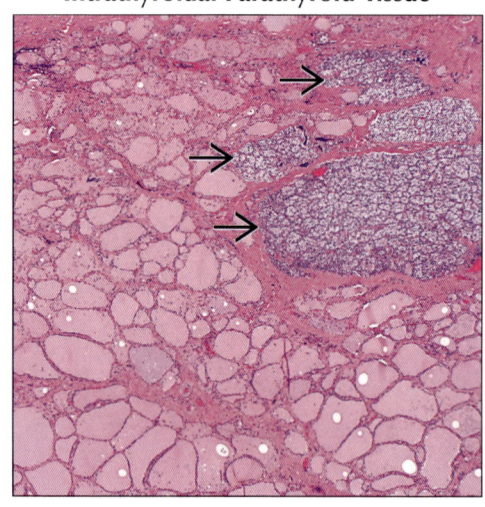

(Left) Thyroid glands generally have very little stroma. Small foci of mature adipose tissue can be seen between follicles in most thyroid glands. Often it is in or near the capsule, but fat can also be present deep in the gland parenchyma ➡. Small collections of chronic inflammatory cells ➡ can be seen in many normal thyroid glands as well. *(Right)* Intrathyroidal ➡ skeletal muscle ➡ is common in the isthmus region. Follicles can also be seen in extrathyroidal skeletal muscle.

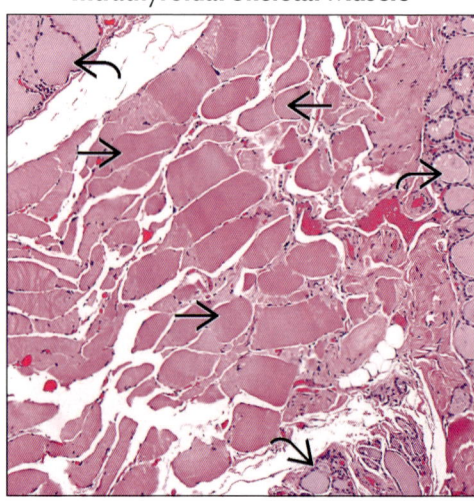

THYROID

Heterotopic Cartilage

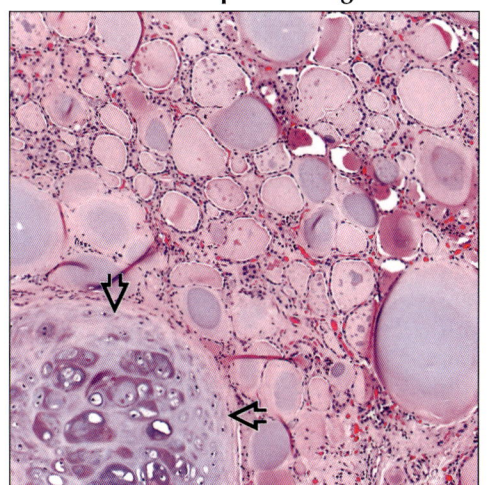

Solid Cell Nest

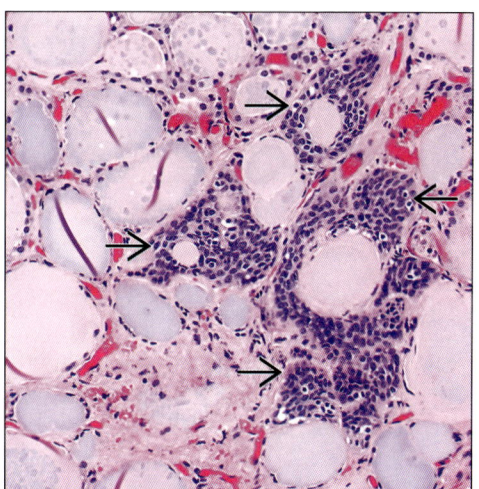

(Left) Intrathyroidal islands of heterotopic mature hyaline cartilage ⇨, presumably of branchial pouch derivation, can be seen in the stroma in about 10% of thyroid glands. *(Right)* Solid cell nests ⇨ are common in thyroid glands and can be found in the mid and upper 1/3 of the lateral lobes, consistent with an ultimobranchial body derivation. They are small multilobed structures composed of uniform basaloid cells. Focal squamous differentiation and cystic change are often seen.

Solid Cell Nest

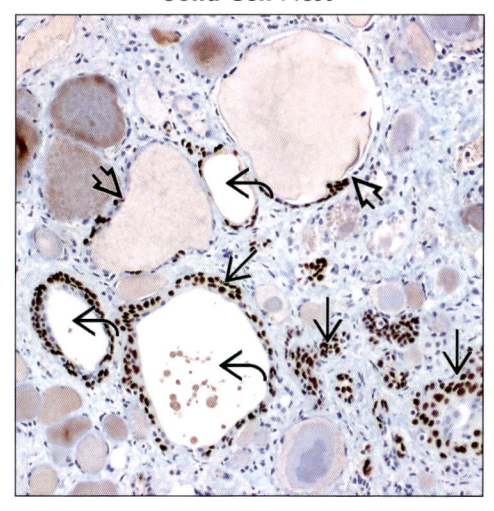

Solid Cell Nest

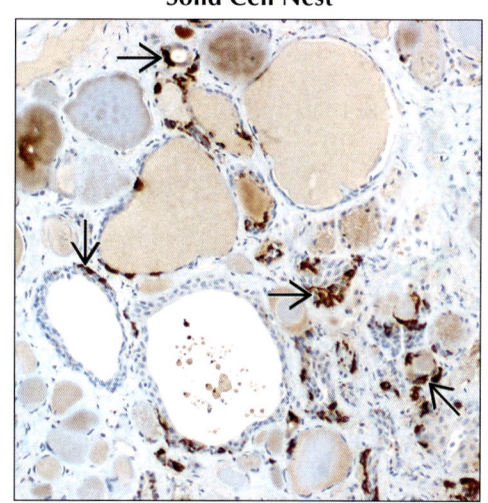

(Left) The basaloid cells are thought to be basal or stem cells. This is supported by strong nuclear reactivity for p63 ⇨, a marker of basal/stem cells in stratified epithelia. Note the cystic areas ⇨ and mixed follicles ⇨ in this solid cell nest. The cystic areas can enlarge, resulting in clinically significant cysts. *(Right)* Some solid cell nests contain a small component of calcitonin-positive C cells ⇨, supporting the embryologic link of C cells and solid cell nests.

C-Cell Cluster

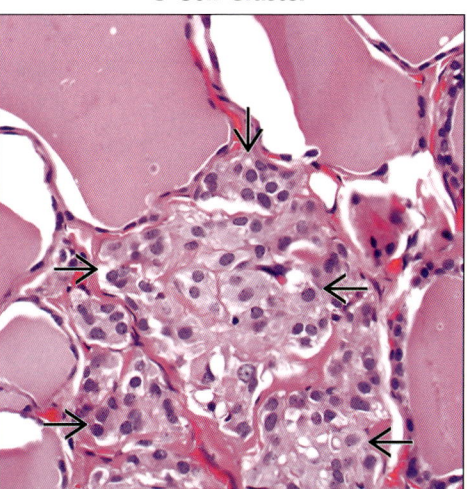

C-Cell Cluster

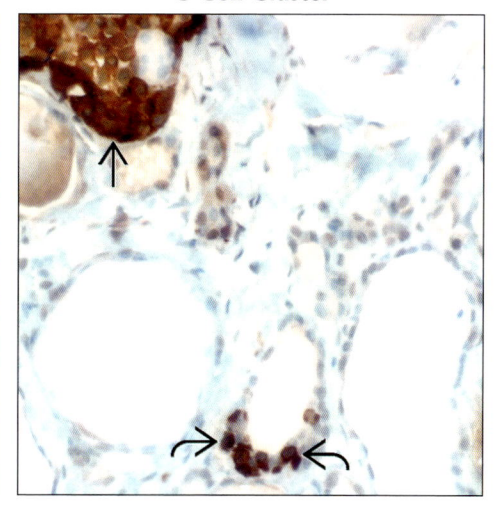

(Left) C cells are normally present in the mid and upper 1/3 of the lateral lobes. They are difficult to identify on routine H&E stains under normal conditions. They are easily identified under hyperplastic conditions such as this C-cell nodule ⇨ from a MEN2 patient. The cells are larger than follicular cells and have abundant pale eosinophilic cytoplasm. *(Right)* Calcitonin stains can be used to identify C cells, such as those in this cluster ⇨ and an adjacent follicle ⇨.

PARATHYROID

Key Facts

Macroscopic Anatomy
- Most people (90-95%) have 4 parathyroid glands: Paired superior and inferior glands
  - Number varies from 2-12, including supernumerary and ectopic glands
  - Intrathyroidal (3%) and intrathymic (10%) are common ectopic locations
- Small (4-6 mm long, 3-4 mm wide, 1-2 mm thick), yellow-tan, lentiform glands typically abutting posterior thyroid capsule
  - Each gland weighs ~ 30-40 mg but can weigh up to 80 mg; inferior glands slightly larger
  - Covered by delicate fibrous capsule with small surface vessels
- Location variable, but most (75%) superior glands lie posterior to mid-superior thyroid poles; inferior gland locations more variable, but most (50%) lie lateral to lower thyroid poles
- Embryologically, paired superior glands originate from the more caudal 4th branchial pouches (endoderm), along with lateral thyroid lobes and parafollicular C cells
- Paired inferior glands originate from the more cephalad 3rd branchial pouches along with thymus gland
  - Longer descent and co-migration with thymus explain the more variable location and incidence of intrathymic inferior parathyroid glands

Microscopic Anatomy
- Thinly encapsulated with fibrous septae extending into parenchyma dividing gland into vague lobules
- Stroma comprised of mature adipocytes and fibroconnective tissue with rich vascular supply
  - Amount of adipose increases with age; although variable, most adult parathyroid glands contain 20-40% stromal adipose
  - Adipose to parenchymal cell ratio used to roughly correlate functional status; hyperfunctioning glands have less stromal adipose
  - Proportion of adipose variably distributed throughout glands and not uniform or predictable
- Chief cells: Parenchymal cells that synthesize and secrete parathyroid hormone
  - Small (6-8 μm) polygonal cells with pale amphophilic, finely vacuolated cytoplasm and round central nuclei with coarse chromatin and small nucleoli
  - Arranged in small nests and thin cords and separated by stromal adipose tissue
  - Cells are intimately associated with delicate capillary network
  - Some areas with acinar or follicular differentiation containing eosinophilic secretions can be seen
  - Chief cells are positive for cytokeratin, chromogranin A, and parathyroid hormone; hyperfunctioning glands tend to have reduced chromogranin A and parathyroid hormone staining due to degranulation
  - Contain glycogen and intracellular lipid; fat stains (e.g., oil red O) can be used to roughly assess gland function as hyperfunctioning glands have reduced intracytoplasmic lipid
- Oxyphil (oncocytic cells)
  - Larger (12-20 μm) chief cells that are fewer in number and have abundant, granular eosinophilic cytoplasm; typically arranged in small nodules
  - Number increases with age, similar to oncocytic change in some other organs (i.e., salivary gland)
  - Ultrastructurally, contain numerous irregular mitochondria similar to other oncocytes
- Clear cells are less common and represent chief cells with abundant cytoplasmic glycogen
- Unencapsulated parathyroid tissue can be seen in soft tissue adjacent to parathyroid glands as well as in skeletal muscle, thyroid gland, and thymus
- Intrathyroidal, intrathymic, and other ectopic areas can be sites of otherwise normal parathyroid glands
- Canals of Kürsteiner may be seen adjacent to some parathyroid glands and likely represent source for many parathyroid cysts

Pitfalls/Artifacts
- Parathyroid with follicular change can mimic thyroid

(Left) Most people (90-95%) have 4 parathyroid glands consisting of paired superior ⇒ and inferior glands ⇒. Most lie posterior to the thyroid gland poles but can also be found in several variant locations. *(Right)* Superior parathyroids arise from the 4th branchial pouch ⇒ along with the primordial lateral thyroids. Inferior parathyroids arise from the 3rd branchial pouch ⇒ along with the thymus ⇒.

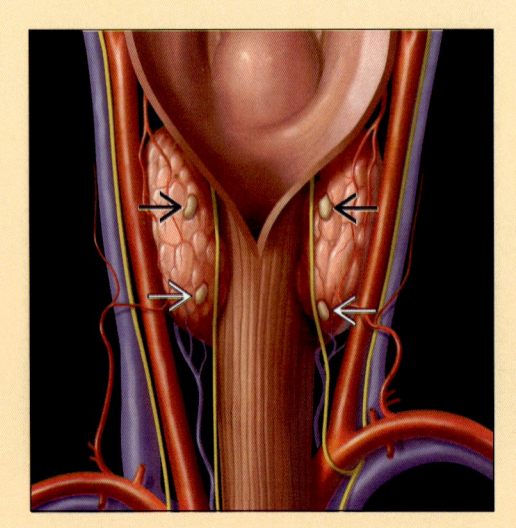

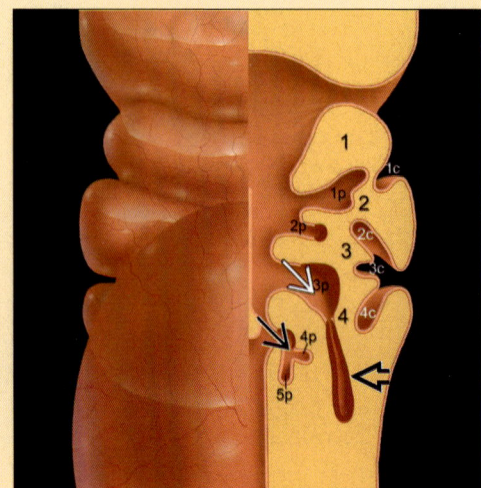

PARATHYROID

Stromal Adipose Tissue

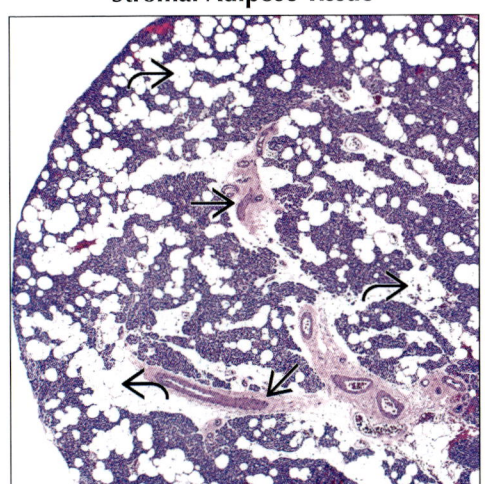

Stromal Adipose Tissue

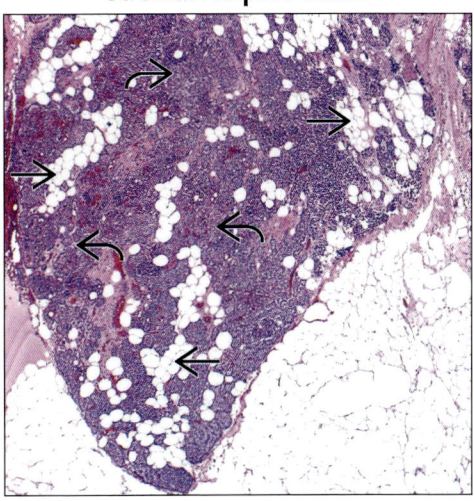

(Left) Stromal adipose increases with age and is sparse in children. Although variable, most normal adult parathyroid glands contain around 40% stromal adipose tissue ➔. Note the vascular pole region containing large arteries and veins extending into septae ➔. *(Right)* This normal parathyroid gland from a euparathyroid individual demonstrates less stromal adipose tissue (~ 20%) ➔, illustrating the marked variation in chief cell cellularity ➔ seen in normal parathyroid glands.

Capsule

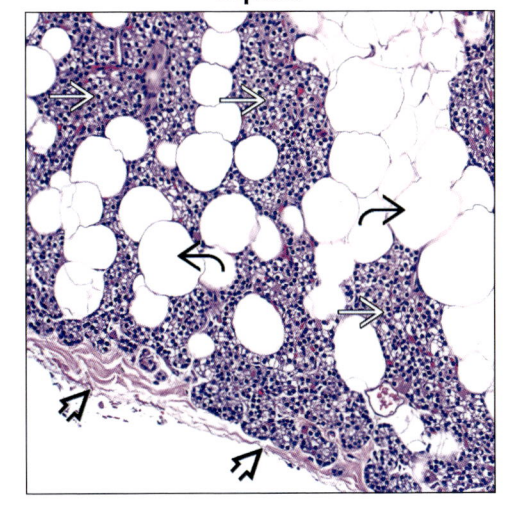

Lobules

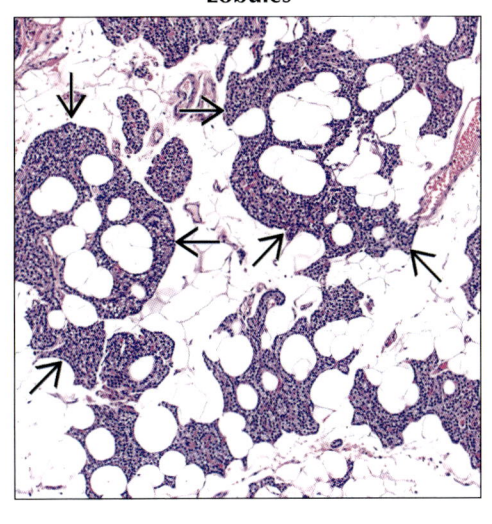

(Left) A delicate fibrous capsule ➔ containing many small intracapsular vessels surrounds normal parathyroid glands. These surface vessels communicate with the vessels in the trabeculae, which receive blood from the hilar (vascular pole) vessels. The chief cells are arranged in nests and cords ➔ and are separated by mature stromal adipocytes ➔. *(Right)* Although well-developed septae are uncommon, the vague lobularity ➔ of the parathyroid can be appreciated at low-power magnification.

Vascular Stroma

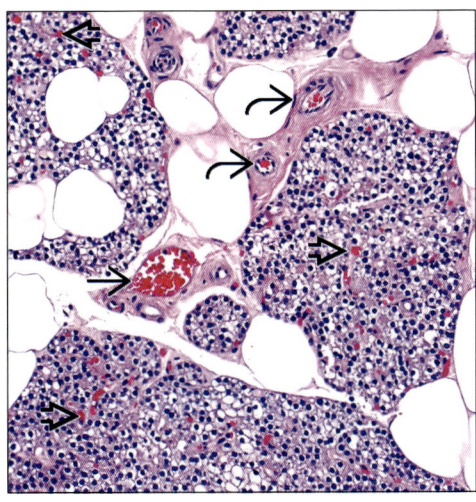

Chief Cells

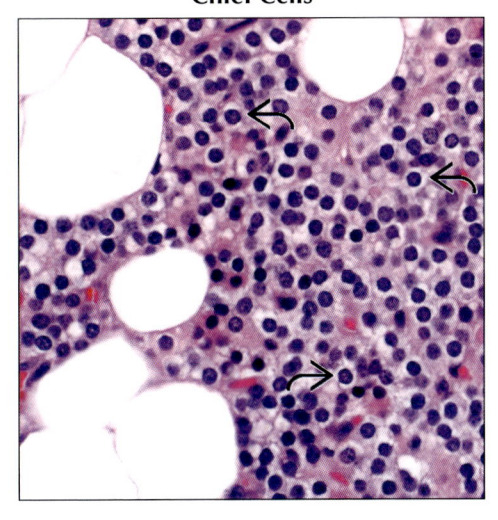

(Left) The fibrous septae contain the vascular supply, including small arterioles ➔ and venules ➔. Numerous small capillaries ➔ surround the chief cells within the lobules. *(Right)* Chief cells ➔ are uniform small cells with pale amphophilic to clear vacuolated cytoplasm. The nuclei are round and small with coarse chromatin and inconspicuous nucleoli. These are the functional cells of the parathyroid, which synthesize and secrete parathyroid hormone in response to hypocalcemia.

PARATHYROID

Parathyroid Hormone

(Left) Calcium metabolism is controlled by a feedback mechanism involving several tissues. Parathyroid hormone (PTH) secretion is stimulated by hypocalcemia and acts to increase serum calcium by resorbing bone and increasing kidney reabsorption and intestinal absorption. PTH also stimulates production of active 1,25(OH)₂ vitamin D3. (Right) Unencapsulated ectopic parathyroid tissue ➔ is commonly seen in tissues adjacent to parathyroid glands, such as this small focus within mature adipose tissue.

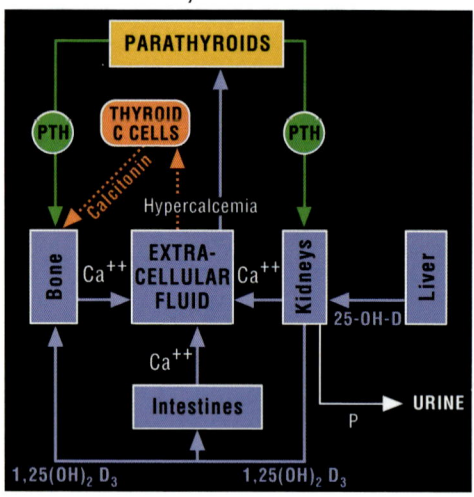

Ectopic Parathyroid Tissue

Intrathymic Parathyroid Gland

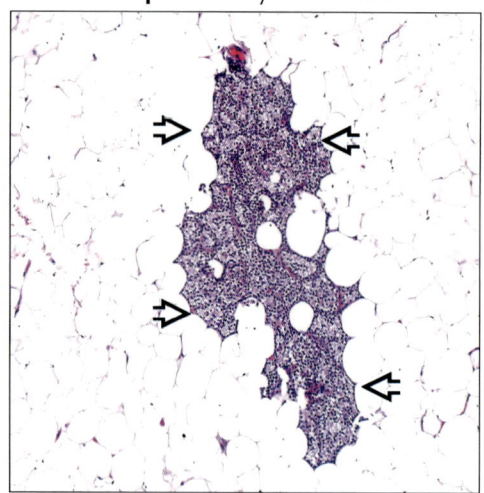

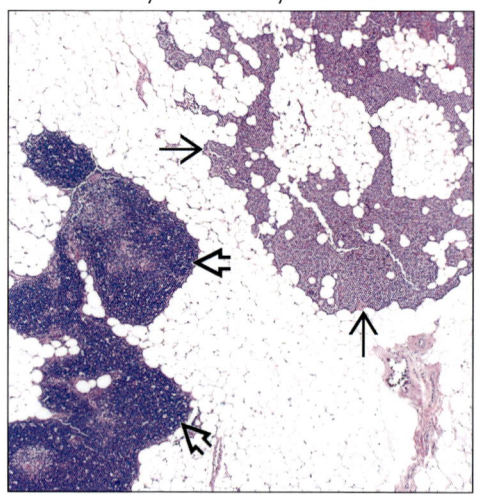

(Left) Ectopic &/or supernumerary inferior parathyroid glands ➔ can be located in the mediastinal thymus ➔ or in cervical thymic extensions. They can also be found higher up in the neck and pericardium. (Right) Oxyphil cells are altered chief cells with abundant, granular, eosinophilic cytoplasm. They have less secretory activity and can be isolated or form small nodules such as this focus ➔. Smaller transitional cells ➔ with eosinophilic cytoplasm can be seen as well.

Oxyphil (Oncocytic) Cells

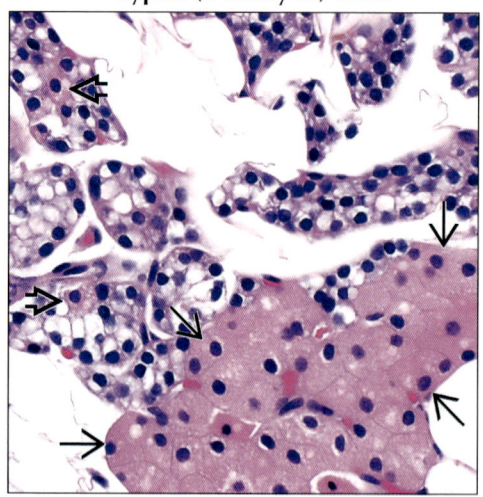

Clear Cells

(Left) Clear cells ➔ are the least common cell type seen in adult parathyroid glands. They also represent altered chief cells, but their cytoplasm is clear due to accumulation of cytoplasmic glycogen. (Right) Although uncommon, follicular ➔ (or acinar) change can be seen in both normal and hyperfunctioning glands. This is characterized by chief cells lining a lumen typically filled with dense eosinophilic secretion ➔. When extensive, this can mimic thyroid gland tissue.

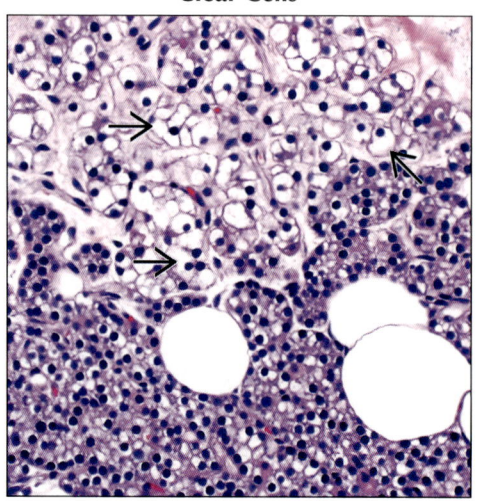

Follicular Change

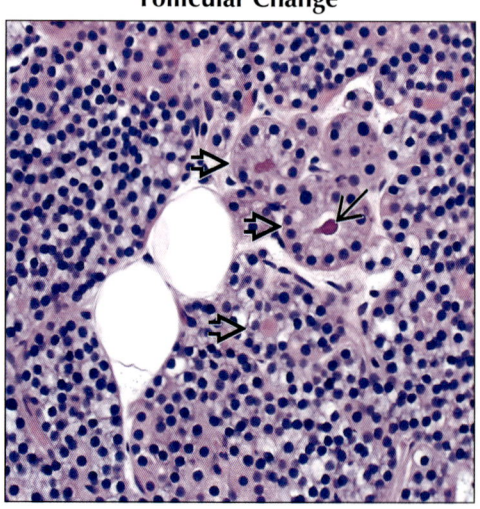

PARATHYROID

Parathyroid Hormone

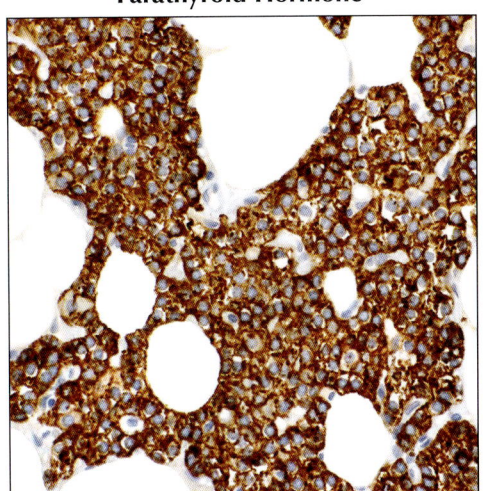

Chromogranin

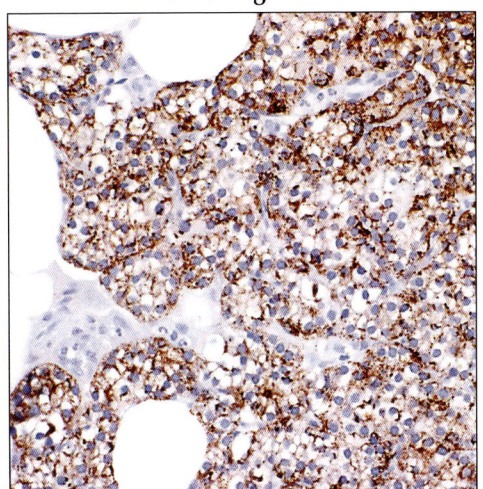

(Left) Chief cells demonstrate strong granular staining for parathyroid hormone (PTH). The granular staining pattern is a result of the PTH protein being stored in cytoplasmic neurosecretory granules. Reduced intensity of PTH staining is seen in hyperfunctioning glands due to neurosecretory degranulation. *(Right)* Although not specific, chromogranin is also positive in chief cells with a granular pattern similar to that of PTH. Chromogranin is colocalized with PTH in the neurosecretory granules.

Intracellular Lipid

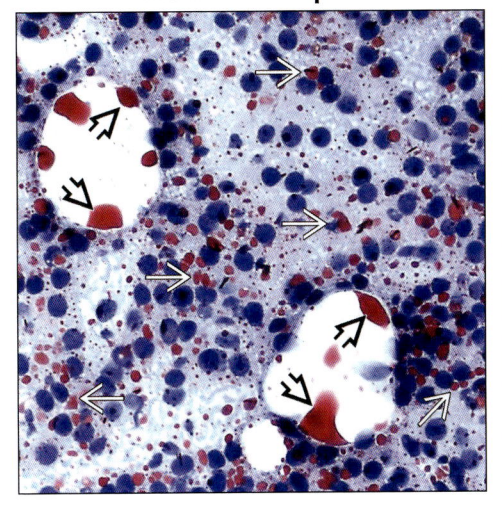

Parathyroid Microcyst

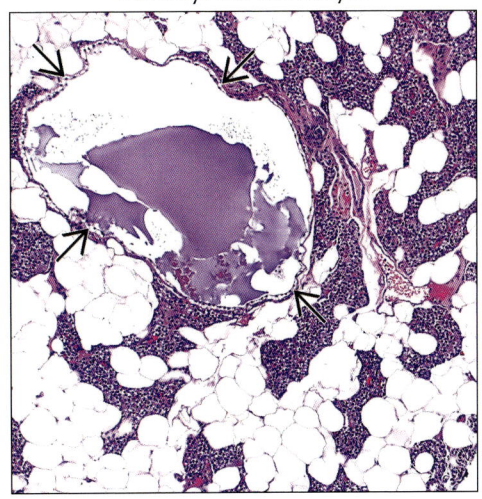

(Left) Chief cells contain intracytoplasmic lipid droplets ➡, which can be highlighted by using fat stains on frozen sections, such as this oil red O stain. The amount of cytoplasmic lipid is roughly inversely proportional to secretory activity and is decreased in hyperparathyroid conditions. Note the mature fat cells with lipid droplets ➡. *(Right)* Not uncommonly, small cysts ➡ lined by clear cuboidal cells can be seen within or adjacent to normal or abnormal parathyroid glands.

Canals of Kürsteiner

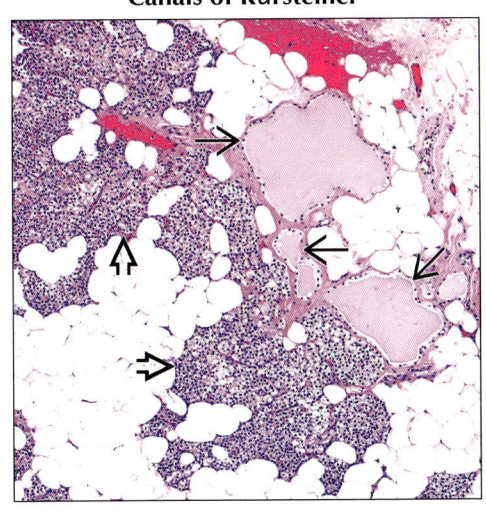

Canals of Kürsteiner

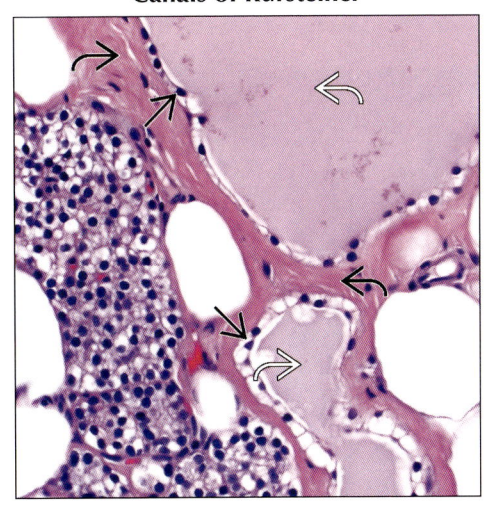

(Left) Canals of Kürsteiner ➡ are occasionally found adjacent to otherwise normal parathyroid glands ➡. These likely represent rudimentary glandular structures derived from branchial endoderm. They account for incidental microcysts as well as most clinically evident parathyroid cysts. *(Right)* The canals are surrounded by sclerotic stroma ➡ and have lumina filled with eosinophilic secretions ➡. They are lined by low cuboidal cells with clear cytoplasm ➡, and they are PTH negative.

PINEAL GLAND

Key Facts

Macroscopic Anatomy
- Small, unpaired endocrine organ providing circadian and seasonal biorhythm control
- Midline location (quadrigeminal cistern) within loose connective tissue of velum interpositum
  - Stalk attached to diencephalon, posterior wall of 3rd ventricle
- Primary vascular supply is medial posterior choroidal artery (lacks blood-brain barrier)

Microscopic Anatomy
- Regular lobules of cellular cords/follicles, separated by connective tissue septa (leptomeninges)
- Pinealocytes-epithelioid cells arranged in pineocytic rosettes
  - Large lobated nuclei, sharply defined nucleoli
  - Photosensory and neuroendocrine derivation
- Interstitium/stroma
  - Loose neuroglial stroma between cords of pinealocytes, in perivascular areas
  - Astrocytes have elongated nuclei and long, GFAP-positive cytoplasmic processes
  - Investing leptomeninges (vellum interpositum)
- Corpora arenacea, or calcium and phosphate salt concretions

Pitfalls/Artifacts
- Cellularity and gland-like histology may mimic epithelioid neoplasm
- Difficult to cytologically distinguish normal from well-differentiated pineocytoma

Age Variation
- Gland enlarges until 1-2 years of age
- Gliosis, cystic change, increasing corpora arenacea occur with age

(Left) Graphic of a horizontal section through the pineal region viewed from above, corpus callosum removed, shows the pineal gland ⇨, superior colliculus ⇨, inferior colliculus ⇨, 3rd ventricle ⇨, internal cerebral veins ⇨, and vein of Galen ⇨. *(Right)* Pinealocytes are arranged in vague pineocytic rosettes ⇨. These rosettes phenotypically correspond to the histologic derivation of pinealocytes from photosensory and neuroendocrine origins.

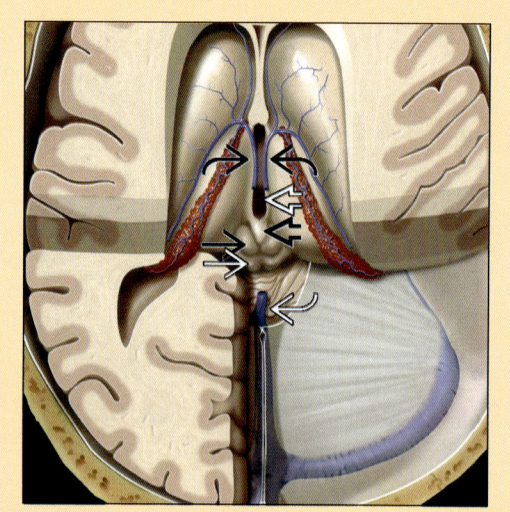

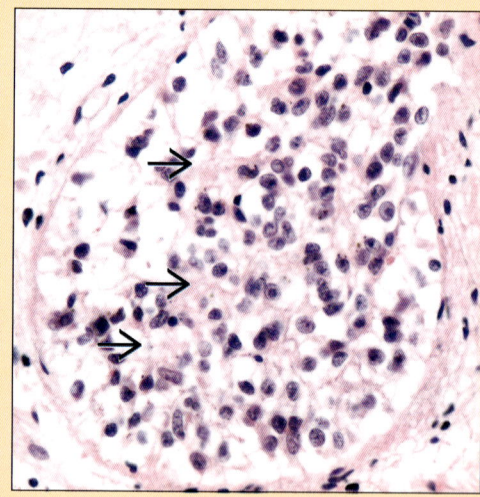

(Left) Superolateral view of a transected brain shows the pineal gland ⇨ located behind the 3rd ventricle ⇨ and above the superior colliculus ⇨. The pineal gland is pine cone-shaped, measuring 5-8 mm and weighing 100-180 mg. (Courtesy M. Nielsen, MS.) *(Right)* Low-power view shows the pineal gland ⇨ and the paired internal cerebral veins ⇨, located superiorly/dorsally. Anteriorly/rostrally is the pineal recess of the 3rd ventricle ⇨, which often contains choroid plexus.

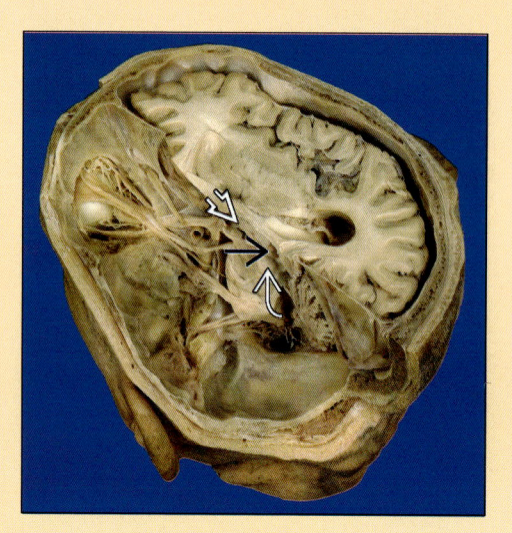

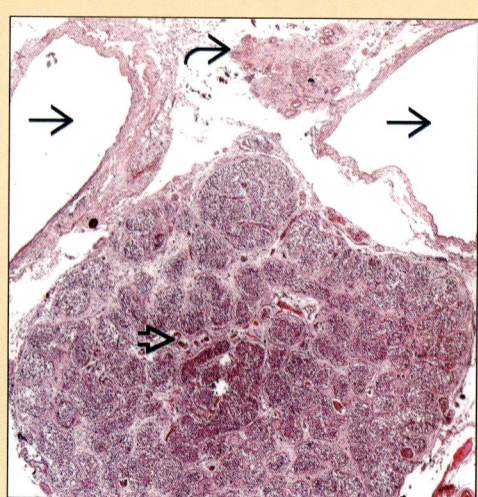

PINEAL GLAND

Lobular Architecture

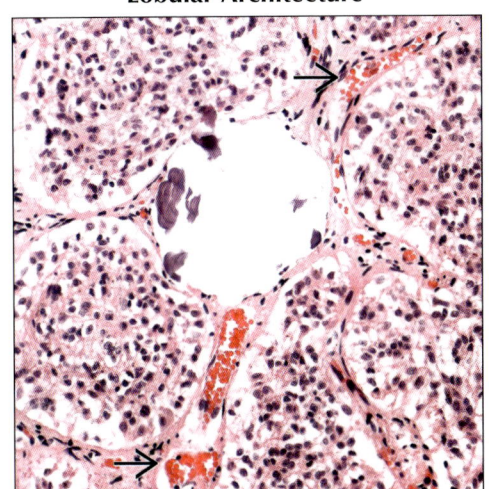

Pinealocytes

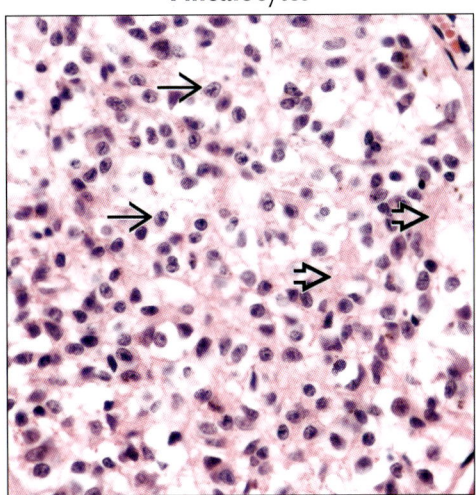

(Left) Regular lobules of cellular cords and follicles are separated by connective tissue septa ⇨. The septa are formed by leptomeninges originating in the overlying pia mater. They contain blood vessels and unmyelinated postganglionic nerve fibers that will form connections with pinealocytes. (Right) Epithelioid pinealocytes ⇨ have large, lobated nuclei and prominent nucleoli. Loose neuroglial stroma ⇨ composed of astrocytes is present in between the cords.

Synaptophysin

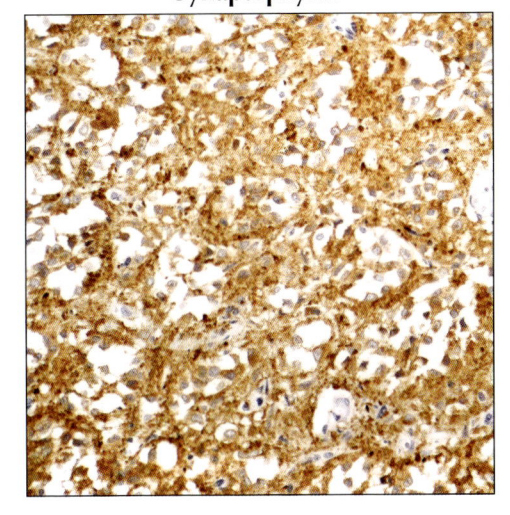

Corpora Arenacea

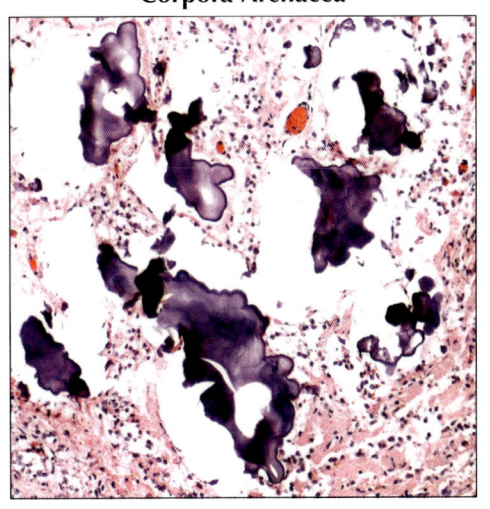

(Left) Pinealocytes are strongly synaptophysin positive. An immunohistochemical stain for GFAP would stain the intervening neuroglial stroma and indigenous astrocytes, and would highlight the lobular architecture. (Right) The large, purple, mineralized concretions in the pineal gland are termed corpora arenacea, acervuli cerebri, or "brain sand." These calcium and phosphate salt precipitations increase after puberty and are almost ubiquitous with older age; they highlight the midline location of the pineal gland on plain radiographic images.

Leptomeninges

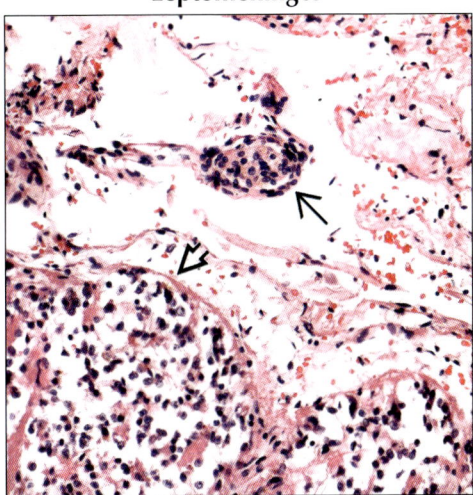

Choroid Plexus

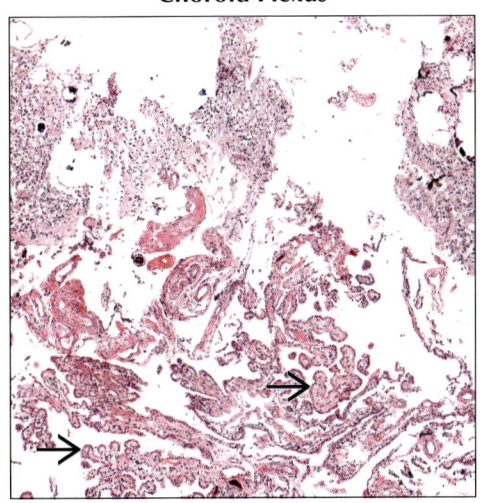

(Left) High-power H&E section shows arachnoid cell nests ⇨ in the investing leptomeninges (connective tissue or velum interpositum) that surround pineal gland lobules ⇨. These nests are the presumed source of pineal region meningiomas. (Right) Low-power H&E section shows tufts of choroid plexus ⇨, which is often found in the ependyma-lined suprapineal recess of the 3rd ventricle. The surrounding loose connective tissue, derived from leptomeninges, is termed velum interpositum.

PITUITARY

Key Facts

Macroscopic Anatomy
- Small, bean-shaped organ measuring 1-1.5 cm, weighing 0.5-0.7 g
- Located centrally at base of brain, within saddle-shaped cavity of sphenoid bone (sella turcica)
  - Close to optic chiasm and cavernous sinuses
- Pituitary stalk connects it to hypothalamus and carries
  - Releasing/inhibitory hormones/factors (through portal vascular system) to adenohypophysis
  - Axonal processes of nerve cell bodies (from hypothalamic nuclei) to neurohypophysis

Anterior Pituitary Lobe (Adenohypophysis)
- 80% of pituitary; composed of pars distalis (anterior), pars intermedia, and pars tuberalis (proximal)
- Embryologically derived from Rathke pouch, which is cranial extension of oral cavity roof (ectoderm)
- Various cell types admixed, arranged in nests/acini
  - Each produces 1 hormone (except gonadotrophs)
  - Immunohistochemical stains for each hormone can help distinguish among cell types
- Surrounded by stellate (sustentacular) cells and capillary-rich, fibroblast-derived reticulin network
- **Somatotrophs (50% of all cells, lateral location)**
  - Acidophilic; produce growth hormone (GH)
  - Stimulation: GH-releasing hormone (GHRH)
  - Inhibition: GH-inhibiting hormone (somatostatin)
- **Lactotrophs (15-20%, posterolateral location)**
  - Acidophilic/chromophobic; produce prolactin (PRL)
  - Inhibition: PRL-inhibitory factor (dopamine)
- **Corticotrophs (15-20%, central mucoid wedge)**
  - Basophilic, PAS-positive; produce proopiomelanocortin (POMC), which is precursor of ACTH, MSH, endorphins/enkephalins, and β-lipotropins
  - Stimulation: Corticotropin-releasing hormone (CRH)
- **Thyrotrophs (5%, anterior central location)**
  - Pale basophilic, PAS-positive; produce thyroid-stimulating hormone (TSH)
  - Stimulation: Thyrotropin-releasing hormone (TRH)
- **Gonadotrophs (10%, evenly distributed)**
  - Basophilic, PAS-positive; produce luteinizing hormone (LH), follicle-stimulating hormone (FSH)
  - Stimulation: Gonadotropin-releasing hormone (GnRH)

Posterior Pituitary Lobe (Neurohypophysis)
- Embryologically derived from caudal outpouching of 3rd ventricle floor/diencephalon (neuroectoderm)
- Composed of pars nervosa and infundibulum
- In contrast to anterior lobe, supplied by arterial blood (superior and inferior hypophyseal arteries)
- Unmyelinated axons and modified, GFAP-positive glial cells (pituicytes) in delicate stroma
- Axons with granular terminal expansions (Herring bodies) store 2 hypothalamic peptide hormones
  - Antidiuretic hormone (vasopressin) and oxytocin
  - Released into systemic (venous) circulation

Pitfalls/Artifacts
- Lateral adenohypophysis is mostly somatotrophs; monotonous appearance mimics adenoma, especially on frozen section or small specimens
- Central adenohypophysis is mostly corticotrophs and often arranged in nodules; also mimics adenoma
- Salivary gland rests
- Incidental Rathke cleft remnant/cyst is common (30%)
- Crooke hyaline: Perinuclear keratin accumulation

Age Variation
- Corticotrophs in posterior lobe ("basophil invasion") should not be mistaken for adenoma
  - Surrounded by axons of neurohypophysis
- Interstitial fibrosis, amyloid deposits, lymphocytosis
- Granular cell nests/tumorlets in stalk or posterior lobe

Metaplasia
- Squamous metaplasia can be seen, especially of gonadotrophs and corticotrophs (pars tuberalis)

Hyperplasia
- Anterior pituitary can enlarge 30% during pregnancy (lactotroph cell hyperplasia)

(Left) Lateral view shows the pituitary gland, consisting of anterior ⇨ and posterior ⇨ lobes, lying within the saddle-shaped cavity of sphenoid bone ⇨ (sella turcica). The pituitary stalk ⇨ connects the pituitary gland to the hypothalamus. (Right) The anterior lobe (adenohypophysis) contains admixed acidophilic ⇨, basophilic ⇨, and chromophobic ⇨ cells arranged in acini. Capillaries ⇨ and sustentacular cells ⇨ make up the surrounding stroma.

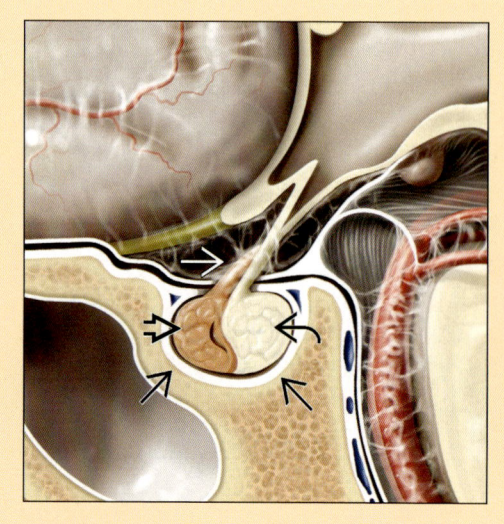

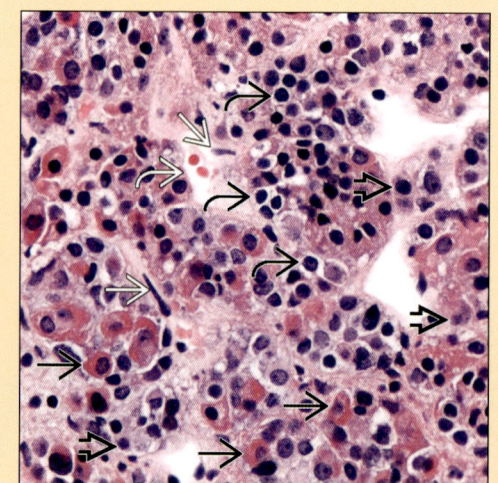

PITUITARY

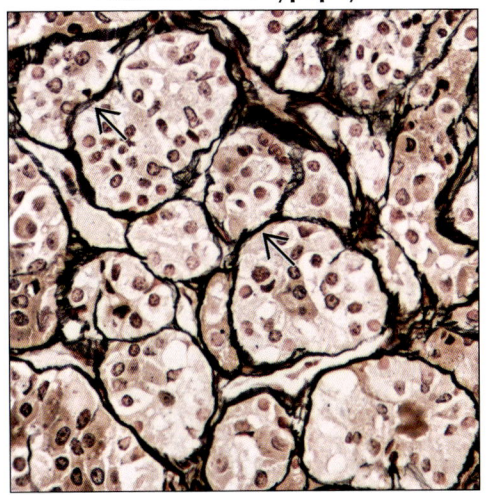

Normal Adenohypophysis
Normal Adenohypophysis

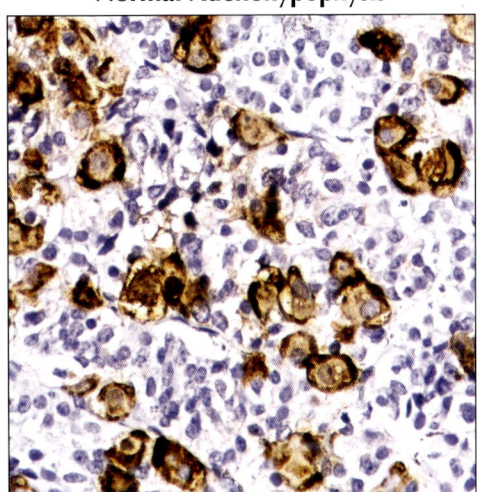

(Left) A reticulin stain highlights the intricate, capillary-rich reticulin stroma ➔ surrounding each acinus of the normal adenohypophysis, in contrast with pituitary adenomas, which generally lack this reticulin network. *(Right)* Corticotroph cells of the anterior pituitary stain with an immunohistochemical stain against ACTH. Each hormone-producing cell of the pituitary can be highlighted in this way with the corresponding antibody immunostain.

Fibrosis and Lymphocytosis
"Basophil Invasion"

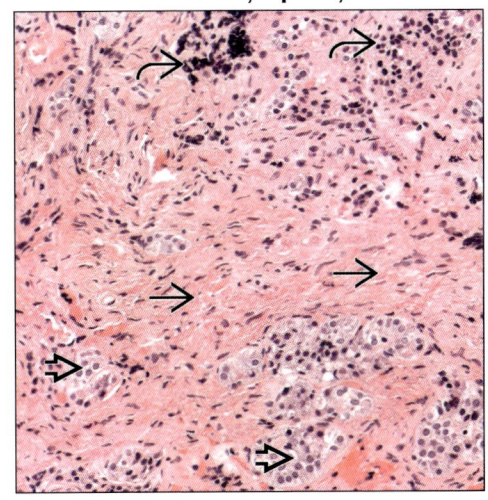

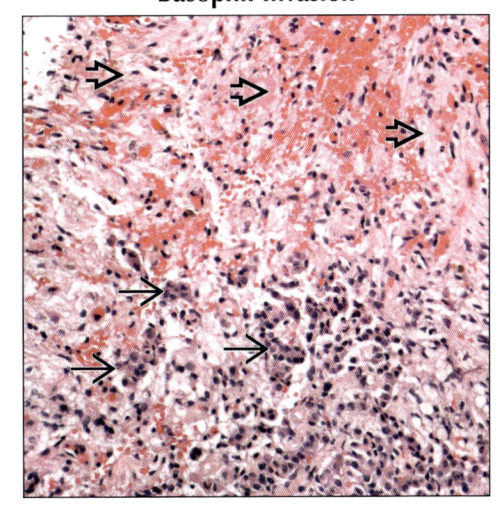

(Left) This photograph shows interstitial fibrosis ➔ of the stroma surrounding the acinar epithelium of anterior pituitary ➔, as well as collections of lymphocytes ➔. Both of these changes are commonly seen in the pituitary gland with advancing age. *(Right)* This population of basophilic corticotroph cells ➔ from the anterior pituitary are infiltrating among the neuronal processes of the posterior lobe (neurohypophysis) ➔. This is not indicative of a neoplastic process.

Normal Neurohypophysis
Salivary Gland Rest

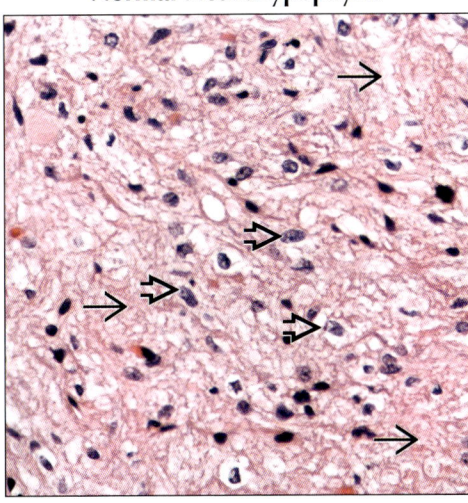

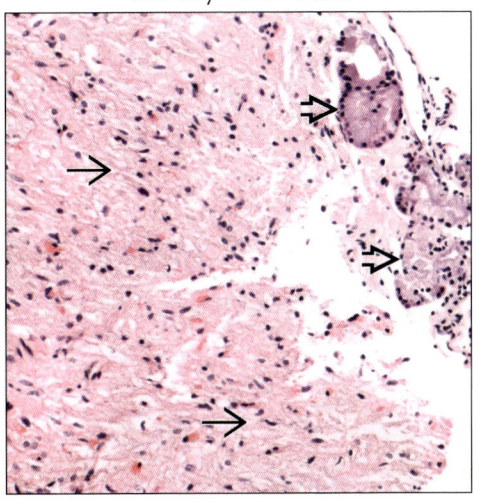

(Left) The posterior pituitary lobe is composed of neuropil ➔ (a network of unmyelinated axons of nerve cell bodies in hypothalamic nuclei) and pituicytes ➔ (modified glial cells with elongated nuclei that stain for GFAP). *(Right)* Salivary gland rests ➔ are common, especially at the junction of the neurohypophysis ➔ and pituitary stalk. They should not be confused with a neoplastic process.

SELECTED REFERENCES

ADRENAL GLAND

1. Anderson JR et al: Ectopic adrenal tissue in adults. Postgrad Med J. 56(661):806-8, 1980
2. Dobbie JW: Adrenocortical nodular hyperplasia: the ageing adrenal. J Pathol. 99(1):1-18, 1969
3. Studzinski GP et al: Observations on the weight of the human adrenal gland and the effect of preparations of corticotropin of different purity on the weight and morphology of the human adrenal gland. J Clin Endocrinol Metab. 23:248-54, 1963

PARAGANGLIA

1. Maniar KP et al: Incidental prostatic paraganglia in radical prostatectomy specimens: a diagnostic pitfall. Int J Surg Pathol. 19(6):772-4, 2011
2. Rode J et al: Paraganglial cells of urinary bladder and prostate: potential diagnostic problem. J Clin Pathol. 43(1):13-6, 1990
3. Coupland RE: The natural history of the chromaffin cell--twenty-five years on the beginning. Arch Histol Cytol. 52(Suppl):331-41, 1989
4. Zak FG et al: The Paraganglionic Chemoreceptor System. Physiology, Pathology, and Clinical Medicine. New York: Springer-Verlag, 1983

THYROID

1. Harach HR: Palpation thyroiditis resembling C cell hyperplasia. Usefulness of immunohistochemistry in their differential diagnosis. Pathol Res Pract. 189(4):488-90, 1993
2. Katoh R et al: Nature and significance of calcium oxalate crystals in normal human thyroid gland. A clinicopathological and immunohistochemical study. Virchows Arch A Pathol Anat Histopathol. 422(4):301-6, 1993
3. Hoyes AD et al: Anatomy and development of the thyroid gland. Ear Nose Throat J. 64(7):318-33, 1985
4. Nadig J et al: C-cell in vestiges of the ultimobranchial body in human thyroid glands. Virchows Arch B Cell Pathol. 27(2):189-91, 1978

PARATHYROID

1. Carney JA: Salivary heterotopia, cysts, and the parathyroid gland: branchial pouch derivatives and remnants. Am J Surg Pathol. 24(6):837-45, 2000
2. Iwasaki A et al: Quantitative analysis of stromal fat content of human parathyroid glands associated with thyroid diseases using computer image analysis. Pathol Int. 45(7):483-6, 1995
3. Utsunomiya H et al: Immunolocalization of parathyroid hormone in human parathyroid glands with special references to microwave antigen retrieval. Endocr Pathol. 6(3):223-7, 1995
4. Akerström G et al: Surgical anatomy of human parathyroid glands. Surgery. 95(1):14-21, 1984
5. Dufour DR et al: The normal parathyroid revisited: percentage of stromal fat. Hum Pathol. 13(8):717-21, 1982

PINEAL GLAND

1. Fèvre-Montange M et al: Histopathology of tumors of the pineal region. Future Oncol. 6(5):791-809, 2010
2. De Girolami U et al: Pathology of tumors of the pineal region. Rev Neurol (Paris). 164(11):882-95, 2008
3. Fuller N et al: Central nervous system. In Mills S: Histology for Pathologists. 3rd ed. Philadelphia: Lippincott Williams & Wilkins. 273-319, 2007

PITUITARY

1. Lopes M et al: Pituitary and sellar region. In Mills S: Histology for Pathologists. 3rd ed. Philadelphia: Lippincott Williams & Wilkins. 322-44, 2007
2. Asa SL et al: Molecular basis of pituitary development and cytogenesis. Front Horm Res. 32:1-19, 2004
3. Bozzola M et al: Development of the pituitary and its abnormalities. J Pediatr Endocrinol Metab. 12 (Suppl 1):319-27, 1999

INDEX

Locators refer to Section:page number.

A

Acinar cell, 1:16
Acral skin, 2:2, 3
Acrosyringium, 2:2, 4
Adaptive immune system. *See* Immune system overview.
Adipose tissue, 3:10–13
   age variation, 3:10
   anatomy, 3:10
   brown fat, 3:10, 12
   fat necrosis, 3:10, 13
   fatty replacement
      parathyroid gland, 3:13
      thymus, 3:13
   fetal fat, 3:11
   histology, 1:28
   hyperplasia, 3:10
   images, 3:11–13
   Lochkern, 3:10, 12
   metaplasia, 3:10
   pitfalls/artifacts, 3:10
   S100 protein in white fat, 3:11
   white adipose tissue, normal, 3:11
   white fat
      anatomy, 3:10
      atrophy, 3:13
      in omentum, 3:11
Adnexal structures, 2:10–13
   age variation, 2:10
   anagen-phase hair follicle, cross section, 2:11
   anatomy, 2:10
   apocrine glands, 2:10, 13
   bulb and suprabulbar region of vellus follicle, 2:11
   CK20(+) Merkel cells in hair follicle, 2:12
   eccrine glands, 2:10
      and ducts, 2:13
   follicular ostia, 2:12
   hair bulb cross section, 2:11
   hair follicles, 2:10, 11–12
   images, 2:11–13
   infundibular region of follicles with Demodex, 2:12
   metaplasia, 2:10
   pitfalls/artifacts, 2:10
   sebaceous glands, 2:10, 11–12
   telogen-phase hair follicle cross section, 2:11
   vellus follicle with sebaceous glands, 2:12
Adrenal gland, 14:2–5
   adrenal capsule, 14:4
   adrenal cortex, 1 and 3 weeks after birth, 14:5
   adrenal medulla, 14:4–5
   age variation, 14:2
   anatomy, 14:2
   central adrenal vein, 14:5
   cortical-medullary junction, 14:4
   hyperplasia, 14:2
   images, 14:3–5
   zona fasciculata, 14:3
   zona glomerulosa, 14:3
   zona reticularis, 14:3
Alcian blue/hyaluronidase stain, 1:2
Alcian blue/PAS stain, 1:2
Alcian blue stain
   pH 1.0, 1:2
   pH 2.5, 1:2
Antibodies, in immunofluorescence, 1:4
Anus and anal canal, 10:28–31
   AIN in transition zone, 10:31
   anal glands, 10:31
   anatomy, 10:28
   anogenital sweat glands, 10:29
   apocrine glands, 10:29
   colorectal and transition zones, 10:30
   eccrine glands, 10:29
   images, 10:29–31
   lamina propria, 10:29
   perianal nevus, 10:31
   perianal skin, 10:29
   pitfalls/artifacts, 10:28
   squamous zone, 10:30
   transition zone, 10:30, 31
Apocrine glands
   anus and anal canal, 10:29
   integument, 2:10, 13
   neurovascular bundle and apocrine glands, dermis, 2:8
Appendix, 10:24–27
   age variation, 10:24
   anatomy, 10:24
   diverticulum, 10:27
   endometriosis, 10:27
   epithelium, 10:25
   fibrous obliteration of the tip, 10:27
   ganglion cells, 10:26

INDEX

hyperplasia, 10:24
images, 10:25–27
intraluminal mucin, 10:27
lamina propria, 10:24, 25
lymphoid tissue, 10:25
mesoappendix, 10:27
mucosa, 10:24
muscularis mucosa, 10:24, 25–26
muscularis propria, 10:24, 26
neural elements, 10:26
pitfalls/artifacts, 10:24
serosa, 10:24, 26
submucosa, 10:24, 26
surface hyperplastic changes, 10:27
Arachnoid cyst, 5:11
Arachnoid mater, 5:10, 11
Arteries, 4:12–15
    adventitia and periadventitial tissue, 4:13
    age variation, 4:12
    anatomy, 4:12
    arterioles, 4:13
    arteriovenous malformation, 4:19
    atherosclerotic plaque, 4:14
    chronic medial dissection, 4:15
    elastic arteries, 4:12, 14–15
    images, 4:13–15
    layers, 4:12
    medial calcific (Mönkeberg-type) sclerosis, 4:15
    muscular arteries, 4:12, 13–14
    pitfalls/artifacts, 4:12
    tangential sectioning artifact, 4:14
    vasculitis, 4:15
Arteriovenous malformation, 4:19
Atrioventricular node
    anatomy, 4:8
    high magnification: trichrome, 4:11
    tissue block, 4:9–10
    trichrome, 4:11
Atrioventricular valves, 4:6, 7
Auditory canal
    external, 7:31
    internal, 7:33
Auerbach plexus
    small intestine, 10:14, 17
    stomach, 10:12
Autoimmune disease, and major histocompatibility complex, 6:5

B

B lymphocytes, 6:4
Basal lamina, of cells, 1:13, 19
Basic histological techniques. See Histological techniques, basic.
Basophil
    innate immune system function, 6:3
    peripheral blood, 6:23, 24

Bile ducts
    accessory, 11:13
    anatomy, 11:2
    images, 11:4
Biliary system. See Hepatobiliary tract and pancreas.
Biliary tract, extrahepatic, 11:14–15
Bladder, 12:16–21
    adventitia, 12:19
    anatomy, 12:16
    cystitis cystica, 12:20
    cystitis glandularis, 12:20
        with intestinal metaplasia, 12:21
    glycogenated squamous epithelium, 12:19
    images, 12:17–21
    inverted papilloma, 12:21
    lamina propria, 12:18
    metaplasia, 12:16
    muscularis mucosae, 12:18
    muscularis propria, 12:19
    normal urothelium, 12:17
    paraganglia, 12:21
    pitfalls/artifacts, 12:16
    tangential sectioning, 12:17
    transurethral resection of bladder tumor, 12:18
    umbrella, 12:17
    von Brunn nests, 12:20
Bone and cartilage, 3:2–7
    age variation, 3:2
    anatomy, 3:2
    Canal of Volkmann, 3:2
    cancellous (trabecular) bone, 3:3
    chondrocytes, 3:2, 7
    cortical (compact) bone, 3:3
    fracture callus, 3:7
    Haversian system, 3:2, 4
    hyaline cartilage, 3:2, 6–7
    images, 3:3–7
    lamellar bone, 3:2, 3–4
    osteoblasts, 3:2, 5
    osteoclasts, 3:2, 6
    osteocytes, 3:2, 6
    periosteum, 3:2, 3
    pitfalls/artifacts, 3:2
    woven bone, 3:2, 5
Bone marrow, 6:14–21
    age variation, 6:14
    anatomy, 6:14
    aspirate smear
        clumping, 6:20
        macrophage, 6:15
    aspiration artifact, 6:20
    bone marrow aspirate, 6:15
        newborn and infant, 6:21
    clot section, 6:15
    core biopsy, 6:15, 20
        adequate and inadequate, 6:21

INDEX

    adolescent male, 6:21
    infant, 6:21
    middle-aged woman, 6:21
    skin in, 6:20
erythroblasts, 6:14, 17
erythroid colony, 6:17
fat cell, 6:18
gelatinous transformation, 6:20
granulocytic cells, 6:16
hematogones, 6:21
hematopoiesis in, 6:5, 14
images, 6:15–23
macrophages, 6:17
    aspirate smear, 6:15
mast cell, 6:18
megakaryocytes, 6:14, 17
osteoblasts, 6:19
osteoclasts, 6:19
paratrabecular granulocytic precursor cells, 6:16
pitfalls/artifacts, 6:14
plasma cells, 6:18
previous biopsy site, 6:20
Bone tissue, histology, 1:28
Brain. *See* Central nervous system.
Breast, 9:2–8
    age variation, 9:2
    anatomy, 9:2
    calponin immunohistochemistry, 9:4
    CD-34 immunohistochemistry, 9:6
    cytokeratin 7 and CK5/6 with p63
        immunohistochemistry, 9:4, 5, 6
    embryologic/fetal development, 9:2
    estrogen receptor immunohistochemistry, 9:6
    images, 9:3–7
    interlobular mammary ducts, 9:5
    Ki-67 immunohistochemistry, 9:6
    lactiferous sinuses, 9:4
    mammary duct system, 9:5, 6
    mastectomy, prophylactic subcutaneous, 9:3
    menopause, 9:7
    nipple
        gross evaluation, 9:3
        and lactiferous duct, 9:4
        sections for microscopy, 9:3
    nipple/areolar complex, 9:3
    physiologic function, 9:2
    post-lactation involution, 9:7
    pregnancy and lactation, 9:7
    squamous/columnar junction, 9:4
    TDLU (terminal ductal lobular units), 9:2, 5, 6
Bronchial-associated lymphoid tissue (BALT), 8:7
Brown fat
    anatomy, 3:10
    images, 3:12
    thymus gland, 6:27

C

Calcium stain (von Kossa), 1:3
Cancellous (trabecular) bone, 3:2, 3
Capillaries, 4:16–19
    age variation, 4:16
    anatomy, 4:16
    cerebral cortical capillaries, 4:17
    fenestrations in glomerular capillaries, 4:18
    images, 4:17–18
    organizing granulation tissue, 4:17
    pulmonary alveolar capillaries, 4:17
    renal medulla capillaries, 4:17
Carbohydrate stains, 1:2–3
    Alcian blue (pH 1.0), 1:2
    Alcian blue (pH 2.5), 1:2
    Alcian blue/hyaluronidase, 1:2
    Alcian blue/PAS, 1:2
    colloidal iron, 1:3
    mucicarmine, 1:2
    PAS (periodic acid-Schiff), 1:2
        with diastase, 1:2
Cardiac conduction system, 4:8–11
    age variation, 4:8
    anatomy, 4:8
    atrioventricular node, 4:8, 9–11
    heart, superior oblique view, 4:9
    His bundle and bundle branches
        anatomy, 4:8
        trichrome, 4:11
    images, 4:9–11
    left atrium and ventricle, opened, 4:9–10
    left bundle branch: trichrome, 4:11
    left ventricular outflow tract, 4:10
    pitfalls/artifacts, 4:8
    Purkinje cell, 4:9–11
    right atrium and ventricle, opened, 4:10
    sinoatrial (sinus) node
        anatomy, 4:8
        excised tissue block, 4:9
        high magnification, 4:10
        trichrome stained and cross section, 4:9
Cardiac valves, 4:6–7
    age variation, 4:6
    anatomy, 4:6
    atrioventricular valves, 4:6, 7
    fibrosa, 4:6
    images, 4:7
    pitfalls/artifacts, 4:6
    semilunar (ventriculoarterial) valve, 4:6, 7
    spongiosa, 4:6
    tendinous cord, 4:7
    tricuspid valve annulus, 4:5
    ventricularis, 4:6
Cardiomyocytes, 4:3
Cartilage. *See* Bone and cartilage.
Cells, 1:12–19
    cell adhesion, 1:13

INDEX

desmosomes (macula adherens), 1:13, 18
    hemidesmosomes, 1:13
cytoplasm, 1:12–13
    cell membrane specializations, 1:13
    endoplasmic reticulum, 1:12–13
    Golgi apparatus, 1:13
    lysosomes, 1:13, 16
    mitochondria, 1:13
cytoskeleton, 1:13
    centrioles, 1:13, 16
    intermediate filaments, 1:13
    microtubules, 1:13
    thick filaments, 1:13
    thin filaments (actin), 1:13
extracellular substances, 1:13
    basal lamina, 1:13, 19
    collagen, 1:13, 19
    elements of, 1:12
images, 1:14–19
membrane, 1:12, 14
membrane-bound organelles, 1:12
non-membrane-bound organelles, 1:12
nucleus, 1:12, 14
    chromatin, 1:12
    chromosomes, 1:12
    cytoplasmic interactions, 1:12, 14
    nucleolus, 1:12, 14
organization, 1:12
Central nervous system, 5:6–9
  age variation, 5:6
  anatomy, 5:6
  brain, anatomy, 5:6
  cerebellar cortex layers, 5:7
  cerebral cortex layers, 5:7
  coronal brain section, 5:7
  GFAP-positive astrocyte, 5:9
  images, 5:7–9
  lipofuscin accumulation, 5:9
  Purkinje cell, 5:7
  senile (neuritic) plaque, 5:9
  spinal cord
    anatomy, 5:6
    central canal, 5:8
    cervical, 5:8
    gray matter, 5:8
    lumbosacral, 5:8
    thoracic, 5:8
    white matter, 5:8
  substantia nigra neurons, 5:9
  synaptophysin-positive neuron, 5:9
  white matter axons, 5:9
Centrioles of cytoskeleton, 1:13, 16
Cervix. See Uterus.
Chondrocytes, 3:2, 7
Choroid plexus, 5:12–13
  age variation, 5:12
  anatomy, 5:12
  images, 5:13
  pitfalls/artifacts, 5:12
Chromatin, in nucleus, 1:12
Chromosomes, 1:12
Circulatory system, 4:2–20
  arteries, 4:12–15
  capillaries, veins, and lymphatics, 4:16–19
  cardiac conduction system, 4:8–11
  cardiac valves, 4:6–7
  heart, 4:2–5
Collagen, extracellular, 1:13, 19
Collecting ducts. See Kidney.
Colloidal iron stain, 1:3
Complement system, innate immune system function, 6:3
Connective tissue, 3:8–9
  anatomy, 3:8
  histology, 1:21–22, 28–29
  images, 3:9
  pitfalls/artifacts, 3:8
Connective tissue stains, 1:3
  elastic stain, 1:3
  Masson trichrome, 1:3
  pentachrome stain, 1:3
  reticulin stain, 1:3
Copper (rhodanine) stain, 1:3
Corpus luteum. See Ovary.
Cortical (compact) bone, 3:3
Cystitis cystica, 12:20
Cystitis glandularis
  bladder, 12:20, 21
  ureter and renal pelvis, 12:14
Cytoplasm, 1:12–13
Cytoplasmic staining. See Nuclear and cytoplasmic staining.
Cytoskeleton. See Cells.

D

Dendritic cells, innate immune system function, 6:2
Dermis, 2:6–9
  age variation, 2:6
  anatomy, 2:6
  blood vessels
    and collagen bundles, 2:8
    and lymphatics, 2:8
  deep dermal nerve, 2:9
  deep dermis, 2:8
  hyperplasia, 2:6
  images, 2:7–9
  interface between papillary and reticular dermis, 2:7
  mast cells, 2:9
  melanin pigment, 2:7
  neurovascular bundle
    and apocrine glands, 2:8
    deep, 2:8

INDEX

Pacinian corpuscle, 2:9
papillary dermis, 2:6, 7
pilar muscles, 2:9
pitfalls/artifacts, 2:6
reticular dermis, 2:6, 7–8
sebaceous gland and pilar muscles, 2:9
severe solar elastosis, 2:7
stromal cells, 2:6
Desmosomes (macula adherens), 1:13, 18
Duodenum, 10:14
Dura mater, 5:10, 11

E

Ear, 7:30–33
anatomy, 7:30
auricular cartilage, 7:31
ceruminous glands, 7:31
cholesteatoma and chronic otitis media, 7:32
endolymphatic sac, 7:33
external auditory canal, 7:31
external ear, 7:30
images, 7:31–33
inner ear, 7:30
internal auditory canal, 7:33
lobule, 7:31
mastoid air cells, 7:33
middle ear, 7:30, 32
middle ear ossicle (incus), 7:32
ossicles, 7:32–33
pitfalls/artifacts, 7:30
tympanic cavity, 7:32
tympanic membrane, 7:31
tympanosclerosis, 7:31
Eccrine glands
anus and anal canal, 10:29
integument, 2:10, 13
Ectopic tissue
cartilage, in tonsil, 7:28
gallbladder, 11:10, 13
parathyroid tissue, 14:14
tonsillar, on tongue, 7:25
Elastic stain, 1:3
Electron microscopy, 1:8–11
assessment of clinical samples, 1:8–9
images, 1:10–11
specimen handling, 1:8
specimen processing, 1:8
terminology, 1:8
Endocardium, 4:3
Endocervix. *See* Uterus.
Endocrine system, 14:2–20
adrenal gland, 14:2–5
paraganglia, 14:6–7
parathyroid, 14:12–15
pineal gland, 14:16–17
pituitary, 14:18–19
thyroid, 14:8–11

Endometrium. *See* Uterus.
Endoplasmic reticulum, 1:12–13
free ribosomes and rER, 1:15
rough endoplasmic reticulum, 1:14
smooth ER (sER), 1:15
Enzymes, 1:3
Eosinophil
innate immune system function, 6:3
peripheral blood, 6:23
Epidermis, 2:2–5
acral skin, 2:2, 3
acrosyringium, 2:2, 4
age variation, 2:2
anatomy, 2:2
cell types, 2:2
focal parakeratosis, 2:3
follicular ostia, 2:2, 4
hyperplasia, 2:2
images, 2:3–5
keratinocytes, 2:2
Langerhans cells
CD1a immunohistochemistry stain for, 2:5
definition, 2:2
intraepidermal, 2:5
melan-A immunohistochemistry in sun-damaged skin, 2:5
melanin pigment, 2:2
melanocytes, 2:2, 4–5
Merkel cells, 2:2
millaria crystallina, 2:5
PAS stain, 2:5
normal epidermis and superficial dermis, 2:3
PAS stain, 2:3
pigmented skin, 2:4
pitfalls/artifacts, 2:2
rete ridges, 2:2
stratified squamous epithelium, 2:2
Epididymis, 12:52, 57–58
Epiglottis, 7:41
Epimysium, 3:16
Epithelial markers, 1:3
Epithelium, histology
classification, 1:20
morphology, 1:20
polarity and specialized structures, 1:21
structure and function, 1:20
Epithelium, squamous. *See* Squamous epithelium.
Esophagus, 10:2–7
adventitia, 10:2, 6
anatomy, 10:2
food matter, 10:4
ganglion cells, 10:6
glycogenic acanthosis, 10:4
heterotopia, 10:3
images, 10:3–7
interstitial cells of Cajal, 10:6
intestinal metaplasia, 10:7

INDEX

lamina propria, 10:2, 4
metaplasia, 10:2
muscularis mucosa, 10:2, 4–5
muscularis propria, 10:2, 5–6
myenteric plexus, 10:6
oral flora, 10:4
pancreatic acinar metaplasia, 10:7
pitfalls/artifacts, 10:2
squamocolumnar junction, 10:2, 7
squamous epithelium, 10:3
submucosa, 10:2, 4–5
submucosal glands, 10:5
External ear. See Ear.
Extracellular matrix, histology, 1:22
Extracellular substances
  basal lamina, 1:13, 19
  collagen, 1:13, 19
  elements of, 1:12
Extrahepatic biliary tract, 11:14–15
  anatomy, 11:14
  images, 11:15
  metaplasia, 11:14
  pitfalls/artifacts, 11:14
Eye and ocular adnexa, 7:2–11
  age variation, 7:2
  anatomy, 7:2
  canal of Schlemm, 7:4
  choroid, 7:7
  ciliary body, 7:6–7, 10
  conjunctiva, 7:5–6
  cornea, 7:3
  corneoscleral limbus, 7:3–4
  eyelid, 7:10–11
  eyelid glands, 7:10
  images, 7:3–11
  iris, 7:6
  lacrimal ducts, 7:11
  lens, 7:6, 9–10
  optic nerve, 7:8–9
  orbital soft tissue, 7:11
  retina, 7:8
  Schwalbe ring, 7:5
  sclera, 7:4
  vitreous, 7:10

F

Fallopian tube, 13:24–29
  age variation, 13:24
  ampulla, 13:24, 25
  anatomy, 13:24
  artifact, tangential sectioning, 13:28
  atrophy, 13:29
  broad ligament, 13:24
  decidual change, 13:28
  endosalpingiosis, 13:29
  epithelium, 13:24, 26
  fimbriated end, 13:24, 26
  hydrosalpinx, 13:29
  hyperplasia, 13:24
  images, 13:25–29
  isthmus, 13:24, 25
  mesonephric remnant, 13:28
  metaplasia, 13:24
  mid-portion, 13:25
  outermost mesothelial cell layer, 13:24
  paratubal cyst, 13:26–27
  pitfalls/artifacts, 13:24
  reactive mesothelium, 13:28
  squamous metaplasia, 13:27
  stroma, 13:24
  tubal pregnancy, 13:28
  Walthard rest, 13:24, 27–28
Fat stains, 1:3
Fat tissue. See Adipose tissue.
Fatty replacement
  parathyroid gland, 3:13
  skeletal muscle, 3:17
  thymus, 3:13
Female genital tract. See Genital tract, female.
Feulgen stain, 1:2
Filaments, of cytoskeleton, 1:13
Follicles
  hair follicles, 2:10, 11–12
  lymph node
    neoplastic follicle, 6:7
    primary follicle, 6:6
    secondary follicle, 6:6, 7
  ovarian follicles, 13:33–34, 36–37
Follicular ostia
  adnexal structures, 2:12
  epidermis, 2:2, 4
Fontana-Masson stain, 1:3
Formalin-fixed, paraffin-embedded tissue, in immunofluorescence, 1:4
Fresh tissue, in immunofluorescence, 1:4

G

Gallbladder, 11:10–13
  accessory bile ducts, 11:13
  anatomy, 11:10
  ducts of Luschka, 11:10, 13
  ectopic tissues, 11:10, 13
  epithelium, 11:11
  ganglion cells, 11:10, 12
  gastric metaplasia, 11:13
  images, 11:11–13
  intestinal metaplasia, 11:13
  lamina propria, 11:11
  metaplasia, 11:10
  mucosa, 11:10, 11
  mucous glands, 11:10, 12
  muscularis, 11:12
  perimuscular connective tissue, 11:12

INDEX

pitfalls/artifacts, 11:10
Rokitansky-Aschoff sinuses, 11:13
Ganglion cells
   appendix, 10:26
   esophagus, 10:6
   gallbladder, 11:10, 12
   large intestine, 10:20
   myenteric ganglionitis, 5:5
   prostate, 12:32
Gastrointestinal system. *See* Tubular gut and peritoneum.
Genital tract, female, 13:2–45. *See also* Genitourinary tract.
   fallopian tube, 13:24–29
   ovary, 13:30–39
   placenta, 13:40–45
   urethral anatomy, 12:22, 25
   urethral squamous metaplasia, 12:25
   uterus, 13:10–23
   vagina, 13:6–9
   vulva, 13:2–5
Genital tract, male. *See also* Genitourinary tract.
   penis, 12:48–51
   prostate: benign glandular and stromal histology, 12:38–47
   prostate: regional anatomy with histologic correlates, 12:28–37
   prostatic urethra (verumontanum), 12:23
   testis and associated excretory ducts, 12:52–59
   urethral anatomy, 12:22, 23, 24
Genitourinary tract, 12:2–27
   bladder, 12:16–21
   kidney, 12:2–11
   ureter and renal pelvis, 12:12–15
   urethra, 12:22–27
Gingivae, 7:14–15
   age variation, 7:14
   anatomy, 7:14
   images, 7:15
Glands, histology, 1:21, 26–27
Glomerulus. *See* Kidney.
Golgi apparatus, 1:13
Granule stains, 1:3
Granules, cellular, 1:16

H

Hair follicles, 2:10, 11–12
Hassall corpuscles, thymus gland, 6:27
Haversian system, 3:2, 4
Head and neck, 7:2–49
   ear, 7:30–33
   eye and ocular adnexa, 7:2–11
   gingivae, 7:14–15
   larynx, 7:40–43
   major salivary glands, 7:44–47
   minor salivary glands, 7:16–17
   nose and paranasal sinuses, 7:34–37
   oral mucosae, 7:12–13
   pharynx, 7:38–39
   teeth, 7:18–21
   tongue, 7:22–25
   tonsils/adenoids, 7:26–29
Heart, 4:2–5
   age variation, 4:2
   anatomy, 4:2
   atrial myocardium, 4:4
   cardiac conduction system, 4:8–11
   cardiac valves, 4:6–7
   cardiomyocytes, 4:3
   contraction band artifact, 4:5
   electron microscopy assessment of specimens, 1:9
   endocardium, 4:2, 3
   hydrophilic polymer gel embolus, 4:5
   hyperplasia, 4:2
   images, 4:3–5
   intramyocardial vessels, 4:5
   lipofuscin (brown atrophy), 4:3
   myocardium
      anatomy, 4:2
      atrial, 4:4
      infant, 4:4
      ventricular, 4:4
   myocyte hypertrophy, 4:4
   papillary muscle tip, 4:5
   pitfalls/artifacts, 4:2
   sarcomere ultrastructure, 4:3
   subendocardial (ischemic) vacuolation, 4:4
   tricuspid valve annulus, 4:5
Hematopoietic and immune systems, 6:2–28
   bone marrow, 6:14–21
   immune system overview, 6:2–5
   lymph nodes, 6:6–9
   peripheral blood, 6:22–25
   spleen, 6:10–13
   thymus, 6:26–27
Hematopoietic/lymphoid markers, 1:3
Hematoxylin and eosin stain, 1:2
Hemidesmosomes, 1:13
Hepatobiliary tract and pancreas, 11:2–23
   extrahepatic biliary tract, 11:14–15
   gallbladder, 11:10–13
   liver, 11:2–9
   pancreas, 11:18–21
   Vaterian system, 11:16–17
Heterotopic tissue
   cartilage, in thyroid gland, 14:11
   pancreatic, in stomach, 10:13
Histochemical staining. *See also* Stains, special.
   definition, 1:2
Histological techniques, basic, 1:2–31
   cells, 1:12–19
   electron microscopy, 1:8–11
   general categories of immunohistochemical antibodies and examples, 1:3

INDEX

histology. *See* Histology.
immunofluorescence, 1:47
special stains and immunohistochemistry of normal tissues, 1:2–3
Histology, 1:20–32
   adipose tissue, 1:28
   bone, 1:28
   cardiac muscle, 1:29
   cartilage, 1:29
   cells, 1:20
   columnar tissue
      simple, 1:25
      stratified, 1:25
   connective tissue, 1:21–22, 28–29
   cuboidal tissue
      simple, 1:24
      stratified, 1:25
   definition, 1:20
   diffuse neuroendocrine system, 1:28
   endocrine gland, 1:27
   epithelium, 1:20–21, 24–25
   extracellular matrix, 1:22
   ganglia, 1:29
   glands, 1:21, 26–27
   images, 1:24–29
   mixed glands, 1:27
   mucous glands, 1:26
   muscle, 1:22, 27, 29
   myoepithelium, 1:27
   nerve, 1:22, 29
   organ systems, 1:22–23
   peripheral nerve, 1:29
   pseudostratified tissue, 1:25
   sebaceous exocrine gland, 1:26
   serous glands, 1:26
   skeletal muscle, 1:29
   smooth muscle, 1:29
   squamous tissue
      simple, 1:24
      stratified, 1:24
   stains. *See also* Stains, special.
      guides to chapters, 1:30–32
   tissues, 1:20–22
   transitional tissue, 1:25
HLA disease associations, 6:5
Hormones, examples, 1:3
Hyaline cartilage, 3:2, 6–7
Hyponychium, 2:14, 15

I

Ileum, 10:14, 17
Immune system overview, 6:2–5. *See also* Hematopoietic and immune systems.
   adaptive immune system components, 6:4
      B lymphocytes, 6:4
      lymphoid tissues, 6:4
      T lymphocytes, 6:4
   bone marrow. *See* Bone marrow.
   clinical implications, 6:4–5
      MHC and autoimmune disease, 6:4–5
      MHC and transplantation, 6:4–5
   HLA disease associations, 6:5
   immunoglobulin classes, basic characteristics, 6:5
   innate immune system components, 6:2–4
      basophils, 6:3
      complement system, 6:3
      dendritic cells, 6:2
      eosinophils, 6:3
      macrophages, 6:3
      major histocompatibility complex, 6:3–4
      mast cells, 6:3
      natural killer cells, 6:3
      neutrophils, 6:3
   lymphoid organs. *See* Lymph nodes; Spleen.
   thymus in, 6:5
Immunofluorescence, 1:4–7
   assessment of clinical specimens, 1:5
   images, 1:6–7
   methodology, 1:4
Immunoglobulin classes, 6:5
Immunohistochemical antibodies and examples, 1:3
Immunohistochemical staining, definition, 1:2
Immunohistochemical stains. *See also* Stains, special.
   guide to chapters, 1:30–31
Innate immune system. *See* Immune system overview.
Inner ear. *See* Ear.
Integument, 2:2–16
   adnexal structures, 2:10–13
   dermis, 2:6–9
   epidermis, 2:2–5
   nail, 2:14–15
Intestines. *See* Large intestine; Small intestine.
Introduction to histology and basic techniques. *See* Histological techniques, basic.
Islets of Langerhans, 11:18, 19–20

J

Jejunum, 10:14, 16

K

Keratinocytes. *See* Epidermis.
Kidney, 12:2–11. *See also* Ureter and renal pelvis.
   afferent & efferent arterioles, 12:10
   age variation, 12:2
   anatomy, 12:2
   artery and arteriole, 12:10
   CD31, capillaries, 12:5, 10
   collecting ducts
      AE1/AE3, 12:8

INDEX

 anatomy, 12:2
 distal tubules and: EMA, 12:7
 EMA, 12:8
 H&E, 12:8
cortex
 anatomy, 12:2
 normal, 12:3
 proximal tubules, 12:6
cytokeratin 7, distal tubules and collecting ducts, 12:8
dendritic cells, resident, 12:11
distal tubular epithelial cell: EM, 12:7
distal tubules
 anatomy, 12:2
 and collecting ducts: EMA, 12:7
 convoluted, 12:7
 EMA, 12:7
dolichos biflorus, 12:8
glomerular capillaries
 normal: EM, 12:5
 schematic, 12:5
glomerular filtration barrier: EM, 12:5
glomerular podocytes
 CD10, 12:5
 foot process and slit diaphragm complex, 12:5
glomerulus, normal
 anatomy, 12:2
 H&E, 12:4
 Jones methenamine silver, 12:4
 Masson trichrome, 12:4
 PAS, 12:4
 pediatric, 12:4
 schematic, 12:4
images, 12:3–11
intercalated cell: EM, 12:9
interlobular artery, 12:9
juxtaglomerular apparatus, 12:2
loop of Henle, 12:2, 7
lymphatics and lymphatic vessels, 12:11
lymphatics in renal sinus, 12:11
macula densa, 12:7
medulla
 anatomy, 12:2
 images, 12:3
 Masson trichrome, 12:8
nephrons with blood supply, schematic, 12:3
nerves, 12:9
peritubular capillary: EM, 12:10
peritubular capillary network, 12:10
pitfalls/artifacts, 12:2
principal cell: EM, 12:9
proximal tubular epithelial cell: EM, 12:6
proximal tubules
 anatomy, 12:2
 CD10, 12:6
 cortex, 12:6
 H&E, 12:6
 PAS, 12:6
renal artery, 12:9
specimens
 electron microscopy assessment, 1:8–9, 10
 immunofluorescence assessment, 1:5, 6
vascular bundle: Alpha smooth muscle actin, 12:10

L

Lamellar bone, 3:2, 3–4
Lamina propria
 anus and anal canal, 10:29
 appendix, 10:24, 25
 bladder, 12:18
 esophagus, 10:2, 4
 gallbladder, 11:11
 oral mucosae, 7:13
 small intestine, 10:14, 16
 stomach, 10:8, 10
 ureter and renal pelvis, 12:13
 vagina, 13:6, 8
Langerhans cells
 CD1a immunohistochemistry stain for, 2:5
 definition, 2:2
 intraepidermal, 2:5
Large intestine, 10:18–23
 anatomy, 10:18
 artifactual epithelial telescoping, 10:23
 artifactual mucosal hemorrhage, 10:23
 bifid crypt, 10:23
 columnar epithelium, 10:19
 endocrine cells, 10:19
 endoscope trauma, 10:23
 hyperplastic mucosal changes, 10:22
 images, 10:19–23
 intraepithelial lymphocytes, 10:21–22
 luminal debris, 10:22
 lymph node, 10:20
 melanosis coli, 10:22–23
 metaplasia, 10:18
 muciphages, 10:22
 mucosa, 10:18, 19
 mucosa-associated lymphoid tissue (MALT), 10:19
 muscularis propria, 10:20
 myenteric plexus with ganglion cells, 10:20
 Paneth cells, 10:19
 pitfalls/artifacts, 10:18
 pneumatosis, 10:21
 pseudolipomatosis, 10:21
 reactive MALT, 10:19
 rectal histiocytes (muciphages), 10:22
 serosa, 10:20
 submucosa, 10:20
 tangential sectioning, 10:21

INDEX

tissue cauterization, 10:21
vegetable material, 10:23
Larynx, 7:40–43
  age variation, 7:40
  anatomy, 7:40
  aryepiglottic fold, 7:41
  arytenoid cartilage, 7:41
  cartilages, 7:40, 41
  epiglottis, 7:40, 41
  glottis, 7:40
  images, 7:41–43
  lymphoid aggregate, 7:43
  metaplasia, 7:40
  Reinke space, 7:42
  saccular cyst, 7:43
  saccule, 7:43
  subglottis, 7:40, 43
  thyroid cartilage, 7:43
  true vocal cord, 7:40, 42
  ventricle and saccule, 7:42
  vocal cord ligament, 7:42
  vocal cords, 7:42
Lipofuscin
  accumulation, in central nervous system, 5:9
  granules, in cell, 1:16, 17
  heart, 4:3
  liver, 11:8
Liver, 11:2–9
  age variation, 11:2
  anatomy, 11:2
  bile caniculi, 11:2, 5
  bile ducts
    anatomy, 11:2
    images, 11:4–5
    interlobular, 11:4
  bile ductules, 11:2, 4
  bridging mimic, 11:9
  central vein, 11:6
  centrilobular zone/zone 3, 11:3
  changes with aging, 11:9
  copper, 11:8
  extramedullary hematopoiesis, 11:9
  hemosiderin, 11:8
  hepatocyte glycogen, 11:3
  hepatocytes, 11:2, 5–6
  images, 11:3–9
  Kupffer cells, 11:7
  lipofuscin, 11:8
  midlobular zone/zone 2, 11:3
  normal lobule, 11:3
  periportal zone/zone 1, 11:3
  pitfalls/artifacts, 11:2
  portal tracts, 11:2, 3–4
  reticulin framework, 11:6
  sinusoids, 11:2, 6, 7
  space of Disse, 11:7
  stellate cells, 11:8
  subcapsular artifact, 11:9
  surgical hepatitis, 11:9
Lung, 8:4–9
  age variation, 8:4
  alveolar epithelium, 8:6
  alveolar macrophages, 8:6
  alveoli, 8:6
  anatomy, 8:4
  anthracosis, 8:9
  asthma, 8:5
  atelectasis, 8:7–8
  bone marrow embolus, 8:8
  bronchi, 8:4, 5
  bronchial-associated lymphoid tissue (BALT), 8:7
  calcification, 8:9
  ciliated pseudostratified columnar epithelium, 8:5
  corpora amylacea, 8:9
  focal foreign body giant cell reaction, 8:8
  hemorrhage, artifactual, 8:8
  images, 8:5–9
  immunofluorescence assessment, 1:5, 7
  interlobular septae, 8:6
  lobar bronchioles, 8:5
    and arteries, 8:5
  macrophages, 8:6–7
  megakaryocytes, 8:9
  meningothelial nodule, 8:9
  metaplastic ossification, 8:9
  peribronchiolar metaplasia, 8:8
  peripheral emphysematous changes, 8:7
  pitfalls/artifacts, 8:4
  pneumocytes, 8:6
  pseudolipoid artifact, 8:8
  vasculature, 8:4, 5
  visceral pleura, 8:7
Lymph nodes, 6:6–9
  anatomy, 6:6
  Bcl-2 immunostain, 6:8
  CD3 immunostain, 6:8
  CD20 immunostain, 6:8
  germinal center, 6:7
  hyperplasia, 6:6
  images, 6:7–9
  immune function of, 6:5
  Ki-67 immunostain, 6:8
  mantle zone, 6:6
  marginal zone, 6:6
  medullary region, 6:6, 9
  neoplastic follicle, 6:7
  paracortex, 6:6, 9
  paracortical hyperplasia, 6:9
  pitfalls/artifacts, 6:6
  primary follicle, 6:6
  secondary follicle, 6:6, 7
  sinuses, 6:9
  subcapsular sinus, 6:9

INDEX

thoracic lymph node, 6:9
tingible body macrophages, 6:7
Lymphatics, 4:16–19
   age variation, 4:16
   anatomy, 4:16
   comparison of vein, lymphatic, and artery, 4:18
   pulmonary lymphatics, 4:19
Lymphoid tissue
   adaptive immune system function, 6:4
   appendix, 10:25
   bronchial-associated lymphoid tissue (BALT), 8:7
   mucosa-associated lymphoid tissue (MALT), 10:19
      reactive, 10:19
   stomach, 10:13
Lysosomes, 1:13, 16

M

Macrophages
   alveolar macrophages, 8:6
   bone marrow, 6:15, 17
   innate immune system function, 6:3
   lung, 8:6–7
   subamniotic macrophages, placenta, 13:42
   tingible body macrophages, lymph nodes, 6:7
Major histocompatibility complex
   autoimmune disease and, 6:4–5
   innate immune system function, 6:3–4
   transplantation and, 6:4–5
Major salivary glands. *See* Salivary glands, major.
Male genital tract. *See* Genital tract, male.
Mallory PTAH (phosphotungstic acid) stain, 1:3
Masson trichrome stain, 1:3
Mast cells
   bone marrow, 6:18
   dermis, 2:9
   granules, 1:16
   innate immune system function, 6:3
Matrix
   enamel matrix of teeth, 7:19, 21
   nail, 2:14, 15
Megakaryocytes
   bone marrow, 6:17
   lung, 8:9
Melan-A immunohistochemistry, in sun-damaged skin, 2:5
Melanin pigment, definition, 2:2
Melanocyte markers, 1:3
Melanocytes
   anatomy, 2:2
   epidermis, 2:4–5
   nail, 2:15
Membrane, cellular, 1:12, 14
Membrane-bound organelles, 1:12
Meninges, 5:10–11
   age variation, 5:10
   anatomy, 5:10
   arachnoid mater, 5:10, 11
   dura mater, 5:10, 11
   images, 5:11
   pia mater, 5:10, 11
   pitfalls/artifacts, 5:10
Mesonephric remnant
   cervix, 13:14
   fallopian tube, 13:28
   prostate gland, 12:43
Mesothelium, 8:10–11
   anatomy, 8:10
   images, 8:11
   pitfalls/artifacts, 8:10
Methenamine silver stain, 1:3
Methyl green-pyronin Y stain, 1:2
MHC. *See* Major histocompatibility complex.
Microtubules, cytoskeleton, 1:13
Microvilli, 1:13
Middle ear. *See* Ear.
Mineral stains, 1:3
Minor salivary glands, 7:16–17
Mitochondria, 1:13
Mucicarmine stain, 1:2
Mucins, 1:3
Mucosa-associated lymphoid tissue (MALT), 10:19
   reactive, 10:19
Mucosal specimens
   oral, immunofluorescence, 1:5
   sinonasal, electron microscopy assessment, 1:9, 10
   small intestine, electron microscopy assessment, 1:9, 10
Müllerian remnants, vagina, 13:9
Muscle, skeletal, 3:14–17
   age variation, 3:14
   anatomy, 3:14
   atrophic fibers, 3:17
   cells, 1:17, 18
   contractile filaments, 1:17
   cross striations, 3:15
   embryonic and fetal muscle, 3:15
   epimysium and perimysium, 3:14, 16
   fatty replacement, 3:17
   hyperplasia, 3:14
   images, 3:15–17
   innervation, 3:16
   metaplasia, 3:14
   pitfalls/artifacts, 3:14
   regenerating muscle fiber, 3:17
   sarcomeres, 3:16
   transverse section, 3:15
   ultrastructure, 3:15–16
Muscle cells
   skeletal muscle, 1:17
   smooth muscle, 1:18
Muscle markers, 1:3

INDEX

Muscle stains, 1:3
Muscles
   electron microscopy assessment, 1:9, 11
   histology, 1:22, 27, 29
   myoepithelium, 1:27
Muscularis mucosa
   appendix, 10:24, 25–26
   bladder, 12:18
   esophagus, 10:2, 4–5
   small intestine, 10:16
   stomach, 10:8, 10
Muscularis propria
   appendix, 10:24, 26
   bladder, 12:19
   esophagus, 10:2, 5–6
   gallbladder, 11:12
   large intestine, 10:20
   small intestine, 10:14, 17
   stomach, 10:8, 11
   vagina, 13:9
Musculoskeletal system, 3:2–18
   adipose tissue, 3:10–13
   bone and cartilage, 3:2–7
   connective tissue, 3:8–9
   skeletal muscle, 3:14–17
Myocardium. *See* Heart.
Myoepithelial markers, 1:3
Myoepithelium, histology, 1:27

N

Nail, 2:14–15
   age variation, 2:14
   anatomy, 2:14
   hyperplasia, 2:14
   hyponychium, 2:14, 15
   images, 2:15
   matrix, 2:14, 15
   melanocytes, 2:15
   nail bed, 2:14
   nail plate, 2:14
   pitfalls/artifacts, 2:14
   proximal nail fold, 2:14, 15
Natural killer cells, innate immune system function, 6:3
Neoplasm specimens, electron microscopy assessment, 1:9, 11
Nerve stains, 1:3
   Cajal stain, 1:3
   luxol fast blue stain, 1:3
   Mallory PTAH (phosphotungstic acid), 1:3
   silver nitrate, 1:3
   Weil stain, 1:3
Nerves
   histology, 1:22, 29
   specimens, electron microscopy assessment, 1:9, 11

Nervous system, 5:2–14
   central nervous system, 5:6–9
   choroid plexus, 5:12–13
   meninges, 5:10–11
   peripheral nervous system, 5:2–5
Neural markers, 1:3
Neuroendocrine cells, histology, 1:28
Neuroendocrine granules and centriole, 1:16
Neuroendocrine markers, 1:3
Neutrophil
   innate immune system function, 6:3
   peripheral blood, 6:23, 24
Nipple. *See* Breast.
Non-membrane-bound organelles, 1:12
Nose and paranasal sinuses, 7:34–37
   anatomy, 7:34
   cell types, 7:34
   glands of Bowman, 7:37
   images, 7:35–37
   olfactory epithelium, 7:37
   olfactory region, 7:34, 36
   paranasal sinus, 7:34, 37
   paranasal sinus ostia, 7:37
   respiratory region, 7:34, 36
   Schneiderian mucosa, 7:35
   secretory duct, 7:37
   septal cartilage, 7:36
   turbinate bone, 7:35
   turbinates, 7:34, 35
   vestibule, 7:36
      anatomy, 7:34
      respiratory transition, 7:36
Nuclear and cytoplasmic staining, 1:2
   Feulgen stain, 1:2
   hematoxylin and eosin, 1:2
   methyl green-pyronin Y, 1:2
   Romanowsky (Wright, Giemsa), 1:2
Nuclear elements of cells, 1:12, 14
Nucleolus, 1:12, 14

O

Ocular adnexa. *See* Eye and ocular adnexa.
Oil red O stain, 1:3
Oncocytes, 1:17
Oncocytoma, 1:17
Oral mucosae, 7:12–13
   age variation, 7:12
   anatomy, 7:12
   images, 7:13
   immunofluorescence assessment, 1:5
Organelles
   membrane-bound, 1:12
   non-membrane-bound, 1:12
Osteoblasts
   bone, 3:2, 5
   bone marrow, 6:19

INDEX

Osteoclasts
   bone, 3:2, 6
   bone marrow, 6:19
Osteocytes, 3:2, 6
Ovary, 13:30–39
   age variation, 13:30
   anatomy, 13:30
   atrophic, 13:39
   corpora albicans, 13:35
   corpora fibrosa, 13:37
   corpus luteum, 13:34–36
      hemorrhagic, 13:35
      involuting, 13:35
      menstruation, 13:35
      pregnancy, 13:36
   cortex, 13:30
   cortical inclusion cyst, 13:37
   cortical inclusion gland, 13:38
   endometriosis, 13:38–39
   follicle cyst, 13:37
   follicles
      involuting, 13:36–37
      mature, 13:34
      preantral, 13:34
      primordial, 13:33
   hemorrhagic corpus luteum, 13:35
   hilar vessels, 13:31
   hilum
      anatomy, 13:30
      nerve, 13:31
   hilus cells, 13:31–32
      pigment, 13:32
      Reinke crystal, 13:31
   hyaline scar, 13:37
   hyperplasia, 13:30
   images, 13:31–39
   medulla, 13:30
   medullary vessels, 13:31
   metaplasia, 13:30
   pitfalls/artifacts, 13:30
   rete ovarii, 13:32
   stroma, 13:32–33
      endosalpingiosis, 13:33
      fat, 13:33
      hyperplasia, 13:39
      luteinized cells, 13:33
   surface adhesion, 13:38
   surface epithelium, 13:30, 37
   surface papillation, 13:38
   theca interna and externa, 13:34
   Walthard rest, 13:38
   Wolffian ducts, 13:32

P

Pancreas, 11:18–21
   acini, 11:18, 19
   age variation, 11:18
   anatomy, 11:18
   connective tissue, 11:18, 21
   ducts, 11:18, 21
   endocrine cells, 11:18
   focal acinar transformation, 11:21
   heterotopic pancreas, in stomach, 10:13
   images, 11:19–21
   interlobular ducts, 11:18, 21
   intrapancreatic fat, 11:20
   islets of Langerhans, 11:18, 19–20
   nerves, 11:21
   pancreatic ducts, 11:20
   pitfalls/artifacts, 11:18
Paneth cells
   large intestine, 10:19
   small intestine, 10:15
Papillary dermis, 2:6, 7
Paraffin-embedded tissue, in immunofluorescence, 1:4
Paraganglia, 14:6–7
   age variation, 14:6
   anatomy, 14:6
   hyperplasia, 14:6
   images, 14:7
   pitfalls/artifacts, 14:6
Paranasal sinuses. *See* Nose and paranasal sinuses.
Parathyroid glands, 14:12–15
   anatomy, 14:12
   canals of Kürsteiner, 14:12, 15
   capsule, 14:13
   chief cells, 14:12, 13
   chromogranin, 14:15
   clear cells, 14:14
   ectopic parathyroid tissue, 14:14
   follicular change, 14:14
   images, 14:13–15
   intracellular lipid, 14:15
   intrathymic parathyroid gland, 14:14
   lobules, 14:13
   oxyphil (oncocytic) cells, 14:12, 14
   parathyroid hormone, 14:14, 15
   parathyroid microcyst, 14:15
   pitfalls/artifacts, 14:12
   stroma, 14:13
   stromal adipose tissue, 14:13
   vascular stroma, 14:13
Parotid gland
   anatomy, 7:44
   images, 7:45–46
   intraparotid lymph node, 7:46
   main parotid (Stensen) duct, 7:46
   oncocytic metaplasia, 7:47
   periparotid lymph node, 7:46
PAS (periodic acid-Schiff) stain, 1:2
   with diastase, 1:2
Penis, 12:48–51
   anatomy, 12:48
   Buck fascia, 12:48, 50

INDEX

corpora cavernosa, 12:49
corpus spongiosum, 12:48, 49–50
dartos, 12:48, 51
foreskin, 12:48, 51
glans, 12:48, 50–51
images, 12:49–51
penile urethra, 12:24
tunica albuginea, 12:48, 49
Pentachrome stain, 1:3
Perimysium, 3:16
Periodic acid-Schiff stain. See PAS (periodic acid-Schiff) stain.
Periosteum, 3:2, 3
Peripheral blood, 6:22–25
    age variation, 6:22
    agglutination, 6:24
    anatomy, 6:22
    basophil, 6:23
        partial degranulation, 6:24
    cryoglobulin, 6:24
    eosinophil, 6:23
    feather edge, 6:25
    hyperplasia, 6:22
    images, 6:23–25
    monocyte, 6:23
    neutrophils, 6:23
        toxic, 6:24
    newborn blood, 6:25
    normal blood, 6:23
        4-month-old infant, 6:25
    normal lymphocyte, infant, 6:25
    normal white blood cells, 6:23
    pitfalls/artifacts, 6:22
    platelets, 6:24
Peripheral nervous system, 5:2–5
    anatomy, 5:2
    connective tissue sheaths, 5:2
    dorsal spinal root (sensory) ganglion, 5:3
    images, 5:3–5
    myenteric ganglionitis, 5:5
    non-neuronal (satellite) cells, 5:2
    normal peripheral nerve, 5:3–5
    organization, 5:2
    peripheral nerve tumor, 5:5
    pitfalls/artifacts, 5:2
    types of neurons, 5:2
Peritoneal membranes, 10:32–33
    anatomy, 10:32
    images, 10:33
    pitfalls/artifacts, 10:32
Pharynx, 7:38–39
    anatomy, 7:38
    hypopharynx, 7:39
    images, 7:39
    oropharyngeal mucosa, 7:39
    Thornwaldt duct cyst, 7:39
    tonsil, 7:39
    uvula, 7:39

Phosphotungstic acid-hematoxylin (PTAH) stain, 1:3
    Mallory PTAH (phosphotungstic acid) stain, 1:3
Pia mater, 5:10, 11
Pigment stains, 1:3
Pineal gland, 14:16–17
    age variation, 14:16
    anatomy, 14:16
    images, 14:17
    pitfalls/artifacts, 14:16
Pinocytotic vesicles, 1:13
Pituitary gland, 14:18–19
    age variation, 14:18
    anatomy, 14:18
        anterior pituitary lobe (adenohypophysis), 14:18
        posterior pituitary lobe (neurohypophysis), 14:18
    hyperplasia, 14:18
    images, 14:19
    metaplasia, 14:18
    pitfalls/artifacts, 14:18
Placenta, 13:40–45
    age variation, 13:40
    amnion, 13:42
        anatomy, 13:40
        and chorion, 13:42
        squamous metaplasia, 13:43
    amniotic membrane, 13:40
    anatomy, 13:40
    calcification, 13:45
    chorion, 13:42
        and amnion, 13:40
        superficial layers, 13:40
    decidua, 13:45
    decidualized endometrium, 13:45
    diamniotic monochorionic membranes, 13:43
    fetal blood elements, 13:43
    images, 13:41–45
    implantation site, 13:45
    membrane: sclerotic villi, 13:42
    metaplasia, 13:40
    perivillous fibrin, 13:45
    placental disk, 13:40
    subamniotic clefts, 13:42
    subamniotic macrophages, 13:42
    umbilical cord
        allantoic remnant, 13:41
        anatomy, 13:40
        hemorrhage, 13:41
        omphalomesenteric duct remnant, 13:41
    villi, 13:40, 44
        immature, 13:43, 44
        sclerotic, 13:42
        secondary, 13:44
        tertiary, 13:44–45
Plasma cells, 1:15

INDEX

Prostate: Benign glandular and stromal histology, 12:38–47
  age variation, 12:38
  anatomy, 12:38
  architecture, 12:39
  atrophy
    cystic, 12:41–42
    partial, 12:42
    sclerotic, 12:43
    simple, 12:41
  basal cell hyperplasia, 12:41
  benign prostatic hyperplasia, 12:40
  cell layers, 12:38
  clear cell cribriform hyperplasia, 12:43
  Cowper gland, 12:38, 45
  ejaculatory duct, 12:45
  extraprostatic tissues, 12:47
  glands, 12:39
  hyperplasia, 12:38
  images, 12:39–47
  inflammatory changes, 12:44
  mesonephric remnants, 12:43
  metaplasia, 12:38
  nuclei/cytoplasm, 12:39
  pitfalls/artifacts, 12:38
  post-atrophic hyperplasia, 12:42–43
  prominent basal cells, 12:41
  seminal vesicle, 12:38, 46
  stroma, 12:38
  stromal hyperplasia, 12:40
Prostate: Regional anatomy with histologic correlates, 12:28–37
  age variation, 12:28
  anatomy, 12:28
  anterior prostate, 12:33
  anterior soft tissue, 12:33
  apical cross section, 12:29
  apical prostate, 12:29
  bladder neck, 12:37
    true, 12:37
  central zone, 12:34
  ejaculatory duct, 12:35
    paired, 12:35
  extraprostatic tissue, posterolateral, 12:32
  ganglion, 12:32
  hyperplasia, 12:28
  images, 12:29–37
  metaplasia, 12:28
  mid-level section, 12:30
  mid-prostate peripheral zone, 12:30
  mid-prostate transition zone, 12:31
  periurethral prostate, 12:31
  pitfalls/artifacts, 12:28
  prostate tissue near bladder base, 12:37
  seminal vesicles, 12:36
  superior prostate cross section, 12:34
  transition zone, 12:31
  transition zone boundary with peripheral zone, 12:31
Proximal nail fold, 2:14, 15
Prussian blue stain, 1:3
PTAH (phosphotungstic acid-hematoxylin) stain, 1:3
  Mallory PTAH (phosphotungstic acid) stain, 1:3
Purkinje cell
  cardiac conduction system, 4:9–11
  central nervous system, 5:7

R

Renal pelvis. *See* Ureter and renal pelvis.
Respiratory system, 8:2–12
  lung, 8:4–9
  mesothelium, 8:10–11
  trachea, 8:2–3
Rete ovarii, 13:32
Rete ridges, epidermis, 2:2
Rete testis, 12:52, 56–57
Reticular dermis, 2:6, 7–8
Reticulin stain, 1:3
Romanowsky (Wright, Giemsa) stains, 1:2

S

Sagittal sinus, superior, 5:11
Salivary gland ducts and acini, 1:16
Salivary glands, major, 7:44–47
  age variation, 7:44
  anatomy, 7:44
  images, 7:45–47
  intraparotid lymph node, 7:46
  main parotid (Stensen) duct, 7:46
  myoepithelial cells, 7:46
  parotid gland
    anatomy, 7:44
    images, 7:45–46
    oncocytic metaplasia, 7:47
  periparotid lymph node, 7:46
  pitfalls/artifacts, 7:44
  sebaceous glands, 7:46
  serous demilunes, 7:47
  sublingual gland
    anatomy, 7:44
    images, 7:45, 47
  submandibular gland
    anatomy, 7:44
    images, 7:45, 47
Salivary glands, minor, 7:16–17
  anatomy, 7:16
  Blandin and Nunn glands, 7:17
  excretory ducts, 7:17
  images, 7:17
  mucous acinus and intercalated duct, 7:17
  mucous cells, 7:17
  von Ebner glands, 7:17

INDEX

Sarcomeres
    heart, 4:3
    skeletal muscle, 3:16
Scanning electron microscopy. *See* Electron microscopy.
Sebaceous exocrine gland, histology, 1:26
Sebaceous glands
    adnexal structures, 2:10, 11–12
    dermis, 2:9
    major salivary glands, 7:46
Semilunar (ventriculoarterial) valves, 4:6, 7
Seminal vesicle, prostate gland, 12:36, 38, 46
Seminiferous tubules, 12:52, 54
Silver nitrate stain, 1:3
Sinoatrial (sinus) node
    anatomy, 4:8
    excised tissue block, 4:9
    high magnification, 4:10
    trichrome stained and cross section, 4:9
Sinonasal mucosa specimens, electron microscopy assessment, 1:9, 10
Skeletal muscle. *See* Muscle, skeletal.
Skin. *See also* Integument.
    immunofluorescence assessment, 1:5, 7
Slide storage, in immunofluorescence, 1:4
Small intestine, 10:14–17
    age variation, 10:14
    anatomy, 10:14
    artifactual villous blunting, 10:17
    Auerbach plexus, 10:14, 17
    Brunner glands, 10:16
    brush border, 10:15
    crypts, 10:14, 15
    duodenum, 10:14
    endocrine cells, 10:16
    epithelium, 1:19
    ileocecal valve, 10:17
    ileum, 10:14, 17
    images, 10:15–17
    intraepithelial lymphocytes, 10:15
    jejunum, 10:14, 16
    lacteals, 10:15
    lamina propria, 10:14, 16
    mucosa, 10:15
    mucosal specimens, electron microscopy assessment, 1:9, 10
    muscularis mucosa, 10:16
    muscularis propria, 10:14, 17
    Paneth cells, 10:15
    Peyer patches, 10:17
    pitfalls/artifacts, 10:14
    submucosa, 10:14, 16
Special stains. *See* Stains, special.
Spermatocytes, primary, 12:55–56
Spinal cord. *See* Central nervous system.
Spleen, 6:10–13
    age variation, 6:10
    anatomy, 6:10
    CD3 immunostain, 6:13
    CD20 immunostain, 6:13
    congestion, 6:13
    cords and sinuses, 6:12
    factor VIII immunostain, 6:13
    images, 6:11–13
    immune function of, 6:5
    perifollicular zone, 6:10, 11
    pitfalls/artifacts, 6:10
    red pulp, 6:12–13
        anatomy, 6:10
        capillary, 6:12
        red and white pulp, 6:10
        sinuses, 6:12
    reticulin stain, 6:13
    sinuses, 6:12
    vasculature, 6:10
    white pulp, 6:11
        anatomy, 6:10
        follicles, 6:11
        red and white pulp, 6:11
Squamous epithelium
    glycogenated, bladder, 12:19
    histology, images, 1:24–25
    intercellular bridges, image, 1:18
    stratified, epidermis, 2:2
    tonofilaments, 1:18
Squamous metaplasia
    amnion, 13:43
    endocervix, 13:12
    fallopian tube, 13:27
    placenta, 13:43
    tongue, 7:25
    trachea, 8:3
    urethra
        female, 12:25
        keratinizing, 12:26
Stains, special, 1:2–3
    carbohydrate stains, 1:2–3
    connective tissue stains, 1:3
    fat stains, 1:3
    histochemical staining, definition, 1:2
    immunohistochemical staining, definition, 1:2
    immunohistochemical stains, guide to chapters, 1:30–31
    miscellaneous stains, 1:3
    muscle stains, 1:3
    nerve stains, 1:3
    nuclear and cytoplasmic staining, 1:2
    pigments, minerals, and granules, 1:3
    special stains, guide to chapters, 1:32
    terminology, 1:2
Stomach, 10:8–13
    age variation, 10:8
    anatomy, 10:8
    antrum, 10:8, 11
    Auerbach plexus, 10:12

INDEX

cardia, 10:8, 10
endocrine cells, 10:9
heterotopic pancreas, 10:13
images, 10:9–13
lamina propria, 10:8, 10
lymphoid tissue, 10:13
metaplasia, 10:8, 13
mucous neck cells, 10:9
muscularis mucosa, 10:8, 10
muscularis propria, 10:8, 11
oxyntic mucosa, 10:11
pitfalls/artifacts, 10:8
pits, 10:9
pit/surface epithelium, 10:9
proton pump inhibitor effect, 10:13
pseudo-signet ring cells, 10:13
pylorus, 10:13
submucosa, 10:8, 12
subserosa, 10:8, 12
transitional mucosa, 10:11
Stroma
    endocervix, 13:12
    endometrial polyp, 13:18
    fallopian tube, 13:24
    ovary, 13:32–33
        hyperplasia, 13:39
    parathyroid glands, 14:13
    prostate gland. *See* Prostate: Benign glandular and stromal histology.
    uterus
        endometrial stroma, 13:10
        proliferative stroma, 13:16
Stromal adipose tissue
    parathyroid glands, 14:13
    thyroid gland, 14:10
Stromal cells
    dermis, 2:6
    vulva, 13:4
Subarachnoid space, 5:11
Sublingual salivary gland, 7:44, 45, 47
Submandibular salivary gland, 7:44, 45, 47
Submucosa
    appendix, 10:24, 26
    esophagus, 10:2, 4–5
    large intestine, 10:20
    oral mucosae, 7:13
    small intestine, 10:14, 16
    stomach, 10:8, 12
Sudan black B stain, 1:3

T

T lymphocytes
    adaptive immune system function, 6:4
    CD4 T lymphocytes, 6:4
    CD8 T lymphocytes, 6:4
    maturation in thymus, 6:5
    regulatory T lymphocytes, 6:4
    T-cell receptors, 6:4
Teeth, 7:18–21
    age variation, 7:18
    anatomy, 7:18
    cementum, 7:18
    crown, 7:18
    cusp of canine tooth, 7:19
    dentin, 7:18, 21
    enamel
        anatomy, 7:18
        graphic SEM image, 7:21
    enamel matrix, 7:19, 21
    images, 7:19–21
    major components, 7:19
    normal full dentition, 7:19
    periodontal ligament, 7:18, 20
    pitfalls/artifacts, 7:18
    pulp, 7:18, 20
    radiographic image, 7:19
    root
        anatomy, 7:18
        apex, 7:20
Testis and associated excretory ducts, 12:52–59
    adrenal cortical rest, 12:59
    age variation, 12:52
    anatomy, 12:52
    efferent ductules, 12:52, 57
    epididymis, 12:52, 57–58
    images, 12:53–59
    interstitium, 12:52, 53
    Leydig cells, 12:54
    outer surface, 12:53
    outermost testicular capsule, 12:52
    peritubular fibrosis, 12:59
    prepubertal testis, 12:59
    Reinke crystals, 12:54
    rete testis, 12:52, 56–57
    scrotum, 12:52
    seminiferous tubules, 12:52, 54
    Sertoli cells, 12:55
    spermatids, 12:56
    spermatocytes, primary, 12:55–56
    spermatogonia, 12:55
    testicular appendages, 12:59
    tunica albuginea, 12:52, 53
    tunica vaginalis, 12:52, 53
    tunica vasculosa, 12:52, 53
    vas deferens, 12:52, 58
Thymus, 6:26–27
    age variation, 6:26
    anatomy, 6:26
    hyperplasia, 6:26
    images, 6:27
    pitfalls/artifacts, 6:26
    T-cell maturation in, 6:5
Thyroid gland, 14:8–11
    anatomy, 14:8

INDEX

capsule and extracapsular thyroid tissue, 14:9
C-cell cluster, 14:11
colloid calcium oxalate crystals, 14:10
follicular epithelial cells, 14:9
heterotopic cartilage, 14:11
images, 14:9–11
incidental nodules, 14:9
intrathyroidal parathyroid tissue, 14:10
intrathyroidal skeletal muscle, 14:10
palpation thyroiditis, 14:8, 10
resorption vacuoles, 14:9
Sanderson polster, 14:9
solid cell nest, 14:11
stromal adipose tissue, 14:10
thyroid hormone synthesis, 14:9
Toluidine blue stain, 1:3
Tongue, 7:22–25
    anatomy, 7:22
    circumvallate papillae, 7:22, 24
    ectopic tonsil, 7:25
    filiform papillae
        anatomy, 7:22
        bacterial colonization, 7:23
    foliate papillae, 7:22, 24
    fungiform papillae, 7:22, 23–24
    fusiform papillae, 7:23
    images, 7:23–25
    mucous glands, 7:25
    muscle, 7:23
    parenchyma, 7:23
    pitfalls/artifacts, 7:22
    squamous metaplasia, 7:25
    taste buds, 7:22, 24
    ventral tongue, 7:25
    von Ebner glands, 7:25
Tonofilaments, 1:18
Tonsils/adenoids, 7:26–29
    age variation, 7:26
    anatomy, 7:26
    CD3 immunohistochemistry, 7:27
    CD20 immunohistochemistry, 7:27
    ectopic cartilage, 7:28
    ectopic tonsil, on tongue, 7:25
    images, 7:27–29
    lingual tonsils, 7:26, 28–29
    lymphoepithelium, 7:27
    palatine tonsils, 7:26, 27, 28
    pharyngeal tonsil, 7:26, 29, 39
    pitfalls/artifacts, 7:26
    sulfur granules, 7:28
Trachea, 8:2–3
    anatomy, 8:2
    images, 8:2
    metaplasia, 8:2
    pitfalls/artifacts, 8:2
Transmission electron microscopy. *See* Electron microscopy.
Transplant allografts, immunofluorescence assessment, 1:5, 7
Transplantation, and major histocompatibility complex, 6:4–5
Transport media, in immunofluorescence, 1:4
Tubular gut and peritoneum, 10:2–35
    anus and anal canal, 10:28–31
    appendix, 10:24–27
    esophagus, 10:2–7
    large intestine, 10:18–23
    peritoneal membranes, 10:32–33
    small intestine, 10:14–17
    stomach, 10:8–13
Tympanic membrane. *See* Ear.

U

Umbilical cord. *See* Placenta.
Ureter and renal pelvis, 12:12–15
    anatomy, 12:12
    cystitis glandularis, 12:14
    images, 12:13–15
    major and minor calyces, 12:12
    minor calyx over renal papilla, 12:15
    pitfalls/artifacts, 12:12
    renal calyx, 12:15
    renal papilla, 12:12, 14
    renal pelvis, 12:12, 15
    subepithelial connective tissue/lamina propria, 12:13
    ureter with von Brunn nests, 12:14
    von Brunn nests, 12:14
Urethra, 12:22–27
    anatomy, 12:22
    female urethral anatomy, 12:22, 25
    hyperplasia, 12:22
    images, 12:23–27
    intestinal metaplasia, 12:26
    intraepithelial glandular cells, 12:27
    male urethral anatomy, 12:22, 23–24
    metaplasia, 12:22
    mucinous intraepithelial cells, 12:26
    penile urethra, 12:24
    periurethral/paraurethral glands ducts, 12:27
    pitfalls/artifacts, 12:22
    prostatic urethra (verumontanum), 12:23
    squamous metaplasia
        female, 12:25
        keratinizing, 12:26
    urethral ducts, 12:27
    urothelium, 12:23
    von Brunn nests, 12:26
Uterus, 13:10–23
    adenomyosis, 13:22
    age variation, 13:10
    anatomy, 13:10
    arcuate arteries, 13:22

INDEX

Arias-Stella effect, 13:20
atrophic polyp, 13:21–22
cervix
    decidua, 13:11
    and lower uterine segment, 13:14
    mesonephric remnant, 13:14
    transformation zone, 13:11
ectocervix, 13:10, 11
endocervical glands, 13:11
endocervix, 13:10
    microglandular hyperplasia, 13:13
    Nabothian cyst, 13:13
    squamous metaplasia, 13:12
    stroma, 13:12
    tubal metaplasia, 13:12
    tunnel clusters, 13:13
endometrial glands, 13:10
endometrial stroma
    anatomy, 13:10
    proliferative, 13:16
endometritis, chronic, 13:15
endometrium
    anovulatory, 13:21
    atrophic, 13:21
    atrophic polyp, 13:21–22
    breakdown, 13:18
    ciliated cells, 13:18
    decidualized, 13:19
    disordered proliferative, 13:21
    early secretory, 13:16
    interval phase, 13:16
    late secretory, 13:17
    layers, 13:15
    lymphoid aggregate, 13:15
    menstrual, 13:17–18
    polyp, 13:18–19
    proliferative, 13:15
    secretory, 13:16–19
endomyometrium: irregular junction, 13:15
exfoliation artifact, 13:23
fragmentation and pseudocrowding, 13:23
hormone effects, 13:23
images, 13:11–23
implantation site, 13:20
lower uterine segment, 13:10, 14
metaplasia, 13:10
myometrium
    anatomy, 13:10
    superficial, 13:22
Nabothian cyst, endocervix, 13:13
pitfalls/artifacts, 13:10
predecidua, 13:17
proliferative gland, 13:16
serosa, 13:10, 22
serosal adhesion, 13:23
spiral arterioles, 13:17
telescoping artifact, 13:23
transformation zone, 13:10

V

Vagina, 13:6–9
    age variation, 13:6
    anatomy, 13:6
    distal vaginal wall, 13:9
    epithelium, 13:7
    images, 13:7–9
    lamina propria, 13:6, 8
    metaplasia, 13:6
    mucosa, 13:7
    Müllerian remnants, 13:9
    muscularis, 13:9
    pitfalls/artifacts, 13:6
    rectovaginal septum, 13:9
    Wolffian duct remnants, 13:9
Vas deferens, 12:52, 58
Vascular markers, 1:3
Vaterian system, 11:16–17
Veins, 4:16–19
    age variation, 4:16
    anatomy, 4:16
    arteriovenous malformation, 4:19
    comparison of vein, lymphatic, and artery, 4:18
    high endothelial venules, 4:18
    medium-sized vein, 4:17, 18
    pulmonary vein and venules, 4:19
    small vein and muscular artery, 4:18
Venules, 4:16, 18, 19
Villi, placental. See Placenta.
Vocal cord. See Larynx.
von Brunn nests
    bladder, 12:20
    ureter and renal pelvis, 12:14
    urethra, 12:26
Vulva, 13:2–5
    anatomy, 13:2
    Bartholin duct, 13:5
    Bartholin glands, 13:2, 5
    images, 13:3–5
    labia majora, 13:2, 3–4
    labia minora, 13:2, 4
    mammary-like anogenital glands, 13:2, 5
    metaplasia, 13:2
    pitfalls/artifacts, 13:2
    stromal cells, 13:4

W

Walthard rest
    fallopian tube, 13:24, 27–28
    ovary, 13:38
White fat, 3:10, 11–13
Woven bone, 3:2, 5